Tumors and Tumor-like Conditions of the Lung and Pleura

Tumors and Tumor-like Conditions of the Lung and Pleura

CESAR A. MORAN, MD

Professor and Deputy Chair
Director of Thoracic Pathology
Department of Pathology
The University of Texas
M. D. Anderson Cancer Center
Houston, Texas

SAUL SUSTER, MD

Professor and Chairman
Department of Pathology
Medical College of Wisconsin
Milwaukee, Wisconsin

SAUNDERS

ELSEVIER

SAUNDERS
ELSEVIER

1600 John F. Kennedy Blvd.
Ste 1800
Philadelphia, PA 19103-2899

TUMORS AND TUMOR-LIKE CONDITIONS OF THE LUNG AND PLEURA

ISBN: 978-1-4160-3624-1

Library of Congress Cataloging-in-Publication Data
Moran, Cesar.
Tumors and tumor-like conditions of the lung and pleura / Cesar A. Moran, Saul Suster.—1st ed.
p. ; cm.
Includes bibliographical references.
ISBN 978-1-4160-3624-1
1. Lungs—Tumors. 2. Lungs—Pleura. I. Suster, Saul. II. Title.
[DNLM: 1. Lung Neoplasms—diagnosis. 2. Diagnostic Imaging—methods. 3. Pleural Neoplasms—diagnosis. WF 658 M829t 2010]
RC280.L8M625 2010
616.99'424—dc22

2010001329

Publishing Director: Bill Schmitt
Developmental Editor: Katie DeFrancesco
Project Manager: David Saltzberg
Design Direction: Lou Forgione

Printed in the United States

Last digit is the print number: 9 8 7 6 5 4 3 2 1

To our families
Susan, Jenny, Elisa Jean, Dana, Kate, and David
for their continuous support

CONTRIBUTORS

EDITH M. MAROM, MD
Professor of Diagnostic Radiology
Department of Diagnostic Imaging
The University of Texas
M. D. Anderson Cancer Center
Houston, Texas
Chapter 1: Imaging Tumors of the Lung and Pleura

DAVID J. STEWART, MD
Professor and Deputy Chair
Department of Thoracic and Head and Neck Oncology
The University of Texas
M. D. Anderson Cancer Center
Houston, Texas
Chapter 14: Clinical Management of Lung Cancer

GARRETT L. WALSH, MD
Professor of Surgery
Department of Thoracic Surgery
The University of Texas
M. D. Anderson Cancer Center
Houston, Texas
Chapter 2: Staging of Thoracic Malignancies: A Surgeon's Perspective

PREFACE

This textbook gives surgical pathologists a practical approach to the diagnosis of the different tumors and tumor-like conditions that may affect the lung and pleura. The book has been arranged and subdivided based on the different families of tumors that may seed those structures. When important, historical background is provided so that the surgical pathologist becomes more familiar with the different terminologies used over the years. Current concepts and definitions are also presented so that their importance and the difficulties they may pose to the surgical pathologist are apparent. The text focuses on the morphologic approach to the different tumoral conditions and the use of ancillary methods to corroborate the morphologic diagnosis. When appropriate, important advanced studies, such as molecular pathology information, are also provided.

Additionally, the text provides important radiologic, surgical, and oncologic information that must be considered when dealing with the different conditions presented. In presenting these components, which are essential to understanding the pathology of the lung and pleura, we are indebted to Edith Marom, MD, for her contribution on diagnostic imaging; Garrett L. Walsh, MD, for his contribution on surgical staging, and to David J. Stewart, MD, for his contribution on the clinical management of lung cancer. They provide important information that is of great benefit to all involved in the diagnosis and treatment of patients with lung and/or pleural lesions.

This textbook will be useful not only to surgical pathologists but also to oncologists, surgeons, and radiologists who want to get better acquainted with the diverse histologies that may be present in the lung and pleura. Additionally, we hope this text enhances communication among all the different specialties involved in the treatment of patients with tumors of the lung and pleura.

Cesar A. Moran, MD
Saul Suster, MD

CONTENTS

1

Imaging Tumors of the Lung and Pleura

Edith M. Marom

In the past few decades, the use of computers has revolutionized imaging, with the introduction of technologies such as computed tomography (CT), magnetic resonance imaging (MRI), ultrasonography, positron emission tomography (PET), and, more recently, PET-CT, which integrates anatomic (morphologic) and physiologic aspects of imaging. With the ever-greater subspecialization of the different areas of practice within medical oncology—surgical oncology, radiation oncology, and diagnostic radiology—and the expanding use of picture archiving systems, radiologist and clinician may encounter each other only rarely, if at all. Optimal patient outcomes, however, require careful planning of imaging for diagnosis, staging, and follow-up, best achieved through direct communication between the clinician and the radiologist. This chapter presents a general overview of lung and pleural tumor imaging, with an emphasis on the strengths and weaknesses of specific techniques in evaluating different tumor types, to help in selection of the ideal imaging modality for each patient.

PRIMARY MALIGNANT LUNG TUMORS

Screening

Despite new diagnostic techniques, the overall 5-year survival rate for patients with lung cancer, the leading cause of cancer death, remains approximately 15%, and most patients still present with advanced disease.[1] This high death rate is presumed to reflect a combination of difficulty in detecting early-stage disease and lack of significant curative treatment. Abrogating cigarette smoking would be highly effective in reducing the prevalence of lung cancer but would not abolish it altogether, because effecting lifestyle change in an entire population is very difficult; moreover, previous smokers would still be at risk for lung cancer. Detection of the disease at the stage at which cure or control is possible is the theoretical rationale for screening for lung cancer.

Because tumors of the lungs are encased by the rib cage, early diagnosis by physical examination is not possible. Chest radiographs are ideal for demonstrating pulmonary abnormalities that differ significantly from the surrounding structures in density. The lungs contain air, the density of which differs significantly from the soft tissue density of tumor. Early screening studies for lung cancer, therefore, used chest radiography, which fulfills the criteria for a suitable screening test by being simple to perform, inexpensive, painless, and relatively safe, with relatively limited radiation exposure.[2] Nonrandomized, uncontrolled screening studies in the 1950s[3–6] gave way to nonrandomized, controlled trials,[7,8] which showed that persons in the screened group were more likely to have lung cancer detected in the early stages, were more likely to have resectable disease, and enjoyed better survival rates. No clear reduction in lung cancer–associated mortality, however, was documented.

Although survival (number of persons alive after diagnosis of the disease relative to the total number of persons diagnosed with the disease) is commonly reported in screening trials, this statistic can be misleading because it is subject to lead time, study duration, and overdiagnosis biases. An impact on mortality rather than survival is therefore sought, to validate potential screening methods.[9] Accordingly, in the 1970s, four major randomized, controlled trials looked at approximately 37,000 male smokers[10–13] and found that chest radiograph screening yielded no change in mortality. In the screened cohort, patients demonstrated higher 5-year survival rates but no reduction in the number of advanced cancers (i.e., no stage shift). A follow-up study more than 20 years after the Mayo Lung Project confirmed no significant difference in lung cancer mortality.[14] Because of its failure to reduce lung cancer mortality, chest radiograph screening for lung cancer was not recommended.

In the late 1990s, the issue of screening began to reemerge because of the ongoing debate about the validity of the findings on chest radiograph studies and in light of revolutionary developments in CT that enabled detection of pulmonary nodules smaller than 1 cm, in one breath-hold, with a reduced radiation dose to the patient—low-dose CT (LDCT). The studies of lung cancer screening with CT conducted so far have been single-arm studies without a comparative group, or 1-year feasibility randomized, controlled trials.[15] These studies showed that chest CT scans have greater sensitivity than chest radiographs for the detection of pulmonary nodules (Fig. 1-1). Noncalcified nodules could be detected in as many as two thirds of the persons screened, all of whom underwent follow-up or workup to exclude malignancy, but 99% of these nodules were benign.[16] Nodules that remained suspect for lung cancer after workup or follow-up required resection. Nevertheless, more than one third of the nodules resected were associated with benign conditions.[16,17]

Despite the published 10-year survival rate of 88% for patients with stage I disease,[18] and the increased likelihood that cancers detected by LDCT would be operable, LDCT yielded no decreases in the number of advanced lung cancers detected or in the number of deaths from lung cancers compared with predictive historical models of an unscreened population.[19]

More recently, the National Lung Screening Trial (NLST) was launched to directly assess whether screening with LDCT is effective for early detection of lung cancer. NLST compared the effectiveness of two screening tests, LDCT and chest radiograph, on net lung cancer–specific mortality in persons who were at high risk for the development of the disease. Between September 2002 and April 2004, the trial accrued 34,614 participants, who underwent annual imaging. The trial involves follow-up questionnaires administered over 6 to 8 years and thus is still monitoring these patients; prevalence data have not yet been published. In the meantime, patients are encouraged to wait for the results of the NLST, or to be screened as part of a randomized, controlled trial, because it has not been shown that screening with LDCT is effective in reducing mortality.

Early Detection: Solitary Pulmonary Nodule

A solitary pulmonary nodule (SPN), defined as a nodule less than 3 cm in greatest dimension surrounded by lung (see Fig. 1-1), is a common incidental radiologic finding. Its incidence has increased with the growing use of chest CT over the past few decades and in screening studies in asymptomatic populations. Because of concern about lung cancer, further evaluation of such nodules often is suggested. The goal of imaging is to differentiate between nodules that are benign and those that are malignant, so that patients who require surgery are correctly identified; the mean postoperative mortality rate after lung cancer resection in the United States is 5%.[20]

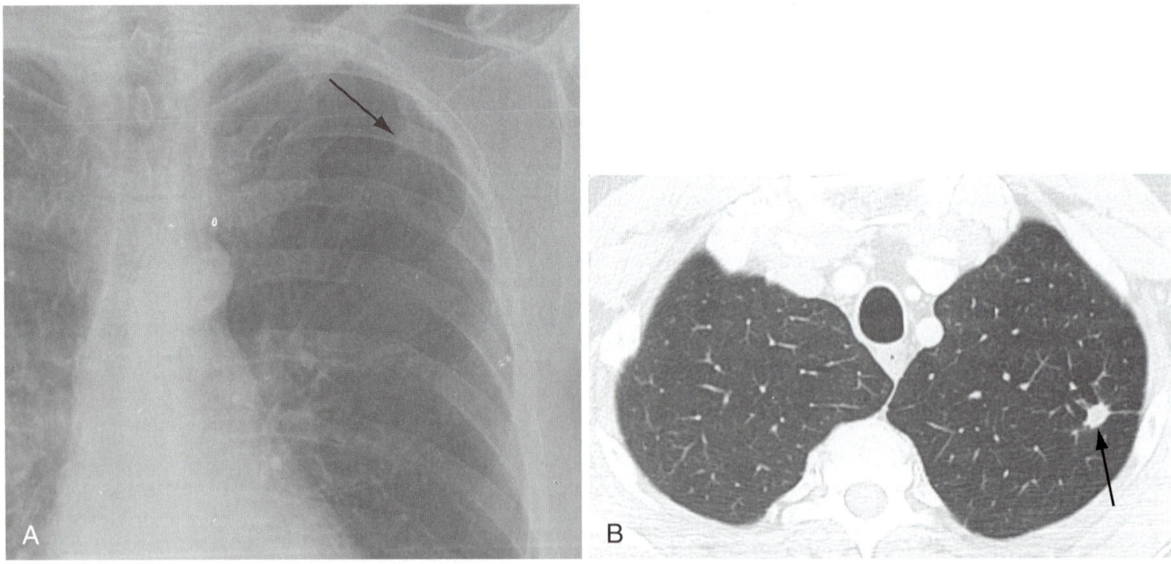

Figure 1-1 **A**, Incidental nodule in a 67-year-old man was discovered on a routine chest radiograph. The small nodule is barely visualized because it is superimposed on ribs *(arrow)*. **B**, Contrast-enhanced chest CT scan shows a spiculated 1.3-cm nodule *(arrow)*. Transthoracic needle biopsy revealed respiratory epithelial cells and histiocytes in a background of extensive necrosis but no malignancy. The nodule nearly completely disappeared without therapy over a period of 3 years, confirming the benign diagnosis.

Chest Radiography

Evaluation of the SPN entails several steps. When a nodule is large enough to be seen on a chest radiograph, this study will be the first step in the investigation. Chest radiography is inexpensive, delivers very little radiation to the patient, and provides an image that often can be compared easily with preexisting radiographs. The initial determination is whether the nodule is indeed within the lung, because mimics of pulmonary nodules are numerous, such as rib fracture, bone island, skin lesion, or overlapping normal structures (see Fig. 1-1). Review of old films or old CT scans is the most cost-efficient way to assess an SPN. If no old images are available, shallow oblique images, fluoroscopy, or chest CT scan can be used.

Once the nodule has been confirmed to be within the lung, it should be assessed for features suggesting benign origin. The ability of chest radiography to discern between malignant and benign pulmonary nodules remains limited, however. Numerous studies in the 1940s and 1950s attempted to address this issue as the use of chest radiography increased exponentially. Before the advent of CT, positive preoperative diagnosis of asymptomatic SPN was rare; early exploratory thoracotomy was strongly urged for patients with these nodules.[21,22] Although larger nodules are more likely to be malignant, no size criterion allows exclusion of malignancy.[23] Two methods of distinguishing benign from malignant nodules were developed, both of which are in use today: documentation of stability of the nodule over a period of 2 years and identification of benign-appearing calcifications. Both methods are problematic: Stability was not found by robust and scientifically valid evidence to be a reliable criterion; the original data from the 1950s suggested a positive predictive value of 65% for benignity.[24] Identifying calcifications on radiographs as benign was shown by a later study to be a subjective judgment.[25]

Computed Tomography

In the absence of a chest radiograph from at least 2 years previously to provide a baseline for judging SPN stability, patients are referred for chest CT scan. CT is superior to chest radiography in establishing the margins and, more important, the internal characteristics of the pulmonary nodule. Spiculated margins are highly suggestive of, although not pathognomonic for, a malignant nodule (Fig. 1-2). This feature can reflect the presence of fibrosis in surrounding lung parenchyma, direct infiltration of the cancer into adjacent lung parenchyma, or localized lymphangitic spread.[26,27] In a study looking at 634 nodules, 50 of 53 (94%) that exhibited diffuse spiculation and 134 of 165 (81%) that showed focal spiculation were primary lung carcinomas.[28] On the other hand, 8 of the 66 (12%) smoothly marginated, nonlobulated nodules were primary lung cancer, 6 (1%) represented a solitary metastasis, and 52 (87%) were benign. Lobulation (Fig. 1-3) implies uneven growth, which often is associated with malignancy,[23] but it is not useful in distinguishing benign from malignant nodules. Of 350 smoothly marginated lobulated nodules, 91 (26%) were primary lung cancer, 57 (16%) were metastatic disease, and 202 (58%) were benign.[28]

With its ability to evaluate the internal characteristics of the SPN, CT revolutionized investigation of these findings. With its improved contrast resolution, elimination

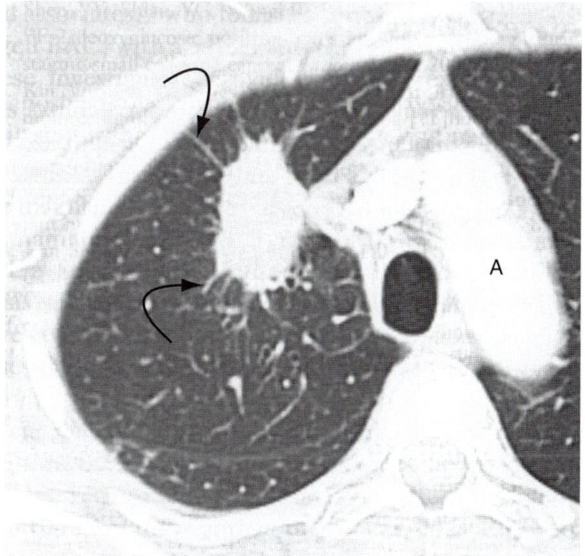

Figure 1-2 Adenocarcinoma with spiculations in a 61-year-old woman. Contrast-enhanced chest CT scan at the level of the transverse aorta (A) demonstrates a 2.8-cm nodule with spiculations *(arrows)*.

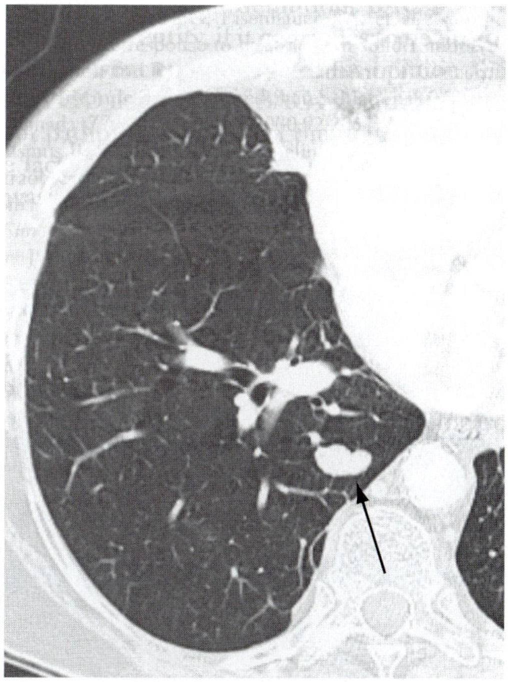

Figure 1-3 Adenocarcinoma with lobulation in a 79-year-old woman. Contrast-enhanced chest CT scan shows a lobulated 1.9 × 1-cm nodule *(arrow)*.

of overlapping structures, and slicing into thin sections, obvious calcifications can be visualized readily. For a nodule to be considered benign, obvious calcifications must be of the benign type. Characteristics of benign calcification include central, diffuse solid (Fig. 1-4), and lamination (Fig. 1-5) patterns and a popcorn-like appearance (Fig. 1-6). Solid, central, and laminated calcification patterns typically result from a remote infection with histoplasmosis or tuberculosis (see Figs. 1-4 and 1-5). The popcorn-like calcification pattern is seen with hamartomas (see Fig. 1-6). For a nodule to be considered benign, it should display one of these four patterns of calcification and should exhibit no other features worrisome for malignancy. If calcifications are eccentric or if a nodule is bilobate, irregular, or spiculated or abuts a central bronchus, it should not be considered benign despite the presence of benign-appearing calcifications, because essentially benign calcifications can be engulfed by malignancy.[28] In addition, because pulmonary metastatic disease from osteosarcoma or chondrosarcoma can manifest as benign-appearing calcified nodules, the calcification pattern cannot be used to differentiate benign from malignant nodules in patients with a history of one of these cancers. In such patients, benignity is established by long-term nodule stability. Another type of calcification, the sandlike, amorphous form, is seen in 6% of lung cancers imaged by CT.[29] Such calcifications can be seen

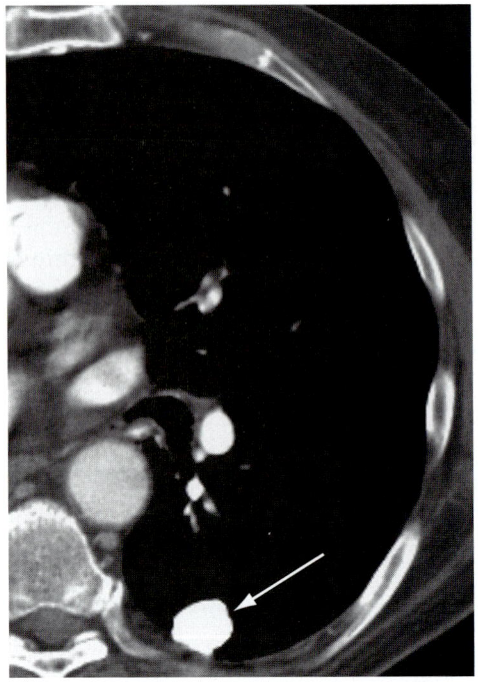

Figure 1-4 The patient was a 73-year-old man who had undergone right lower lobectomy for squamous cell lung cancer 2 years previously. Contrast-enhanced chest CT scan shows a benign, heavily and diffusely calcified nodule in the left lower lobe *(arrow)*. Note that calcification is denser than contrast in the vessels. The nodule proved to be stable on future imaging.

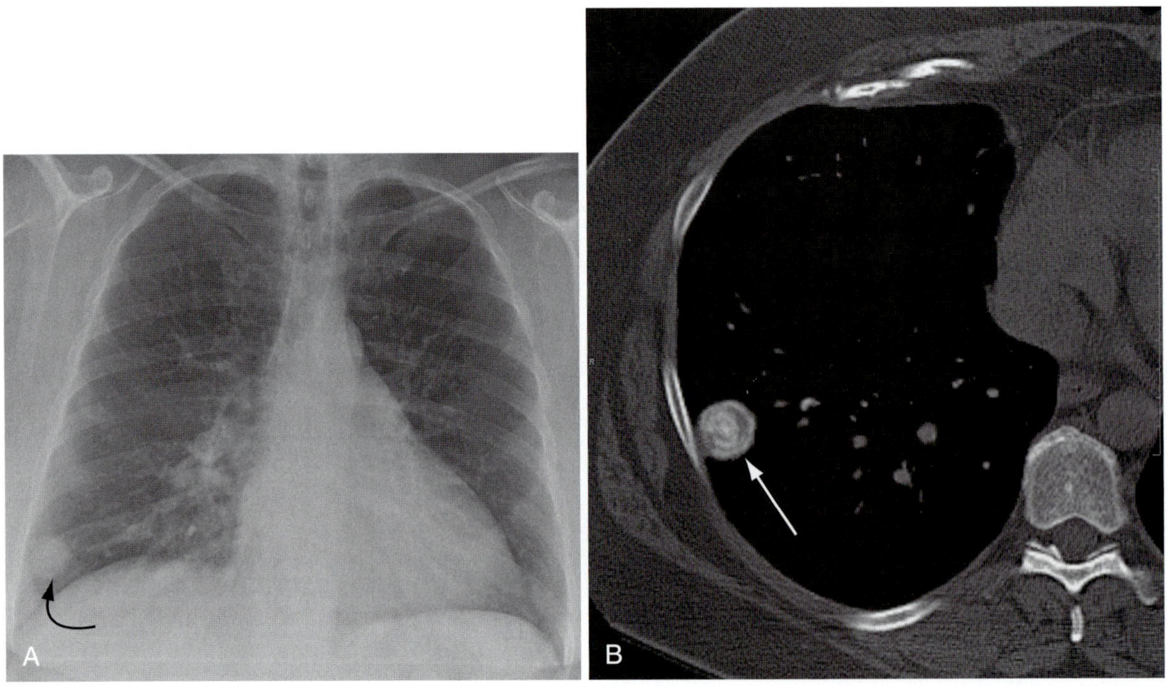

Figure 1-5 **A**, Incidental nodule *(arrow)* was discovered on a routine chest radiograph in a 47-year-old woman. **B**, Non–contrast-enhanced chest CT scan demonstrates laminated calcifications typical for previous infection with histoplasmosis *(arrow)*. The nodule remained stable at 5-year follow-up evaluation by chest CT *(not shown)*.

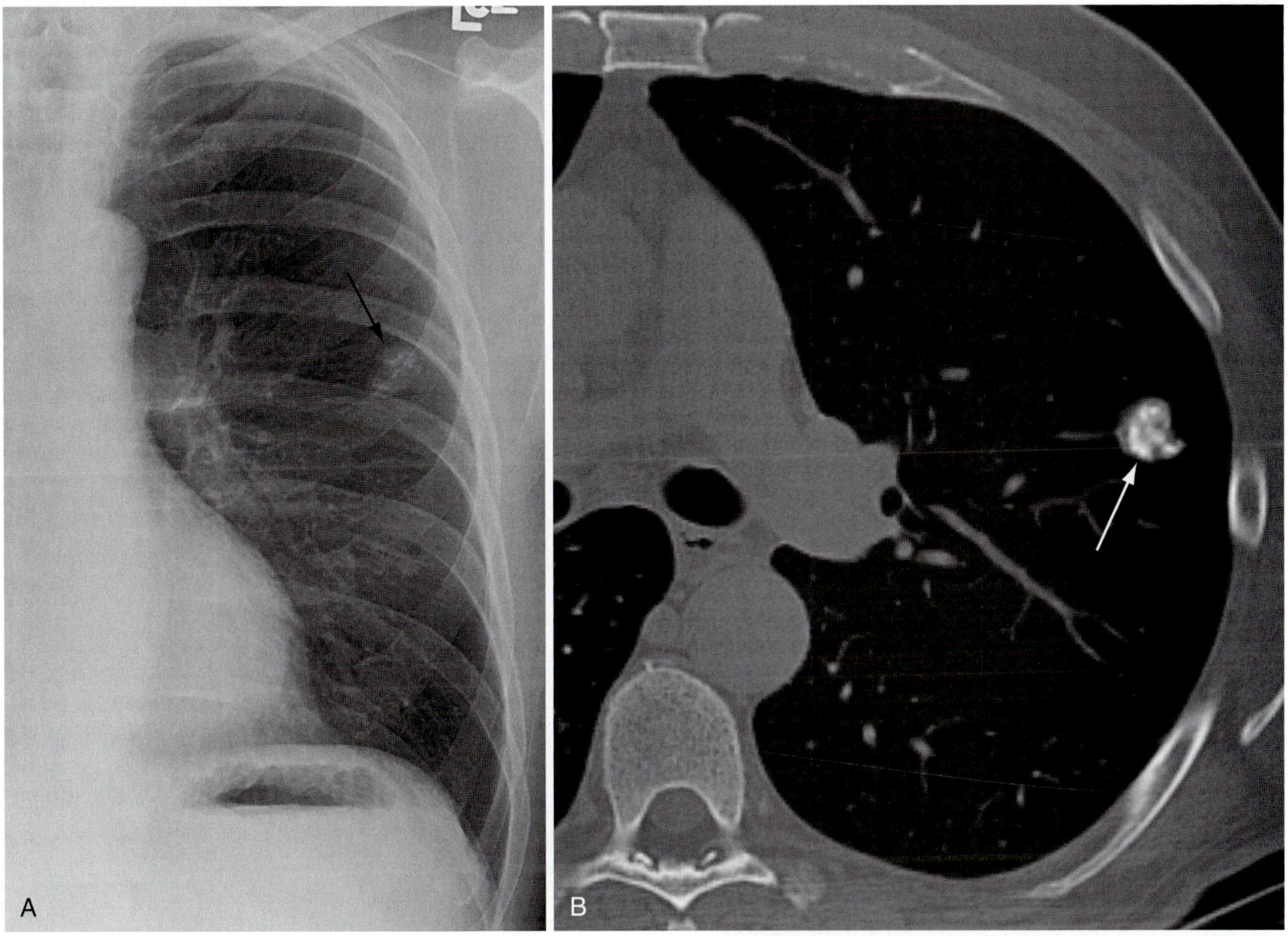

Figure 1-6 Treated non–small cell lung cancer of the right lung in a 59-year-old man. Left upper lobe nodule shows popcorn-like calcifications *(arrow)* on the chest radiograph (**A**) and non–contrast-enhanced chest CT scan (**B**), consistent with a pulmonary hamartoma. This nodule remained stable at 7-year follow-up evaluation by chest CT *(not shown)*.

in both benign and malignant disease and thus are not be useful in diagnosis (Fig. 1-7).

Although most nodules detected by CT are not obviously calcified, CT scans can objectively measure density with Hounsfield units (HU). In some previous attempts to identify subtle calcifications, not obvious to the human eye, measurements of density in HU were used to establish a threshold above which nodules were to be considered calcified and therefore benign.[30,31] These attempts were based on historical studies showing that malignancies with calcifications had been identified on radiographs in less than 1% of patients.[32–34] The assumption was that increased CT sensitivity would lead to identification of more benign nodules, with no false negatives, thereby reducing the number of futile thoracotomies. Subsequently, however, more than 10% of nodules evaluated as having a density higher than the established threshold of 185 HU (above which nodules should have been benign) were found to be malignant. This threshold was abandoned because it did not reliably distinguish between benign and malignant nodules.[31]

Fat is readily recognized on CT scans. A well-demarcated nodule containing fat and having a density between −40 and −120 HU is considered benign, usually a hamartoma (Fig. 1-8). A nodule consisting of fat alone or in combination with calcifications is seen in 60% of hamartomas on thin-section (using 2-mm slices) CT scans.[35] Such a nodule, even if slow-growing (with a doubling time longer than 2 years), is considered to represent a hamartoma. Popcorn-type calcification is a typical finding in hamartoma, although other benign-type calcifications can be seen as well. A third of hamartomas do not contain calcifications or fat on CT scan and remain indeterminate nodules.

The presence of an air bronchogram within a pulmonary nodule is rare (6%) in benign nodules, but this pattern is readily identified by CT scan (Fig. 1-9). Such an appearance is almost always associated with lung cancer of all cell types but is seen most commonly in adenocarcinoma (with or without bronchioloalveolar features).[36] CT scan also can differentiate among solid nodules, those with a ground-glass appearance (in which the lung vessels can

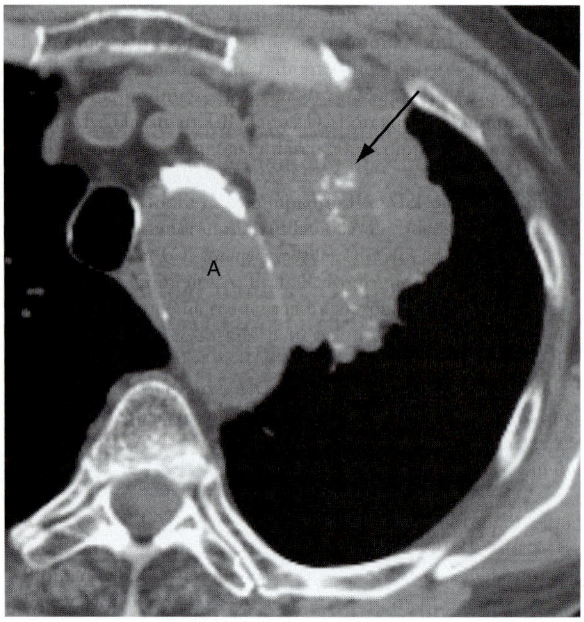

Figure 1-7 Adenocarcinoma of the left upper lobe in a 71-year-old woman. Non–contrast-enhanced chest CT scan at the level of the transverse aorta (A) shows a lobulated mass with amorphous calcifications within it *(arrow)*.

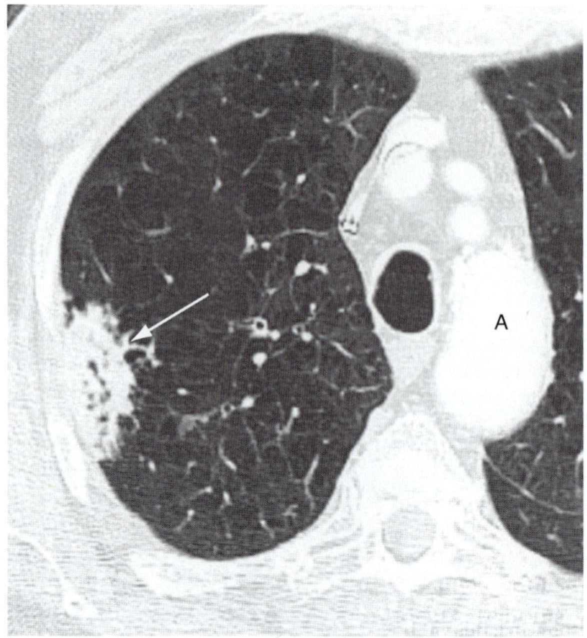

Figure 1-9 The patient was an 82-year-old man who underwent follow-up CT because of a prior history of gastrointestinal stromal tumor. Contrast-enhanced chest CT at the level of the transverse aorta (A) shows a new right upper lobe consolidated mass *(arrow)*. Tubular black structures within the mass represent the air bronchogram. Examination of a biopsy specimen *(not shown)* proved this to represent an adenocarcinoma of lung origin.

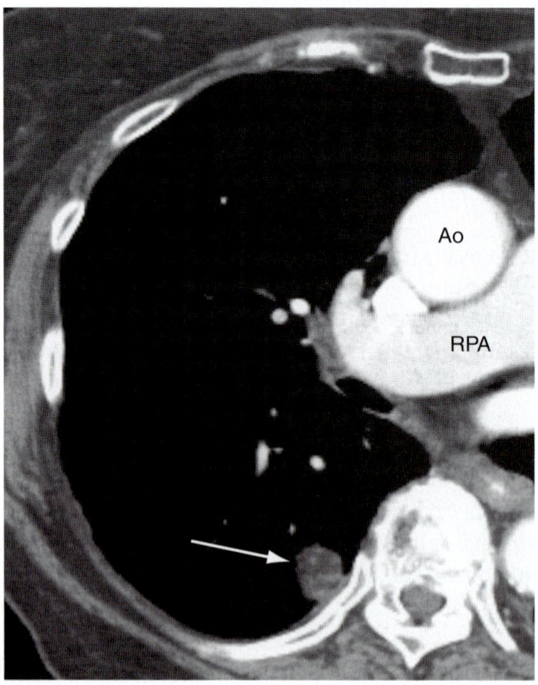

Figure 1-8 The patient was an 80-year-old woman in whom imaging was performed as follow-up for treated esophageal cancer. Contrast-enhanced chest CT scan shows a 2-cm nodule in the right lower lobe *(arrow)*. The nodule is of mixed attenuation and contains fat that is similar in CT appearance to the subcutaneous fat, with attenuation of −80 HU, consistent with a hamartoma. The nodule showed no significant growth at 4-year follow-up evaluation by chest CT *(not shown)*. Ao, aorta; RPA, right pulmonary artery.

be seen through the nodule), and mixed-pattern nodules, which combine a solid portion and ground-glass portion (Fig. 1-10). The malignancy rate is highest for mixed-pattern nodules (63%) and is higher for ground-glass nodules (18%) than for solid nodules (7%).[37]

Despite the superior sensitivity of CT over radiography for detection of benign nodules by identifying fat and calcium, a majority of nodules investigated by the initial CT scan remain indeterminate. The vessels supplying tumors differ both quantitatively and qualitatively from those supplying benign growths and tend to be more "leaky." This inherent difference in blood supply between malignant and benign nodules can be shown by changes in HU values in the pulmonary nodule after intravenous contrast injection. This method, in which the indeterminate nodule is imaged at intervals before and after intravenous contrast administration, was perfected by Swensen and associates.[38,39] Absence of significant lung nodule enhancement (density of 15 HU or less) on CT is suggestive of benignity. Although the method has only 77% accuracy and 58% specificity, it does identify 98% of malignant nodules and therefore is useful in guiding follow-up or intervention.

The CT features described here will identify those patients who have nodules with benign features that do not require follow-up (benign calcifications or fat), those who would benefit from an immediate biopsy, and those who

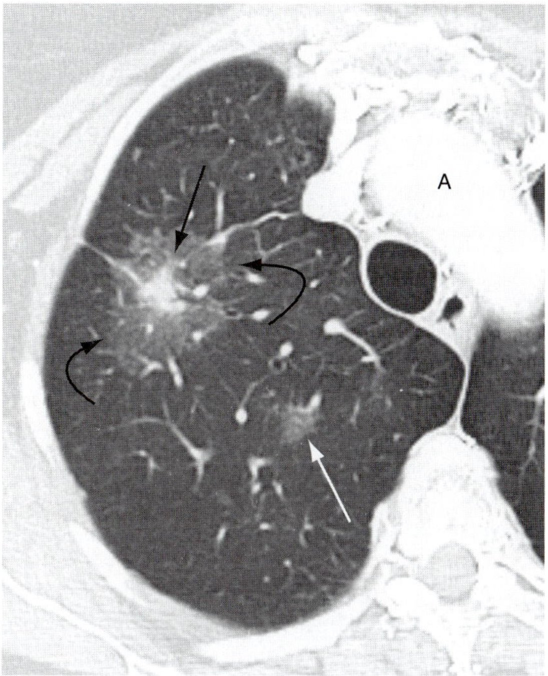

Figure 1-10 Multifocal bronchioloalveolar cell carcinoma in a 68-year-old woman. Contrast-enhanced chest CT scan at the level of the transverse aorta (A) shows one focus of her cancer to be a nodule with a ground-glass appearance *(white arrow)* and another focus as a mass of mixed attenuation: ground-glass opacity *(curved arrows)* with a solid center *(black straight arrow)*.

would benefit from CT monitoring of the nodule to assess its growth. The determination takes into account not only patient risk factors such as age and smoking exposure but also the CT features statistically recognized to be strongly associated with malignancy (e.g., large size, spiculation, mixed solid and ground-glass appearance). Of note, however, stability over a 2-year period is not an invariably valid criterion for benignity. In general, this criterion applies to nodules that are solid and larger than 1 cm.

Reliable detection of growth in nodules smaller than 1 cm can be difficult. For a nodule to double its volume, its diameter must increase by approximately 25%. It is difficult, even with CT, to visually detect the doubling of a 4-mm nodule, which is a change in diameter from 4 mm to 5 mm. Thus, small lung tumors can double in volume yet appear stable. Even computerized volume measurements, rather than diameter measurements, are not invariably accurate with such small nodules, which can appear to change size with differences in inspiratory effort and slice selection.[40] Nodules with a ground-glass appearance or with a mixed solid and ground-glass pattern are detected by CT scan, not by chest radiograph, and a stability criterion for benignity, such as the 2-year stability rule used with nodules detected by chest radiograph, has not been established for such nodules on CT. In fact, such nodules, which often are detected incidentally or by screening chest CT studies, can have very long doubling times. In a screening study in Japan,[41] the mean doubling time for ground-glass-pattern malignant nodules was 813 ± 375 days, for mixed ground-glass and solid tumors 457 ± 260 days, and for solid tumors 149 ± 125 days. In fact, 20% of the nodules in this study had doubling times exceeding 2 years, and these tended to be of the ground-glass type or mixed type. Thus, when a nodule smaller than 1 cm is monitored by CT to establish its benign nature, the follow-up period should be longer than 2 years.

Magnetic Resonance Imaging

The *contrast* resolution of MRI is superior to that of CT. This feature is exploited once cancer is diagnosed, because MRI is superior for evaluation of soft tissue involvement by cancer, such as in determining chest wall or nerve involvement. However, MRI does not serve effectively in early identification of lung cancer. Identifying pulmonary nodules smaller than 1 cm is hampered by the inferior *spatial* resolution of MRI, which is particularly poor in the lungs, as a consequence of characteristics both of the lungs themselves, such as low proton density and numerous air-tissue interfaces, and of the examination, such as motion artifacts from respiratory and cardiac motion. Dynamic contrast-enhanced MRI has been shown in small studies to have sensitivity rates for differentiation of malignant from benign SPNs that were comparable with those obtained with dynamic contrast-enhanced CT, but the nodules investigated usually were larger than the incidental nodules discovered by CT.[42–44]

Positron Emission Tomography

PET imaging with ^{18}F-fluorodeoxyglucose (FDG) has emerged as an additional tool for evaluation of the SPN. FDG-PET is a physiologic imaging modality, with poor spatial resolution in comparison with morphologic imaging modalities such as chest CT or radiograph. This technique assesses use of glucose by different body structures based on the preferential uptake of ^{18}F-FDG by metabolically active tissue. Because many cancers, including non–small cell lung cancer (NSCLC), have a higher metabolic rate than that of surrounding normal tissue, they accumulate ^{18}F-FDG more intensely and therefore appear "hot" on PET images. For nodules that are indeterminate on CT investigation, PET scan can help identify patients who may benefit from immediate biopsy. Initial studies showed that FDG-PET was effective in the differentiation of benign from malignant pulmonary lesions, and several early reports suggested that PET examinations reduce the number of patients with indeterminate nodules who undergo unnecessary thoracotomy, with overall sensitivity, specificity, and accuracy estimated to be 96%, 88%, and 94%, respectively.[45–51] PET is neither uniformly specific nor sensitive, however, particularly if the abnormality is small. Nodules smaller than 1 cm are not measured accurately and sometimes fall below the resolution of the PET scan.[52,53]

Although the combination of PET with a CT scan, or *integrated PET-CT*, has been shown to provide significantly greater specificity than that for either study alone,[54] the quantification of FDG uptake with use of CT for attenuation correction can introduce an artifact related to different breathing states in the CT and PET scans. FDG uptake in nodules, particularly those in the lower lungs, which suffer greater motion from the breathing cycle, will then erroneously appear to be lower than is actually the case.[55]

Cell type also influences FDG uptake. Indolent cancers, such as carcinoid tumors, well-differentiated adenocarcinomas, or bronchioloalveolar cell carcinoma (BAC), demonstrate less FDG activity than that seen in other NSCLCs and in some cases show no increased FDG activity.[48,53,56–60] The typical features of some of these cancers, such as proximity to a bronchus as is common with carcinoid tumors or the consolidative or ground-glass nodule in some BACs, are taken into account in interpreting the results of the PET-CT scan. The negative PET result thus serves as a tool, not a definite marker of benignity. If biopsy is deferred, the SPN with the negative PET result is monitored with serial chest CT scans for growth of the lesion. The data gathered thus far indicate that PET-negative nodules are indolent cancers; accordingly, this approach should not adversely affect patient outcome.[53]

The positive predictive value of PET in most patients is high (90% if the patient is older than 60 years).[61,62] False-positive studies of the primary lesion (a positive FDG-PET result with a lesion that proves to be benign) have been reported with infectious and inflammatory processes such as tuberculosis, histoplasmosis, and rheumatoid nodules.[50,61–66] Lesions with increased FDG uptake, however, should be considered malignant until proven otherwise and should be managed accordingly.

Imaging of Lung Cancer Subtypes

Imaging cannot replace histologic sampling of lung masses, but certain subtypes of lung cancer can manifest with typical imaging features.

Squamous cell carcinoma typically originates centrally, so the presenting manifestation frequently is postobstructive pneumonia or atelectasis, which is readily identified on the chest radiograph[34,67,68] (Fig. 1-11). Less common manifestations are mucoid impaction, bronchiectasis, and hyperinflation.[34,68,69] Approximately one third of squamous cell carcinomas arise beyond the segmental bronchi.[34,68] Squamous cell carcinomas are more likely to cavitate than the other histologic subtypes of lung cancer.[68] Cavitation occurs in 10% to 30% of these cancers and is more common in large peripheral masses and poorly differentiated tumors.[68] Because most squamous cell carcinomas grow slowly and become symptomatic because of their central location, extrathoracic metastases are encountered less commonly in imaging at presentation.[68]

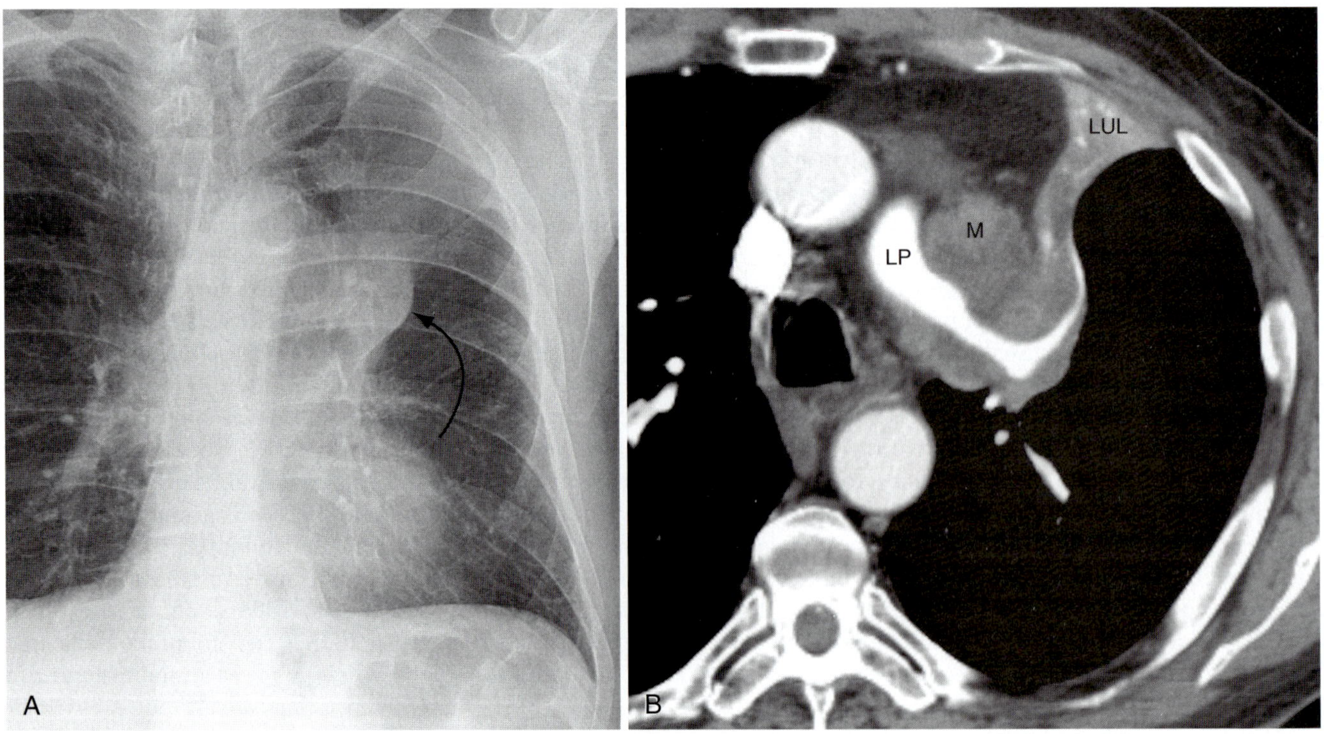

Figure 1-11 Newly diagnosed poorly differentiated squamous cell lung cancer in a 71-year-old man. **A**, Chest radiograph at presentation shows a central left hilar mass *(arrow)*. The hazy opacity above the arrow represents the collapsed left upper lobe. **B**, Contrast-enhanced chest CT scan at the level of the left pulmonary artery (LP) shows the central mass (M) encasing and narrowing the left pulmonary artery, causing left upper lobe (LUL) collapse.

Adenocarcinomas typically manifest as peripheral SPNs (see Fig. 1-9). Historically, nodules have been described as typically having soft tissue attenuation and an irregular or spiculated margin.[34,68] With the expanding use of CT and screening studies, however, an increasing number of adenocarcinomas manifest as nodules with a ground-glass appearance on CT or with mixed ground-glass and solid components (see Fig. 1-10). A correlation has been found between these CT appearances and the classification proposed by Noguchi and coworkers, whereby small (2 cm or less in greatest dimension) peripheral adenocarcinomas are classified into six types based on tumor growth patterns: type A, localized BAC; type B, localized BAC with foci of structural collapse of alveoli; type C, localized BAC with active fibroblastic proliferation; type D, poorly differentiated adenocarcinoma; type E, tubular adenocarcinoma; and type F, papillary adenocarcinoma with a compressive growth pattern.[70–72] Ground-glass attenuation of nodular opacities has been reported to be more frequent in types A to C than in types D to F, whereas soft tissue attenuation is more frequent in types B to F.[70] The soft tissue attenuation component tends to be absent or less than a third of the opacity with type A and greater in extent (more than two thirds) in types D to F. Mixed nodules, with both ground-glass and solid components, have a higher likelihood of being invasive and of higher stage than nodules with a pure ground-glass appearance.[73,74]

Although BAC is known to manifest with the unusual appearance of consolidation, this presentation is seen in only 30% of the cases; the rest of these tumors manifest as SPNs (43%) or multiple nodules (30%).[75] The SPNs are usually peripherally located and can remain stable in size for many years, with doubling times greater than 2 years. They can be of the ground-glass type or mixed type,[70,76] with cystic changes or cavitation occurring rarely, in up to 7%.[77,78] When a nodule exhibits multiple small, focal low-attenuation regions (pseudocavitation) or air bronchograms, the diagnosis of BAC should be suspected.[27,75,78,79] On PET-CT scans, BAC can show low FDG activity, lower than expected for malignancy.[57,80,81]

Large cell carcinoma usually manifests as a peripheral, poorly marginated large mass (larger than 7 cm in greatest dimension).[34,67,68,82–84] Although growth typically is rapid, cavitation is uncommon.

The most common presentation of carcinoid tumors is that of a central endobronchial mass, with or without atelectasis or consolidation, or, less commonly, a well-demarcated pulmonary nodule.[85,86] The tumors usually are less than 3 cm in diameter (Fig. 1-12), although occasionally they may be as large as 10 cm.[85,87–89] Calcification is seen in 25% of carcinoids by CT.[86] Carcinoids can show low FDG uptake on PET-CT studies, lower than expected for malignancies.[53,56,90]

The primary tumor of small cell lung cancer (SCLC) typically is small, in a central location, and associated with marked hilar and mediastinal adenopathy, frequently with engulfment of the primary lesion until it is no longer identifiable[34,67,83,91] (Fig. 1-13). With the increased use of CT and screening CT scans, the number of SCLCs encountered as early, small peripheral SPNs without intrathoracic adenopathy has increased. In the literature, detection of such early disease was reported in only 5% of the cases.[91,92]

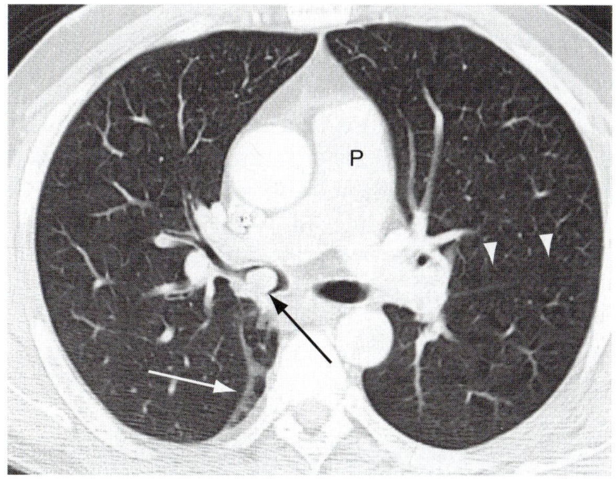

Figure 1-12 The patient was a 47-year-old man who presented with a new cough. Contrast-enhanced chest CT scan shows a nodule *(black arrow)* within the bronchus intermedius, causing some atelectasis of the right lower lobe, as depicted by the displacement of the right major fissure *(white arrow)*. Compare the normal position of the left major fissure *(white arrowheads)*. Nodule was removed endobronchially and proved to represent carcinoid. P, main pulmonary artery.

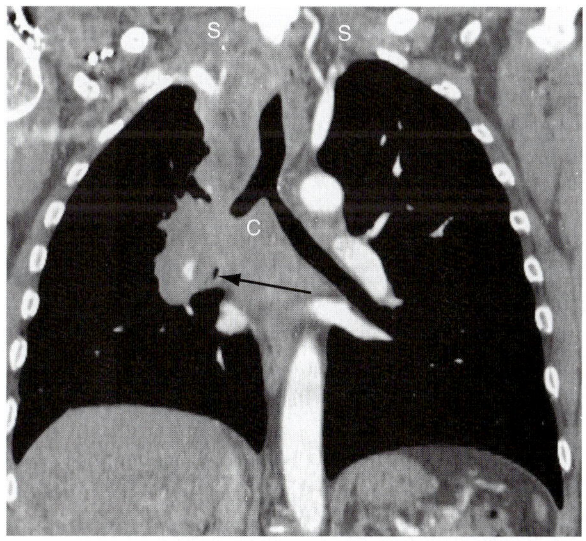

Figure 1-13 Newly diagnosed small cell lung cancer in a 52-year-old man. Coronal contrast-enhanced chest CT scan shows conglomerate lymphadenopathy involving the right hilum, subcarinal region (C), and bilateral paratracheal regions extending to involve the bilateral supraclavicular regions (S). This process obliterates the right main bronchus and significantly narrows the right lower lobe bronchus *(arrow)*. Note that the primary cancer cannot be differentiated from the extensive lymphadenopathy.

Staging

Non–Small Cell Lung Cancer

Accurate staging of lung cancer is important in determining disease management and prognosis. The primary goal of radiologic staging is to distinguish disease that is potentially resectable (stages I to IIIA) from nonresectable disease (stages IIIB and IV). The current TNM staging system assesses the primary tumor (T), spread into local lymph nodes (N), and distant spread, or metastasis (M). This system originally was designed for conventional anatomic assessment and does not take into account information from FDG-PET scans, although the PET data currently are being integrated into this staging system, and the use of this modality is described in this section. The TNM system proposed in 1997 is in current use (Tables 1-1 and 1-2).[93] A proposed revision to this TNM staging system was published recently[94] and has been implemented in some academic centers, but it has not yet been fully implemented in all clinical practices (Tables 1-3 and 1-4).

TABLE 1-1 NON–SMALL CELL LUNG CANCER: TUMOR-NODE-METASTASIS (TNM) DESCRIPTORS IN INTERNATIONAL STAGING SYSTEM FOR LUNG CANCER—6TH EDITION

Primary Tumor (T)	
TX	Primary tumor cannot be assessed *or* Tumor proven by the presence of malignant cells in sputum or bronchial washings but not visualized by imaging or bronchoscopy
T0	No evidence of primary tumor
Tis	Carcinoma in situ
T1	Tumor ≤ 3 cm in greatest dimension, surrounded by lung or visceral pleura, without bronchoscopic evidence of invasion more proximal than the lobar bronchus* (i.e., not in the main bronchus)
T2	Tumor with any of the following features of size or extent: >3 cm in greatest dimension Involves main bronchus, ≥2 cm distal to the carina Invades the visceral pleura Associated with atelectasis or obstructive pneumonitis that extends to the hilar region but does not involve the entire lung
T3	Tumor of any size that directly invades any of the following: chest wall (including superior sulcus tumors), diaphragm, mediastinal pleura, parietal pericardium *or* Tumor in the main bronchus < 2 cm distal to the carina, but without involvement of the carina, or tumor associated with atelectasis or obstructive pneumonitis of the entire lung
T4	Tumor of any size that invades any of the following: mediastinum, heart, great vessels, trachea, esophagus, vertebral body, carina *or* Tumor with a malignant pleural or pericardial effusion,† or with satellite tumor nodule(s) within the ipsilateral primary tumor lobe of the lung
Regional Lymph Nodes (N)	
NX	Regional lymph nodes cannot be assessed
N0	No regional lymph node metastasis
N1	Metastasis to ipsilateral peribronchial and/or ipsilateral hilar lymph nodes, and intrapulmonary nodes involved by direct extension of the primary tumor
N2	Metastasis to ipsilateral mediastinal and/or subcarinal lymph node(s)
N3	Metastasis to contralateral mediastinal, contralateral hilar, ipsilateral or contralateral scalene, or supraclavicular lymph node(s)
Distant Metastasis (M)	
MX	Presence of distant metastasis cannot be assessed
M0	No distant metastasis
M1	Distant metastasis present‡

*The uncommon superficial tumor of any size with its invasive component limited to the bronchial wall, which may extend proximal to the main bronchus, also is classified T1.

†Most pleural effusions associated with lung cancer are due to tumor. In a few patients, however, abundant cytopathologic evidence indicates that the effusion is not related to the tumor; in such cases, the effusion should be excluded as a staging element and the patient's disease should be staged T1, T2, or T3. Disease associated with pericardial effusion is classified according to the same rules.

‡Separate metastatic tumor nodule(s) in the ipsilateral non–primary tumor lobe(s) of the lung also are classified M1.

From Mountain CF. Revisions in the International System for Staging Lung Cancer. *Chest.* 1997;111:1710–1717; used with permission.

TABLE 1-2 NON–SMALL CELL LUNG CANCER: STAGE GROUPING BY TUMOR-NODE-METASTASIS (TNM) SUBSETS IN INTERNATIONAL SYSTEM FOR STAGING LUNG CANCER—6TH EDITION*

Stage	TNM Subset
0	Carcinoma in situ
IA	T1N0M0
IB	T2N0M0
IIA	T1N1M0
IIB	T2N1M0
	T3N0M0
IIIA	T3N1M0
	T1N2M0
	T2N2M0
	T3N2M0
IIIB	T4N0M0
	T4N1M0
	T4N2M0
	T1N3M0
	T2N3M0
	T3N3M0
	T4N3M0
IV	Any T any N M1

*Staging is not relevant for occult carcinoma, designated TXN0M0.
From Mountain CF. Revisions in the International System for Staging Lung Cancer. *Chest.* 1997;111:1710–1717; used with permission.

Although consensus on the optimal imaging modality for the staging of lung cancer is elusive, evidence-based guidelines were published by American Society of Clinical Oncology (ASCO) in 2004.[95] Initial evaluation is recommended to include a chest radiograph and a contrast-enhanced chest CT scan that encompasses the adrenal glands and liver. A PET scan is recommended for further evaluation in cases in which CT provides no evidence of metastatic disease. This recommendation is based on the fact that FDG-PET imaging improves nodal and distant metastatic staging and frequently alters staging to a degree that changes management.[96–101] The use of integrated PET-CT scanners has further enhanced the accuracy of staging of NSCLC, because these two studies, when performed together, complement each other by overcoming the lack of spatial resolution inherent in the PET scan and the lack of physiologic information inherent in the CT scan. These studies, in combination with clinical and laboratory findings, are then used to determine the necessity of additional imaging studies, as discussed later in this section.

Primary Tumor (T Status)

The T status is defined by the primary cancer's size, location, and invasion into surrounding structures. Because of the inferior spatial resolution of the PET scan, it is not used for T staging, which takes into account morphologic features alone. This restriction holds despite evidence that the amount of FDG uptake does correlate with prognosis,[102–105] and that patients whose primary tumor has higher FDG avidity, even if early-stage, have a shorter survival. The proposed staging system[94] includes changes to T status: T1 has been subcategorized as T1a, for tumors 2 cm or less in greatest dimension, or T1b, for tumors more than 2 to 3 cm or less in greatest dimension; T2 has been subcategorized as T2a, for tumors more than 3 to 5 cm or less in size, or T2, for tumors associated with certain other factors (see Table 1-1) and 5 cm or less in size, or T2b, for tumors more than 5 to 7 cm or less in size; T2 tumors larger than 7 cm have been reclassified as T3; T4 tumors with additional nodule(s) in the same lobe have been reclassified as T3; M1 tumors with additional nodule(s) in the same lung have been reclassified as T4; and T4 pleural dissemination has been reclassified as M1.

CT is the best overall imaging modality for determining the T stage, which usually is size-dependent. CT can readily identify features of more advanced T stage, such as gross chest wall involvement with rib destruction or bulging chest wall abnormality. CT is inaccurate, however, for identifying subtle chest wall involvement, such as involvement of the parietal pleura rather than tumor merely abutting the structure. In one study, the sensitivity of CT in distinguishing T3–T4 tumors from T0–T2 tumors was 63% and specificity was 84%.[106] Some subtle CT criteria suggestive of chest wall invasion are obliteration of the extrapleural fat plane, tumor-pleura contact extent greater than 3 cm in length, higher ratio of tumor-pleura contact extent to tumor height, and formation of an obtuse angle between tumor and pleura.[107] Despite the superior contrast resolution of MRI, its accuracy in identifying chest wall invasion is insufficient and similar to that of CT.[106,108] Although ultrasound imaging has a very limited role in the evaluation of patients with NSCLC, because the air within the lungs interferes with sound wave transmission, it affords better soft tissue resolution than that obtained with CT and has the advantage of providing real-time imaging throughout the respiratory cycle. For detection of chest wall involvement, ultrasound imaging is superior to CT, with a sensitivity of 89% (compared with 40% for CT) and similar specificity, approaching 100%.[109]

For detection of direct mediastinal involvement, CT and MRI findings suggestive of subtle invasion of the mediastinum are tumor contact extent greater than 3 cm with mediastinum, angle of contact with aorta greater than 90 degrees, and lack of mediastinal fat between the mass and mediastinal structures.[110–112] Although MRI was found in one study to be superior to CT in identifying direct mediastinal involvement,[106] accuracy of both modalities in assessment of mediastinal involvement was disappointing, with a sensitivity of 55% for CT and 64% for MRI.[113]

TABLE 1-3 NON-SMALL CELL LUNG CANCER: TUMOR-NODE-METASTASIS (TNM) DESCRIPTORS IN PROPOSED INTERNATIONAL STAGING SYSTEM FOR LUNG CANCER—7TH EDITION

Descriptor	Definition
T (Primary Tumor)	
TX	Primary tumor cannot be assessed
	or
	Tumor proven by the presence of malignant cells in sputum or bronchial washings but not visualized by imaging or bronchoscopy
T0	No evidence of primary tumor
Tis	Carcinoma in situ
T1	Tumor ≤ 3 cm in greatest dimension, surrounded by lung or visceral pleura, without bronchoscopic evidence of invasion more proximal than the lobar bronchus (i.e., not in the main bronchus)*
T1a	Tumor ≤ 2 cm in greatest dimension
T1b	Tumor > 2 cm, but ≤3 cm in greatest dimension
T2	Tumor > 3 cm, but ≤7 cm in greatest dimension
	or
	Tumor with any of the following features (T2 tumors with these features are classified T2a if ≤5 cm in size)
	Involves main bronchus, ≥2 cm distal to the carina
	Invades visceral pleura
	Associated with atelectasis or obstructive pneumonitis that extends to the hilar region but does not involve the entire lung
T2a	Tumor > 3 cm, but ≤5 cm in greatest dimension
T2b	Tumor > 5 cm, but ≤7 cm in greatest dimension
T3	Tumor > 7 cm in greatest dimension
	or
	Tumor that directly invades any of the following: chest wall (including superior sulcus tumors), diaphragm, phrenic nerve, mediastinal pleura, parietal pericardium
	or
	Tumor in the main bronchus < 2 cm distal to the carina but without involvement of the carina, or associated with atelectasis or obstructive pneumonitis of the entire lung or separate tumor nodule(s) in the same lobe
T4	Tumor of any size that invades any of the following: mediastinum, heart, great vessels, trachea, recurrent laryngeal nerve, esophagus, vertebral body, carina
	or
	Tumor with separate tumor nodule(s) in a different ipsilateral lobe
N (Regional Lymph Nodes)	
NX	Regional lymph nodes cannot be assessed
N0	No regional lymph node metastasis
N1	Metastasis in ipsilateral peribronchial and/or ipsilateral hilar lymph nodes and intrapulmonary nodes, including involvement by direct extension
N2	Metastasis in ipsilateral mediastinal and/or subcarinal lymph node(s)
N3	Metastasis in contralateral mediastinal, contralateral hilar, ipsilateral or contralateral scalene, or supraclavicular lymph node(s)
M (Distant Metastasis)	
MX	Distant metastasis cannot be assessed
M0	No distant metastasis
M1	Distant metastasis
M1a	Separate tumor nodule(s) in a contralateral lobe; tumor with pleural nodules or malignant pleural (or pericardial) effusion†
M1b	Distant metastasis

*The uncommon superficial spreading tumor of any size with its invasive component limited to the bronchial wall, which may extend proximally to the main bronchus, is also classified as T1.

†Most pleural (and pericardial) effusions with lung cancer are due to tumor. In a few patients, however, findings on multiple cytopathologic examinations of pleural (pericardial) fluid are negative for tumor, and the fluid is nonbloody and is not an exudate. Where these elements and clinical judgment dictate that the effusion is not related to the tumor, the effusion should be excluded as a staging element and the patient's disease should be classified as T1, T2, T3, or T4.

From Goldstraw P, Crowley J, Chansky K, et al. International Association for the Study of Lung Cancer International Staging Committee participating institutions. The IASLC Lung Cancer Staging Project: proposals for the revision of the TNM stage groupings in the forthcoming (seventh) edition of the TNM classification of malignant tumours. *J Thorac Oncol*. 2007;8:706–714; used with permission.

TABLE 1-4 NON–SMALL CELL LUNG CANCER: STAGE GROUPING BY TUMOR-NODE-METASTASIS (TNM) SUBSETS AND OTHER PROPOSED CHANGES IN INTERNATIONAL STAGING SYSTEM FOR LUNG CANCER—7TH EDITION

Previous T/M Descriptor	Proposed T/M	N0	N1	N2	N3
T1 (≤2 cm)	T1a	IA	IIA	IIIA	IIIB
T1 (>2–3 cm)	T1b	IA	IIA	IIIA	IIIB
T2 (≤5 cm)	T2a	IB	**IIA**	IIIA	IIIB
T2 (>5–7 cm)	T2b	**IIA**	IIB	IIIA	IIIB
T2 (>7 cm)	T3	**IIB**	**IIIA**	IIIA	IIIB
T3 invasion		IIB	IIIA	IIIA	IIIB
T4 (same lobe nodules)		**IIB**	**IIIA**	**IIIA**	IIIB
T4 (extension)	T4	**IIIA**	**IIIA**	IIIB	IIIB
M1 (ipsilateral lung)		**IIIA**	**IIIA**	**IIIB**	**IIIB**
T4 (pleural effusion)	M1a	**IV**	**IV**	**IV**	**IV**
M1 (contralateral lung)		IV	IV	IV	IV
M1 (distant)	M1b	IV	IV	IV	IV

Listings in **bold** indicate a change from the sixth edition for a particular TNM category.
From Goldstraw P, Crowley J, Chansky K, et al. International Association for the Study of Lung Cancer International Staging Committee participating institutions. The IASLC Lung Cancer Staging Project: proposals for the revision of the TNM stage groupings in the forthcoming (seventh) edition of the TNM classification of malignant tumours. *J Thorac Oncol.* 2007;8:706–714; used with permission.

The superb soft tissue contrast resolution and multiplanar capability of MRI are ideally used for evaluation of superior sulcus tumors. In a retrospective study of 143 patients with superior sulcus tumors, longer survival was associated with surgery in the absence of nodal disease.[114] An absolute contraindication to surgery is tumor invasion of the brachial plexus roots or trunks above the level of the T1 nerve root. The similarity of the brachial plexus to its surrounding structures, its superior-inferior orientation, and its small size make it almost impossible to evaluate accurately in the axial plane. It is, however, readily identified in the sagittal plane by MRI.[115] Although NSCLC T4 lesions, such as those involving the vertebral body, generally are considered unresectable, superior sulcus tumors that involve less than 50% of the vertebral body may be resectable, often with the aid of the neurosurgical team.[116–118] At the time of imaging, MRI can determine whether the carotid artery and the vertebral artery are involved by tumor; such involvement is a relative contraindication to surgery. MRI also can determine if the contralateral vessels are severely affected by atherosclerotic disease, in which case surgery may not be an option.[119] In addition to determining resectability, imaging plays a vital role in selecting the most appropriate surgical approach. Posteriorly located tumors are amenable to resection through a posterolateral incision, but tumors that involve the trunks of the brachial plexus or the subclavian vessels usually require an anterior approach.

Over the years, different MRI sequences have been developed to overcome flow artifacts and to improve vascular and cardiac images in motion. MRI is used to assess whether the tumor directly involves the heart and, if it does, to what extent. It has been shown that in a select group of patients with T4 lesions involving the heart (Fig. 1-14), a trimodality approach (chemotherapy and concomitant radiotherapy plus surgery) improved survival. Patients who underwent tumor resection had a significantly better 5-year survival rate than that in patients who did not: 38% versus 5.6%.[120]

In the current staging system, disease presenting as a malignant pleural effusion falls into the T category

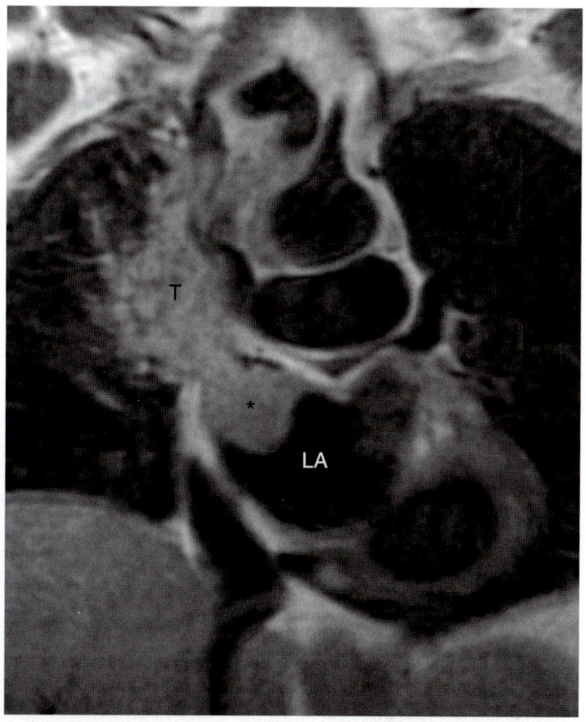

Figure 1-14 Newly diagnosed poorly differentiated adenocarcinoma of the right upper lobe in a 64-year-old woman. Coronal view on MRI study of the heart, double inversion recovery sequence, demonstrates the right upper lobe tumor (T) invading the left atrium (LA) through the orifice of the right superior pulmonary vein. *Tumor within the left atrium.

of staging, as T4 disease; in the proposed new system, such cases should fall into the M category of disease.[94] Unfortunately, it is frequently difficult to establish the diagnosis of a malignant pleural effusion, because fluid obtained at thoracentesis is positive for malignancy in only 66% of patients,[121] and the pleura does not always show nodularity on CT imaging. Imaging with PET is helpful, but studies on the accuracy of PET in establishing the diagnosis of a malignant effusion are few, with reported sensitivities of 92% to 100%, specificities of 67% to 71%, negative predictive values of 100%, and positive predictive values of 63% to 79%.[122,123] PET scans for pleural malignancy should be interpreted with caution and in conjunction with the CT scan, as inflammation after talc pleurodesis can last for years, and show increased FDG uptake in the absence of malignant cells[124] (Fig. 1-15). A negative PET result can be useful, however, in confirming the absence of pleural metastatic disease, particularly when the results of thoracentesis are also negative.

Nodal Disease (N Status)

The proposed new staging system includes no changes in nodal staging (see Tables 1-1 and 1-3). The role of the chest radiograph in the nodal staging of NSCLC is usually minor, as it is usually insensitive to mild and modest nodal enlargement. Bulky bilateral adenopathy dictates a diagnosis of stage IIIB. If the patient is too ill or is unwilling to undergo treatment, this should suffice for staging. For the majority of patients, however, more accurate staging is needed.

CT scanning is routinely used for noninvasive staging of the lymph nodes. The sole criterion for differentiating benign from malignant lymph nodes, by CT or by MRI, is size. The most widely used criterion for identifying a malignant lymph node is a short axis diameter greater than 1 cm.[125] This criterion was chosen as a fine balance between sensitivity and specificity, in order to minimize false-negative evaluations. Numerous studies have looked at the performance of CT in distinguishing benign and malignant lymph nodes in patients with NSCLC. A large study that pooled lymph node data for 5111 patients from 43 different studies found that the sensitivity of CT for detecting metastases in the mediastinal lymph nodes was 51% and the specificity 86%. Similarly, two meta-analyses showed sensitivity rates of 61% to 64% and specificities of 74% to 79%.[126,127] The accuracies of CT and MRI in detecting nodal metastases are similar: the accuracy of CT ranges from 56% to 82% and that of MRI from 50% to 82%.[106,113,128–131] Such poor performance is due to the fact that normal-sized lymph nodes may harbor tumor and that nodal enlargement may be a response to a benign reactive process.[132,133] Recent attempts to abandon the size criteria for malignancy in favor of MRI examination of internal characteristics of the lymph node, such as high signal intensity, eccentric cortical thickening, or obliterated fatty hilum, have shown similar disappointing results, with accuracy rates of 70% to 73%.[134,135]

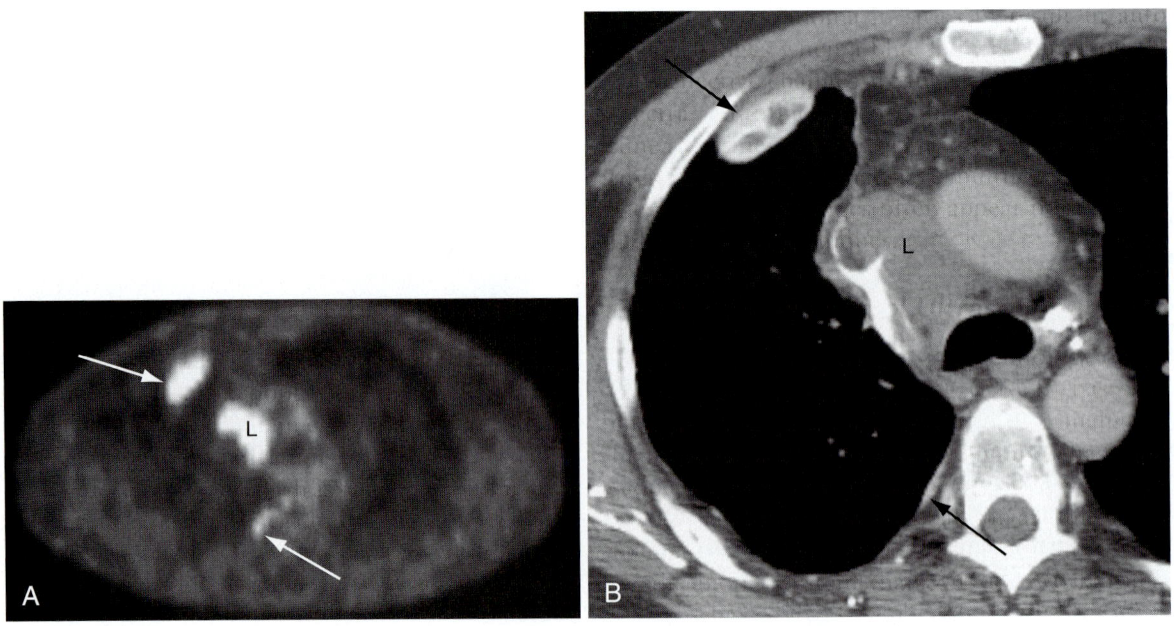

Figure 1-15 Mediastinal lymph node recurrence 2 years after right upper lobectomy for non–small cell lung cancer in a 56-year-old man. **A**, Axial PET scan demonstrates uptake within the right paratracheal lymph node (L), reflecting recurrence. Focal high FDG activity is apparent within the two regions in the pleura that were initially suspicious for pleural metastatic disease *(white arrows)*. **B**, Corresponding contrast-enhanced chest CT study, however, shows that the focal FDG-avid regions within the pleura correspond to high-density pleural abnormalities *(black arrows)*, consistent with activity from the inflammatory response to talc pleurodesis. The patient had undergone talc pleurodesis for persistent air leak after his lobectomy 2 years before these images were obtained.

The accuracy of PET is superior to that of CT in nodal staging, but the results should be interpreted with caution and in conjunction with CT findings. Non-neoplastic inflammatory processes also show increased FDG activity. As with the pulmonary nodule, PET is less accurate in the evaluation of lymph nodes smaller than 10 mm. In a pooled analysis of multiple studies in which a total of 2865 patients were evaluated, the sensitivity and specificity of PET for identifying metastatic lymph nodes were 74% and 85%, respectively.[136] In a meta-analysis of 17 studies comprising 833 patients, the overall sensitivity of PET for detecting nodal metastases was 83% and the specificity was 92%, whereas the sensitivity and specificity of chest CT were 59% and 78%, respectively.[137] Integrated PET-CT improves nodal staging over that achieved with PET alone.[96,138] In the presence of enlarged lymph nodes, PET and PET-CT become less specific and less accurate but more sensitive in detecting nodal metastatic spread.[139–143] In one meta-analysis, the median sensitivity and specificity of PET scans were 100% and 78%, respectively, in patients with enlarged lymph nodes.[127] The reduced specificity in the presence of enlarged lymph nodes means that almost one fourth of patients diagnosed with metastatic lymph nodes actually had no nodal metastasis but rather a reactive or inflammatory lymphadenopathy.

Because of these limitations, ASCO recommends that a confirmatory biopsy be performed in cases of FDG-avid mediastinal lymph nodes, so that patients with operable disease will not be denied curative surgery.[95] A PET scan is justified even when the initial chest CT scan confirms highly suspect mediastinal lymph nodes. The PET scan may influence the site of biopsy by identifying a previously unsuspected location of metastatic disease (which may upstage the disease) or a location that is safer to biopsy. In patients whose mediastinal lymph nodes are smaller than 1 cm, approximately 20% will show false-negative findings on PET scans; in a meta-analysis, the sensitivity and specificity of PET were 82% and 93%, respectively.[127] Although PET demonstrates all lymph node stations, whereas mediastinoscopic or transbronchial lymph node biopsy is unable to sample all lymph node stations, biopsy remains the most accurate preoperative measure for identifying occult metastatic disease in mediastinal lymph nodes smaller than 1 cm.

Distant Metastases (M Status)

The purpose of staging is to detect metastatic disease, particularly at the common metastatic sites for NSCLC—the adrenal glands, liver, brain, and bone—with the goal of preventing nontherapeutic thoracotomy. In the recently proposed revision to the TNM staging system, M status has been divided into M1a for metastases within the thoracic cavity and M1b for extrathoracic metastatic disease. The M1a category includes malignant pleural effusions and malignant pleural nodules, previously designated T4, and metastatic pulmonary nodules to the contralateral lung.[94]

Beyond the initial chest CT scan, little consensus has emerged regarding the optimal noninvasive staging for NSCLC. When patients are found to have early disease (stage I or II) by the initial chest CT examination, with no clinical symptomatology, the yield for imaging for additional metatatic disease is low.[144–146] Although some proponents advise further extrathoracic staging for tumors whose histologic type is associated with a higher likelihood of extrathoracic metastasis at the time of presentation, such as adenocarcinoma or large cell carcinoma,[144,145,147,148] this approach was not found to be productive in a large series of patients with early-stage lung cancer.[146] In addition, results of each imaging modality should be interpreted with caution, because biopsy of each suspected metastatic site is not feasible, and results often rely on follow-up or comparison with other imaging modalities. In a study examining biopsy specimens of normal-appearing adrenal glands in patients with NSCLC staged by chest CT scan, 12% of the glands were found to harbor metastatic disease. A more recent study that compared autopsy results with findings on CT scan of the adrenal glands obtained within 90 days before death showed that CT detected only 20% of the metastatic adrenal glands. This low sensitivity was considered to be due to the lack of substantial structural change in many of these adrenal glands.[149]

On the basis of these findings, recent guidelines of the American College of Chest Physicians[150] and the latest ASCO recommendations[95] recommend PET scanning for staging but also further imaging in accordance with to symptomatology or for abnormal lesions that remain indeterminate after the initial investigations with PET and CT. Except in the brain, PET has a higher sensitivity and specificity than CT or bone scan in detecting metastatic disease.[151–153] In a study of 303 patients, the sensitivity and specificity for detection of M1 disease by PET were 83% and 90%, respectively.[98] An average of 15% of patients have unexpected distant metastases detected by PET,[101] and in 20% of patients, findings on PET imaging preclude nontherapeutic thoracotomy.[98,99] PET scanning has the advantage of imaging the entire body with one examination and assessing areas not covered by conventional imaging, such as the skin, muscles, and pelvis, for detection of unusual metastatic foci.

The adrenal glands are the most common site of metastasis in patients with NSCLC,[154,155] and adrenal metastasis can occur as an isolated site in as many as 6% of patients.[156] Adrenal masses are found in as many as 20% of patients at initial presentation, yet a majority are benign.[154,155,157–166] CT or MRI features suggesting that an adrenal nodule is malignant include size greater than 3 cm, poorly defined margins, an irregularly enhancing rim, invasion of adjacent structures, and high signal intensity on T2-weighted MRI sequences.[167] When CT shows an adrenal nodule with density measured as 10 HU or less, a confident diagnosis of adrenal adenoma is made. This finding has 98% sensitivity but only 71% specificity,[168] because 30% of adenomas do not contain a sufficient amount of lipid to be measurable by CT.[169] In these cases, an effective choice is MRI using chemical shift analysis to differentiate a benign from a malignant nodule.[170-172] Results of chemical shift analysis (with MRI) and HU measurement (with CT) can include errors when the adrenal gland nodule is small.

PET imaging is excellent in establishing that an adrenal nodule is benign. Although early studies suggested that the accuracy of PET in determining the nature of an adrenal mass was 100%,[153,172] further experience with PET scanning has shown that, although the sensitivity and specificity are high at 100% and 80% to 90%, respectively, increased FDG uptake can be seen in adenomas.[152,173] Greater accuracy is obtained when an adrenal nodule is found to have greater FDG activity than that of the liver, rather than using a specific standardized uptake value (SUV) as a threshold[174] (Fig. 1-16). Because uptake can be high in adenomas, ASCO recommends that an isolated adrenal mass on an ultrasound image, CT scan, or FDG-PET scan be biopsied to rule out metastatic disease if the lesion is otherwise considered to be potentially resectable.

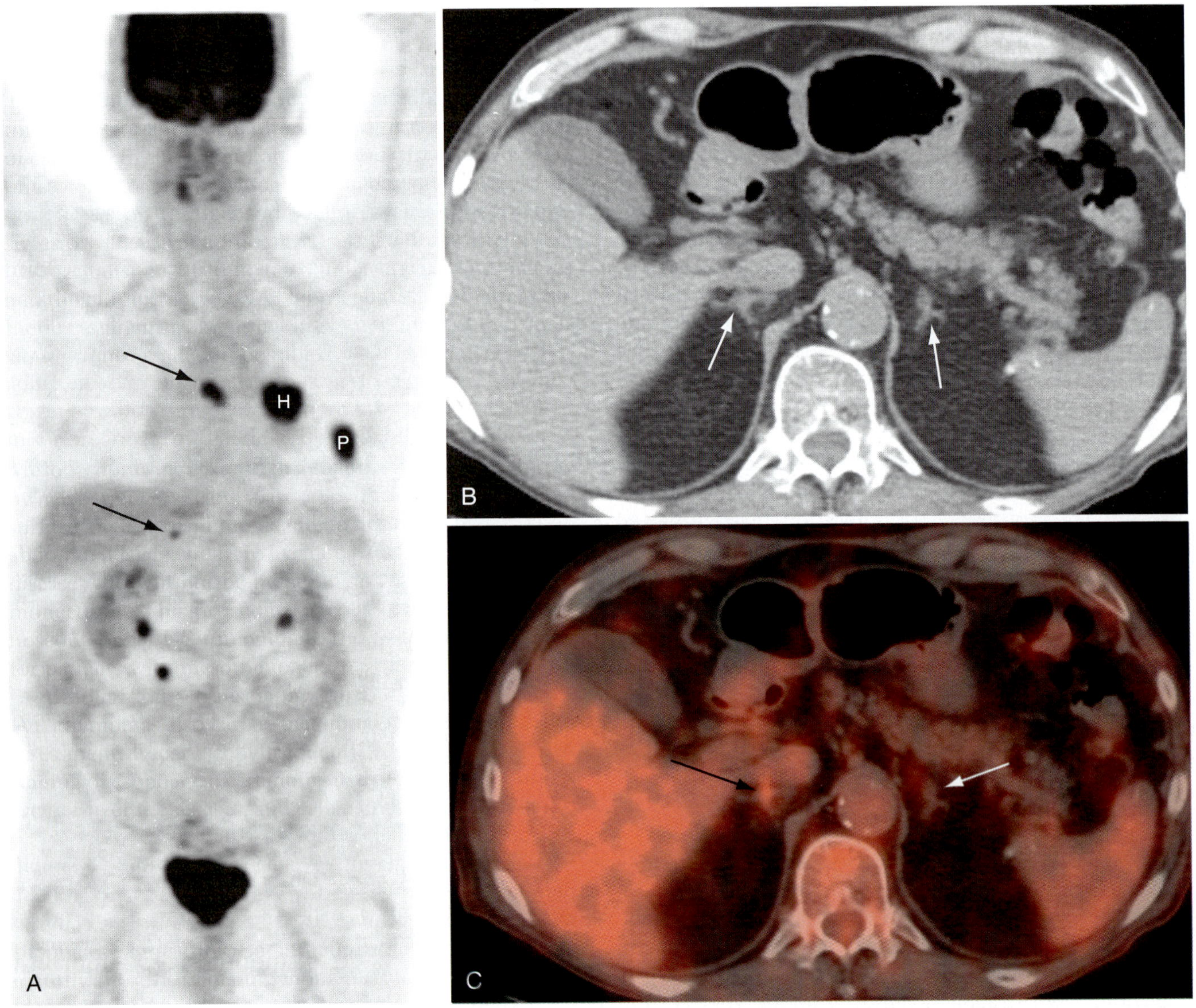

Figure 1-16 Non–small cell lung cancer in an 83-year-old man. **A**, PET coronal maximum intensity projection image shows FDG uptake in the primary cancer (P) and in right hilar (H) and subcarinal *(upper arrow)* lymph nodes. Uptake also is evident above the right kidney, corresponding to the right adrenal region *(lower arrow)*. **B**, Corresponding CT scan shows mild fullness in both adrenal glands *(white arrows)*. **C**, Fused PET-CT image shows FDG uptake in the right adrenal gland *(black arrow)*, biopsy-proven to represent metastatic disease. The left non–FDG-avid adrenal gland *(white arrow)* proved to be stable for 1 year.

Although NSCLC frequently metastasizes to the liver, it is unusual for the liver to be an isolated site of disease, particularly in the absence of metastatic disease to regional lymph nodes. In most cases, therefore, the finding of liver metastases does not significantly alter management of the disease.[175] One meta-analysis found that only 3% of asymptomatic patients with NSCLC will have liver metastases on CT scan. Although PET has been found to detect liver metastases with accuracy rates ranging between 92% and 100%,[153,157,176] with only rare false-positive findings, the data from available studies are limited and were not compared with results of systematic biopsies or state-of-the-art liver imaging. When a liver lesion is suspected to represent metastatic disease by any imaging modality, it needs to be confirmed with biopsy if the disease is considered to be potentially resectable.[95]

Routine evaluation for brain metastases in asymptomatic patients presenting with newly diagnosed NSCLC remains controversial and is not universally recommended by ASCO.[95] When brain CT is performed in asymptomatic patients staged for NSCLC, the median prevalence of brain metastases is 3% (range, 0% to 21%),[144,177–184] with a median predictive value of a negative clinical evaluation of 97%, whereas when brain CT is performed in both symptomatic and asymptomatic patients, the prevalence of brain metastases is 14% (range, 6% to 32%).[185–193] Asymptomatic brain metastases are more commonly found in patients with advanced intrathoracic disease.[148,194] The detection rate for patients with stage I or II disease is 4% with imaging by CT or MRI, whereas a detection rate of 11.4% has been reported for those with stage III disease.[184] Although MRI can detect smaller and more numerous brain metastases,[184] no studies have been conducted showing that MRI is better than CT at identifying patients with metastases from NSCLC. Consequently, ASCO recommends that either CT or MRI is acceptable for imaging for brain metastases. Either study should be performed in patients who have neurologic signs or symptoms, as well as in asymptomatic patients with stage III disease who are being considered for aggressive local therapy such as thoracotomy or irradiation.[95] PET is not recommended for imaging of brain metastases: PET performs poorly in the evaluation of brain metastases because FDG avidly accumulates in the gray matter, limiting detectability of metastatic disease, which usually occurs in the same region. Sensitivity for detection of brain metastases by PET can be as low as 60%.[153]

Although patients with skeletal metastases usually are symptomatic or have laboratory abnormalities indicating bone metastases,[192] 27% of asymptomatic patients in one study were found to have skeletal metastases.[195] However, false-positive abnormalities on technetium-99m methylene diphosphonate bone scintigraphy are numerous, owing to the frequency of degenerative and traumatic skeletal changes. PET scanning is superior to bone scintigraphy in identifying skeletal metastases: PET not only is able to view marrow metastases that typically are not detected by bone scintigraphy but also yields few false-positive results. The specificity, sensitivity, negative predictive value, positive predictive value, and accuracy of PET scanning in the assessment of bone metastases all exceed 90%.[151,153,195,196] Accordingly, ASCO's position is that bone scintigraphy is optional in patients who have evidence of bone metastases by PET scanning, unless suggestive symptomatology is noted in regions not imaged by PET. Because of the possibility of false-positive uptake with both PET and bone scintigraphy, patients who are operative candidates are required to have histologic confirmation or corroboration by morphologic imaging (plain radiography, CT, or MRI) of a lesion that will increase the stage of their disease.[95]

To summarize staging for NSCLC, imaging with a chest CT scan that includes the adrenal glands is routine. If disease does not appear to be metastatic, further staging with PET or PET-CT is recommended.[95] Biopsy of suspect mediastinal lymph nodes (i.e., those larger than 1 cm or with increased FDG activity) is needed for confirmation of nodal disease. Patients with locally advanced disease who are to undergo aggressive therapy (surgery or irradiation) should undergo dedicated brain imaging (MRI or contrast-enhanced CT) even if they are asymptomatic. Additional imaging, such as brain imaging for early disease or dedicated bone imaging (plain film, scintigraphy, or MRI) is performed if the patient is symptomatic, or to clarify equivocal imaging findings on the initial PET and CT studies. When a metastatic focus is found that would change clinical management, such as one metastatic lesion in a patient whose disease is otherwise resectable, it should be verified with biopsy.

Small Cell Lung Cancer

Compared with imaging studies of NSCLC, studies on the usefulness of imaging in the staging of SCLC are few. This lack may be related to the dismal prognosis for the disease, to the fact that the great majority of patients are treated nonsurgically, or to the simplified method of dichotomous staging developed by the Veterans Administration Lung Cancer Study Group.[197] According to this method, limited disease includes tumors confined to the hemithorax of origin, the mediastinum, and/or the supraclavicular lymph nodes. In extensive disease, tumor spreads beyond those limited sites. Most patients presenting with SCLC have disseminated disease at initial staging.[198] Since the common sites of metastatic disease are the liver, bone, bone marrow, brain, and retroperitoneal lymph nodes, many of the patients with metastatic disease are identified at the initial staging chest CT scan, but there is no concensus as to the routine use of imaging modalities in this disease.

Multiple studies are routine, including bone marrow aspiration, brain MRI, CT of the chest and abdomen, and bone scintigraphy.[199] Attempts have been made to image the entire body with one imaging modality and eliminate the multiplicity of studies. Although this can be done with MRI, it has not gained popularity.[198] Lately, attempts have been made to popularize staging with PET or PET-CT, but this was not embraced in the management guidelines issued recently by the American College of Chest Physicians,[199] mainly because a majority of these studies investigated fewer than 50 patients and lacked reference standards to verify staging accuracy.[200–205] As in NSCLC, PET-CT is more accurate than chest CT staging alone and is inferior to conventional imaging when assessing for brain metastases.[200–208] Most recent reports suggest that staging with PET entails a change in management in 8% to 16% of patients with SCLC.[207,208]

Extensive assessment for bone metastases (i.e., bone marrow aspiration, bone scintigraphy, and MRI) is not performed for asymptomatic patients with limited disease. It is usually reserved for patients with extensive disease because isolated bone metastases and bone marrow metastases are not common.[197,209,210]

Brain metastases, on the other hand, are common at presentation. Because they are seen at presentation in as many as 24% of asymptomatic patients who undergo contrast-enhanced brain MRI, such imaging has been advocated by many experts as part of routine staging.[198,211]

Liver metastases and retroperitoneal lymph node metastases usually are asymptomatic yet are common at presentation of SCLC.[197,209] Staging should therefore include the entire liver, and imaging for this purpose should be performed with intravenous contrast, by either CT or MRI.

Follow-up Evaluation

Assessing Response to Chemotherapy

Accurately assessing a cancer's response to chemotherapy is important clinically, for individual patients (both surgical and nonsurgical candidates) and for trials assessing the efficacy of novel anticancer therapies. In patients with potentially resectable lung cancer receiving chemoradiotherapy, evaluating the response of the tumor to therapy is important in assessing the efficacy of treatment and predicting the long-term prognosis. This information is of potential value in helping to determine which patients will benefit most from surgery and which patients may require additional nonsurgical treatment. In patients who are not surgical candidates, or whose disease is not responding to therapy, potentially toxic and expensive chemotherapeutic drugs may be changed or discontinued. Small differences in patients' response rates can affect the outcome of phase I and II clinical trials, which may dictate which new drugs are introduced to the market. Accordingly, uniform, reproducible, and accurate response criteria are essential.

Traditionally, response to therapy has been assessed by measuring tumor volume. Because calculation of tumor volume is cumbersome, simplified methods have been applied over the years that are correct for spherical tumors. Response criteria proposed in 1979 after a meeting on the Standardization of Reporting Results of Cancer Treatment were widely accepted.[212] These criteria, known as the World Health Organization (WHO) criteria for reporting the results of cancer treatment, are based largely on tumor measurements in two dimensions—the two longest perpendicular diameters in the axial plane that are perpendicular to each other. In 1994, the WHO criteria were reviewed, and revised guidelines known as Response Evaluation Criteria in Solid Tumors (RECIST) were proposed. These guidelines recommended determination of treatment response using a single measurement of the largest tumor diameter in the axial plane.[213]

Measurements using the WHO and RECIST criteria can be inaccurate for nonspherical tumors and for tumors with indistinct margins. When these criteria were proposed, a generalized assumption was that they would allow accuracy and reproducibility of measurements performed by different readers. The accuracy of the criteria has been questioned, however, because a recent study demonstrated great interobserver variability in the measurement of tumors, potentially leading to incorrect interpretations of tumor response. Consistency in measured diameters was improved when the same reader performed serial tumor measurements—a protocol that can be implemented in clinical trials but is not always feasible in routine daily practice.[214]

PET imaging after the initiation of chemotherapy or radiotherapy can assess the response of the primary tumor to treatment by detecting a reduction in metabolic activity of the primary mass,[215,216] a favorable prognostic indicator of survival for both patients with NSCLC and those with SCLC.[42,200,217–221] In a prospective study in 60 patients with stage III NSCLC who underwent neoadjuvant chemoradiotherapy before surgical resection, a restaging PET study performed 2 weeks after induction therapy was able to predict the pathologic response in the primary tumor, determined at subsequent surgery, with a sensitivity of 86% and a specificity of 81%.[215] In another prospective study in 57 patients with locally advanced NSCLC who underwent restaging PET imaging after only one cycle of platinum-based chemotherapy, a fall in SUV_{max} of 20% or greater in the primary tumor was an independent predictor of long-term survival.[220] Median survival duration was 252 days in responders but only 151 days in nonresponders. Because SUV is only a semiquantitive measurement affected by multiple technical factors, small changes in SUV are considered insignificant.

In 1999, after reviewing FDG-PET oncology studies, the European Organization for Research and Treatment of Cancer PET study group published universal guidelines for determination of tumor response that have been applied to studies.[222] These have been implemented in daily practice and some study designs, but have not yet been implemented into the RECIST guidelines.[223] These guidelines define complete metabolic response as complete resolution of FDG activity in the tumor; partial metabolic response as a decrease of SUV by 15% to 25% after one chemotherapy cycle, or a decrease of greater than 25% after more than one chemotherapy cycle; stable metabolic disease as an increase in SUV of less than 25% or decrease of SUV of less than 15%; and progressive disease as an increase in SUV by more than 25%.

Some issues with PET imaging in the evaluation of tumor response remain unresolved. The ideal timing of the study has not yet been demonstrated, because inflammatory response from therapy, such as associated with radiation therapy, increases FDG activity as well. FDG-PET does not appear to offer any advantages over CT for lymph node staging or for predicting the pathologic response after neoadjuvant treatment of NSCLC.[215,224] In patients who have received neoadjuvant therapy before planned surgical resection, clearance of all tumor from mediastinal lymph nodes is important for a favorable outcome after subsequent surgery.[225,226] Repeat invasive nodal sampling by mediastinoscopy is difficult owing to the extensive mediastinal fibrosis that results from neoadjuvant therapy, which also reduces the diagnostic yield of material obtained by endoscopic fine needle aspiration. Unfortunately, results with both CT and PET have been disappointing in use of these modalities for detection of viable residual tumor and fibrotic lymph nodes after neoadjuvant chemotherapy. Further studies are needed before PET can be used routinely for assessment of tumor response.

Detection of Recurrence after Definitive Treatment

The 2003 ASCO recommendations for the treatment of NSCLC[95] did not see a role for routine imaging in asymptomatic patients after curative treatment of NSCLC, because no rigorous randomized, controlled trials of lung cancer follow-up were conducted to show that early detection of recurrence in asymptomatic patients would significantly prolong survival. A prospective study aggressively monitoring 192 patients postoperatively with chest radiographs every 3 months and with chest CT scans and bronchoscopy every 6 months found a 71% recurrence rate; 26% of the recurrences were in asymptomatic patients.[227] The 3-year survival rate was 13% in all patients but 31% in patients whose recurrence was detected while they were asymptomatic. These results do not take into account the lead time bias, which is known to influence survival. Large retrospective series in which traditional morphologic imaging was used for follow-up monitoring have questioned the benefits of aggressive surveillance.[228–230]

At present, no published findings assessing the effect of early detection of recurrence by PET on survival are available. Detection of recurrent disease using morphologic imaging such as CT can be hampered by the effects of treatment, both surgery and irradiation, which often leave parenchymal scars, fibrosis, pleural thickening, or effusions, any of which may simulate recurrent disease.

PET imaging has been shown to be more useful than conventional imaging for diagnosing tumor recurrence, and findings can lead to major changes in management in as many as 63% of patients with suspected relapse.[231–233] Several prospective studies have shown a sensitivity of 98% to 100% and a specificity of 62% to 92% for the detection of recurrent malignancy after definitive treatment with surgery, chemotherapy, or radiotherapy.[215,231,234,235] Specificity of PET for detection of malignant disease is lower than at initial staging because post-therapeutic inflammation is FDG-avid, especially in the first few months after radiation therapy. This pitfall can be overcome only by careful inspection of both PET and CT images. Diffuse FDG uptake is suggestive of the inflammation associated with radiation therapy,[200] whereas focal uptake is more suggestive of recurrence. Waiting 3 to 6 months for the inflammatory response to subside will permit detection of the focal residual FDG uptake of recurrence. For improved detection earlier on, careful inspection of the CT images may be helpful in identifying typical inflammatory changes. Findings that suggest recurrence of disease on a post-treatment PET scan should be confirmed by biopsy, to avoid treatment errors.

Uncommon Primary Pulmonary Malignancies

Some histologic subtypes of primary lung cancer are rare but typically have radiologic features that may suggest their histologic traits, as discussed next.

Sarcomatoid Carcinoma

Carcinomas with pleomorphic, sarcomatoid, or sarcomatous elements are rare. On radiologic images, these neoplasms can manifest either as large peripheral masses or as polypoid endobronchial lesions with atelectasis or postobstructive pneumonia.[236–239] Calcification and cavitation are uncommon, but necrosis and hemorrhage can manifest as areas of heterogeneous attenuation on CT scan[237–239] (Fig. 1-17). Hilar or mediastinal adenopathy is uncommon.[238] Pleural effusion can result from local invasion.[237] Metastases involve sites similar to those of lung cancer: lung, liver, bones, adrenal glands, and brain.[239]

The typical appearance of pulmonary blastoma is a large (2.5 to 26 cm in diameter), well-marginated peripheral mass.[240–243] Multiple masses, cavitation, and calcification are rare.[243] Local invasion of the mediastinum and of the pleura occurs in 8% and 25% of cases, respectively.[241] Metastases to hilar and mediastinal lymph nodes are present in 30% of the cases after resection.[241] Extrathoracic metastases are common and have a distribution similar to that of lung cancer.[241,244]

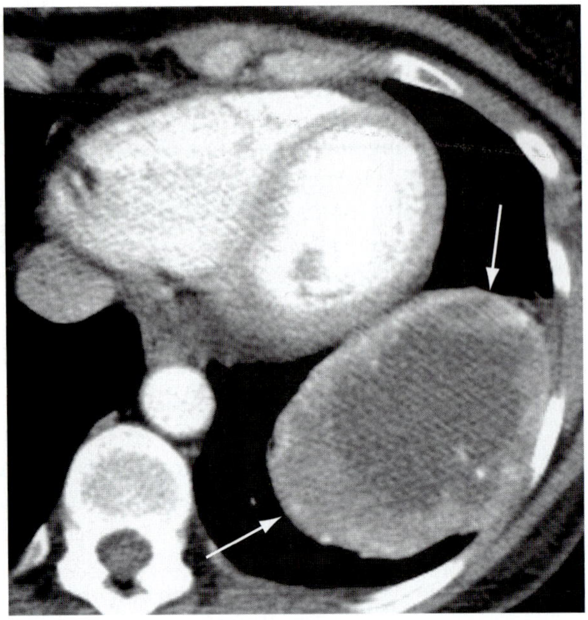

Figure 1-17 The patient was a 49-year-old asymptomatic woman who was discovered to have a left lung mass on a chest radiograph obtained for evaluation for clubbing of the fingers. Contrast-enhanced chest CT scan demonstrated a 9-cm mass *(arrows)*. Note the heterogeneity of the tumor with peripheral contrast enhancement and a large central low-attenuation region consistent with necrosis. Pathologic examination revealed sarcomatoid malignant neoplasm.

Neoplasms of the Tracheobronchial Glands

Neoplasms of the tracheobronchial glands only rarely manifest as a peripheral pulmonary nodule, which usually is located in the central airways. Of note, these neoplasms frequently are missed on chest radiographs, because the tracheal air column and proximal bronchi often constitute a "blind spot" for many radiologists. This limitation suggests the importance of CT imaging, which readily demonstrates the airways, in an adult patient who presents with new-onset "asthma."

Up to 80% of adenoid cystic carcinomas are confined to the trachea or main bronchi (Fig. 1-18), but 10% to 15% may manifest as a peripheral pulmonary nodule.[245-248] The typical radiologic appearance is that of an endotracheal or endobronchial mass, usually lobulated or polypoid, encroaching on the airway lumen. Masses can be circumferential and may manifest as diffuse stenosis.[249] A less common manifestation is a peripheral lung nodule or mass.[246,248] Although metastatic spread from adenoid cystic carcinoma has a distribution similar to that of metastatic spread from NSCLC,[248] such spread occurs late, because this tumor exhibits slow, progressive local growth.[246] Patients with this cancer, therefore, usually are considered to be surgical candidates, and CT is used for surgical planning. Although CT readily demonstrates the extratracheal extent of these tumors, it underestimates the longitudinal extent of the tumor.[250] This limitation is related in part to technical factors, which can be addressed by imaging the tumor with thin slices and reconstruction in different planes, but also to the tendency of the tumor to infiltrate beneath the mucosa, which is not identifiable by CT.

Mucoepidermoid carcinomas typically arise in the main or lobar bronchi but, in rare instances, may be located in the trachea and periphery of the lung.[251-253] They usually are slow-growing, low-grade neoplasms with a benign clinical course, although some have high-grade features with a more aggressive clinical course.[253-255] These two forms have a similar radiographic appearance, however, and cannot be distinguished from each other.[253] The tumor manifests as a central endobronchial mass; less common presentations include a polypoid intraluminal tracheal nodule and peripheral pulmonary nodule or mass.

Mesenchymal Malignant Tumors of the Lung

Spindle cell sarcomas (malignant fibrous histiocytoma, hemangiopericytoma, fibrosarcoma, leiomyosarcoma, synovial sarcoma) are the most common primary pulmonary sarcomas.[256-259] On radiologic images, they are more commonly located in the periphery of the lung, although central and endobronchial masses are reported.[257,258,260-262] Tumors as large as 25 cm in diameter have been reported at presentation, probably reflecting this sarcoma's slow growth rate and tendency to metastasize late. The tumor typically is sharply marginated and occasionally calcified.[256-258,260,263] Cavitation is uncommon, although heterogeneous attenuation resulting from necrosis within the mass may be seen on CT scan.[256,263] The rich vascularity of hemangiopericytomas in the lung can be appreciated on CT, MRI, and ultrasound imaging, but this tumor cannot be distinguished from other sarcomas, which can contain similar-looking vascularity. Features suggesting rich vascularity include feeding arteries, which can be visualized directly by CT or MR angiography, as well as indirect signs such as avid enhancement on contrast-enhanced chest CT or MRI, and evidence of hemorrhage; high attenuation on unenhanced chest CT scan and hyperintense areas on both T1- and T2-weighted images at MRI.[262,264,265]

Primary lung sarcomas with a vascular origin (angiosarcomas, epithelioid hemangioendotheliomas) are rare primary tumors of the lungs.[258,266,267] Angiosarcomas of the lung are described as multiple bilateral nodules, but most probably are metastatic, and a primary elsewhere has to be excluded.[258] Pulmonary epithelioid hemangioendothelioma usually manifests radiologically as multiple, 1- to 2-cm bilateral pulmonary nodules, although single nodules and unilateral distribution have been reported in approximately one fourth of affected patients.[266,268,269] Irregular thickening of the bronchovascular bundles and

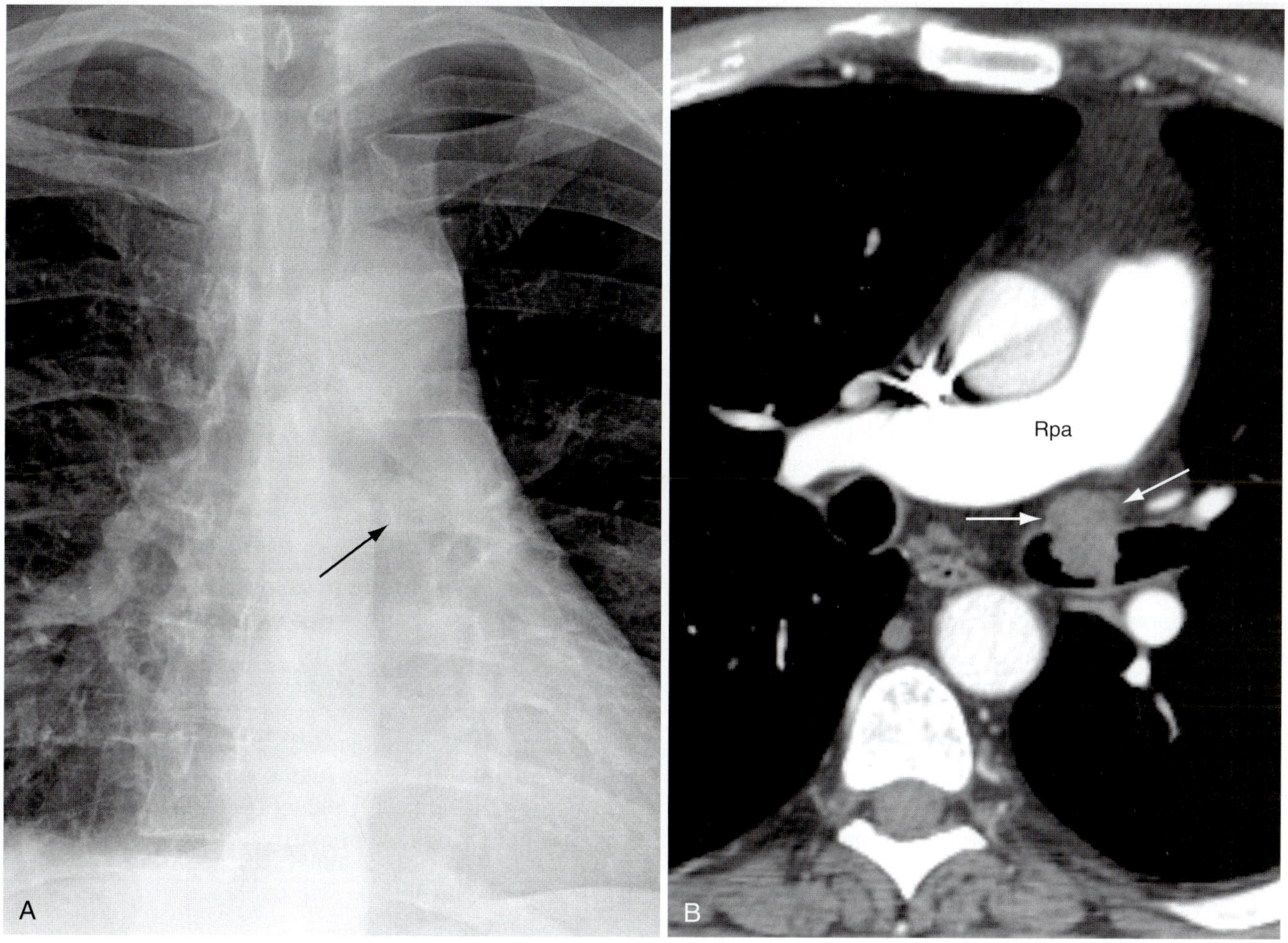

Figure 1-18 Adenoid cystic carcinoma of the left bronchus in a 48-year-old man presenting with pneumonia. **A**, On a 1-month follow-up radiograph after resolution of pneumonia, the left endobronchial abnormality is very difficult to see *(arrow)*. **B**, Contrast-enhanced chest CT scan at the level of the right pulmonary artery (Rpa) confirms a left bronchial mass *(arrows)* involving the extrabronchial soft tissues, with near-complete obliteration of the left bronchial lumen.

perilobular structures due to lymphangitic spread and associated multiple pulmonary nodules as well as multiple small peripheral nodules seen bilaterally on high-resolution CT scans also have been described.[270] Calcification is rarely detected but is common on histologic examination.[268,269] Although primary lung sarcoma usually is an indolent tumor, the presence of hemorrhagic pleural effusion is a poor prognostic sign.[266]

Primary Lymphoma of Lung

The radiologic findings in primary lymphoma of the lung may vary according to the criteria used to define this disease. Perhaps the most widely accepted criterion for this definition is monoclonal lymphoid proliferation, without extrathoracic lymphoma sites at presentation or for at least 3 months after diagnosis. Some investigators restrict the diagnosis to pulmonary parenchymal disease only, whereas others include hilar adenopathy with or without mediastinal adenopathy.[271–277] The parenchymal manifestations of the disease include solitary nodule or mass, multiple nodules or masses, focal or multifocal consolidation, reticulonodular opacities, and atelectasis.[272,278–282] Hilar adenopathy is rare, and pleural effusions occur in 7% to 25% of the patients.[272,279,283]

SECONDARY MALIGNANT LUNG TUMORS

Although metastasis to the lung can occur along multiple routes, through pulmonary or bronchial arteries, lymphatics, or airways, the radiologic manifestations of such disease demonstrate considerable overlap. The four patterns of metastatic disease to the lung parenchyma are parenchymal nodules, interstitial thickening (lymphangitic carcinomatosis), tumor emboli with or without pulmonary hypertension or infarction, and airway obstruction from endobronchial tumor.

Parenchymal nodules constitute the most common manifestation of metastatic disease to the lung and usually are multiple, with lower lobe predominance.[284] Although the increasing use of multidetector helical (spiral) CT with decreasing slice thickness has led to increased sensitivity for the detection of pulmonary metastatic disease, specificity is low, and many of the nodules identified are benign. When nodules are new, growing, and multiple in a patient with a primary malignancy, they are more likely to represent metastatic disease. When the diagnosis is in doubt, biopsy is considered for the largest nodule. Small nodules (less than 4 mm in greatest dimension) in a patient with malignancy should be monitored to assess for growth. Such nodules are too small for accurate assessment with PET scanning.

Solitary metastases to the lung are uncommon, occurring in 2% to 10% of patients presenting with an SPN.[21,28,285] Their prevalence is dependent on the type of imaging: More than one additional nodule was identified on CT scan in 32% of cases in which only one nodule was observed on a chest radiograph.[286] Certain primary malignancies are more likely to manifest with metastatic disease to the lung in the form of a solitary nodule: sarcoma, carcinoma of the colon, kidney, testicle, or breast, and melanoma.[21,287,288] No reliable radiologic criteria have been found to distinguish an SPN that is a primary malignancy from metastatic disease,[28,285] because their imaging features overlap.

When multiple pulmonary nodules are present, they usually are well demarcated, although they may have irregular margins, as is seen more commonly with adenocarcinoma.[289] The nodules may vary in size, ranging from large cannonball metastases, as seen in sarcomas, to multiple, small 1-mm nodules, to a miliary pattern, as seen in thyroid cancer. Some unusual patterns of metastatic nodules have been recognized. Cavitation in metastatic nodules, as detected by chest radiograph, is seen in approximately 4% of metastatic cases, most commonly those of squamous cell histology.[290,291] On CT, however, cavitation is seen in 9% of metastatic nodules at equal frequencies for adenocarcinoma and squamous cell histologic subtypes.[292] Metastatic sarcoma also can cavitate, which accounts for pneumothorax on presentation.[293,294] As already stated, heavily calcified pulmonary nodules are considered to be benign. This rule does not apply, however, to primary osteosarcoma or chondrosarcoma, because calcification and ossification can occur in pulmonary metastases from these primaries.[293] Calcification in pulmonary metastases from other primary malignancies is much less common but has been reported with synovial sarcoma, giant cell tumor of the bone, and carcinomas of the colon, ovary, breast, and thyroid.[293,295–297] The CT *halo sign*, which is a solid nodule surrounded by ground-glass opacities (opacities through which the pulmonary vessels can be seen on the scan), suggests peritumoral hemorrhage,[289] but this possibility should be distinguished from other processes that have this appearance, such as invasive fungal infections, BAC, and lymphoma.[298–300]

Lymphangitic carcinomatosis is uncommon but usually occurs from primary tumors arising from lung, breast, stomach, pancreas, prostate, cervix, or thyroid.[293,301] Chest radiographic findings may mimic those in pulmonary edema, from which it must be distinguished, and include thickened bronchovascular markings and interlobular septal thickening and, in some cases, pleural effusions.[302,303] As many as 50% of patients with pathologically proven lymphangitic carcinomatosis have a normal-appearing chest radiograph.[304,305] In one study, the rate of confident diagnosis of lymphangitic carcinomatosis rose from 54% when based on clinical information and chest radiograph alone to 92% with the addition of chest CT, whereas without imaging, no case was confidently diagnosed.[306] Lymphangitic carcinomatosis typically manifests on thin-section CT with thickening of the interlobular septa and peribronchovascular bundles and preservation of the normal lung architecture.[303,307] This pattern of interstitial thickening gives a CT appearance characterized by polygonal shapes with a central dot (Fig. 1-19). This feature in association with nodularity of the interlobular septa is pathognomonic for this condition, because such nodularity is not seen with pulmonary edema.[308] When no nodularity is seen, the nondependent distribution and asymmetry may help distinguish lymphangitic carcinomatosis from pulmonary edema. Approximately 30% of patients with lymphangitic carcinomatosis present with pleural effusions and 40% with mediastinal or hilar adenopathy.[303]

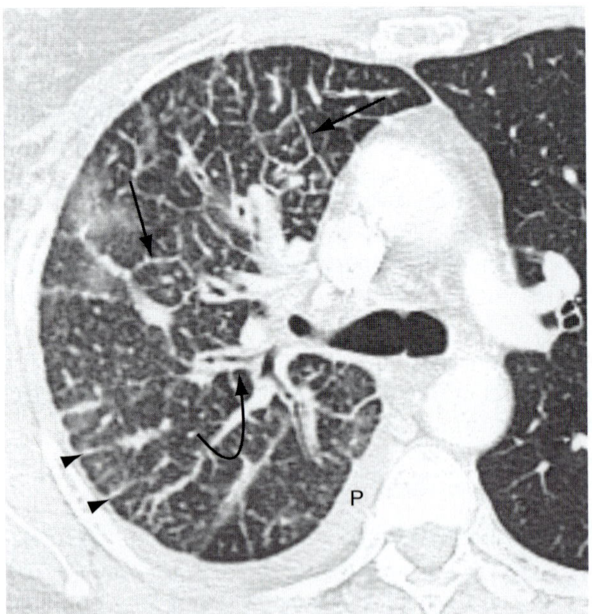

Figure 1-19 Non–small cell lung cancer and lymphangitic carcinomatosis of the right lung in a 53-three-year-old woman. Contrast-enhanced chest CT scan shows nodular thickening of the interlobular septa at the periphery of the lung *(arrowheads)* and peribronchovascular thickening *(curved arrow)*, as well as polygonal shapes *(straight arrows)* with a central dot, which represent the thickened interlobular septa encasing the secondary pulmonary lobule, with thickened interstitium surrounding the central pulmonary arteriole. P, pleural effusion.

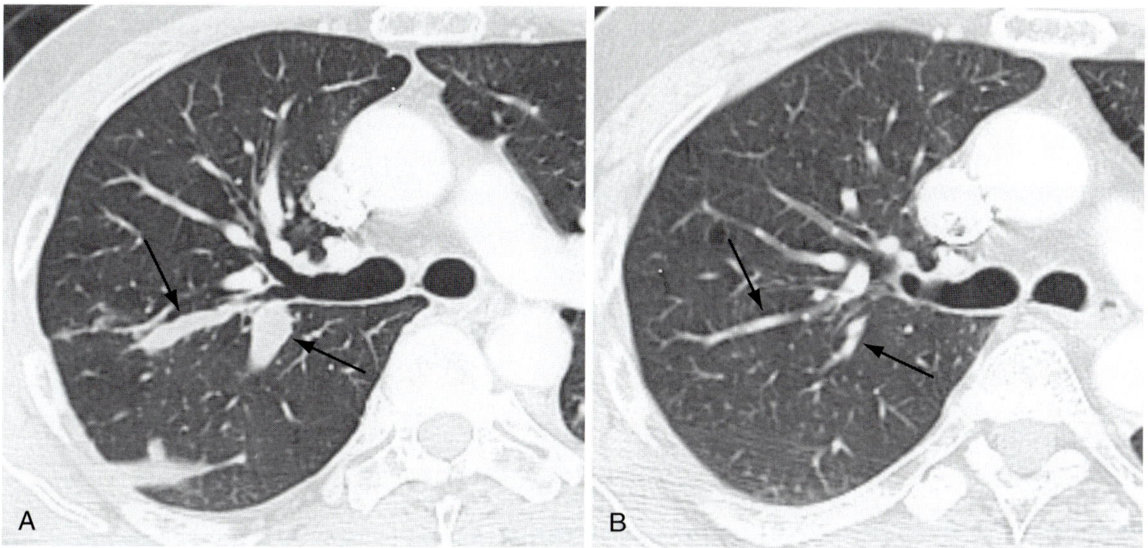

Figure 1-20 Chondrosarcoma metastatic to the lungs in a 54-year-old man. **A**, Contrast-enhanced chest CT scan demonstrates beading of pulmonary arteries *(arrows)* from pulmonary arterial tumor emboli. These changes progressed over a 1-year period. **B**, Initial chest CT scan obtained 16 months earlier shows the corresponding vessels before metastatic lung involvement.

Tumor emboli are rarely identified by imaging despite being observed microscopically in as many as 26% of cancer patients at autopsy.[309,310] This may be related to the fact that they usually are located in small or medium-sized arteries, which makes radiologic diagnosis difficult.[311] Tumors frequently associated with pulmonary tumor emboli are hepatomas, breast and renal cell carcinomas, gastric and prostatic cancers, and choriocarcinomas.[310,311] On CT scan, tumor emboli are seen as dilatation or beading of the subsegmental arteries (Fig. 1-20), which may be accompanied by peripheral wedge-shaped areas of attenuation due to infarction.[312–314] A "tree-in-bud" appearance (i.e., branching peripheral centrilobular opacities) has been described as a manifestation of pulmonary tumor embolism.[315,316]

Endobronchial metastasis is rare, but the origin most frequently is carcinoma of the breast, colorectum, or kidney or melanoma.[317–322] Plain radiographic findings are secondary to the bronchial obstruction and include atelectasis, postobstructive pneumonitis, and air trapping. On CT scans, the metastatic lesion typically is seen as a polypoid endobronchial soft tissue mass.[323]

PRIMARY MALIGNANT PLEURAL TUMORS

Mesothelioma

Imaging plays an integral part in the diagnosis, staging, and response assessment of mesothelioma. The disease poses challenges in imaging because of its complex three-dimensional configuration. Treatment, whether radical surgery or conservative, is dependent on stage, which also is dependent on accurate imaging delineation of this tumor. Typically, mesothelioma manifests as a unilateral pleural mass with a moderate to large pleural effusion. It is a locally aggressive tumor that rarely metastasizes to distant sites; nevertheless, most patients present with advanced-stage disease and expire within 1 year of presentation.[324–331]

Diagnostic Evaluation

Chest Radiographs

Usually, malignant pleural mesothelioma (MPM) is detected first on the chest radiograph, which typically demonstrates a unilateral pleural abnormality with a moderate to large effusion.[332–336] In 45% to 60% of patients, mesothelioma manifests as a smooth, lobular pleural mass that infiltrates the pleural space and fissures.[332–334] As the tumor grows, it typically encases the lung, causing ipsilateral shift of the mediastinum with narrowing of intercostal spaces[336] (Fig. 1-21).

Signs of local invasion on plain radiographs are osseous destruction and periosteal reaction of the ribs.[333,336,337] Because the disease abuts the ipsilateral mediastinum and hilum, lymph node involvement is rarely assessed with chest radiography. Metastatic disease to the lungs may produce pulmonary nodules or thickening of the interlobular septa[336,338,339] but is uncommon at presentation. Contralateral pleural abnormalities usually are associated with asbestos-related pleural disease, although in rare cases they can be due to pleural metastases.

Computed Tomography

The examination of choice for the initial evaluation of MPM is contrast-enhanced multidetector chest CT, which has superseded MRI as the primary modality for

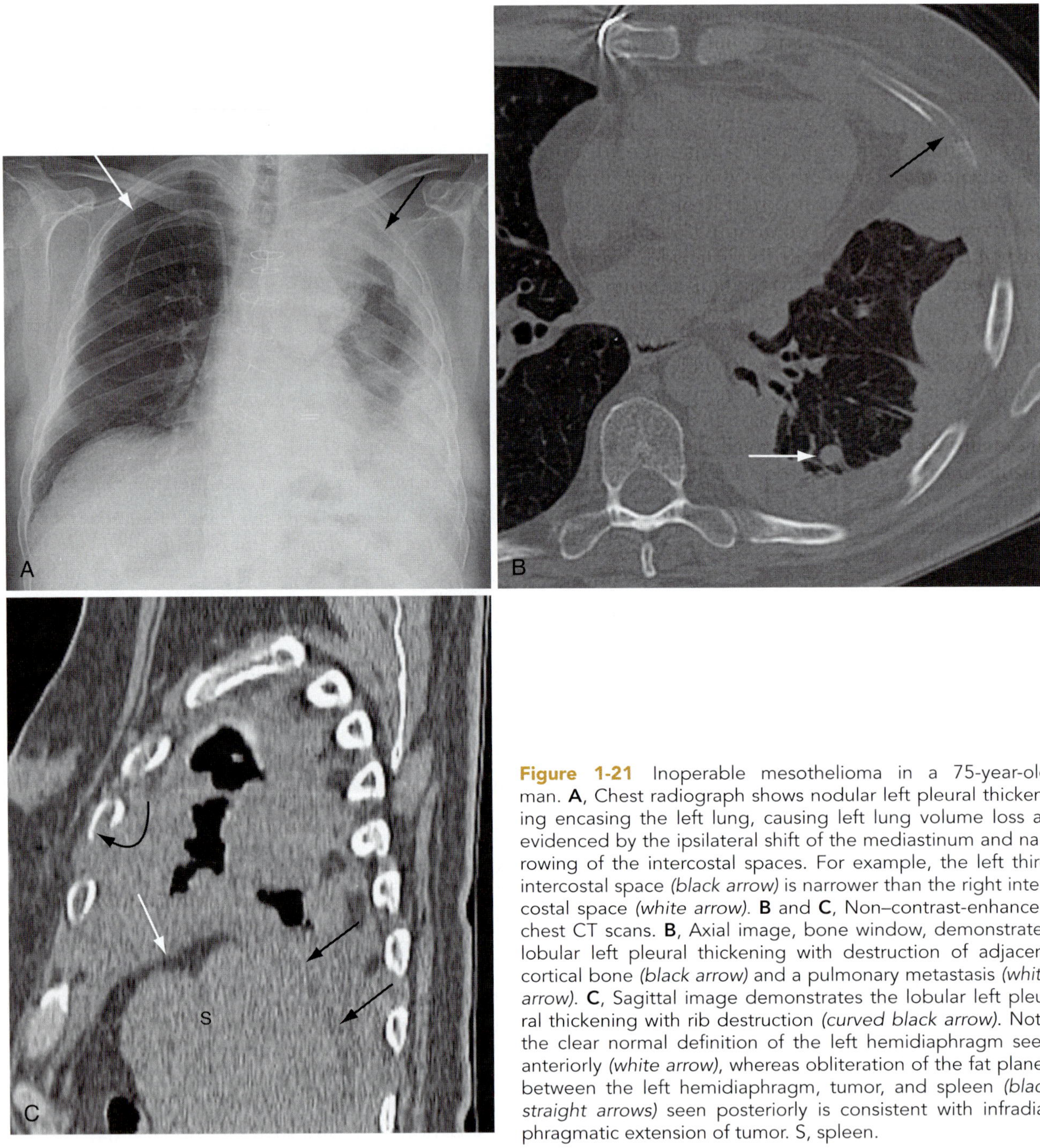

Figure 1-21 Inoperable mesothelioma in a 75-year-old man. **A**, Chest radiograph shows nodular left pleural thickening encasing the left lung, causing left lung volume loss as evidenced by the ipsilateral shift of the mediastinum and narrowing of the intercostal spaces. For example, the left third intercostal space *(black arrow)* is narrower than the right intercostal space *(white arrow)*. **B** and **C**, Non–contrast-enhanced chest CT scans. **B**, Axial image, bone window, demonstrates lobular left pleural thickening with destruction of adjacent cortical bone *(black arrow)* and a pulmonary metastasis *(white arrow)*. **C**, Sagittal image demonstrates the lobular left pleural thickening with rib destruction *(curved black arrow)*. Note the clear normal definition of the left hemidiaphragm seen anteriorly *(white arrow)*, whereas obliteration of the fat planes between the left hemidiaphragm, tumor, and spleen *(black straight arrows)* seen posteriorly is consistent with infradiaphragmatic extension of tumor. S, spleen.

determining the T status of patients with these tumors. An earlier study using an older CT technique showed that CT assessment of diaphragmatic invasion was somewhat limited by the constraints of axial imaging.[340] With today's imaging techniques, however, using thin-section as well as routine coronal and sagittal reconstructions, gross diaphragmatic invasion can be visualized directly, rather than relying solely on indirect signs. To ensure that the entire pleura is evaluated, care must be taken to initiate the scan from the thoracic inlet to the level of the L3 vertebral body.[341] Occasionally, more caudal imaging is needed if bulky tumor has caused lower deflection of the hemidiaphragm.

The vast majority of patients have pleural effusions and nodular pleural thickening, usually with lower zone predominance. Although the abnormal, nodular, and enhancing pleura usually is appreciated readily, this may not be the case early in the disease course or after surgical intervention for pleurodesis. Moreover, the pattern of disease often cannot be distinguished from that with metastatic disease to the pleura. Therefore, definitive diagnosis requires biopsy. Later in the disease course, the tumor grows circumferentially around the lung.[191,336,342–346] Aggressive tumors can invade local structures. Tumors invading the chest wall obscure and infiltrate extrapleural fat and intercostal muscles, displace ribs, and may destroy adjacent bone (see Fig. 1-21).[342,345,347] Occasionally, CT scan demonstrates focal chest wall invasion at the previous biopsy site, surgical scar, or chest tube tract.[339] Direct mediastinal extension can cause infiltration of fat planes, but tumors may invade local mediastinal structures such as great vessels, esophagus, or trachea. Such local invasion suggests that the soft tissue mass surrounds more than 50% of the structure.[339,340] Pericardial MPM invasion is suggested by nodular pericardial thickening, which may be accompanied by pericardial effusion. In assessment of diaphragmatic invasion, a clear fat plane between the inferior diaphragmatic surface and the adjacent abdominal organs and a smooth diaphragmatic contour suggest that the tumor does not extend through the diaphragm.[340]

CT has its limitations in the evaluation of mesothelioma. Because of the complex shape of the pleura, differentiating abnormal pleura from adjacent pleural effusion or collapsed adjacent lung can be inaccurate. This limitation is complicated by the fact that by the time the staging CT scan is performed, many patients have undergone invasive biopsy attempts or pleurodesis, resulting in inflammatory or fibrotic changes that can mimic malignancy.

Magnetic Resonance Imaging

MRI usually is reserved for assessment of patients with potentially resectable disease in whom initial chest CT scan findings are equivocal for chest wall, pericardial, or diaphragmatic invasion. The marked enhancement of this tumor after administration of gadolinium-based contrast, in combination with the multiplanar imaging capability of MRI, is particularly useful for delineating multifocal chest wall invasion and transdiaphragmatic invasion.[348] Because MRI examinations usually take considerable time, imaging is tailored to a specific problematic location and not to searching for distant metastatic disease.

The signal intensity of MPM typically is the same or slightly greater than that of the adjacent chest wall muscle on T1-weighted images and moderately greater on T2-weighted images. Administration of contrast yields intense enhancement of involved pleural tissue.

On MRI, as on CT, loss of normal fat planes, gross extension into mediastinal fat, and tumor surrounding more than 50% of a mediastinal structure all suggest tumor invasion.[340]

PET Imaging

MPM foci on PET are FDG-avid.[349–354] The poor spatial resolution of PET imaging limits its utility as the sole imaging modality for MPM. The use of integrated PET-CT imaging, which coregisters anatomic and functional data, ameliorates the limitations.[355] PET-CT has been shown to improve the localization of regions with increased FDG activity and the accuracy of staging in patients with MPM.[355] PET does not, however, overcome the limitations of other imaging modalities in the evaluation of minute foci of transdiaphragmatic invasion. The major strength of PET is in delineating metastatic spread, undetected by morphologic imaging, to lymph nodes and distant sites. Moreover, PET can predict survival in mesothelioma when the entire extent of pleural disease is assessed using total glycolytic volume but not when disease foci are assessed with SUV_{max}.[356]

Staging

For distinguishing patients who would benefit from surgical resection from those needing palliative treatment, the recently proposed International Mesothelioma Interest Group staging system for MPM has been gaining acceptance[357] (Tables 1-5 and 1-6). The presence of advanced locoregional primary tumor (T4), N2 or N3 disease (mediastinal, internal mammary, and supraclavicular lymph nodes), or M1 disease precludes surgery. Because the extent of local tumor and regional lymph node status are factors in selecting patients for potentially curative resection, although current imaging modalities are suboptimal in determining these clinical characteristics, extended surgical staging is offered to potential surgical candidates. Such staging includes mediastinal nodal biopsies at locations suggested by the imaging findings, which can be performed using mediastinoscopy, transbronchial biopsy, or transthoracic needle biopsy, as well as laparoscopy and peritoneal lavage for exclusion of transdiaphragmatic involvement.[357]

Primary Tumor

The emphasis in imaging the T stage is on distinguishing between tumors that are resectable from those that are not.[358] In patients with locally advanced tumor, radiologic imaging usually is directed at distinguishing T3 disease, which is a solitary focus of chest wall involvement, involvement of the endothoracic fascia, mediastinal fat extension, or nontransmural pericardial involvement, from nonresectable T4 disease, which is diffuse tumor extension or multiple chest wall foci; direct extension to the mediastinal organs, spine, internal pericardial surface, or contralateral pleura; or transdiaphragmatic invasion (see Fig. 1-21). Many of these T stage differentiating factors are pathologic features, often minute or at the microscopic level, which cannot be detected by current imaging techniques.

In a study comparing the accuracy of MRI and nonhelical CT in evaluation of MPM,[348] MRI and CT were found to be of nearly equivalent diagnostic accuracy in overall staging of this cancer, at approximately 50% to 65%. The only significant differences in accuracy

TABLE 1-5 MALIGNANT PLEURAL MESOTHELIOMA, DIFFUSE: NEW TUMOR-NODE-METASTASIS (TNM) INTERNATIONAL STAGING SYSTEM

T—Primary Tumor	
T1a	Tumor limited to ipsilateral parietal pleura, including mediastinal and diaphragmatic pleura; no involvement of visceral pleura
T1b	Tumor involving ipsilateral parietal pleura, including mediastinal and diaphragmatic pleura; scattered foci of tumor also involving visceral pleura
T2	Tumor involving each ipsilateral pleural surface with at least one of the following features: Involvement of diaphragmatic muscle Confluent visceral pleural tumor (including fissures) or extension of tumor from visceral pleura into underlying pulmonary parenchyma
T3	Locally advanced but potentially resectable tumor; tumor involving all of ipsilateral pleural surfaces with at least one of the following: Involvement of endothoracic fascia Extension into mediastinal fat Solitary, completely resectable focus of tumor extending into soft tissues of chest wall Nontransmural involvement of pericardium
T4	Locally advanced technically unresectable tumor; tumor involving all of ipsilateral pleural surfaces with at least one of the following: Diffuse extension or multifocal masses of tumor in chest wall, with or without associated rib destruction Direct transdiaphragmatic extension of tumor to peritoneum Direct extension of tumor to contralateral pleura Direct extension of tumor to one or more mediastinal organs Direct extension of tumor into spine Tumor extending through to internal surface of pericardium with or without pericardial effusion, or tumor involving myocardium
N—Lymph Nodes	
NX	Regional lymph nodes not assessable
N0	No regional lymph node metastases
N1	Metastases in ipsilateral bronchopulmonary or hilar lymph nodes
N2	Metastases in subcarinal or ipsilateral mediastinal lymph nodes, including ipsilateral internal mammary nodes
N3	Metastases in contralateral mediastinal, contralateral internal mammary, and ipsilateral or contralateral supraclavicular lymph nodes
M—Metastases	
MX	Distant metastases not assessable
M0	No distant metastases
M1	Distant metastases present

From Truong MT, Marom EM, Erasmus JJ. Preoperative evaluation of patients with malignant pleural mesothelioma: role of integrated CT-PET imaging. *J Thorac Imaging.* 2006;21:146–153; used with permission.

TABLE 1-6 MALIGNANT PLEURAL MESOTHELIOMA: STAGE GROUPING BY TUMOR-NODE-METASTASIS (TNM) DESCRIPTORS IN INTERNATIONAL STAGING SYSTEM

Stage	TNM Subset
Ia	TlaNOMO
Ib	TlbNOMO
II	T2NOMO
IIII	Any T3M0
	Any N1M0
	Any N2M0
IV	Any T4
	Any N3
	Any M1

From Truong MT, Marom EM, Erasmus JJ. Preoperative evaluation of patients with malignant pleural mesothelioma: role of integrated CT-PET imaging. *J Thorac Imaging.* 2006;21:146–153; used with permission.

between CT and MRI were in two categories: invasion of the diaphragm (CT accuracy 55%, MRI 82%; $P = 0.01$) and invasion of endothoracic fascia or a single chest wall focus (CT accuracy 46%, MRI 69%; $P = 0.05$).

Owing to the poor spatial resolution of PET, the sensitivity for correct T staging using PET alone is 19%.[350] With the use of modern multidetector CT scanners, in combination with PET scanning in integrated PET-CT scanners, the accuracy of T staging is greater than was previously published for nonhelical CT and PET scanning, with a sensitivity for detection of T4 disease of 67%.[355]

Because of the limitations in evaluating minute and microscopic invasion with imaging, the role of imaging in T4 disease is simply to identify visible disease, whereas accurate staging of apparent T3 disease requires extensive surgical staging with laparoscopy. In a study assessing the value of laparoscopy before surgical treatment of MPM, 9% of the patients (10 of 109) were found to have diaphragmatic invasion or peritoneal metastases; these disease manifestations were identified by cross-sectional imaging in only 3% (3 of 109).[359]

Nodal Disease

Hilar lymph node enlargement (N1 disease) usually cannot be differentiated from the primary tumor in MPM because the primary tumor engulfs that region directly. More important is for imaging to correctly identify mediastinal and supraclavicular involvement, because survival is poor in patients with mediastinal, supraclavicular, or internal mammary nodal metastases.[225,360] Thus, patients with N2 or N3 disease are precluded from curative resection.

As already discussed, nodal status is determined by size of nodes on CT or MRI scans; nodes larger than 1 cm suggest metastatic involvement. Using this criterion, the accuracy of determining N status for MPM is approximately 50% for both CT and MRI.[348,361] PET scanning cannot replace the need for aggressive mediastinal lymph node staging. The sensitivity for detecting nodal metastatic disease is poor, being only 11% for PET alone and 38% for integrated PET-CT.[350,355] PET plays an important role, however, in the staging of mediastinal lymph nodes, because the pattern of lymphatic spread of MPM is unpredictable relative to other intrathoracic tumors. In MPM, PET serves as a guiding tool, directing the biopsy needle to the most suspect lymph node, because aggressive biopsy, whether performed using mediastinoscopy or by transesophageal or transbronchial routes, cannot access all lymph nodes.[225,349,352,353] This limitation may explain the poor sensitivity of mediastinoscopy (36%) for N2 disease as compared with intraoperative findings in one study.[359] Yet another study found the overall nodal staging sensitivity of mediastinoscopy to be 80%.[361] Thus, sampling of all FDG-avid lymph nodes may be necessary to improve preoperative staging in patients considered for extrapleural pneumonectomy.

Metastatic Disease

Historically, distant hematogenous spread of MPM was considered rare, yet it has been reported that distant metastasis may be the initial site of recurrence following extrapleural pneumonectomy.[360] It is possible that, in such cases, metastatic disease existed at presentation but was not detected by imaging methods used at that time. With the increasing use of PET-CT for the staging of MPM, distant hematogenous disease evidently is more common than was formerly believed.[362,363] Such disease can be focal or diffuse, with involvement of the brain, lung, bone, adrenal gland, peritoneum, abdominal lymph nodes, and abdominal wall. The major strength of PET is in its ability to detect hematogenous metastatic disease, which is not detectable by the other routine imaging modalities.[350,353,355] The use of PET alone in the staging of MPM identified 11% of patients with extrathoracic metastatic disease, precluding them from surgery.[353] PET-CT identified extrathoracic metastases that were undetected by clinical and morphologic imaging in 24% of patients with MPM.[355]

To summarize, CT, MRI, and PET-CT all can be used for staging of mesothelioma, but because of their suboptimal accuracy in T and N staging of this cancer, and because of the morbidity and mortality associated with extrapleural pneumonectomy, extended surgical staging is still needed for patients with MPM being evaluated for resection. The use of PET-CT in routine staging of patients with MPM can lead to more appropriate selection of patients for extrapleural pneumonectomy, predominantly by highlighting previously unsuspected sites of extrathoracic metastatic disease.

Follow-up

Traditionally, response to chemotherapy is assessed by its effect on the size of tumor. Because measuring tumor volume is cumbersome, assessment of response to chemotherapy has evolved from measuring the two-dimensional cross-sectional area—the WHO approach[212]—to measuring the one-dimensional longest diameter—the RECIST approach.[213,364] These approaches are most accurate with roughly spherical tumors and thus are not appropriate for the monitoring of mesothelioma.[365] Modifications of the RECIST criteria have been established to evaluate MPM by measuring tumor diameter perpendicular to the chest wall or mediastinum.[366] The modified method is not only tedious (and therefore not practicable for routine use in clinical practice) but also is subject to significant interobserver variability[367] and, moreover, is mathematically inaccurate.[367] Because tumor volume has been shown to correlate with survival better than does tumor thickness in mesothelioma,[368] automated and semiautomated measurement techniques are being developed and show promise.[367,369,370] Independent computer differentiation of tumor from normal tissues is problematic in MPM, however, because the tumor abuts the chest wall, which on imaging appears similar to the tumor itself.

FDG-PET imaging is increasingly being used to monitor patients treated for MPM. Early studies showed that PET can predict survival before initiation of therapy.[371–373] Low SUV was found to be associated with better survival, whereas high SUV was associated with a risk of death up to three times higher.[350,372] Only two prospective studies document the use of PET in evaluation of the tumor response to chemotherapy. Although both studies show that PET predicts prolonged survival in patients with a better metabolic response, different methods were used to determine this response. In one study, a decrease in SUV_{max} after two doses of chemotherapy was assessed.[374] In 20 patients undergoing chemotherapy for MPM, early metabolic response, defined as a decrease of 25% or more in tumor FDG uptake as measured by SUV, was associated with longer time to tumor progression. Patients with an early metabolic response had a median time to tumor progression of 14 months, whereas it was 7 months for those who did not have an early metabolic response. No correlation was found between time to tumor progression and response to therapy evaluated by CT. In the other study, in which 20 patients were assessed after one dose of chemotherapy, quantitative volume-based FDG activity was measured to obtain the total glycolytic volume, which reflects total metabolically active tumor burden.[356] The total glycolytic volume was predictive of survival ($P = 0.015$). Neither a reduction in the SUV_{max} ($P = 0.097$) nor CT scan ($P = 0.131$) demonstrated a statistically significant association with patient survival.

Improved imaging techniques are needed for assessment of disease extent and evaluation of treatment response. Anatomic (morphologic) imaging modalities such as CT and MRI are suboptimal for this assessment, which is further complicated after therapy, because active tumor can have morphologic characteristics similar to those of reparative tissue changes or scars. At present, early imaging with FDG-PET shows some promise but will need to be verified with larger studies. Animal studies are under way investigating the possible use of monoclonal antibodies targeted to mesothelioma, such as mesothelin.[375,376] Such strategies would not only improve tumor identification but also provide a mechanism for targeted therapy in the future.

Localized Fibrous Tumor of the Pleura

Although localized fibrous tumor of the pleura usually is benign, malignant forms have been described. Histologic distinction between the benign and malignant forms may be difficult or impossible; however, some imaging features are seen more commonly in malignant disease.

Chest Radiographs

Both malignant and benign forms of the disease can be slow-growing and manifest as an incidental mass discovered on routine chest radiography. Studies of patients with localized fibrous tumor of the pleura published between 1942 and 1972 reported that 72% of patients were symptomatic at presentation, whereas studies published between 1973 and 1980 reported symptoms in only 54% of patients. This decrease in the prevalence of symptoms in patients with localized fibrous tumor of the pleura may relate to more widespread imaging of asymptomatic populations and the resultant detection of a larger number of incidental tumors.[377] These lesions are sharply defined, smooth or somewhat lobulated masses of homogeneous density ranging in diameter from 1 to 40 cm.[377–379] In a large series assessing localized fibrous tumor of the pleura, nearly 80% occupied the lower hemithorax, a third (encompassing both benign and malignant forms) occupied more than one half of a hemithorax, and 91% had at least one well-defined border[377] (Fig. 1-22). When the lesion is small, up to approximately 4 cm, the typical imaging appearance of extraparenchymal growths can be seen, because the growth forms obtuse angles with the chest wall. When the tumor is larger, however, establishing the site of origin of disease is more difficult. No feature on plain radiographs reliably distinguishes benign from malignant tumor.

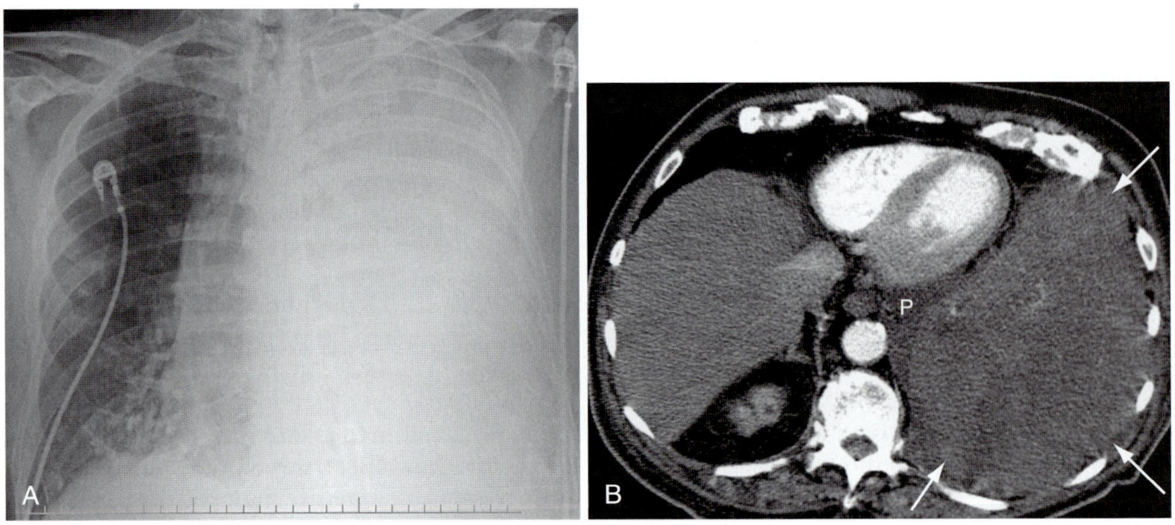

Figure 1-22 The patient was a 92-year-old man who presented with shortness of breath. **A**, Portable chest radiograph shows complete opacification of the left hemithorax with shift of the mediastinum to the right. **B**, Contrast-enhanced chest CT scan shows a 20-cm heterogeneous mass *(arrows)* occupying the major portion of the left hemithorax, associated with a pleural effusion (P). The mass was surgically removed and found to represent a malignant fibrous tumor of the pleura.

Computed Tomography

Localized fibrous tumors of the pleura typically displace rather than invade thoracic organs, thereby causing compressive atelectasis. Features that are suggestive of a malignant form of localized fibrous tumor of the pleura are an ipsilateral effusion, tumor size larger than 10 cm, and central necrosis (manifested as low attenuation) (see Fig. 1-22).[377,379] Low-attenuation regions are seen in 100% of the malignant tumors but also in 35% of the benign tumors.[377] These tumors avidly enhance; homogeneous enhancement typically is seen in the benign form of disease but not in the malignant form. Heterogeneous enhancement after intravenous contrast injection is universal in the malignant form of disease (100%) but is not uncommon in the benign form (60%).[377] Calcification is described in 7% to 26% of cases and usually is reported in large lesions in association with necrosis.[377,379,380] Chest wall involvement is rare but can be seen with both benign and malignant forms. In a series of 78 cases of localized fibrous tumor of the pleura, 17 malignant and 61 benign, chest wall involvement with the benign lesions was seen as rib sclerosis, whereas such involvement with the malignant forms was seen as tumor spread to soft tissue.[377]

Magnetic Resonance Imaging

The MRI features of localized fibrous tumor of the pleura reflect the histologic findings and the amount of fibrous tissue, necrosis, and hemorrhage. Usually the tumor has predominant low or intermediate signal intensity on both T1- and T2-weighted images,[377,381–385] which is reflective of the fibrous collagenous tissue, although high and heterogeneous signal intensity on T2-weighted images, from necrosis and cystic or myxoid degeneration, has been described. Intense enhancement after intravenous injection of gadolinium-based contrast material is typical. Although the multiplanar imaging of MRI has been beneficial in demonstrating the relationship of the tumor to the diaphragm for preoperative planning, thin-section multidetector CT recently has been replacing MRI because it demonstrates the vascular pedicle of the tumor as an aid to surgical resection.[386]

Positron Emission Tomography

To date, only two reports, together comprising seven patients, have been published on the use of FDG-PET imaging of localized fibrous tumor of the pleura. These initial studies showed that all four of the malignant tumors that were assessed by PET scan showed increased FDG activity, whereas all three of the benign tumors did not. Further studies are needed to assess the true sensitivity and specificity of FDG-PET in discrimination of the malignant form from the benign form of localized fibrous tumor of the pleura.[387,388]

SECONDARY MALIGNANT PLEURAL TUMORS

The tumors that most often cause malignant pleural effusions are carcinomas of the lung, breast, ovary, and stomach, and lymphoma. Not all pleural metastases manifest with a pleural effusion. An autopsy series of 191 patients with malignancy found that 29% of them had metastatic disease to the pleura, and that only approximately half of those had an accompanying pleural effusion.[389] Metastatic disease to the pleura can manifest on the different imaging modalities as pleural nodularity, which is highly suggestive of malignancy, or as a nonspecific pleural effusion. Identification of a malignant pleural effusion at the time of initial staging is a poor prognostic sign that renders the disease inoperable. The etiology of the pleural effusion may be a process other than metastatic disease, however, including reactive fluid collection or infection. Cytologic analysis of malignant pleural effusion fluid identifies the malignancy in only approximately two thirds of the cases.[121] Moreover, repeat thoracocentesis identifies a positive specimen in only another 30% of cases.[390] Similarly, biochemical analysis of the pleural fluid fails to accurately differentiate between benign and malignant effusion.[391–393]

Thoracoscopy has an excellent diagnostic yield (greater than 95%)[394] but is invasive and requires a trained surgical staff and appropriate facilities. Morphologic imaging, including CT and MRI, cannot be relied on exclusively for the diagnosis of a malignant pleural effusion, because empyemas and parapneumonic effusions can at times have similar imaging characteristics.[395–397] Chest radiographic findings with a pleural effusion are variable. The malignant pleural effusion can be large, opacifying the entire hemithorax, or of moderate or small size, and the pleural fluid be loculated or free flowing. It is not possible to differentiate on the chest radiograph whether the lobularity is due to loculations of pleural fluid or to soft tissue nodularity; therefore, imaging with ultrasound, CT, or MRI is added for further characterization. Presence of multiple pleural nodules or nodular pleural thickening is typical of malignant pleural effusions, whether imaged by ultrasonography, CT, or MRI, and is seen almost exclusively in malignant effusions. The absence of such features on these studies does not exclude metastatic disease, however, because the metastatic pleural nodules may be too small to identify by imaging.[395]

The real accuracy of the different imaging modalities in identifying malignant pleural disease is unknown. Data for studies assessing the accuracy of imaging in identifying malignant pleural disease are from highly selected groups of patients, because comparison with cytologic findings is not accurate. CT and MRI give a better overview of the entire pleural surface than ultrasound imaging and are not operator-dependent. Studies investigating the role of CT in the differentiation of benign from malignant pleural thickening in the absence of pleural fluid have found that the following features are highly specific for malignant pleural disease: circumferential thickening (100% specificity); pleural nodularity (94%); parietal pleural thickening greater than 1 cm (94%); and mediastinal pleural involvement (88%).[345] In a study evaluating 50 surgical candidates with early-stage NSCLC, the value of preoperative thoracoscopy and CT was assessed in determing the T status.[395] Thoracoscopic staging was more accurate than CT staging: It ruled out malignant pleural effusion in seven (14%) patients with radiologically obvious effusion and identified radiologically inapparent malignant pleural effusion in three (6%) patients. In this study, errors in thoracoscopic staging resulted in no inappropriate operations. Errors in CT staging, however, would have resulted in operations unlikely to help the patient, or would have inappropriately excluded patients from surgery. Thoracoscopic staging was more accurate than CT staging in this cohort of patients with NSCLC and negative mediastinoscopic findings.

It has been shown that FDG-PET scanning is an accurate diagnostic tool in differentiating benign from malignant pleural effusion in patients with malignant disease, with sensitivity rates ranging between 88% and 100% and specificity rates of 71% to 94%.[122,123,398–401] In a study of 92 patients with NSCLC and pleural abnormalities,[123] the sensitivity, specificity, positive predictive value, negative predictive value, and accuracy of FDG-PET in detection of pleural involvement were 100%, 71%, 63%, 100%, and 80%. When findings on CT performed separately were combined with PET findings, the specificity increased from 71% to 76%, the positive predictive value increased from 63% to 67%, and the accuracy increased from 80% to 84%. The relatively low specificity and positive predictive value were a result of false-positive increased FDG uptake in cases of infection.

Of note, foci of pleural FDG uptake should be inspected carefully on corresponding CT images. Lungs that have undergone talc pleurodesis (see Fig. 1-15) can show increased FDG activity due to inflammation, which can persist for years. This typical CT appearance is characterized by pleural thickening associated with increased attenuation corresponding with areas of talc deposition. This CT pattern, therefore, should prompt consideration of a benign cause, rather than tumor, for the FDG "abnormalities."[124]

Pleural nodularity identified by any imaging modality is highly suggestive of metastatic disease. Although early studies with PET and PET-CT show that PET scanning is highly accurate for identification of malignant pleural effusion, reports confirming similar efficacy in the absence of any morphologic abnormality have not yet been published.

CONCLUSIONS

Imaging plays an integral role in detection, staging, and follow-up evaluation of malignancies of the lung and pleura. New modalities are emerging, and the hybrid techniques that combine functional and morphologic imaging show promise. Molecular-based modalities under development are expected to improve the imaging of these malignancies and to enable incorporation of treatment. As these modalities evolve, close communication between the treating clinician and the radiologist is important to ensure selection of the ideal imaging modalities for each clinical scenario.

REFERENCES

1. Gloeckler Ries LA, Reichman ME, Lewis DR, Hankey BF, Edwards BK. Cancer survival and incidence from the Surveillance, Epidemiology, and End Results (SEER) program. *Oncologist*. 2003;8:541–552.
2. Hulka BS. Cancer screening. Degrees of proof and practical application. *Cancer*. 1988;62:1776–1780.
3. Hayata Y, Funatsu H, Kato H, Saito Y, Sawamura K, Furose K. Results of lung cancer screening programs in Japan. *Recent Results Cancer Res*. 1982;82:163–173.
4. Lilienfield A, Archer PG, Burnett CH, Chamberlain EW, Davis D, Davis RL. An evaluation of radiographic and cytologic screening for early detection of lung cancer: a cooperative pilot study of the American Cancer Society and the Veterans Administration. *Cancer Res*. 1966;26:2083–2121.
5. Nash FA, Morgan JM, Tomkins JG. South London Lung Cancer Study. *BMJ*. 1968;2:715–721.
6. Weiss W, Boucot KR. The Philadelphia Pulmonary Neoplasm Research Project. Early roentgenographic appearance of bronchogenic carcinoma. *Arch Intern Med*. 1974;134:306–311.
7. Brett GZ. The value of lung cancer detection by six-monthly chest radiographs. *Thorax*. 1968;23:414–420.
8. Wilde JA. 10-year follow-up of semi-annual screening for early detection of lung cancer in the Erfurt County, GDR. *Eur Respir J*. 1989;2:656–662.
9. Black WC, Welch HG. Screening for disease. *AJR Am J Roentgenol*. 1997;168:3–11.
10. Flehinger BJ, Melamed MR. Current status of screening for lung cancer. *Chest Surg Clin N Am*. 1994;4:1–15.
11. Fontana RS, Sanderson DR, Taylor WF, et al. Early lung cancer detection: results of the initial (prevalence) radiologic and cytologic screening in the Mayo Clinic study. *Am Rev Respir Dis*. 1984;130:561–565.
12. Frost JK, Ball Jr WC, Levin ML, et al. Early lung cancer detection: results of the initial (prevalence) radiologic and cytologic screening in the Johns Hopkins study. *Am Rev Respir Dis*. 1984;130:549–554.
13. Kubik A, Polak J. Lung cancer detection. Results of a randomized prospective study in Czechoslovakia. *Cancer*. 1986;57:2427–2437.
14. Marcus PM, Bergstralh EJ, Fagerstrom RM, et al. Lung cancer mortality in the Mayo Lung Project: impact of extended follow-up. *J Natl Cancer Inst*. 2000;92:1308–1316.
15. Black C, de Verteuil R, Walker S, et al. Population screening for lung cancer using computed tomography, is there evidence of clinical effectiveness? A systematic review of the literature. *Thorax*. 2007;62:131–138.
16. Swensen SJ, Jett JR, Hartman TE, et al. Lung cancer screening with CT: Mayo Clinic experience. *Radiology*. 2003;226:756–761.
17. Wilson DO, Weissfeld JL, Fuhrman CR, et al. The Pittsburgh Lung Screening Study (PLuSS): outcomes within 3 years of a first CT scan. *Am J Respir Crit Care Med*. 2008;178(9):956–961.

18. Henschke CI, Yankelevitz DF, Libby DM, Pasmantier MW, Smith JP, Miettinen OS. Survival of patients with stage I lung cancer detected on CT screening. *N Engl J Med.* 2006;355:1763–1771.
19. Bach PB, Jett JR, Pastorino U, Tockman MS, Swensen SJ, Begg CB. Computed tomography screening and lung cancer outcomes. *JAMA.* 2007;297:953–961.
20. Goodney PP, Lucas FL, Stukel TA, Birkmeyer JD. Surgeon specialty and operative mortality with lung resection. *Ann Surg.* 2005;241:179–184.
21. Steele JD. The solitary pulmonary nodule. Report of a cooperative study of resected asymptomatic solitary pulmonary nodules in males. *J Thorac Cardiovasc Surg.* 1963;46:21–39.
22. Walske BR. The solitary pulmonary nodule: a review of 217 cases. *Dis Chest.* 1966;49:302–304.
23. Gurney JW. Determining the likelihood of malignancy in solitary pulmonary nodules with Bayesian analysis. Part I. Theory. *Radiology.* 1993;186:405–413.
24. Yankelevitz DF, Henschke CI. Does 2-year stability imply that pulmonary nodules are benign? *AJR Am J Roentgenol.* 1997;168:325–328.
25. Berger WG, Erly WK, Krupinski EA, Standen JR, Stern RG. The solitary pulmonary nodule on chest radiography: can we really tell if the nodule is calcified? *AJR Am J Roentgenol.* 2001;176:201–204.
26. Heitzman ER, ed. *The Lung: Radiologic-Pathologic Correlations.* St. Louis: CV Mosby; 1984.
27. Zwirewich CV, Vedal S, Miller RR, Muller NL. Solitary pulmonary nodule: high-resolution CT and radiologic-pathologic correlation. *Radiology.* 1991;179:469–476.
28. Siegelman SS, Khouri NF, Leo FP, Fishman EK, Braverman RM, Zerhouni EA. Solitary pulmonary nodules: CT assessment. *Radiology.* 1986;160:307–312.
29. Mahoney MC, Shipley RT, Corcoran HL, Dickson BA. CT demonstration of calcification in carcinoma of the lung. *AJR Am J Roentgenol.* 1990;154:255–258.
30. Siegelman SS, Zerhouni EA, Leo FP, Khouri NF, Stitik FP. CT of the solitary pulmonary nodule. *AJR Am J Roentgenol.* 1980;135:1–13.
31. Swensen SJ, Harms GF, Morin RL, Myers JL. CT evaluation of solitary pulmonary nodules: value of 185-H reference phantom. *AJR Am J Roentgenol.* 1991;156:925–929.
32. Byrd RB, Miller WE, Carr DT, Payne WS, Woolner LB. The roentgenographic appearance of squamous cell carcinoma of the bronchus. *Mayo Clin Proc.* 1968;43:327–332.
33. Lehar TJ, Carr DT, Miller WE, Payne WS, Woolner LB. Roentgenographic appearance of bronchogenic adenocarcinoma. *Am Rev Respir Dis.* 1967;96:245–248.
34. Theros EG. Caldwell Lecture: varying manifestation of peripheral pulmonary neoplasms: a radiologic-pathologic correlative study. *AJR Am J Roentgenol.* 1977;1976 128:893–914.
35. Siegelman SS, Khouri NF, Scott Jr WW, et al. Pulmonary hamartoma: CT findings. *Radiology.* 1986;160:313–317.
36. Kui M, Templeton PA, White CS, Cai ZL, Bai YX, Cai YQ. Evaluation of the air bronchogram sign on CT in solitary pulmonary lesions. *J Comput Assist Tomogr.* 1996;20:983–986.
37. Henschke CI, Yankelevitz DF, Mirtcheva R, McGuinness G, McCauley D, Miettinen OS. CT screening for lung cancer: frequency and significance of part-solid and nonsolid nodules. *AJR Am J Roentgenol.* 2002;178:1053–1057.
38. Swensen SJ, Morin RL, Schueler BA, et al. Solitary pulmonary nodule: CT evaluation of enhancement with iodinated contrast material—a preliminary report. *Radiology.* 1992;182:343–347.
39. Swensen SJ, Viggiano RW, Midthun DE, et al. Lung nodule enhancement at CT: multicenter study. *Radiology.* 2000;214:73–80.
40. Bankier AA, O'Donnell CR, Boiselle PM. Quality initiatives. Respiratory instructions for CT examinations of the lungs: a hands-on guide. *Radiographics.* 2008;28:919–931.
41. Hasegawa M, Sone S, Takashima S, et al. Growth rate of small lung cancers detected on mass CT screening. *Br J Radiol.* 2000;73:1252–1259.
42. Awaya H, Matsumoto T, Honjo K, Miura G, Emoto T, Matsunaga N. A preliminary study of discrimination among the components of small pulmonary nodules by MR imaging: correlation between MR images and histologic appearance. *Radiat Med.* 2000;18:29–38.
43. Cronin P, Dwamena BA, Kelly AM, Bernstein SJ, Carlos RC. Solitary pulmonary nodules and masses: a meta-analysis of the diagnostic utility of alternative imaging tests. *Eur Radiol.* 2008;18(9):1840–1856.
44. Schaefer JF, Vollmar J, Schick F, et al. Solitary pulmonary nodules: dynamic contrast-enhanced MR imaging—perfusion differences in malignant and benign lesions. *Radiology.* 2004;232:544–553.
45. Conti PS, Lilien DL, Hawley K, Keppler J, Grafton ST, Bading JR. PET and [18F]-FDG in oncology: a clinical update. *Nucl Med Biol.* 1996;23:717–735.
46. Gould MK, Maclean CC, Kuschner WG, Rydzak CE, Owens DK. Accuracy of positron emission tomography for diagnosis of pulmonary nodules and mass lesions: a meta-analysis. *JAMA.* 2001;285:914–924.
47. Gupta NC, Frank AR, Dewan NA, et al. Solitary pulmonary nodules: detection of malignancy with PET with 2-[18F]-fluoro-2-deoxy-D-glucose. *Radiology.* 1992;184:441–444.
48. Gupta NC, Maloof J, Gunel E. Probability of malignancy in solitary pulmonary nodules using fluorine-18-FDG and PET. *J Nucl Med.* 1996;37:943–948.
49. Hubner KF, Buonocore E, Gould HR, et al. Differentiating benign from malignant lung lesions using "quantitative" parameters of FDG PET images. *Clin Nucl Med.* 1996;21:941–949.
50. Patz Jr EF, Lowe VJ, Hoffman JM, et al. Focal pulmonary abnormalities: evaluation with F-18 fluorodeoxyglucose PET scanning. *Radiology.* 1993;188:487–490.
51. Scott WJ, Schwabe JL, Gupta NC, Dewan NA, Reeb SD, Sugimoto JT. Positron emission tomography of lung tumors and mediastinal lymph nodes using [18F]fluorodeoxyglucose. The Members of the PET-Lung Tumor Study Group. *Ann Thorac Surg.* 1994;58:698–703.
52. Kernstine KH, Grannis Jr FW, Rotter AJ. Is there a role for PET in the evaluation of subcentimeter pulmonary nodules? *Semin Thorac Cardiovasc Surg.* 2005;17:110–114.
53. Marom EM, Sarvis S, Herndon 2nd JE, Patz Jr EF. T1 lung cancers: sensitivity of diagnosis with fluorodeoxyglucose PET. *Radiology.* 2002;223:453–459.
54. Jeong SY, Lee KS, Shin KM, et al. Efficacy of PET/CT in the characterization of solid or partly solid solitary pulmonary nodules. *Lung Cancer.* 2008;61(2):186–194.
55. Pan T, Mawlawi O, Nehmeh SA, et al. Attenuation correction of PET images with respiration-averaged CT images in PET/CT. *J Nucl Med.* 2005;46:1481–1487.
56. Erasmus JJ, McAdams HP, Patz Jr EF, Coleman RE, Ahuja V, Goodman PC. Evaluation of primary pulmonary carcinoid tumors using FDG PET. *AJR Am J Roentgenol.* 1998;170:1369–1373.
57. Higashi K, Ueda Y, Seki H, et al. Fluorine-18-FDG PET imaging is negative in bronchioloalveolar lung carcinoma. *J Nucl Med.* 1998;39:1016–1020.
58. Kim BT, Kim Y, Lee KS, et al. Localized form of bronchioloalveolar carcinoma: FDG PET findings. *AJR Am J Roentgenol.* 1998;170:935–939.
59. Lowe VJ, Fletcher JW, Gobar L, et al. Prospective investigation of positron emission tomography in lung nodules. *J Clin Oncol.* 1998;16:1075–1084.
60. Prauer HW, Weber WA, Romer W, Treumann T, Ziegler SI, Schwaiger M. Controlled prospective study of positron emission tomography using the glucose analogue [18F]fluorodeoxyglucose in the evaluation of pulmonary nodules. *Br J Surg.* 1998;85:1506–1511.

61. Fletcher JW, Kymes SM, Gould M, et al. A comparison of the diagnostic accuracy of ^{18}F-FDG PET and CT in the characterization of solitary pulmonary nodules. *J Nucl Med.* 2008;49:179–185.
62. Marom EM, Erasmus JJ, Patz EF. Lung cancer and positron emission tomography with fluorodeoxyglucose. *Lung Cancer.* 2000;28:187–202.
63. Dewan NA, Gupta NC, Redepenning LS, Phalen JJ, Frick MP. Diagnostic efficacy of PET-FDG imaging in solitary pulmonary nodules. Potential role in evaluation and management. *Chest.* 1993;104:997–1002.
64. Kubota K, Matsuzawa T, Fujiwara T, et al. Differential diagnosis of lung tumor with positron emission tomography: a prospective study. *J Nucl Med.* 1990;31:1927–1932.
65. Quint LE, Francis IR, Wahl RL, Gross BH, Glazer GM. Preoperative staging of non-small-cell carcinoma of the lung: imaging methods. *AJR Am J Roentgenol.* 1995;164:1349–1359.
66. Strauss LG, Conti PS. The applications of PET in clinical oncology. *J Nucl Med.* 1991;32:623–648.
67. Rosado-de-Christenson ML, Templeton PA, Moran CA. Bronchogenic carcinoma: radiologic-pathologic correlation. *Radiographics.* 1994;14:429–446.
68. Sider L. Radiographic manifestations of primary bronchogenic carcinoma. *Radiol Clin North Am.* 1990;28(3):583–597.
69. Woodring JH. Unusual radiographic manifestations of lung cancer. *Radiol Clin North Am.* 1990;28:599–618.
70. Kishi K, Homma S, Kurosaki A, et al. Small lung tumors with the size of 1 cm or less in diameter: clinical, radiological, and histopathological characteristics. *Lung Cancer.* 2004;44:43–51.
71. Noguchi M, Morikawa A, Kawasaki M, et al. Small adenocarcinoma of the lung. Histologic characteristics and prognosis. *Cancer.* 1995;75:2844–2852.
72. Takashima S, Li F, Maruyama Y, et al. Discrimination of subtypes of small adenocarcinoma in the lung with thin-section CT. *Lung Cancer.* 2002;36:175–182.
73. Kondo T, Yamada K, Noda K, Nakayama H, Kameda Y. Radiologic-prognostic correlation in patients with small pulmonary adenocarcinomas. *Lung Cancer.* 2002;36:49–57.
74. Suzuki K, Kusumoto M, Watanabe S, Tsuchiya R, Asamura H. Radiologic classification of small adenocarcinoma of the lung: radiologic-pathologic correlation and its prognostic impact. *Ann Thorac Surg.* 2006;81:413–419.
75. Lee KS, Kim Y, Han J, Ko EJ, Park CK, Primack SL. Bronchioloalveolar carcinoma: clinical, histopathologic, and radiologic findings. *Radiographics.* 1997;17:1345–1357.
76. Gandara DR, Aberle D, Lau D, et al. Radiographic imaging of bronchioloalveolar carcinoma: screening, patterns of presentation and response assessment. *J Thorac Oncol.* 2006;1:S20–S26.
77. Strollo DC, Rosado-de-Christenson ML, Franks TJ. Reclassification of cystic bronchioloalveolar carcinomas to adenocarcinomas based on the revised World Health Organization Classification of Lung and Pleural Tumours. *J Thorac Imaging.* 2003;18:59–66.
78. Weisbrod GL, Towers MJ, Chamberlain DW, Herman SJ, Matzinger FR. Thin-walled cystic lesions in bronchioalveolar carcinoma. *Radiology.* 1992;185:401–405.
79. Okubo K, Mark EJ, Flieder D, et al. Bronchoalveolar carcinoma: clinical, radiologic, and pathologic factors and survival. *J Thorac Cardiovasc Surg.* 1999;118:702–709.
80. Aquino SL, Halpern EF, Kuester LB, Fischman AJ. FDG-PET and CT features of non-small cell lung cancer based on tumor type. *Int J Mol Med.* 2007;19:495–499.
81. Tsunezuka Y, Shimizu Y, Tanaka N, Takayanagi T, Kawano M. Positron emission tomography in relation to Noguchi's classification for diagnosis of peripheral non-small-cell lung cancer 2 cm or less in size. *World J Surg.* 2007;31:314–317.
82. Byrd RB, Carr DT, Miller WE, Payne WS, Woolner LB. Radiographic abnormalities in carcinoma of the lung as related to histological cell type. *Thorax.* 1969;24:573–575.
83. Filderman AE, Shaw C, Matthay RA. Lung cancer. Part I: Etiology, pathology, natural history, manifestations, and diagnostic techniques. *Invest Radiol.* 1986;21:80–90.
84. Shin MS, Jackson LK, Shelton Jr RW, Greene RE. Giant cell carcinoma of the lung. Clinical and roentgenographic manifestations. *Chest.* 1986;89:366–369.
85. Garcia-Yuste M, Matilla JM, Cueto A, et al. Typical and atypical carcinoid tumours: analysis of the experience of the Spanish Multi-centric Study of Neuroendocrine Tumours of the Lung. *Eur J Cardiothorac Surg.* 2007;31:192–197.
86. Zwiebel BR, Austin JH, Grimes MM. Bronchial carcinoid tumors: assessment with CT of location and intratumoral calcification in 31 patients. *Radiology.* 1991;179:483–486.
87. McCaughan BC, Martini N, Bains MS. Bronchial carcinoids. Review of 124 cases. *J Thorac Cardiovasc Surg.* 1985;89:8–17.
88. Muller NL, Miller RR. Neuroendocrine carcinomas of the lung. *Semin Roentgenol.* 1990;25:96–104.
89. Valli M, Fabris GA, Dewar A, Hornall D, Sheppard MN. Atypical carcinoid tumour of the lung: a study of 33 cases with prognostic features. *Histopathology.* 1994;24:363–369.
90. Chong S, Lee KS, Kim BT, et al. Integrated PET/CT of pulmonary neuroendocrine tumors: diagnostic and prognostic implications. *AJR Am J Roentgenol.* 2007;188:1223–1231.
91. Urschel JD. Surgical treatment of peripheral small cell lung cancer. *Chest Surg Clin N Am.* 1997;7:95–103.
92. Govindan R, Ihde DC. Practical issues in the management of the patient with small cell lung cancer. *Chest Surg Clin N Am.* 1997;7:167–181.
93. Mountain CF. Revisions in the International System for Staging Lung Cancer. *Chest.* 1997;111:1710–1717.
94. Goldstraw P, Crowley J, Chansky K, et al. The IASLC Lung Cancer Staging Project: proposals for the revision of the TNM stage groupings in the forthcoming (seventh) edition of the TNM classification of malignant tumours. *J Thorac Oncol.* 2007;2:706–714.
95. Pfister DG, Johnson DH, Azzoli CG, et al. American Society of Clinical Oncology treatment of unresectable non-small-cell lung cancer guideline: update 2003. *J Clin Oncol.* 2004;22:330–353.
96. Lardinois D, Weder W, Hany TF, et al. Staging of non-small-cell lung cancer with integrated positron-emission tomography and computed tomography. *N Engl J Med.* 2003;348:2500–2507.
97. Pieterman RM, van Putten JW, Meuzelaar JJ, et al. Preoperative staging of non-small-cell lung cancer with positron-emission tomography. *N Engl J Med.* 2000;343:254–261.
98. Reed CE, Harpole DH, Posther KE, et al. Results of the American College of Surgeons Oncology Group Z0050 trial: the utility of positron emission tomography in staging potentially operable non-small cell lung cancer. *J Thorac Cardiovasc Surg.* 2003;126:1943–1951.
99. van Tinteren H, Hoekstra OS, Smit EF, et al. Effectiveness of positron emission tomography in the preoperative assessment of patients with suspected non-small-cell lung cancer: the PLUS multicentre randomised trial. *Lancet.* 2002;359:1388–1393.
100. Vansteenkiste JF, Stroobants SG, De Leyn PR, et al. Lymph node staging in non-small-cell lung cancer with FDG-PET scan: a prospective study on 690 lymph node stations from 68 patients. *J Clin Oncol.* 1998;16:2142–2149.
101. Verhagen AF, Bootsma GP, Tjan-Heijnen VC, et al. FDG-PET in staging lung cancer: how does it change the algorithm? *Lung Cancer.* 2004;44:175–181.
102. Ahuja V, Coleman RE, Herndon J, Patz Jr EF. The prognostic significance of fluorodeoxyglucose positron emission tomography imaging for patients with nonsmall cell lung carcinoma. *Cancer.* 1998;83:918–924.
103. Berghmans T, Dusart M, Paesmans M, et al. Primary tumor standardized uptake value (SUV_{max}) measured on fluorodeoxyglucose positron emission tomography (FDG-PET) is of prognostic value for survival in non-small cell lung cancer (NSCLC): a systematic review and meta-analysis (MA) by the European Lung Cancer

Working Party for the IASLC Lung Cancer Staging Project. *J Thorac Oncol.* 2008;3:6–12.

104. Goodgame B, Pillot GA, Yang Z, et al. Prognostic value of preoperative positron emission tomography in resected stage I non-small cell lung cancer. *J Thorac Oncol.* 2008;3:130–134.
105. Hanin FX, Lonneux M, Cornet J, et al. Prognostic value of FDG uptake in early stage non-small cell lung cancer. *Eur J Cardiothorac Surg.* 2008;33:819–823.
106. Webb WR, Gatsonis C, Zerhouni EA, et al. CT and MR imaging in staging non-small cell bronchogenic carcinoma: report of the Radiologic Diagnostic Oncology Group. *Radiology.* 1991;178:705–713.
107. Ratto GB, Piacenza G, Frola C, et al. Chest wall involvement by lung cancer: computed tomographic detection and results of operation. *Ann Thorac Surg.* 1991;51:182–188.
108. Padovani B, Mouroux J, Seksik L, et al. Chest wall invasion by bronchogenic carcinoma: evaluation with MR imaging. *Radiology.* 1993;187:33–38.
109. Bandi V, Lunn W, Ernst A, Eberhardt R, Hoffmann H, Herth FJ. Ultrasound vs. CT in detecting chest wall invasion by tumor: a prospective study. *Chest.* 2008;133:881–886.
110. Glazer HS, Kaiser LR, Anderson DJ, et al. Indeterminate mediastinal invasion in bronchogenic carcinoma: CT evaluation. *Radiology.* 1989;173:37–42.
111. Herman SJ, Winton TL, Weisbrod GL, Towers MJ, Mentzer SJ. Mediastinal invasion by bronchogenic carcinoma: CT signs. *Radiology.* 1994;190:841–846.
112. McLoud TC. CT of bronchogenic carcinoma: indeterminate mediastinal invasion. *Radiology.* 1989;173:15–16.
113. Martini N, Heelan R, Westcott J, et al. Comparative merits of conventional, computed tomographic, and magnetic resonance imaging in assessing mediastinal involvement in surgically confirmed lung carcinoma. *J Thorac Cardiovasc Surg.* 1985;90:639–648.
114. Komaki R, Roth JA, Walsh GL, et al. Outcome predictors for 143 patients with superior sulcus tumors treated by multidisciplinary approach at the University of Texas M. D. Anderson Cancer Center. *Int J Radiat Oncol Biol Phys.* 2000;48:347–354.
115. Bruzzi JF, Komaki R, Walsh GL, et al. Imaging of non-small cell lung cancer of the superior sulcus: part 1: anatomy, clinical manifestations, and management. *Radiographics.* 2008;28:551–560.
116. Bilsky MH, Vitaz TW, Boland PJ, Bains MS, Rajaraman V, Rusch VW. Surgical treatment of superior sulcus tumors with spinal and brachial plexus involvement. *J Neurosurg.* 2002;97:301–309.
117. Gandhi S, Walsh GL, Komaki R, et al. A multidisciplinary surgical approach to superior sulcus tumors with vertebral invasion. *Ann Thorac Surg.* 1999;68:1778–1784; discussion 1784–1775.
118. York JE, Walsh GL, Lang FF, et al. Combined chest wall resection with vertebrectomy and spinal reconstruction for the treatment of Pancoast tumors. *J Neurosurg.* 1999;91:74–80.
119. Dartevelle P, Macchiarini P. Surgical management of superior sulcus tumors. *Oncologist.* 1999;4:398–407.
120. Galetta D, Cesario A, Margaritora S, et al. Enduring challenge in the treatment of nonsmall cell lung cancer with clinical stage IIIB: results of a trimodality approach. *Ann Thorac Surg.* 2003;76:1802–1808; discussion 1808–1809.
121. The American Thoracic Society and The European Respiratory Society. Pretreatment evaluation of non-small-cell lung cancer. *Am J Respir Crit Care Med.* 1997;156:320–332.
122. Erasmus JJ, McAdams HP, Rossi SE, Goodman PC, Coleman RE, Patz EF. FDG PET of pleural effusions in patients with non-small cell lung cancer. *AJR Am J Roentgenol.* 2000;175:245–249.
123. Schaffler GJ, Wolf G, Schoellnast H, et al. Non-small cell lung cancer: evaluation of pleural abnormalities on CT scans with ^{18}F FDG PET. *Radiology.* 2004;231:858–865.
124. Kwek BH, Aquino SL, Fischman AJ. Fluorodeoxyglucose positron emission tomography and CT after talc pleurodesis. *Chest.* 2004;125:2356–2360.
125. Glazer GM, Gross BH, Quint LE, Francis IR, Bookstein FL, Orringer MB. Normal mediastinal lymph nodes: number and size according to American Thoracic Society mapping. *AJR Am J Roentgenol.* 1985;144:261–265.
126. Dwamena BA, Sonnad SS, Angobaldo JO, Wahl RL. Metastases from non-small cell lung cancer: mediastinal staging in the 1990s—meta-analytic comparison of PET and CT. *Radiology.* 1999;213:530–536.
127. Gould MK, Kuschner WG, Rydzak CE, et al. Test performance of positron emission tomography and computed tomography for mediastinal staging in patients with non-small-cell lung cancer: a meta-analysis. *Ann Intern Med.* 2003;139:879–892.
128. Klein JS, Webb WR. The radiologic staging of lung cancer. *J Thorac Imaging.* 1991;7:29–47.
129. Musset D, Grenier P, Carette MF, et al. Primary lung cancer staging: prospective comparative study of MR imaging with CT. *Radiology.* 1986;160:607–611.
130. Staples CA, Muller NL, Miller RR, Evans KG, Nelems B. Mediastinal nodes in bronchogenic carcinoma: comparison between CT and mediastinoscopy. *Radiology.* 1988;167:367–372.
131. Webb WR. MR imaging in the evaluation and staging of lung cancer. *Semin Ultrasound CT MR.* 1988;9:53–66.
132. Gdeedo A, Van Schil P, Corthouts B, Van Mieghem F, Van Meerbeeck J, Van Marck E. Prospective evaluation of computed tomography and mediastinoscopy in mediastinal lymph node staging. *Eur Respir J.* 1997;10:1547–1551.
133. McLoud TC, Bourgouin PM, Greenberg RW, et al. Bronchogenic carcinoma: analysis of staging in the mediastinum with CT by correlative lymph node mapping and sampling. *Radiology.* 1992;182:319–323.
134. Kim HY, Yi CA, Lee KS, et al. Nodal metastasis in non-small cell lung cancer: accuracy of 3.0-T MR imaging. *Radiology.* 2008;246:596–604.
135. Yi CA, Shin KM, Lee KS, et al. Non-small cell lung cancer staging: efficacy comparison of integrated PET/CT versus 3.0-T whole-body MR imaging. *Radiology.* 2008;248:632–642.
136. Toloza EM, Harpole L, McCrory DC. Noninvasive staging of non-small cell lung cancer: a review of the current evidence. *Chest.* 2003;123:137S–146S.
137. Birim O, Kappetein AP, Stijnen T, Bogers AJ. Meta-analysis of positron emission tomographic and computed tomographic imaging in detecting mediastinal lymph node metastases in nonsmall cell lung cancer. *Ann Thorac Surg.* 2005;79:375–382.
138. Antoch G, Stattaus J, Nemat AT, et al. Non-small cell lung cancer: dual-modality PET/CT in preoperative staging. *Radiology.* 2003;229:526–533.
139. Al-Sarraf N, Gately K, Lucey J, Wilson L, McGovern E, Young V. Lymph node staging by means of positron emission tomography is less accurate in non-small cell lung cancer patients with enlarged lymph nodes: analysis of 1,145 lymph nodes. *Lung Cancer.* 2008;60:62–68.
140. de Langen AJ, Raijmakers P, Riphagen I, Paul MA, Hoekstra OS. The size of mediastinal lymph nodes and its relation with metastatic involvement: a meta-analysis. *Eur J Cardiothorac Surg.* 2006;29:26–29.
141. Dietlein M, Weber K, Gandjour A, et al. Cost-effectiveness of FDG-PET for the management of potentially operable non-small cell lung cancer: priority for a PET-based strategy after nodal-negative CT results. *Eur J Nucl Med.* 2000;27:1598–1609.
142. Scott WJ, Shepherd J, Gambhir SS. Cost-effectiveness of FDG-PET for staging non-small cell lung cancer: a decision analysis. *Ann Thorac Surg.* 1998;66:1876–1883; discussion 1883–1875.
143. Spiro SG, Porter JC. Lung cancer—where are we today? Current advances in staging and nonsurgical treatment. *Am J Respir Crit Care Med.* 2002;166:1166–1196.
144. Grant D, Edwards D, Goldstraw P. Computed tomography of the brain, chest, and abdomen in the preoperative assessment of non-small cell lung cancer. *Thorax.* 1988;43:883–886.

145. Silvestri GA, Lenz JE, Harper SN, Morse RA, Colice GL. The relationship of clinical findings to CT scan evidence of adrenal gland metastases in the staging of bronchogenic carcinoma. *Chest.* 1992;102:1748–1751.
146. Tanaka K, Kubota K, Kodama T, Nagai K, Nishiwaki Y. Extrathoracic staging is not necessary for non-small-cell lung cancer with clinical stage T1–2 N0. *Ann Thorac Surg.* 1999;68:1039–1042.
147. Figlin RA, Piantadosi S, Feld R. Intracranial recurrence of carcinoma after complete surgical resection of stage I, II, and III non-small-cell lung cancer. *N Engl J Med.* 1988;318:1300–1305.
148. Robnett TJ, Machtay M, Stevenson JP, Algazy KM, Hahn SM. Factors affecting the risk of brain metastases after definitive chemoradiation for locally advanced non-small-cell lung carcinoma. *J Clin Oncol.* 2001;19:1344–1349.
149. Allard P, Yankaskas BC, Fletcher RH, Parker LA, Halvorsen Jr RA. Sensitivity and specificity of computed tomography for the detection of adrenal metastatic lesions among 91 autopsied lung cancer patients. *Cancer.* 1990;66:457–462.
150. Silvestri GA, Gould MK, Margolis ML, et al. Noninvasive staging of non-small cell lung cancer: ACCP evidenced-based clinical practice guidelines (2nd edition). *Chest.* 2007;132:178S–201S.
151. Bury T, Barreto A, Daenen F, Barthelemy N, Ghaye B, Rigo P. Fluorine-18 deoxyglucose positron emission tomography for the detection of bone metastases in patients with non-small cell lung cancer. *Eur J Nucl Med.* 1998;25:1244–1247.
152. Erasmus JJ, Patz Jr EF, McAdams HP, et al. Evaluation of adrenal masses in patients with bronchogenic carcinoma using ^{18}F-fluorodeoxyglucose positron emission tomography. *AJR Am J Roentgenol.* 1997;168:1357–1360.
153. Marom EM, McAdams HP, Erasmus JJ, et al. Staging non-small cell lung cancer with whole-body PET. *Radiology.* 1999;212:803–809.
154. Englemen RM, McNamara WL. Bronchogenic carcinoma: a statistical review of two hundred twenty four autopsies. *J Thorac Surg.* 1954;27:227–237.
155. Mathews MJ, Kanhouwa S, Pickren J, Robinette D. Frequency of residual and metastatic tumor in patients undergoing curative surgical resection for lung cancer. *Cancer Treat Rep (Part 3).* 1973;4:63–67.
156. Postmus PE, Brambilla E, Chansky K, et al. The IASLC Lung Cancer Staging Project: proposals for revision of the M descriptors in the forthcoming (seventh) edition of the TNM classification of lung cancer. *J Thorac Oncol.* 2007;2:686–693.
157. Bury T, Dowlati A, Paulus P, et al. Whole-body ^{18}FDG positron emission tomography in the staging of non-small cell lung cancer. *Eur Respir J.* 1997;10:2529–2534.
158. Bury T, Dowlati A, Paulus P, Hustinx R, Radermecker M, Rigo P. Staging of non-small-cell lung cancer by whole-body fluorine-18 deoxyglucose positron emission tomography. *Eur J Nucl Med.* 1996;23:204–206.
159. Erasmus JJ, Munden RF. The role of integrated computed tomography positron-emission tomography in esophageal cancer: staging and assessment of therapeutic response. *Semin Radiat Oncol.* 2007;17:29–37.
160. Ettinghausen SE, Burt ME. Prospective evaluation of unilateral adrenal masses in patients with operable non-small-cell lung cancer. *J Clin Oncol.* 1991;9:1462–1466.
161. Nielsen Jr ME, Heaston DK, Dunnick NR, Korobkin M. Preoperative CT evaluation of adrenal glands in non-small cell bronchogenic carcinoma. *AJR Am J Roentgenol.* 1982;139:317–320.
162. Oliver Jr TW, Bernardino ME, Miller JI, Mansour K, Greene D, Davis WA. Isolated adrenal masses in nonsmall-cell bronchogenic carcinoma. *Radiology.* 1984;153:217–218.
163. Pagani JJ. Normal adrenal glands in small cell lung carcinoma: CT-guided biopsy. *AJR Am J Roentgenol.* 1983;140:949–951.
164. Pagani JJ. Non-small cell lung carcinoma adrenal metastases. Computed tomography and percutaneous needle biopsy in their diagnosis. *Cancer.* 1984;53:1058–1060.
165. Pagani JJ, Bernardino ME. Incidence and significance of serendipitous CT findings in the oncologic patient. *J Comput Assist Tomogr.* 1982;6:268–275.
166. Sparup J, Friis M, Brenoe J, et al. Computed tomography and the TNM classification of lung cancer. *Scand J Thorac Cardiovasc Surg.* 1990;24:207–211.
167. Mayo-Smith WW, Boland GW, Noto RB, Lee MJ. State-of-the-art adrenal imaging. *Radiographics.* 2001;21:995–1012.
168. Boland GW, Lee MJ, Gazelle GS, Halpern EF, McNicholas MM, Mueller PR. Characterization of adrenal masses using unenhanced CT: an analysis of the CT literature. *AJR Am J Roentgenol.* 1998;171:201–204.
169. Pena CS, Boland GW, Hahn PF, Lee MJ, Mueller PR. Characterization of indeterminate (lipid-poor) adrenal masses: use of washout characteristics at contrast-enhanced CT. *Radiology.* 2000;217:798–802.
170. Schwartz LH, Ginsberg MS, Burt ME, Brown KT, Getrajdman GI, Panicek DM. MRI as an alternative to CT-guided biopsy of adrenal masses in patients with lung cancer. *Ann Thorac Surg.* 1998;65:193–197.
171. Outwater EK, Siegelman ES, Huang AB, Birnbaum BA. Adrenal masses: correlation between CT attenuation value and chemical shift ratio at MR imaging with in-phase and opposed-phase sequences. *Radiology.* 1996;200:749–752.
172. Boland GW, Goldberg MA, Lee MJ, et al. Indeterminate adrenal mass in patients with cancer: evaluation at PET with 2-[F-18]-fluoro-2-deoxy-D-glucose. *Radiology.* 1995;194:131–134.
173. Yun M, Kim W, Alnafisi N, Lacorte L, Jang S, Alavi A. ^{18}F-FDG PET in characterizing adrenal lesions detected on CT or MRI. *J Nucl Med.* 2001;42:1795–1799.
174. Caoili EM, Korobkin M, Brown RK, Mackie G, Shulkin BL. Differentiating adrenal adenomas from nonadenomas using ^{18}F-FDG PET/CT: quantitative and qualitative evaluation. *Acad Radiol.* 2007;14:468–475.
175. Patz Jr EF, Erasmus JJ, McAdams HP, et al. Lung cancer staging and management: comparison of contrast-enhanced and nonenhanced helical CT of the thorax. *Radiology.* 1999;212:56–60.
176. Hustinx R, Paulus P, Jacquet N, Jerusalem G, Bury T, Rigo P. Clinical evaluation of whole-body ^{18}F-fluorodeoxyglucose positron emission tomography in the detection of liver metastases. *Ann Oncol.* 1998;9:397–401.
177. Butler AR, Leo JS, Lin JP, Boyd AD, Kricheff II. The value of routine cranial computed tomography in neurologically intact patients with primary carcinoma of the lung. *Radiology.* 1979;131:399–401.
178. Cole Jr FH, Thomas JE, Wilcox AB, Halford 3rd HH. Cerebral imaging in the asymptomatic preoperative bronchogenic carcinoma patient: is it worthwhile? *Ann Thorac Surg.* 1994;57:838–840.
179. Jacobs L, Kinkel WR, Vincent RG. 'Silent' brain metastasis from lung carcinoma determined by computerized tomography. *Arch Neurol.* 1977;34:690–693.
180. Jennings EC, Aungst CW, Yatco R. Asymptomatic patients with primary carcinoma; computerized axial tomography study. *N Y State J Med.* 1980;80:1096–1098.
181. Kormas P, Bradshaw JR, Jeyasingham K. Preoperative computed tomography of the brain in non-small cell bronchogenic carcinoma. *Thorax.* 1992;47:106–108.
182. Osada H, Kojima K, Tsukada H, Nakajima Y, Imamura K, Matsumoto J. Cost-effectiveness associated with the diagnosis and staging of non-small-cell lung cancer. *Jpn J Thorac Cardiovasc Surg.* 2001;49:1–10.
183. Osada H, Nakajima Y, Taira Y, Yokote K, Noguchi T. The role of mediastinal and multi-organ CT scans in staging presumable surgical candidates with non-small-cell lung cancer. *Jpn J Surg.* 1987;17:362–368.
184. Yokoi K, Kamiya N, Matsuguma H, et al. Detection of brain metastasis in potentially operable non-small cell lung cancer: a comparison of CT and MRI. *Chest.* 1999;115:714–719.

185. Bilgin S, Yilmaz A, Ozdemir F, Akkaya E, Karakurt Z, Poluman A. Extrathoracic staging of non-small cell bronchogenic carcinoma: relationship of the clinical evaluation to organ scans. *Respirology*. 2002;7:57–61.
186. Crane JM, Nelson MJ, Ihde DC, et al. A comparison of computed tomography and radionuclide scanning for detection of brain metastases in small cell lung cancer. *J Clin Oncol.* 1984;2:1017–1024.
187. Habets JM, van Oosterhout AG, ten Velde GP, Wilmink JT, Twijnstra A. Diagnostic value of CT in the detection of brain metastasis in small cell lung cancer patients. *J Belge Radiol.* 1992;75:179–181.
188. Hooper RG, Tenholder MF, Underwood GH, Beechler CR, Spratling L. Computed tomographic scanning of the brain in initial staging of bronchogenic carcinoma. *Chest*. 1984;85:774–776.
189. Johnson DH, Windham WW, Allen JH, Greco FA. Limited value of CT brain scans in the staging of small cell lung cancer. *AJR Am J Roentgenol.* 1983;140:37–40.
190. Levitan N, Hong WK, Byrne RE, et al. Role of computerized cranial tomography in the staging of small cell carcinoma of the lung. *Cancer Treat Rep*. 1984;68:1375–1377.
191. Mintz BJ, Tuhrim S, Alexander S, Yang WC, Shanzer S. Intracranial metastases in the initial staging of bronchogenic carcinoma. *Chest*. 1984;86:850–853.
192. Salvatierra A, Baamonde C, Llamas JM, Cruz F, Lopez-Pujol J. Extrathoracic staging of bronchogenic carcinoma. *Chest*. 1990;97:1052–1058.
193. Tarver RD, Richmond BD, Klatte EC. Cerebral metastases from lung carcinoma: neurological and CT correlation. Work in progress. *Radiology*. 1984;153:689–692.
194. Earnest FT, Ryu JH, Miller GM, et al. Suspected non-small cell lung cancer: incidence of occult brain and skeletal metastases and effectiveness of imaging for detection–pilot study. *Radiology*. 1999;211:137–145.
195. Schirrmeister H, Arslandemir C, Glatting G, et al. Omission of bone scanning according to staging guidelines leads to futile therapy in non-small cell lung cancer. *Eur J Nucl Med Mol Imaging*. 2004;31:964–968.
196. Hsia TC, Shen YY, Yen RF, Kao CH, Changlai SP. Comparing whole body ^{18}F-2-deoxyglucose positron emission tomography and technetium-99m methylene diophosphate bone scan to detect bone metastases in patients with non-small cell lung cancer. *Neoplasma*. 2002;49:267–271.
197. Darling GE. Staging of the patient with small cell lung cancer. *Chest Surg Clin N Am.* 1997;7:81–94.
198. Jelinek JS, Redmond 3rd J, Perry JJ, et al. Small cell lung cancer: staging with MR imaging. *Radiology*. 1990;177:837–842.
199. Samson DJ, Seidenfeld J, Simon GR, et al. Evidence for management of small cell lung cancer: ACCP evidence-based clinical practice guidelines (2nd edition). *Chest*. 2007;132:314S–323S.
200. Blum R, MacManus MP, Rischin D, Michael M, Ball D, Hicks RJ. Impact of positron emission tomography on the management of patients with small-cell lung cancer: preliminary experience. *Am J Clin Oncol.* 2004;27:164–171.
201. Bradley JD, Dehdashti F, Mintun MA, Govindan R, Trinkaus K, Siegel BA. Positron emission tomography in limited-stage small-cell lung cancer: a prospective study. *J Clin Oncol.* 2004;22:3248–3254.
202. Brink I, Schumacher T, Mix M, et al. Impact of [^{18}F]FDG-PET on the primary staging of small-cell lung cancer. *Eur J Nucl Med Mol Imaging*. 2004;31:1614–1620.
203. Kamel EM, Zwahlen D, Wyss MT, Stumpe KD, von Schulthess GK, Steinert HC. Whole-body ^{18}F-FDG PET improves the management of patients with small cell lung cancer. *J Nucl Med.* 2003;44:1911–1917.
204. Schumacher T, Brink I, Mix M, et al. FDG-PET imaging for the staging and follow-up of small cell lung cancer. *Eur J Nucl Med.* 2001;28:483–488.
205. Shen YY, Shiau YC, Wang JJ, Ho ST, Kao CH. Whole-body ^{18}F-2-deoxyglucose positron emission tomography in primary staging small cell lung cancer. *Anticancer Res.* 2002;22:1257–1264.
206. Kut V, Spies W, Spies S, Gooding W, Argiris A. Staging and monitoring of small cell lung cancer using [^{18}F]fluoro-2-deoxy-D-glucose-positron emission tomography (FDG-PET). *Am J Clin Oncol.* 2007;30:45–50.
207. Niho S, Fujii H, Murakami K, et al. Detection of unsuspected distant metastases and/or regional nodes by FDG-PET [corrected] scan in apparent limited-disease small-cell lung cancer. *Lung Cancer*. 2007;57:328–333.
208. Vinjamuri M, Craig M, Campbell-Fontaine A, Almubarak M, Gupta N, Rogers JS. Can positron emission tomography be used as a staging tool for small-cell lung cancer? *Clin Lung Cancer*. 2008;9:30–34.
209. Abrams J, Doyle LA, Aisner J. Staging, prognostic factors, and special considerations in small cell lung cancer. *Semin Oncol.* 1988;15:261–277.
210. Stahel RA, Mabry M, Skarin AT, Speak J, Bernal SD. Detection of bone marrow metastasis in small-cell lung cancer by monoclonal antibody. *J Clin Oncol.* 1985;3:455–461.
211. Hochstenbag MM, Twijnstra A, Wilmink JT, Wouters EF, ten Velde GP. Asymptomatic brain metastases (BM) in small cell lung cancer (SCLC): MR-imaging is useful at initial diagnosis. *J Neurooncol.* 2000;48:243–248.
212. Miller AB, Hoogstraten B, Staquet M, Winkler A. Reporting results of cancer treatment. *Cancer*. 1981;47:207–214.
213. Therasse P, Arbuck SG, Eisenhauer EA, et al. New guidelines to evaluate the response to treatment in solid tumors. European Organization for Research and Treatment of Cancer, National Cancer Institute of the United States, National Cancer Institute of Canada. *J Natl Cancer Inst.* 2000;92:205–216.
214. Erasmus JJ, Gladish GW, Broemeling L, et al. Interobserver and intraobserver variability in measurement of non-small-cell carcinoma lung lesions: implications for assessment of tumor response. *J Clin Oncol.* 2003;21:2574–2582.
215. Ryu JS, Choi NC, Fischman AJ, Lynch TJ, Mathisen DJ. FDG-PET in staging and restaging non-small cell lung cancer after neoadjuvant chemoradiotherapy: correlation with histopathology. *Lung Cancer*. 2002;35:179–187.
216. Ichiya Y, Kuwabara Y, Sasaki M, et al. A clinical evaluation of FDG-PET to assess the response in radiation therapy for bronchogenic carcinoma. *Ann Nucl Med.* 1996;10:193–200.
217. Dooms C, Verbeken E, Stroobants S, Nackaerts K, De Leyn P, Vansteenkiste J. Prognostic stratification of stage IIIA-N2 non-small-cell lung cancer after induction chemotherapy: a model based on the combination of morphometric-pathologic response in mediastinal nodes and primary tumor response on serial 18-fluoro-2-deoxy-glucose positron emission tomography. *J Clin Oncol.* 2008;26:1128–1134.
218. Mac Manus MP, Hicks RJ, Matthews JP, et al. Positron emission tomography is superior to computed tomography scanning for response-assessment after radical radiotherapy or chemoradiotherapy in patients with non-small-cell lung cancer. *J Clin Oncol.* 2003;21:1285–1292.
219. Mac Manus MP, Hicks RJ, Matthews JP, Wirth A, Rischin D, Ball DL. Metabolic (FDG-PET) response after radical radiotherapy/chemoradiotherapy for non-small cell lung cancer correlates with patterns of failure. *Lung Cancer*. 2005;49:95–108.
220. Weber WA, Petersen V, Schmidt B, et al. Positron emission tomography in non-small-cell lung cancer: prediction of response to chemotherapy by quantitative assessment of glucose use. *J Clin Oncol.* 2003;21:2651–2657.
221. Nahmias C, Hanna WT, Wahl LM, Long MJ, Hubner KF, Townsend DW. Time course of early response to chemotherapy in non-small cell lung cancer patients with ^{18}F-FDG PET/CT. *J Nucl Med.* 2007;48:744–751.

222. Young H, Baum R, Cremerius U, et al. Measurement of clinical and subclinical tumour response using [18F]-fluorodeoxyglucose and positron emission tomography: review and 1999 EORTC recommendations. European Organization for Research and Treatment of Cancer (EORTC) PET Study Group. *Eur J Cancer.* 1999;35:1773–1782.
223. Eisenhauer EA, Therasse P, Bogaerts J, et al. New response evaluation criteria in solid tumors: revised RECIST guideline (version 1.1). *Eur J Cancer.* 2009;45(2):228–247.
224. Ohtsuka T, Kotsuka Y, Yagyu K, Furuse A, Oka T. Tuberculous pseudoaneurysm of the thoracic aorta. *Ann Thorac Surg.* 1996;62:1831–1834.
225. Sugarbaker DJ, Flores RM, Jaklitsch MT, et al. Resection margins, extrapleural nodal status, and cell type determine postoperative long-term survival in trimodality therapy of malignant pleural mesothelioma: results in 183 patients. *J Thorac Cardiovasc Surg.* 1999;117:54–63; discussion 63–55.
226. Voltolini L, Luzzi L, Ghiribelli C, Paladini P, Di Bisceglie M, Gotti G. Results of induction chemotherapy followed by surgical resection in patients with stage IIIA (N2) non-small cell lung cancer: the importance of the nodal down-staging after chemotherapy. *Eur J Cardiothorac Surg.* 2001;20:1106–1112.
227. Westeel V, Choma D, Clement F, et al. Relevance of an intensive postoperative follow-up after surgery for non-small cell lung cancer. *Ann Thorac Surg.* 2000;70:1185–1190.
228. Gilbert S, Reid KR, Lam MY, Petsikas D. Who should follow up lung cancer patients after operation? *Ann Thorac Surg.* 2000;69:1696–1700.
229. Berenguer J, Allende MC, Lee JW, et al. Pathogenesis of pulmonary aspergillosis. Granulocytopenia versus cyclosporine and methylprednisolone-induced immunosuppression. *Am J Respir Crit Care Med.* 1995;152:1079–1086.
230. Haddad FJ, Younes RN, Gross JL, Deheinzelin D. Pleurodesis in patients with malignant pleural effusions: talc slurry or bleomycin? Results of a prospective randomized trial. *World J Surg.* 2004;28:749–753; discussion 753–744.
231. Hicks RJ, Kalff V, MacManus MP, et al. The utility of (18)F-FDG PET for suspected recurrent non-small cell lung cancer after potentially curative therapy: impact on management and prognostic stratification. *J Nucl Med.* 2001;42:1605–1613.
232. Keidar Z, Haim N, Guralnik L, et al. PET/CT using ^{18}F-FDG in suspected lung cancer recurrence: diagnostic value and impact on patient management. *J Nucl Med.* 2004;45:1640–1646.
233. Roberts KB, Manus MP, Hicks RJ, et al. PET imaging for suspected residual tumour or thoracic recurrence of non-small cell lung cancer after pneumonectomy. *Lung Cancer.* 2005;47:49–57.
234. Bury T, Corhay JL, Duysinx B, et al. Value of FDG-PET in detecting residual or recurrent nonsmall cell lung cancer. *Eur Respir J.* 1999;14:1376–1380.
235. Inoue T, Kim EE, Komaki R, et al. Detecting recurrent or residual lung cancer with FDG-PET. *J Nucl Med.* 1995;36:788–793.
236. Ishida T, Tateishi M, Kaneko S, et al. Carcinosarcoma and spindle cell carcinoma of the lung. Clinicopathologic and immunohistochemical studies. *J Thorac Cardiovasc Surg.* 1990;100:844–852.
237. Kim KI, Flint JD, Muller NL. Pulmonary carcinosarcoma: radiologic and pathologic findings in three patients. *AJR Am J Roentgenol.* 1997;169:691–694.
238. Nappi O, Glasner SD, Swanson PE, Wick MR. Biphasic and monophasic sarcomatoid carcinomas of the lung. A reappraisal of 'carcinosarcomas' and 'spindle-cell carcinomas.' *Am J Clin Pathol.* 1994;102:331–340.
239. Wick MR, Ritter JH, Humphrey PA. Sarcomatoid carcinomas of the lung: a clinicopathologic review. *Am J Clin Pathol.* 1997;108:40–53.
240. Boldrini R, Devito R, Diomedi-Camassei F, et al. Pulmonary blastomas of childhood: histologic, immunohistochemical, ultrastructural aspects and therapeutic considerations. *Ultrastruct Pathol.* 2005;29:493–501.
241. Francis D, Jacobsen M. Pulmonary blastoma. *Curr Top Pathol.* 1983;73:265–294.
242. Liman ST, Altinok T, Topcu S, et al. Survival of biphasic pulmonary blastoma. *Respir Med.* 2006;100:1174–1179.
243. Weisbrod GL, Chamberlain DW, Tao LC. Pulmonary blastoma, report of three cases and a review of the literature. *Can Assoc Radiol J.* 1988;39:130–136.
244. LeMense GP, Reed CE, Silvestri GA. Pulmonary blastoma: a rare lung malignancy. *Lung Cancer.* 1996;15:233–237.
245. Allen MS. Malignant tracheal tumors. *Mayo Clin Proc.* 1993;68:680–684.
246. Conlan AA, Payne WS, Woolner LB, Sanderson DR. Adenoid cystic carcinoma (cylindroma) and mucoepidermoid carcinoma of the bronchus. Factors affecting survival. *J Thorac Cardiovasc Surg.* 1978;76:369–377.
247. Dalton ML, Gatling RR. Peripheral adenoid cystic carcinoma of the lung. *South Med J.* 1990;83:577–579.
248. Gallagher CG, Stark R, Teskey J, Kryger M. Atypical manifestations of pulmonary adenoid cystic carcinoma. *Br J Dis Chest.* 1986;80:396–399.
249. McCarthy MJ, Rosado-de-Christenson ML. Tumors of the trachea. *J Thorac Imaging.* 1995;10:180–198.
250. Spizarny DL, Shepard JA, McLoud TC, Grillo HC, Dedrick CG. CT of adenoid cystic carcinoma of the trachea. *AJR Am J Roentgenol.* 1986;146:1129–1132.
251. Trentini GP, Palmieri B. Mucoepidermoid tumor of the trachea. *Chest.* 1972;62:336–338.
252. Turnbull AD, Huvos AG, Goodner JT, Foote Jr FW. Mucoepidermoid tumors of bronchial glands. *Cancer.* 1971;28:539–544.
253. Yousem SA, Hochholzer L. Mucoepidermoid tumors of the lung. *Cancer.* 1987;60:1346–1352.
254. Klacsmann PG, Olson JL, Eggleston JC. Mucoepidermoid carcinoma of the bronchus: an electron microscopic study of the low grade and the high grade variants. *Cancer.* 1979;43:1720–1733.
255. Spencer H. Bronchial mucous gland tumours. *Virchows Arch A Pathol Anat Histol.* 1979;383:101–115.
256. Katz DS, Lane MJ, Leung AN, Marcus FS, Sakata MK. Primary malignant pulmonary hemangiopericytoma. *Clin Imaging.* 1998;22:192–195.
257. Moran CA, Suster S, Abbondanzo SL, Koss MN. Primary leiomyosarcomas of the lung: a clinicopathologic and immunohistochemical study of 18 cases. *Mod Pathol.* 1997;10:121–128.
258. Suster S. Primary sarcomas of the lung. *Semin Diagn Pathol.* 1995;12:140–157.
259. Zeren H, Moran CA, Suster S, Fishback NF, Koss MN. Primary pulmonary sarcomas with features of monophasic synovial sarcoma: a clinicopathological, immunohistochemical, and ultrastructural study of 25 cases. *Hum Pathol.* 1995;26:474–480.
260. Attanoos RL, Appleton MA, Gibbs AR. Primary sarcomas of the lung: a clinicopathological and immunohistochemical study of 14 cases. *Histopathology.* 1996;29:29–36.
261. Janssen JP, Mulder JJ, Wagenaar SS, Elbers HR, van den Bosch JM. Primary sarcoma of the lung: a clinical study with long-term follow-up. *Ann Thorac Surg.* 1994;58:1151–1155.
262. Yousem SA, Hochholzer L. Primary pulmonary hemangiopericytoma. *Cancer.* 1987;59:549–555.
263. Halle M, Blum U, Dinkel E, Brugger W. CT and MR features of primary pulmonary hemangiopericytomas. *J Comput Assist Tomogr.* 1993;17:51–55.
264. Lorigan JG, David CL, Evans HL, Wallace S. The clinical and radiologic manifestations of hemangiopericytoma. *AJR Am J Roentgenol.* 1989;153:345–349.
265. Yilmaz E, Akkoclu A, Kargi A, et al. Radiography, Doppler sonography, and MR angiography of malignant pulmonary hemangiopericytoma. *AJR Am J Roentgenol.* 2003;181:1079–1081.
266. Bagan P, Hassan M, Le Pimpec Barthes F, et al. Prognostic factors and surgical indications of pulmonary epithelioid

hemangioendothelioma: a review of the literature. *Ann Thorac Surg*. 2006;82:2010–2013.

267. Weiss SW, Ishak KG, Dail DH, Sweet DE, Enzinger FM. Epithelioid hemangioendothelioma and related lesions. *Semin Diagn Pathol*. 1986;3:259–287.
268. Dail DH, Liebow AA, Gmelich JT, et al. Intravascular, bronchiolar, and alveolar tumor of the lung (IVBAT). An analysis of twenty cases of a peculiar sclerosing endothelial tumor. *Cancer*. 1983;51:452–464.
269. Ross GJ, Violi L, Friedman AC, Edmonds PR, Unger E. Intravascular bronchioloalveolar tumor: CT and pathologic correlation. *J Comput Assist Tomogr*. 1989;13:240–243.
270. Sakamoto N, Adachi S, Monzawa S, et al. High resolution CT findings of pulmonary epithelioid hemangioendothelioma: unusual manifestations in 2 cases. *J Thorac Imaging*. 2005;20:236–238.
271. Bragg DG, Chor PJ, Murray KA, Kjeldsberg CR. Lymphoproliferative disorders of the lung: histopathology, clinical manifestations, and imaging features. *AJR Am J Roentgenol*. 1994;163:273–281.
272. Cordier JF, Chailleux E, Lauque D, et al. Primary pulmonary lymphomas. A clinical study of 70 cases in nonimmunocompromised patients. *Chest*. 1993;103:201–208.
273. Fiche M, Caprons F, Berger F, et al. Primary pulmonary non-Hodgkin's lymphomas. *Histopathology*. 1995;26:529–537.
274. Nicholson A, Harris N. Marginal zone B-cell lymphoma of the mucosa-associated lymphoid tissue (MALT) type. In: Travis WD, Arambilla E, Muller-Hermelink HK, Harris CC, eds. *World Health Organization Classification of Tumours: Tumours of the Lung, Pleura, Thymus and Heart*. Lyon, France: IARC Press; 2004:88–90.
275. Ramani S, Karnad AB. Primary pulmonary non-Hodgkin's lymphoma. *South Med J*. 1995;88:243–245.
276. Saltzstein SL. Pulmonary malignant lymphomas and pseudolymphomas: classification, therapy, and prognosis. *Cancer*. 1963;16:928–955.
277. Toh HC, Ang PT. Primary pulmonary lymphoma—clinical review from a single institution in Singapore. *Leuk Lymphoma*. 1997;27:153–163.
278. King LJ, Padley SP, Wotherspoon AC, Nicholson AG. Pulmonary MALT lymphoma: imaging findings in 24 cases. *Eur Radiol*. 2000;10:1932–1938.
279. Koss MN. Pulmonary lymphoid disorders. *Semin Diagn Pathol*. 1995;12:158–171.
280. Lee KS, Kim Y, Primack SL. Imaging of pulmonary lymphomas. *AJR Am J Roentgenol*. 1997;168:339–345.
281. Li G, Hansmann ML, Zwingers T, Lennert K. Primary lymphomas of the lung: morphological, immunohistochemical and clinical features. *Histopathology*. 1990;16:519–531.
282. O'Donnell PG, Jackson SA, Tung KT, Hassan B, Wilkins B, Mead GM. Radiological appearances of lymphomas arising from mucosa-associated lymphoid tissue (MALT) in the lung. *Clin Radiol*. 1998;53:258–263.
283. Kennedy JL, Nathwani BN, Burke JS, Hill LR, Rappaport H. Pulmonary lymphomas and other pulmonary lymphoid lesions. A clinicopathologic and immunologic study of 64 patients. *Cancer*. 1985;56:539–552.
284. Crow J, Slavin G, Kreel L. Pulmonary metastasis: a pathologic and radiologic study. *Cancer*. 1981;47:2595–2602.
285. Primack SL, Lee KS, Logan PM, Miller RR, Muller NL. Bronchogenic carcinoma: utility of CT in the evaluation of patients with suspected lesions. *Radiology*. 1994;193:795–800.
286. Peuchot M, Libshitz HI. Pulmonary metastatic disease: radiologic-surgical correlation. *Radiology*. 1987;164:719–722.
287. Clagett OT, Woolner LB. Surgical treatment of solitary metastatic pulmonary lesion. *Med Clin North Am*. 1964;48:939–943.
288. Toomes H, Delphendahl A, Manke HG, Vogt-Moykopf I. The coin lesion of the lung. A review of 955 resected coin lesions. *Cancer*. 1983;51:534–537.
289. Hirakata K, Nakata H, Haratake J. Appearance of pulmonary metastases on high-resolution CT scans: comparison with histopathologic findings from autopsy specimens. *AJR Am J Roentgenol*. 1993;161:37–43.
290. Chaudhuri MR. Cavitary pulmonary metastases. *Thorax*. 1970;25:375–381.
291. Dodd GD, Boyle JJ. Excavating pulmonary metastases. *Am J Roentgenol Radium Ther Nucl Med*. 1961;85:277–293.
292. Seo JB, Im JG, Goo JM, Chung MJ, Kim MY. Atypical pulmonary metastases: spectrum of radiologic findings. *Radiographics*. 2001;21:403–417.
293. Libshitz HI, North LB. Pulmonary metastases. *Radiol Clin North Am*. 1982;20:437–451.
294. Patel AM, Ryu JH. Angiosarcoma in the lung. *Chest*. 1993;103:1531–1535.
295. Franchi M, La Fianza A, Babilonti L, et al. Serous carcinoma of the ovary: value of computed tomography in detection of calcified pleural and pulmonary metastatic implants. *Gynecol Oncol*. 1990;39:85–88.
296. Hall FM, Frank HA, Cohen RB, Ezpeleta ML. Ossified pulmonary metastases from giant cell tumor of bone. *AJR Am J Roentgenol*. 1976;127:1046–1047.
297. Jimenez JM, Casey SO, Citron M, Khan A. Calcified pulmonary metastases from medullary carcinoma of the thyroid. *Comput Med Imaging Graph*. 1995;19:325–328.
298. Gaeta M, Blandino A, Scribano E, Minutoli F, Volta S, Pandolfo I. Computed tomography halo sign in pulmonary nodules: frequency and diagnostic value. *J Thorac Imaging*. 1999;14:109–113.
299. Kim Y, Lee KS, Jung KJ, Han J, Kim JS, Suh JS. Halo sign on high resolution CT: findings in spectrum of pulmonary diseases with pathologic correlation. *J Comput Assist Tomogr*. 1999;23:622–626.
300. Primack SL, Hartman TE, Lee KS, Muller NL. Pulmonary nodules and the CT halo sign. *Radiology*. 1994;190:513–515.
301. Filderman AE, Coppage L, Shaw C, Matthay RA. Pulmonary and pleural manifestations of extrathoracic malignancies. *Clin Chest Med*. 1989;10:747–807.
302. Levin B. Subpleural interlobular lymphectasia reflecting metastatic carcinoma. *Radiology*. 1959;72:682–688.
303. Munk PL, Muller NL, Miller RR, Ostrow DN. Pulmonary lymphangitic carcinomatosis: CT and pathologic findings. *Radiology*. 1988;166:705–709.
304. Janower ML, Blennerhassett JB. Lymphangitic spread of metastatic cancer to the lung. A radiologic-pathologic classification. *Radiology*. 1971;101:267–273.
305. Sadoff L, Grossman J, Weiner H. Lymphangitic pulmonary metastases secondary to breast cancer with normal chest x-rays and abnormal perfusion lung scans. *Oncology*. 1975;31:164–171.
306. Grenier P, Chevret S, Beigelman C, Brauner MW, Chastang C, Valeyre D. Chronic diffuse infiltrative lung disease: determination of the diagnostic value of clinical data, chest radiography, and CT and Bayesian analysis. *Radiology*. 1994;191:383–390.
307. Stein MG, Mayo J, Muller N, Aberle DR, Webb WR, Gamsu G. Pulmonary lymphangitic spread of carcinoma: appearance on CT scans. *Radiology*. 1987;162:371–375.
308. Ren H, Hruban RH, Kuhlman JE, et al. Computed tomography of inflation-fixed lungs: the beaded septum sign of pulmonary metastases. *J Comput Assist Tomogr*. 1989;13:411–416.
309. Kane RD, Hawkins HK, Miller JA, Noce PS. Microscopic pulmonary tumor emboli associated with dyspnea. *Cancer*. 1975;36:1473–1482.
310. Winterbauer RH, Elfenbein IB, Ball Jr WC. Incidence and clinical significance of tumor embolization to the lungs. *Am J Med*. 1968;45:271–290.
311. Chan CK, Hutcheon MA, Hyland RH, Smith GJ, Patterson BJ, Matthay RA. Pulmonary tumor embolism: a critical review of clinical, imaging, and hemodynamic features. *J Thorac Imaging*. 1987;2:4–14.

312. Kang CH, Choi JA, Kim HR, Oh YH, Kim HK, Kang EY. Lung metastases manifesting as pulmonary infarction by mucin and tumor embolization: radiographic, high-resolution CT, and pathologic findings. *J Comput Assist Tomogr.* 1999;23:644–646.
313. Kim AE, Haramati LB, Janus D, Borczuk A. Pulmonary tumor embolism presenting as infarcts on computed tomography. *J Thorac Imaging.* 1999;14:135–137.
314. Shepard JA, Moore EH, Templeton PA, McLoud TC. Pulmonary intravascular tumor emboli: dilated and beaded peripheral pulmonary arteries at CT. *Radiology.* 1993;187:797–801.
315. Franquet T, Gimenez A, Prats R, Rodriguez-Arias JM, Rodriguez C. Thrombotic microangiopathy of pulmonary tumors: a vascular cause of tree-in-bud pattern on CT. *AJR Am J Roentgenol.* 2002;179:897–899.
316. Tack D, Nollevaux MC, Gevenois PA. Tree-in-bud pattern in neoplastic pulmonary emboli. *AJR Am J Roentgenol.* 2001;176:1421–1422.
317. Albertini RE, Ekberg NL. Endobronchial metastasis in breast cancer. *Thorax.* 1980;35:435–440.
318. Amer E, Guy J, Vaze B. Endobronchial metastasis from renal adenocarcinoma simulating a foreign body. *Thorax.* 1981;36:183–184.
319. Braman SS, Whitcomb ME. Endobronchial metastasis. *Arch Intern Med.* 1975;135:543–547.
320. Jariwalla AG, Seaton A, McCormack RJ, Gibbs A, Campbell IA, Davies BH. Intrabronchial metastases from renal carcinoma with recurrent tumour expectoration. *Thorax.* 1981;36:179–182.
321. Sutton Jr FD, Vestal RE, Creagh CE. Varied presentations of metastatic pulmonary melanoma. *Chest.* 1974;65:415–419.
322. Zias EA, Owen RP, Borczuk A, Reichel J, Frater RW. An unusual presentation of metastatic colon cancer to the lung. *Chest.* 1998;113:244–246.
323. Marom EM, Goodman PC, McAdams HP. Focal abnormalities of the trachea and main bronchi. *AJR Am J Roentgenol.* 2001;176:707–711.
324. Alberts AS, Falkson G, Goedhals L, Vorobiof DA, Van der Merwe CA. Malignant pleural mesothelioma: a disease unaffected by current therapeutic maneuvers. *J Clin Oncol.* 1988;6:527–535.
325. De Pangher Manzini V, Brollo A, Franceschi S, De Matthaeis M, Talamini R, Bianchi C. Prognostic factors of malignant mesothelioma of the pleura. *Cancer.* 1993;72:410–417.
326. Fusco V, Ardizzoni A, Merlo F, et al. Malignant pleural mesothelioma. Multivariate analysis of prognostic factors on 113 patients. *Anticancer Res.* 1993;13:683–689.
327. Herndon JE, Green MR, Chahinian AP, Corson JM, Suzuki Y, Vogelzang NJ. Factors predictive of survival among 337 patients with mesothelioma treated between 1984 and 1994 by the Cancer and Leukemia Group B. *Chest.* 1998;113:723–731.
328. Huncharek M, Kelsey K, Mark EJ, et al. Treatment and survival in diffuse malignant pleural mesothelioma; a study of 83 cases from the Massachusetts General Hospital. *Anticancer Res.* 1996;16:1265–1268.
329. Ong ST, Vogelzang NJ. Chemotherapy in malignant pleural mesothelioma. A review. *J Clin Oncol.* 1996;14:1007–1017.
330. Tammilehto L, Maasilta P, Kostiainen S, Appelqvist P, Holsti LR, Mattson K. Diagnosis and prognostic factors in malignant pleural mesothelioma: a retrospective analysis of sixty-five patients. *Respiration.* 1992;59:129–135.
331. Yates DH, Corrin B, Stidolph PN, Browne K. Malignant mesothelioma in south east England: clinicopathological experience of 272 cases. *Thorax.* 1997;52:507–512.
332. Antman KH. Clinical presentation and natural history of benign and malignant mesothelioma. *Semin Oncol.* 1981;8:313–320.
333. Heller RM, Janower ML, Weber AL. The radiological manifestations of malignant pleural mesothelioma. *Am J Roentgenol Radium Ther Nucl Med.* 1970;108:53–59.
334. Solomon A. Radiological features of diffuse mesothelioma. *Environ Res.* 1970;3:330–338.
335. Taylor RA, Johnson LP. Mesothelioma: current perspectives. *West J Med.* 1981;134:379–383.
336. Wechsler RJ, Rao VM, Steiner RM. The radiology of thoracic malignant mesothelioma. *Crit Rev Diagn Imaging.* 1984;20:283–310.
337. Steiner RM, Cooper MW, Brodovsky H. Rib destruction: a neglected finding in malignant mesothelioma. *Clin Radiol.* 1982;33:61–65.
338. Hillerdal G. Pleural plaques and risk for bronchial carcinoma and mesothelioma. A prospective study. *Chest.* 1994;105:144–150.
339. Miller BH, Rosado-de-Christenson ML, Mason AC, Fleming MV, White CC, Krasna MJ. From the archives of the AFIP. Malignant pleural mesothelioma: radiologic-pathologic correlation. *Radiographics.* 1996;16:613–644.
340. Patz Jr EF, Shaffer K, Piwnica-Worms DR, et al. Malignant pleural mesothelioma: value of CT and MR imaging in predicting resectability. *AJR Am J Roentgenol.* 1992;159:961–966.
341. Benamore RE, O'Doherty MJ, Entwisle JJ. Use of imaging in the management of malignant pleural mesothelioma. *Clin Radiol.* 2005;60:1237–1247.
342. Kawashima A, Libshitz HI. Malignant pleural mesothelioma: CT manifestations in 50 cases. *AJR Am J Roentgenol.* 1990;155:965–969.
343. Leung AN, Muller NL, Miller RR. CT in differential diagnosis of diffuse pleural disease. *AJR Am J Roentgenol.* 1990;154:487–492.
344. Mirvis S, Dutcher JP, Haney PJ, Whitley NO, Aisner J. CT of malignant pleural mesothelioma. *AJR Am J Roentgenol.* 1983;140:665–670.
345. Ng CS, Munden RF, Libshitz HI. Malignant pleural mesothelioma: the spectrum of manifestations on CT in 70 cases. *Clin Radiol.* 1999;54:415–421.
346. Rabinowitz JG, Efremidis SC, Cohen B, et al. A comparative study of mesothelioma and asbestosis using computed tomography and conventional chest radiography. *Radiology.* 1982;144:453–460.
347. Wong RJ, Lin DT, Schoder H, et al. Diagnostic and prognostic value of [(18)F]fluorodeoxyglucose positron emission tomography for recurrent head and neck squamous cell carcinoma. *J Clin Oncol.* 2002;20:4199–4208.
348. Heelan RT, Rusch VW, Begg CB, Panicek DM, Caravelli JF, Eisen C. Staging of malignant pleural mesothelioma: comparison of CT and MR imaging. *AJR Am J Roentgenol.* 1999;172:1039–1047.
349. Benard F, Sterman D, Smith RJ, Kaiser LR, Albelda SM, Alavi A. Metabolic imaging of malignant pleural mesothelioma with fluorodeoxyglucose positron emission tomography. *Chest.* 1998;114:713–722.
350. Flores RM, Akhurst T, Gonen M, Larson SM, Rusch VW. Positron emission tomography defines metastatic disease but not locoregional disease in patients with malignant pleural mesothelioma. *J Thorac Cardiovasc Surg.* 2003;126:11–16.
351. Gerbaudo VH, Sugarbaker DJ, Britz-Cunningham S, Di Carli MF, Mauceri C, Treves ST. Assessment of malignant pleural mesothelioma with (18)F-FDG dual-head gamma-camera coincidence imaging: comparison with histopathology. *J Nucl Med.* 2002;43:1144–1149.
352. Nanni C, Castellucci P, Farsad M, et al. Role of ^{18}F-FDG PET for evaluating malignant pleural mesothelioma. *Cancer Biother Radiopharm.* 2004;19:149–154.
353. Schneider DB, Clary-Macy C, Challa S, et al. Positron emission tomography with f18-fluorodeoxyglucose in the staging and preoperative evaluation of malignant pleural mesothelioma. *J Thorac Cardiovasc Surg.* 2000;120:128–133.
354. Zubeldia J, Abou-Zied M, Nabi H. 11. Evaluation of patients with known mesothelioma with ^{18}F-fluorodeoxyglucose and PET. Comparison with computed tomography. *Clin Positron Imaging.* 2000;3:165.

355. Erasmus JJ, Truong MT, Smythe WR, et al. Integrated computed tomography–positron emission tomography in patients with potentially resectable malignant pleural mesothelioma: staging implications. *J Thorac Cardiovasc Surg.* 2005;129:1364–1370.
356. Francis RJ, Byrne MJ, van der Schaaf AA, et al. Early prediction of response to chemotherapy and survival in malignant pleural mesothelioma using a novel semiautomated 3-dimensional volume-based analysis of serial ^{18}F-FDG PET scans. *J Nucl Med.* 2007;48:1449–1458.
357. Truong MT, Marom EM, Erasmus JJ. Preoperative evaluation of patients with malignant pleural mesothelioma: role of integrated CT-PET imaging. *J Thorac Imaging.* 2006;21:146–153.
358. Rusch VW. A proposed new international TNM staging system for malignant pleural mesothelioma from the International Mesothelioma Interest Group. *Lung Cancer.* 1996;14:1–12.
359. Rice DC, Erasmus JJ, Stevens CW, et al. Extended surgical staging for potentially resectable malignant pleural mesothelioma. *Ann Thorac Surg.* 2005;80:1988–1992; discussion 1992–1983.
360. Rusch VW, Venkatraman E. The importance of surgical staging in the treatment of malignant pleural mesothelioma. *J Thorac Cardiovasc Surg.* 1996;111:815–825; discussion 825–816.
361. Schouwink JH, Kool LS, Rutgers EJ, et al. The value of chest computed tomography and cervical mediastinoscopy in the preoperative assessment of patients with malignant pleural mesothelioma. *Ann Thorac Surg.* 2003;75:1715–1718; discussion 1718–1719.
362. Erasmus JJ, Truong MT, Smythe WR, et al. Integrated computed tomography-positron emission tomography in patients with potentially resectable malignant pleural mesothelioma: staging implications. *J Thorac Cardiovasc Surg.* 2005;129(6):1364–1370.
363. Rice DC, Stevens CW, Correa AM, et al. Outcomes after extrapleural pnemonectomy and intensity-modulated radiation therapy for malignant pleural mesothelioma. *Ann Thorac Surg.* 2007;84(5):1685–1692; discussion 1692–1693.
364. James K, Eisenhauer E, Christian M, et al. Measuring response in solid tumors: unidimensional versus bidimensional measurement. *J Natl Cancer Inst.* 1999;91:523–528.
365. Mazumdar M, Smith A, Schwartz LH. A statistical simulation study finds discordance between WHO criteria and RECIST guideline. *J Clin Epidemiol.* 2004;57:358–365.
366. Byrne MJ, Nowak AK. Modified RECIST criteria for assessment of response in malignant pleural mesothelioma. *Ann Oncol.* 2004;15:257–260.
367. Armato 3rd SG, Oxnard GR, MacMahon H, et al. Measurement of mesothelioma on thoracic CT scans: a comparison of manual and computer-assisted techniques. *Med Phys.* 2004;31:1105–1115.
368. Pass HI, Temeck BK, Kranda K, Steinberg SM, Feuerstein IR. Preoperative tumor volume is associated with outcome in malignant pleural mesothelioma. *J Thorac Cardiovasc Surg.* 1998;115:310–317; discussion 317–318.
369. Armato 3rd SG, Oxnard GR, Kocherginsky M, Vogelzang NJ, Kindler HL, MacMahon H. Evaluation of semiautomated measurements of mesothelioma tumor thickness on CT scans. *Acad Radiol.* 2005;12:1301–1309.
370. Zhao B, Schwartz L, Flores R, et al. Automated segmentation of mesothelioma volume on CT scan. In: Fitzpatrick JM, Reinhardt JM, eds. *Medical Imaging 2005: Image Processing.* San Diego, CA: SPIE Press; 2005:866–871.
371. Flores RM. The role of PET in the surgical management of malignant pleural mesothelioma. *Lung Cancer.* 2005;49(Suppl 1): S27–S32.
372. Flores RM, Akhurst T, Gonen M, et al. Positron emission tomography predicts survival in malignant pleural mesothelioma. *J Thorac Cardiovasc Surg.* 2006;132:763–768.
373. Steinert HC, Santos Dellea MM, Burger C, Stahel R. Therapy response evaluation in malignant pleural mesothelioma with integrated PET-CT imaging. *Lung Cancer.* 2005;49(Suppl 1): S33–S35.
374. Ceresoli GL, Chiti A, Zucali PA, et al. Early response evaluation in malignant pleural mesothelioma by positron emission tomography with [^{18}F]fluorodeoxyglucose. *J Clin Oncol.* 2006;24:4587–4593.
375. Chang K, Pastan I, Willingham MC. Isolation and characterization of a monoclonal antibody, K1, reactive with ovarian cancers and normal mesothelium. *Int J Cancer.* 1992;50:373–381.
376. Hassan R, Wu C, Brechbiel MW, Margulies I, Kreitman RJ, Pastan I. [111]Indium-labeled monoclonal antibody K1: biodistribution study in nude mice bearing a human carcinoma xenograft expressing mesothelin. *Int J Cancer.* 1999;80:559–563.
377. Rosado-de-Christenson ML, Abbott GF, McAdams HP, Franks TJ, Galvin JR. From the archives of the AFIP: localized fibrous tumor of the pleura. *Radiographics.* 2003;23:759–783.
378. Desser TS, Stark P. Pictorial essay: solitary fibrous tumor of the pleura. *J Thorac Imaging.* 1998;13:27–35.
379. Ferretti GR, Chiles C, Choplin RH, Coulomb M. Localized benign fibrous tumors of the pleura. *AJR Am J Roentgenol.* 1997;169:683–686.
380. Sandvliet RH, Heysteeg M, Paul MAA. large thoracic mass in a 57-year-old patient. Solitary fibrous tumor of the pleura. *Chest.* 2000;117:897–900.
381. Dynes MC, White EM, Fry WA, Ghahremani GG. Imaging manifestations of pleural tumors. *Radiographics.* 1992;12:1191–1201.
382. George JC. Benign fibrous mesothelioma of the pleura: MR findings. *AJR Am J Roentgenol.* 1993;160:204–205.
383. Harris GN, Rozenshtein A, Schiff MJ. Benign fibrous mesothelioma of the pleura: MR imaging findings. *AJR Am J Roentgenol.* 1995;165:1143–1144.
384. Tateishi U, Nishihara H, Morikawa T, Miyasaka K. Solitary fibrous tumor of the pleura: MR appearance and enhancement pattern. *J Comput Assist Tomogr.* 2002;26:174–179.
385. Tublin ME, Tessler FN, Rifkin MD. US case of the day. Solitary fibrous tumor of the pleura (SFTP). *Radiographics.* 1998;18:523–525.
386. Usami N, Iwano S, Yokoi K. Solitary fibrous tumor of the pleura: evaluation of the origin with 3D CT angiography. *J Thorac Oncol.* 2007;2:1124–1125.
387. Hara M, Kume M, Oshima H, et al. F-18 FDG uptake in a malignant localized fibrous tumor of the pleura. *J Thorac Imaging.* 2005;20:118–119.
388. Kohler M, Clarenbach CF, Kestenholz P, et al. Diagnosis, treatment and long-term outcome of solitary fibrous tumours of the pleura. *Eur J Cardiothorac Surg.* 2007;32:403–408.
389. Rodriguez-Panadero F, Borderas Naranjo F, Lopez Mejias J. Pleural metastatic tumours and effusions. Frequency and pathogenic mechanisms in a post-mortem series. *Eur Respir J.* 1989;2:366–369.
390. Light RW, Erozan YS, Ball Jr WC. Cells in pleural fluid. Their value in differential diagnosis. *Arch Intern Med.* 1973;132:854–860.
391. Burgess LJ, Maritz FJ, Taljaard JJ. Comparative analysis of the biochemical parameters used to distinguish between pleural transudates and exudates. *Chest.* 1995;107:1604–1609.
392. Ceyhan BB, Demiralp E, Celikel T. Analysis of pleural effusions using flow cytometry. *Respiration.* 1996;63:17–24.
393. Metintas M, Ozdemir N, Solak M, et al. Chromosome analysis in pleural effusions. Efficiency of this method in the differential diagnosis of pleural effusions. *Respiration.* 1994;61:330–335.
394. Menzies R, Charbonneau M. Thoracoscopy for the diagnosis of pleural disease. *Ann Intern Med.* 1991;114:271–276.
395. Arenas-Jimenez J, Alonso-Charterina S, Sanchez-Paya J, Fernandez-Latorre F, Gil-Sanchez S, Lloret-Llorens M. Evaluation of CT findings for diagnosis of pleural effusions. *Eur Radiol.* 2000;10:681–690.
396. Falaschi F, Battolla L, Mascalchi M, et al. Usefulness of MR signal intensity in distinguishing benign from malignant pleural disease. *AJR Am J Roentgenol.* 1996;166:963–968.

397. Shiono T, Yoshikawa K, Takenaka E, Hisamatsu K. MR imaging of pleural and peritoneal effusion. *Radiat Med.* 1993;11:123–126.
398. Duysinx B, Nguyen D, Louis R, et al. Evaluation of pleural disease with 18-fluorodeoxyglucose positron emission tomography imaging. *Chest.* 2004;125:489–493.
399. Gupta NC, Rogers JS, Graeber GM, et al. Clinical role of F-18 fluorodeoxyglucose positron emission tomography imaging in patients with lung cancer and suspected malignant pleural effusion. *Chest.* 2002;122:1918–1924.
400. Kramer H, Pieterman RM, Slebos DJ, et al. PET for the evaluation of pleural thickening observed on CT. *J Nucl Med.* 2004;45:995–998.
401. Toaff JS, Metser U, Gottfried M, et al. Differentiation between malignant and benign pleural effusion in patients with extra-pleural primary malignancies: assessment with positron emission tomography–computed tomography. *Invest Radiol.* 2005;40:204–209.

2

Staging of Thoracic Malignancies: A Surgeon's Perspective

Garrett L. Walsh

The best hope for cure for most patients with malignancies involving the chest cavity lies with surgery. Complete resection of all gross disease with clear microscopic margins is the optimal surgical outcome, and the result is termed an *R0 resection*. Occasionally, despite the surgeon's best efforts, microscopic positive margins remain. This result is described as an *R1 resection*. In such instances, the patient will require adjuvant local therapy, such as radiation therapy, to deal with the residual microscopic disease. A resection that leaves gross disease in the chest is an *R2 resection*—the worst possible outcome, with several deleterious effects: Any benefit from the surgery is counteracted by the morbidity and hospital stay related to the failed operation, with absolutely no improvement in long-term survival. The attempted resection may have additional negative impact on survival by delaying definitive treatment (chemotherapy or radiation therapy) until the patient has recovered sufficiently from the surgery, or can even result in premature death (i.e., perioperative mortality). Moreover, the immunosuppressive effects of a major operation and a general anesthetic procedure are well recognized and may contribute to the rapid disease progression seen in some patients after a failed attempted resection. An extensive dissection with the ultimate finding of unresectable disease also can interfere with the blood supply to the tumor or with local lymph system drainage, impairing subsequent delivery of chemotherapeutic agents to the lesions, and rendering the dissected tissues relatively hypoxic, with decreased ability of delivered radiation energy to sterilize the tissues. The psychological effects on a patient who undergoes an "open and close" procedure (in which the disease unexpectedly is recognized to be beyond surgical cure) also can significantly impair further treatment efforts. For all of these reasons, the importance of accurate and appropriate preoperative staging in patients with thoracic malignancies cannot be overemphasized. The aim of the surgical evaluation is to maximize R0 resections, minimize the number of R1 results, and ideally completely eliminate R2 attempts.

As discussed later on, preoperative clinical staging takes place in three phases:

- Clinical assessment and ordering of appropriate diagnostic tests
- Radiographic review
- Interventional staging procedures, when indicated

The thoracic surgeon must evaluate a tumor by two criteria: (1) its local invasiveness (T status) and (2) the biologic aggressiveness of the tumor (N and M status). The surgeon initially casts a broad net, looking for metastatic disease, and then focuses the evaluation on the N and finally the T status. Imaging techniques have helped a great deal in elucidating the anatomy of the primary tumor, but radiographic and nuclear medicine techniques have been less accurate in evaluating the biologic spread of the tumor. This chapter describes how thoracic surgeons approach the patient with a thoracic malignancy and use staging interventions to determine whether or not an exploration of the chest cavity will be of benefit.[1]

TUMOR-NODE-METASTASIS AND STAGE GROUPINGS

The original tumor-node-metastasis (TNM) descriptors for lung cancer are listed in Table 1-1. The original staging system for lung cancer was developed by Dr. Clifton Mountain using the M.D. Anderson Cancer Center database and by Dr. Naruke from Japan, with a combined institutional experience of nearly 5000 patients.[2] This staging system divided lung cancer into clinical and pathologic stages. Five stages of lung cancer were defined, with four T descriptors and four N descriptors, resulting in 16 subgroupings, as follows: stage I (T1N0 and T2N0), stage II (T1N1 and T2N1), stage IIIA (any T3 or any N2: T3N0, T3N1, T3N2, T1N2, and T2N2), stage IIIB (any T4 and any N3: T4N0, T4N1, T4N2, T4N3, T1N3, T2N3, T3N3), and stage IV (any T plus any N, with M1 disease). As required for all staging systems, a reassessment was performed 10 years after the original implementation. The resulting minor refinements and modifications, published in 1997,[3] included the following:

1. Stage I and stage II were divided into two subcategories, IA and IB and IIA and IIB, in recognition of the effect of the size of the tumor (T1 or T2) on survival.
2. T3N0 was moved into a IIB category, based on the favorable survival statistics of these patients compared with other patients in the IIIA category.
3. A satellite lesion in the same lobe, which previously moved up the T descriptor by one grouping, was now considered to represent T4 disease.

Now at the second-decade mark, the International Association for the Study of Lung Cancer (IASLC) has revised the system for a second time, based on long-term data for more than 100,000 patients. This revision further refines and permits better prognostication for patients with lung cancer and allows a more accurate comparison between patients in clinical trial outcomes and enrollments.[4-7] A summary of the changes proposed in the IASLC system, to be adopted in 2009, follows:

- T1 (3 cm or less in greatest dimension) tumors will be further subclassified into T1a (2 cm or less) and T1b (larger than 2 cm up to 3 cm).
- T2 tumors will be subclassified into T2a (larger than 3 to 5 cm in greatest dimension) and T2b (larger than 5 to 7 cm).
- T2 tumors greater than 7 cm will be reclassified as T3.
- Satellite T4 nodules in the same lobe will be reclassified as T3.
- Nodules in an ipsilateral lung will be down-classified from M1 disease to T4 disease.
- Pleural effusions, which have always been classified as T4, will be up-classified to M1a.
- M disease will be subclassified into M1a and M1b, with M1a denoting nodules in the contralateral lung, pleural nodules, or malignant pleural or pericardial effusions.
- M1b will designate distant metastases.

No changes in the nodal descriptors have been implemented between the three versions of the classification system. However, a new anatomic nodule map is prepared to clarify differences between the current Asian and Western nomenclatures with groupings of nodes into zones.[8,9]

The staging of small cell carcinoma of the lung previously used a dichotomous staging system of limited versus extensive disease, with *limited* defined as that confined to the chest and *extensive* as presence of extrathoracic disease. The stage groupings for non-small cell lung cancer seem to work reasonably well for small cell carcinoma and will be adopted as a more universal staging system.

SURGICAL GUIDELINES

As a general rule, surgery is always indicated for stage I and stage II disease, provided that the patient has sufficient cardiopulmonary reserve to tolerate the resection. Patients with T3N0 and T4N0 lesions are still evaluated for potential curative intent (i.e., for feasibility of R0 resection); however, extended resection of more than just the lung tissue is required for these T3 and T4 tumors. Such tumors can involve chest wall, diaphragm, pericardium, mediastinal vascular structures, carina, vertebral body, and even the heart itself. The surgical morbidity and perioperative mortality will be increased, but the risks and benefits must be weighed and individualized for each patient on the basis of the tumor's anatomic characteristics and the patient's comorbidities.

Nodal disease must be evaluated separately and is a major factor in the final surgical equation. Surgeons work backwards to try to rule out N3 and then N2 disease, to identify patients as candidates for surgery after involvement of mediastinal nodes has been ruled out. Patients with N1 and N0 disease, regardless of their T status, are considered to be potential surgical candidates.

Patients with proven N3 disease (supraclavicular or contralateral mediastinal nodal disease) are not surgical candidates. Patients with N2 disease (involvement of ipsilateral mediastinal nodes) have very poor results with surgery alone. This category represents the most complex gray area in decision making regarding treatment for lung cancer. N2 disease is quite heterogeneous and can range in extent from microscopic disease encapsulated in a single node at a solitary nodal station to advanced bulky N2 multistation disease with extracapsular spread. Neoadjuvant chemotherapy followed by surgery may be of benefit in very limited disease, as in the former instance, but has no role to play in the latter instance. The patient with bulky disease or extracapsular spread is treated with definitive chemotherapy combined with radiation therapy given either sequentially or concurrently as indicated by the patient's medical condition and age. The patient with N2 disease that is not recognized preoperatively and is discovered on the final pathology review requires adjuvant treatment in the postoperative setting.

N1 disease is less frequently diagnosed radiographically preoperatively. Recent advances in endoscopic bronchial ultrasound imaging permit sampling of nodes contained within the hilum. N0 disease is diagnosed by exclusion. Patients with N1 and N0 disease are considered to be potential candidates for R0 resections.

STAGING PHASE I: CLINICAL ASSESSMENT AND DIAGNOSTIC TESTING

Despite significant advances in radiographic imaging, including the use of PET scanning, the clinical evaluation by the surgeon remains crucial in the ultimate selection of patients who will benefit from surgery. The initial history and review of systems must focus on symptoms of potentially locally advanced or systemic disease. Asymptomatic patients in whom the tumor is discovered on routine imaging usually for unrelated problems often have the best chance of having localized disease. The vast majority of patients, however, present with signs and symptoms usually related to more locally advanced or metastatic disease. Paraneoplastic presentations, including Eaton-Lambert syndrome and hypertrophic pulmonary osteoarthropathy, may mimic systemic disease but can be reversed with resection of the primary localized tumor.

Presence of cough, often dry and nonproductive, can signify an endobronchial lesion—possible in a lobar airway (T2) or the main bronchial airway within 2 cm of the carina (T3), or involving the carina or trachea proper (T4). In addition, stimulation of the cough receptors that surround the trachea or the bronchial tree by either the primary tumor or involved lymph nodes can induce coughing. Fever with a cough implies a proximal airway obstruction and distal pneumonitis. The obstruction can result from intrinsic airway involvement or extrinsic compression.

Tumors that extend to the pain sensitive parietal pleura (T3) can manifest with pleuritic chest pain, a pleural rub, or constant discomfort. Extension of tumors into the chest wall proper (also T3 disease) usually are associated with greater discomfort that typically is constant and not easily relieved by any movement or shift in body position, including sitting and standing. The location of pain often is classic in superior sulcus tumors—interscapular pain with radiation down the medial aspect of the arm with the involvement of the intercostal brachial nerve. Extension into the spine (T4 disease) can result in pain that may be aggravated by axial loading with weight bearing as the integrity and support of the spine are progressively destroyed by the tumor. Destruction of the vertebral body can result in its collapse with retropulsion of the bone into the spinal canal, with worsening neurologic symptoms (gait disturbance, bowel and bladder dysfunction) from direct compression of the spinal cord within the dural sac. Extension into the neural foramen can have a similar effect with spinal cord compression.

The mediastinal extension of tumors can cause a variety of signs and symptoms. Voice hoarseness is an extremely important symptom and often signifies unresectable disease. This can occur either from direct involvement of the tumor or with nodal disease. With left-sided lesions, the recurrent nerve typically is involved in the aortopulmonary window from station #5 lymph nodes or tumor extension beneath the aortic arch. Demonstration of left vocal cord paralysis by means of simple indirect laryngoscopy is all that is required to confirm advanced disease, unlikely to be helped by surgery. On the right, the recurrent nerve comes off on a more oblique angle as the vagus nerve passes over the right subclavian artery and "recurs" where the innominate artery divides into the right carotid and right subclavian arteries. Such involvement can occur with high, medially positioned right upper lobe lung tumors or high paratracheal nodal disease.

Involvement of mediastinal structures is defined as T4 disease in describing the primary tumor with its direct involvement. Structures that can be involved include the superior vena cava, often manifesting with signs and symptoms of superior vena cava syndrome. This presentation can be subtle in the beginning, with some blurring of vision, early-morning facial edema, headaches, and prominence of some veins on the neck or chest.

The pericardium (T3) can be resected en bloc with a tumor, but direct involvement of the heart (T4) is a more advanced presentation. In such cases, the patient can present with a dysrhythmia or signs of a pericardial effusion and tamponade. The aorta can be invaded, in which case usually severe localized pain from nerve fibers in the aortic adventitia will help to make the diagnosis. Although imaging studies often cannot clearly delineate aortic wall involvement, the presence of severe pain (either anterior or posterior in the interscapular region) is a very strong indicator of locally advanced disease beyond the confines of the lung. Other mediastinal structures include the trachea and the esophagus. A cough immediately after swallowing liquids usually indicates a tracheoesophageal fistula—an example of an advanced lesion usually treated with palliative intent only.

Evidence of metastatic disease must be detected by a detailed and focused review of signs and symptoms. Recent onset of a headache, a new hip or back pain, unexplained weight loss, and anorexia are all important clinical features that warrant further investigation. Paraneoplastic presentations are often seen and must be separated from mechanical symptoms from metastatic disease.

The physical examination can be quite helpful. Palpation of the supraclavicular fossa for nodal disease is the single most important aspect of the physical examination for staging. Small firm nodes—which often are too small to be picked up by PET imaging and would be too small to exceed the 1-cm threshold for the radiologist to comment on a computed tomography (CT) scan—are best discovered on physical examination by an experienced clinician. Auscultatory findings of a localized wheeze or stridor often indicate advanced disease. Diminished breath sounds can mean proximal obstruction or a pleural effusion. Shift of the trachea can mean either lobar or total volume loss on the affected side. An irregular cardiac rhythm or distended neck veins can indicate pericardial involvement with tamponade. Distended collateral veins on the chest or engorgement of neck veins may indicate a superior vena cava obstruction. Pain on percussion of the thoracic or lumbar spine or pain with movement of the hip may signify localized metastatic disease involving bones. The neurologic findings of a Horner's syndrome may signify involvement of the thoracic sympathetic plexus with secondary lid droop and meiosis.

Brain metastases can manifest in myriad ways, depending on the location of the metastatic lesion or lesions. In a patient without neurologic signs or symptoms, however, MRI has less than a 5% chance of finding an occult metastatic lesion.

Physiologic testing of the patient often can be done in the clinic. In general, a patient who can climb a flight of stairs can tolerate a lobectomy. The ability to climb two flights is required for a pneumonectomy. Although these are relatively crude measures of exercise performance, they have stood up well over the past 50 years or so to even more sophisticated exercise testing, including exercise oxygen consumption testing. Pulmonary function tests include spirometry and diffusion capacity testing; nuclear xenon split perfusion and ventilation function tests are used when spirometry demonstrates a forced expiratory volume in 1 second (FEV_1) below 70%. Such testing permits calculation of a predicted postoperative FEV_1. A minimum of 33% of predicted based on the patient's age and height has served well as the lower limit of postoperative function, to avoid rendering the patient a respiratory cripple from the resection. Exercise oxygen consumption testing is performed when the predicted FEV_1 is less than 40%. Remarkably, some patients with good cardiac function and good peripheral muscle utilization of oxygen can tolerate a resection with marginal pulmonary function.

Cardiac workup often is performed in patients with a history of cardiac disease, stent placement, or cardiac valvular or coronary bypass operations. The physiologic demands from a pulmonary resection on the patient are greater than those from a routine open heart procedure. As a result, the perioperative mortality after lung surgery is greater than after cardiac surgery. After cardiac surgery, the mechanical cardiac defects are usually corrected, so the patient should be in better functional status postoperatively than preoperatively. When a cancer operation is performed, however, the tumor and otherwise normal-functioning lung must be removed. As a result, the patient will have less physiologic reserve postoperatively than preoperatively. Again, this observation emphasizes the importance of accurate preoperative staging, to limit surgery to those who will be benefited.

Patients should abstain from cigarette smoking for a minimum of 2 to 3 weeks before an operation is performed, to improve their mucociliary clearance in the postoperative setting, thereby avoiding the cascading complications of sputum retention, airway occlusion, atelectasis, and pneumonia. Several weeks are required, because an immediate reactive bronchorrhea results from the immediate cessation of smoking.

The appropriate radiologic tests for a patient with lung cancer include a standard chest radiograph, a CT scan of the chest including the upper abdomen (to look for adrenal metastases), and a brain MRI study if the patient has relevant symptoms or the primary tumor is large or central or is associated with nodal disease. Positron emission tomography (PET) scans or integrated CT-PET scans, when available, have become routine in the evaluation of all patients with lung cancer. A focused radiographic examination is done to evaluate any suspicious area identified by PET scanning. Similarly, any new bone-related symptom in a patient necessitates spot films of the region to help differentiate between degenerative bone lesions and metastatic disease.[10]

STAGING PHASE II: RADIOGRAPHIC REVIEW

When reviewing a radiograph, the surgeon must evaluate independently the primary tumor and the extent of nodal disease. The primary tumor is evaluated to see if it can be resected en bloc without breaching the tumor. First, a hypothetical, uninterrupted line must be drawn around the tumor and the adjacent or involved anatomic structures. The surgeon must assess the anatomic extent required to obtain such a negative margin, if this can be reconstructed, and the potential physiologic impact of such a resection on the patient. The more extensive the resection, the greater the risks of the procedure. A lobectomy for a small T1 lesion in an otherwise healthy patient carries a perioperative mortality rate of 1% or less. A right pneumonectomy, however, in a patient older than 70 years of age has been associated with a mortality rate of 10% or higher in some series. Clearly, procedures that entail extensive chest wall resections, carinal resections, and vascular reconstructions with the occasional use of circulatory bypass techniques will result in greater morbidity and mortality than more limited resections.

The surgeon must decide when the surgical risks of the procedure and the postoperative course exceed the benefits of the procedure based on the patient's age, symptomatology, and comorbidities. These risks must be weighed closely against the anticipated long-term survival of the patient if an R0 resection can be accomplished. For instance, with direct invasion of the left atrium by a lung cancer without nodal disease (T4N0), complete removal can result in a 25% 5-year survival rate. If the surgical mortality rate exceeds 25%, then there is no role for surgery. If, however, the procedure can be accomplished with a perioperative mortality rate of 5% to 10%, then surgery may be worth the risk. This risk must be balanced by the expected survival rate if a nonsurgical option is chosen. If the surgery carries a 10% mortality rate and the 5-year survival rate with chemotherapy and radiation therapy is 20%, then the nonsurgical option in this patient will afford the best long-term chance of survival. If the same patient has proven N2 disease on preoperative assessment, then the 5-year survival rate even with successful surgery is less than 5%. Surgery is therefore not indicated in this setting, even if the surgical mortality rate for the procedure is only 5%. Nonsurgical management (chemotherapy and radiation therapy) is indicated in such cases. Improved staging even if achieved using invasive procedures (which can be accomplished with fairly low morbidity and virtually no risk of death) can avoid major procedures and is both cost-effective and less traumatic to the patient.

Nodal disease is best assessed by size criteria (larger than 1 cm in short-axis dimension), number of nodes, and station distribution of the nodal enlargement, and recently with PET imaging. PET is quite sensitive but lacks specificity; this limitation is compounded by presence or history of granulomatous conditions such as histoplasmosis. Tissue confirmation of PET positivity is important before selection of the treatment algorithm for the patient. Disease in these patients can easily be overstaged by false-positive PET interpretations.[11–13]

Due to the high sensitivity of PET scans, a patient with a small peripheral lung cancer with negative findings on PET scan of the mediastinum can proceed directly to thoracotomy for resection if the patient is otherwise healthy. The chance of finding an occult N2 node in such cases is less than 5%.

STAGING PHASE III: INTERVENTIONAL STAGING PROCEDURES

The third and final phase of preoperative staging consists of appropriate interventional staging procedures, each of which has specific indications, advantages, and limitations. The following techniques are discussed: transthoracic needle aspiration (TTNA), bronchoscopy (rigid and flexible), laser fluorescence bronchoscopy, navigational bronchoscopy, endobronchial ultrasound imaging (EBUS), endoscopic ultrasound imaging (EUS), mediastinoscopy and video-assisted mediastinoscopy, video-assisted thoracoscopy (VATS), laparoscopy, and the Chamberlain procedure.

Transthoracic Needle Aspiration

The ability of interventional radiologists to place a small needle or core biopsy needle in virtually any place in the chest is extremely helpful in preoperative staging for patients with thoracic malignancies. On-site, real-time cytopathologic review has made several procedures much more sensitive, thereby avoiding unnecessary repeat biopsies, and can limit the need for further testing should the results of the first pass be positive. If the patient presents de novo for workup and the diagnosis is unknown, initial biopsy of a clinically enlarged mediastinal node, rather than the primary tumor, can be very useful. If malignancy is confirmed through this mediastinal node biopsy, a diagnosis and stage have been established with one pass of the needle. As described earlier, if the nodes are enlarged, the contralateral node is preferentially biopsied to confirm N3 disease, which would identify the patient as having disease unresectable for cure. If findings are negative, then an ipsilateral N2 node is sampled next. Adrenal biopsy can demonstrate pathologic findings in keeping with lung cancer histology at the first pass and confirm M1b disease in one procedure only. The interventional radiologist can reach small 5-mm peripheral lesions and mediastinal disease, even if it requires a transsternal approach or going through the superior vena cava into a mediastinal node. Virtually any conceivable needle path can be used to biopsy a lesion.

A pneumothorax can result in 10% to 15% of the patients, more commonly in those with emphysema. In most cases this can be treated with immediate placement of a small chest tube. An overnight stay may be required with typically prompt sealing of the air leak. Some prolonged air leaks can result but are rare. Transient hemoptysis can occur but is almost always of small volume and self-limited. Injury to an intercostal artery can occur and may require operative repair. A rare complication of a central air embolism has been reported as a result of a tract created between the aerated pulmonary parenchyma and a pulmonary vein during the procedure.

Bronchoscopy

Rigid Bronchoscopy

The rigid bronchoscope is rarely used for diagnostic or staging purposes in patients with peripherally situated bronchogenic tumors. Rigid bronchoscopy can be used with central tumors to determine whether the trachea is fixed in position or is moveable. This technique is especially helpful in the assessment of primary airway tumors, permitting determination of the length of tracheal involvement and temporary "coring out" of tumor in patients who present with stridor and partial airway obstruction. It is an essential tool for the thoracic surgeon when major hemoptysis is a presenting manifestation of a thoracic malignancy. Mediastinal tumors, such as thymomas, may manifest with significant airway compression, and a rigid scope may be critical to control the airway in these patients, especially if they are given muscle paralytics during the procedure. Rigid bronchoscopy is performed with the patient under general anesthesia.

Flexible Bronchoscopy

Advances in endoscopic equipment, with charge-coupled device (CCD) camera chips at the end of flexible scopes, have permitted the development of smaller scopes, which are less traumatic to the patient, resulting in superb magnified images. This improvement allows outpatient procedures using topical anesthesia and light sedation only. Many instruments can be passed through the working channel of the scope to permit biopsy under direct vision. Therapeutic interventions also can be safely performed, including airway dilation for strictures, control of bleeding with laser and argon plasma coagulators, debulking procedures, and stent placement.

From a staging perspective, subtle mucosal changes can be appreciated with the superior optics and magnification afforded by flexible scopes. Submucosal spread from the primary tumor or extrinsic, malignant nodal involvement can be detected. Gross or subtle distortion of the central airways can be appreciated. Splaying of the primary or secondary carinas can signify extensive nodal involvement. Small and larger fistulas between the esophagus and the airway can be detected. Using CT scans and observed changes in the airways to direct needle placement, direct transbronchial Wang needle biopsy can be performed, without necessarily requiring ultrasound guidance, although the yield is lower than with ultrasound-guided biopsy. Direct involvement of the airway or extrinsic compression can be recognized in all 18 named and numbered bronchopulmonary segments and beyond. Smaller scopes permit an even more distal examination of the airway. Complications are rare and usually are related to lidocaine toxicity such as seizures, from airway mucosal absorption of the topical anesthetic, or excessive sedation from the benzodiazepams or narcotics used to sedate the patient. Reversal agents occasionally are required, as is transient mask ventilation if the patient's oxygen saturation drops. Complications from the bronchoscopy may include epistaxis if the nasal passage is chosen as the route for scope insertion, transient hemoptysis from biopsy sites, laryngospasm, or a sore throat from the procedure. Aspiration is always a potential risk in the unsecured airway. The biopsy forceps are small, so complications are rare. Pneumothorax can result from a peripheral lung biopsy or a Wang needle aspiration.

Navigational Bronchoscopy

Recent advances in CT scanning, coupled with the use of global positioning system (GPS) technology and steerable catheters, have permitted the development of navigational bronchoscopy systems that permit a directed biopsy of peripheral lesions previously not reachable with any degree of reliability by standard bronchoscopy. Previously, fluoroscopy was required in the anteroposterior and lateral views to facilitate localization and biopsy of a peripheral lesion. This technique often was a hit-or-miss process.

Using navigational bronchoscopy, a route to the lesion is developed through the review of the CT images. Airway landmarks are used to direct the catheter to the target lesion. Defined points are registered at the time of the bronchoscopy and matched to the preplanned CT scan route. As the endoscopist selects the path to the lesion, landmarks are shown on the real-time endoscopic route. Once the limits of the scope are reached, a steerable catheter goes beyond the tip of the scope, again using radiology guidance to the target lesion. Onscreen guidance helps the operator decide at which angle to steer the catheter until the target lesion is in the center. At this point, the biopsy is performed.[14–16]

Laser Fluorescence Bronchoscopy

Subtle changes to the mucosa of the airway in the development of carcinoma in situ can result in autofluorescence changes when a blue light is shined on the airway and reflective changes are magnified in the red and green spectra. Autofluorescence bronchoscopy permits real-time assessment of the airway and can be helpful in identifying patients who may have multifocal disease, in which the pathologic changes often appear normal under white light imaging techniques.[17–23]

Endoscopic Bronchial Ultrasound Imaging

Over the past several years, the technology of endoscopic bronchial ultrasound imaging (EBUS) has significantly changed the staging of intrathoracic malignancies for many thoracic surgeons.[23–25] Olympus has developed a scope, slightly larger than the typical diagnostic bronchoscope, that has an inflatable balloon and ultrasound probe to image the airway and the surrounding structures. A needle biopsy system that exits the working channel at an angle is coupled to the ultrasound imaging device. Lymph nodes are demonstrated as hyperechoic round to oval masses in the typical anatomic locations. Doppler imaging is used to distinguish a mediastinal vessel (aorta, pulmonary artery, azygos vein, innominate artery) from the lymph nodes. Under ultrasound guidance, the needle is passed several times through the node, and immediate cytopathologic analysis confirms sufficient lymphoid tissue and can quickly diagnose carcinoma. Noncancer diagnoses such as sarcoidosis can be made quickly. Nodes at virtually every nodal station except #5 and #6 and #8 and #9 can be reached. EBUS has the advantage over mediastinoscopy in that hilar nodes in the #11 and #12 locations also can be reached. Sampling subcarinal and paratracheal nodes is fairly straightforward.[26]

The hardest part of this procedure is getting through the wall of the trachea. Often a point between the cartilaginous rings must be selected. Many surgeons prefer to perform this procedure with the patient under general anesthesia to minimize the respiratory motion of the airway, especially when lymph nodes less than 1 cm in size are the target. Small nodes in the 4- to 6-mm range can be biopsied when they are running along the wall of the tracheobronchial tree. The procedure is well tolerated and often is performed through a single-lumen endotracheal tube or a laryngeal mask airway.

Complications are rare, although a pneumothorax can occur with biopsy of these nodes. The patient may require a general anesthetic, as procedures can last up to 1 hour in duration if multiple stations are sampled. Bleeding complications are extremely unlikely, because the needle is very small.

As the imaging qualities improve with second- and third-generation scopes and the needle systems improve, the need for mediastinoscopy in the future can be expected to be greatly reduced. In my own thoracic practice, the assessment of the mediastinum already has shifted to these techniques. Interventional pulmonologists also have been involved a great deal more often in nodal staging for bronchogenic malignancies. The limitations still remain prolonged duration of the procedure, the requirement for general anesthesia to minimize movement of airway structures, and the initial and maintenance expense of the scope and the ultrasound probe, which can easily be damaged and often costs $20,000 or more to repair.[27–31]

Endoscopic Ultrasound Imaging

A radial probe attached to an esophagoscope can be used to evaluate lymph nodes in the paraesophageal and inferior pulmonary ligament regions. This technology is termed endoscopic ultrasound imaging (EUS). Although rare, direct invasion of the esophagus by a lung cancer can be assessed using the esophagoscope.[32,33] Subcarinal nodes can also be biopsied by EBUS using the bronchoscope passed into the esophagus at the end of the standard airway examination.

Mediastinoscopy

Standard mediastinoscopy has been used for nearly 50 years to assess the lymph nodes in the upper, paratracheal, and subcarinal locations. This procedure initially required a simple light directed down a rigid scope. Subsequent advances in optics placed the fiberoptic lights and the fiberoptics for the camera down the side of the scope, which has resulted in video-mediastinoscopy. These improvements now permit a magnified image of the operative field to be viewed on a television monitor. Better imaging and optics have made modern video-mediastinoscopy a much safer procedure and one that can more easily be taught to thoracic surgical residents.[34]

The procedure requires use of a general anesthetic, a small suprasternal neck incision, and dissection along the pretracheal plane, beneath the innominate artery. Nodes can be rapidly biopsied from the 2L and 2R positions, the 4R and 4L positions, and the nodal station #7 (subcarinal). Nodes along the right and left main bronchi also can be biopsied. The procedure can be performed in less than 15 minutes and allows larger nodal samples to be obtained, which can help in the diagnosis of small cell and lymphoma pathology. An on-site immediate cytopathologic review for the adequacy of the specimen is not required.

An extended mediastinoscopy is an infrequently performed technique in which the nodes at stations #5 and #6 are biopsied by passing the scope through the anterior mediastinal compartment and along the arch of the aorta to the aortopulmonary window.[35–39]

The advantages of mediastinoscopy are the speed of sampling of the nodes, the improved specimens obtained, and the more robust nature of the scope, which permits hundreds of procedures to be done without need for repair. The disadvantages include the need for general anesthesia, some neck swelling from the dissection, often a sore throat, and the rare but real risk of injury to mediastinal structures including major vessels (innominate artery, azygos vein, pulmonary artery, aorta), injury to the trachea or right upper lobe bronchus, injury to the esophagus, which can be biopsied along its anterior wall during removal of 4L nodes or subcarinal nodes, or injury to nerves such as the left recurrent nerve as it courses in the left tracheoesophageal groove but recurs close to the takeoff of the left main bronchus. Although death from this procedure is extremely rare, major vessel injury may require an emergency sternotomy or thoracotomy to repair the injury. "Redo" mediastinoscopy after induction therapy may be indicated.[40] Virtual mediastinoscopy using integrated CT-PET shows potential.[41]

Video-Assisted Thoracoscopy

Availability of 5-mm and 10-mm scopes with 0-degree and 30-degree lenses permits a thorough examination of the entire hemithorax. In patients in whom analysis of pleural fluid sampled at initial thoracentesis yielded negative findings, a VATS procedure performed to rule out pleural implants before thoracotomy can be helpful. The entire parietal pleura, visceral pleura, and mediastinal and diaphragmatic surfaces can be examined. The aortopulmonary and prevascular nodes (stations #5 and #6, respectively) can be approached from the left using this procedure.[42] The subcarinal nodes and paraesophageal and inferior pulmonary ligament nodes also can be sampled or dissected. In some centers, minimally invasive techniques have become the preferred method for pulmonary dissection and resection. Small anterior access incisions, coupled with the excellent optics of the thoracoscopic telescopes, permit the use of standard surgical instruments, without the need to spread the ribs. As a result, postoperative pain is diminished. Most routine anatomic dissections can be performed, including lobectomies and segmentectomies, without the need to do a formal, rib-spreading procedure. The short-term functional results (shoulder girdle motion, return to work, pain control) are excellent, and the long-term survival results are comparable to those achieved with standard open procedures.

Chamberlain Procedure

The Chamberlain procedure is a limited open thoracotomy anterior approach, often with resection of a portion of cartilage of the second or third rib. This approach permits biopsy of the prevascular and aortopulmonary window nodes on the left and some nodes anterior to the superior vena cava on the right.

Care must be taken to avoid injury to the vagus nerves and the phrenic nerves. VATS procedures give better cosmetic results in women, in which an anterior chest incision is to be avoided, if possible.

Laparoscopy

Mesothelioma can extend through the diaphragm. In my own experience, use of laparoscopy to examine the undersurface of the diaphragm and to perform a diagnostic abdominal lavage helps to exclude patients with advanced disease who will not be helped by an extrapleural pneumonectomy. This procedure is coupled with a mediastinoscopy or EBUS to complete the preoperative staging for patients with mesothelioma.[43]

Although rare, transdiaphragmatic extension of stage IVA thymomas also can be diagnosed with a laparoscopic assessment. Laparoscopy frequently has been used in the staging of esophageal carcinoma to evaluate for malignant ascites, liver metastases, and celiac nodal disease.[44–46]

SUMMARY

In practice, the thoracic surgeon uses various tools to identify those patients in whom an R0 resection is most likely and who have the best chance of long-term survival. The initial step in preoperative staging for thoracotomy is a careful review of the broad scope of clinical and radiographic findings in an attempt to exclude early on those patients who are medically inoperable because of limited cardiopulmonary reserve or in whom stage IV disease is suspected on the basis of evidence from a focused history identifying metastatic symptoms, CT-PET imaging, or brain imaging. The next level of scrutiny is to identify unresectable T4 disease or N3 nodal disease. This distinction is accomplished through either imaging or directed biopsy. N2 disease is next ruled out through mediastinoscopy, EBUS, EUS, VATS, or Chamberlain approaches. Patients who have potentially "limited, resectable" N2 are considered for induction protocols. The remaining patients with N1 and N0 disease and resectable T1, T2, or T3 disease are considered for surgery. The optimal approach in this group is to use noninvasive imaging techniques first and then proceed with the least to most invasive staging diagnostic tests. If this algorithm is followed, intraoperative surprises resulting in R2 resections or in "open and close" procedures should be rare. The importance of accurate staging is essential for patients with thoracic malignancies. In the future, biologic marker assays will complement and probably replace many of the radiographic and invasive procedures described in this chapter.

REFERENCES

1. Detterbeck FC, Tanoue LT, Boffa DJ. Anatomy, biology and concepts, pertaining to lung cancer stage classification. *J Thorac Oncol.* 2009;4(4):437–443.
2. Mountain CF. A new international staging system for lung cancer. *Chest.* 1986;89:225S–233S.
3. Mountain CF. Revisions in the International System for Staging Lung Cancer. *Chest.* 1997;111(6):1710–1717.
4. Rami-Porta R, Crowley JJ, Goldstraw P. The revised TNM staging system for lung cancer. *Ann Thorac Cardiovasc Surg.* 2009;15(1):4–9.
5. Travis WD. Reporting lung cancer pathology specimens. Impact of the anticipated 7th edition TNM classification based on recommendations of the IASLC Staging Committee. *Histopathology.* 2009;54(1):3–11.
6. Groome PA, Bolejack V, Crowley JJ, et al. The IASLC Lung Cancer Staging Project: validation of the proposals for revision of the T, N, and M descriptors and consequent stage groupings in the forthcoming (seventh) edition of the TNM classification of malignant tumours. *J Thorac Oncol.* 2007;2(8):694–705.
7. Rusch VW, Crowley J, Giroux DJ, et al. The IASLC Lung Cancer Staging Project: proposals for the revision of the N descriptors in the forthcoming seventh edition of the TNM classification for lung cancer. *J Thorac Oncol.* 2007;2(7):603–612.
8. Rusch VW, Asamura H, Watanabe H, Giroux DJ, Rami-Porta R, Goldstraw P. The IASLC lung cancer staging project: a proposal for a new international lymph node map in the forthcoming seventh edition of the TNM classification for lung cancer. *J Thorac Oncol.* 2009;4(5):568–577.
9. Pisters KM, Darling G. The IASLC Lung Cancer Staging Project: "the nodal zone." *J Thorac Oncol.* 2007;2(7):583–584.
10. Groth SS, Whitson BA, Maddaus MA. Radiographic staging of mediastinal lymph nodes in non–small cell lung cancer patients. *Thorac Surg Clin.* 2008;18(4):349–361.
11. Poeppel TD, Krause BJ, Heusner TA, Boy C, Bockisch A, Antoch G. PET/CT for the staging and follow-up of patients with malignancies. *Eur J Radiol.* 2009;70(3):382–392.
12. Sorensen JB, Ravn J, Loft A, Brenoe J, Berthelsen AK. Preoperative staging of mesothelioma by ^{18}F-fluoro-2-deoxy-D-glucose positron emission tomography/computed tomography fused imaging and

mediastinoscopy compared to pathological findings after extrapleural pneumonectomy. *Eur J Cardiothorac Surg.* 2008;34(5):1090–1096.
13. Plathow C, Staab A, Schmaehl A, et al. Computed tomography, positron emission tomography, positron emission tomography/computed tomography, and magnetic resonance imaging for staging of limited pleural mesothelioma: initial results. *Invest Radiol.* 2008;43(10):737–744.
14. Weiser TS, Hyman K, Yun J, Litle V, Chin C, Swanson SJ. Electromagnetic navigational bronchoscopy: a surgeon's perspective. *Ann Thorac Surg.* 2008;85(2):S797–S801.
15. Summers RM. Navigational aids for real-time virtual bronchoscopy. *AJR Am J Roentgenol.* 1997;168(5):1165–1170.
16. Makris D, Scherpereel A, Leroy S, et al. Electromagnetic navigation diagnostic bronchoscopy for small peripheral lung lesions. *Eur Respir J.* 2007;29(6):1187–1192.
17. Lam B, Wong MP, Fung SL, et al. The clinical value of autofluorescence bronchoscopy for the diagnosis of lung cancer. *Eur Respir J.* 2006;28(5):915–919.
18. Jeremy GP, Banerjee AK, Read CA, et al. Surveillance for the detection of early lung cancer in patients with bronchial dysplasia. *Thorax.* 2007;62(1):43–50.
19. Herth FJ, Eberhardt R, Ernst A. The future of bronchoscopy in diagnosing, staging and treatment of lung cancer. *Respiration.* 2006;73(4):399–409.
20. Ikeda N, Honda H, Hayashi A, et al. Early detection of bronchial lesions using newly developed videoendoscopy-based autofluorescence bronchoscopy. *Lung Cancer.* 2006;52(1):21–27.
21. Herth FJ, Ernst A, Becker HD. Autofluorescence bronchoscopy—a comparison of two systems (LIFE and D-Light). *Respiration.* 2003;70(4):395–398.
22. Pasic A, Vonk-Noordegraaf A, Risse EK, Postmus PE, Sutedja TG. Multiple suspicious lesions detected by autofluorescence bronchoscopy predict malignant development in the bronchial mucosa in high risk patients. *Lung Cancer.* 2003;41(3):295–301.
23. Kusunoki Y, Imamura F, Uda H, Mano M, Horai T. Early detection of lung cancer with laser-induced fluorescence endoscopy and spectrofluorometry. *Chest.* 2000;118(6):1776–1782.
24. Gilbert S, Wilson DO, Christie NA, et al. Should endobronchial ultrasonography be part of the thoracic surgeon's armamentarium? *J Thorac Cardiovasc Surg.* 2009;137(2):413–418.
25. Melloni G, Casiraghi M, Bandiera A, et al. Transbronchial needle aspiration in lung cancer patients suitable for operation with positive mediastinal positron emission tomography. *Ann Thorac Surg.* 2009;87(2):373–378.
26. Gu P, Zhao YZ, Jiang LY, Zhang W, Xin Y, Han BH. Endobronchial ultrasound–guided transbronchial needle aspiration for staging of lung cancer: a systematic review and meta-analysis. *Eur J Cancer.* 2009;45(8):1389–1396.
27. Navani N, Spiro SG, Janes SM. EBUS-TBNA for the mediastinal staging of non–small cell lung cancer. *J Thorac Oncol.* 2009;4(6):776–777.
28. Adams K, Shah P, Edmonds L, Lim E. Test performance or endobronchial ultrasound and transbronchial needle aspiration biopsy for mediastinal staging in patients with lung cancer: systematic review and meta-analysis. *Thorax.* 2009;64(9):757–762.
29. Medford AR, Bennett JA, Free CM, Agrawal S. Mediastinal staging procedures in lung cancer: EBUS, TBNA and mediastinoscopy. *Curr Opin Pulm Med.* 2009;15(4):334–342.
30. Navani N, Spiro SG, Janes SM. Mediastinal staging of NSCLC with endoscopic and endobronchial ultrasound. *Nat Rev Clin Oncol.* 2009;6(5):278–286.
31. Groth SS, Whitson BA, D'Cunha J, Maddaus MA, Alsharif M, Andrade RS. Endobronchial ultrasound–guided fine-needle aspiration of mediastinal lymph nodes: a single institution's early learning curve. *Ann Thorac Surg.* 2008;86(4):1104–1109.
32. Stigt JA, Oostdijk AH, Timmer PR, Shahin GM, Boers JE, Groen HJ. Comparison of EUS-guided fine needle aspiration and integrated PET-CT in restaging after treatment for locally advanced non-small cell lung cancer. *Lung Cancer.* 2009;66(2):198–204.
33. Schipper P, Schoolfield M. Minimally invasive staging of N2 disease: endobronchial ultrasound/transesophageal endoscopic ultrasound, mediastinoscopy, and thoracoscopy. *Thorac Surg Clin.* 2008;18(4):363–379.
34. Leschber G, Sperling D, Klemm W, Merk J. Does video-mediastinoscopy improve the results of conventional mediastinoscopy? *Eur J Cardiothorac Surg.* 2008;33(2):289–293.
35. Thomsen RW. Mediastinoscopy and video-assisted thoracoscopic surgery: anesthetic pitfalls and complications. *Semin Cardiothorac Vasc Anesth.* 2008;12(2):128–132.
36. Annema JT, Tournoy KG, Rabe KF. Lung cancer staging with minimally invasive endoscopic techniques. *JAMA.* 2008;299(21):2510–2511.
37. Witte B, Neumeister W, Huertgen M. Does endoesophageal ultrasound-guided fine-needle aspiration replace mediastinoscopy in mediastinal staging of thoracic malignancies? *Eur J Cardiothorac Surg.* 2008;33(6):1124–1128.
38. Wallace MB, Pascual JM, Raimondo M, et al. Minimally invasive endoscopic staging of suspected lung cancer. *JAMA.* 2008;299(5):540–546.
39. Ernst A, Feller-Kopman D, Herth FJ. Endobronchial ultrasound in the diagnosis and staging of lung cancer and other thoracic tumors. *Semin Thorac Cardiovasc Surg.* 2007;19(3):201–205.
40. Marra A, Hillejan L, Fechner S, Stamatis G. Remediastinoscopy in restaging of lung cancer after induction therapy. *J Thorac Cardiovasc Surg.* 2008;135(4):843–849.
41. Shiono H, Okumura M, Sawabata N, et al. Virtual mediastinoscopy for safer and more accurate mediastinal exploration. *Ann Thorac Surg.* 2007;84(3):995–999.
42. Cerfolio RJ, Bryant AS, Eloubeidi MA. Accessing the aortopulmonary window (#5) and the paraaortic (#6) lymph nodes in patients with non–small cell lung cancer. *Ann Thorac Surg.* 2007;84(3):940–945.
43. Rice DC, Erasmus JJ, Stevens CW, et al. Extended surgical staging for potentially resectable malignant pleural mesothelioma. *Ann Thorac Surg.* 2005;80(6):1988–1992.
44. Krasna MJ, Jiao X, Sonett JR, et al. Thoracoscopic and laparoscopic lymph node staging in esophageal cancer: do clinicopathological factors affect the outcome? *Ann Thorac Surg.* 2002;73(6):1710–1713.
45. Luketich JD, Schauer P, Landreneau R, et al. Minimally invasive surgical staging is superior to endoscopic ultrasound in detecting lymph node metastases in esophageal cancer. *J Thorac Cardiovasc Surg.* 1997;114(5):817–821.
46. Krasna MJ, Flowers JL, Attar S, McLaughlin J. Combined thoracoscopic/laparoscopic staging of esophageal cancer. *J Thorac Cardiovasc Surg.* 1996;111(4):800–806.

3

Non–Small Cell Carcinomas of the Lung

Epithelial neoplasms are by far the most common primary malignancies in the lung. Worldwide, lung cancer is the leading cause of illness and death in patients with neoplastic disease as reflected in morbidity and mortality rates for this population. Environmental hazards, including tobacco use, have been conclusively linked to the development of pulmonary carcinoma. Recently, several important features have been observed in the epidemiology of lung cancer, including an increased frequency among African-American men compared with white men, and an increased frequency of squamous cell carcinoma among white women compared with African-American women. Histopathologically, adenocarcinoma appears to be the most common lung cancer diagnosis; squamous cell carcinoma appears to be more commonly associated with tobacco use.[1–8] In 2007, Wahbah and associates[9] demonstrated that adenocarcinoma diagnoses have become far more frequent over the past 3 decades: In 1980, adenocarcinomas in both men and women accounted for approximately 29% of the cases, and squamous cell carcinoma accounted for approximately 39%. By 2003, adenocarcinomas had increased to represent 40% of cases, whereas squamous cell carcinomas had decreased to 29%. In a Japanese study from 1958 to 1997, the investigators determined that the average age at death from lung cancer is 71.6 years for males and 73 years for females.[10] Regardless of the histologic type and ethnic group affected, the survival rate after 5 years is poor; as better techniques for early detection are developed, however, survival rates may be expected to improve.

CLINICAL ASPECTS

Non–small cell carcinomas of the lung are by far the most common malignant tumors, usually appearing in the sixth and seventh decades of life. The study by Wahbah and colleagues[9] reported the average age at diagnosis for patients with lung carcinoma to be 59 years for both men and women. The patient's symptomatology will depend largely on the anatomic location and the size of the tumor. Tumors that are centrally located are more likely to manifest earlier in the clinical course, typically with signs and symptoms of pulmonary obstruction such as cough, dyspnea, wheezing, hemoptysis, and pneumonia. Tumors that are located in the periphery of the lung will not cause symptoms until they reach a relatively large size. Some clinical signs and symptoms may be correlated with a particular type of tumor—for example, bronchorrhea (expectoration of large amounts of mucus) most commonly is seen in bronchioloalveolar carcinoma (BAC).[10] Depending on the extent of the tumor within the thorax, clinical manifestations may include pleuritic pain, the Pancoast syndrome, or superior vena cava syndrome.[10,11] Paraneoplastic syndromes such as inappropriate secretion of antidiuretic hormone, Cushing's syndrome, or acromegaly also may be associated with some non–small cell carcinomas of the lung.[10–12] Infectious processes such as tuberculosis and other primary pulmonary conditions such as pulmonary fibrosis and bronchiectasis also have been reported in association with these tumors.[13–15]

HISTOPATHOLOGIC CLASSIFICATION

The histopathologic classification of non–small cell carcinomas of the lung can be extensive. Table 3-1 presents a histopathologic classification based on the different growth patterns that have been described for these tumors. For some of these growth patterns, a rather specific clinical behavior has been recognized. An important point to keep in mind, however, is that the staging of non–small cell carcinomas is paramount in assessing outcome. Therefore, although it is important to properly classify a tumor from its histopathologic features, it also is crucial to demonstrate all of the features necessary for accurate staging of the tumor.

SQUAMOUS CELL CARCINOMA

Squamous cell carcinoma is currently less common than adenocarcinoma; however, squamous cell carcinoma is more commonly associated with tobacco use. Unlike adenocarcinoma, squamous cell carcinoma may show a progressive disease pattern, ranging from mild dysplasia (atypia) to carcinoma in situ to invasive squamous cell carcinoma.

Clinical Features

After diagnosis of dysplasia or squamous cell carcinoma in situ of the lung, in most cases a clearly identifiable tumor mass is absent. The great majority of patients come to medical attention because of a history of tobacco use or human papillomavirus infection. Some patients may provide a history of cough and respiratory difficulty.

TABLE 3-1 HISTOPATHOLOGIC CLASSIFICATION OF NON–SMALL CELL CARCINOMAS
Squamous cell carcinoma
Bronchioloalveolar carcinoma
Adenocarcinoma
Large cell carcinoma
Adenosquamous carcinoma
Lymphoepithelioma-like carcinoma
Rhabdoid carcinoma
Sarcomatoid/pleomorphic carcinoma

Histologic Features

Squamous Cell Dysplasia/Carcinoma In Situ

Although no foolproof mechanism has been found to distinguish between mild and moderate dysplasia on histopathologic grounds, and because such distinction may be rather arbitrary, a reasonable approach is to follow criteria similar to those used for other organ systems, such as the uterine cervix. In many cases, however, the diagnosis of high-grade dysplasia is synonymous with that of carcinoma in situ.

Mild Dysplasia

The diagnosis of mild dysplasia is made when cellular atypia is observed at, or just above, the basal cell layer. The nuclei may be hyperchromatic, and mitotic figures may be observed. No mitotic activity or cellular atypia is found in the midportion of the mucosa, which may show normal maturation.

Moderate Dysplasia

For a diagnosis of moderate dysplasia, the findings are similar to those of mild dysplasia; however, the cellular atypia and mitotic activity are not limited to the lower portion of the mucosa. In addition, the cellular atypia may be more pronounced and mitotic figures may be seen in the midportion of the mucosa. Normal maturation may still be identified in the upper portion of the mucosa, however.

Severe Dysplasia/Carcinoma In Situ

Severe dysplasia and carcinoma in situ are intrinsically associated conditions and represent the same pathologic process. Histologically, the mucosa shows full-thickness involvement: The cellular changes and mitotic figures occupy the entire mucosa; maturation is essentially absent, atypical mitotic figures may be seen at any level, and cellular atypia is much more pronounced (Fig. 3-1A). In some cases, the process may extend to the endobronchial glands; such extension, however, does not imply that the process is invasive (Fig. 3-1B). Careful evaluation is needed in cases with marked chronic inflammation, which may either obscure the true nature of the process or mimic an invasive neoplasm. In some unusual cases of in situ squamous cell carcinoma, changes may be observed in the epithelium that are histologically similar to those caused by Paget's disease (Fig. 3-1C). Although this pagetoid change may be extensive, it is still possible to find areas of more conventional squamous cell differentiation.

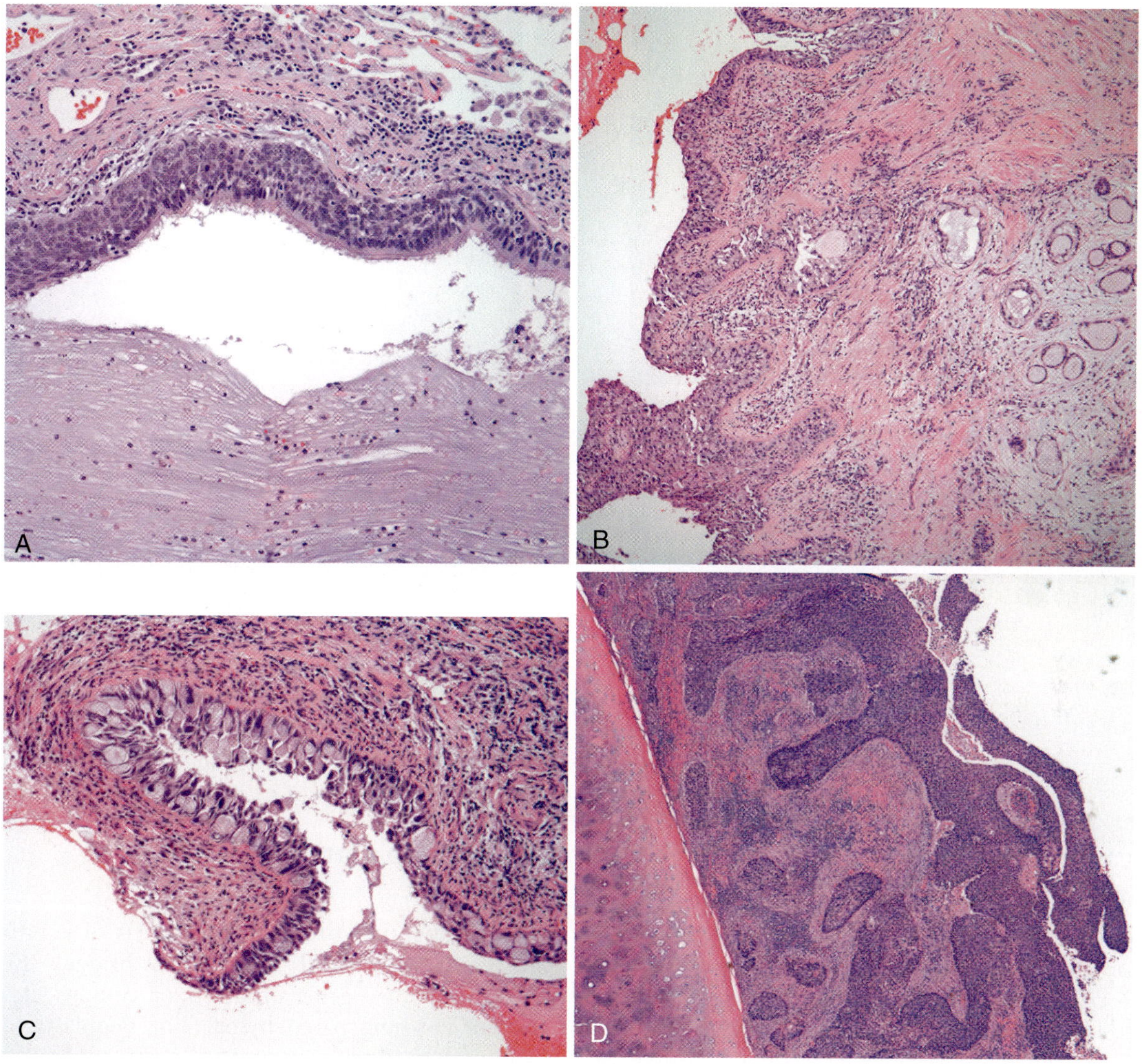

Figure 3-1 **A**, Low-power view of a squamous cell carcinoma in situ. Note the transition from dysplasia (ciliated epithelium is still present) to carcinoma in situ. **B**, In situ squamous cell carcinoma with glandular extension. **C**, In situ squamous cell carcinoma with pagetoid-like appearance. **D**, The squamous cell carcinoma in situ component predominates, with areas of invasion.

Invasive Squamous Cell Carcinoma

Traditionally, squamous cell carcinomas have been classified as well-, moderately, or poorly differentiated. Most of the factors influencing this classification involve the presence of either keratinization or intercellular bridges. Therefore, the closer a tumor mimics normal squamous epithelium, the better the grade of differentiation will be.

Clinical Features

As with other non–small cell carcinomas, patients may complain of cough, dyspnea, hemoptysis, or thoracic pain. Presence of such signs and symptoms generally reflects the anatomic location of the tumor. Tumors that are centrally located are more likely to produce signs and symptoms associated with obstruction, whereas tumors that are in the periphery of the lung are more likely to produce thoracic pain, owing to the large size they may attain.

Macroscopic Features

Squamous cell carcinomas may be seen as polypoid tumors obstructing the lumen of the airway (Fig. 3-2). As they reach a larger size, they may be seen extrinsically pushing into airway structures. Squamous cell carcinomas may be observed in the periphery of the lung, in a subpleural location (Fig. 3-3), or infiltrating the pleura with direct invasion into the soft tissues of the chest wall.

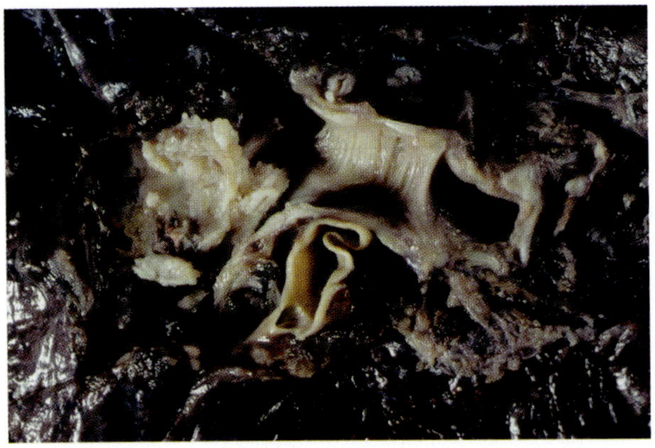

Figure 3-2 Squamous cell carcinoma with a polypoid growth pattern.

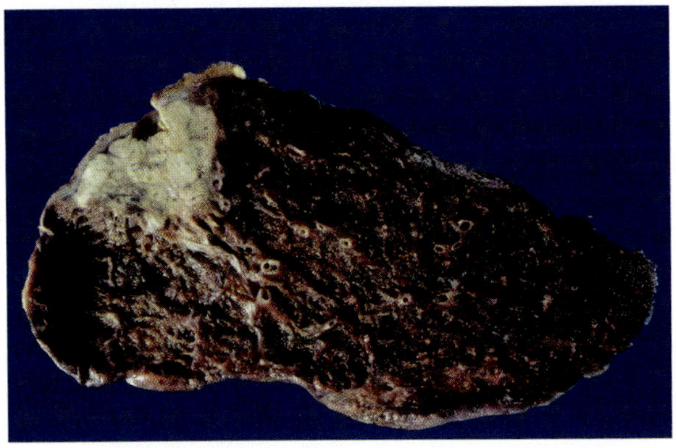

Figure 3-3 Peripheral squamous cell carcinoma. The tumor is in a subpleural location.

Tumor size may range from smaller than 1 cm to larger than 10 cm in greatest dimension. These tumors are white-tan and well demarcated, but not encapsulated. The cut surface may be homogeneous or show extensive areas of necrosis or hemorrhage. In some instances the tumor takes the form of a cavitary tumor mass (Fig. 3-4).

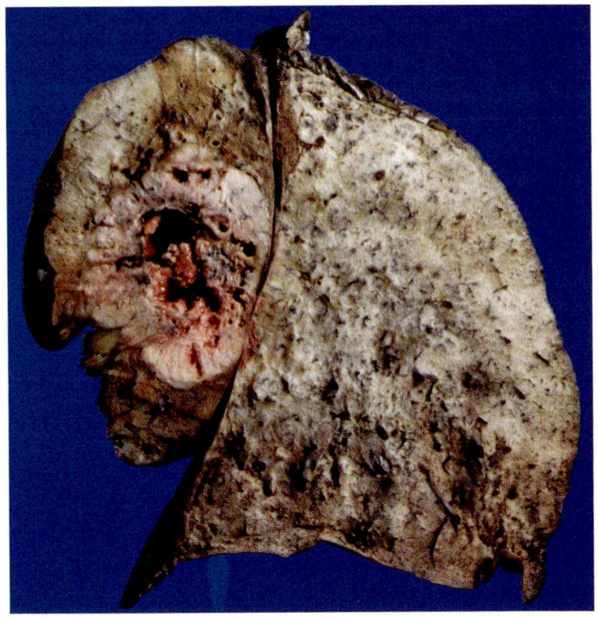

Figure 3-4 Squamous cell carcinoma showing cavitary changes and necrosis.

Well-Differentiated Squamous Cell Carcinoma

Well-differentiated tumors show areas of keratinization and easily identifiable intercellular bridges (Fig. 3-5). The tumor may grow in sheets or ribbons, destroying the normal lung parenchyma. The neoplastic cells are oval, with moderate amounts of eosinophilic cytoplasm,

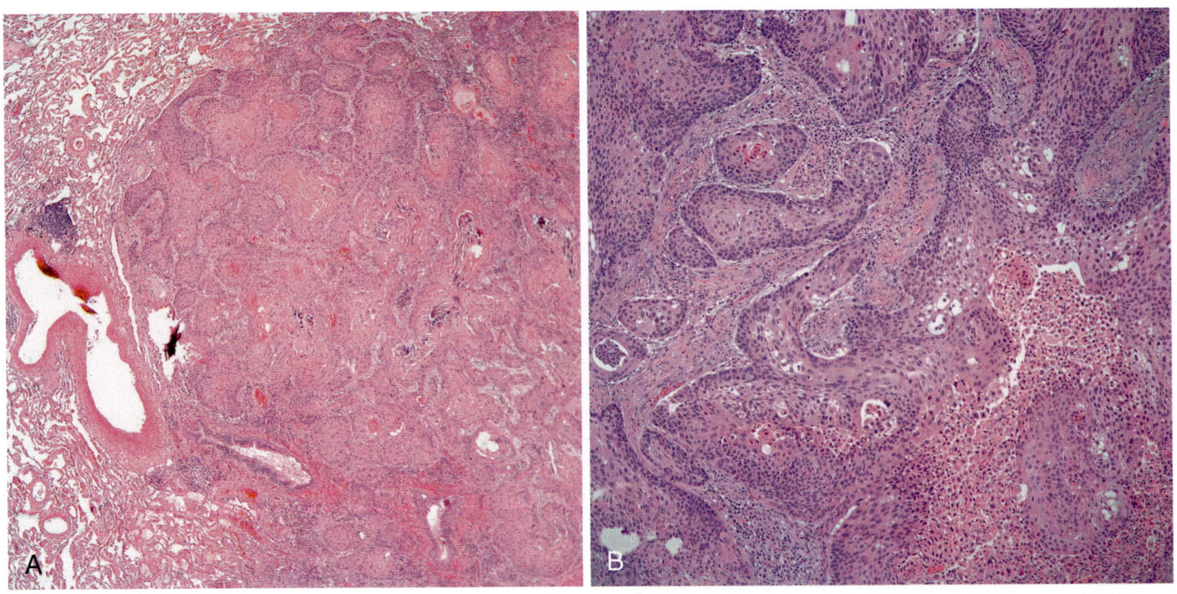

Figure 3-5 Well-differentiated squamous cell carcinoma. **A,** Tumor is destroying normal lung parenchyma. **B,** High-power view showing extensive areas of keratinization.

small nuclei, and inconspicuous nucleoli. Mitotic figures are present and can be numerous. Areas of necrosis or hemorrhage usually are absent or may be only focally present.

Moderately Differentiated Squamous Cell Carcinoma

Moderately differentiated tumors may still show areas in which either keratinization or intercellular bridges can be identified. However, more extensive areas of hemorrhage and necrosis, which may obscure the true nature of the neoplasm, also may be observed. Mitotic figures and cellular pleomorphism are more prominent (Fig. 3-6).

Poorly Differentiated Squamous Cell Carcinoma

Poorly differentiated squamous cell carcinomas have a tendency to grow in sheets, in which definitive evidence of squamous differentiation may be lacking. Extensive necrosis and hemorrhage may be present. The presence of cellular pleomorphism and mitotic activity is marked. In focal areas, however, it may still be possible to find unequivocal areas showing squamous cell differentiation (Fig. 3-7).

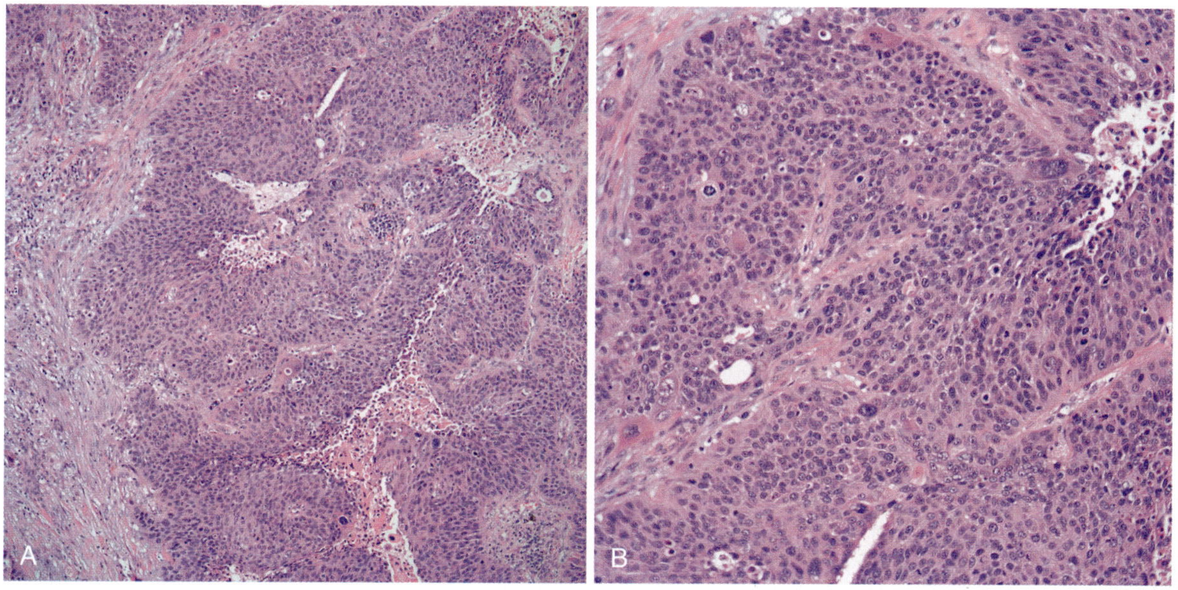

Figure 3-6 **A**, Moderately differentiated squamous cell carcinoma with focal desmoplastic reaction. **B**, High-power view showing tumor cells with more nuclear atypia and increased mitotic activity.

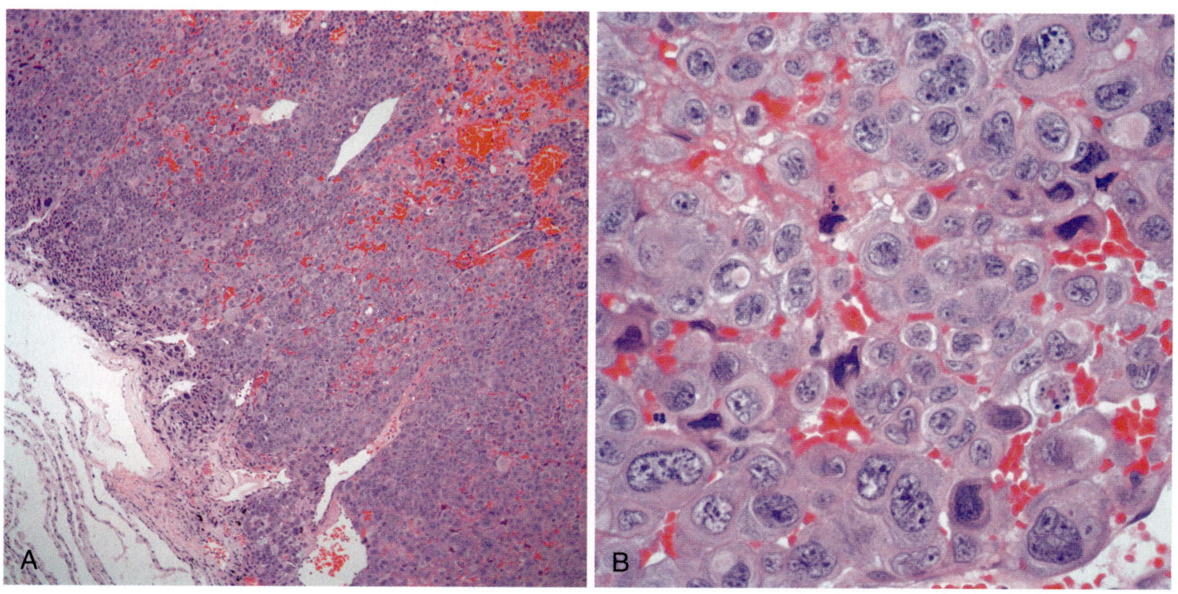

Figure 3-7 **A**, Poorly differentiated squamous cell carcinoma. Sheets of neoplastic cells can be seen. **B**, High-power view. Focal areas of squamous differentiation can still be recognized.

TABLE 3-2 HISTOPATHOLOGIC GROWTH PATTERNS OF SQUAMOUS CELL CARCINOMA

Exophytic
Cystic
Small cell–like
Spindle cell
Basaloid
Adenoid-like
Ameloblastic-like
Clear cell
Granular-like
Syringomatous-like

Histologic Variants

Squamous cell carcinomas show a variety of different growth patterns, which are summarized in Table 3-2 and illustrated throughout the chapter (Figs. 3-8 to 3-16). Some of the more important variants that have been presented in the literature are described next.

Exophytic

The unusual exophytic variant of squamous cell carcinoma also is known as Sherwin tumor in honor of one of the first investigators to assess this particular growth pattern. Sherwin and colleagues[16] documented the existence of this neoplasm after reviewing the cases of 85 patients diagnosed with squamous cell carcinoma. These workers isolated nine patients between 50 and 74 years of age in whom the tumor resembled an exophytic neoplasm. These patients all had undergone resection of the tumor; those who were treated with pneumonectomy had a more favorable outcome than those who were treated with lobectomy. Histologically, the tumors grew in an exophytic manner, obstructing the airway. They were of the well-differentiated grade, and none of the patients had metastasis to lymph nodes. The investigators noted that this type of squamous cell carcinoma may potentially have a more favorable outcome than other, more infiltrative variants.

Dulmet-Brender and associates[17] also presented their experience with 34 cases collected over 35 years and concluded that these tumors are almost always of the T1N0 stage at presentation. In their experience, however, the prognosis was not any better than it would be for another non–small cell carcinoma at the same stage. These workers concluded that these tumors were not a more common squamous cell carcinoma detected at an earlier stage, but rather that they represented a distinct variant.

More recently, Cooper and associates[18] documented a similar occurrence in a 75-year-old woman. The initial chest radiographic appearance was unremarkable, but an endobronchial tumor became evident on computed tomography (CT) scan. On resection of the mass, a papillary endobronchial neoplasm that did not extend into the adjacent lung parenchyma was found.

Histologically, all of these lesions appear to have the same characteristics: an exophytic tumor with squamous appearance, in some cases with extensive keratinization. In some areas, the tumor may acquire a papillary growth pattern in which the papillary projections show only a thin line of fibroconnective tissue, with no invasion. The most important histologic characteristic is the limited behavior of the tumor; it extends exophytically into the lumen without invasion into the bronchial wall. Rarely, the endobronchial glands also may show extension, but bronchial wall invasion should not be observed. The papillary fronds show cellular atypia, nuclear pleomorphism, and mitotic activity with some atypical mitotic figures.

Although the diagnosis of exophytic squamous cell carcinoma should not pose a problem from a histologic standpoint, some other lesions that manifest in similar fashion may be considerations in the differential diagnosis. In 1969, Laubscher[19] described a tumor referred to as "solitary squamous cell papilloma." Histologically, the tumor is a keratinizing, noninvasive squamous cell neoplasm that, based on the illustrations provided, shares some features with the cases described by Sherwin and colleagues.[16] The existence of noninvasive papillary neoplastic disease, such as solitary condylomatous papilloma and lower respiratory tract papillomatosis, is well recognized in the literature. These lesions will show squamous epithelium with some evidence of maturation remaining and in focal areas may demonstrate areas of transition between squamous and nonsquamous epithelium.[20–22]

Cystic

The cystic variant usually is recognized from the gross appearance of the tumor. It is characterized by prominent cystically dilated spaces, which may be filled with necrotic or inflammatory debris. In the periphery of the tumor, strands of squamous cell carcinoma, which may resemble buds or ribbons, are typical features. Usually, these tumors are well differentiated and have undergone cystic and necrotic changes (see Fig. 3-8).

Small Cell

The small cell growth pattern is unusual and represents a very small percentage of squamous cell carcinomas. Currently, no single series of cases has been presented in the literature; most reports are of single anecdotal cases described in textbooks.[23] Histologically, the tumor shows a proliferation of small cells with oval nuclei and inconspicuous nucleoli. Unlike in true small cell carcinomas, the chromatin displayed in the small cell variant of squamous cell carcinoma is not the typical "salt and pepper" type; rather, a smoother type of scant cytoplasm is observed (see Fig. 3-9). In cases in which a transbronchial

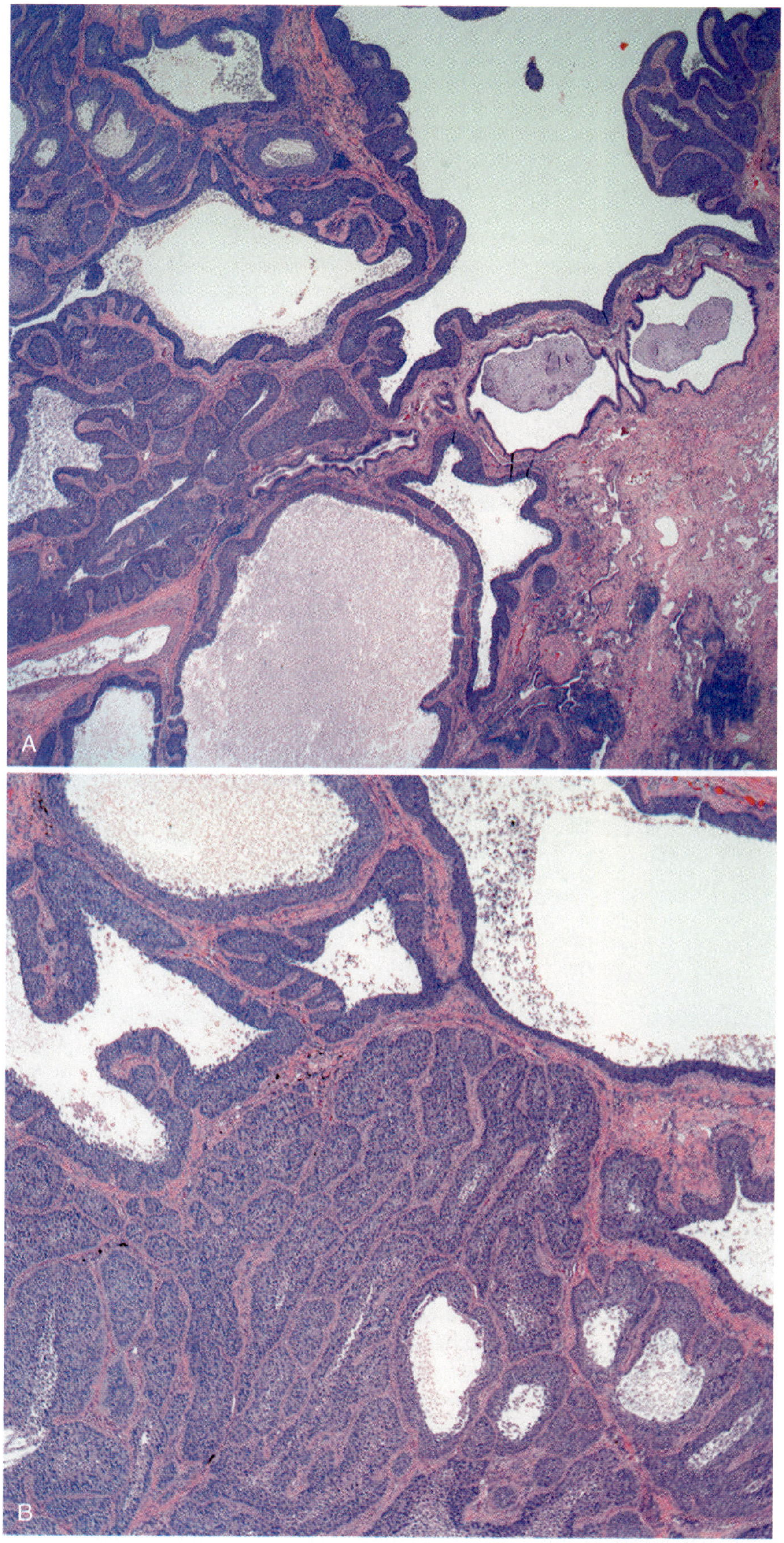

Figure 3-8 **A**, Squamous cell carcinoma with prominent cystic changes. **B**, Cystic squamous cell carcinoma with areas of solid tumor.

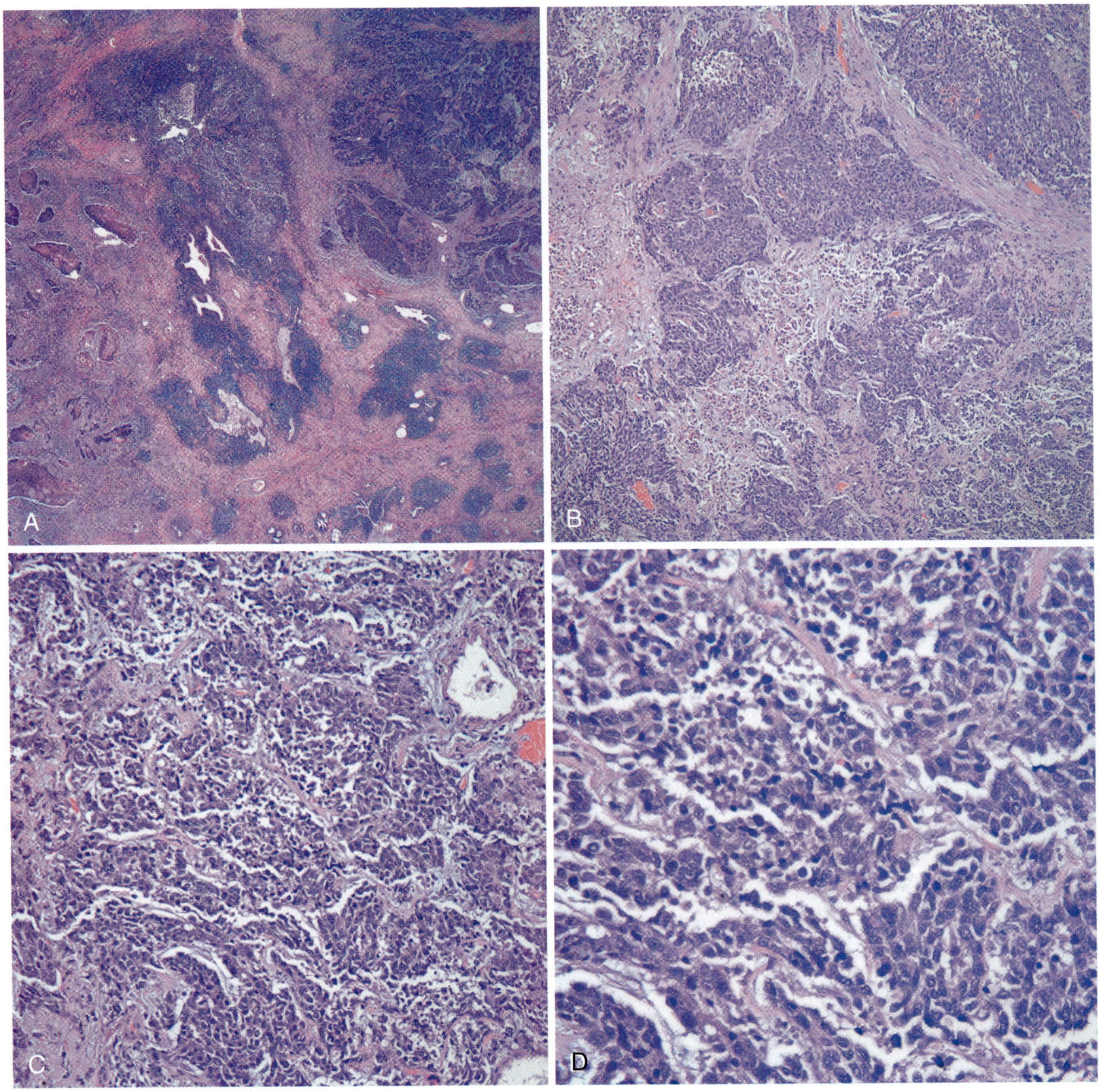

Figure 3-9 Small cell variant of squamous cell carcinoma. **A**, It is still possible to identify focal areas of conventional squamous cell carcinoma. **B**, Low-power view. Note the haphazard distribution of the tumor. **C**, Intermediate-power view showing islands of tumor cells with a vaguely neuroendocrine pattern. **D**, High-power view showing tumor cells with scant cytoplasm, round to oval nuclei, and the presence of nucleoli.

biopsy has been performed, the finding of squamous cell carcinoma in situ should raise clinical suspicion for the small cell variant. When squamous cell carcinoma in situ is not evident, it is important to identify areas in which the tumor may show focal keratinization or other clues to squamous cell differentiation. In more complicated cases, the use of immunohistochemical studies may be helpful. The small cell variant of squamous cell carcinoma may show positive staining for keratin 5/6 and p63, with negative staining for neuroendocrine markers; however, some squamous cell carcinomas also may show focal positive staining for some of the neuroendocrine markers—namely, synaptophysin.

Spindle Cell

The spindle cell growth pattern also is rather unusual and can be confused with other spindle cell neoplasms, especially sarcomas. It is characterized by fascicles of fusiform cells with elongated nuclei and inconspicuous nucleoli, increased mitotic figures, and atypical mitotic figures (see Fig. 3-10). The tumor may show interlacing fascicles of cells mimicking sarcomas. In focal areas, however, keratin pearls, single cell keratinization, or frank focus of keratinization may be observed. Currently, the use of immunohistochemical studies including immunostaining for epithelial markers such as broad-spectrum keratin,

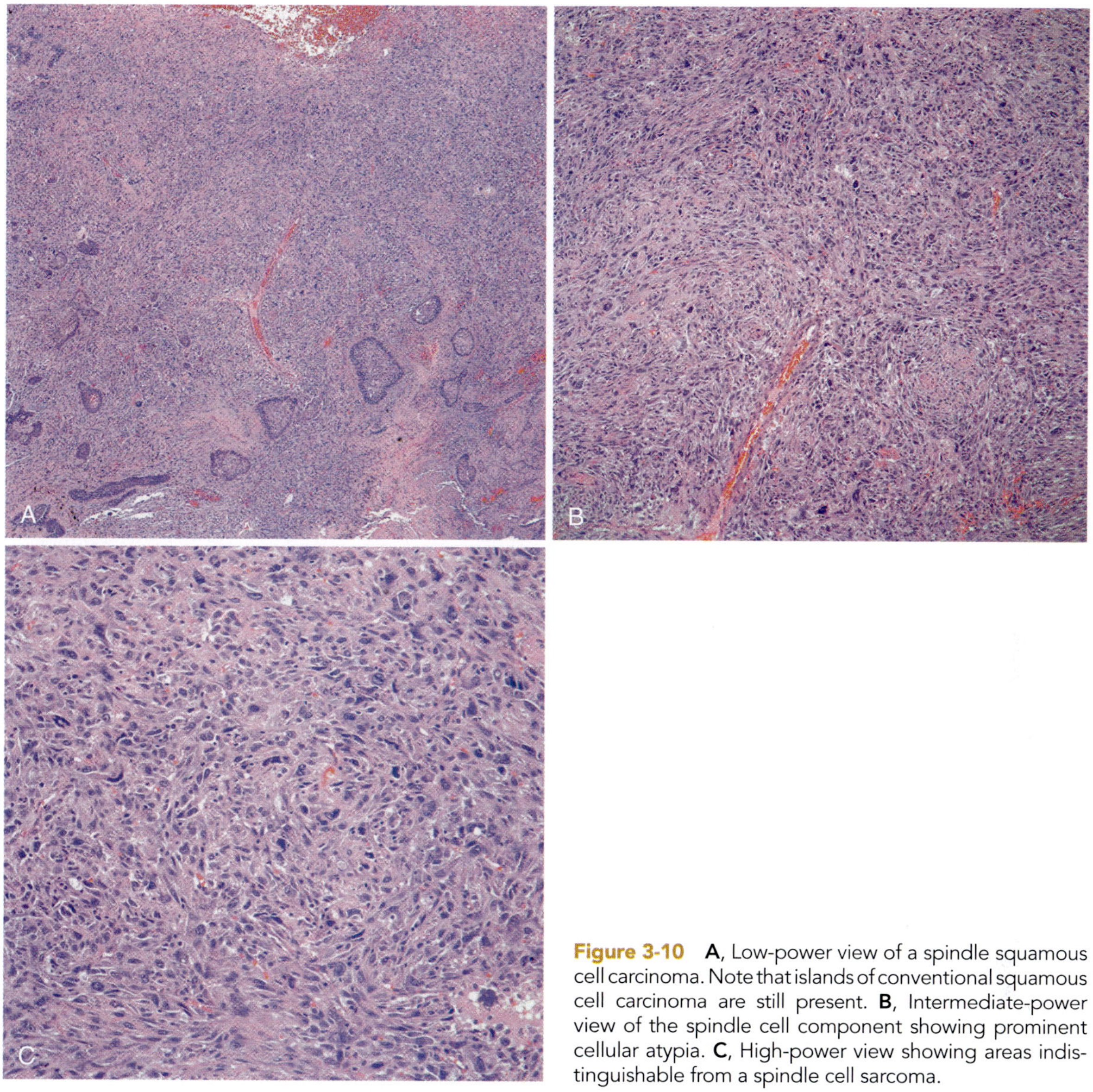

Figure 3-10 **A**, Low-power view of a spindle squamous cell carcinoma. Note that islands of conventional squamous cell carcinoma are still present. **B**, Intermediate-power view of the spindle cell component showing prominent cellular atypia. **C**, High-power view showing areas indistinguishable from a spindle cell sarcoma.

low-molecular-weight keratin, keratin 5/6, or p63 may help in distinguishing these tumors from primary pulmonary sarcomas. Electron microscopic studies also may be useful, because spindle cell carcinomas may manifest epithelial differentiation with the presence of intercellular junctions and tonofilaments.[24]

Basaloid

The basaloid growth pattern is an unusual variant of squamous cell carcinoma and resembles that seen in basal cell carcinomas of the skin. The tumor cells are arranged in islands, with palisading of the nuclei (see Fig. 3-11). Mitotic figures are numerous, and nuclear atypia is prominent. The cells may acquire a fusiform appearance, with elongated nuclei and inconspicuous nucleoli. In some cases, areas of keratinizatin are present, whereas in others, the squamous cell differentiation may be subtler. Because this basaloid pattern may be present in other tumors, such as neuroendocrine carcinomas or the so-called basaloid carcinomas of the lung, it is important to ensure that the tumor under investigation represents a true basaloid squamous cell carcinoma.

Immunohistochemical and Molecular Features

Currently, the literature describes numerous immunohistochemical markers that may have the potential to distinguish squamous cell carcinomas from other types of non–small cell carcinomas, including keratin 5/6, p63, and thyroid transcription factor-1 (TTF-1).[25,26] Immunostaining for these markers is particularly useful in cases in which the patient has a history of squamous cell carcinoma of extrathoracic origin, and the lung biopsy seems to show

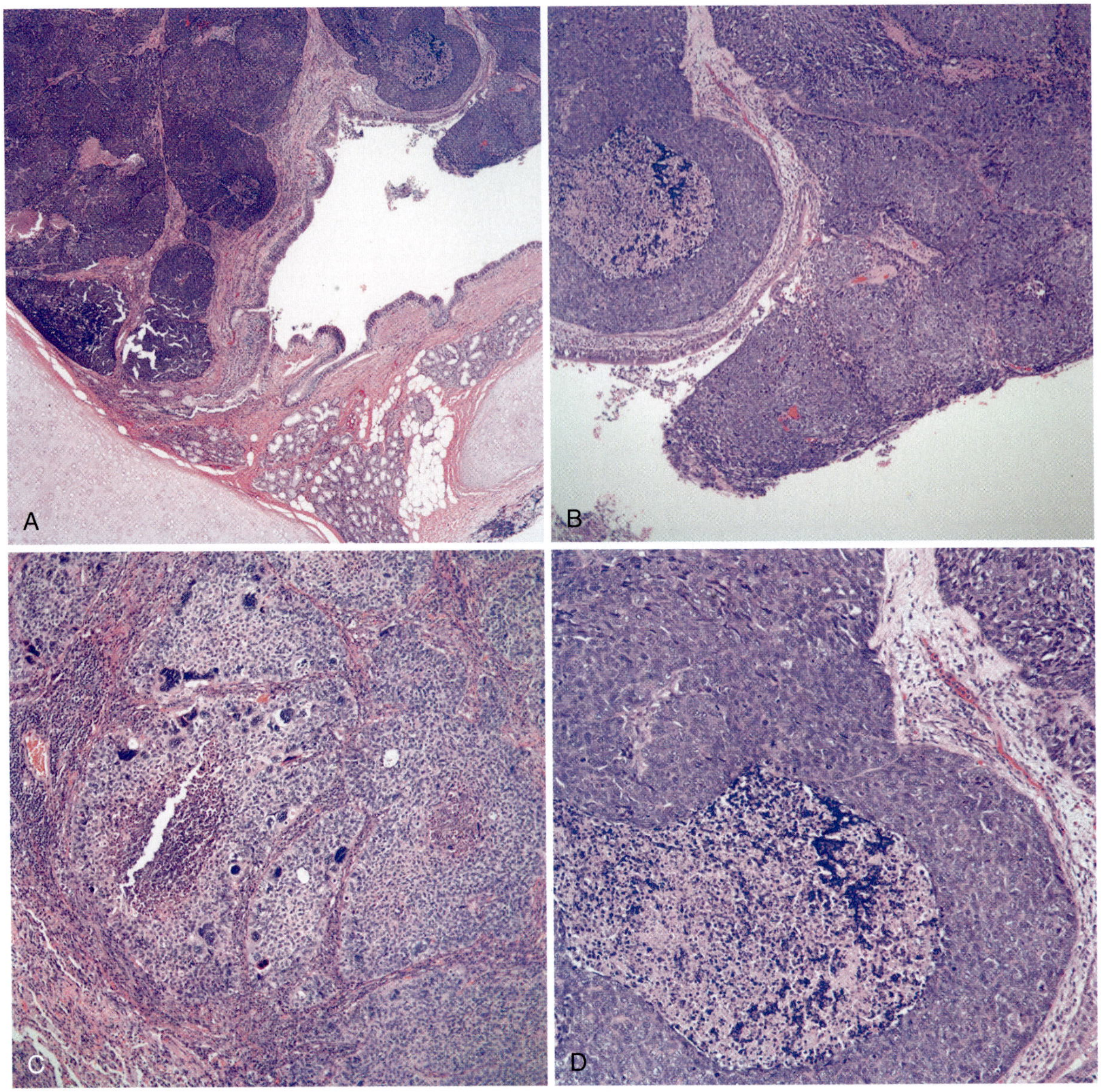

Figure 3-11 **A**, Low-power view of a basaloid squamous cell carcinoma. The tumor is centrally located. **B**, Basaloid squamous cell carcinoma showing areas of invasive and in situ carcinoma. **C**, Basaloid squamous cell carcinoma showing a small component of malignant multinucleated giant cells. **D**, High-power view showing prominent nuclear atypia and increased mitotic activity.

another non–small cell carcinoma. Also, when a patient with a previous carcinoma of the lung presents with a different pulmonary neoplasm, these markers may be used to determine whether the tumor is a recurrence or a separate primary lung neoplasm. Other immunohistochemical markers have shown positive staining in squamous cell carcinomas, including CD117; however, the significance of the positive staining is not yet clear.[27]

Yoshino[28] performed molecular studies in 22 cases of squamous cell carcinomas of the lung and found that loss of heterozygosity (LOH) was more frequently observed in squamous cell carcinomas than in adenocarcinomas of the lung, and that LOH tends to be associated with tobacco use. In a comparative genomic hybridization analysis, Chujo and coworkers[29] encountered over-representation of the long arm of chromosome 3 (3q) in squamous cell carcinomas of the lung and concluded that an increased copy number at 3q may contribute to the development of squamous cell carcinoma of the lung.

BRONCHIOLOALVEOLAR CARCINOMA

Many controversial issues associated with the diagnosis of bronchioloalveolar carcinoma (BAC) have emerged. Multiple definitions have been applied to this tumor over the years, and the interpretation of these definitions varies

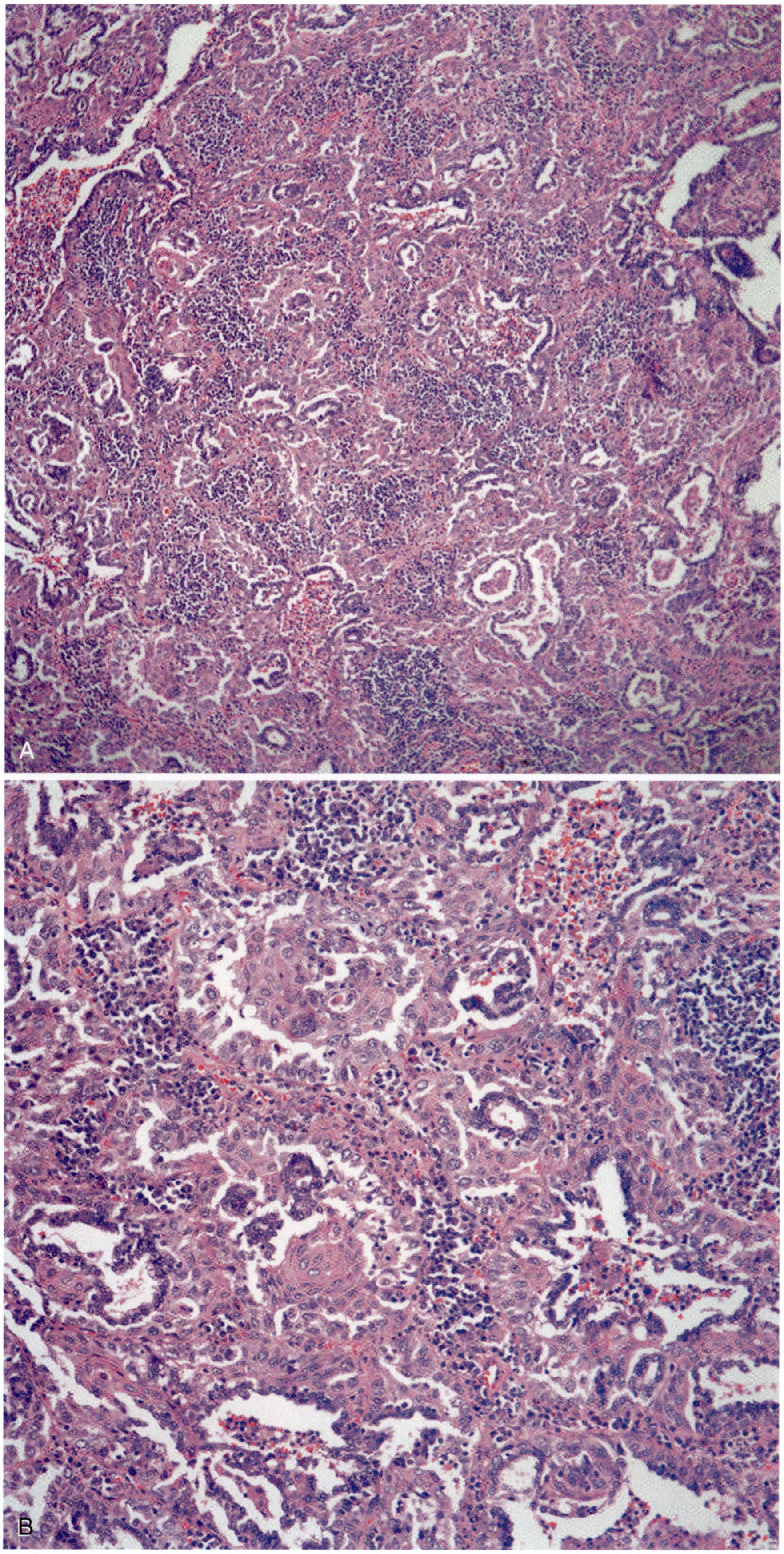

Figure 3-12 **A**, Low-power view of a squamous cell carcinoma with adenoid-like features. **B**, Intermediate-power view showing areas that mimic adenocarcinoma.

Continued

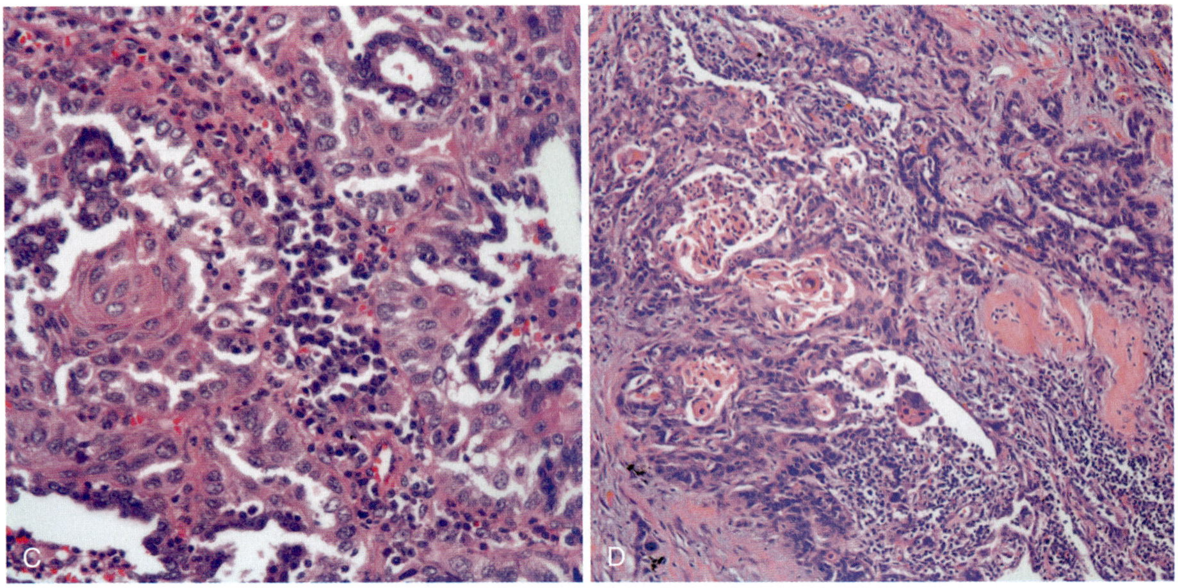

Figure 3-12—cont'd **C** and **D**, High-power views showing areas of more conventional squamous cell carcinoma with focal keratinization.

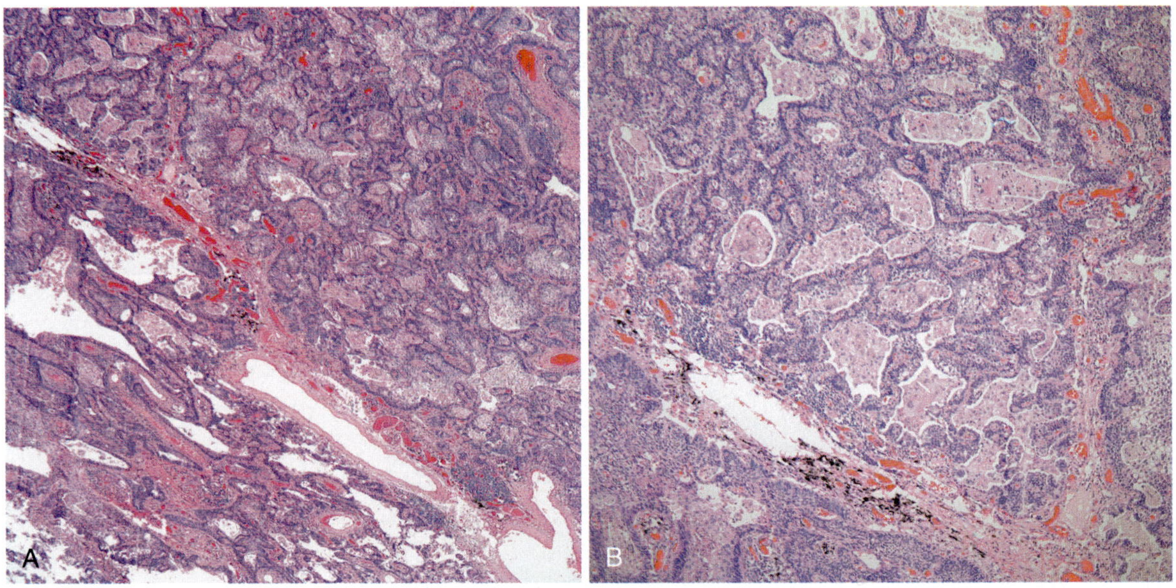

Figure 3-13 **A**, Squamous cell carcinoma with an ameloblastic-like growth pattern composed of anastomosing ribbons of tumor cells. **B**, High-power view showing areas of keratinization.

from individual to individual. The currently accepted definition of BAC is considerably different from those of previous decades. This definition is so restrictive that BAC can now be considered to be adenocarcinoma in situ. Many years ago, the descriptions of BAC were much broader; in fact, most of the series presented in the literature on BAC have described tumors that had metastasized, or that had involved other thoracic structures.

Historical Aspects

In 1876, Malassez[30] was the first to describe a primary pulmonary neoplasm with an unusual alveolar pattern of growth. In Malassez's description, the tumor appeared to be multinodular and therefore was named "Cancer Encephaloide of the Lung (Epithelioma)." Twenty-seven years later, Musser[31] described a similar tumor under the designation "Primary Cancer of the Lung." Both of these descriptions are essentially similar in terms of histopathology; however, the gross features were quite different. Malassez described a multinodular tumor replacing lung parenchyma, whereas Musser described a diffuse process, similar to an infectious process such as bronchopneumonia. These two representations demonstrate what are currently acknowledged to be the two main growth patterns of BAC. The presence of metastatic disease was noted in both of these descriptions.

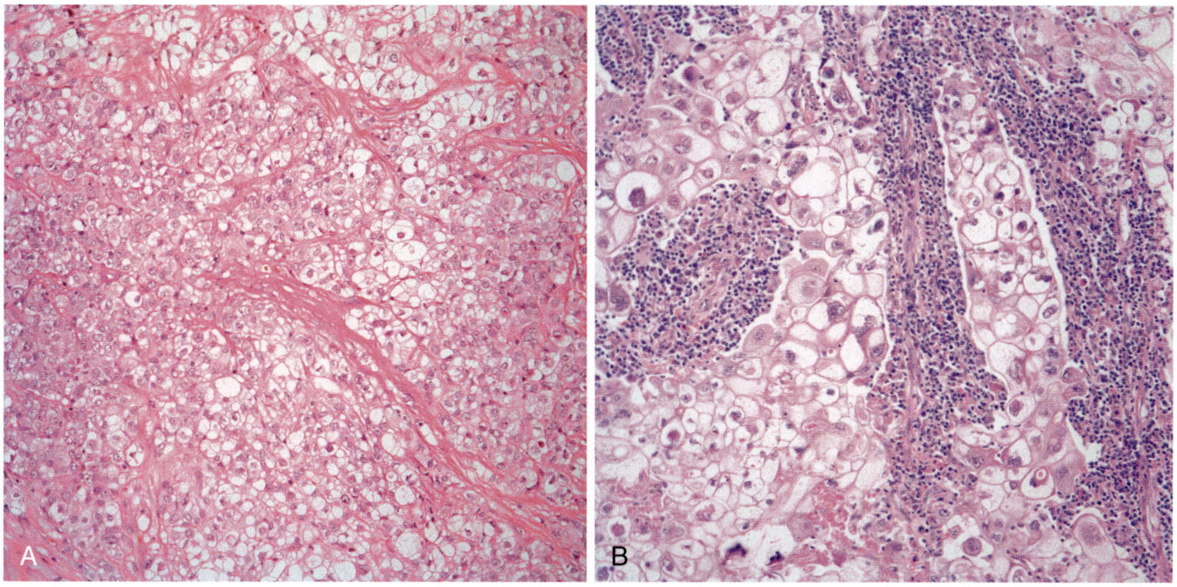

Figure 3-14 **A**, Squamous cell carcinoma with clear cell change. **B**, High-power view showing clear cells admixed with inflammatory reaction.

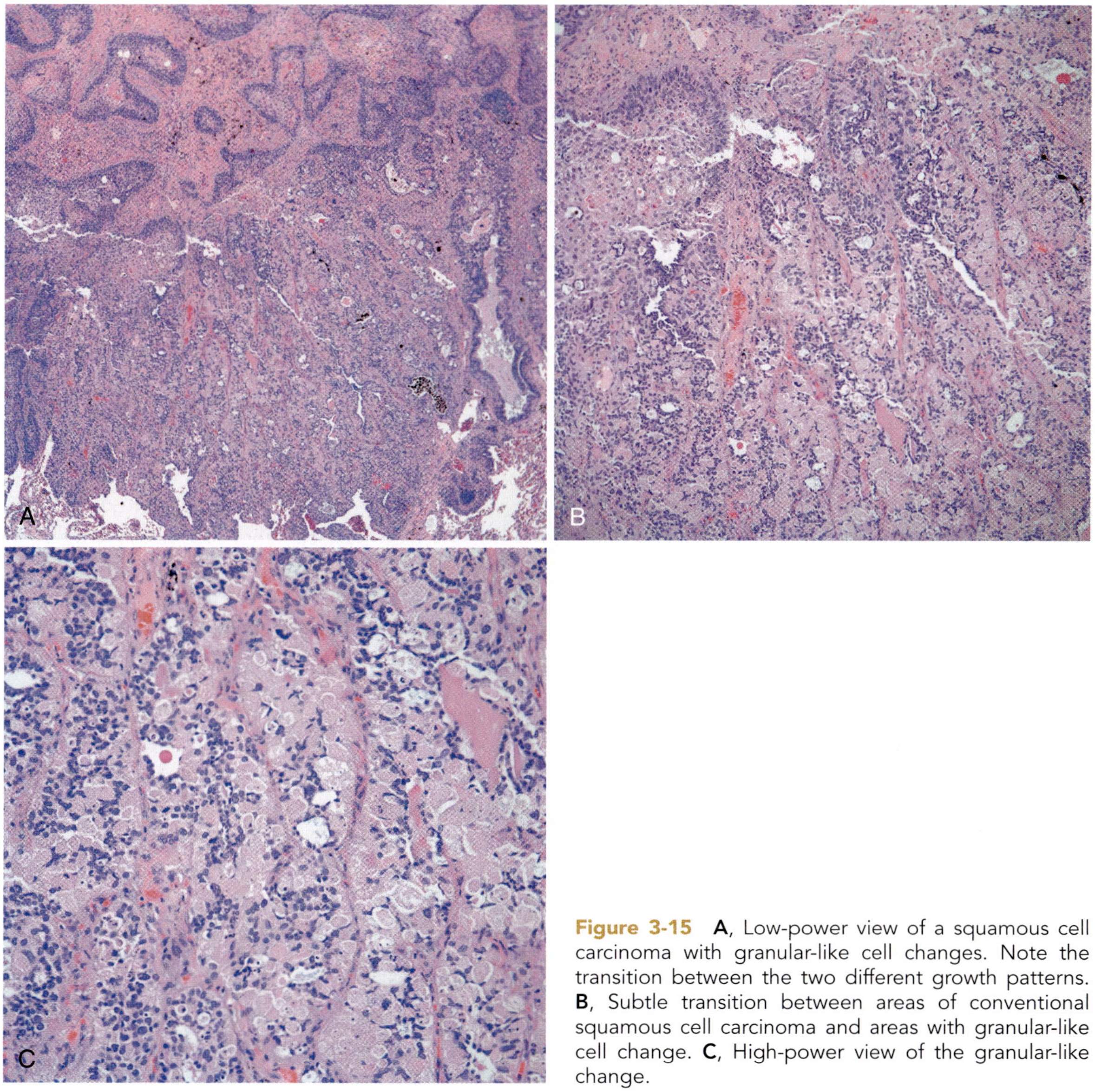

Figure 3-15 **A**, Low-power view of a squamous cell carcinoma with granular-like cell changes. Note the transition between the two different growth patterns. **B**, Subtle transition between areas of conventional squamous cell carcinoma and areas with granular-like cell change. **C**, High-power view of the granular-like change.

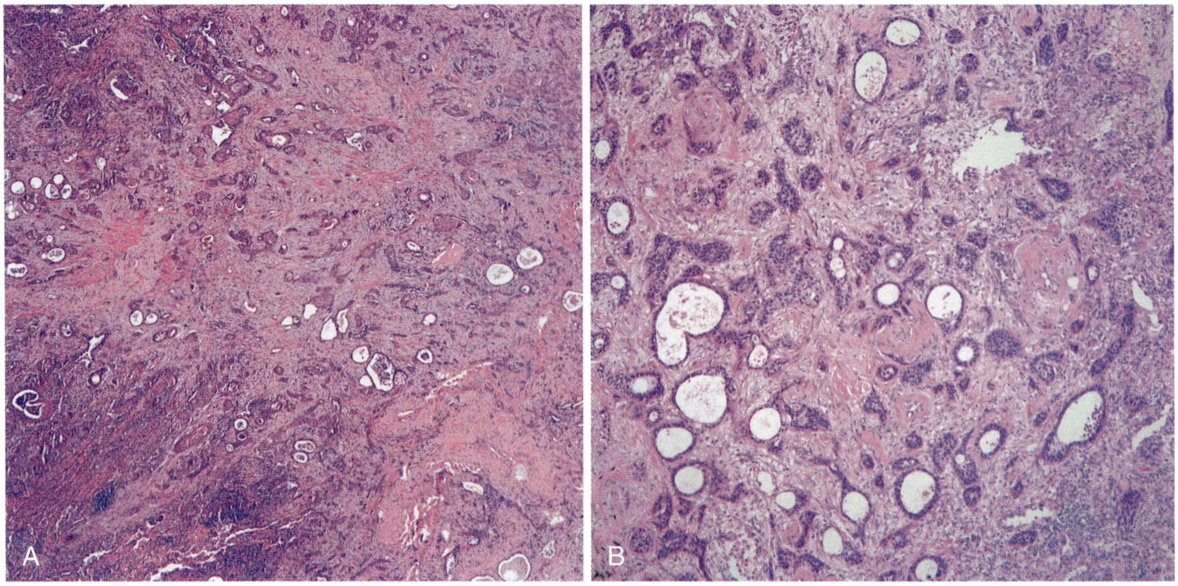

Figure 3-16 Squamous cell carcinoma with syringomatous-like changes. **A**, Low-power view. **B**, High-power view. The syringomatous-like component is similar to that seen in adnexal neoplasms.

During the first half of the 20th century, a sizable number of cases with histopathologic and macroscopic characteristics similar to those described by Malassez and Musser were presented in the literature.[32–40] The gross features of these cases were either multinodular or diffuse; histopathologically, the tumors showed the alveolar lining replaced either by columnar or low cuboidal cellular proliferation. Numerous terms were used to describe this neoplasm, including alveolar cell cancer, primary multiple carcinoma, multiple nodular carcinoma, diffuse lung carcinoma, alveolar carcinoma, carcinosis, carcinomatoides alveogenica multicentrica, alveolar cell tumor, and pulmonary alveolar adenomatosis.

Among these early investigators, the main point of debate centered on the existence of alveolar epithelium. Those who denied the existence of alveolar epithelium did not believe that epithelial neoplasm could arise from alveolar structures, whereas those who supported the existence of alveolar epithelium were ready to classify these neoplasms as alveolar carcinomas. Nevertheless, the concept of a tumor growing along alveolar structures remained. Almost all of the cases described during the first half of the 20th century involved tumors that extended beyond the lung parenchyma. In a majority of cases, tumors seeding the pleura or peribronchial lymph nodes, or tumors outside of the thoracic cavity, were documented. Despite the discussion surrounding alveolar epithelium, some researchers suggested a possible infectious origin for these tumors, likening them to similar tumors seen in sheep (the so-called Jaagsiekte). As a result of the lack of consensus on whether these tumors originated from alveolar epithelium or from finer terminal bronchioles, the term *bronchioloalveolar carcinoma* was established.

Definition

In 1960, Liebow[41] not only coined the term *bronchioloalveolar carcinoma* but also provided a definition for the diagnosis of this neoplasm. Liebow defined BAC as a well-differentiated adenocarcinoma and distinguished it from "ordinary" adenocarcinoma on the basis of lack of evidence regarding the cell of origin. In addition, Liebow identified three main forms of this neoplasm: single nodular, disseminated nodular, and diffuse. He also noted that the tumor is capable of invading lymph nodes, pleura, and extrathoracic organs—a feature that is observed in greater than 50% of autopsy cases.[41] In Liebow's opinion, the tumors may have a long dormancy or slow growth, particularly those presenting as isolated nodules. He also pointed out that 50% of patients present with bilateral disease. In 1980, the Armed Forces Institute of Pathology[42] defined BAC as "a lesion with relatively bland cytologic features that arises in the periphery of the lung and spreads on the walls of the distal air spaces." In the second published series of the Armed Forces Institute of Pathology (1995),[23] the definition is that of a subset of adenocarcinoma, common and distinctive enough to warrant separation from the other subtypes. In the two most recent publications of the World Health Organization (WHO),[43,44] the tumor is defined as an adenocarcinoma with bronchioloalveolar pattern and no evidence of stromal, vascular, or pleural invasion. On the basis of these publications, it is apparent that the definition of BAC has changed to the point at which diagnosis is possible only by complete examination of the entire tumor in question, and not on biopsy material.

Analysis of the Literature

The literature on bronchioloalveolar carcinoma is filled with controversy, and many of the studies that address the controversial issues have only generated more debate. In 1955, Overholt and colleagues[45] reported a study of 15 patients treated surgically, 11 of whom had no evidence of metastasis at follow-up. Of note, however, these workers also documented the development of metastatic disease to the brain in one patient and ipsilateral disease in another two patients. Belgrad[46] and Munnel[47] and their coworkers also made a similar claim in a study of patients with localized disease. According to both groups of investigators, surgery may have eradicated these patients' tumors. However, Belgrad and colleagues[46] also acknowledged that for tumors characterized by diffuse involvement of a lobe, the prognosis may not be as good. On the other hand, Watson and Farpour[48] studied 265 patients in whom the clinical behavior of the tumor was, in some cases, more aggressive. In their series, 82 patients showed metastatic disease on autopsy, and only 16 of 82 patients who were treated with excisional surgery survived more than 5 years. Other researchers have questioned the validity of the BAC diagnosis, arguing that BAC represents a pattern rather than a specific entity, because many tumors of extrathoracic origin can metastasize to the lung in a manner indistinguishable from that characteristic of pulmonary BAC.[49,50] In a study of 30 cases of BAC, Bennett and Sasser[50] concluded that there is no morphologic, histogenetic, or clinical basis to separate "bronchioloalveolar carcinoma" from adenocarcinoma of the lung. Contrary to that opinion, Delarue and colleagues[51] presented their views in a reappraisal of bronchioloalveolar carcinoma, and insisted on considering BAC a specific clinicopathologic entity. These workers' criteria for the diagnosis of BAC were as follows: (1) absence of primary adenocarcinoma elsewhere; (2) absence of intrinsic tumor of bronchogenic origin; (3) peripheral location involving alveolar ducts and sacs; and (4) unaffected interstitium. However, they noted that metastatic adenopathies and malignant pleural effusions may occur. The overall survival rate for the 74 patients studied was 34% at 3 years. Marco and Galy[52] presented their experience with BAC in 29 patients, separated into three main groups depending on the extent of their disease. Group 3 was composed of patients with pleural and lymph node involvement.

Over the years, some researchers have focused on differentiating BAC from conventional adenocarcinoma, whereas others have attempted to further divide BAC into subcategories.[53–55] Singh and associates[55] have argued that in addition to the peripheral lesion recognized as BAC, two other subtypes also may occur: the Clara cell and the type II pneumocyte subtypes. Other investigators have supported this opinion and have stated that BAC and peripheral bronchogenic adenocarcinoma are derived from secretory cells that resemble bronchiolar Clara cells, thereby separating them from conventional bronchogenic adenocarcinoma.[56] Some workers also have attempted to correlate histopathologic features of BAC with survival. In a study of 34 cases in which BAC was separated into type 1 and type 2 tumors, Manning and coworkers[57] stated that type 1 BAC is associated with mucus production and is most likely to be multicentric, whereas type 2 BAC does not show much mucus production and is most likely to be solitary. These investigators observed a 5-year survival rate of 72% for patients with the nonmucinous type (type 2), whereas patients with the mucinous type (type 1) had a 25% 5-year survival rate. Clayton[58] arrived at a somewhat different conclusion in a study of 45 cases of BAC, finding that aerogenous spread had occurred in 24 of 36 nonmucinous tumors, and that at 5 years, these patients either had died from their disease or were alive with metastasis, whereas in 12 nonmucinous tumors without aerogenous spread, the 5-year survival rate was 61%. Clayton also found that smaller tumors carried a better prognosis, and that the presence of alveolar spread, rather than cell type, was the most important feature to predict prognosis.

In a 21-year retrospective study, Thomas and coworkers[59] concluded that BAC is a valid term that represents a heterogeneous population of tumors; they argued that BAC should be retained as a term describing a growth pattern. In their experience, BAC carries a bad prognosis, which may be attributed to the fact that many patients are asymptomatic until the disease is advanced and inoperable. In a large study between 1968 and 1986, Elson and associates[60] accumulated 193 cases of BAC, of which only 39 were selected as pure BAC. The type of material available for review in this study was unclear, however, and it is likely that the specimens were mixed among cytology smears, biopsy, and surgical resection. Thus, it is difficult to determine the validity of the designation "pure BAC."

In 1991, Daly and colleagues[61] of the Mayo Clinic presented a study of 134 patients with BAC. Ten of the patients described (7.5%) had lymph node metastasis, and although the great majority were stage I, several cases in stages II, IIIA, and IIIB also were included. The survival rate for patients who were T1N0M0 at 5 years was 90%, in contrast with patients who were T2, N0, M0, for whom the survival rate was 55%. These workers concluded that BAC has a unique natural history, which is more influenced by local neoplastic process than by lymph node metastases. From the same institution, Feldman and associates[62] presented a study of 25 patients with metastatic BAC in which the response to chemotherapy was compared with that in patients with conventional adenocarcinoma. These investigators concluded that the chemotherapeutic response and the median rates of disease progression were similar in both groups and further stated that metastatic BAC is an aggressive disease that is associated with poor prognosis, similar to metastatic conventional adenocarcinoma of the lung. A similar experience was reported by Breathnach and colleagues[63] in their study of 28 cases of BAC in stages IIIB and IV. In this particular report, patients with advanced BAC were more likely to have bilateral disease but were at lower risk for development of brain metastasis. In another study from Taiwan, the investigators collected 50 cases of BAC, including patients in different stages of disease. These workers concluded that BAC frequently manifests with lymphatic spread or systemic metastasis at diagnosis, and that in most cases patients with localized BAC fare better than those with the diffuse type of BAC.[64] Also, Fujimoto and associates[65] presented a study of 53 cases of BAC and found no difference in survival between patients who underwent resection for BAC and those who were operated on for non-BAC. Of note, however, these investigators found that patients with stage IV BAC had a better response to chemotherapy than that observed in patients with non-BAC tumors.

BAC has been perceived as a tumor of increasing frequency in younger persons, females, and nonsmokers,[66,67] with a reported incidence as high as 14%. Read and coworkers[68] presented an epidemiologic study of BAC over 2 decades (1979 to 1998) based on analysis of the SEER database and concluded that despite the apparent increase in BAC, this tumor represents less than 4% of all primary non–small cell carcinomas of the lung. In a different analysis of SEER database, Raz found that BAC is not associated with younger mean age at diagnosis and that the tumor is not associated with an age younger than 50 years at diagnosis.[69] As suggested by some investigators, BAC may have an environmental etiology other than tobacco use.[67] In addition, BAC in children is believed to carry a better prognosis, although the tumor is rare in the pediatric age group.[70]

More recent literature on BAC, using the latest definition by the WHO, also has provided conflicting information. In a study focusing on the survival and recurrence of BAC stage I disease, Breathnach and coworkers[71] found a 5-year survival rate for patients with BAC of 83%, as opposed to 63% for those with other types of adenocarcinoma. Rena and associates[72] described similar findings in a study of 28 patients with stage I pure BAC, reporting a 5-year disease-free rate of 81% and a long-term survival rate of 86%, as opposed to the 5-year disease-free survival rate of 51% and long-term survival rate of 71% for conventional adenocarcinoma. Although these investigators claim that the WHO criteria were followed in these cases, 20 patients were diagnosed using fine needle aspiration biopsy, which is not permitted under the WHO's current criteria. In a study of 20 cases of BAC, Gaeta and coworkers[73] focused on pattern of recurrence after surgical resection, concluding that diffuse BAC may develop from previous focal carcinoma, and that the mucinous type is the one most likely to become diffuse. In this study, the investigators included three different types of BAC: mucinous, nonmucinous, and mixed adenocarcinomas with prominent bronchioloalveolar pattern. A study by Ebright and associates,[74] however, concluded that the most important predictors of survival in BAC are clinical pattern and pathologic stage, rather than degree of invasion as seen on histologic examination.

In 2006, Travis and colleagues[75] investigated the relevance of the WHO histopathologic criteria for the diagnosis of BAC. According to these workers, the existing evidence indicates that patients with solitary, small, peripheral BACs have a 100% survival at 5 years. They argue that the basis for the newly proposed classification of BAC is derived from a study by Noguchi and associates[76] on the histologic characteristics and prognosis of small adenocarcinomas of the lung. In this study, the investigators reported 236 cases of resected peripheral adenocarcinomas of the lung in which the lesions were no more than 2 cm in greatest diameter. They separated the cases into different types designated A to F, and the ones belonging to types A and B were coded as localized BAC. Foci of structural collapse of alveoli were present in the type B cases but not the type A cases. The cases in the A and B groups together amounted to 28 (14 cases of each category). Closer analysis of the data showed that although general information is provided for the 236 case studies, the investigators did not provide a specific tumor size for types A and B, instead stating that "they are usually larger than 1 cm"—thus leaving open the possibility that some of these lesions may have been less than 1 cm. In addition, even though the investigators claimed that no lymph node metastasis was present in any of the 28 cases of localized BAC, they also stated that 3 of 34 (not the 28 cases specified) showed pleural involvement whereas 2 of 34 (again, not the initial 28 cases) showed vascular involvement.

Travis and colleagues[75] also cite a study conducted by Zell and coworkers[77] as evidence of the clinical impact of the WHO criteria on the diagnosis of BAC. In this study, Zell and coworkers presented a retrospective analysis of data from the population-based Cancer Surveillance Programs of three Southern California counties from 1995 to 2003, analyzing cases diagnosed as BAC before and after May 1999, when the WHO published the new criteria for the diagnosis of BAC. The investigators found that the overall survival period for patients with BAC diagnosed after 1999 was 53 months; before May 1999, it had been 32 months. At time of presentation, 48%

of the patients had localized disease, 26% had regional spread, and 24% had metastatic disease. Furthermore, patients with BAC were found to have a "significantly" prolonged median overall survival (42 months), with 1-year survival rate of 69%, 2-year survival rate of 58%, and 5-year survival rate of 41%. When patients were stratified by extent of disease, the overall median survival rate for patients with localized disease was 98 months. The investigators also found that the incidence of BAC had increased from 5% before 1999 to 5.5% after 1999, raising the possibility that despite the WHO's restrictive new criteria, the incidence of BAC was actually increasing.

Zell and coworkers[77] also found that before the latest version of the WHO criteria, from January 1995 to May 1999, the 1-year survival rate was 66.5% and the 2-year survival rate was 54%. From June 1999 to December 2003, however, the 1-year survival rate was 72.5% and the 2-year survival rate was 63.3%. It is this 6% to 9% difference that the proponents of the WHO criteria use to support the current criteria for the diagnosis of BAC. Of the 1909 patients with a histologically confirmed diagnosis of BAC and complete TNM staging identified by Zell and coworkers[78] in 2007, 627 patients (33%—probably the same cohort of patients used in this group's previous publication) were found to have stage I disease, and 572 (30%) had stage II disease. Basing their analysis on current criteria established by the WHO, these investigators demonstrated that patients with stage I disease had a 1-year survival rate of 94% and a 5-year survival rate of 65%, and patients with stage II disease had a 1-year survival rate of 89% and a 5-year survival rate of 45%. This study has the benefit of a larger population than Noguchi's,[76] which claimed a 100% survival rate. The Zell investigators[78] did assert, however, that survival had improved in patients in late stages of disease, a claim that would seem to contradict the WHO criteria, which limits the diagnosis of BAC to tumors that do not show pleural, lymphatic, and interstitial involvement. Even so, it is of great interest to review the stated survival rates in earlier publications on BAC, before the current WHO criteria took effect.

Grover and colleagues[79] summarized the experience of the Lung Cancer Study Group by collecting a large series of 235 tumors diagnosed as pure BAC between the years 1977 and 1988. These workers concluded that the mortality rate for patients with BAC stage I (T1N0) was 7% per year, or approximately 35% at 5 years. These data support the findings of Zell and coworkers,[77] rather than those of Noguchi.[76] More recently, Garfield and colleagues[80] raised concerns about the current definition of BAC, mainly in cases with multifocal involvement, and stated that the current definition is inapplicable for patients with stage IIIB and stage IV disease. Similar concerns also were raised by Damhuis and associates,[81] who found an unfavorable prognosis for tage I BAC, with a 5-year survival rate of 24%. Although these investigators provided possible explanations for this rather poor outcome, they concluded that the current definition makes it difficult to establish the diagnosis of BAC before surgery, and they question whether the diagnosis of "BAC with invasive component" should be maintained.

Dissatisfaction with the WHO criteria for the diagnosis of BAC has been expressed by several groups of investigators.[82,83] In an ultrastructural analysis of 155 cases of BAC, Sidhu and colleagues[82] stated that the unique characteristic of BAC is its cell type, and that the extent of lepidic growth, degree of differentiation, and degree of stromal desmoplasia cannot be used as definitional requirements. These workers further characterized the current definition of the WHO as a form of *in situ adenocarcinoma*, in which BAC is defined as a pattern rather than an entity, being accepted as an entity only when the lesion is not invasive. The current criteria negate the notion that BAC has the potential to spread and makes the staging of tumor pathology impractical. Thus, under this current definition, BAC may become an extremely rare entity, if it continues to be diagnosed at all.[82] Hajdu[70] went even farther in his opinion about the current WHO definition of BAC by stating that when "a group of pathologists changed the definition of BAC, it was de facto implied that BAC is carcinoma in situ and that invasive BAC does not exist."

Gross Features

Three main presentations for BAC are recognized:

Localized: In this form of the disease, a peripheral mass is present in the lung parenchyma, which may be indistinguishable from any other non–small cell carcinoma in the lung. Usually these tumors are smaller than 3 cm in greatest diameter and do not show areas of necrosis or hemorrhage. They are well-defined tumors without encapsulation. The cut surface appears homogeneous and is tan in color.

Multinodular: In this presentation, the tumor involves extensive areas of the lung parenchyma in a miliary fashion, almost mimicking metastatic disease. The nodules are of variable size but usually are less than 1 cm in greatest diameter. This type of presentation may involve a lobe or the entire lung parenchyma (Fig. 3-17).

Diffuse: This presentation is similar in appearance to a pneumonic process. The tumor involves extensive areas of lung parenchyma that may encompass one lobe or the entire lung parenchyma. No tumor masses or nodules are identified in this form of the disease, and the appearance is that of a non-neoplastic process (Fig. 3-18).

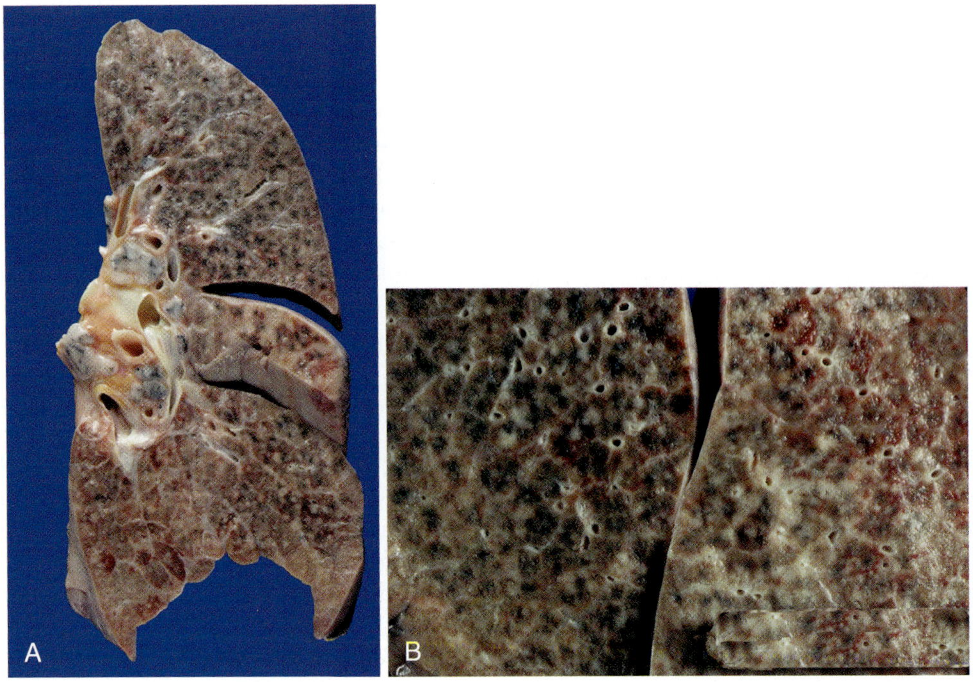

Figure 3-17 Bronchioloalveolar carcinoma, gross specimen. **A**, Numerous small nodules are distributed throughout the entire lung parenchyma. **B**, High-power view.

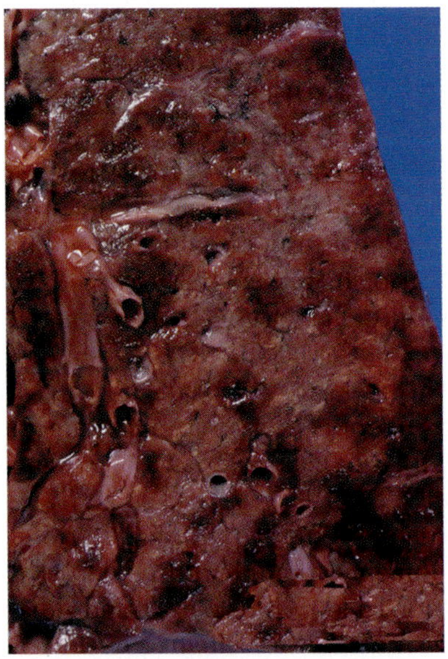

Figure 3-18 Bronchioloalveolar carcinoma, pneumonic type. Note the absence of a pulmonary mass or nodules.

Histologic Features

The histopathologic features of BAC echo those of its gross appearance. In the *nodular* form of the tumor, an almost intact, normal-appearing lung parenchyma is seen at light microscopy. Closer inspection, however, reveals areas in which the alveolar walls are being replaced by either a low cuboidal or a cylindrical type of epithelium, entirely or partly lining the alveolar wall and reminiscent of the outline of the normal alveolar wall (Figs. 3-19 to 3-21). The tumor does not show increased mitotic activity or cellular pleomorphism with nuclear atypia. The proliferation is rather bland but is distinct from the normal alveolar lining.

The *multinodular* pattern of BAC resembles a metastatic tumor in terms of the extensive "skip" areas of normal lung parenchyma. The tumor nodules appear to be discretely affecting extensive areas of the lung parenchyma, but in a nodular pattern rather than as a continuous process (Fig. 3-22). A low cuboidal or columnar type of mucinous epithelium lines the alveoli; in some areas, it is possible to identify normal alveoli that are filled with an acellular mucinous material. Mitotic figures and cellular pleomorphism with nuclear atypia are not common; nor are necrosis and hemorrhage.

The *diffuse* pattern of BAC is almost invariably of the mucinous type. In this pattern, two important features may be easily identifiable: extensive areas in which the alveoli are filled with mucinous material containing mucinophages, and the presence of alveoli that are being replaced by a columnar mucinous type of epithelium (Fig. 3-23). At low magnification, this pattern can be easily misread as a pneumonic process; thus, it is referred to as the pneumonic type.

Differential Diagnosis

The most important consideration in the differential diagnosis for BAC is atypical adenomatous hyperplasia. The histopathologic characteristics of these two lesions

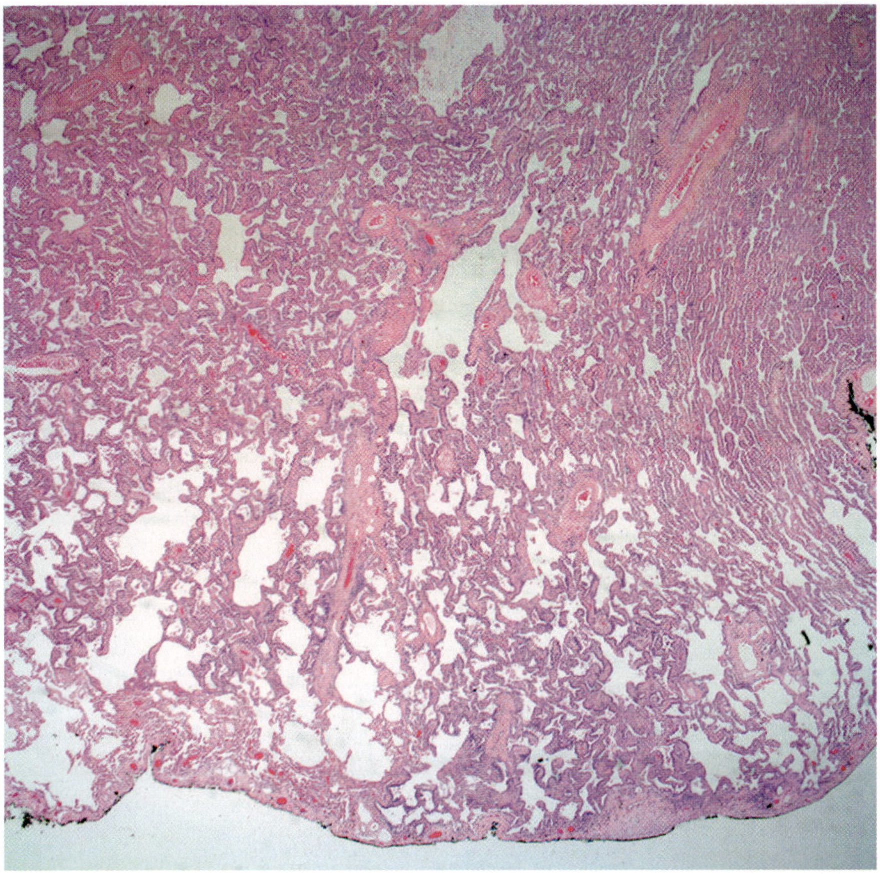

Figure 3-19 Bronchioloalveolar carcinoma appearing as a small peripheral nodule, without involvement of the pleura.

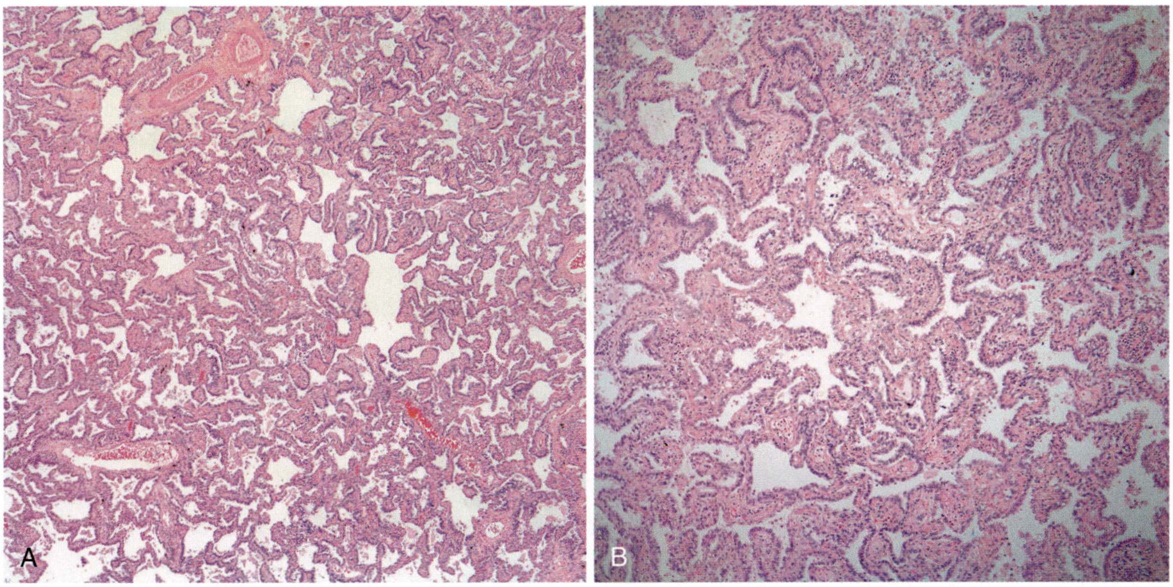

Figure 3-20 **A**, Bronchioloalveolar carcinoma showing a well-defined pattern lining the alveolar walls. **B**, Note the absence of interstitial involvement.

are very similar, and in many situations the only way to separate them is strictly by size. Atypical adenomatous hyperplasia is defined as a lesion of no more than 0.5 cm in greatest diameter. In small core needle biopsy specimens, however, the distinction between these two conditions on histologic grounds may prove to be very difficult. One other lesion that may be important to include in the differential diagnosis is papillary adenoma of type II pneumocytes.[84] This lesion is exceedingly rare and occurs in a central location.

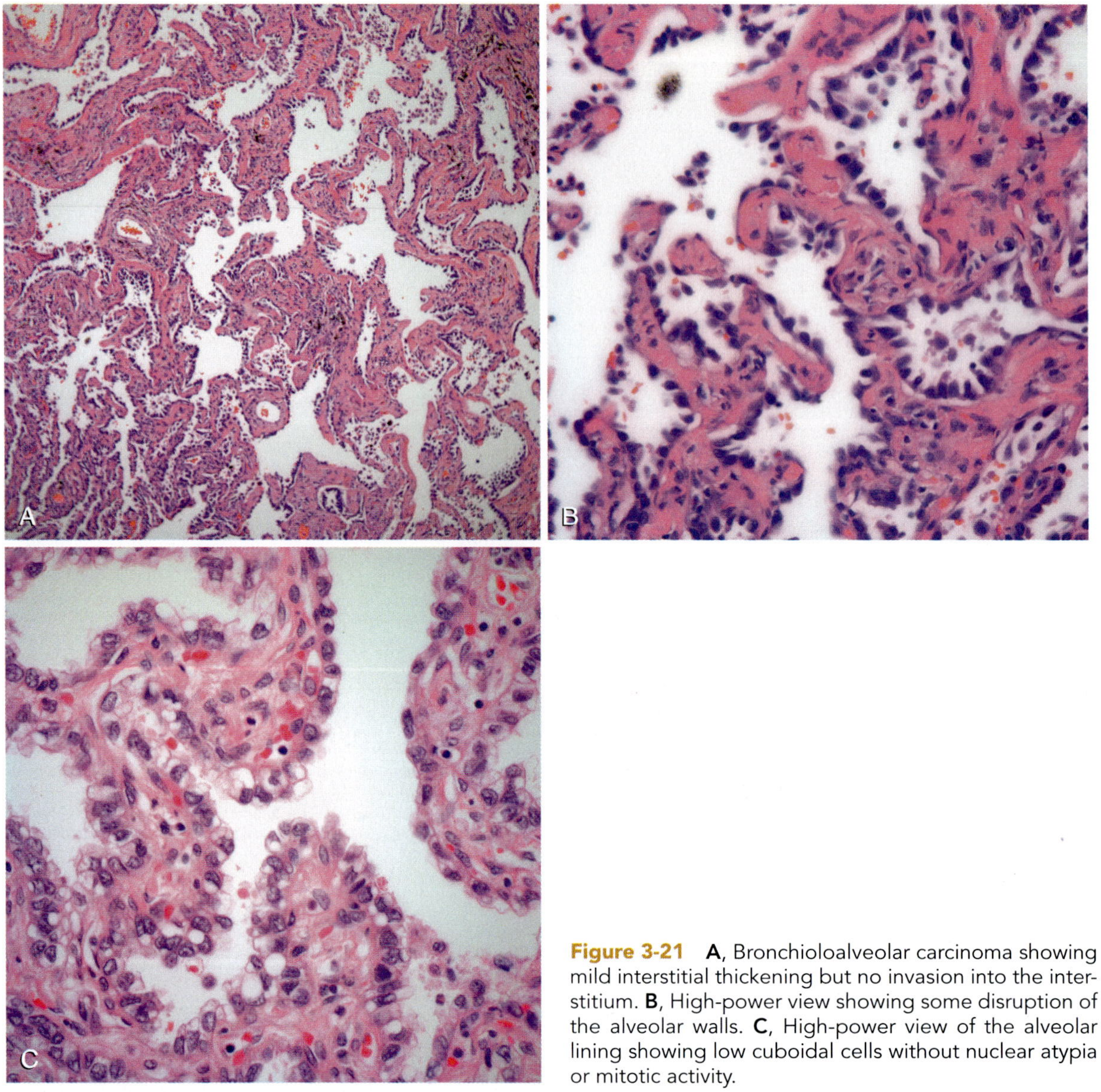

Figure 3-21 **A**, Bronchioloalveolar carcinoma showing mild interstitial thickening but no invasion into the interstitium. **B**, High-power view showing some disruption of the alveolar walls. **C**, High-power view of the alveolar lining showing low cuboidal cells without nuclear atypia or mitotic activity.

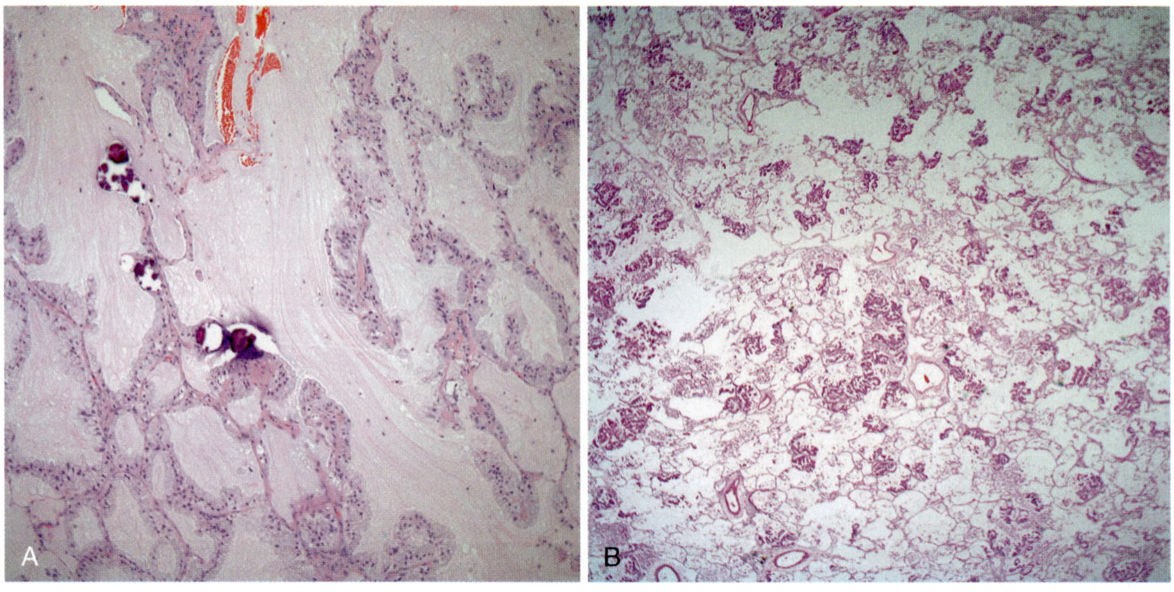

Figure 3-22 **A**, Mucinous bronchioloalveolar carcinoma (BAC) showing extensive deposition of mucoid intra-alveolar material and focal calcifications. **B**, Mucinous BAC showing areas of normal lung parenchyma and numerous small tumor nodules.

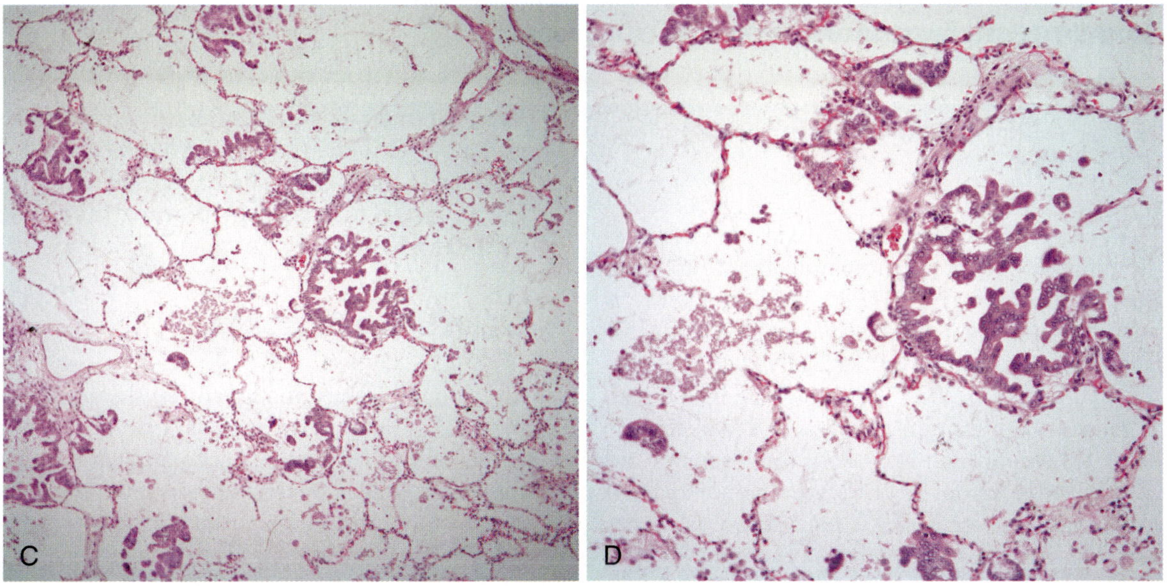

Figure 3-22—cont'd **C**, Mucinous BAC showing areas of normal alveoli and alveoli that are being replaced by neoplastic epithelium. **D**, High-power view of a neoplastic process lining the alveolar wall.

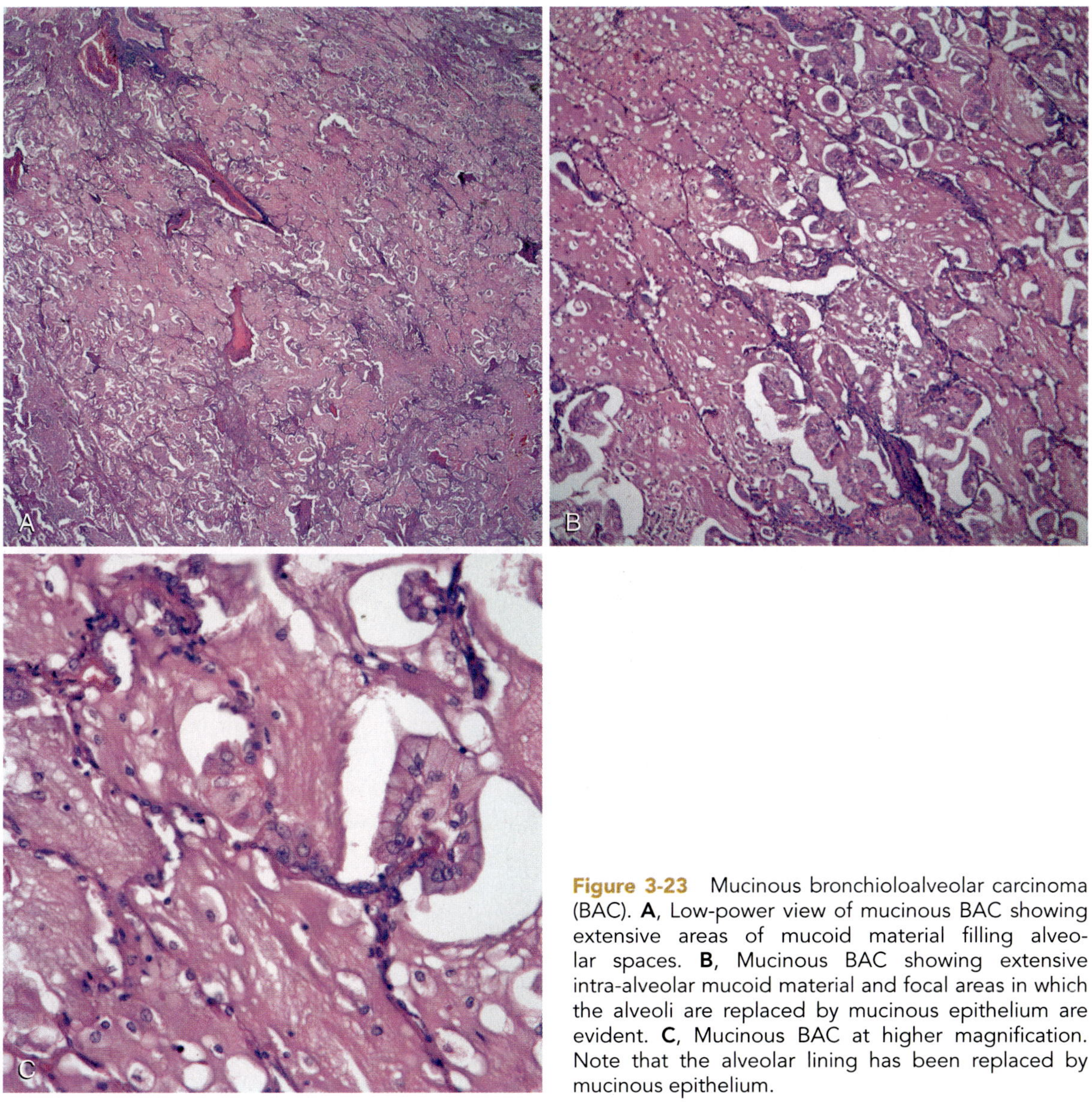

Figure 3-23 Mucinous bronchioloalveolar carcinoma (BAC). **A**, Low-power view of mucinous BAC showing extensive areas of mucoid material filling alveolar spaces. **B**, Mucinous BAC showing extensive intra-alveolar mucoid material and focal areas in which the alveoli are replaced by mucinous epithelium are evident. **C**, Mucinous BAC at higher magnification. Note that the alveolar lining has been replaced by mucinous epithelium.

ATYPICAL ADENOMATOUS HYPERPLASIA

Atypical adenomatous hyperplasia (AAH) is currently defined by the WHO as an adenomatous lesion no more than 0.5 cm in diameter (Fig. 3-24). AAH frequently is associated with lung adenocarcinoma with a bronchioloalveolar component, and histologically, AAH may be indistinguishable from BAC.[85,86] In a study of 3641 resections for lung adenocarcinoma, Koga and colleagues[84] found that AAH was present in 57% of these tumors and proposed that these lesions may be a precursor of lung adenocarcinoma, specifically BAC. Of interest, Morandi and associates[87] attempted to correlate the genetic relationship among atypical adenomatous hyperplasia, BAC, and adenocarcinoma, concluding that AAH and the associated cancer are genetically independent, and that less frequently, AAH foci may represent an early spread of cells from the main tumor, rather than a precursor tumor.

ADENOCARCINOMA

Adenocarcinomas are malignant epithelial tumors characterized by the presence of glandular differentiation. Depending on the degree of glandular differentiation, adenocarcinomas are grouped into three histopathologic grades: well-, moderately, and poorly differentiated. Traditionally, four major growth patterns have been

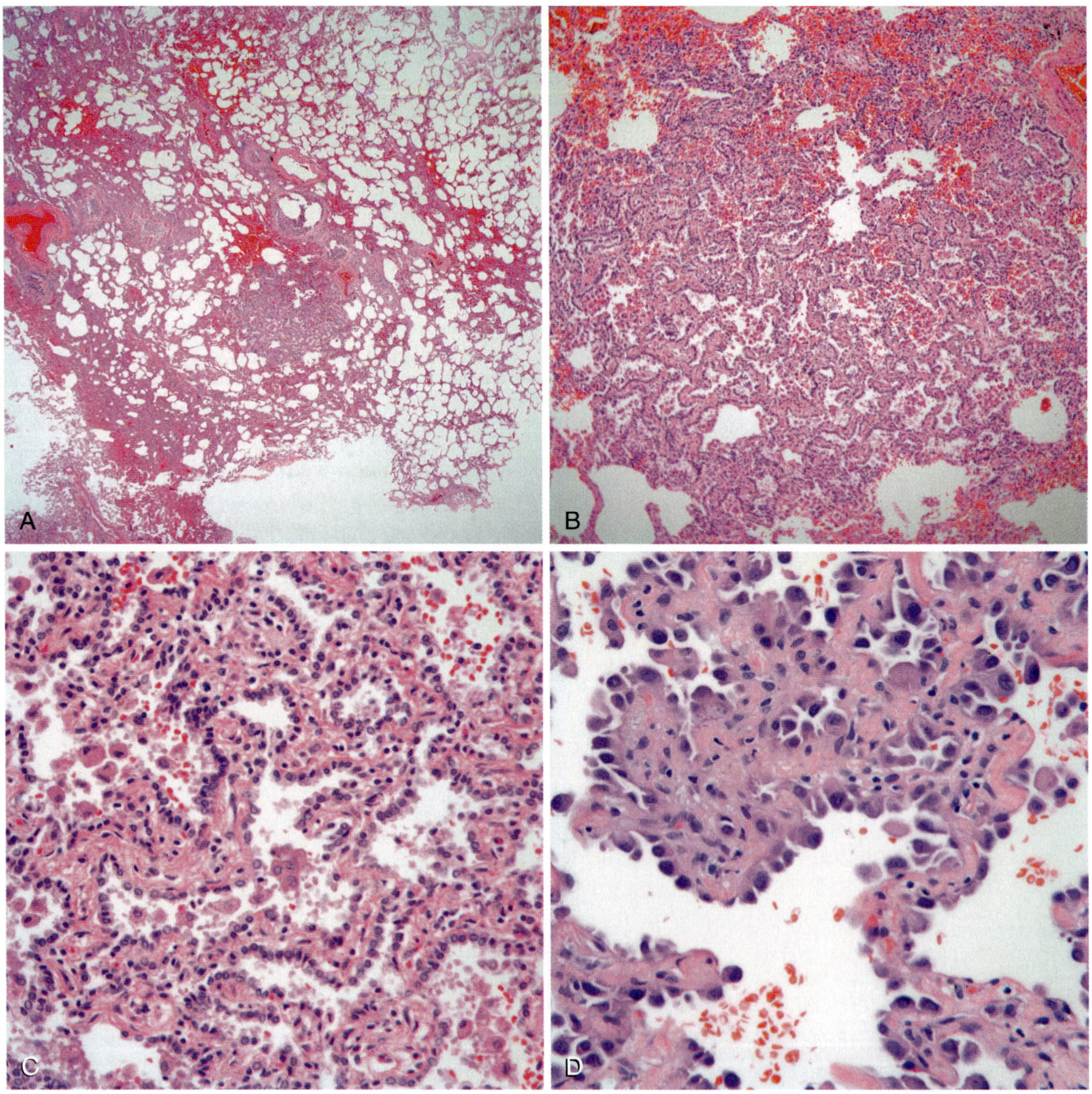

Figure 3-24 Atypical adenomatous hyperplasia (AAH). **A**, Low-power view. Note the small diameter of the lesion (less than 5 cm). **B**, Intermediate-power view showing pattern similar to that of bronchioloalveolar carcinoma. **C**, At this magnification, the features of AAH are indistinguishable from those of bronchioloalveolar carcinoma. **D**, High-power view showing nuclear atypia.

recognized: acinar, solid, papillary, and bronchioloalveolar. Depending on the degree of differentiation, the intracellular mucin or the intraglandular mucinous content may vary. In well-differentiated adenocarcinomas, the glandular malignant component may show intraluminal collections of mucinous material, whereas in solid component and poorly differentiated tumors, the presence of mucin is more evident at the intracellular level. In these cases, histochemical stains such as mucicarmine may help to properly identify the mucinous content. Ultrastructural studies may reveal Clara cell granules in peripheral lung adeocarcinomas; Ogata and Endo[88] suggest that peripheral adenocarcinomas may show Clara cell differentiation regardless of the histologic growth pattern. Hirata and colleagues[89] suggest that bronchial gland cell–type adenocarcinoma occurs more often in younger patients than in older patients (mean age, 50 years).

Some researchers[90] have classified adenocarcinomas by means of cellular morphology and anatomic site, rather than by histologic differentiation, dividing them into parenchymal adenocarcinomas, bronchial adenocarcinomas, and adenocarcinomas of uncertain origin. To some extent, these classifications correlate with the degree of differentiation of a particular tumor. In many instances, however, tumors will display varied histologic patterns ranging from well- to poorly differentiated. In small biopsy specimens, it may be impossible to assess the full spectrum of histologic variability.

Gross Features

Adenocarcinomas may manifest as central or peripheral tumors. Tumor size may range from 0.5 cm to larger than 10 cm in greatest dimension. These tumors appear to be well delimited but not encapsulated and are grayish to light brown in color (Fig. 3-25). Areas of hemorrhage or necrosis may be present. When located centrally, the tumor may compress airway structures or in some cases actually obstruct the airway (Fig. 3-26). Peripheral tumors may have the same macroscopic characteristics as those of central tumors but appear to be in a subpleural location. In some instances, puckering or retraction of the pleura may be present (Fig. 3-27). In this setting, it is important to consider the possibility of gross pleural invasion, because tumors smaller than 3 cm with pleural invasion are placed in a different staging category. Inking the pleural surface is recommended in order to properly evaluate it under light microscopic examination.

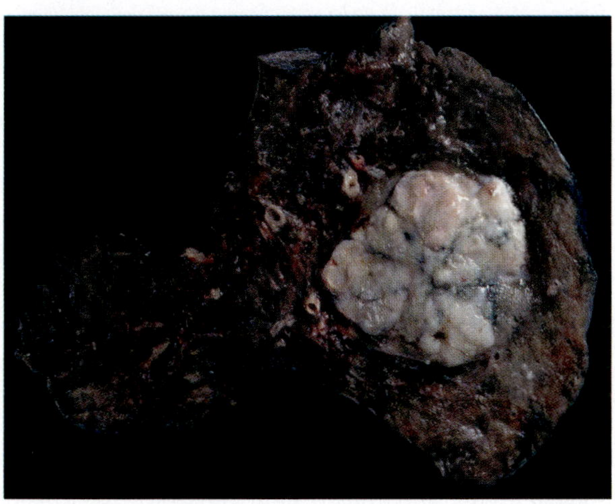

Figure 3-25 Peripheral adenocarcinoma. Note the well-circumscribed tumor and the distance from the pleural surface.

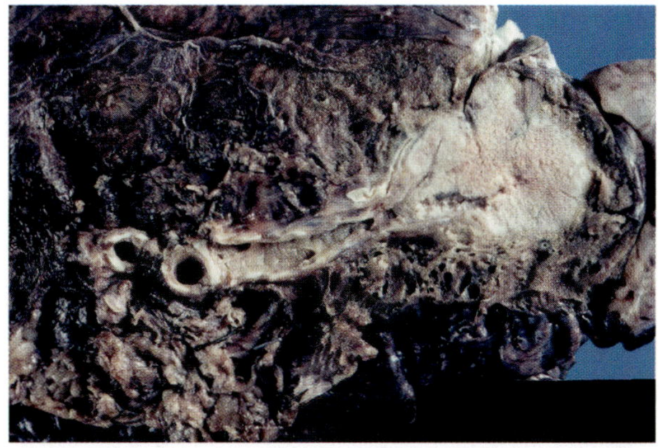

Figure 3-26 Central adenocarcinoma involving airway structures.

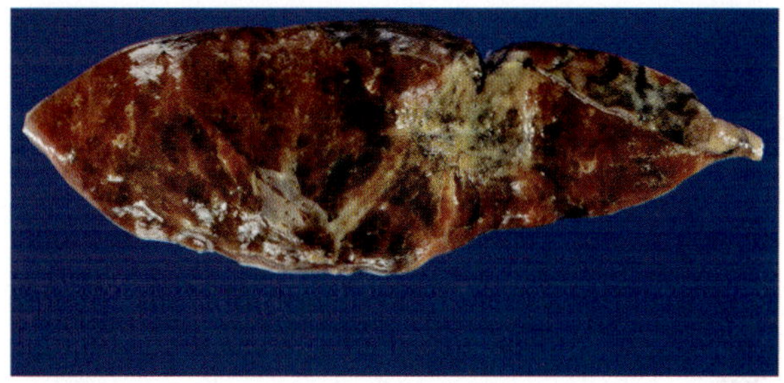

Figure 3-27 Peripheral adenocarcinoma showing puckering of the pleural surface.

Although in most instances lung carcinomas manifest as a solitary tumor, in a study of 50 cases of consecutive adenocarcinomas, Miller and colleagues[91] documented that 12% were in fact multiple adenocarcinomas. It is important to assess the size of the adjacent nodules in this setting. If the lesions are smaller than 0.5 cm in diameter and display the proper histologic features, they may be classified as atypical adenomatous hyperplasia; however, if the nodules are larger than 0.5 cm, the possibility of multifocal adenocarcinoma must be considered.

Histopathologic Features

Histopathologic findings will reflect the degree of tumor differentiation.

Well-differentiated adenocarcinoma: At low-power magnification, well-differentiated adenocarcinoma appears as an atypical glandular proliferation replacing normal lung parenchyma (Figs. 3-28 to 3-34). These

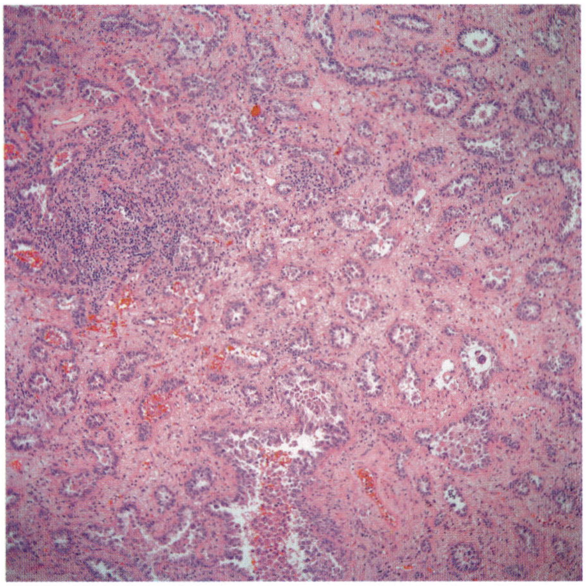

Figure 3-28 Well-differentiated adenocarcinoma showing a fairly homogeneous proliferation of glandular structures.

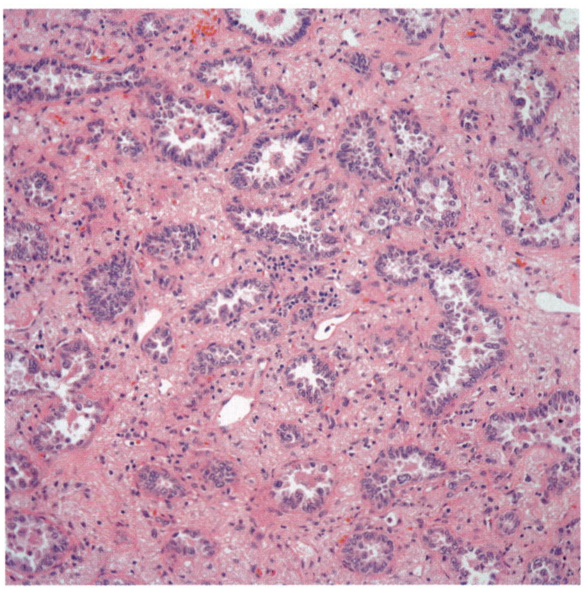

Figure 3-29 Atypical glandular proliferation destroying normal lung parenchyma.

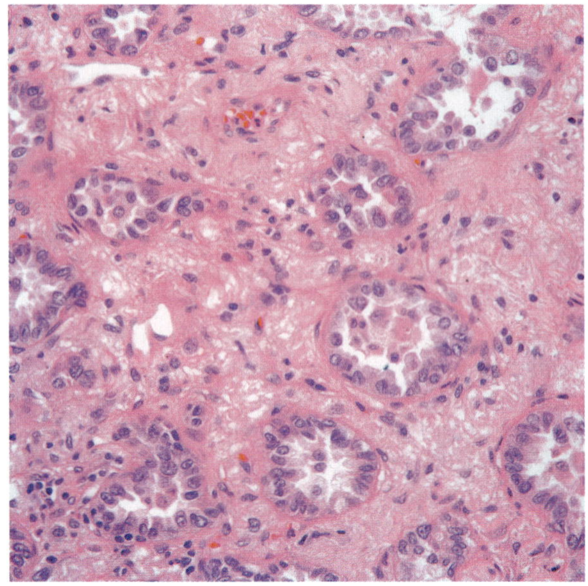

Figure 3-30 Glandular proliferation showing destruction of normal architecture. Note the bland appearance of the glandular component.

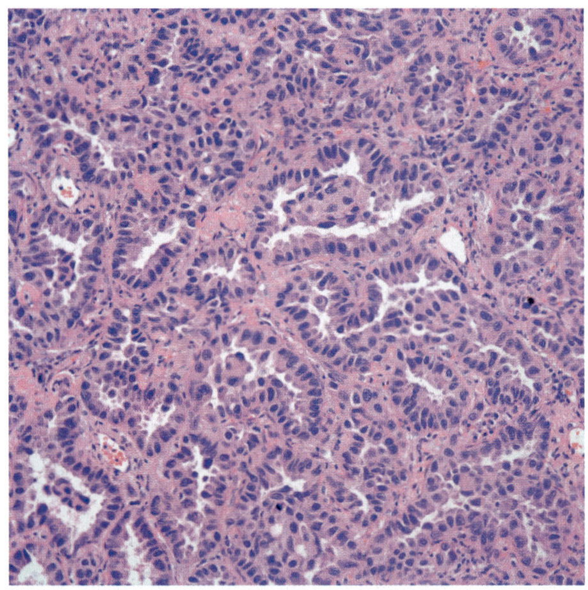

Figure 3-31 Well-differentiated adenocarcinoma showing a glandular proliferation with more atypical cytologic features than present in Figures 3-28 to 3-30.

tumors are well defined but not encapsulated, and the glandular appearance is relatively easily identified by light microscopy. The malignant glands are composed of columnar or mucinous epithelium, with round to oval cells, ample cytoplasm, round nuclei, and prominent nucleoli. In some well-differentiated tumors, the cytologic features of the neoplastic glandular proliferation are bland, with virtual absence of mitotic activity. In others, mitotic figures are present, and areas of hemorrhage and necrosis may be conspicuous. The glandular proliferation may be embedded in dense areas of fibrocollagenous tissue. The acinar and the papillary growth patterns commonly are seen in well-differentiated adenocarcinomas.

Moderately differentiated adenocarcinoma: As in well-differentiated tumors, the glandular formation is apparent; however, the formation or partial formation of variably sized glandular structures also may be observed. The cellular component may exhibit more prominent nuclear atypia, and mitotic figures are more readily identifiable (Figs. 3-35 to 3-40). Areas of necrosis or hemorrhage may be present, as may areas of inflammatory

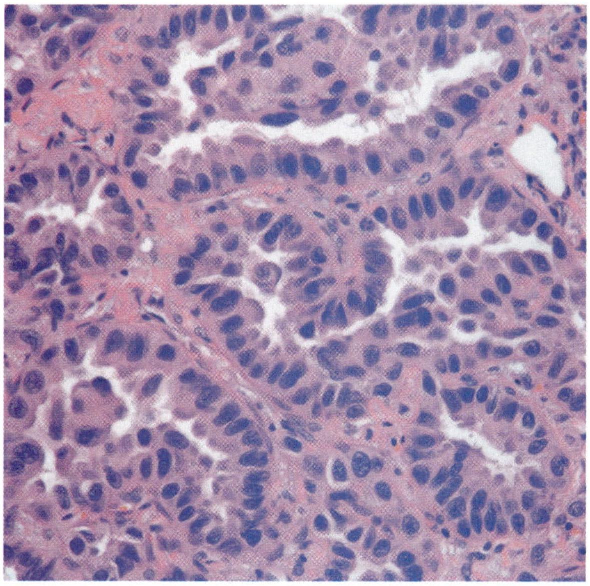

Figure 3-32 A well-differentiated adenocarcinoma at higher magnification, showing increased nuclear atypia and scattered mitotic figures.

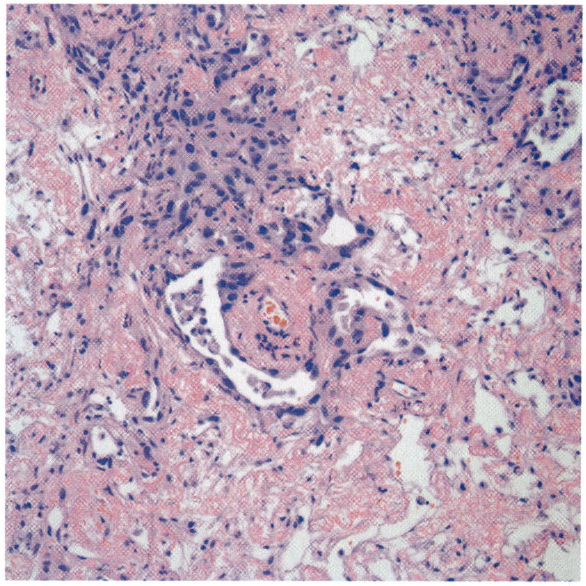

Figure 3-34 High-power view showing atypical glands with focal solid focus of adenocarcinoma.

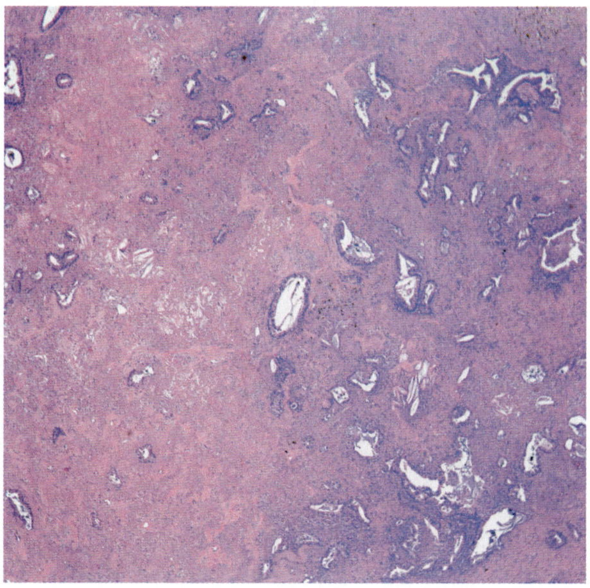

Figure 3-33 Low-power view of a well-differentiated adenocarcinoma showing atypical glands embedded in a dense collagenous stroma (so-called scar carcinoma).

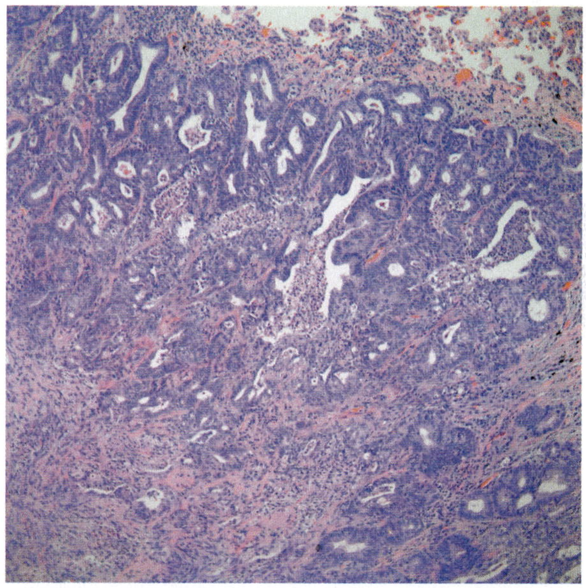

Figure 3-35 Moderately differentiated adenocarcinoma. The tumor is sharply circumscribed from lung parenchyma.

reaction. The acinar and papillary growth patterns often are observed with this degree of differentiation.

Poorly differentiated adenocarcinoma: These tumors are characterized by the presence of sheets of neoplastic cells with only focal areas of glandular differentiation (Figs. 3-41 to 3-49). The solid growth pattern, in which focal areas of abortive glandular formation are present, is most commonly observed in tumors of this histologic grade. High-power magnification of the malignant cellular component may display cells with ample cytoplasm, round to oval nucleus, and prominent nucleolus. The cells may show vacuolization of the cytoplasm, and in such cases the use of histochemical studies, such as mucicarmine, may be helpful to demonstrate the presence of intracellular mucin. Areas of more conventional glandular differentiation also may be observed, which will assist in the classification of the tumor as adenocarcinoma.

The most important data used in lung carcinoma staging are the size of the tumor, the presence of pleural

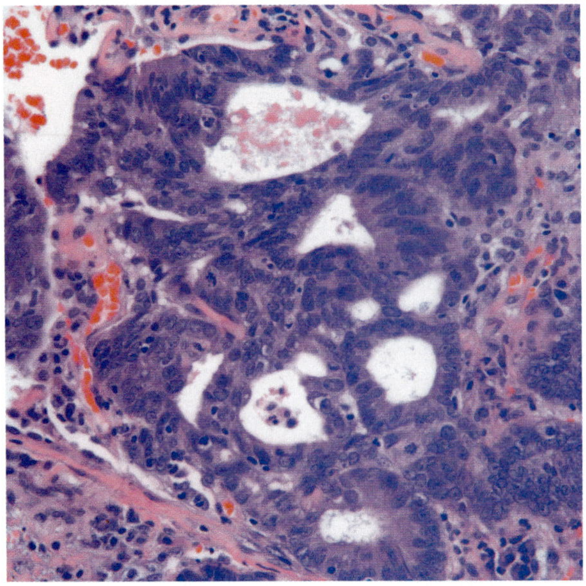

Figure 3-36 Moderately differentiated adenocarcinoma showing prominent nuclear atypia. Mitotic figures are readily apparent.

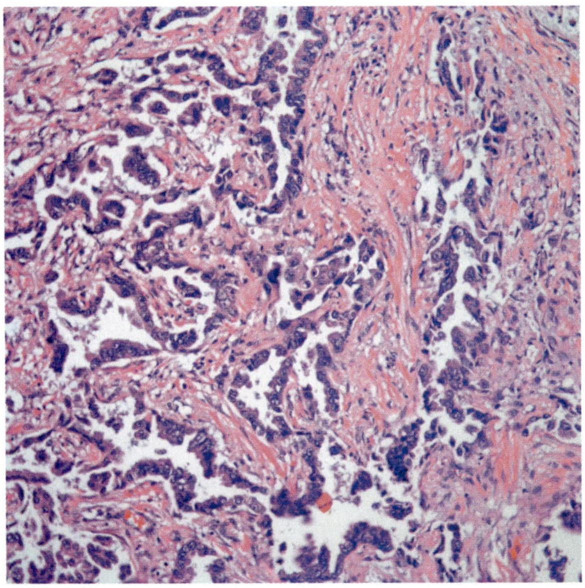

Figure 3-37 Moderately differentiated adenocarcinoma. Glands of different sizes and incomplete gland formation embedded in fibrous tissue can be seen.

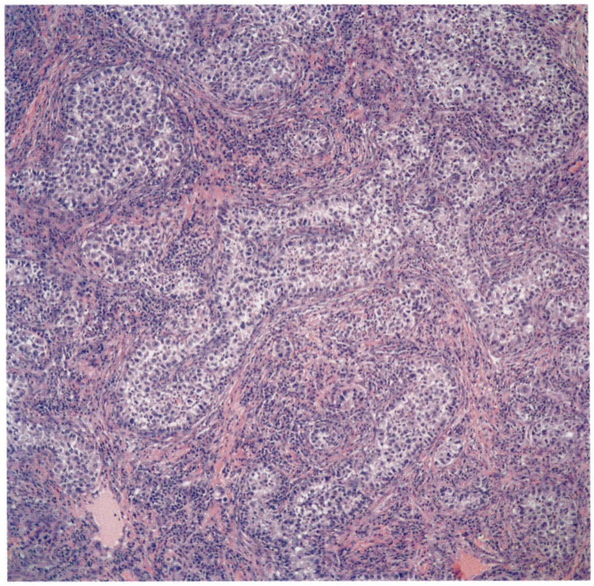

Figure 3-38 Moderately differentiated adenocarcinoma showing an acinar growth pattern.

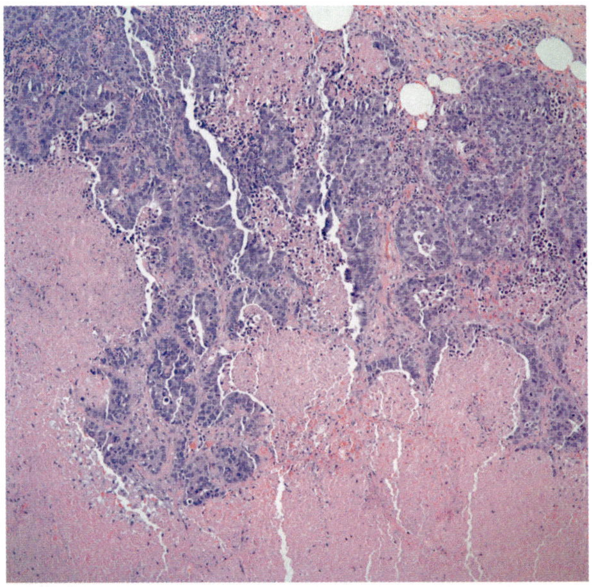

Figure 3-39 Moderately differentiated adenocarcinoma with areas of necrosis.

involvement (Figs. 3-50 and 3-51), and the involvement of lymph nodes. Even though modern radiographic techniques provide very important and valid information regarding the size of tumors, it is still the responsibility of the pathologist to determine tumor size by gross examination. The gross evaluation also is crucial in determining pleural involvement. Subsequent to lobectomy or pneumonectomy, all possible lymph nodes must be dissected in order to determine the proper stage.

Although adenocarcinomas traditionally are conceptualized as tumors forming glandular structures, they may display a wide array of cellular components. This variability can make classification highly problematic, especially when limited material is provided for evaluation. Some of these features have been used to identify specific variants of adenocarcinoma[92] (described later; Table 3-3). Table 3-4 summarizes some of the more unusual features that may be encountered in adenocarcinomas (Figs. 3-52 to 3-69).

Immunohistochemical Features

Pulmonary adenocarcinomas may show positive staining for many carcinomatous epitopes, including

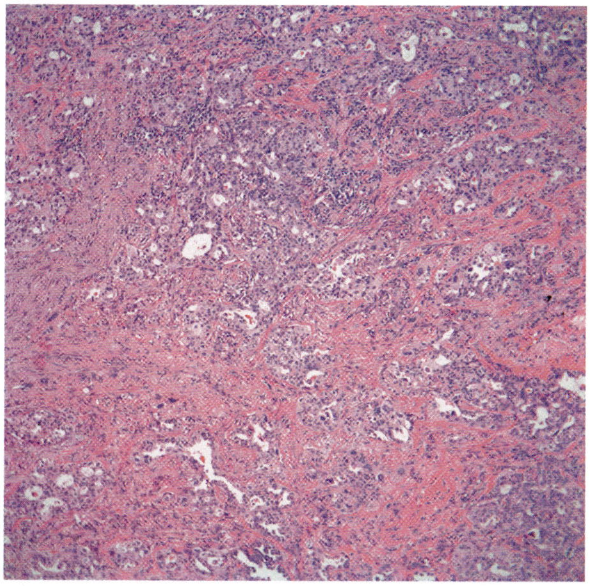

Figure 3-40 Moderately differentiated adenocarcinoma with an acinar growth pattern. Note that it is still possible to identify glandular differentiation.

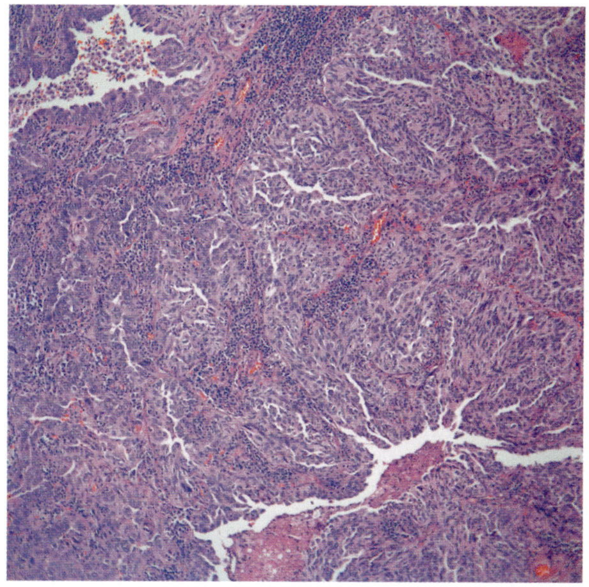

Figure 3-42 Solid pattern of adenocarcinoma showing cellular atypia.

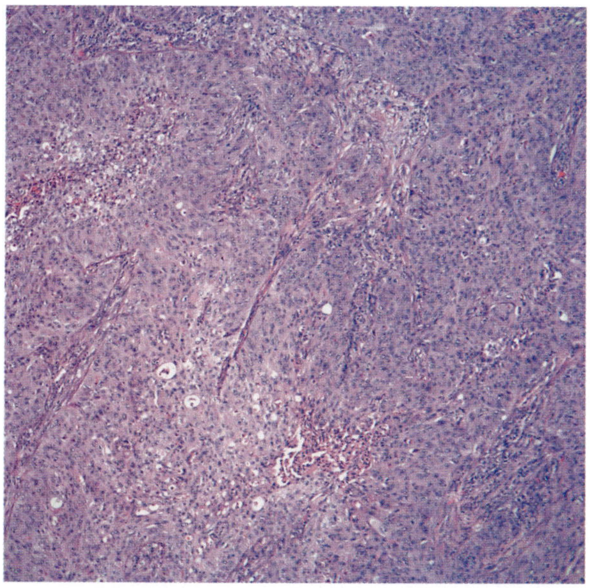

Figure 3-41 Poorly differentiated adenocarcinoma with a solid growth pattern.

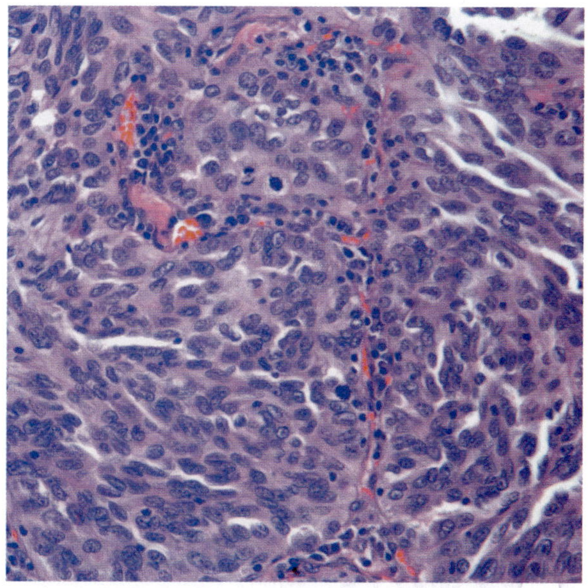

Figure 3-43 Higher-power view of a poorly differentiated adenocarcinoma showing cellular atypia and mitotic activity.

carcinoembryonic antigen (CEA), B72.3, CD15 (Leu M1), BER-EP4, broad-spectrum keratin, low-molecular-weight keratin (CAM 5.2), keratin 7, surfactant protein, PE-10, and TTF-1. In some cases keratin 20 also may show positive staining in primary lung tumors. Depending on the clinical setting, other immunohistochemical studies may be used to rule out the possibility of an extrapulmonary malignancy. In a study of estrogen and progesterone receptors in lung adenocarcinomas by Dabbs and coworkers,[93] 56% of bronchioloalveolar carcinomas and 80% of adenocarcinomas with no special type show positive nuclear staining with the estogen receptor clone 6F11, whereas no staining was seen with the 1D5 clone. The investigators reported no staining for progesterone receptors.

Table 3-5 presents a practical approach to the use of immunohistochemical studies in patients with adenocarcinoma of the lung, depending on the clinical circumstances.

Molecular Biology

Over the past decade, many important discoveries have led to marked improvement in the management

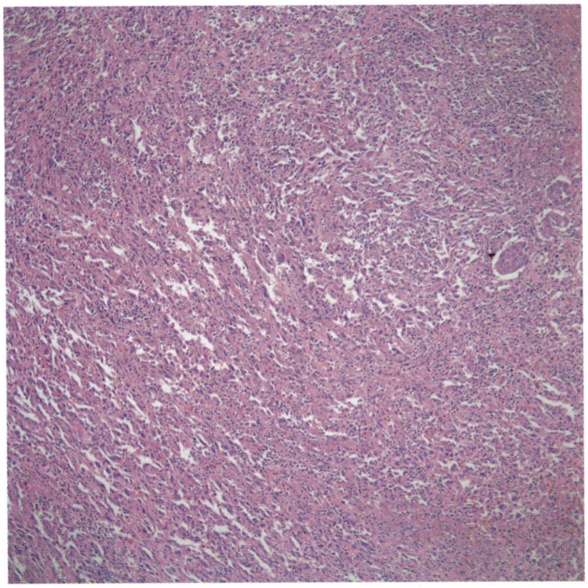

Figure 3-44 Poorly differentiated adenocarcinoma with a solid growth pattern. Only focal areas of glandular differentiation are present.

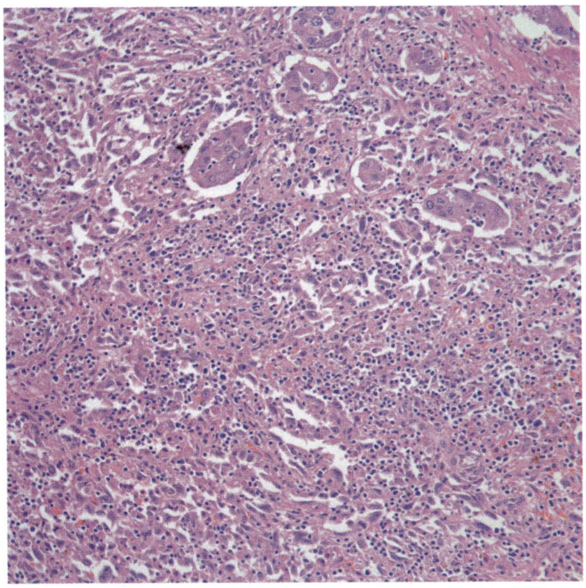

Figure 3-45 Higher-power view of a poorly differentiated adenocarcinoma. Note the focal areas of neoplastic glandular structures.

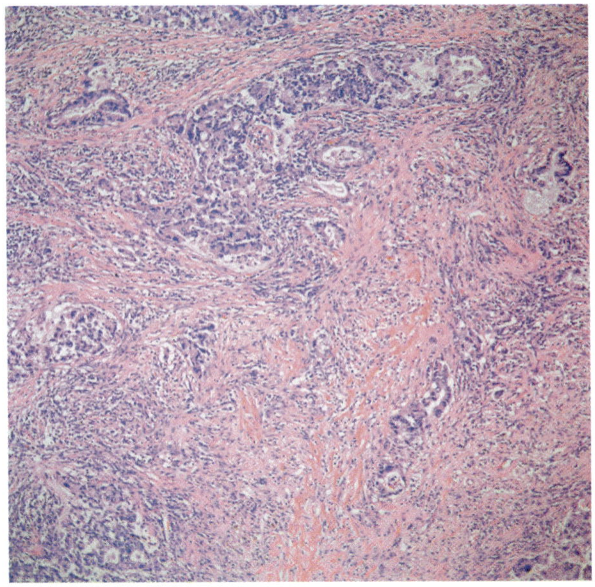

Figure 3-46 Poorly differentiated adenocarcinoma showing areas of solid and glandular growth pattern.

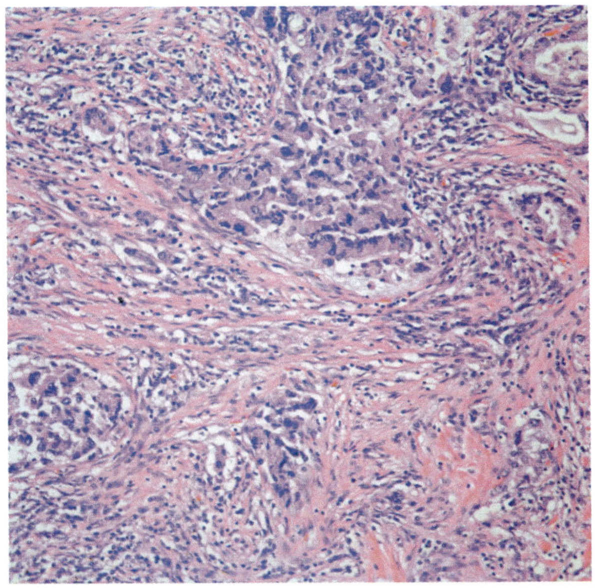

Figure 3-47 High-power view of glandular component of poorly differentiated adenocarcinoma, showing incomplete formation of glandular structures.

of patients with adenocarcinoma.[94–102] One of the most crucial has focused on the epidermal growth factor receptor (EGFR). A mutation in the tyrosine kinase (TK) domain of the EGFR gene appears to occur in some adenocarcinomas, which seem to respond better to treatments targeting this abnormality. Although additional genetic and epigenetic changes have been observed, their application in daily clinical practice awaits further study. Several studies have identified clinical and pathologic features that may represent independent predictors of response to EGFR TK inhibitors, such as adenocarcinoma histologic type, Asian background, female gender, and nonsmoker status. Currently, EGFR mutations involving the TK domain have been reported exclusively in lung carcinoma. These mutations appear to be of four different types, affecting exons 18, 19, 20, and 21 (Figs. 3-70 and 3-71). As indicated by our own clinical observations, adenocarcinoma appears to show the highest incidence of mutations among all non–small cell carcinomas.

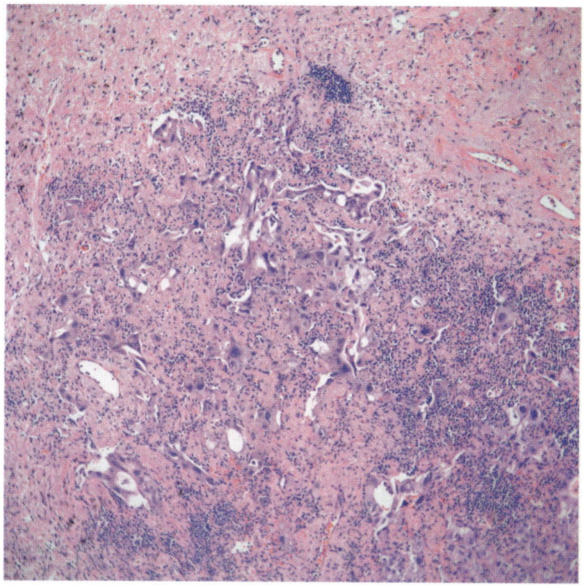

Figure 3-48 Poorly differentiated adenocarcinoma with areas of collagenization.

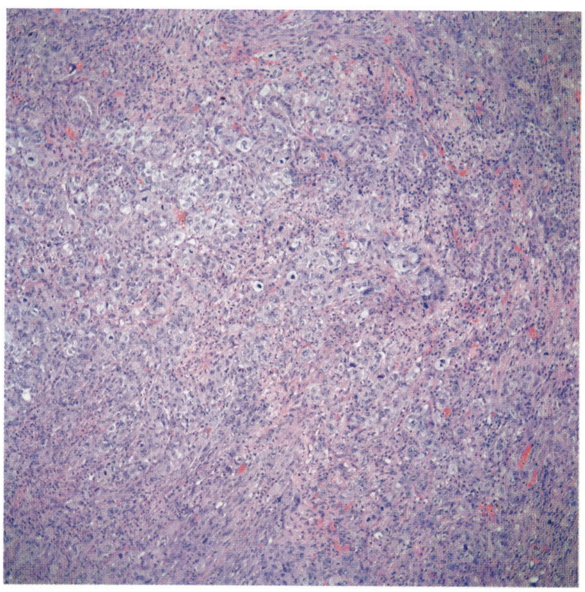

Figure 3-49 Solid areas of poorly differentiated adenocarcinoma. Note the marked nuclear atypia and mitotic activity.

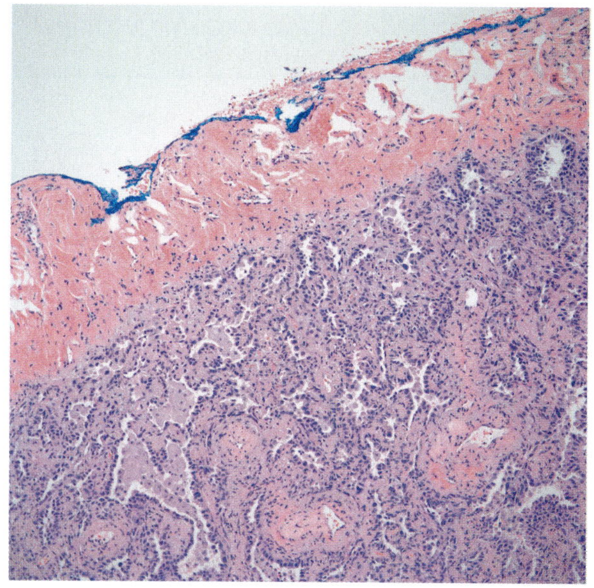

Figure 3-50 Pulmonary adenocarcinoma without pleural involvement.

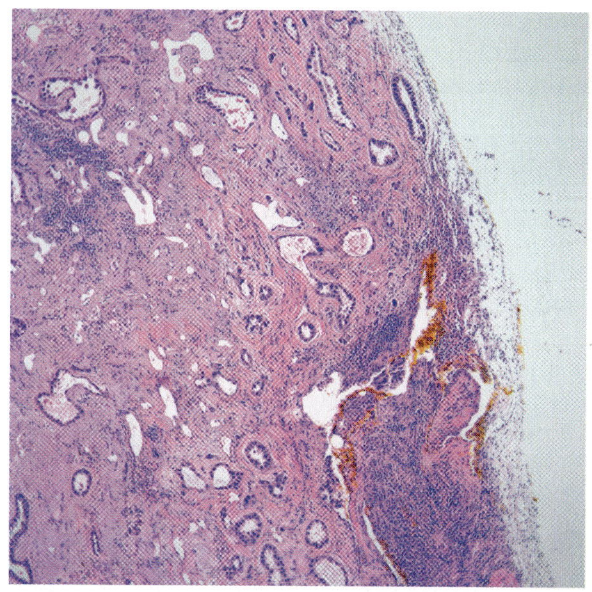

Figure 3-51 Pulmonary adenocarcinoma with pleural involvement.

Mucin-Rich ("Colloid") Adenocarcinoma

Primary lung neoplasms displaying extensive areas of mucin are uncommon, and in many cases these tumors represent metastatic lesions from known or occult gastrointestinal, ovarian, breast, or genitourinary neoplasms. In recent years, the proper classification of these tumors has been controversial, and even in the current WHO classification[31] for tumors of the lung, pleura, mediastinum, and heart, a definitive solution has not been agreed upon. The debate centers on the existence of benign mucinous neoplasms, coded under designations such as mucinous cystadenoma of the lung. Some investigators contend that these tumors are best described as low-grade mucinous carcinomas of the lung,[103] and that they are part of the histopathologic spectrum that mucinous tumors may exhibit. To gain an appreciation of this spectrum, careful analysis of the previous designations that have been used to code mucin-rich adenocarcinomas of the lung is essential.

TABLE 3-3 HISTOPATHOLOGIC GROWTH PATTERNS IN PRIMARY ADENOCARCINOMA OF THE LUNG

Mucinous (so-called) colloid carcinoma
Papillary adenocarcinoma
Micropapillary adenocarcinoma
Papillary carcinoma with morular component
Signet ring cell adenocarcinoma
Secretory endometrioid–like adenocarcinoma
Hepatoid

TABLE 3-4 UNUSUAL HISTOPATHOLOGIC FEATURES OF ADENOCARCINOMAS

Adenomatoid-like
Cribriform
Intestinal-like
Embryonal carcinoma–like
Prominent syncytial giant cell component
Warthin tumor–like
Granulomatous
Ciliated epithelium
Clear cell*

*Clear cell change can be seen in adenocarcinoma, squamous cell carcinoma, or large cell carcinoma. Accordingly, it is not considered to represent a specific neoplasm.

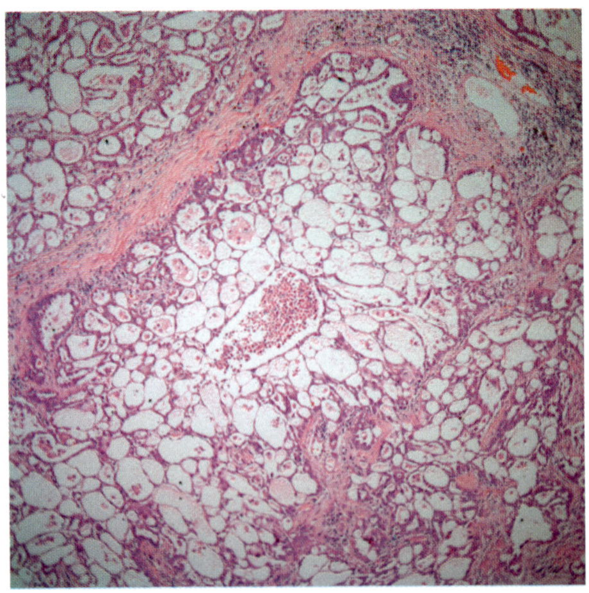

Figure 3-52 Adenocarcinoma with prominent adenomatoid-like features.

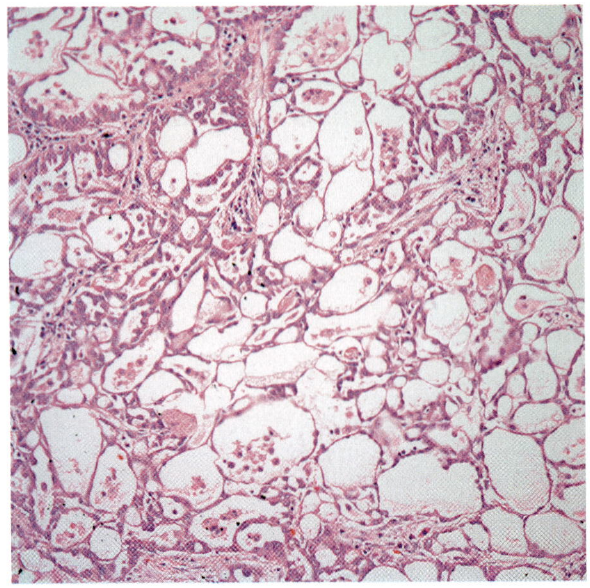

Figure 3-53 High-power view of an adenocarcinoma with adenomatoid-like features. Note the absence of nuclear atypia or mitotic activity.

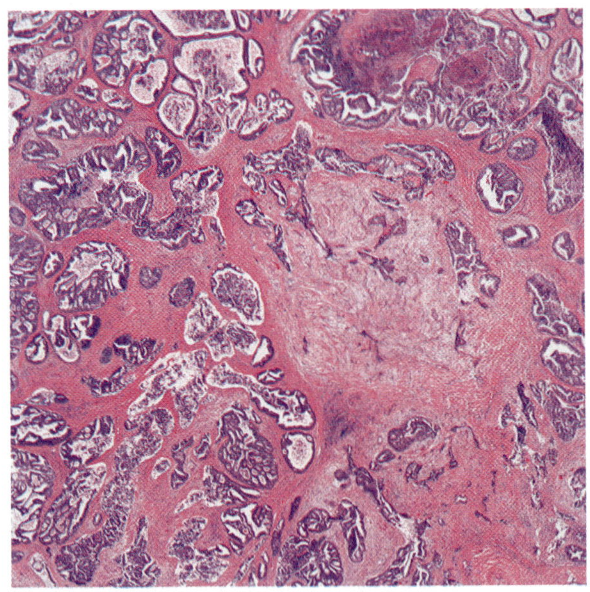

Figure 3-54 Adenocarcinoma with prominent cribriform growth pattern.

Mucinous Cystadenoma

Introduced by Kragel and associates[104] in 1990, so-called "mucinous cystadenoma" is one of the earliest designations provided for these tumors. These workers described two 62-year-old patients, a man and a woman, who were found to have a solitary lung tumor on radiographic examination. Both tumors were located in the right middle lobe, and surgical resection was performed. On gross examination, both tumors were noted to be cystic, and histopathologic features included abundant mucin production with the presence of columnar epithelium.

In 1991, Traub[105] contested that the same tumor had been described previously under the designation of multilocular cystic carcinoma. Kragel and associates[104] argued that the tumors described by Traub would be better

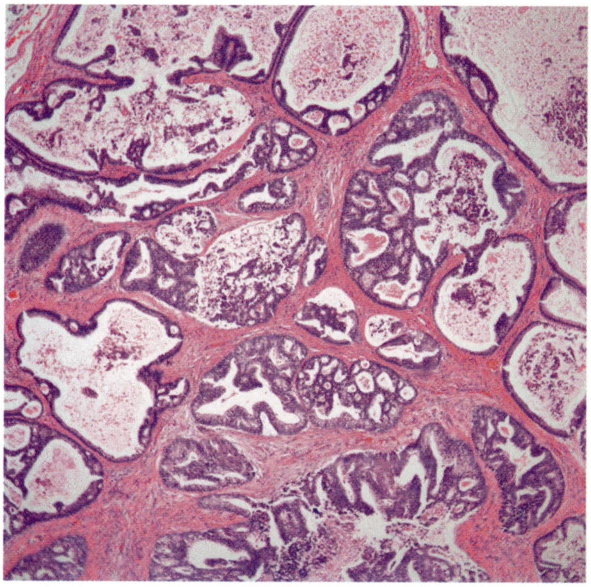

Figure 3-55 Cribriform growth pattern in a primary lung adenocarcinoma.

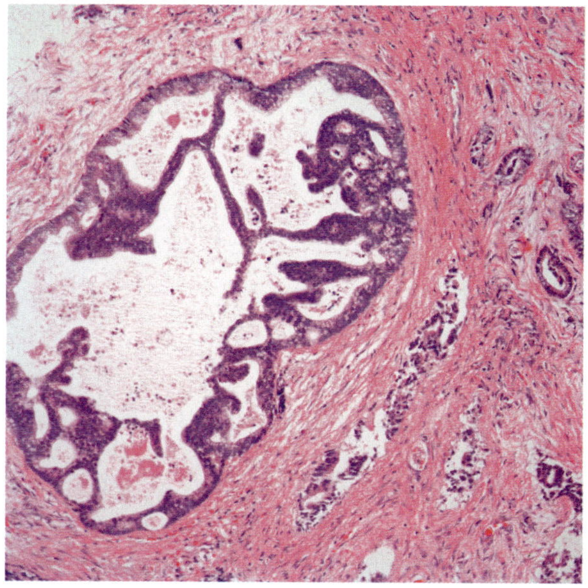

Figure 3-56 Closer view of a cribriform adenocarcinoma of the lung. Note the presence of the so-called Roman bridges pattern.

classified as the mucinous variant of BAC. Although this particular entity is distinguished as a specific tumor in the latest version of the WHO criteria, most investigators consider it to be part of the spectrum of mucinous carcinomas of the lung.

Pulmonary Mucinous Cystic Tumor

This term *pulmonary mucinous cystic tumor* was introduced by Dixon and coworkers[106] in a case report of a 59-year-old man who had a pulmonary mass for 11 years

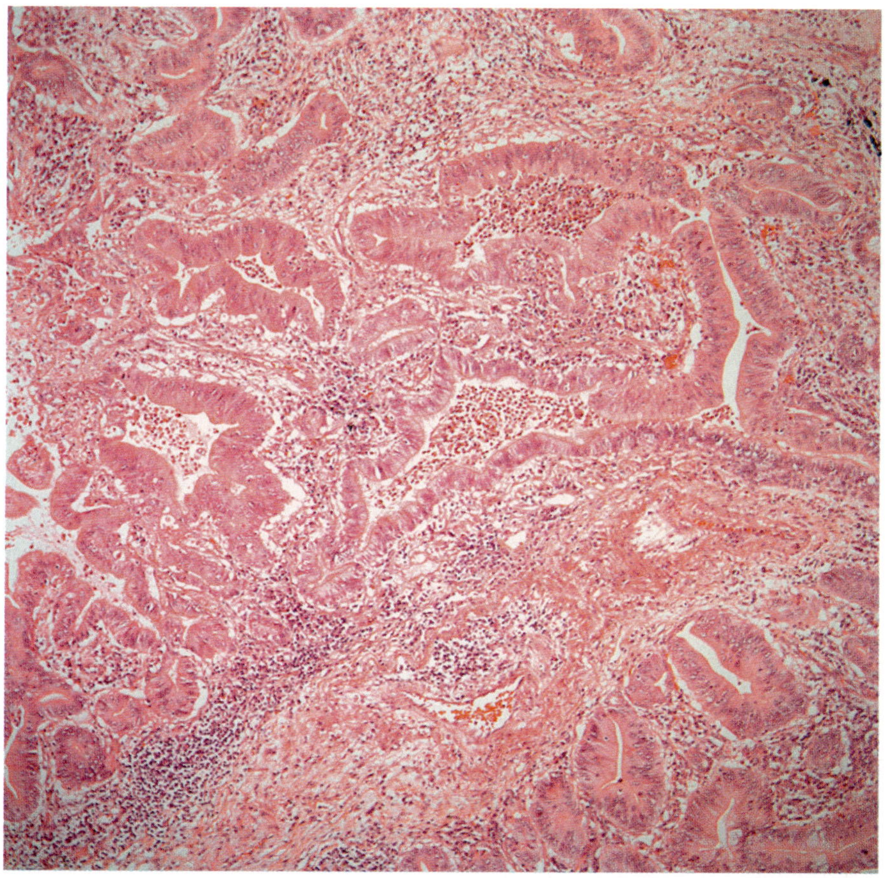

Figure 3-57 Low-power view of an otherwise conventional cribriform adenocarcinoma.

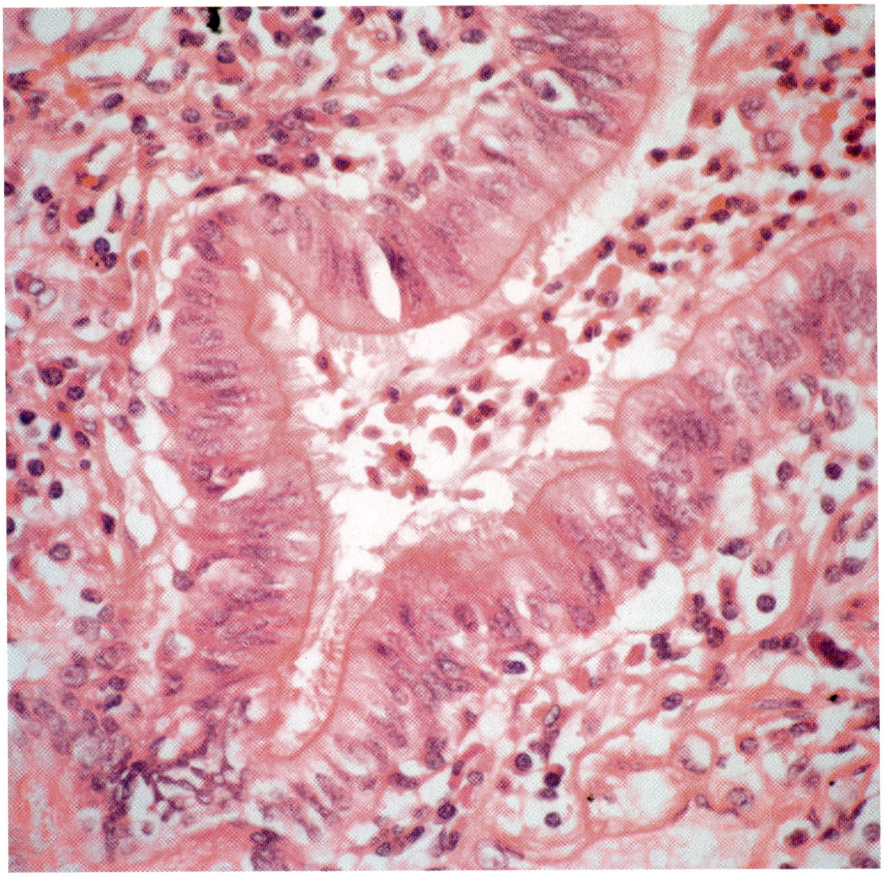

Figure 3-58 High-power view of the tumor in Figure 3-57 showing the presence of ciliated neoplastic glands.

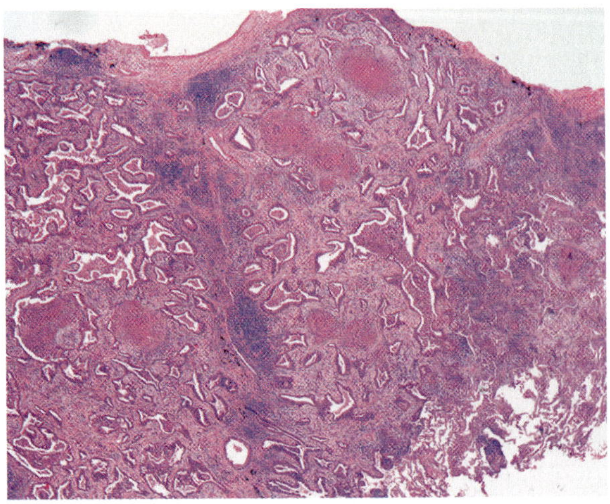

Figure 3-59 Low-power view of an adenocarcinoma with granulomatous component.

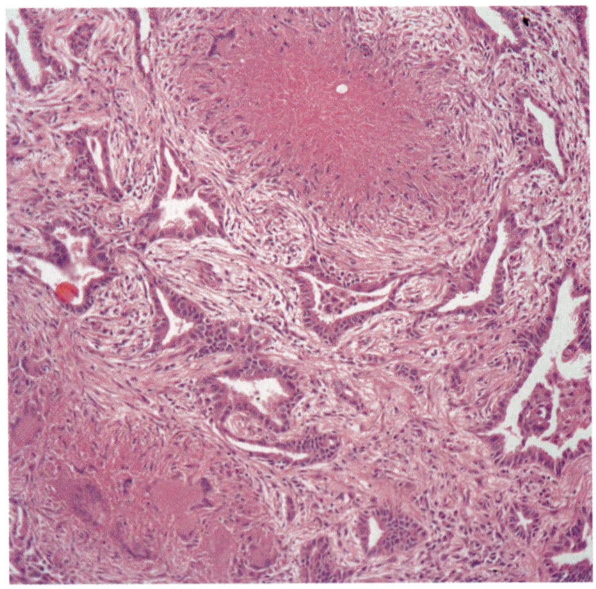

Figure 3-60 The tumor from Figure 3-59 at higher magnification. Neoplastic glands can be seen in close proximity to caseous granulomatous inflammation.

before resection. Surgical resection of the tumor was performed, and the tumor mass was described as cystic. Histologically, the description of the tumor is similar to that by Traub and Kragel.[104,105] In this case, however, Dixon and coworkers mention the presence of an atypical glandular component. They avoid the term "carcinoma" and regard the reported neoplasm as an indolent lesion with a favorable prognosis based on negative findings after a clinical follow-up period of 5 years.

Higashima and associates[107] described cases similar to Dixon and coworkers'[106] but interpreted them differently. The tumors reported by Higashima's group show similar gross and microscopic features but were designated "cystic mucinous adenocarcinoma of the lung."

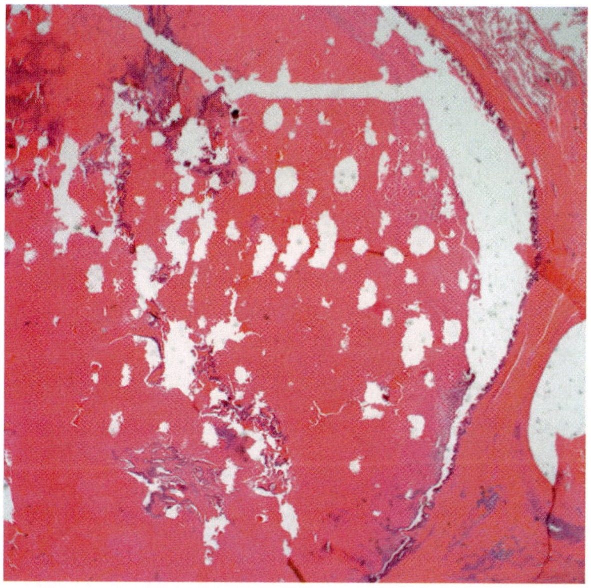

Figure 3-61 Adenocarcinoma showing large, cystically dilated glands with central necrosis and free-floating malignant glands.

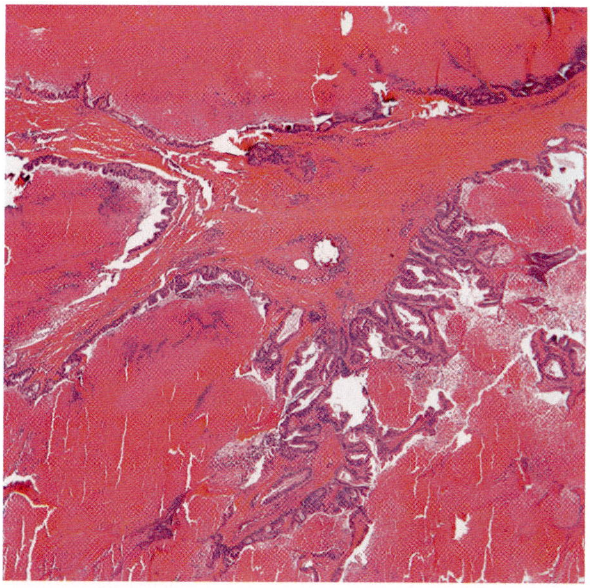

Figure 3-62 High-power view of the malignant glands from Figure 3-61, which are composed of a rather tall mucinous epithelium similar to that seen in gastrointestinal tumors.

These workers concluded that the tumors represented a mucus-producing variant of adenocarcinoma of the lung, distinct from previously described mucinous tumors such as mucinous cystadenoma.

Davison[108] described a similar case in a 69-year-old woman with a peripheral lung nodule that was found incidentally during a routine physical examination. The gross and microscopic features were essentially the same as those previously reported under the terms *cystadenoma*, *mucinous tumor*, and *cystic mucinous*

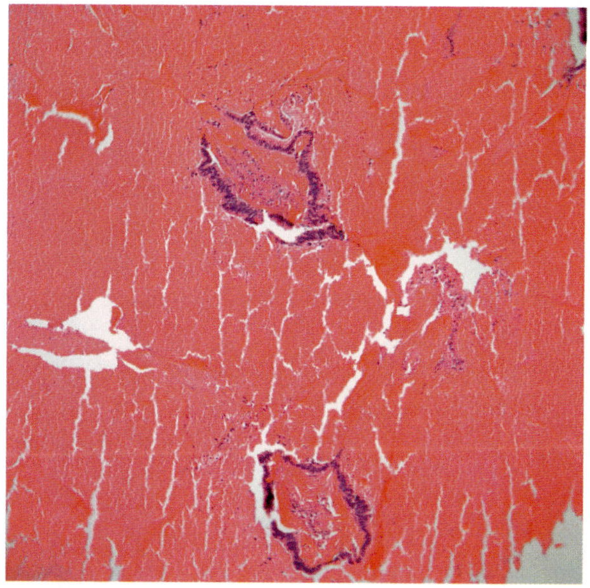

Figure 3-63 Adenocarcinoma. High-power view of necrotic areas containing the malignant glandular component. This feature mimics metastasis from gastrointestinal origin.

adenocarcinoma. Davison described a solid focus of well-differentiated adenocarcinoma and thus opted for the designation of adenocarcinoma arising in a mucinous cystadenoma of the lung. This report raises the possibility that mucin-rich carcinomas may arise from a benign mucinous cystadenoma that subsequently becomes malignant.

Pulmonary Mucinous Cystic Tumors of Borderline Malignancy

In 1991 Graeme-Cook and Mark[109] introduced a new term, *pulmonary mucinous cystic tumors of borderline malignancy*, based on a study of 11 cases of primary mucinous cystic tumors of the lung. The descriptions again reflected the cystic and mucinous nature of these tumors, which in some cases showed a "solid epithelial proliferation." The follow-up report provided, for periods ranging from 1 to 9 years, describes an "indolent" tumor. Despite the fact that these workers considered this tumor "neoplastic," the term "carcinoma" was avoided in favor of "borderline tumor."

Mucinous ("Colloid") Carcinoma

The term *mucinous ("colloid") carcinoma* is the latest designation for the family of mucin-rich neoplasms and attempts to encompass all of the previous descriptions. It was introduced in a 1992[110] study of 24 cases. Clinically, grossly, and microscopically, the tumors demonstrated a mixture of the various features described in previous reports. Areas with a solid epithelial glandular proliferation were observed in some of the cases. The most important contrasting feature presented in this series is that

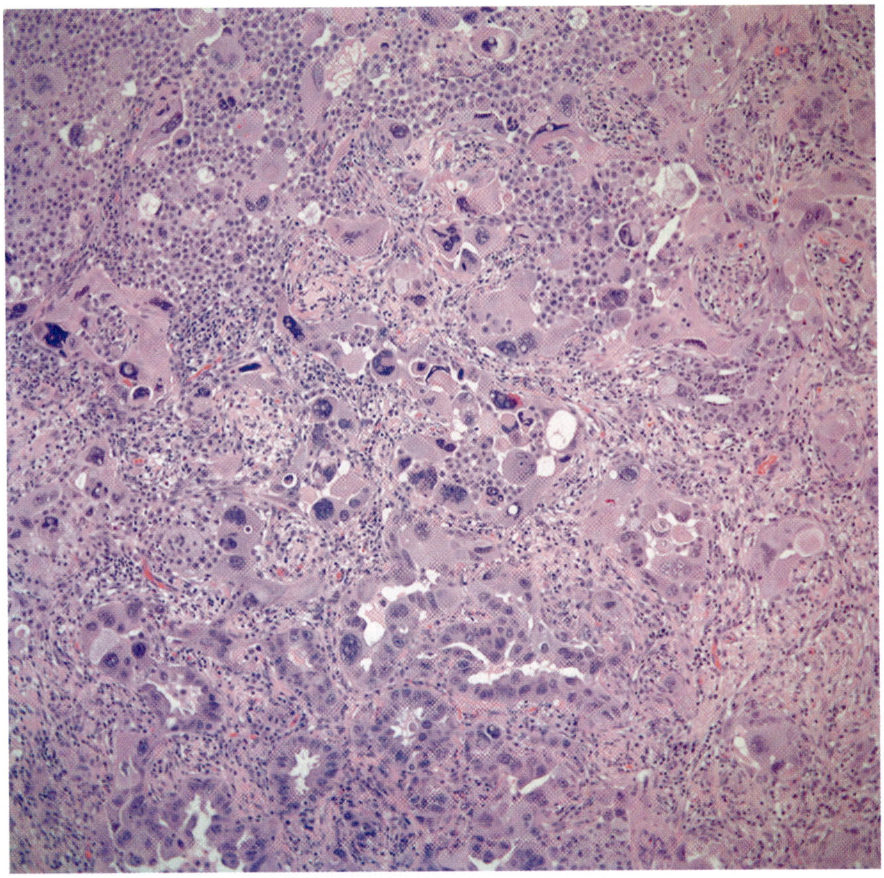

Figure 3-64 Adenocarcinoma containing numerous syncytial-like giant cells.

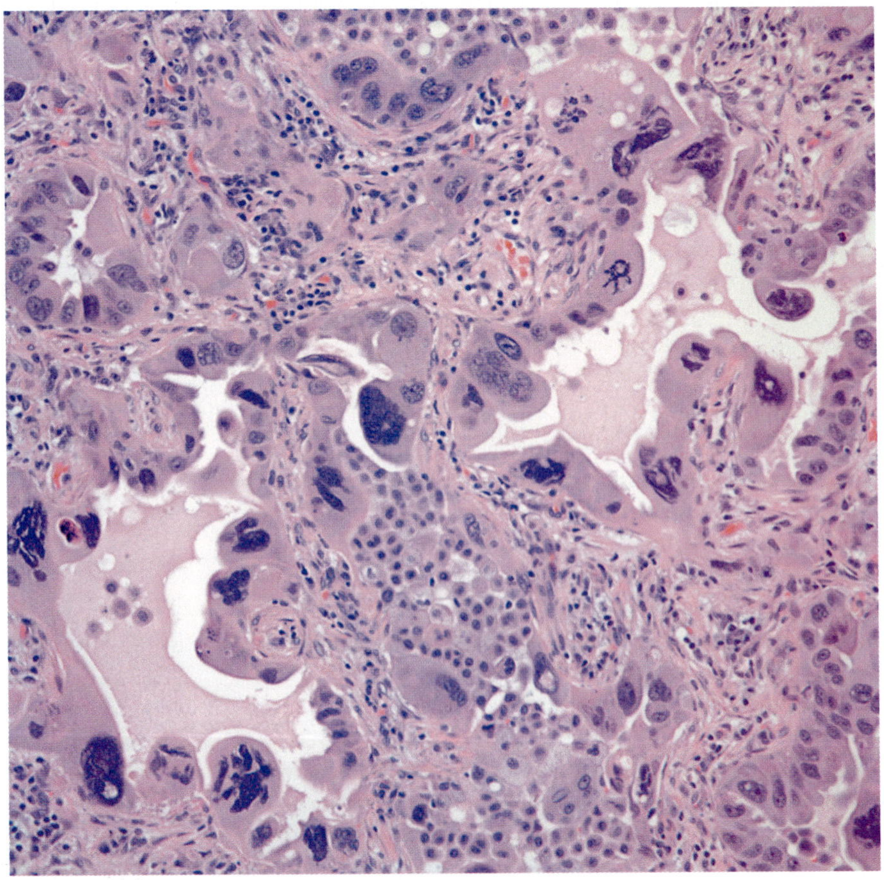

Figure 3-65 Adenocarcinoma. High-power view of multinucleated giant cells displaying prominent atypia and atypical mitotic figures.

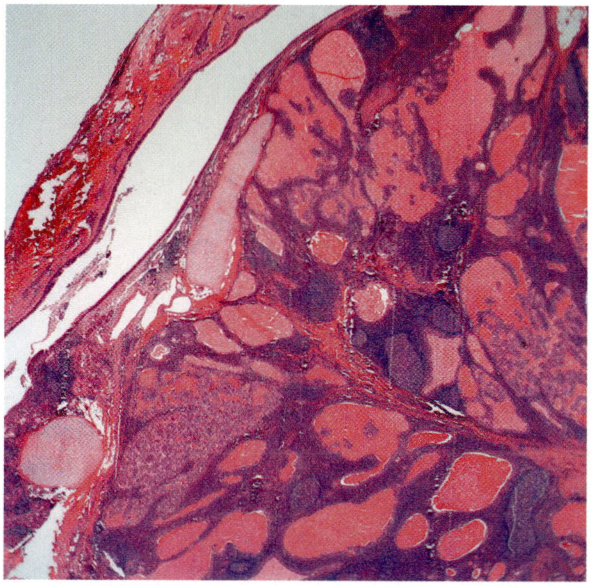

Figure 3-66 Low-power view of an adenocarcinoma mimicking a Warthin's tumor.

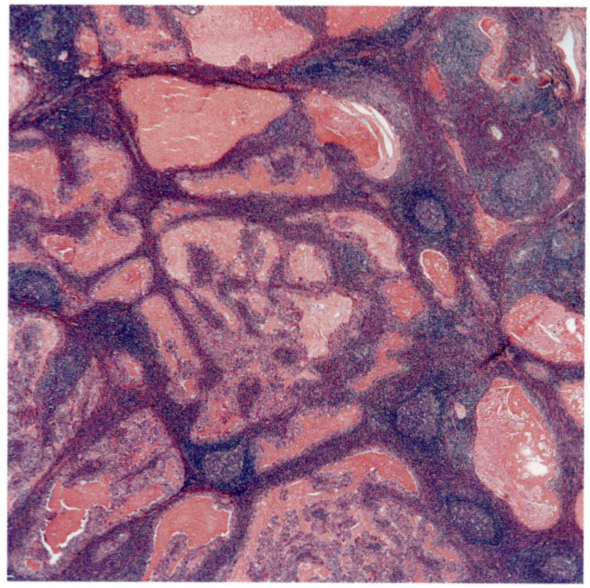

Figure 3-67 Warthin-like adenocarcinoma of the lung showing cystically dilated neoplastic areas associated with prominent lymphocytic component.

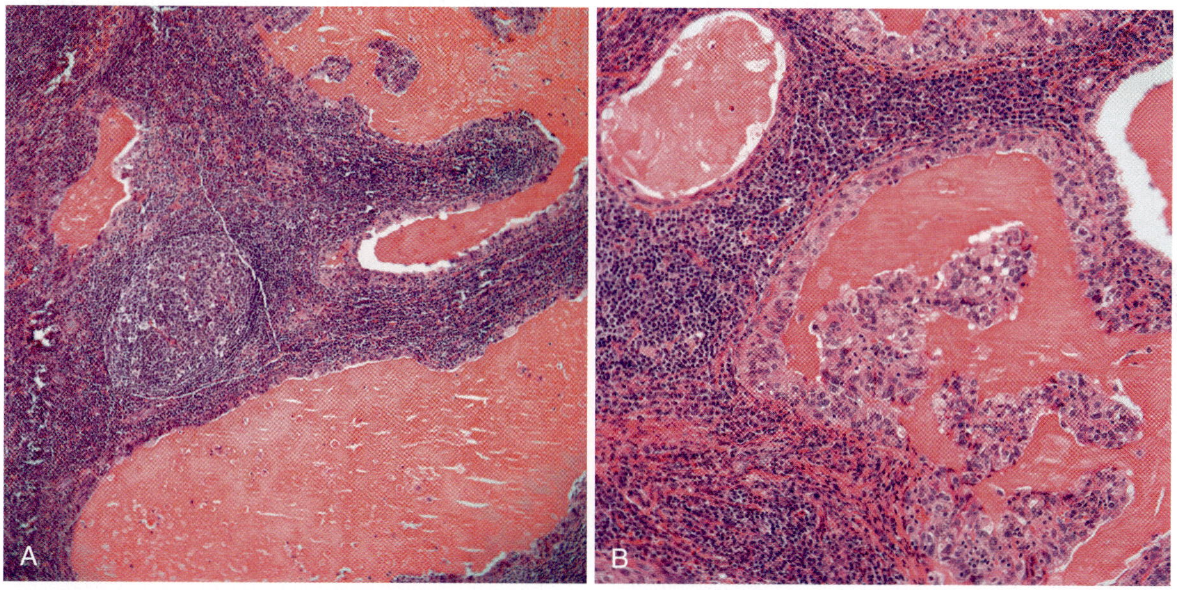

Figure 3-68 **A**, Warthin-like adenocarcinoma of the lung showing hyperplasia of lymphoid component with germinal centers. **B**, High-power view of the malignant epithelial component.

some metastatic lesions, including bone and brain, were encountered during the follow-up period, ranging from 2 to 192 months. Some patients also experienced recurrence of the tumor, whereas for others, the follow-up was uneventful.

It is likely that all of the reports in the literature refer to a single pathologic entity. Clinically, grossly, and histologically, the tumors described display only minor differences, and if it can be accepted that some may be benign, identification of an exact criterion to separate the benign neoplasms from the malignant ones is very difficult. If these tumors are consistently approached as low-grade carcinomas with metastatic potential, however, it becomes crucial that the patient undergo complete surgical resection with close follow-up. At least one of the reported series supports this argument, because some of the patients eventually developed metastatic disease.[110] Accordingly, some workers have advocated that all mucin-rich tumors of the lung be classified as carcinomas of low-grade malignant potential. In cases

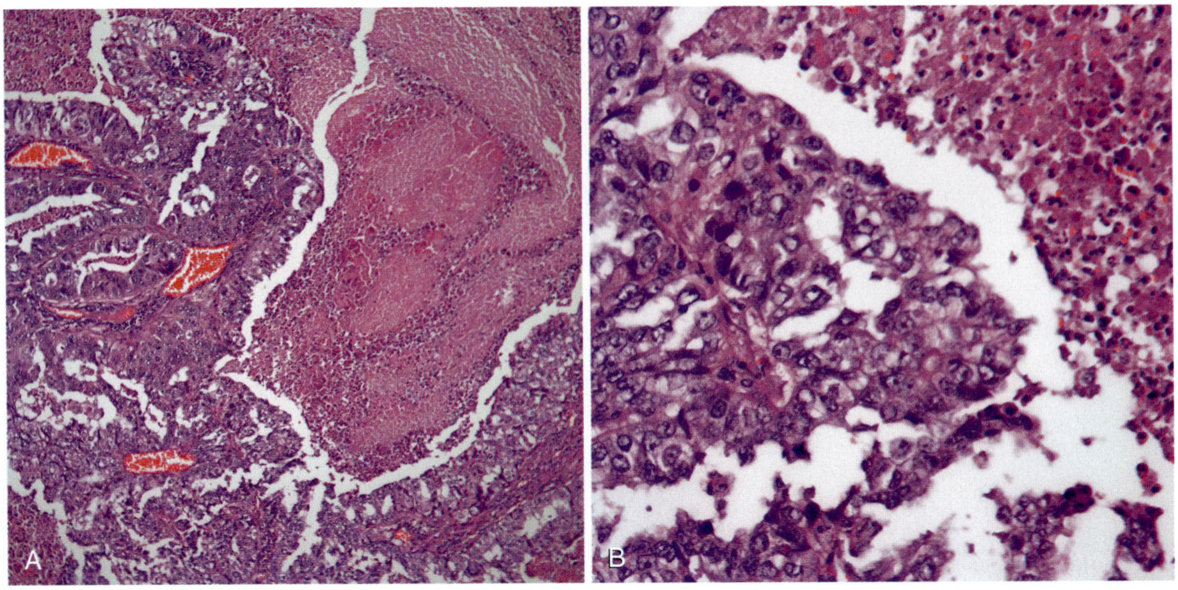

Figure 3-69 **A**, Poorly differentiated adenocarcinoma displaying features that mimic embryonal carcinoma. **B**, High-power view of an embryonal carcinoma–like pulmonary adenocarcinoma. Note the presence of necrosis and cells with prominent nucleoli and nuclear vacuolization.

TABLE 3-5 IMMUNOHISTOCHEMICAL FEATURES OF PULMONARY ADENOCARCINOMAS IN CONTRAST WITH OTHER COMMON METASTATIC LESIONS

Antibody	Lung	Colon	Breast	Endometrium
Pan-keratin	+	+	+	+
TTF-1	+	–	–*	+*,125
Keratin 7	+	–	+	+
Keratin 20	–/+*	+	–	–
CDX-2	–/+	+	–	–
ER	–/+	–	–	+
PR	–	–	–	+
GCDFP	–	–	+	–
CEA	+	+	+	–/+
Mammoglobin	–	–	+	–
Surfactant	+	–	–	–

*In some cases, sporadic cells may show positive staining.
+, positive staining; –, negative staining; –/+, mainly negative, but positive staining may occur in some cases; CEA, carcinoembryonic antigen; ER, estrogen receptor; GCDFP, gross cystic disease fluid protein; PR, progesterone receptor; TTF-1, thyroid transcription factor-1.

in which the tumor is solitary and amenable to complete surgical resection, this may be the only treatment required; however, for those patients who present with widespread pulmonary involvement and advanced clinical staging, the prognosis may be dismal. The most predictive histologic features of malignant potential include the following:

- Solid areas displaying cellular atypia and mitotic activity
- Foci of stromal invasion
- Extensive pulmonary disease

These tumors currently are diagnosed on the basis of clinical and morphologic findings; however, the use of immunohistochemical and ultrastructural studies may be useful to distinguish primary from metastatic disease.

Gross Features

Mucinous tumors of the lung are characterized by a soft mucoid consistency, and cystic structures may be readily identifiable. The tumor sometimes appears as a more solid mass; however, closer inspection should reveal microcystic structures. Size may vary, with some tumors as small as 1 cm and others occurring as large, widely disseminated tumors in the lung parenchyma (Fig. 3-72).

Microscopic Features

The low-power view reveals extensive areas of mucoid material destroying normal lung parenchyma (Figs. 3-73 to 3-77). These may show focal areas with clusters of atypical cells, or single cells with atypical features. In some cases, the low-power view may show a cystic tumor, whereas in other cases, the tumor may display microcystic structures filled with mucoid material. One of the most important features is the presence of a residual alveolar wall, lined by mucus-producing epithelium resembling that of the intestines. The alveolar wall may be focal, and a careful search may be necessary when this feature is not readily visible. Less common findings may include focal solid areas of adenocarcinoma, which can appear either as conventional adenocarcinoma or as adenocarcinoma with papillary features. It is important to

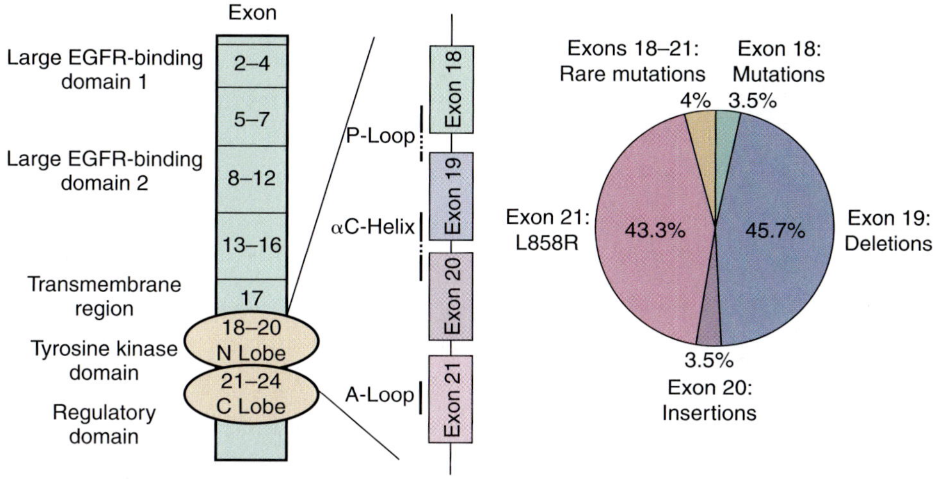

Figure 3-70 Molecular analysis of exons in pulmonary adenocarcinoma. EGFR, epidermal growth factor receptor. (From Prudkin L, Wistuba II. Epidermal growth factor receptor abnormalities in lung cancer. Pathogenetic and clinical implications. *Ann Diagn Pathol.* 2006;10(5):306–315. Used with permission.)

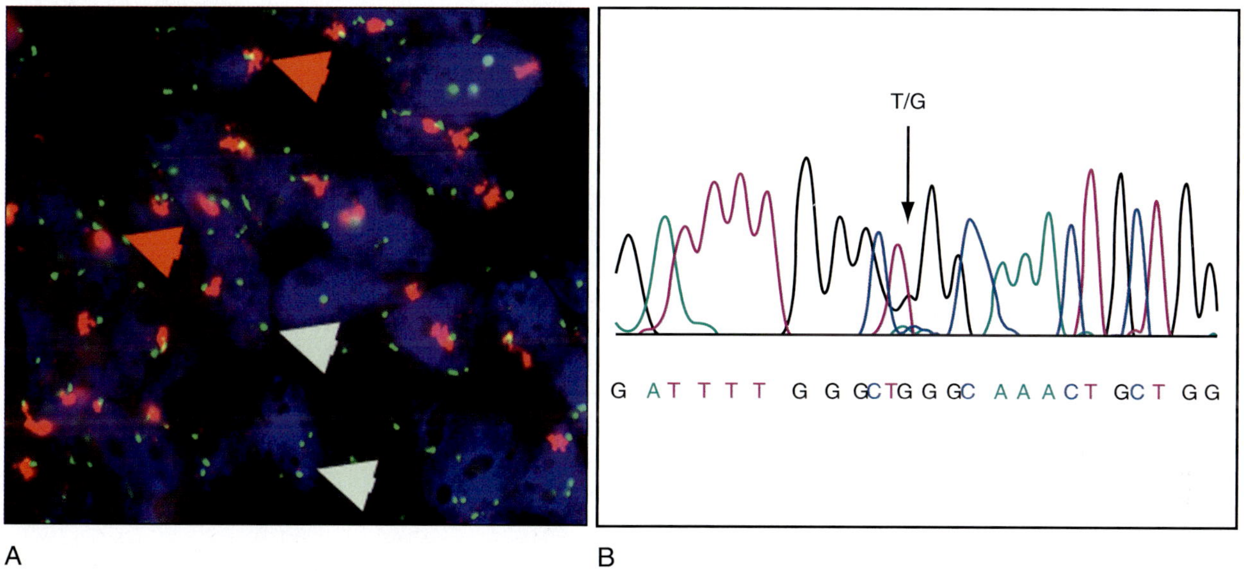

Figure 3-71 Gene amplification in lung adenocarcinoma. **A**, Fluorescence in situ hybridization gene amplification. **B**, Sequencing: Exon L858R 21 mutation. (From Prudkin L, Wistuba II. Epidermal growth factor receptor abnormalities in lung cancer. Pathogenetic and clinical implications. *Ann Diagn Pathol.* 2006;10(5):306–315. Used with permission.)

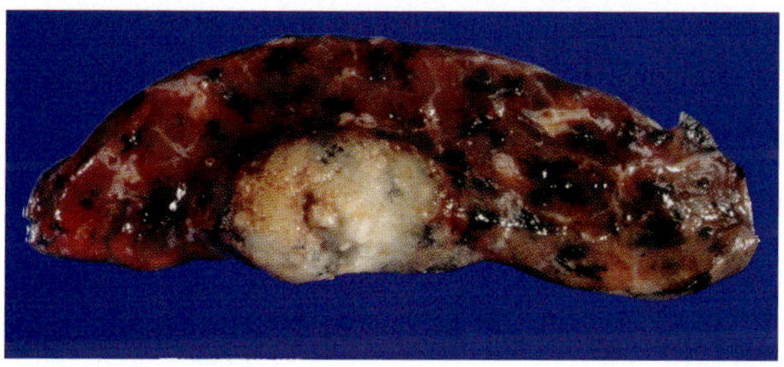

Figure 3-72 Colloid carcinoma of lung. Note the presence of mucoid material at cut surface.

sample these tumors properly, as the most characteristic changes may be present only in focal areas, whereas other areas may show only extensive mucoid material distributed haphazardly in the lung parenchyma, destroying normal architecture.

Immunohistochemical Features

As with any other primary lung adenocarcinoma, the use of TTF-1 and keratin 7 immunostaining may help to demonstrate the epithelial component of the tumor. It is more important, however, to include other stains in the immunohistochemical workup, to assist in ruling out tumors with similar histologic features but different origin. Immunostaining for keratin 20, CDX-2 (caudal type homeobox transcription factor 2), CD10, and gross cystic disease fluid protein (GCDFP) may rule out tumors of gastrointestinal, genitourinary, and breast origin, respectively.

Clinical Behavior

Mucin-rich tumors tend to follow an indolent course, in which patients are treated with complete surgical resection.

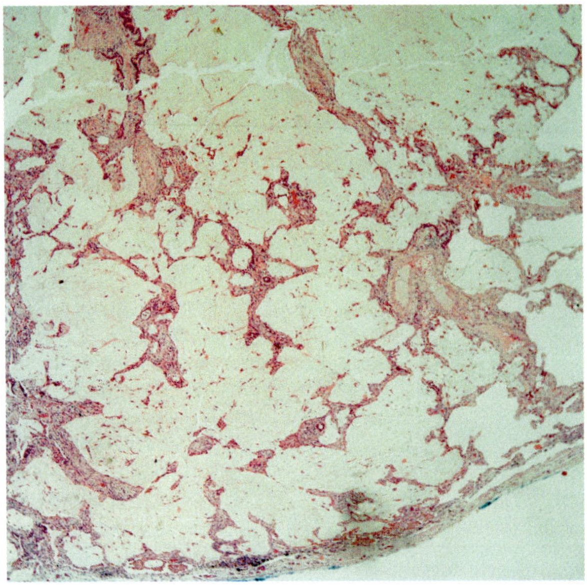

Figure 3-73 Low-power view of a colloid carcinoma destroying the lung parenchyma. Note the subpleural location of the tumor.

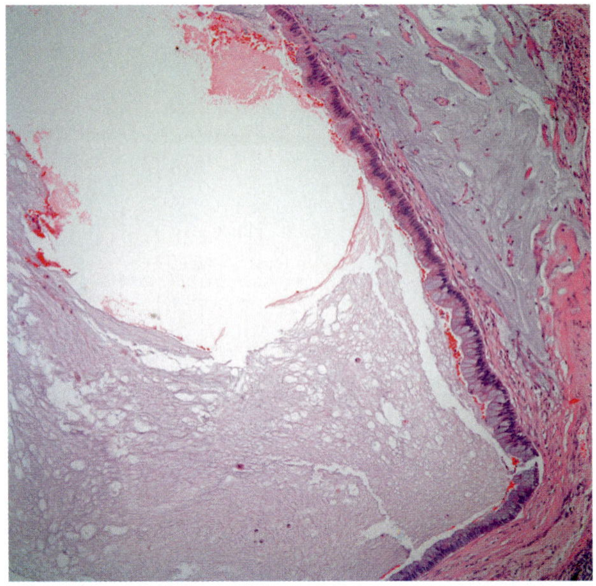

Figure 3-75 Colloid carcinoma showing cystic areas lined by mucinous epithelium.

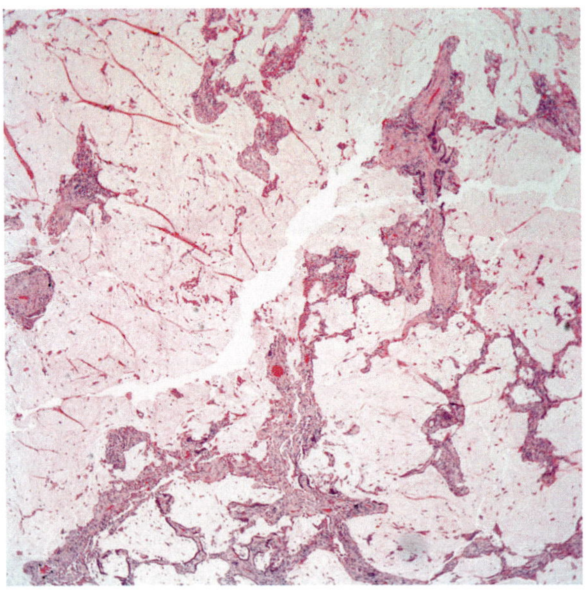

Figure 3-74 Colloid carcinoma showing extensive areas of mucoid material destroying normal lung parenchyma.

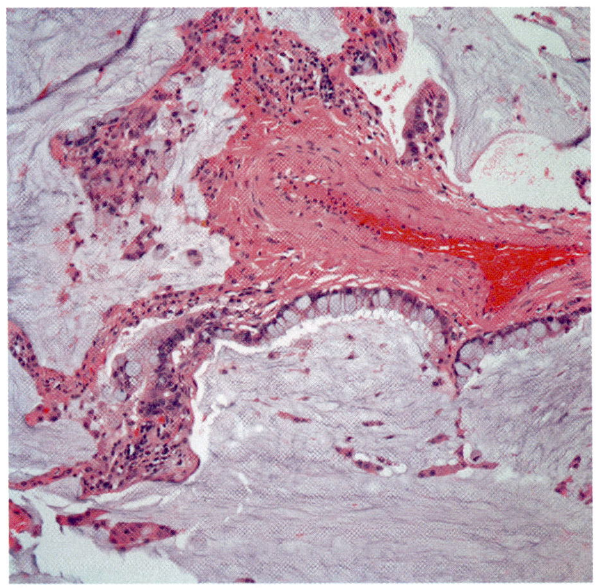

Figure 3-76 Colloid carcinoma showing areas of residual alveoli lined by mucinous epithelium.

In some cases, these tumors can be aggressive, and metastatic disease may be widespread. Stage at the time of diagnosis is the most important criterion used to predict prognosis. For tumors that are small and amenable to complete surgical resection, the course may be indolent, whereas for tumors that are large or have spread outside the lung parenchyma or thoracic cavity, the prognosis is more guarded.

Papillary Adenocarcinoma

Although the earlier literature acknowledges the existence of adenocarcinomas with papillary features, these cases had been grouped under other designations, including variants of BAC, until the late 1990s. Several studies of this growth pattern have calculated that it represents approximately 10% of all adenocarcinomas of the lung.

In 1997, Silver and Askin[111] introduced the term "true" papillary carcinomas of the lung. These workers described 31 patients with primary papillary carcinomas and set parameters for diagnosis, concluding that at least 75% of the tumor should display papillary features in order for it to be coded under this designation. Papillary adenocarcinoma appears to affect men

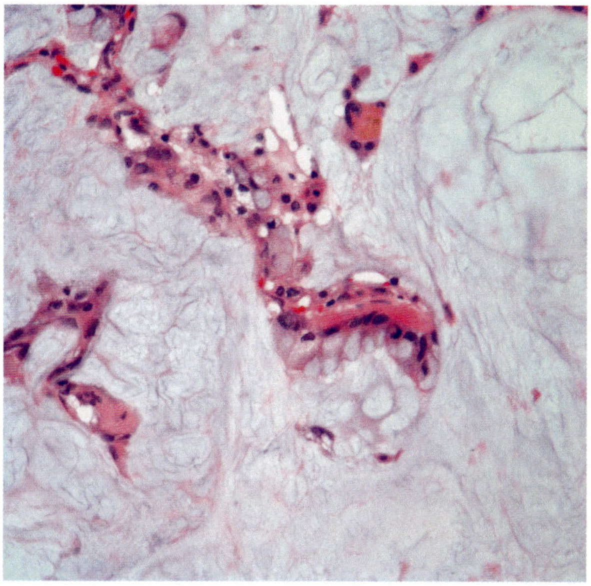

Figure 3-77 Colloid carcinoma with extensive areas of mucoid material, and focal areas in which the alveoli are being replaced by mucinous epithelium.

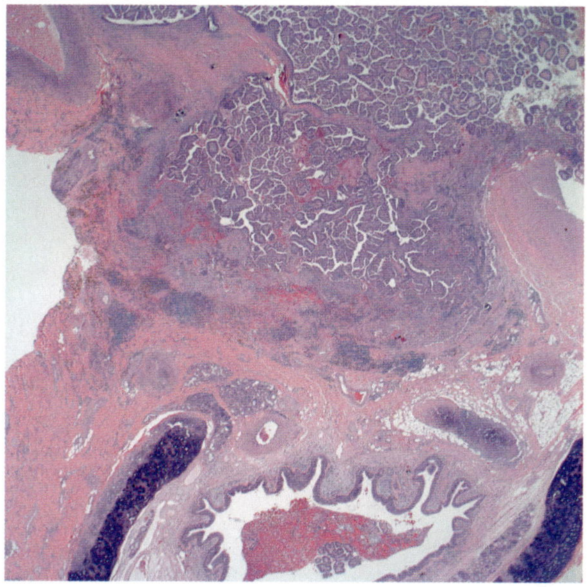

Figure 3-78 Low-power view of a papillary carcinoma.

and women equally, although in some reports a slight predominance in women has been reported.[112] It does not appear to occur in a particular lung or pulmonary segment. The tumor is more common in adults, with a mean age at diagnosis of 64 years. The great majority of these patients will present with a single solitary pulmonary tumor, although in a few cases the tumor may be multifocal. Only a few studies of this variant have been presented in the literature,[111–113] but they all describe a separate clinicopathologic entity that appears to be more aggressive than conventional BAC.

Gross Features

The tumor may manifest in a central or peripheral location, and mass may vary in size from 1 cm to larger than 10 cm in greatest dimension. In gross appearance the tumor is well delimited and light brown in color, and the cut surface may show a homogeneous surface. In some cases, necrosis and hemorrhage are present.

Histologic Features

At low magnification, a papillary neoplasm destroying normal lung parenchyma is visible. In some areas, the papillary pattern may acquire a more complex configuration, with papillary cores of different sizes and lengths (Figs. 3-78 to 3-81). Closer examination of these papillary structures reveals a delicate fibrovascular core lined by neoplastic cells, in which the nuclei are displaced toward the periphery. The nuclei also may show grooves and intranuclear inclusions. Mitotic figures are not common; however, psammoma bodies may be haphazardly distributed in tumoral areas. In some cases, a tumor may display the pattern of a papillary adenocarcinoma but with the cytologic features characteristic of an oncocytic papillary adenocarcinoma (Figs. 3-82 to 3-84).

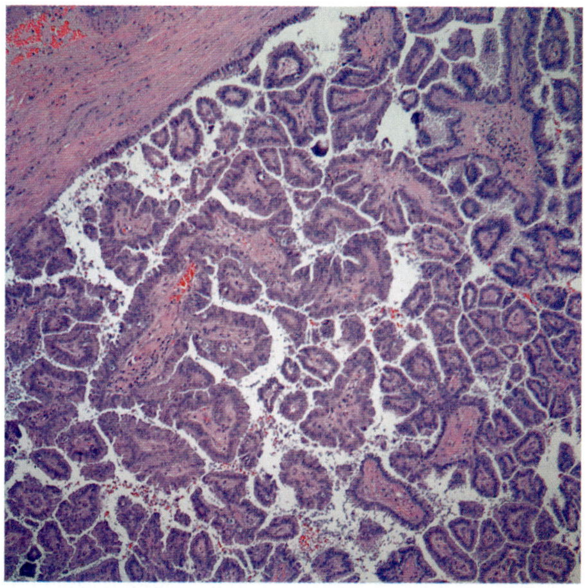

Figure 3-79 Papillary adenocarcinoma showing prominent papillary proliferation, with papillae of different sizes.

Immunohistochemical Features

Immunostaining for keratin 7, TTF-1, and thyroglobulin should be performed in these cases, owing to the predominant papillary growth pattern and the similar histology of several metastatic lesions to the lung.

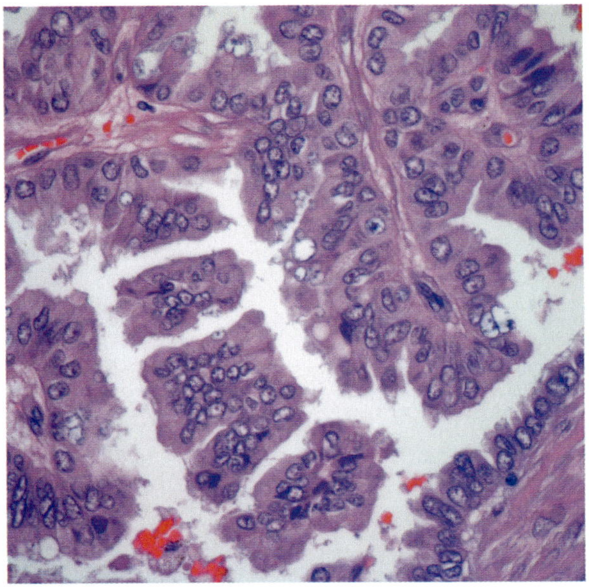

Figure 3-80 High-power view of a papillary adenocarcinoma with cells displaying clearing of the nuclei. Mitotic figures are not very prominent.

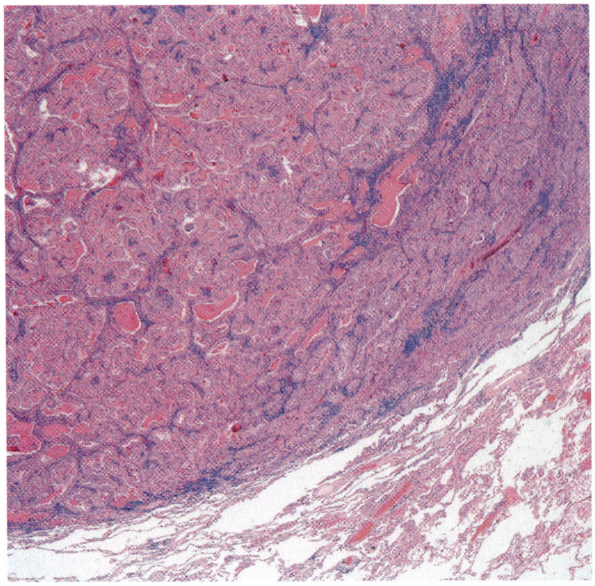

Figure 3-82 Low-power view of an oncocytic papillary adenocarcinoma.

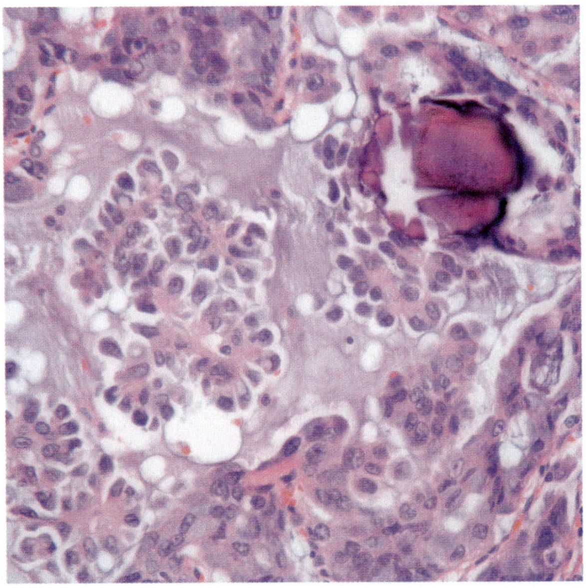

Figure 3-81 Papillary adenocarcinoma showing psammoma bodies.

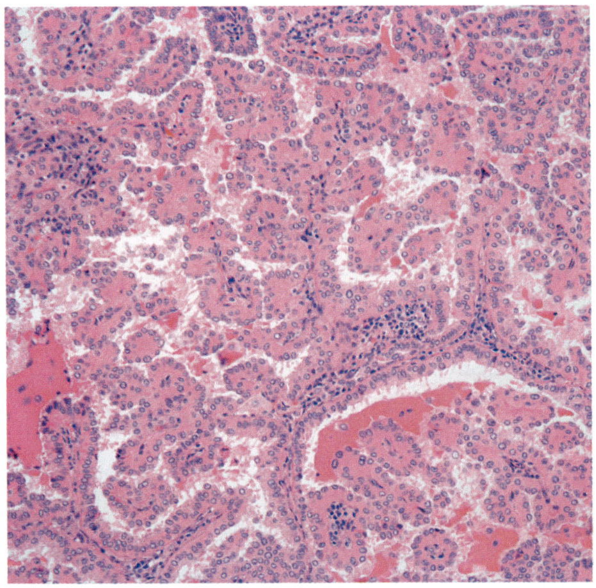

Figure 3-83 Papillary adenocarcinoma with oncocytic change.

Molecular Biology

Despite the relatively low frequency of papillary adenocarcinoma of the lung, molecular biology studies have been performed to determine whether it should be classified as a separate clinicopathologic entity, and to pinpoint differences from other types of lung carcinoma, especially BAC. It has been determined that the rate of occurrence of loss of heterogeneity (LOH) on 3p for papillary adenocarcinoma is approximately 80%, in contrast with 14% for BAC.[112]

Clinical Behavior

The prognosis and survival rate for patients with papillary adenocarcinoma appear to be linked to the clinical staging. In the series presented by Silver and Askin,[111] 75% of the patients experienced a recurrence or were found to have metastatic disease. Patients with early-stage disease at diagnosis tend to fare better; in this series, follow-up (for a mean of 3.4 years) showed that just over 50% of the patients with stage I disease had survived, compared with only 25% of those with stage II disease.

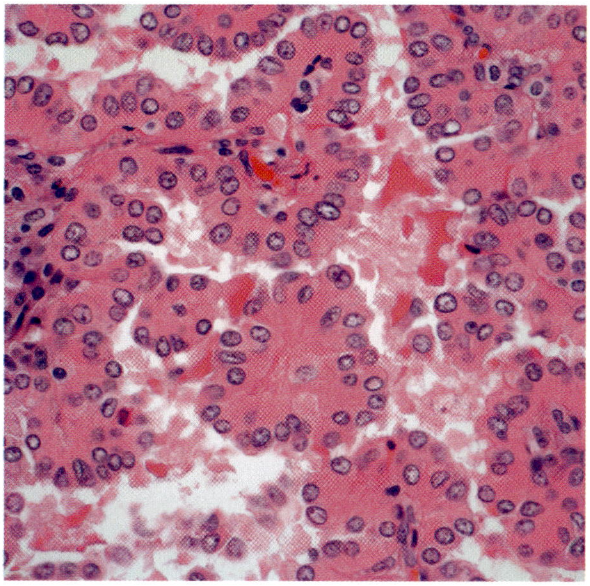

Figure 3-84 High-power magnification of a papillary adenocarcinoma showing prominent oncocytic features.

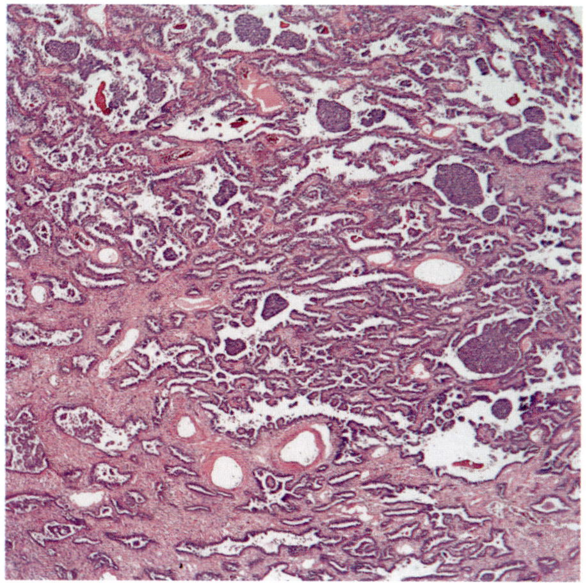

Figure 3-85 Low-power view of a papillary adenocarcinoma with morular component. Note the presence of morules floating in alveolar spaces.

Papillary Adenocarcinoma with Prominent Morular Component

In one series, three cases of the unusual growth pattern of papillary carcinoma known as "papillary adenocarcinoma with prominent morular component" were described in adult patients between the ages of 25 and 68 years.[114] Clinically, these patients presented with clinical signs and symptoms similar to those in any lung carcinoma: cough, dyspnea, and chest pain. No lung or lung segment appears to have a predilection for this tumor.

Gross Features

Size ranges from 2.5 to 3.5 cm in greatest dimension, and the tumor masses are well-defined, soft, and white to tan in color. Evidence of necrosis or hemorrhage is lacking.

Microscopic Features

Like true papillary adenocarcinomas, these tumors have a predominantly papillary architecture. Within the papillary structures, however, small cellular aggregates in the form of "morules" can be detected. These morules are distributed in a haphazard fashion, without attachment to papillary structures (Figs. 3-85 to 3-87). In all of the cases described, areas of conventional adenocarcinoma also were present.

Immunohistochemical Studies

The tumor characteristically shows positive staining for keratin, carcinoembryonic antigen (CEA), and TTF-1 but negative staining for thyroglobulin. TTF-1 staining also is positive in the morular component of the tumor.

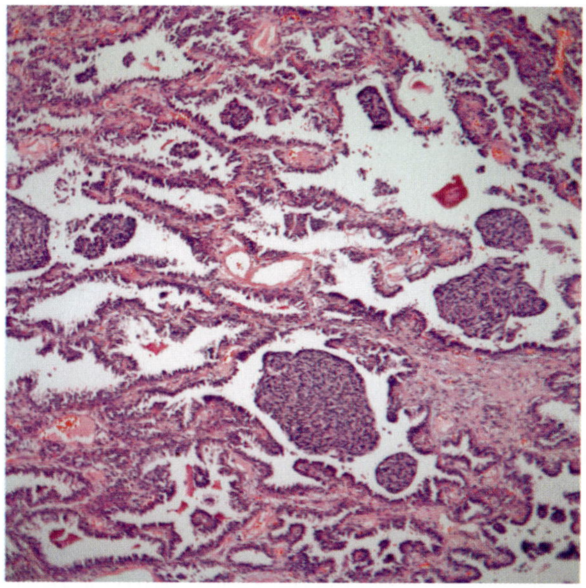

Figure 3-86 High-power view of the morular component in a papillary adenocarcinoma.

Clinical Behavior

All of the patients described underwent surgical resection; however, the follow-up period thus far has been too short to identify a more definitive clinical behavior. It is possible that the clinical behavior is similar to that of true papillary adenocarcinoma.

Micropapillary Adenocarcinoma

The micropapillary variant of adenocarcinoma was first described relatively recently, and only a few series have

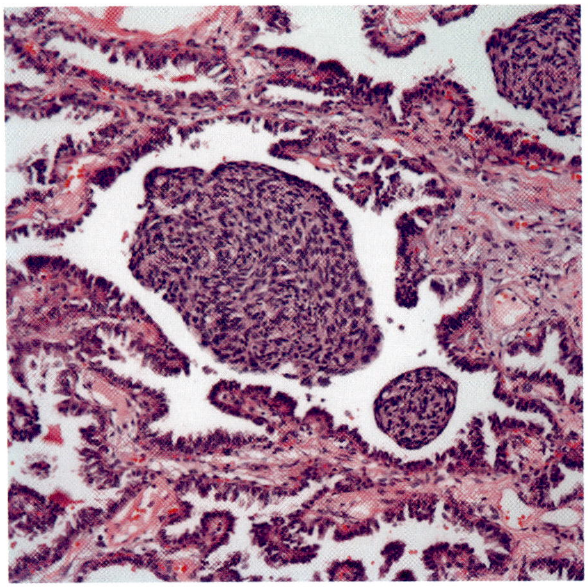

Figure 3-87 Papillary adenocarcinoma. Morules can be seen floating in neoplastic glands without attachment to any structure.

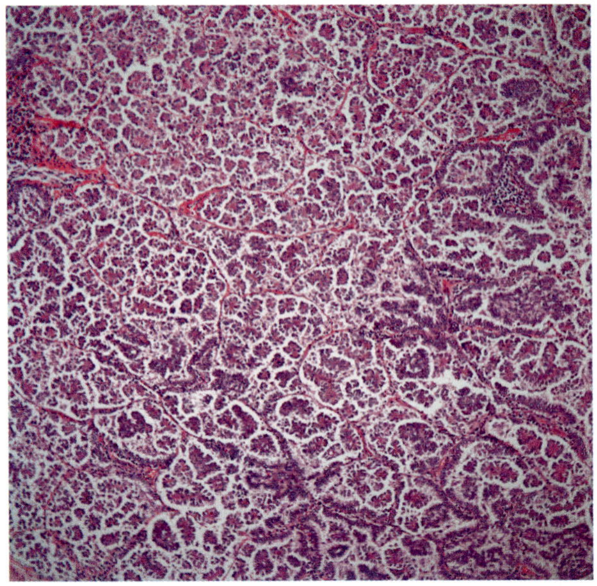

Figure 3-88 Low-power view of micropapillary adenocarcinoma.

been presented in the literature.[115–119] Nevertheless, it is widely accepted that tumors of this variant behave more aggressively than true papillary adenocarcinomas. Metastatic disease has been reported in more than 25% of patients. Therefore, adenocarcinomas must be carefully evaluated for this growth pattern, because its presence indicates possible aggressive clinical behavior. The extent of the micropapillary growth pattern may vary, in some cases appearing rather focal and in others more extensive. Micropapillary features may be associated with any type of adenocarcinoma, and their presence does not reflect the size of the tumor.

Amin and coworkers[115] were the first to report this variant, comparing it with similar tumors in the breast and bladder. In this series of 35 cases, most patients were in late stages of disease (stages III and IV) at clinical presentation. Patients with stage I disease, however, went on to develop metastatic disease in a relatively short period of time, emphasizing the aggressive behavior of these tumors.

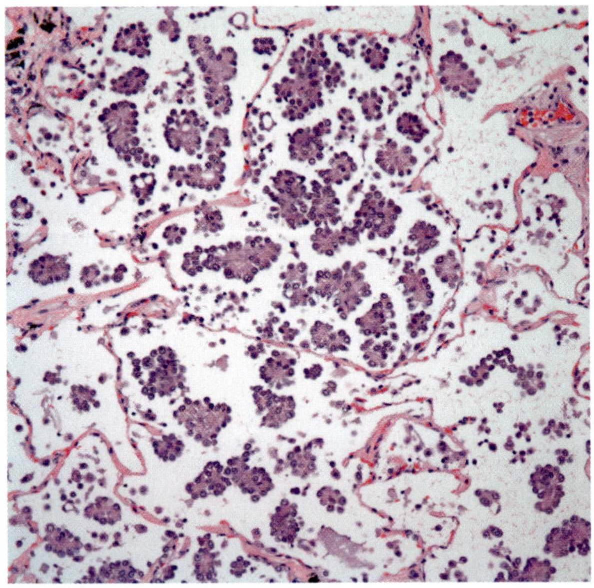

Figure 3-89 Papillary adenocarcinoma. Micropapillae can be seen floating in alveolar spaces.

Microscopic Features

The most important feature distinguishing the papillary from the micropapillary growth patterns is the absence of fibrovascular cores in the micropapillary variant (Figs. 3-88 to 3-90). Micropapillary tumors may display clusters of cells that fill the alveolar spaces and are detached from the lining of the alveolar wall, giving the appearance of free-floating cells. These clusters may vary in size from a few cells to sizable clusters. Micropapillary adenocarcinoma tends to invade vascular spaces, mimicking metastatic disease to the lung. A closer view of the malignant cells will show mild to moderate amounts of amphophilic cytoplasm and round to oval nuclei with inconspicuous nucleoli. Mitotic figures are present but not in large numbers. Although areas of necrosis and hemorrhage may be present, they are not very common.

Immunohistochemical Features

Amin and coworkers[115] conducted immunohistochemical studies in 15 cases, using antibodies for keratin 7, keratin 20, and TTF-1. In 14 of the cases, the tumor showed positive staining for keratin 7, and in 12 cases, positive

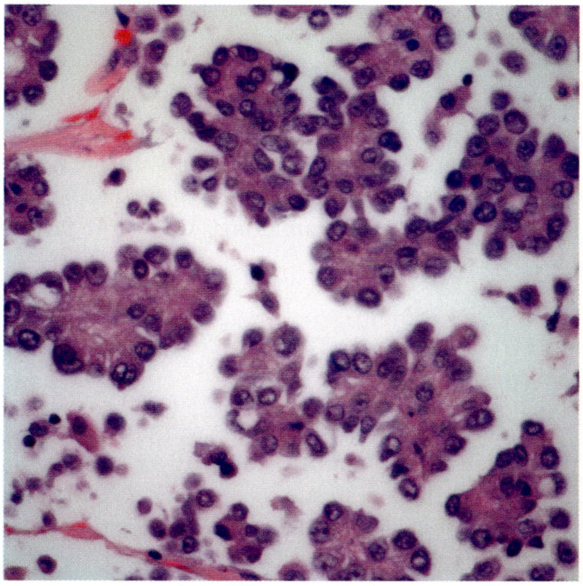

Figure 3-90 Papillary adenocarcinoma. High-power view of micropapillae showing a bland appearance and absence of fibrovascular cores.

staining for TTF-1. Of interest, positive staining for keratin 20 also was seen in 2 cases. Of note, not all of these tumors may show positive staining for TTF-1 or keratin 7. In these cases, good clinical correlation is essential to rule out metastatic lesions to the lung, especially tumors of breast and bladder origin. Thus, it may be necessary to widen the panel of immunohistochemical studies, depending on the circumstances.

Clinical Behavior

As previously stated, micropapillary carcinoma has a tendency to manifest in late stages of disease with metastases to the lymph nodes and pleura, or outside of the thoracic cavity. A majority of the reported cases have been stages III and IV, and the clinical outcome for these patients is related to stage at the time of diagnosis.

Signet Ring Cell Adenocarcinoma

Signet ring cell adenocarcinoma is another unusual variant, and only a few series have been reported.[120–123] No gender predisposition has been documented, and the tumors do not arise in any particular lung or lung segment. The ages of the patients described have ranged from 30 to 75 years. Hayashi[122] concluded that signet ring cell adenocarcinomas are closely related to bronchial gland cell–type adenocarcinoma. Although signet ring cells occasionally may be observed in otherwise conventional adenocarcinomas, in the cases reported, the signet ring cell component has been a predominant feature. Castro and associates[123] included cases in which signet ring cell features made up at least 75% of the tumors. This variant may occur in a central or peripheral location, and clinical signs and symptoms are related to the size and anatomic location of the mass. The tumors are soft and gray in color and sometimes contain areas of hemorrhage and necrosis. Size may vary, ranging from 1 cm to greater than 5 cm in greatest dimension.

Microscopic Features

Two histopathologic growth patterns have been described for signet ring cell adenocarcinoma: acinar and diffuse. In the *acinar* pattern, tumor cells are distributed in small nests separated by thin bands of fibroconnective tissue, which may contain an inflammatory infiltrate (Figs. 3-91 to 3-93). At higher magnification, these nests are seen to be composed of medium-sized cells with clear cytoplasm, and the nuclei are displaced toward the periphery, imparting the signet ring appearance. Nuclear atypia and numerous mitotic figures are not common. In some areas, the tumor cells appear to be filling alveolar spaces. In the *diffuse* pattern, sheets of malignant cells arranged in cords or distributed haphazardly appear to dissect, infiltrate, and destroy areas of normal lung parenchyma. The cytologic features of both growth patterns are similar. Histochemical studies using periodic acid–Schiff (PAS) stain with and without diastase and mucicarmine show strong positive cytoplasmic staining for mucin.

Immunohistochemical Features

Although the cases reported have emphasized the histopathologic growth pattern of signet ring cells, the immunohistochemical studies performed have been limited. Hayashi and associates[122] found that signet ring cell

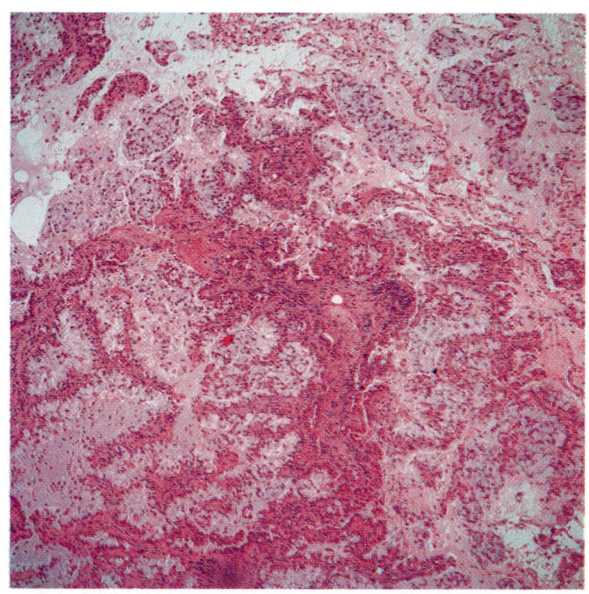

Figure 3-91 Signet ring cell adenocarcinoma of the lung with both acinar and diffuse patterns.

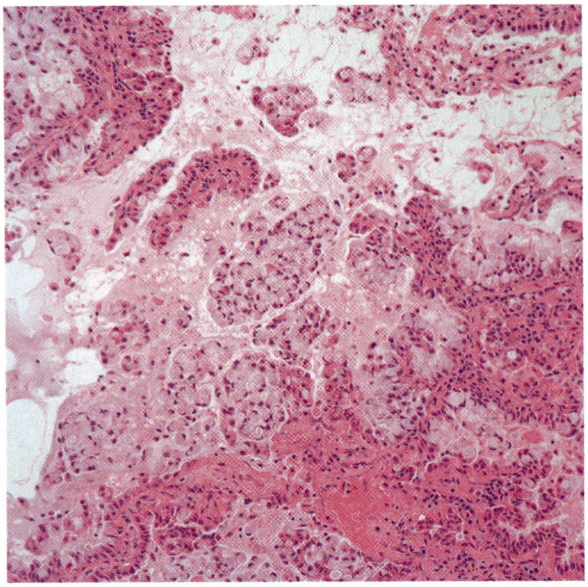

Figure 3-92 Signet ring cell adenocarcinoma showing diffuse growth pattern.

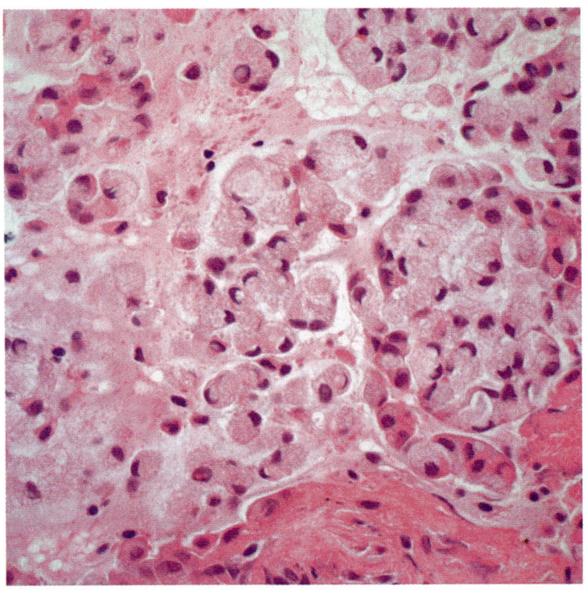

Figure 3-93 High-power view of a signet ring cell adenocarcinoma showing the characteristic cell morphology.

adenocarcinomas of the lung display positive staining for MUC-1 and negative staining for MUC-2, whereas the opposite is true for tumors of gastrointestinal origin. Castro and coworkers[123] performed a limited immunohistochemical study in a few of the cases reported and observed that keratin 7 staining was positive in 50%, TTF-1 showed positive nuclear staining in 100%, and staining for keratin 20 was negative in 100%. When the signet ring cell variant is suspected, the immunohistochemical survey should include keratins 7 and 20, TTF-1 and CDX-2, GCDFP and mammoglobin, to rule out the possibility of a gastrointestinal or breast carcinoma.

Clinical Behavior

As with gastrointestinal tract tumors of similar histologic pattern, these tumors display aggressive clinical behavior. Castro and coworkers[123] reported that 50% of the patients for whom follow-up data were available had died within 12 months. Thus, it is vital to distinguish these tumors from other adenocarcinomas with more favorable histologic features.

"Secretory Endometrioid–Like" Adenocarcinoma

A "secretory endometrioid–like" growth pattern has been recognized recently,[124] and although only a few cases have been reported, the investigators have been able to evaluate many other cases with similar features. These tumors must be regarded as a specific variant of adenocarcinoma in order to distinguish them from fetal adenocarcinoma (pulmonary blastoma, monophasic type)—a distinction that may have important therapeutic considerations. The patients described so far have been adult men and women between the ages of 52 and 81 years. No apparent predilection for any lung or lung segment is recognized. The tumors manifest as central or peripheral lung masses, with clinical signs and symptoms depending on the anatomic location.

Microscopic Features

The low-power view shows a complex glandular proliferation destroying normal lung parenchyma. The glandular architecture is composed of branching tubules and papillae, with a variably dense desmoplastic stroma. Higher magnification reveals a monolayer of cuboidal to columnar cells, ranging in size from medium to large, lining the tubules and papillae. Cytoplasmic clearing, reminiscent of secretory endometrium, is the most striking feature (Figs. 3-94 and 3-95). Areas of necrosis and hemorrhage may alternate in some cases. High mitotic activity and prominent nuclear atypia are not common.

Immunohistochemical Features

Steinhauer[124] reported that these tumors demonstrated positive staining for keratin 7 and TTF-1 and negative staining for keratin 20, Wilms tumor suppressor gene protein-1 (WT-1), chromogranin, and progesterone and estrogen receptors. An important point to keep in mind, however, is that some endometrial and endocervical adenocarcinomas may express TTF-1 in tumor cells.[125]

Clinical Behavior

The clinical behavior of secretory endometrioid–like adenocarcinoma may be closely related to clinical stage at the time of diagnosis.

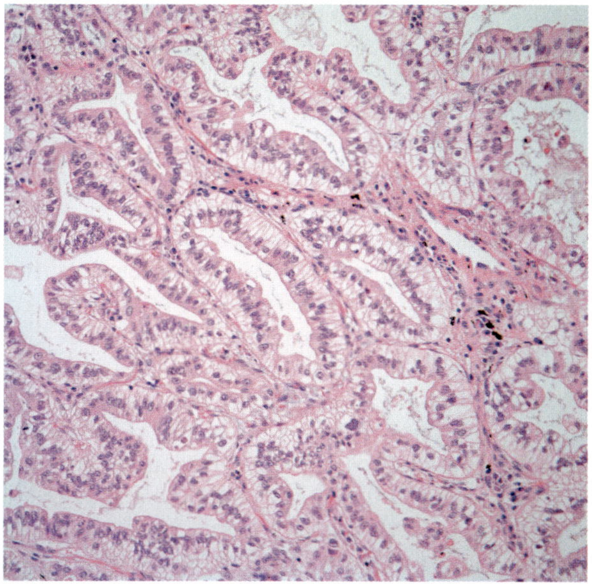

Figure 3-94 Secretory endometrioid–like adenocarcinoma of the lung showing numerous neoplastic glands arranged in a back-to-back pattern.

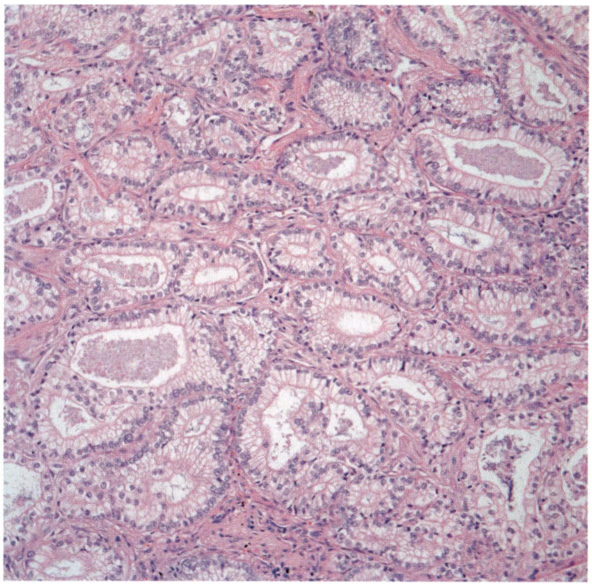

Figure 3-95 Secretory endometrioid–like adenocarcinoma of the lung displaying neoplastic cells with clearing of the cytoplasm.

Hepatoid Adenocarcinoma

The hepatoid histopathologic growth pattern is extremely unusual, and only a few cases have been reported.[126–132] All of these cases have occured in men between the ages of 35 and 82 years. Tumor size ranges from 3 cm to larger than 10 cm in greatest dimension. The production of alpha-fetoprotein is an important feature of this variant.

Microscopic Features

The tumor characteristically displays a neoplastic cellular proliferation arranged in cords or sheets of cells (Figs. 3-96 to 3-98). Higher magnification reveals that these are composed of medium-sized cells with ample eosinophilic cytoplasm and round to oval nuclei, some of which have prominent nucleoli. This cellular proliferation mimics the normal architecture of the liver parenchyma. In some cells, it is possible to identify hyaline globules, which can be more apparent with use of histochemical PAS staining. Necrosis, hemorrhage, and increased mitotic activity are not common in these tumors.

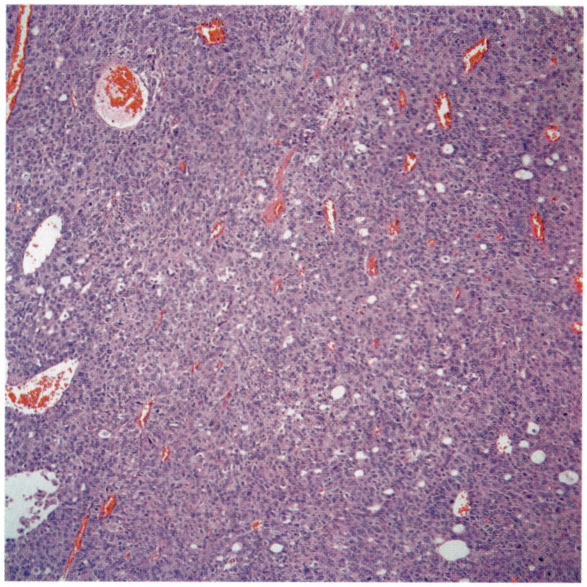

Figure 3-96 Hepatoid adenocarcinoma of the lung showing a solid neoplastic proliferation.

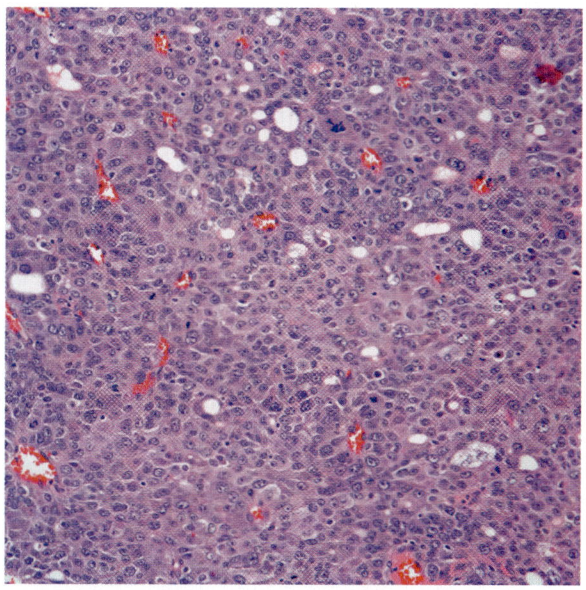

Figure 3-97 Hepatoid adenocarcinoma of the lung displaying medium-sized cells with ample cytoplasm. A few mitotic figures are visible.

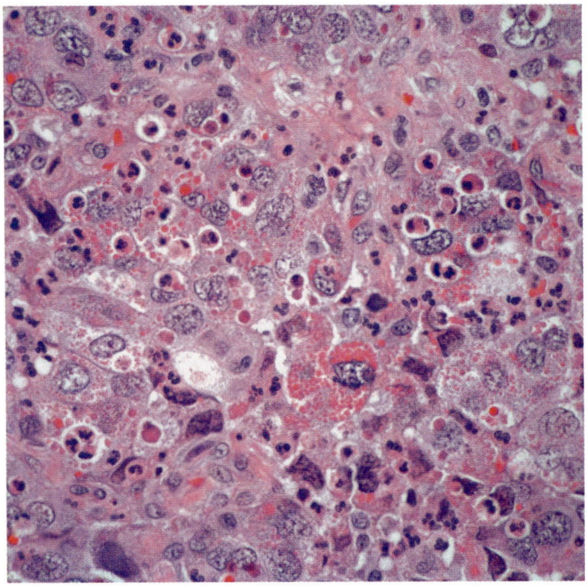

Figure 3-98 Hepatoid adenocarcinoma of the lung showing numerous hyaline extra- and intracellular globules.

Immunohistochemical Features

The most important immunohistochemical feature of hepatoid adenocarcinoma is positive staining for alpha-fetoprotein. Owing to the rarity of these neoplasms, however, more extensive immunohistochemical studies have not been completed.

Clinical Behavior

In the few cases reported, a majority of patients died within 2 years of the initial diagnosis. In some cases, however, the clinical behavior is less aggressive, with survival for longer than 3 years.

LARGE CELL CARCINOMA

By definition, large cell carcinoma is a carcinoma that does not show small cell, adenocarcinoma, or squamous cell differentiation. Large cell carcinoma is not an appropriate diagnosis for every non–small cell carcinoma, however. The use of immunohistochemical studies in small biopsies may reduce the real percentage of cases that are classified as large cell carcinomas. For practical purposes, it may be wise to reserve this diagnosis for cases in which surgical resection confirms that adenocarcinoma and squamous cell carcinoma are definitively absent. In past publications,[133–135] it has been estimated that large cell carcinoma may represent somewhere between 6% and 20% of all lung carcinomas; however, this percentage may be lowered once the current use of ancillary studies is taken into account. It also is important to distinguish large cell carcinoma from the so-called large cell neuroendocrine carcinoma, which must display a neuroendocrine pattern and positive neuroendocrine markers. The diagnosis of large cell carcinoma must be made cautiously, because some "non–small cell carcinomas" may show positive staining for neuroendocrine markers.

In the past, some workers have argued that all "large cell undifferentiated carcinomas of the lung" are actually poorly differentiated adenocarcinomas or squamous cell carcinomas. Churg[133] came to this conclusion after an ultrastructural analysis of seven cases of "large cell carcinoma." Yesner[134] defined large cell carcinoma as a diagnosis of exclusion, arguing that the biology of large cell carcinoma is similar to that of adenocarcinoma, in that both are peripheral in approximately 72% of cases and have similar metastatic patterns. Albain and coworkers,[135] however, found that large cell carcinomas can be either central or peripheral in location and may be more common in female patients. In this particular study, the investigators attempted to divide the cases into two groups demonstrating ultrastructural differentiation toward either adenocarcinoma or squamous cell carcinoma. In 48 cases (approximately one third of the total studied), no such differentiation was encountered. Kodama and associates[136] reported similar findings in an ultrastructural study of 18 cases, only 4 of which did not show any type of differentiation. These studies raise the possibility that the specific diagnosis of large cell carcinoma of the lung is a rare entity, if all of the diagnostic tools currently available are put to use.

Clinical Features

As in other pulmonary carcinomas, clinical signs and symptoms will depend on the anatomic location of the tumor. With central tumors, the patient is more likely to present with signs and symptoms of obstruction, such as hemoptysis, cough, and dyspnea, whereas with large peripheral tumors, the patient may experience chest pain, obstructive pneumonia, or weight loss, among others.

Gross Features

Large cell carcinomas may be located centrally or peripherally and may manifest as a large tumor mass compressing airway structures. The tumors are bulky and light tan in color, and on cut surface they may show areas of necrosis or hemorrhage (Fig. 3-99). They are well defined but not encapsulated and may attain a size larger than 10 cm in greatest dimension, with extensive involvement of lung parenchyma.

Histologic Features

At low magnification, large cell carcinomas display sheets of cells without any particular arrangement. The sheets are composed of a dyscohesive neoplastic cellular

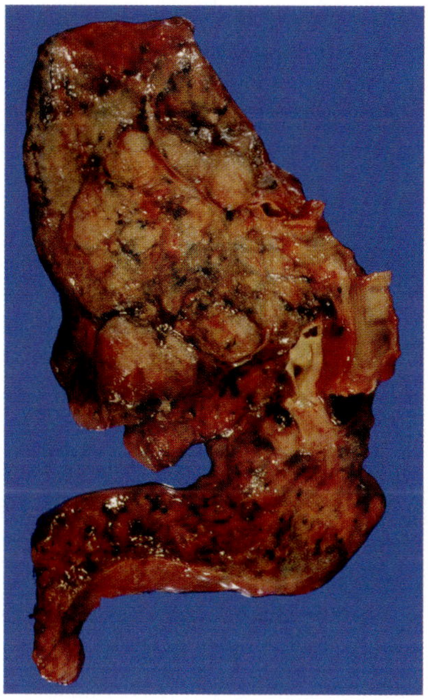

Figure 3-99 Gross specimen of a large cell carcinoma. The tumor occupies extensive areas of lung parenchyma.

proliferation of larger cells with moderate amounts of light eosinophilic cytoplasm, round to oval nuclei, and prominent nucleoli (Fig. 3-100). Mitotic figures and atypical mitoses are commonly seen, as are extensive areas of necrosis or inflammatory exudate. In some cases, osteoclast-like giant cells have been described.[137] Some investigators have observed elaboration and secretion of ectopic gonadotropin by the tumor cells.[138]

Immunohistochemical and Molecular Biology Features

Large cell carcinomas show positive staining for broad-spectrum keratin, low-molecular-weight keratin, keratin 7, and epithelial membrane antigen (EMA). However, they may not show positive staining for TTF-1, p63, and keratin 5/6. Other carcinomatous epitopes that may be useful in distinguishing large cell carcinoma from other malignancies include CEA and CD15.

Zhong and coworkers[139] recently identified the LKB1 mutation in large cell carcinoma of the lung and have argued that the acquired loss of function of the LKB1 mutation may be involved in the pathogenesis of large cell carcinoma.

ADENOSQUAMOUS CARCINOMA

By definition, adenosquamous carcinomas display areas that, by themselves, would be diagnosed as either squamous cell carcinoma or adenocarcinoma on light microscopy. It is likely that many cases that would once have been diagnosed as adenosquamous carcinoma actually represent unusual variants of squamous cell carcinoma with areas of glandular and solid growth patterns. Some tumors may have been incorrectly classified as adenosquamous on the basis of positive mucicarmine staining in solid areas of poorly differentiated squamous cell carcinomas. Thus, accurate evaluation of the incidence of adenosquamous carcinoma is very difficult. Nevertheless, the tumor has been recognized for a number of years as a specific entity with a potentially more aggressive clinical behavior than that observed for conventional squamous cell carcinoma or adenocarcinoma.[140–151] The proportion of either of those components within an adenosquamous carcinoma is debatable and ranges from 5% to 10% in published reports. In practice, they should be present in at least 5% of the entire tumor. This feature may not be obvious in a small biopsy specimen; therefore, the diagnosis of adenosquamous carcinoma is more appropriately left for complete surgical resections.

In 1985, Fitzgibbons and Kern[140] reported a study of 7 cases of adenosquamous cell carcinoma of the lung, and determined that adenosquamous carcinomas represent less than 1% of all lung carcinomas. These workers reviewed 1125 cases of lung carcinoma between the years 1968 and 1984 and identified 21 cases diagnosed as adenosquamous carcinoma; however, only 7 of those 21 cases fulfill the criteria of unequivocal areas of either squamous cell carcinoma or adenocarcinoma. A majority of the tumors were peripheral, and in most cases the predominant tumor was squamous cell carcinoma, either well- or moderately differentiated. The lowest percentage of tumor area recorded for either squamous cell carcinoma or adenocarcinoma was 10%. Although the great majority of cases were diagnosed from material obtained at surgical resection in the form of wedge resection, lobectomy, and pneumonectomy, one case was diagnosed from a biopsy specimen in which the investigators found equal amounts of both components. A majority of the patients had larger tumors (larger than 3 cm in greatest dimension). Using similar criteria, Naunheim and associates[141] studied 20 cases of adenosquamous carcinoma after reviewing 873 cases of lung carcinoma between the years 1974 and 1985 and estimated that adenosquamous carcinoma represents 2.3% of lung carcinomas. Cases diagnosed by biopsy were included, because only 12 of the patients described underwent surgical resection. In two separate studies on adenosquamous carcinoma comprising 103 and 127 patients, respectively, diagnosed with adenosquamous carcinoma between the years 1977 and 1986, Sridhar and colleagues[142,143] estimated the occurrence of adenosquamous carcinoma at 8% of lung carcinomas. Case selection in these studies[142] differed from that in the study by Fitzgibbons and Kern.[140] Sridhar's group[142] included mostly biopsy material (91 cases) and cytology specimens (12 cases) and did not specify criteria for diagnosis. Therefore, it is likely that a sizable

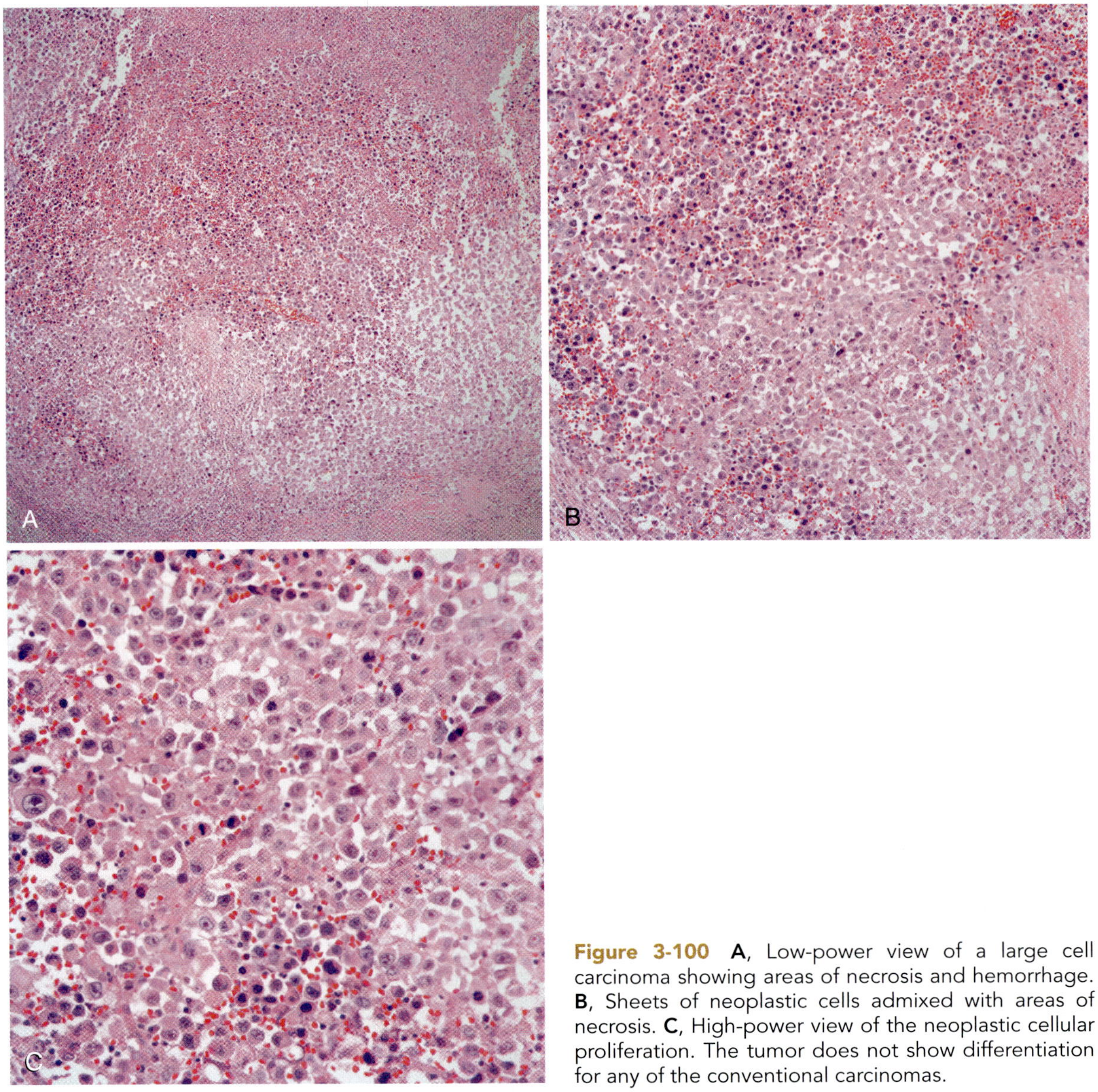

Figure 3-100 **A**, Low-power view of a large cell carcinoma showing areas of necrosis and hemorrhage. **B**, Sheets of neoplastic cells admixed with areas of necrosis. **C**, High-power view of the neoplastic cellular proliferation. The tumor does not show differentiation for any of the conventional carcinomas.

percentage of the cases included may not have been true adenosquamous carcinomas. Takamori and associates[144] presented one of the largest series of adenosquamous carcinomas, identifying 56 cases diagnosed after surgical resection of 2160 surgical resections for lung carcinoma. These workers estimated a 2.6% occurrence and included only cases with a minimum of 5% of the opposite histologic component. They determined that adenosquamous carcinoma displays a more aggressive clinical behavior than that typical for adenocarcinoma or squamous cell carcinoma, particularly in stages I and II.

Clinical Features

Adenosquamous carcinoma manifests with signs and symptoms similar to those of other lung carcinomas, including cough, dyspnea, hemoptysis, pneumonia, chest pain, and weight loss. No particular clinical setting is predictive of a diagnosis of adenosquamous carcinoma.

Gross Features

Like adenocarcinoma or squamous cell carcinoma, adenosquamous carcinoma may manifest as a peripheral or central tumor, which may range in size from 1 cm to larger than 10 cm in greatest dimension. Some reports have noted a more common peripheral location; nevertheless, the tumor may arise in either anatomic location. No specific gross feature has been documented that distinguishes adenosquamous carcinoma from other non–small cell carcinomas.

Histologic Features

As previously stated, adenosquamous carcinoma is characterized by the presence of unequivocal areas of squamous cell carcinoma and adenocarcinoma that, alone, would lead to a diagnosis of the tumor as such (Fig. 3-101). The proportion of either of those components should be at least 5%. The squamous cell component is more likely to be well- or moderately differentiated, with identifiable keratinization and intercellular bridges. Likewise, in the adenocarcinomatous component, glandular or tubular differentiation should still be visible. The two components may merge, and the transition between them will often be subtle, without any abrupt change. When two distinct tumor nodules are visible, one of squamous cell carcinoma and the other of adenocarcinoma, the possibility of two separate tumors should be considered.

Immunohistochemical and Molecular Biology Features

Adenosquamous tumors may show positive immunostaining for the markers that indicate its separate components: p63 and keratin 5/6 in squamous cell carcinomas, and TTF-1 in adenocarcinomas. Staining for CD44, CD44v6, and CD44v7-8 also has been positive in the squamous cell component of adenosquamous carcinoma; however, these antibodies are not reliable in poorly differentiated tumors.[152]

Kanazawa and coworkers[153] compared the genetic alterations of p53 and K-ras chromosomal abnormalities at 9p21 and 9q31-32. These workers found the same mutation of p53 in both components, with p53 overexpression, and suggested a monoclonal transition from squamous cell carcinoma to adenocarcinoma. Kang and

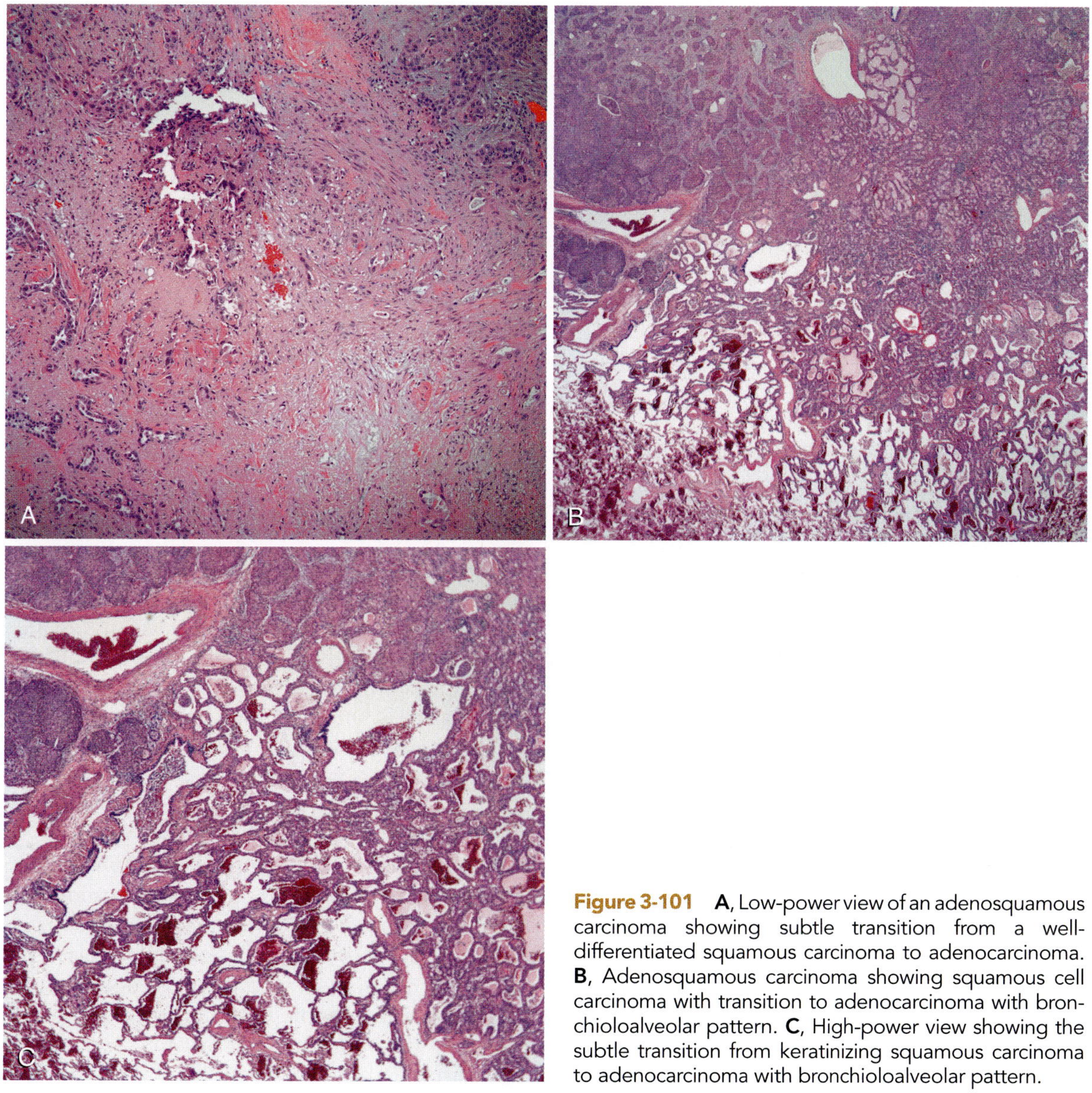

Figure 3-101 **A**, Low-power view of an adenosquamous carcinoma showing subtle transition from a well-differentiated squamous carcinoma to adenocarcinoma. **B**, Adenosquamous carcinoma showing squamous cell carcinoma with transition to adenocarcinoma with bronchioloalveolar pattern. **C**, High-power view showing the subtle transition from keratinizing squamous carcinoma to adenocarcinoma with bronchioloalveolar pattern.

associates[154] studied the mutation status of EGFR kinase domain from exons 18 to 21 in 25 cases of adenosquamous carcinoma and found identical EGFR mutations in both components, suggesting the possibility of monoclonality in the histogenesis of adenosquamous carcinoma. In a single case, however, Liang and colleagues[155] found that trisomy 12 correlates with elevated expression of p21ras.

LYMPHOEPITHELIOMA-LIKE CARCINOMA

Lymphoepithelioma-like carcinoma (LELC) occurs rarely as a primary carcinoma of the lung and is the counterpart of a similar tumor in the head and neck, undifferentiated carcinoma or Schmincke tumor. It also has been described in several other areas within the thoracic cavity, including the thymus, as well as outside of the thoracic cavity.

The real incidence of this tumor as a primary lung carcinoma is difficult to assess, owing to its rarity and demographic distribution. LELC of the lung has been described predominantly in Asian patients, mostly as individual case reports, with only a few small series of cases.[156–164] Begin and colleagues[156] are credited for the first description, in a 40-year-old female nonsmoker of Asian background with a lung tumor that histologically resembled a nasopharyngeal tumor. The immunologic profile was suggestive of EBV infection. Han and coworkers[157] presented one of the largest series, comparing 32 cases of LELC with conventional non–small cell carcinomas of the lung. In Han's series, tumors were more common in men than in women, patient age ranged from 39 to 73 years, and a majority of patients were in early stages of disease (stages I and II). These workers concluded that LELC carries a better prognosis than that for conventional non–small cell carcinomas, even in late-stage disease. Tumor necrosis (>5%) and tumor recurrence were associated with poor prognosis. In their series of 11 cases of LELC, Chan and colleagues[158] reported similar patient demographics and concluded that LELC of the lung may demonstrate variable and possibly aggressive clinical behavior. Butler and associates[159] reported a small series of four cases in adults (three women and one man). Three of the patients were white, and one was of Asian background. These investigators found a more favorable outcome.

Although the great majority of cases described occur in adults, LELC also has been reported in the pediatric age group. Curcio and associates[165] described a case in which an 8-year-old child of Asian background underwent pneumonectomy and chemotherapy for a primary LELC of the lung. In situ hybridization studies demonstrated nuclear positivity for Epstein-Barr virus (EBV)–encoded small RNA-1 (EBER-1) in tumor cells, whereas the adjacent lymphocytes showed negative findings. Other reports have been more focused on the identification of EBV,[166–171] which appears to be strongly associated with the development of LELC in the lung. In most cases in which EBV has been found in association with LELC, the patients are of Asian background. The tumor appears not to be related to tobacco use. In 1991, Gal and colleagues[166] described a single case of LELC of the lung, identifying EBV in the carcinoma cells but not in the lymphoid stroma. These workers concluded that this finding suggests a possible oncogenic relationship between EBV and LELC of the lung. Chen and coworkers[169] performed a study of 127 cases of non–small cell carcinomas of the lung, including LELC (5 cases), and encountered positive nuclear staining for EBER-1 in non–small cell carcinomas other than LELC. Although the intensity of staining was stronger in LELC, squamous cell carcinomas also showed positive staining. These investigators estimated that approximately 8% of non–small cell carcinomas also may show positive staining for EBER-1 but also concluded that EBV infection may play a different role in the tumorigenesis of primary LELC of the lung from that in development of the conventional variants of non–small cell carcinoma.

Castro and associates[170] analyzed the relationship between EBV and LELC of the lung in 6 white patients using in situ hybridization studies and found that all of the cases were negative for EBV, suggesting absence of any relationship between EBV and LELC of the lung in white patients. More recently, Chang and colleagues[171] analyzed 23 cases of pulmonary LELC and documented that a higher EBV serologic grade correlates with a larger tumor size. These investigators also reported that nearly all cases had Bcl-2-oncoprotein expression, and that latent membrane protein-1, p53, and c-erb B-2 expression was low.

Clinical Features

No specific symptomatology is associated with this neoplasm. Patients may present with cough, dyspnea, or hemoptysis or may be completely asymptomatic, and the tumor is detected by chest radiologic examination during routine examination. It appears that at least 50% of the patients are in the early stages of disease (stages I and II) at presentation.

Histologic Features

The hallmark of this neoplasm is a lymphocytic background that at low magnification may mimic an inflammatory reaction. The inflammatory stroma is composed predominantly of mature lymphocytes, but in some cases plasma cells also may be present. Admixed with this lymphocytic or lymphoplasmacytic stroma are sheets of cells growing in ribbons or small islands. The neoplastic cellular proliferation is composed of medium-sized, round to oval cells with indistinct cellular borders and moderate amounts of cytoplasm. The nucleus is round, and vesiculation of the nuclei may be observed. Many cells have prominent nucleoli, and mitotic figures are readily identified (Fig. 3-102). Although necrosis and hemorrhage are not common, they do occur in a small proportion of cases. The neoplastic cellular proliferation often appears to be haphazardly distributed in the lymphoid stroma, without any particular pattern.

Differential Diagnosis

The most important consideration in the differential diagnosis for LELC is metastasis from a primary nasopharyngeal tumor. Because it is similar in histology to LELC, a good clinical history is vital in distinguishing between the two. If a marked lymphocytic stroma is identified, lymphoma also may enter into the differential diagnosis and should be ruled out using immunostaining for markers of epithelial differentiation.

Immunohistochemical Features

Immunostaining for epithelial markers, including keratins and EMA, may be of help in diagnosing LELC. This tumor also shows positive staining for lymphoid markers, including leukocyte common antigen (LCA) and Bcl-2. Perhaps the most important study to perform, although not for diagnostic purposes, is in situ hybridization for EBV, especially for patients of Asian background.

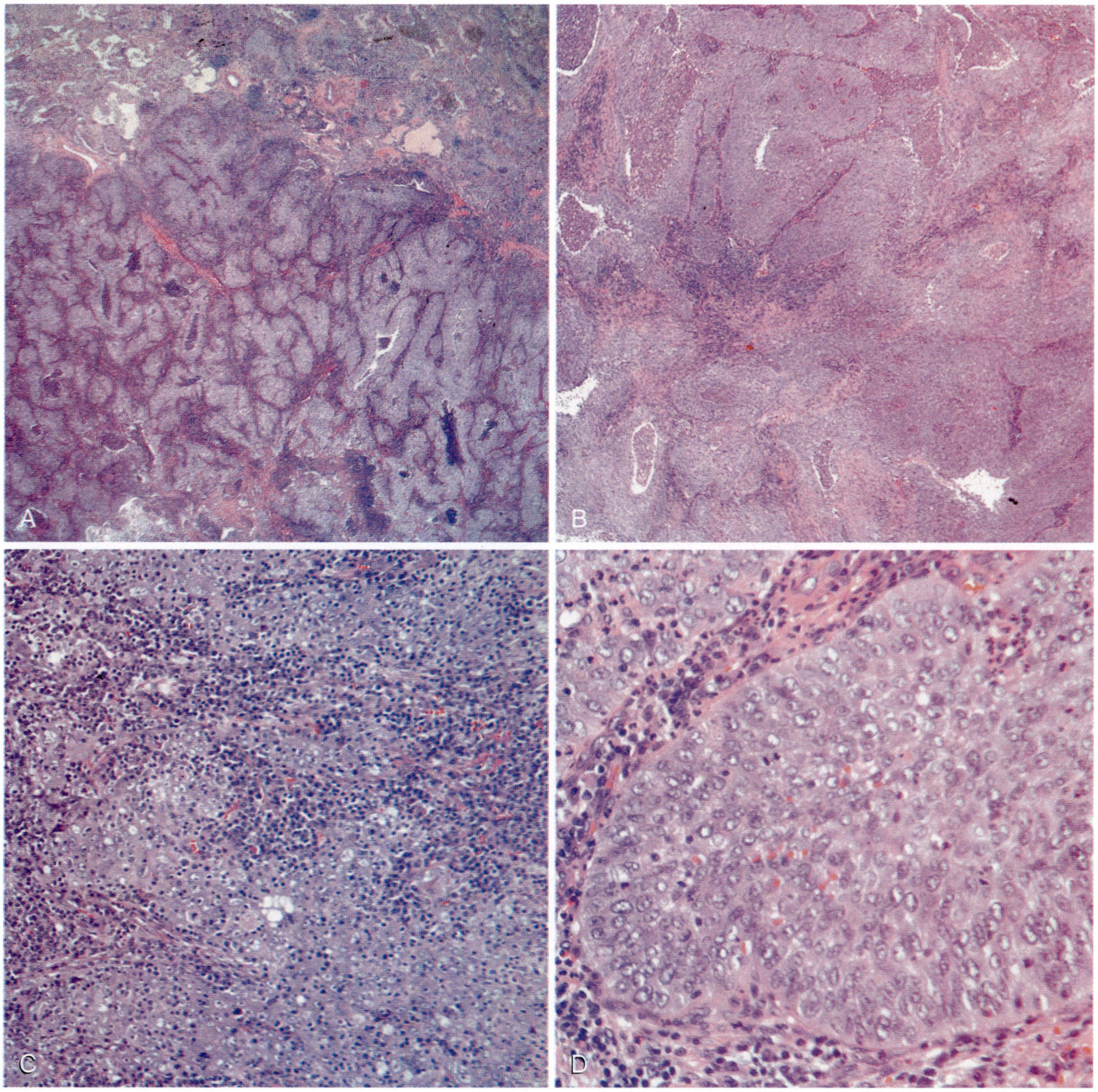

Figure 3-102 Lymphoepithelioma-like carcinoma. **A**, Low-power view showing a well-demarcated tumor. **B**, Tumor islands are admixed with an inflammatory reaction. **C**, Neoplastic cells without any particular arrangement are admixed with inflammatory cells. **D**, High-power view showing tumor cells with prominent nucleoli and increased mitotic activity.

RHABDOID CARCINOMA

Primary lung neoplasms resembling those initially described in the kidney as malignant rhabdoid tumors have been well documented in the literature.[172–182] Malignant rhabdoid tumors appear to occur in a ubiquitous distribution, and those arising outside the kidney have been referred to as "extrarenal rhabdoid tumors" or "pseudorhabdoid tumors." The question of whether rhabdoid carcinoma of the lung is a specific clinicopathologic entity or a growth pattern is beyond the scope of this discusssion.

These tumors are rare as primary lung neoplasms, and although their proper classification is controversial, herein they are regarded as *rhabdoid carcinomas*, rather than the ambiguous designations of "rhabdoid phenotype" and "dedifferentiated carcinoma." Rhabdoid carcinoma should be considered to be a growth pattern arising in a heterogeneous group of tumors, including adenocarcinoma, large cell carcinoma, or neuroendocrine carcinomas. As Wick and colleagues[182] have demonstrated, however, the clinical setting may dictate a particular interpretation. Although by light microscopy, primary lung tumors display the rhabdoid feature in a proportion of no less than 10%, on immunohistochemical studies, the tumor cells may show positive staining for epithelial markers (keratin and EMA), and ultrastructural studies may reveal cytoplasmic accumulation of intermediate filaments or mitochondria. In a majority of cases, however, an additional component of conventional non–small cell carcinoma also is detected, suggesting that this rhabdoid component is a growth pattern, rather than a specific clinicopathologic entity in the lung.

Rubenchik and associates[172] were the first to describe a "rhabdoid tumor" in the lung—an intrapulmonary tumor in a 74-year-old man. The tumor displayed rhabdoid features, and electron microscopy revealed the cytoplasmic intermediate filaments that characterize malignant rhabdoid tumors of the kidney. As more cases have been documented in the lung, it has been noted that most of the time, even when the major portion of the tumor is of the rhabdoid phenotype, the light microscopic features of adenocarcinoma, large cell carcinoma, or sarcomatoid carcinoma can still be identified. Malignant rhabdoid tumors also may show sarcomatoid areas, making diagnosis even more difficult. Because rhabdoid features are associated with other more conventional variants of lung carcinoma, the term *dedifferentiated phenotype* has been proposed for these tumors.[175] Although some investigators have suggested a good prognosis for these tumors, accurate staging at the time of diagnosis is likely to play a more significant role in patient outcomes.

Histologic Features

As its name implies, rhabdoid carcinoma resembles the so-called malignant rhabdoid tumors of the kidney. At low magnification, the destruction of normal lung parenchyma is apparent, and the tumor appears well demarcated but not encapsulated. It has a tendency to grow in sheets of tumor cells, in a dyscohesive or vaguely nested pattern. At high magnification, the neoplastic cells are seen to be large, with abundant eosinophilic cytoplasm and round to oval nuclei. In some cells, the nuclei are located toward the periphery, whereas in others they are more centrally located, with prominent nucleoli (Fig. 3-103). Other unusual features may include a spindle cell (sarcomatous) component or multinucleated giant cells. In some cases, areas of more conventional non–small cell carcinoma may be identified, although they may be focal. The diagnosis of rhabdoid carcinoma can be accomplished in a small biopsy specimen; however, a resected specimen is preferable, so that many sections may be examined for areas of more conventional carcinoma.

Immunohistochemical Features

In a majority of cases, staining for epithelial markers (keratins and EMA) has yielded positive results; however, the positive staining may be focal. CD34, CD56, actin, vimentin, and rarely desmin also may stain positively. Myoglobin staining has not been reported to be positive in rhabdoid carcinomas.

Differential Diagnosis

Because the lung is a common site for metastatic tumors, it is important to address this possibility in diagnosing rhabdoid carcinomas. Malignant melanomas and sarcomas are common metastatic tumors in the lung, and both may display a rhabdoid growth pattern. Immunohistochemical studies, including immunostaining for S-100 protein, HMB-45, melan A, myoglobin, caldesmon, sox2, and others, should be used to rule out this possibility. A good clinical history also is valuable in weighing the possibility of metastatic disease.

SARCOMATOID CARCINOMA AND PLEOMORPHIC CARCINOMA

Sarcomatoid carcinoma and pleomorphic carcinoma are presented together in this section because of their similarity in histopathologic characteristics. Some workers believe that these tumors are two separate clinical entities; others argue that they are part of the spectrum of differentiation of the same tumor. Tumors without a heterologous component as seen on light microscopy (e.g., chondrosarcoma, osteosarcoma, rhabdomyosarcoma) are

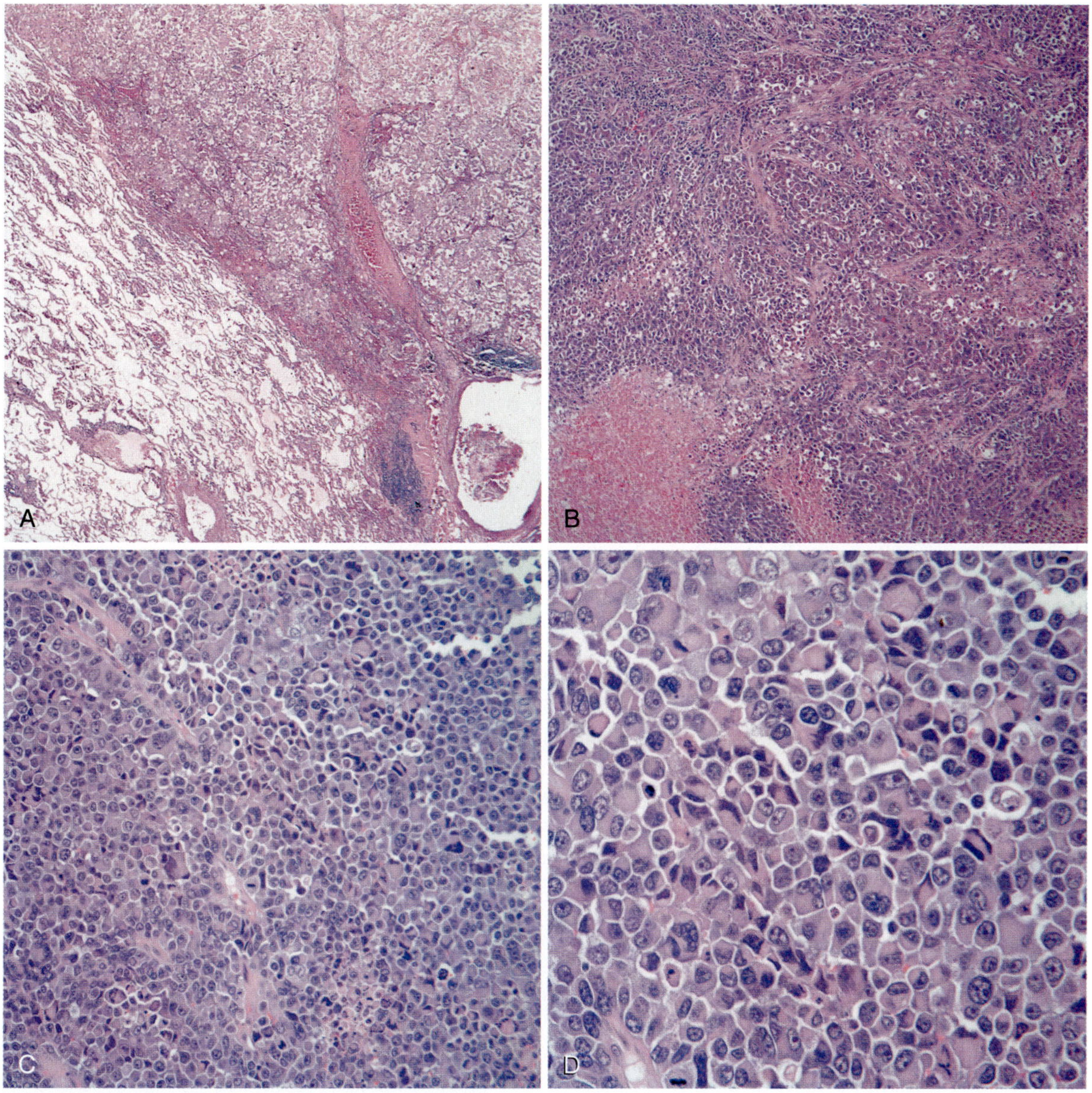

Figure 3-103 **A**, Pulmonary rhabdoid carcinoma. A well-defined tumor mass can be seen. **B**, Rhabdoid carcinoma with areas of necrosis. **C**, Rhabdoid carcinoma with prominent cellular atypia. **D**, High-power view of a rhabdoid carcinoma showing the typical histologic features of larger cells with ample cytoplasm and prominent nucleoli.

not considered here because they are discussed with carcinosarcomas in Chapter 6.

By definition, sarcomatoid/pleomorphic growth pattern designation is reserved for tumors that display a malignant epithelial spindle cell component almost exclusively. The following discussion attempts to differentiate sarcomatoid carcinoma from pleomorphic carcinoma as much as possible. Previously, sarcomatoid carcinoma has been classified as spindle cell carcinoma, carcinoma with pseudosarcomatous stroma, or metaplastic carcinoma, and pleomorphic carcinoma has been described as giant cell carcinoma, sarcomatoid carcinoma, carcinoma with pseudosarcomatous stroma, and pseudosarcomatous carcinoma.

In 1988, Humphrey and associates[183] reported eight cases of pulmonary carcinoma with sarcomatoid component. Although admitting that spindle cell squamous cell carcinoma would be a less controversial diagnosis for these tumors, these workers proposed that pulmonary carcinomas exhibiting evidence of epithelial differentiation in the sarcomatoid component be termed *spindle cell carcinomas*, whereas those in which malignant cartilage, bone, or muscle can be identified should be termed *carcinosarcomas*. Matsui and colleagues[184] reported three cases of spindle cell carcinoma of the lung (two of "monophasic" spindle cell carcinomas and one of adenosquamous carcinoma with spindle cell component), in which the tumors expressed keratin and vimentin in differing degrees.

These investigators concluded that the spindle cell component displays a spectrum of phenotypes originating from squamous cell carcinoma and designated "monophasic" spindle cell carcinoma as an extreme phenotype of squamous cell carcinoma mimicking mesenchymal differentiation.

In a more focused study of sarcomatoid carcinomas of the lung, Ro and coworkers[185] analyzed 14 cases for which they provided more specific criteria for inclusion: (1) the concurrent presence of malignant epithelial and sarcomatoid spindle cell components and (2) positive immunoreactivity for antikeratin antibodies or ultrastructural demonstration of epithelial differentiation in sarcomatoid tumors in which the epithelial component was inconspicuous. The patients were between the ages of 43 and 78 years, and 12 of the 14 patients were men. Histologically, the most common growth pattern in the sarcomatoid component of these tumors was malignant fibrous histiocytoma in 10 cases. Two cases displayed a fibrosarcomatous pattern, and another two showed an unclassified sarcomatous component. A majority of the patients were in late stages of disease (11 patients had stage III or IV disease). On the basis of these findings, the investigators concluded that primary tumors in the lung showing extensive "sarcomatoid" component should be carefully evaluated for epithelial differentiation using immunohistochemical or electron microscopic studies, and that sarcomatoid carcinomas of the lung are aggressive neoplasms that usually manifest in late stages.

The term *pleomorphic carcinoma* was introduced by Fishback and coworkers,[186] in an attempt to encompass all cases previously designated as spindle cell carcinomas or giant cell carcinomas.[187–195] These investigators presented a study of 78 patients, comprising 57 men and 21 women, between the ages of 35 and 83 years (mean, 62 years). Clinically, the patients presented with variable symptomatology including chest pain, cough, and hemoptysis. A small percentage of patients (14%) were asymptomatic. Almost one half of the patients presented with stage I and stage II disease (41% with stage I and 6% with stage II disease); 39% had stage III disease, and 12% had stage IV disease. Histologically, only 22% of the cases studied showed only a spindle or a giant cell component (or both); the remaining tumors showed foci of adenocarcinoma (45%), large cell carcinoma (25%), or squamous cell carcinoma (8%). These workers found that 53 of 69 patients in whom clinical follow-up was available survived no longer than 6 years (mean, 23 months; median, 10 months). In addition, a significant shortening of survival was observed for patients with tumors larger than 5 cm, clinical stage higher than I, and lymph node involvement. The last feature was the single most important prognostic factor, whereas the presence of adenocarcinoma or squamous cell carcinoma did not influence the prognosis. This report demonstrates that spindle cell or giant cell carcinoma may be observed in association with other histologic subtypes besides squamous cell carcinoma.

Some researchers have argued that pleomorphic carcinoma may represent a genetically distinct entity, separate from adenocarcinoma or squamous cell carcinoma. Przygodzki and coworkers[196] performed comparative DNA sequencing and immunohistochemical analysis in 22 cases of pleomorphic carcinoma, 42 cases of squamous cell carcinoma, and 97 cases of adenocarcinoma. These workers found that in pleomorphic carcinoma, p53 mutations were more common in exon 7, whereas in adenocarcinoma and squamous cell carcinoma, p53 mutations were more common in exon 8. In addition, K-ras-2 mutations were present in only a few pleomorphic carcinomas (9%, or 2 of the 22 cases studied), whereas they were more common in adenocarcinoma (36%, or 35 of the 97 cases studied); they were not present at all in squamous cell carcinoma.

Gross Features

No specific gross features are recognized to distinguish sarcomatoid/pleomorphic carcinoma from other non–small cell carcinomas. These tumors can attain a large size, however, and in many series the patients present almost exclusively in late stages of disease. The tumors can occupy large portions of the lung parenchyma, because they can reach more than 10 cm in greatest dimension (Fig. 3-104). On cut surface, they may be tan in color with a homogeneous surface, with or without areas of necrosis or hemorrhage. They can appear in either a central or a peripheral location.

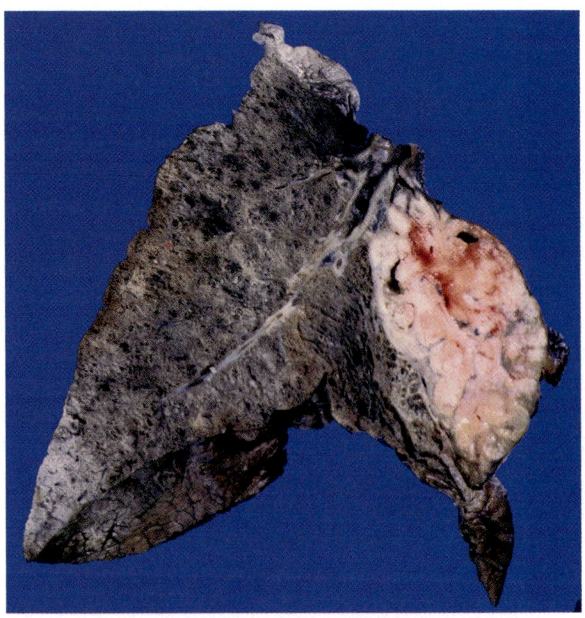

Figure 3-104 Pleomorphic carcinoma of the lung, gross specimen. The tumor displays a tan cut surface with focal areas of hemorrhage.

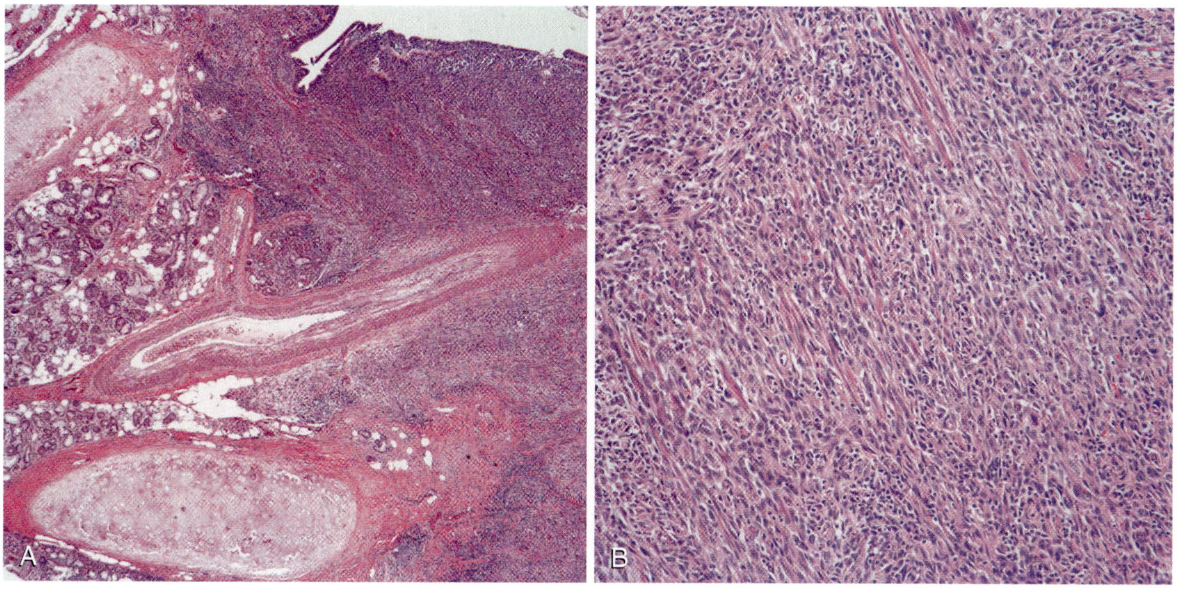

Figure 3-105 **A**, Sarcomatoid carcinoma in a central location, showing a spindle cell proliferation. **B**, Malignant spindle cell proliferation mimicking a sarcoma.

Histologic Features

The most salient histopathologic feature is the presence of a spindle cell proliferation that can be arranged in a fascicular pattern, mimicking any of the conventional sarcomas of soft tissues (Fig. 3-105). The cells are elongated, sometimes displaying a "cigar"-type nucleus and inconspicuous nucleoli. Mitotic figures are easily identifiable, and atypical forms are common, as are areas of necrosis and hemorrhage. In cases that have been reported under the rubric of pleomorphic carcinoma, the tumors display essentially the same histologic characteristics as those described for sarcomatoid carcinomas, except for the additional component of multinucleated malignant giant cells, which can be bi-, tri-, or multinucleated (Fig. 3-106). No heterologous component should be present for this diagnosis, however.

Immunohistochemical and Ultrastructural Features

The use of immunohistochemical studies should help distinguish these tumors from true sarcomas. Positive staining for epithelial markers such as keratins and EMA has been reported in these tumors. On the basis of our own

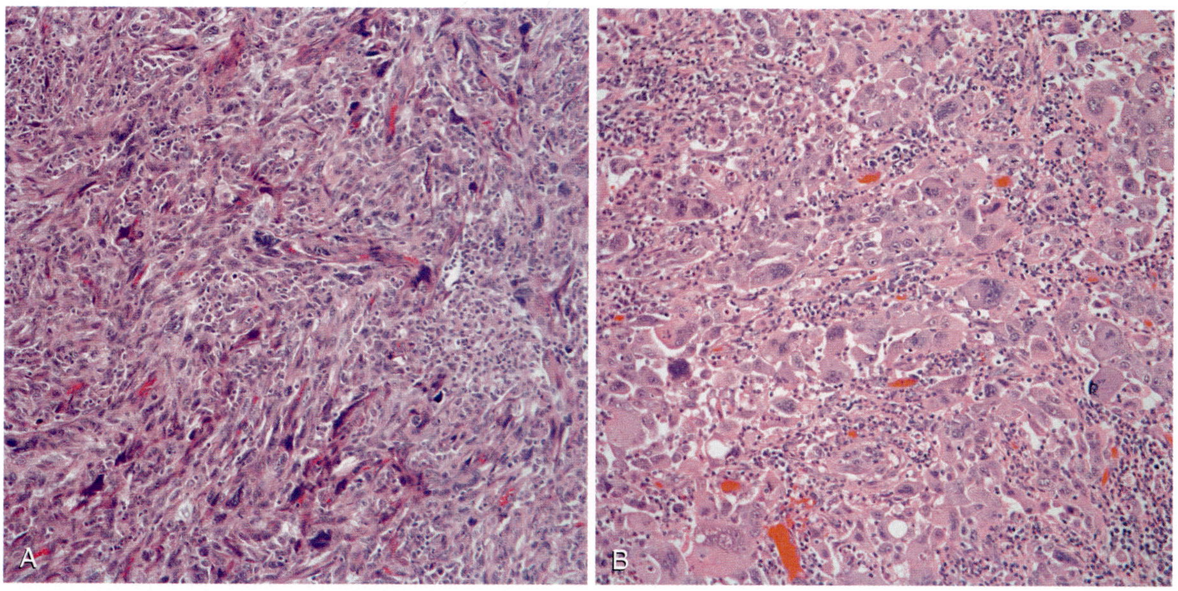

Figure 3-106 **A**, Pleomorphic carcinoma showing spindle cells admixed with multinucleated giant cells. **B**, Pleomorphic carcinoma with marked presence of multinucleated giant cells.
Continued

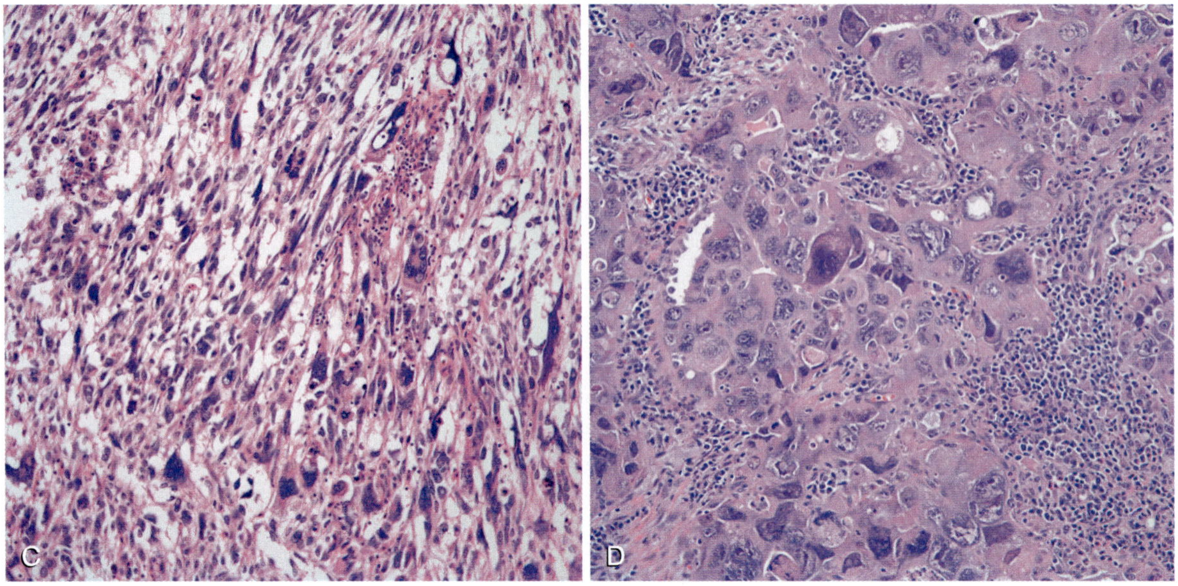

Figure 3-106—cont'd **C**, Pleomorphic carcinoma with dyscohesive spindle cells admixed with multinucleated giant cells. **D**, Pleomorphic carcinoma showing epithelioid areas admixed with malignant multinucleated giant cells.

observations, actin and vimentin also may stain positively. Staining for desmin, myoglobin, caldesmon, and CD31 should be negative. Ultrastructurally, tumor cells may show epithelial differentiation by displaying tonofilaments or desmosomes.

CLEAR CELL CARCINOMA

The presence of a clear cell component in pulmonary carcinomas has been reported in the past. Such clear cell changes, however, do not constitute a specific clinicopathologic entity; rather, clear cells should be considered to be a histopathologic feature that may be present in many tumors, including adenocarcinoma, large cell carcinoma, and squamous cell carcinoma.

As suggested by other investigators,[197,198] the presence of clear cells, in and of itself, does not appear to affect prognosis. Tumors displaying clear cell change should be classified into one of the major groups of lung carcinomas.

REFERENCES

1. Rosado-de-Christenson ML, Templeton PA, Moran CA. Bronchogenic carcinoma: radiologic/pathologic correlation. *Radiographics*. 1994;14:429–446.
2. Travis WD, Travis LB, Devesa SS. Lung cancer. *Cancer*. 1995;75:191–202.
3. Devesa SS, Shaw GL, Blot WJ. Changing patterns of lung cancer incidence by histological type. *Cancer Epidemiol Biomarkers Prev*. 1991;1:29–34.
4. Aronchick JM. Lung cancer: epidemiology and risk factors. *Semin Roentgenol*. 1990;25:5–11.
5. Gritz ER. Lung cancer: now, more than ever, a feminist issue. *CA Cancer J Clin*. 1993;43:197–199.
6. Rubin SA. Lung cancer: past, present, and future. *J Thorac Imaging*. 1991;7:1–8.
7. Garfinkel L, Silverberg E. Lung cancer and smoking trends in the United States over the past 25 years. *CA Cancer J Clin*. 1991;41:137–145.
8. Stanley K, Stjernswärd J. Lung cancer—a worldwide health problem. *Chest*. 1989;96(suppl 1):1S–5S.
9. Wahbah M, Boroumand N, Castro C, El-Zeky F, Eltorky M. Changing trends in the distribution of the histologic types of lung cancer: a review of 4,439 cases. *Ann Diagn Pathol*. 2007;11:89–96.
10. Morita T. A statistical study of lung cancer in the annual of pathological autopsy cases in Japan, from 1958 to 1997, with reference to time trends of lung cancer in the world. *Jpn J Cancer Res*. 2002;93:15–23.
11. Grippi MA. Clinical aspects of lung cancer. *Semin Roentgenol*. 1990;25:12–24.
12. Fraser RG, Paré JAP, Fraser RS, Genereux GP. Neoplastic diseases of the lung. In: Fraser RG, Paré JAP, Paré PD, Fraser RS, Genereux GP, eds. *Diagnosis of Diseases of the Chest*. 3rd ed. Philadelphia: WB Saunders; 1989:1327–1399.
13. Boyars MC. Clinical manifestations of carcinoma of the lung. *J Thorac Imaging*. 1991;7:21–28.
14. Haque AK. Pathology of carcinoma of the lung: an update on current concepts. *J Thorac Imaging*. 1991;7:9–20.
15. Pietra GG. The pathology of carcinoma of the lung. *Semin Roentgenol*. 1990;25:25–33.
16. Sherwin RP, Laforet EG, Strieder JW. Exophytic endobronchial carcinoma. *J Thorac Cardiovasc Surg*. 1962;43:716–730.
17. Dulmet-Brender E, Jaubert F, Huchon G. Exophytic endobronchial epidermoid carcinoma. *Cancer*. 1986;57:1358–1364.
18. Cooper L, Hagenschneider JK, Banky S, Rosado-de-Christenson ML, Suster S. Papillary endobronchial squamous cell carcinoma. *Ann Diagn Pathol*. 2005;9:284–288.
19. Laubscher F. Solitary squamous cell papilloma of bronchial origin. *Am J Clin Pathol*. 1969;52:599–603.
20. Spencer H, Dail DH, Arneaud J. Non-invasive bronchial epithelial papillary tumors. *Cancer*. 1980;45:1486–1497.
21. Trillo A, Guha A. Solitary condylomatous papilloma of the bronchus. *Arch Pathol Lab Med*. 1988;112:731–733.

22. Al-Saleem T, Peale AR, Norris CM. Multiple papillomatosis of the lower respiratory tract. Clinical and pathologic study of eleven cases. *Cancer*. 1968;22:1173–1184.
23. Colby TV, Koss MN, Travis WD. Tumors of the lower respiratory tract. In: *Atlas of Tumor Pathology*. Fascicle 13, Third Series. Washington, DC: Armed Forces Institute of Pathology; 1995:203.
24. Suster S, Huszar M, Herczeg E. Spindle cell squamous carcinoma of the lung. Immunocytochemical and ultrastructural study of a case. *Histopathology*. 1987;11:871–878.
25. Wang BY, Gil J, Kaufman D, Gan L, Kohtz DS, Burstein DE. P63 in pulmonary epithelium, pulmonary squamous neoplasms, and other pulmonary tumors. *Hum Pathol*. 2002;33:921–926.
26. Pelosi G, Pasini F, Olsen Stenholm C, et al. P63 immunoreactivity in lung cancer: yet another player in the development of squamous cell carcinomas? *J Pathol*. 2002;198:100–109.
27. Pelosi G, Barisella M, Pasini F, et al. CD117 immunoreactivity in stage I adenocarcinoma and squamous cell carcinoma of the lung: relevance to prognosis in a subset of adenocarcinoma patients. *Mod Pathol*. 2004;17:711–721.
28. Yoshino I, Osoegawa A, Yohena T, et al. Loss of heterozygosity (LOH) in non-small cell lung cancer: difference between adenocarcinoma and squamous cell carcinoma. *Respir Med*. 2005;99:308–312.
29. Chujo M, Noguchi T, Miura T, Arinaga M, Uchida Y, Tagawa Y. Comparative genomic hybridization analysis detected frequent overrepresentation of chromosome 3q in squamous cell carcinoma of the lung. *Lung Cancer*. 2002;38:23–29.
30. Malassez L. Examen histologique d'un cas de cancer encephaloide du poumon (epithelioma). *Arch Physiologie Normale et Pathologique*. 1876;3:352–372.
31. Musser JH. Primary cancer of the lung. *Univ Pa Med Bull*. 1903;16:289–296.
32. Sweany HC. Case reports, laboratory methods and technical notes—a so-called alveolar cell cancer of the lung. *Arch Pathol*. 1935;19:203–2077.
33. Casilli AR, White HJ. Rare forms of primary malignant lung tumors: report of three types. *Am J Clin Pathol*. 1940;10:623–641.
34. Neubuerger KT, Geever EF. Alveolar cell tumor of the human lung. *Arch Pathol*. 1942;33:551–569.
35. Herbut PA. Bronchiolar origin of "alveolar cell tumor" of the lung. *Am J Pathol*. 1944;20:911–929.
36. Wood DA, Pierson PH. Pulmonary alveolar adenomatosis in man. *Am Rev Tuberc*. 1945;51:205–224.
37. Ikeda K. Alveolar cell carcinoma of the lung. *Am J Clin Pathol*. 1945;15:50–63.
38. Osserman KE, Neuhof H. Mucocellular papillary adenocarcinoma of the lung and lobectomy. *J Thorac Surg*. 1946;15:272–278.
39. Drymalski GW, Thompson JR, Sweany HC. Pulmonary adenomatosis. *Am J Pathol*. 1948;24:1083–1093.
40. Delarue NC, Graham EA. Alveolar cell carcinoma of the lung (pulmonary adenomatosis, Jagziekte?): a multicentric tumor of epithelial origin. *J Thorac Surg*. 1949;18:237–251.
41. Liebow AA. Bronchiolo-alveolar carcinoma. *Adv Intern Med*. 1960;10:329–358.
42. Carter D, Eggleston JC. Tumors of the lower respiratory tract. In: *Atlas of Tumor Pathology*, Fascicle 17, Second Series. Bethesda, MD: Armed Forces Institute of Pathology; 1980.
43. Travis WD, Colby TV, Corrin B, et al. *Histological Typing of Lung and Pleural Tumours (World Health Organization International Histological Classification of Tumours)*. 3rd ed. New York: Springer Verlag; 1999:36.
44. Travis WD, Brambilla E, Muller-Hermelink K, Harris CC. *WHO Classification of Tumours: Pathology and Genetics of Tumours of the Lung, Pleura, Thymus, and Heart*. Lyon, France: IARC Press; 2004.
45. Overholt RH, Meissner WA, Delmonico E. Favorable bronchiolar carcinoma. *Dis Chest*. 1955;27:403–413.
46. Belgrad R, Good CA, Woolner LB. Alveolar-cell carcinoma (terminal bronchiolar carcinoma): a study of surgically excised tumors with special emphasis on localized lesions. *Radiology*. 1962;79:789–798.
47. Munell ER, Lawson RC, Keller DF. Solitary bronchiolar (alveolar cell) carcinoma of the lung. *J Thorac Cardiovasc Surg*. 1966;52:261–270.
48. Watson WL, Farpour A. Terminal bronchiolar or "alveolar cell" cancer of the lung. Two hundred sixty-five cases. *Cancer*. 1966;19:776–780.
49. Rosenblatt MB, Lisa JR, Collier F. Primary and metastatic bronchiolo-alveolar carcinoma. *Dis Chest*. 1967;52:147–152.
50. Bennett DE, Sasser WF. Bronchiolar carcinoma: a valid clinicopathologic entity? A study of 30 cases. *Cancer*. 1969;24:876–887.
51. Delarue NC, Anderson W, Sanders D, Starr J. Bronchiolo-alveolar carcinoma: a reappraisal after 24 years. *Cancer*. 1972;29:90–97.
52. Marco M, Galy P. Bronchioloalveolar carcinoma: clinicopathologic relationships, natural history, and prognosis in 29 cases. *Am Rev Respir Dis*. 1973;107:621–629.
53. Schraufnagel D, Peloquin A, Paré JA, Wang NS. Differentiating bronchioloalveolar carcinoma from adenocarcinoma. *Am Rev Respir Dis*. 1982;125:74–79.
54. Singh G, Katyal SL. Bronchioloalveolar carcinomas: a heterogenous group. *Am Rev Respir Dis*. 1982;126:183–184.
55. Singh G, Katyal SL, Torikata C. Carcinoma of type II pneumocytes: immunodiagnosis of a subtype of "bronchioloalveolar carcinomas." *Am J Pathol*. 1981;102:195–208.
56. Dermer GB. Origin of bronchioloalveolar carcinoma and peripheral bronchial adenocarcinoma. *Cancer*. 1982;49:881–887.
57. Manning JT, Spjut HJ, Tschen JA. Bronchioloalveolar carcinoma: the significance of two histopathologic types. *Cancer*. 1984;54:525–534.
58. Clayton F. Bronchioloalveolar carcinomas. Cell types, patterns of growth, and prognostic correlates. *Cancer*. 1986;57:1555–1564.
59. Thomas JS, Tullett WM, Stack BH. Bronchioloalveolar cell carcinoma: a 21-year retrospective study of cases at the Western Infirmary, Glasgow. *Br J Dis Chest*. 1985;79:132–140.
60. Elson CE, Moore SP, Johnston WW. Morphologic and immunohistochenical studies of bronchioloalveolar carcinoma at Duke University Medical Center, 1968–1986. *Anal Quant Cytol Histol*. 1989;11:261–274.
61. Daly RC, Trastek VF, Pairolero PC, et al. Bronchoalveolar carcinoma: factors affecting survival. *Ann Thorac Surg*. 1991;51:368–377.
62. Feldman ER, Eagan RT, Schaid DJ. Metastatic bronchioloalveolar carcinoma and metastatic adenocarcinoma of the lung: comparison of clinical manifestations, chemotherapeutic responses, and prognosis. *Mayo Clin Proc*. 1992;67:27–32.
63. Breathnach OS, Ishibe N, Williams J, Linnoila RI, Caporaso N, Johnson BE. Clinical features of patients with stage iiib and IV bronchioloalveolar carcinoma of the lung. *Cancer*. 1999;86:1165–1173.
64. Hsu CP, Chen CY, Hsu NY. Bronchioloalveolar carcinoma. *J Thorac Cardiovasc Surg*. 1995;110:374–381.
65. Fujimoto N, Segawa Y, Takigawa N, et al. Clinical investigation of bronchioloalveolar carcinoma: a retrospective analysis of 53 patients in a single institution. *Anticancer Res*. 1999;19:1369–1374.
66. Barkley JE, Green MR. Bronchioloalveolar carcinoma. *J Clin Oncol*. 1996;14:2377–2386.
67. Goodwin LO, Mason JM, Hajdu SI. Gene expression patterns of paired bronchioloaveolar carcinoma and benign lung tissue. *Ann Clin Lab Sci*. 2001;31:369–375.
68. Read WL, Page NC, Tierney RM, Piccirillo JF, Govindan R. The epidemiology of bronchioloalveolar carcinoma over the past two decades: analysis of the SEER database. *Lung Cancer*. 2004;45:137–142.
69. Raz DJ, Jablons DM. Bronchioloalveolar carcinoma is not associated with younger age at diagnosis: an analysis of the SEER database. *J Thorac Oncol*. 2006;1:339–343.

70. Ohye RG, Cohen DM, Caldwell S, Qualman SJ. Pediatric bronchioloalveolar carcinoma: a favorable pediatric malignancy? *J Pediatr Surg.* 1998;33:730–732.
71. Breathnach OS, Kwiatkowski DJ, Finkelstein DM, et al. Bronchioloalveolar carcinoma of the lung: recurrences and survival in patients with stage I disease. *J Thorac Cardiovasc Surg.* 2001;121:42–47.
72. Rena O, Papalia E, Ruffini E, et al. Stage I pure bronchioloalveolar carcinoma: recurrences, survival and comparison with adenocarcinoma of the lung. *Eur J Cardiothorac Surg.* 2003;23:409–414.
73. Gaeta M, Blandino A, Pergolizzi S, et al. Patterns of recurrence of bronchioloalveolar cell carcinoma after surgical resection: a radiological, histological, and immunohistochemical study. *Lung Cancer.* 2003;42:319–326.
74. Ebright MI, Zakowski MF, Martin J, et al. Clinical pattern and pathologic stage but not histologic features predict outcome for bronchioloalveolar carcinoma. *Ann Thorac Surg.* 2002;74:1640–1647.
75. Travis WD, Garg K, Franklin WA, et al. Bronchioloalveolar carcinoma and lung adenocarcinoma: the clinical importance and research relevance of the 2004 World Health Organization pathologic criteria. *J Thorac Oncol.* 2006;1:S13–S19.
76. Noguchi M, Morikawa A, Kawasaki M, et al. Small adenocarcinoma of the lung. Histologic characteristics and prognosis. *Cancer.* 1995;75:2844–2852.
77. Zell JA, Ou SH, Ziogas A, Anton-Culver HA. Epidemiology of bronchioloalveolar carcinoma: improvement in survival after release of the 1999 WHO classification of lung tumors. *J Clin Oncol.* 2005;23:8396–8405.
78. Zell JA, Ignatius Ou SH, Ziogas A, Anton-Culver HA. Validation of the proposed International Association for the Study of Lung Cancer non–small cell lung cancer staging system revisions for advanced bronchioloalveolar carcinoma using data from the California Cancer Registry. *J Thorac Oncol.* 2007;2:1078–1085.
79. Grover FL, Piantadosi S. Recurrence and survival following resection of bronchioloalveolar carcinoma of the lung—the Lung Cancer Study Group experience. *Ann Surg.* 1989;209:779–790.
80. Garfield DH, Cadranel JL, Wislez M, Franklin WA, Hirsch FR. The bronchioloalveolar carcinoma and peripheral adenocarcinomna spectrum of diseases. *J Thorac Oncol.* 2006;1:344–359.
81. Damhuis RA, Schütte PR, Varin OC, van den Berg PM, Heinhuis R, Plaisier PW. Poor results after surgery for bronchioloalveolar carcinoma. *Eur J Surg Oncol.* 2006;32:573–576.
82. Sidhu SG, Wieczorek R, Cassai ND, Zhu CC. The concept of bronchioloalveolar cell adenocarcinoma: redefinition, a critique of the 1999 WHO classification, and an ultrastructural analysis of 155 cases. *Int J Surg Pathol.* 2003;11:89–99.
83. Hajdu SI. The story of bronchioloalveolar carcinoma. *Ann Clin Lab Sci.* 2005;35:336–338.
84. Noguchi M, Kodama T, Shimosato Y, et al. Papillary adenoma of type 2 pneumocytes. *Am J Surg Pathol.* 1986;10:134–139.
85. Koga T, Hashimoto S, Sugio K, et al. Lung adenocarcinoma with bronchioloalveolar component is frequently associated with foci of high-grade atypical adenomatous hyperplasia. *Am J Clin Pathol.* 2002;117:464–470.
86. Travis WD, Linnoila RI, Horowitz M, et al. Pulmonary nodules resembling bronchioloalveolar carcinoma in adolescent cancer patients. *Mod Pathol.* 1988;1:372–377.
87. Morandi L, Asioli S, Cavazza A, Pession A, Damiani S. Genetic relationship among atypical adenomatous hyperplasia, bronchioloalveolar carcinoma, and adenocarcinoma of the lung. *Lung Cancer.* 2007;56:35–42.
88. Ogata T, Endo K. Clara cell granules of peripheral lung cancers. *Cancer.* 1984;54:1635–1644.
89. Hirata H, Noguchi M, Shimosato Y, Uei Y, Goya T. Clinicopathologic and immunohistochemical characteristics of bronchial gland cell type adenocarcinoma of the lung. *Am J Clin Pathol.* 1990;93:20–25.
90. Edwards CW. Pulmonary adenocarcinoma: review of 106 cases and proposed new classification. *J Clin Pathol.* 1987;40:125–135.
91. Miller RR, Nelems B, Evans KG, Müller NL, Ostrow DN. Glandular neoplasia of the lung: a proposed analogy to colonic tumors. *Cancer.* 1988;61:1009–1014.
92. Moran CA. Pulmonary adenocarcinoma: the expanding spectrum of histologic variants. *Arch Pathol Lab Med.* 2006;130:958–962.
93. Dabbs DJ, Landreneau RJ, Liu Y, et al. Detection of estrogen receptor by immunohistochemistry in pulmonary adenocarcinoma. *Ann Thorac Surg.* 2002;73:403–406.
94. Prudkin L, Wistuba II. Epidermal growth factor receptor abnormalities in lung cancer. Pathogenetic and clinical implications. *Ann Diagn Pathol.* 2006;10:306–315.
95. Minna JD, Roth JA, Gazdar A. Focus on lung cancer. *Cancer Cell.* 2002;1:49–52.
96. Kris MG, Natale RB, Herbst RS, et al. Efficacy of gefitinib, an inhibitor of the epidermal growth factor receptor tyrosine kinase, in symptomatic patients with non-small cell lung cancer, a randomized trial. *JAMA.* 2003;290:2149–2158.
97. Fukuoka M, Yano S, Giaccone G, et al. Multi-institutional randomized phase II trial of gefitinib for previously treated patients with advanced non–small lung cancer (the IDEAL 1 Trial). *J Clin Oncol.* 2003;21:2237–2246.
98. Pérez-Soler R, Chachoua A, Hammond LA, et al. Determinants of tumor response and survival with erlotinib in patients with non–small cell lung cancer. *J Clin Oncol.* 2004;22:3238–3247.
99. Miller VA, Kris MG, Shah N, et al. Bronchioloalveolar pathologic subtype and smoking history predict sensitivity to gefitinib in advanced non–small cell lung cancer. *J Clin Oncol.* 2004;22:1103–1109.
100. Shigematsu H, Gazdar AF. Somatic mutations of epidermal growth factor receptor signaling pathway in lung cancers. *Int J Cancer.* 2006;118:257–262.
101. Pao W, Miller V, Zakowski M, et al. EGF receptor gene mutations are common in lung cancers from "never smokers" and are associated with sensitivity of tumors to gefitinib and erlotinib. *Proc Natl Acad Sci U S A.* 2004;101:13306–13311.
102. Lynch TJ, Bell DW, Sordella R, et al. Activating mutations in the epidermal growth factor receptor underlying responsiveness of non–small cell lung cancer to gefitinib. *N Engl J Med.* 2004;350:2129–2139.
103. Moran CA. Mucin-rich tumors of the lung. *Adv Anat Pathol.* 1995;2:299–305.
104. Kragel PJ, Devaney KO, Meth BM, Linnoila I, Frierson Jr HF, Travis WD. Mucinous cystadenoma of the lung. A report of two cases with immunohistochemical and ultrastructural analysis. *Arch Pathol Lab Med.* 1990;114:1053–1056.
105. Traub B. Mucinous cystadenoma of the lung [letter]. *Arch Pathol Lab Med.* 1991;115:740.
106. Dixon AY, Moran JF, Wesselius LJ, McGregor DH. Pulmonary mucinous cystic tumor. Case report with review of the literature. *Am J Surg Pathol.* 1993;17:722–728.
107. Higashiyama M, Doi O, Kodama K, Yokouchi H, Tateishi R. Cystic mucinous adenocarcinoma of the lung. Two cases of cystic variant of mucus-producing lung adenocarcinoma. *Chest.* 1992;101:763–766.
108. Davison AM, Lowe JW, Da Costa P. Adenocarcinoma arising in a mucinous cystadenoma of the lung. *Thorax.* 1992;47:129–130.
109. Graeme-Cook F, Mark EJ. Pulmonary mucinous cystic tumors of borderline malignancy. *Hum Pathol.* 1991;22:185–190.
110. Moran CA, Hochholzer L, Fishback N, Travis WD, Koss MN. Mucinous (so-called colloid) carcinomas of the lung. *Mod Pathol.* 1992;5:634–638.
111. Silver SA, Askin FB. True papillary carcinoma of the lung: a distinct clinicopathologic entity. *Am J Surg Pathol.* 1997;21:43–51.
112. Jian Z, Tomizawa Y, Yanagitani N, Iijima H, Sano T, Nakajima T. Papillary adenocarcinoma of the lung is a more advanced adenocarcinoma than bronchioloalveolar carcinoma that is composed of two distinct histological subtypes. *Pathol Int.* 2005;55:619–625.

113. Aida S, Shimazaki H, Sato K, et al. Prognostic analysis of pulmonary adenocarcinoma subclassification with special consideration of papillary and bronchioloalveolar types. *Histopathology*. 2004;45:468–476.
114. Moran CA, Jagirdar J, Suster S. Papillary lung adenocarcinoma with prominent "morular" component. *Am J Clin Pathol*. 2004;122:106–109.
115. Amin MB, Tamboli P, Merchant SH, et al. Micropapillary component in lung adenocarcinoma: a distinctive histologic feature with possible prognostic significance. *Am J Surg Pathol*. 2002;26:358–364.
116. Makimoto Y, Nabeshima K, Iwasaki H, et al. Micropapillary pattern: a distinct pathological marker to subclassify tumours with a significantly poor prognosis within small peripheral lung adenocarcinoma (≤20 mm) with mixed bronchioloalveolar and invasive subtypes (Noguchi's type C tumours). *Histopathology*. 2005;46:677–684.
117. Kuroda N, Hamaguchi N, Takeuchi E, Ohara M, Hirouchi T, Mizuno K. Lung adenocarcinoma with micropapillary pattern: a clinicopathological study of 25 cases. *APMIS*. 2006;114:381–385.
118. Miyoshi T, Satoh Y, Okumura S, et al. Early-stage lung adenocarcinomas with a micropapillary pattern, a distinct pathologic marker for a significantly poor prognosis. *Am J Surg Pathol*. 2003;27:101–109.
119. Hoshi R, Tsuzuku M, Horai T, Ishikawa Y, Satoh Y. Micropapillary clusters in early-stage lung adenocarcinomas: a distinct cytologic sign of significantly poor prognosis. *Cancer*. 2004;102:81–86.
120. Kish JK, Ro JY, Ayala AG, McMurtrey MJ. Primary mucinous adenocarcinoma of the lung with signet-ring cells: a histochemical comparison with signet-ring cell carcinomas of other sites. *Hum Pathol*. 1989;20:1097–1102.
121. Sarma DP, Hoffmann EO. Primary signet-ring cell carcinoma of the lung. *Hum Pathol*. 1990;21:459–460.
122. Hayashi H, Kitamura H, Nakatani Y, Inayama Y, Ito T, Kitamura H. Primary signet-ring cell carcinoma of the lung: histochemical and immunohistochemical characterization. *Hum Pathol*. 1999;30:378–383.
123. Castro CY, Moran CA, Flieder DG, Suster S. Primary signet ring cell adenocarcinoma of the lung: a clinicopathological study of 15 cases. *Histopathology*. 2001;39:397–401.
124. Steinhauer JR, Moran CA, Suster S. "Secretory endometrioid–like" adenocarcinoma of the lung. *Histopathology*. 2005;47:219–220.
125. Siami K, McCluggage WG, Ordonez NG, et al. Thyroid transcription factor-1 expression in endometrial and endocervical adenocarcinomas. *Am J Surg Pathol*. 2007;31:1759–1763.
126. Ishikura H, Kanda M, Ito M, Nosaka K, Mizuno K. Hepatoid adenocarcinoma: a distinctive histological subtype of alpha-fetoprotein–producing lung carcinoma. *Vich Arch A Pathol Anat Histopathol*. 1990;417:73–80.
127. Arnould L, Drouot F, Fargeot P, et al. Hepatoid adenocarcinoma of the lung: report of a case of an unusual alpha-fetoprotein–producing lung tumor. *Am J Surg Pathol*. 1997;21:1113–1118.
128. Nasu M, Soma T, Fukushima H, Kudo K, Matsubara O. Hepatoid carcinoma of the lung with production of alpha-fetoprotein and abnormal prothrombin: an autopsy case report. *Mod Pathol*. 1997;10:1054–1058.
129. Carlinfante G, Foschini MP, Pasquinelli G, Scotti R, Cavazza A. Hepatoid carcinoma of the lung: a case report with immunohistochemical, ultrastructural and in-situ hybridization findings. *Histopathology*. 2000;37:88–89.
130. Yasunami R, Hashimoto Z, Ogura T, Hirao F, Yamamura Y. Primary lung cancer producing alpha-fetoprotein: a case report. *Cancer*. 1981;47:926–929.
131. Miyake M, Ito M, Taki T, Mitsuoka A, Wada H, Hitomi S. [A case report of two patients with primary lung cancer secreting AFP.]. *Nippon Kyobu Geka Gakkai Zasshi*. 1986;34:914–919.
132. Hayashi Y, Takanashi Y, Ohsawa H, Ishii H, Nakatani Y. Hepatoid adenocarcinoma in the lung. *Lung Cancer*. 2002;38:211–214.
133. Churg A. The fine structure of large cell undifferentiated carcinoma of the lung. Evidence for its relation to squamous cell carcinomas and adenocarcinomas. *Hum Pathol*. 1978;9:143–156.
134. Yesner R. Large cell carcinoma of the lung. *Semin Diagn Pathol*. 1985;2:255–269.
135. Albain KS, True LD, Golomb HM, Hoffman PC, Little AG. Large cell carcinoma of the lung. Ultrastructural differentiation and clinicopathologic correlations. *Cancer*. 1985;56:1618–1623.
136. Kodama T, Shimosato Y, Koide T, Watanabe S, Teshima S. Large cell carcinoma of the lung—ultrastructural and immunohistochemical studies. *Jpn J Clin Oncol*. 1985;15:431–441.
137. Leung CS, Morava-Protzner I. Large cell carcinoma of the lung with osteoclast-like giant cells. *Histopathology*. 1998;32:482–484.
138. Masse SR, Dawson DT, Khaliq A. Ectopic gonadotropin in a case of anaplastic large-cell carcinoma of the lung. *Can Med Assoc J*. 1974;111:253–255.
139. Zhong D, Guo L, de Aguirre I, et al. LKB1 mutation in large cell carcinoma of the lung. *Lung Cancer*. 2006;53:285–294.
140. Fitzgibbons PL, Kern WH. Adenosquamous carcinoma of the lung: a clinical and pathologic study of seven cases. *Hum Pathol*. 1985;16:463–466.
141. Naunheim KS, Taylor JR, Skosey C, et al. Adenosquamous lung carcinoma: clinical characteristics, treatment, and prognosis. *Ann Thorac Surg*. 1987;44:462–466.
142. Sridhar KS, Raub WA, Duncan RC, Hilsenbeck S. The increasing recognition of adenosquamous lung carcinoma (1977–1986). *Am J Clin Oncol*. 1992;356–362.
143. Sridhar KS, Bounassi MJ, Raub Jr W, Richman SP. Clinical features of adenosquamous lung carcinoma in 127 patients. *Am Rev Respir Dis*. 1990;142:19–23.
144. Takamori S, Noguchi M, Morinaga S, et al. Clinicopathologic characteristics of adenosquamous carcinoma of the lung. *Cancer*. 1991;67:649–654.
145. Ishida T, Kaneko S, Yokoyama H, Inoue T, Sugio K, Sugimachi K. Adenosquamous carcinoma of the lung. Clinicopathologic and immunohistochemical features. *Am J Clin Pathol*. 1992;97:678–685.
146. Ghandur-Mnaymneh L, Raub Jr WA, Sridhar KS, Albores-Saavedra J, Gould E, Duncan RC. The accuracy of the histological classification of lung carcinoma and its reproducibility: a study of 75 archival cases of adenosquamous carcinoma. *Cancer Invest*. 1993;11:641–651.
147. Hofmann HS, Knolle J, Neef H. The adenosquamous lung carcinoma: clinical and pathological characteristics. *J Cardiovasc Surg*. 1994;35:543–547.
148. Shimizu J, Oda M, Hayashi Y, Nonomura A, Watanabe Y. A clinicopathologic study of resected cases of adenosquamous carcinoma of the lung. *Chest*. 1996;109:989–994.
149. Hsia JY, Chen CY, Hsu CP, Shai SE, Wang PY. Adenosquamous carcinoma of the lung. Surgical results compared with squamous cell and adenocarcinoma. *Scand Cardiovasc J*. 1999;33:29–32.
150. Nakagawa K, Yasumitsu T, Fukuhara K, Shiono H, Kikui M. Poor prognosis after lung resection for patients with adenosquamous carcinoma of the lung. *Ann Thorac Surg*. 2003;75:1740–1744.
151. Gawrychowski J, Brulinski K, Malinowski E, Papla B. Prognosis and survival after radical resection of primary adenosquamous lung carcinoma. *Eur J Cardiothoracic Surg*. 2005;27:686–692.
152. Ylagan LR, Scholes J, Demopoulos R. CD44: a marker of squamous differentiation in adenosquamous neoplasms. *Arch Pathol Lab Med*. 2000;124:212–215.
153. Kanazawa H, Ebina M, Ino-Oka N, et al. Transition from squamous cell carcinoma to adenocarcinoma in adenosquamous carcinoma of the lung. *Am J Pathol*. 2000;156:1289–1298.
154. Kang SM, Kang HJ, Shin JH, et al. Identical epidermal growth factor receptor mutations in adenocarcinomatous and squamous cell carcinomatous components of adenosquamous carcinoma of the lung. *Cancer*. 2007;109:581–587.

155. Liang JC, Kurzrock R, Gutterman JU, Gallick GE. Trisomy 12 correlates with elevated expression of p21ras in a human adenosquamous carcinoma of the lung. *Cancer Genet Cytogenet.* 1986;23:183–188.
156. Bégin LR, Eskandari J, Joncas J, Panasci L. Epstein-Barr virus related lymphoepithelioma-like carcinoma of lung. *J Surg Oncol.* 1987;36:280–283.
157. Han AJ, Xiong M, Gu YY, Lin SX, Xiong M. Lymphoepithelioma-like carcinoma of the lung with a better prognosis: a clinicopathologic study of 32 cases. *Am J Clin Pathol.* 2001;115:841–850.
158. Chan JK, Hui PK, Tsang WY, et al. Primary lymphoepithelioma-like carcinoma of the lung. A clinicopathologic study of 11 cases. *Cancer.* 1995;76:413–422.
159. Butler AE, Colby TV, Weiss L, Lombard C. Lymphoepithelioma-like carcinoma of the lung. *Am J Surg Pathol.* 1989;13:632–639.
160. Ho JC, Lam WK, Wong MP, et al. Lymphoepithelioma-like carcinoma of the lung: experience with ten cases. *Int J Tuberc Lung Dis.* 2004;8:890–895.
161. Guerrero A, Laflamme M, Agoff SN, Williams WM, Karmy-Jones R. Primary lymphoepithelioma-like carcinoma of the lung. *Can Respir J.* 2001;8:431–433.
162. Frank MW, Shields TW, Joob AW, et al. Lymphoepithelioma-like carcinoma of the lung. *Ann Thorac Surg.* 1997;64:1162–1164.
163. Wöckel W, Höfler HH, Popper HH, Morresi A. Lymphoepithelioma-like carcinoma of the lung. *Pathol Res Pract.* 1995;191:1170–1174.
164. Miller B, Montgomery C, Watne AL, Johnson D, Bailey T, Kowalski R. Lymphoepithelioma-like carcinoma of the lung. *J Surg Oncol.* 1991;48:62–68.
165. Curcio LD, Cohen JS, Grannis FW, Paz IB, Chilcote R, Weiss LM. Primary lymphoepithelioma-like carcinoma of the lung in a child. Report of an Epstein-Barr virus–related neoplasm. *Chest.* 1997;111:250–251.
166. Gal AA, Unger ER, Koss MN, Yen TS. Detection of Epstein-Barr virus in lymphoepithelioma-like carcinoma of the lung. *Mod Pathol.* 1991;4:264–268.
167. Pittaluga S, Wong MP, Chung LP, Loke SL. Clonal Epstein-Barr virus in lymphoepithelioma-like carcinoma of the lung. *Am J Surg Pathol.* 1993;17:678–682.
168. Higashiyama M, Doi O, Kodama K, et al. Lymphoepithelioma-like carcinoma of the lung: analysis of two cases for Epstein-Barr virus infection. *Hum Pathol.* 1995;26:1278–1282.
169. Chen FF, Yan JJ, Lai WW, Jin YT, Su IJ. Epstein-Barr virus–associated nonsmall cell lung carcinoma: undifferentiated "lymphoepithelioma-like" carcinoma as a distinct entity with better prognosis. *Cancer.* 1998;82:2334–2342.
170. Castro CY, Ostrowski ML, Barrios R, et al. Relationship between Epstein-Barr virus and lymphoepithelioma-like carcinoma of the lung: a clinicopathologic study of 6 cases and review of the literature. *Hum Pathol.* 2001;32:863–872.
171. Chang YL, Wu CT, Shih JY, Lee YC. New aspects in clinicopathologic and oncogene studies of 23 pulmonary lymphoepithelioma-like carcinomas. *Am J Surg Pathol.* 2002;26:715–723.
172. Rubenchik I, Dardick I, Auger M. Cytopathology and ultrastructure of primary rhabdoid tumor of the lung. *Ultrastruct Pathol.* 1996;20:355–360.
173. Cavazza A, Colby TV, Tsokos M, Rush W, Travis WD. Lung tumors with rhabdoid phenotype. *Am J Clin Pathol.* 1996;105:182–188.
174. Chetty R, Bhana B, Batitang S, Govender D. Lung carcinomas composed of rhabdoid cells. *Eur J Surg Oncol.* 1997;23:432–434.
175. Miyagi J, Tsuhako K, Kinjo T, Iwamasa T, Hashimoto H, Ishikawa S. Rhabdoid tumour of the lung is a dedifferentiated phenotype of pulmonary adenocarcinoma. *Histopathology.* 2000;37:37–44.
176. Shimazaki H, Aida S, Sato M, Deguchi H, Ozeki Y, Tamai S. Lung carcinoma with rhabdoid cells: a cllinicopathological study and survival analysis of 14 cases. *Histopathology.* 2001;38:425–434.
177. Kaneko T, Honda T, Fukushima M, Haniuda M, Komatsu H, Kodama T. Large cell carcinoma of the lung with rhabdoid phenotype. *Pathol Int.* 2002;52:643–647.
178. Hiroshima K, Shibuya K, Shimamura F, et al. Pulmonary large cell carcinoma with rhabdoid phenotype. *Ultrastruct Pathol.* 2003;27:55–59.
179. Tamboli P, Toprani TH, Amin MB, et al. Carcinoma of lung with rhabdoid features. *Hum Pathol.* 2004;35:8–13.
180. Yilmazbayhan D, Ates LE, Dilege S, Gulluoglu M, Tanju S, Kalayci G. Pulmonary large cell carcinoma with rhabdoid phenotype. *Ann Diagn Pathol.* 2005;9:223–226.
181. Falconieri G, Moran CA, Pizzolitto S, Zidar A, Angione V, Wakely Jr PE. Intrathoracic rhabdoid carcinoma: a clinicopathological immunohistochemical, and ultrastructural study of 6 cases. *Ann Diagn Pathol.* 2005;9:279–283.
182. Wick MR, Ritter JH, Dehner LP. Malignant rhabdoid tumors: a clinicopathologic review and conceptual discussion. *Semin Diagn Pathol.* 1995;12:233–248.
183. Humphrey PA, Scroggs MW, Roggli VL, Shelburne JD. Pulmonary carcinomas with a sarcomatoid element: an immunocytochemical and ultrastructural analysis. *Hum Pathol.* 1988;19:155–165.
184. Matsui K, Kitagawa M. Spindle cell carcinoma of the lung: a clinicopathologic study of three cases. *Cancer.* 1991;67:2361–2367.
185. Ro JY, Chen JL, Lee JS, Sahin AA, Ordóñez NG, Ayala AG. Sarcomatoid carcinoma of the lung. Immunohistochemical and ultrastructural studies of 14 cases. *Cancer.* 1992;69:376–386.
186. Fishback NF, Travis WD, Moran CA, Guinee Jr DG, McCarthy WF, Koss MN. Pleomorphic (spindle/giant cell) carcinoma of the lung. A clinicopathologic correlation of 78 cases. *Cancer.* 1994;73:2936–2945.
187. Razzuk MA, Urschel Jr HC, Albers JE, Martin JA, Paulson DL. Pulmonary giant cell carcinoma. *Ann Thorac Surg.* 1976;21:540–545.
188. Wang NS, Seemayer TA, Ahmed MN, Knaack J. Giant cell carcinoma of the lung. A light and electron microscopic study. *Hum Pathol.* 1976;7:3–16.
189. Bendel WL, Ishak KG. Giant cell carcinoma of the lung: report of two cases. *Am J Clin Pathol.* 1961;35:435–440.
190. Nash AD, Stout AP. Giant cell carcinoma of the lung: report of 5 cases. *Cancer.* 1958;11:369–376.
191. Herman DL, Bullock WK, Waken JK. Giant cell adenocarcinoma of the lung. *Cancer.* 1966;19:1337–1346.
192. Hellstrom HR, Fisher ER. Giant cell carcinoma of the lung. *Cancer.* 1963;16:1080–1088.
193. Shin MS, Jackson LK, Shelton Jr RW, Greene RE. Giant cell carcinoma of the lung. Clinical and roentgenographic manifestations. *Chest.* 1986;89:366–369.
194. Ginsberg SS, Buzaid AC, Stern H, Carter D. Giant cell carcinoma of the lung. *Cancer.* 1992;70:606–610.
195. Addis BJ, Dewar A, Thurlow NP. Giant cell carcinoma of the lung—immunohistochemical and ultrastructural evidence of dedifferentiation. *J Pathol.* 1988;155:231–240.
196. Przygodzki RM, Koss MN, Moran CA, et al. Pleomorphic (giant and spindle cell) carcinoma is genetically distinct from adenocarcinoma and squamous cell carcinoma by K-ras-2 and p53 analysis. *Am J Clin Pathol.* 1996;106:487–492.
197. Katzenstein AL, Prioleau PG, Askin FB. The histologic spectrum and significance of clear-cell change in lung carcinoma. *Cancer.* 1980;45:943–947.
198. Edwards C, Carlile A. Clear cell carcinoma of the lung. *J Clin Pathol.* 1985;38:880–885.

4

Salivary Gland–Type Tumors of the Lung

Primary salivary gland–type tumors of the lung are uncommon tumors that comprise no more than 1% of all lung neoplasms.[1] Because of their rarity as primary lung neoplasms, salivary gland–type tumors may pose problems in interpretation of findings in small biopsy specimens. They often are mistakenly identified as non–small cell carcinomas; however, their clinical behavior can be quite different from that of conventional non–small cell carcinomas. Because of the similar immunohistochemical profile that these tumors may share among themselves and with other conventional non–small cell carcinomas of the lung, an awareness of their occurrence as primary lung tumors is essential for accurate diagnosis and proper clinical management. It can be difficult to make this diagnosis from small transbronchial biopsy specimens, in which a limited amount of material is available for evaluation. Accordingly, in many instances, definitive diagnosis of this tumor type is best accomplished using material obtained at complete surgical resections.

Salivary gland–type tumors in the lung do not follow the same patterns of occurrence as those in the salivary glands. For instance, mixed tumors (pleomorphic adenomas), which are common in the salivary glands, are very uncommon in the lung. The most common salivary gland–type tumors of the lung are of the malignant type, such as mucoepidermoid carcinoma or adenoid cystic carcinoma. Also, at the histopathologic level, some differences may be observed with certain types of tissues. Because salivary gland–type tumors of the lung have no parallel with any tumors of the salivary glands, the diagnosis of salivary gland–type tumors of the lung requires careful clinical, radiologic, and pathologic correlation.

MUCOEPIDERMOID CARCINOMA

Clinical Features

Mucoepidermoid carcinoma (MEC) is the most common salivary gland–type tumor of the lung. It can occur at any age; however, most affected patients are adults.[2–10] Yousem and Hocholzer, in their analysis of a large series of these tumors, reported 58 patients between the ages of 9 and 78 years, with a slight female preponderance. Clinically, patients' signs and symptoms varied in accordance with the size and location of the tumor. Larger tumors in a central location are most likely to produce clinical signs and symptoms, including those related to obstruction, pneumonia, dyspnea, chest pain, and cough. Tumors that are not associated with the airway may produce symptoms when they reach a large size.

Macroscopic Features

MECs are classically described as exophytic endobronchial tumors that can attain a size of up to 5 cm in greatest dimension. They usually are well circumscribed, with a smooth surface (Fig. 4-1). On cut surface, the tumors may be solid or cystic, and in many instances they exhibit both features. No predilection for any lung or lung segment for involvement by these tumors has been documented.

Microscopic Features

Histologically, MECs can be divided into low- and high-grade tumors. The classification as low- or high-grade is based on histopathologic features, such as the presence of necrosis, hemorrhage, cellular atypia, and mitotic activity. Because both histologic variants share similar features, careful evaluation of these neoplasms is important.

In low-grade tumors, the low-power view shows a tumor composed of cystic and solid areas in close association (Fig. 4-2). The cystic component may contain acellular material within the cyst-like structures, which may be mixed with calcifications (Fig. 4-3). Higher magnification shows both components in detail. The solid component is composed of sheets of round to polygonal cells

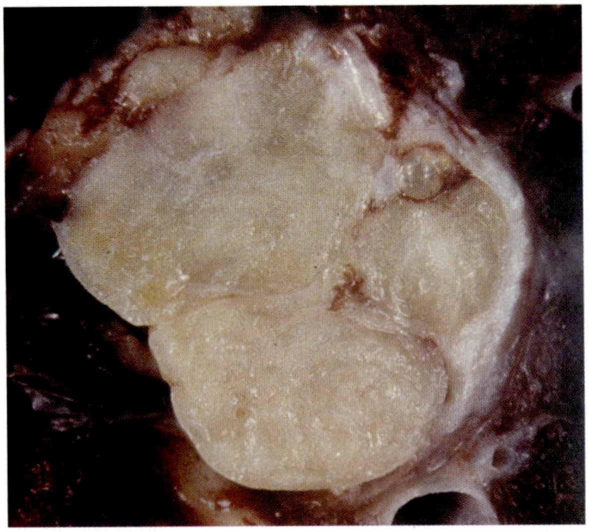

Figure 4-1 Gross specimen of a mucoepidermoid carcinoma. The yellowish tumor is well defined, with a smooth surface.

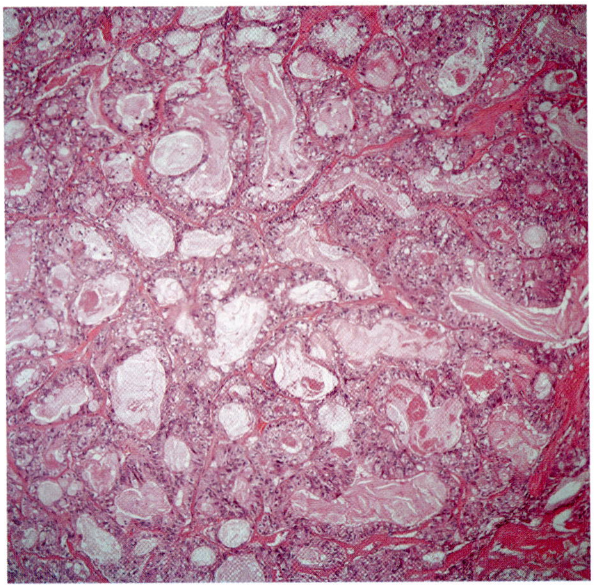

Figure 4-3 Solid component of a mucoepidermoid carcinoma with calcifications.

with distinct cell borders, light eosinophilic cytoplasm, round small nucleus, and inconspicuous nucleoli (Fig. 4-4). In some areas, this solid component may show the presence of sheets of similar cells with clear cytoplasm (intermediate cells) (Fig. 4-5). Mitotic activity and cellular pleomorphism are absent. In some of the cystic areas it is possible to observe the presence of "epidermoid cells" admixed with mucus-secreting cells (so-called mucocytes) (Fig. 4-6). Both of these components may be embedded in, or separated by, bands of fibroconnective tissue (Fig. 4-7), or embedded in an inflammatory background composed predominantly of plasma cells (Fig. 4-8). In some of these tumors, both solid and cystic components may show areas in which the cells acquire a more oncocytic appearance (Fig. 4-9). MECs may show extensive areas of solid component with a glandular-like appearance, in which histochemical staining for mucicarmine may be helpful to demonstrate the presence of mucus-secreting cells (Fig. 4-10). Areas with an exuberant fibroblastic proliferation, so-called sclerosing mucoepidermoid carcinoma, also may be predominant in these tumors. In some MECs, the appearance on low-power magnification may mimic that of a basaloid carcinoma; however, closer examination of the islands of tumor cells will

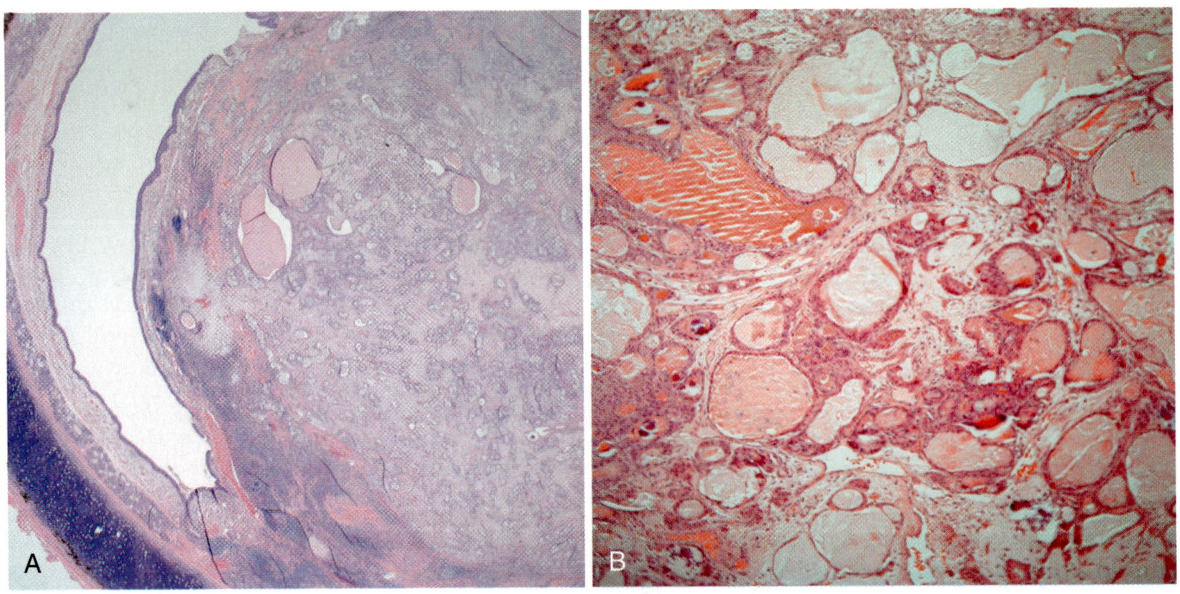

Figure 4-2 **A**, Low-power view of an endobronchial mucoepidermoid carcinoma. **B**, Mucoepidermoid carcinoma with a mixture of cystic and solid areas.

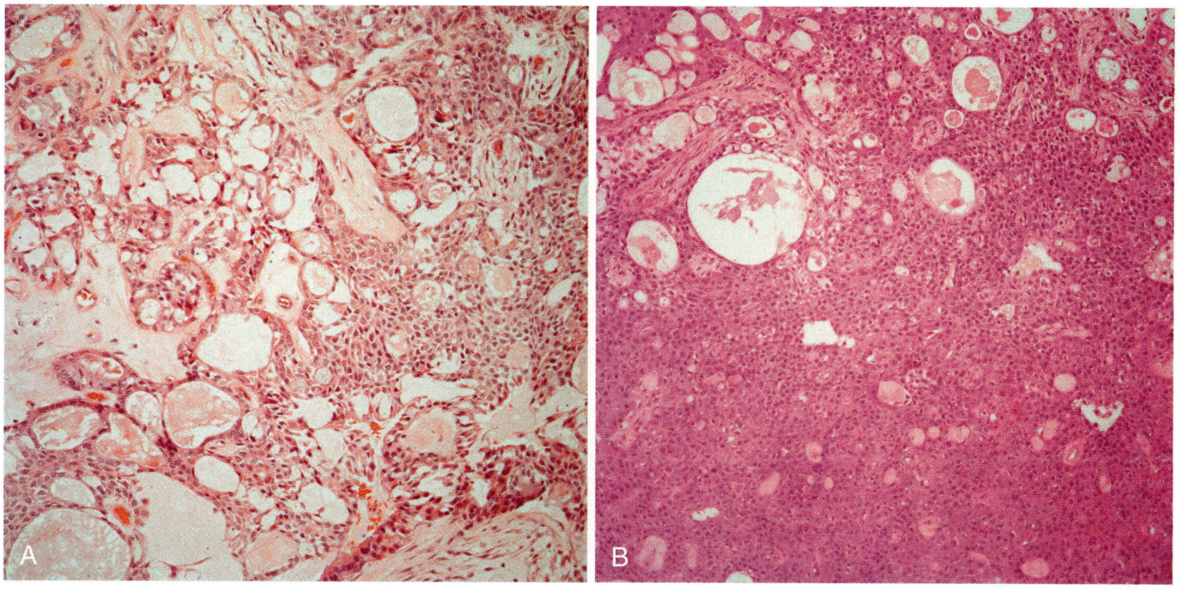

Figure 4-4 Mucoepidermoid carcinoma. **A**, Solid epidermoid component admixed with cystic areas. **B**, Closer view of the epidermoid component showing lack of nuclear atypia or mitotic activity.

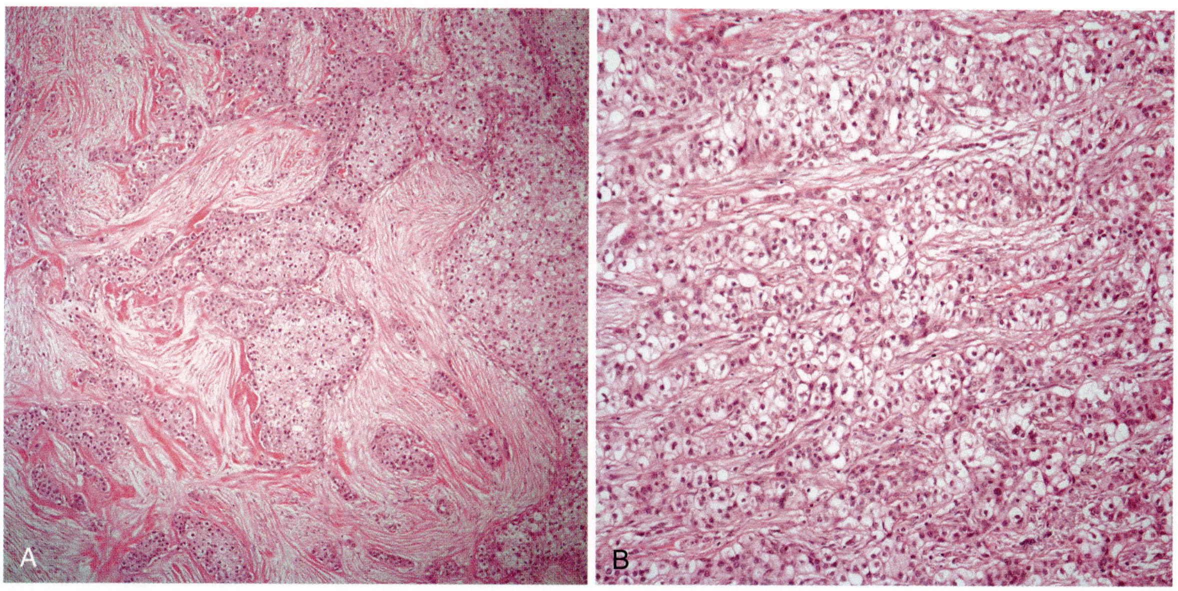

Figure 4-5 Mucoepidermoid carcinoma. **A**, Prominent areas composed of clear cells separated by fibroconnective tissue. **B**, High-power view of clear cells showing the characteristic bland appearance.

disclose the presence of epidermoid elements admixed with mucus-secreting cells (Fig. 4-11). In a minority of cases, the mucus-secreting glands predominate, with little solid component (Fig. 4-12). An important feature of MEC is the absence of keratinization in both solid and cystic components (Fig. 4-13).

High-grade tumors will display areas of necrosis or hemorrhage at low-power magnification. In the high-power view, the tumors will display areas of cytologic atypia in terms of nuclear pleomorphism and mitotic activity (Fig. 4-14). Even in the high-grade neoplasms, however, areas of low-grade differentiation may be encountered.

Immunohistochemical Features

The use of immunohistochemical studies to diagnose or to rule out MEC is limited. The tumor may display immunohistochemical features similar to those of conventional non–small cell carcinomas. Thus, the final interpretation is based largely on morphology alone.

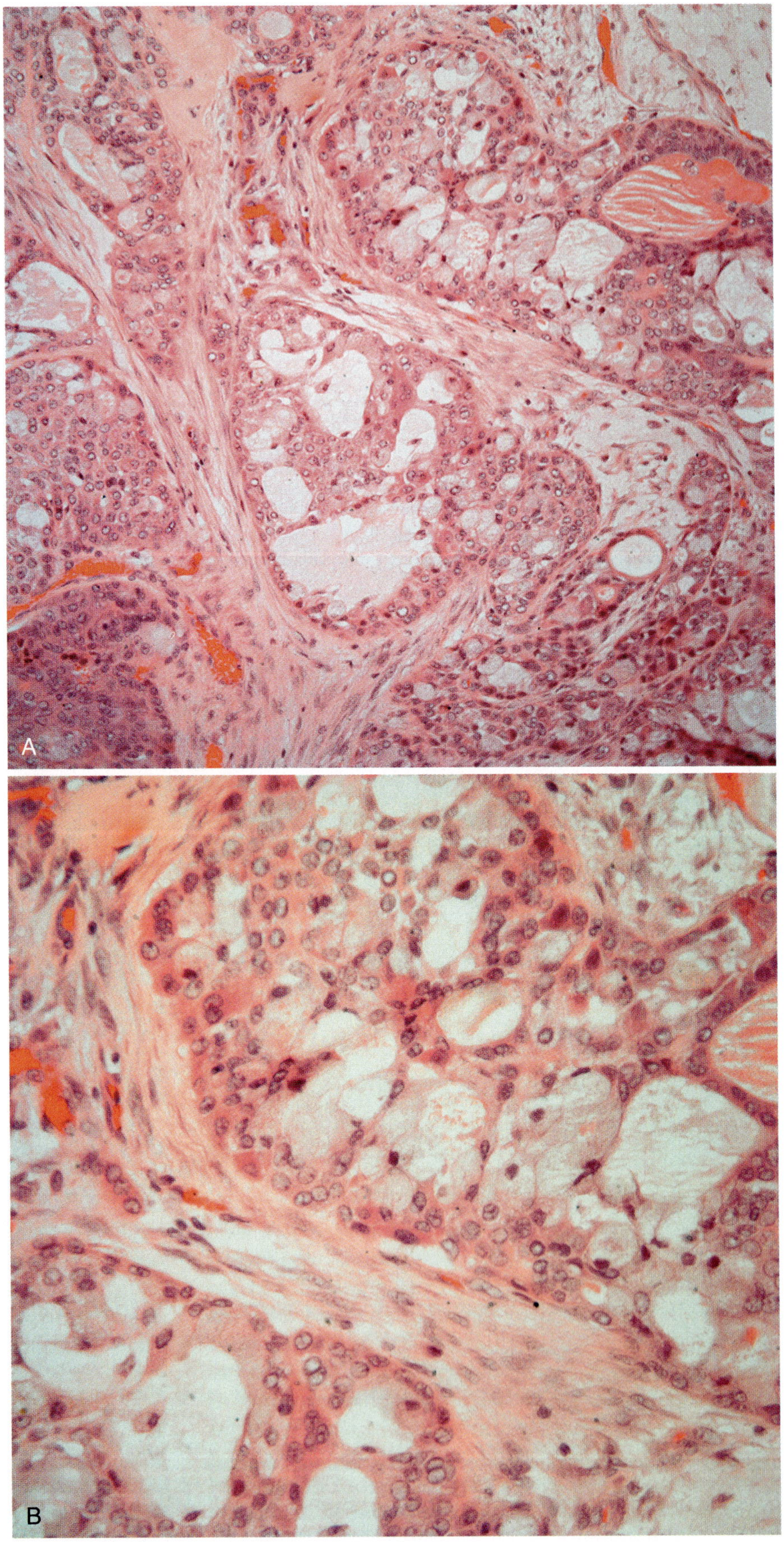

Figure 4-6 Mucoepidermoid carcinoma. **A**, Epidermoid elements admixed with mucus-producing cells. **B**, High-power view showing the mucus-secreting cells (mucocytes).

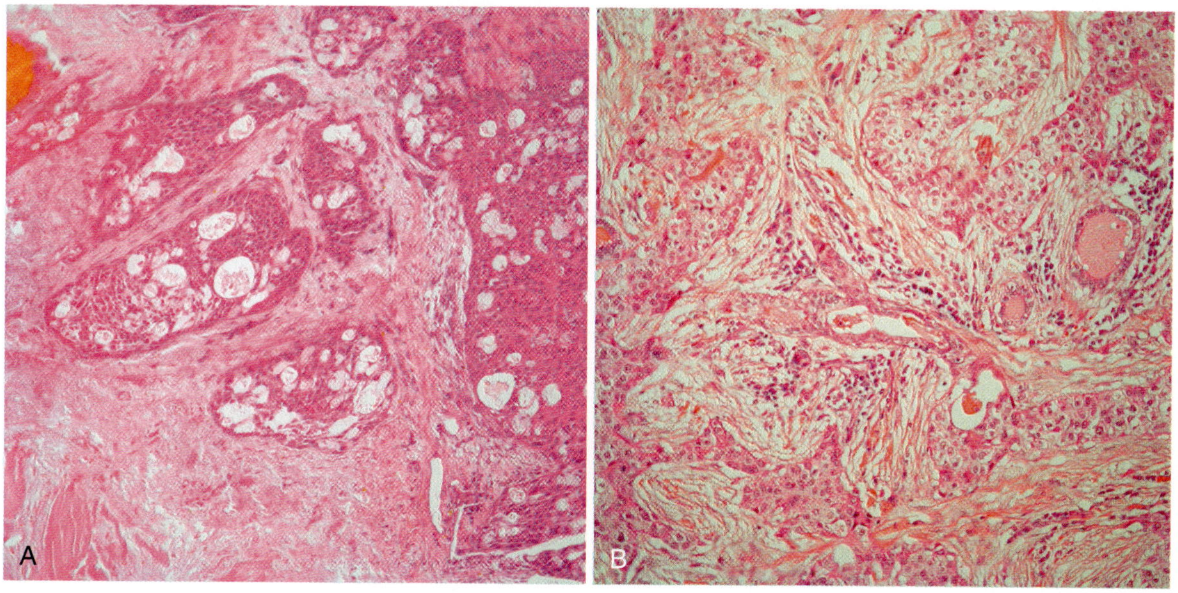

Figure 4-7 Mucoepidermoid carcinoma. **A**, Tumor cells embedded in areas of fibrocollagen. **B**, Haphazard arrangement with areas of fibroconnective tissue separating tumor areas.

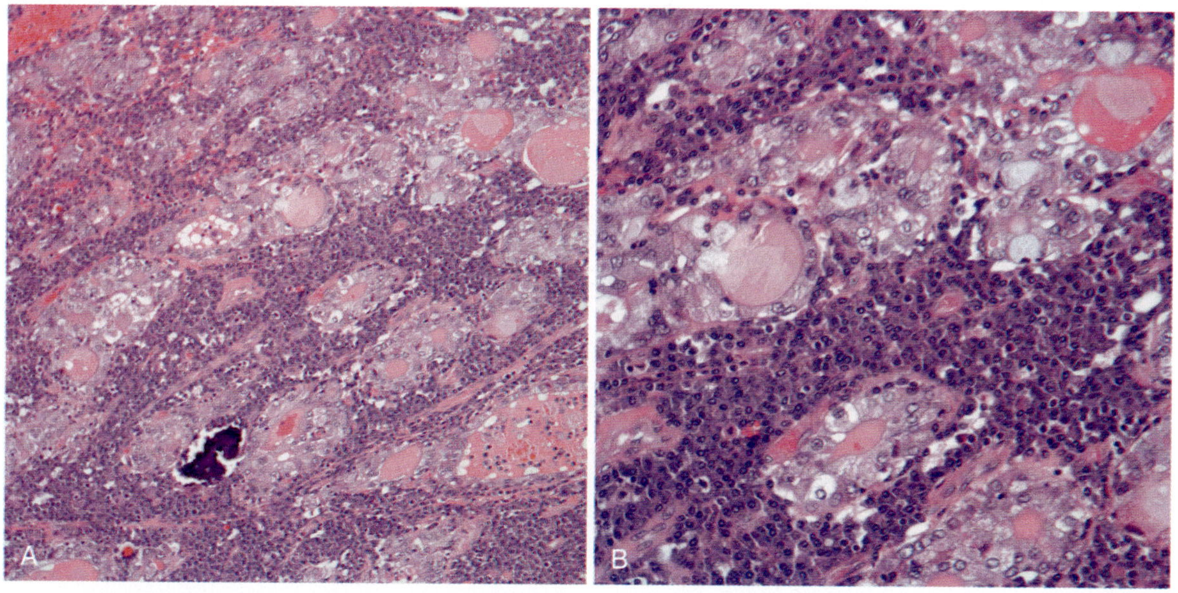

Figure 4-8 **A**, Mucoepidermoid carcinoma with a prominent inflammatory component. **B**, Mucoepidermoid carcinoma with a prominent plasma cell infiltrate.

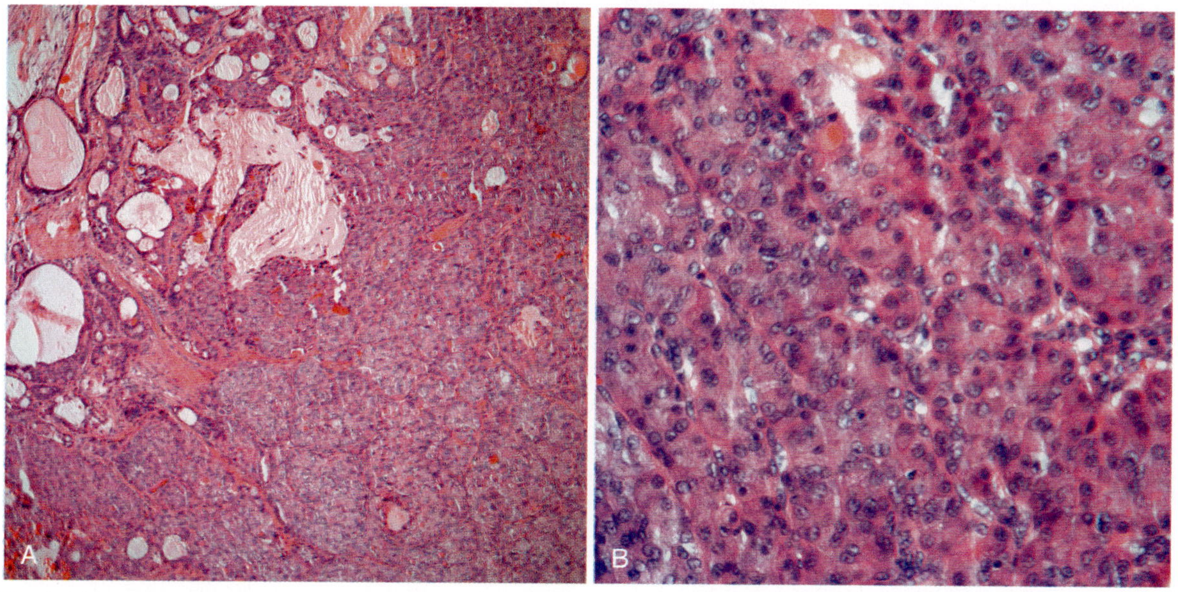

Figure 4-9 **A**, Mucoepidermoid carcinoma with a more solid oncocytic component. **B**, High-power magnification of the oncocytic component.

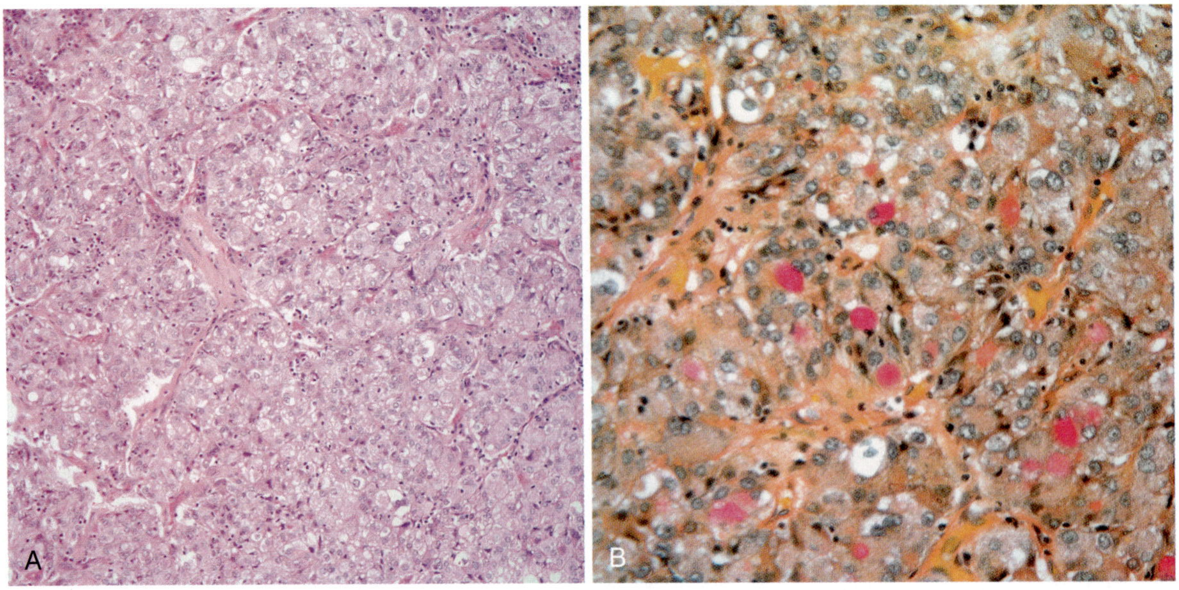

Figure 4-10 **A**, Mucoepidermoid carcinoma with a prominent solid pattern. **B**, Mucicarmine histochemical stain shows numerous mucus-producing cells (mucocytes).

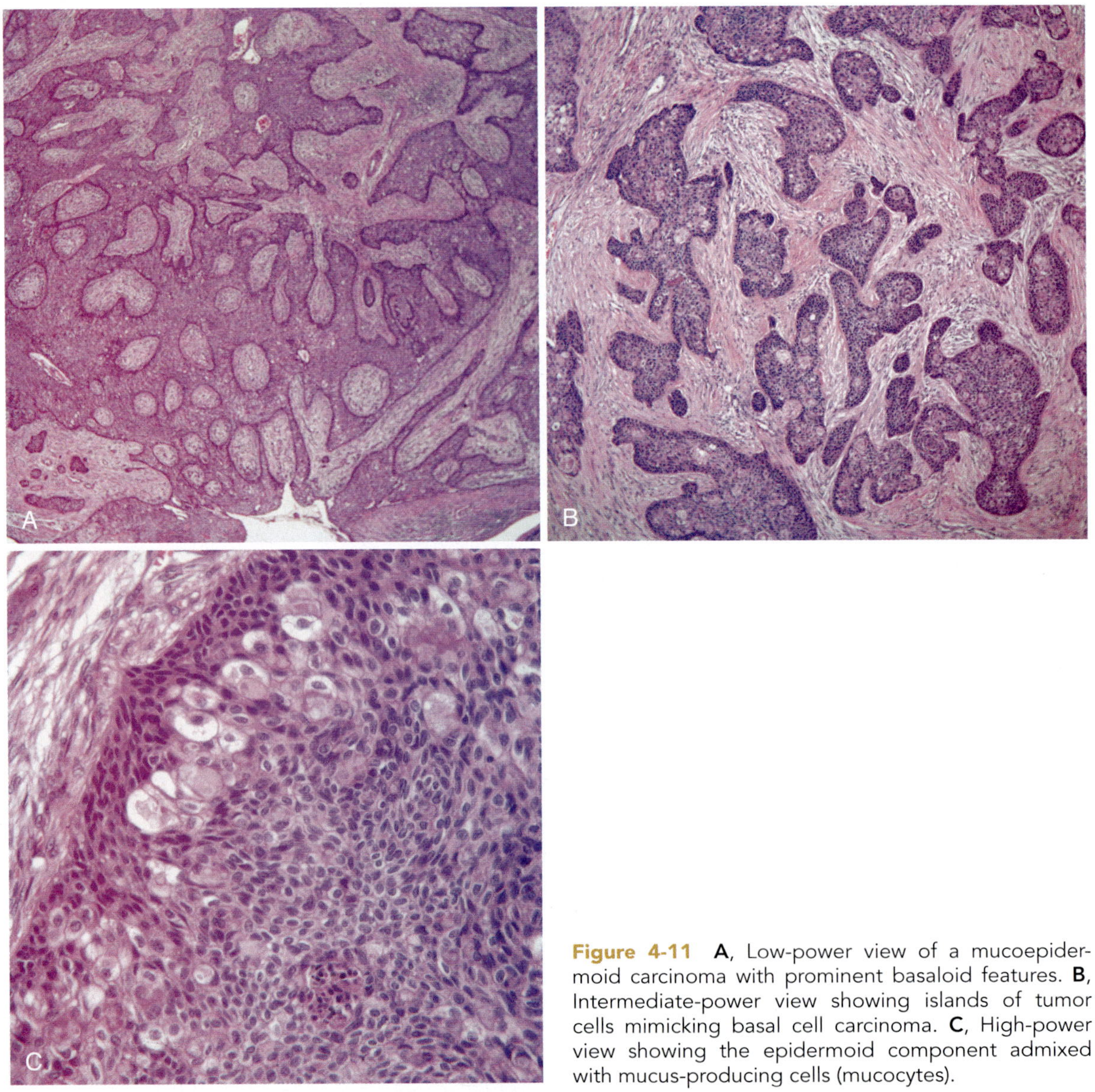

Figure 4-11 **A**, Low-power view of a mucoepidermoid carcinoma with prominent basaloid features. **B**, Intermediate-power view showing islands of tumor cells mimicking basal cell carcinoma. **C**, High-power view showing the epidermoid component admixed with mucus-producing cells (mucocytes).

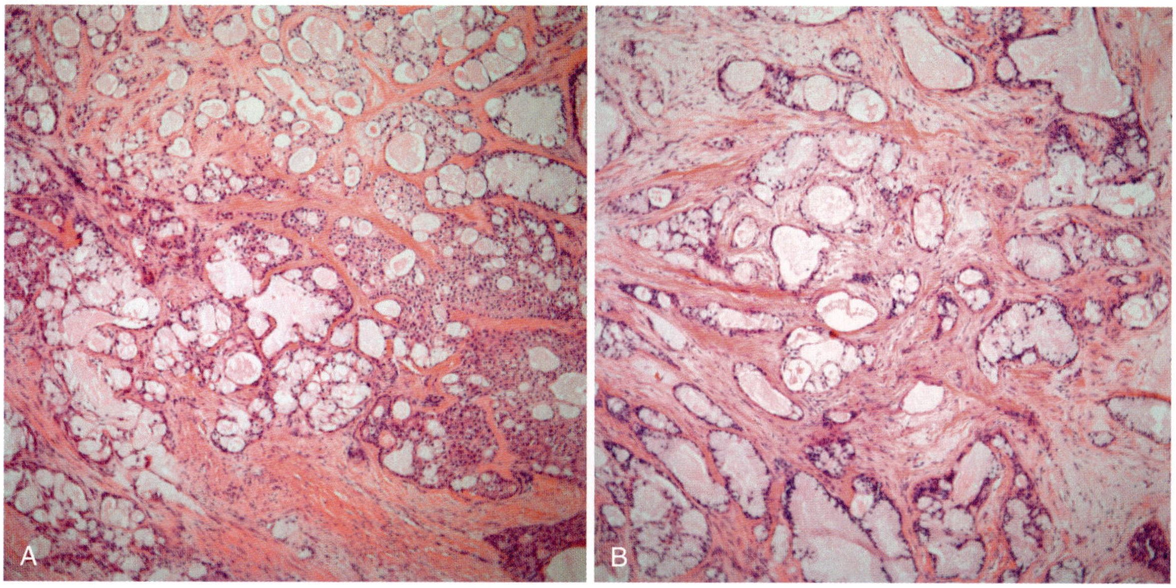

Figure 4-12 **A**, Low-grade mucoepidermoid carcinoma with predominant glandular component and focal solid areas. **B**, Mucoepidermoid carcinoma with a predominant glandular component composed of mucus-producing cells.

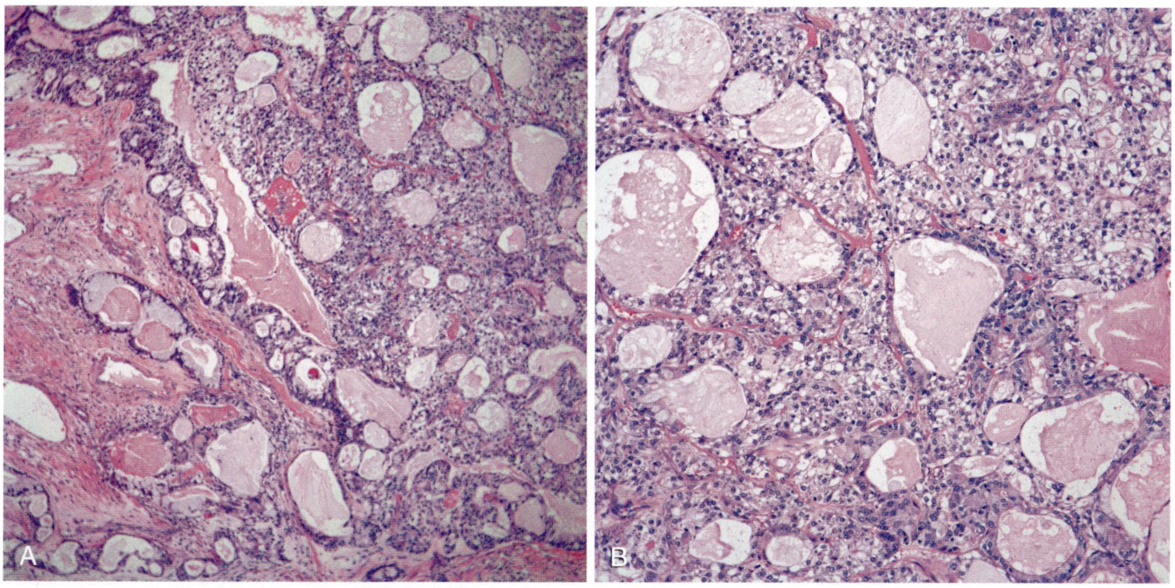

Figure 4-13 **A**, Low-power view of a low-grade mucoepidermoid carcinoma with solid and cystic areas and absence of keratinization. **B**, The same tumor at high-power magnification.

Differential Diagnosis

The scope of the differential diagnosis will depend primarily on the material available for review. In small biopsy specimens, low-grade tumors may pose more diagnostic difficulty. If the tumor shows cystic changes with a glandular appearance, mucous gland adenoma may be the most difficult clinical entity to rule out. If the specimen shows a more solid component, squamous cell carcinoma will be the leading consideration in the differential diagnosis. In the latter case, the presence of keratinization, nuclear atypia, and mitotic activity and presence of an in situ component may lead to a more correct interpretation. The separation of low- and high-grade tumors cannot be accomplished in a small biopsy specimen; this distinction requires careful examination of material obtained at complete surgical resection. Another possibility in the differential diagnosis is adenosquamous carcinoma; for this diagnosis, however, it is imperative to observe unequivocal areas of squamous cell carcinoma admixed with unequivocal areas of adenocarcinoma.

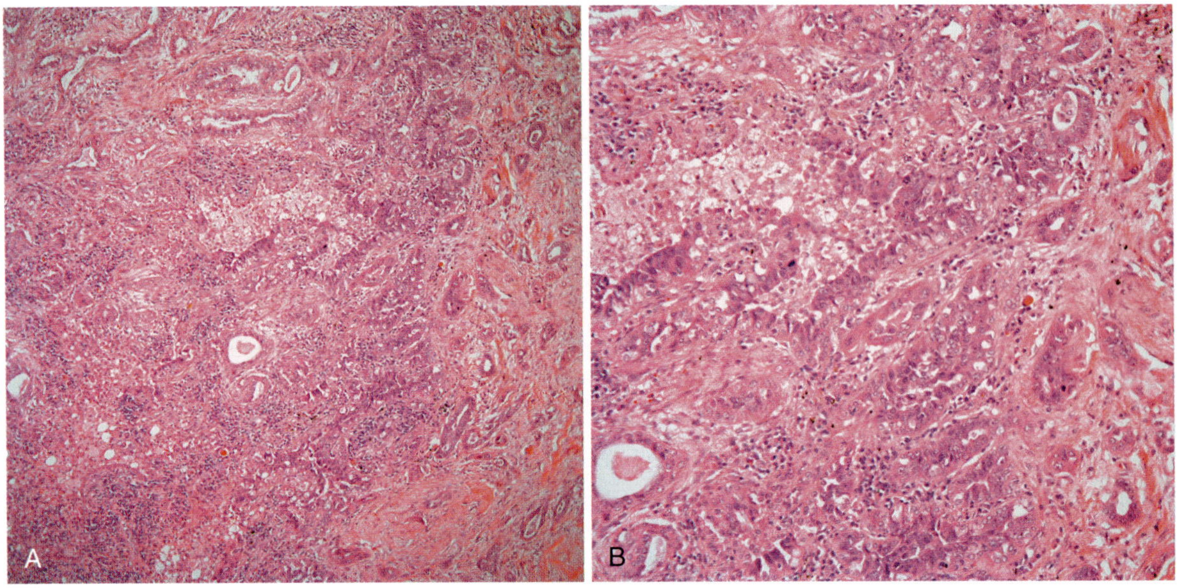

Figure 4-14 **A**, High-grade mucoepidermoid carcinoma showing a disorganized pattern. **B**, Atypical epithelial component with nuclear atypia and mitotic activity.

Clinical Behavior

The behavior of MEC is closely related to the degree of differentiation. Low-grade tumors can be managed surgically, and complete surgical resection is the treatment of choice. When complete surgical resection is not possible, the possibility of recurrence is high, and additional treatment may be considered. Tumors of high-grade histology often display aggressive behavior. In such cases, surgical resection and additional medical options should be considered.

ADENOID CYSTIC CARCINOMA

Clinical Features

Adenoid cystic carcinoma appears to be the second most common tumor in this family of neoplasms.[11–18] Most of the cases described are in adults. In one of the larger series of these tumors, patient ages ranged from 29 to 79 years (mean, 54 years), with a slight predilection for men in a ratio of 2:1.[11] As with other types of salivary gland–type tumors of the lung, when the tumors are centrally located, the patient may present with pulmonary obstructive symptoms, pneumonia, dyspnea, cough, wheezing, or hemoptysis. If the tumor occurs in the periphery of the lung, however, the patient may be asymptomatic.

Macroscopic Features

Most adenoid cystic carcinomas will manifest in a central endobronchial location. The tumors may range from 1 to 4 cm in greatest diameter (Fig. 4-15). They usually are well circumscribed and of soft consistency.

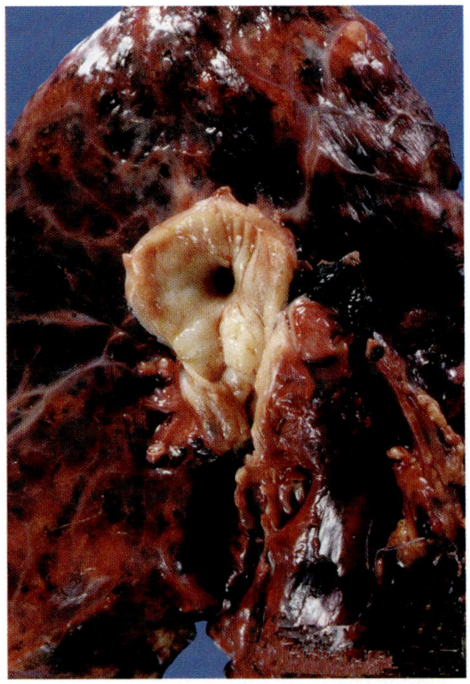

Figure 4-15 Gross image of an endobronchial adenoid cystic carcinoma.

Microscopic Features

Three distinct growth patterns for adenoid cystic carcinoma have been described: cylindromatous, tubular, and solid. The most common growth pattern is the *cylindromatous* pattern, characterized by islands of tumor cells arranged in a jigsaw pattern (Fig. 4-16). Thin bands of fibroconnective tissue separate each one of these islands. At higher magnification, the cystic areas are seen to be lined by two rows of cells, which are composed of

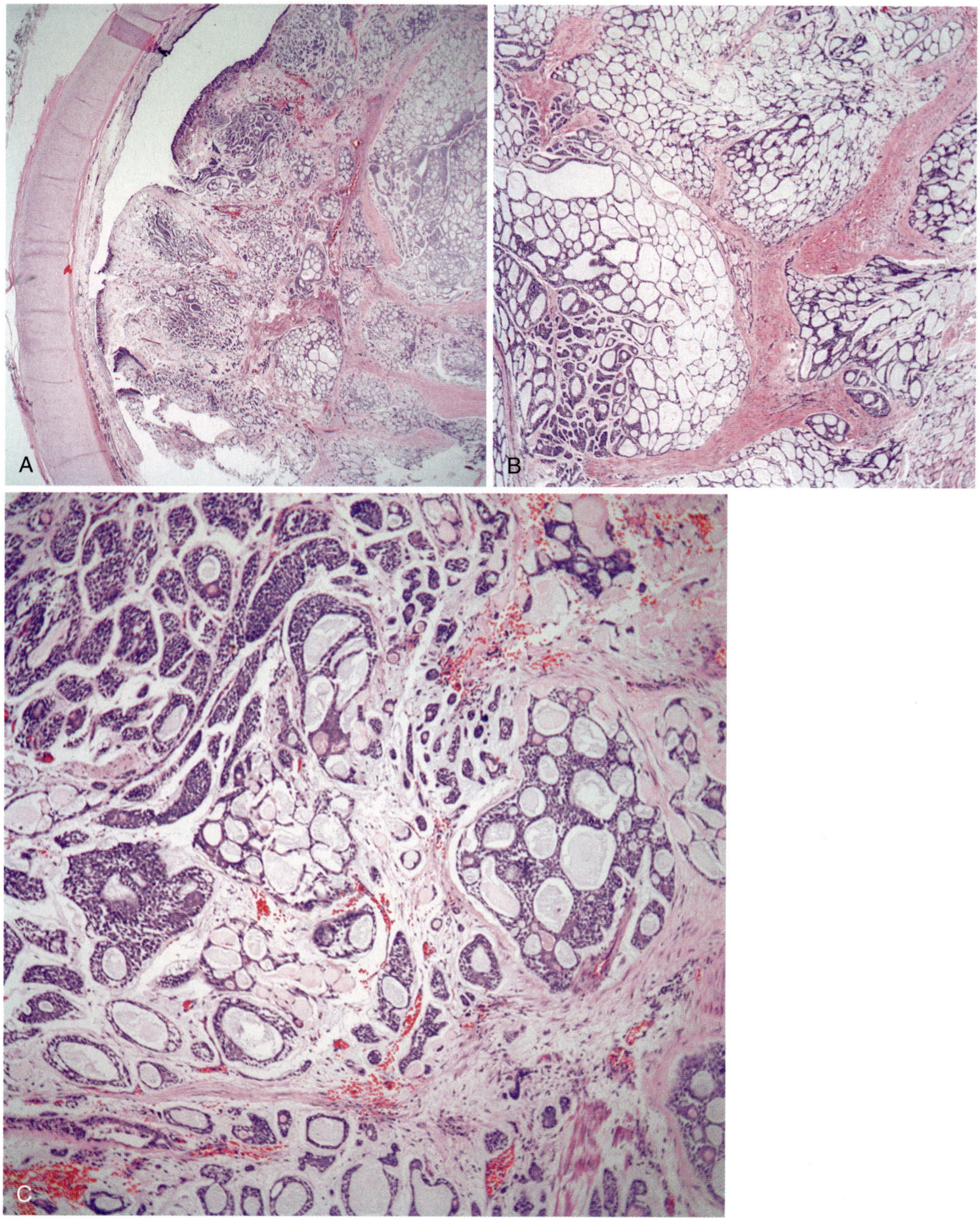

Figure 4-16 **A**, Low-power view of adenoid cystic carcinoma. **B**, Classic cylindromatous growth pattern. **C**, Islands of tumor cells within the classic cylindromatous component.

somewhat smaller cells with scant cytoplasm and round to angulated nuclei (Fig. 4-17). In the lumen of these cystic areas, it frequently is possible to identify acellular material or the presence of extensive areas of hyalinization (Fig. 4-18). Mitotic figures, cellular pleomorphism, necrosis, and hemorrhage usually are absent.

The *tubular* growth pattern characteristically shows neoplastic cells arranged in small, glandular-like "tubules." Cytologically, the tumor cells are similar to those seen in the cylindromatous pattern (Fig. 4-19). In some areas, these "tubules" may merge, giving an image of a solid glandular pattern (Fig. 4-20).

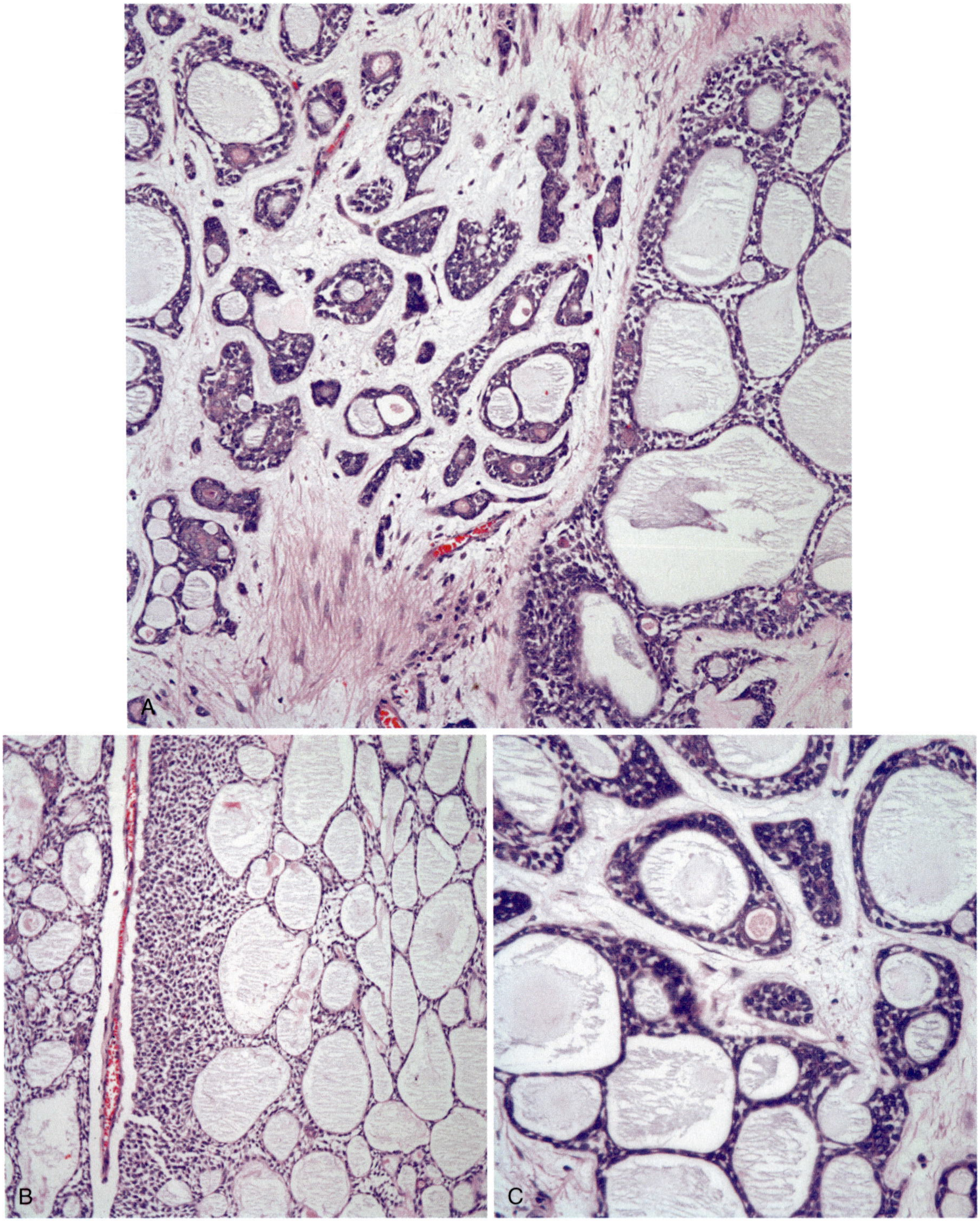

Figure 4-17 Adenoid cystic carcinoma. **A**, Cylindromatous growth pattern composed of cystic structures of different sizes. **B**, Cystic structures admixed with more solid epithelial areas. **C**, Structures composed of two rows of cells. Note the absence of nuclear atypia or mitotic activity.

The *solid* growth pattern is the most unusual of the three and may show cellular atypia and mitotic activity. In this pattern, it is common to observe the presence of delicate collagen bands separating either tubules or dissecting tumor cells (Fig. 4-21). It also is possible to identify areas of more conventional tubular or cylindromatous growth, which makes the identification of this tumor a little easier (Fig. 4-22). Pure tubular or solid adenoid cystic carcinomas are rare, and even though one pattern may be more prominent than the other,

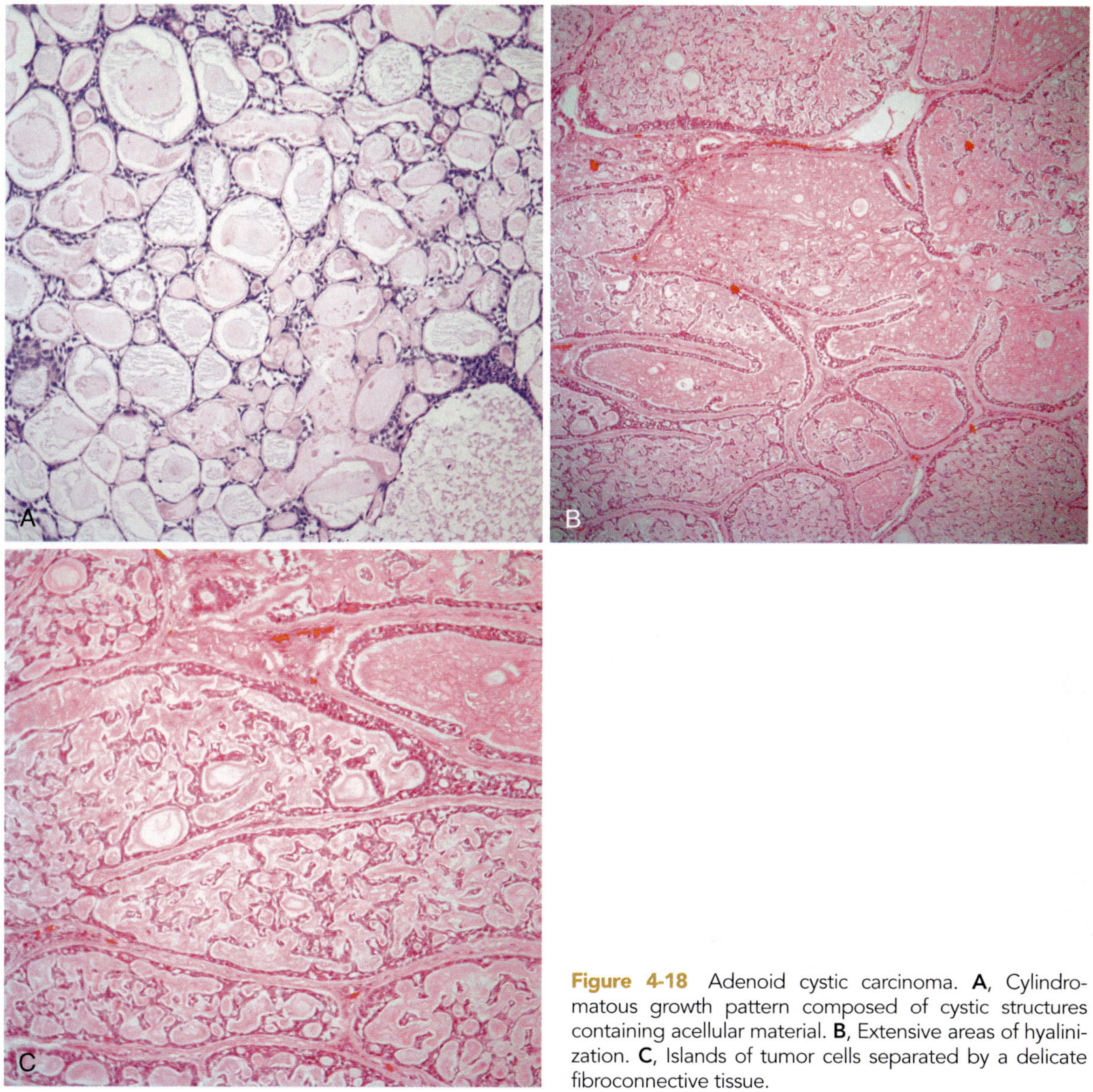

Figure 4-18 Adenoid cystic carcinoma. **A**, Cylindromatous growth pattern composed of cystic structures containing acellular material. **B**, Extensive areas of hyalinization. **C**, Islands of tumor cells separated by a delicate fibroconnective tissue.

observation of the areas of conventional differentiation will lead to a more correct interpretation. An important feature in all three growth patterns is the presence of perineural invasion.

Immunohistochemical Features

Like many other salivary gland–type tumors, adenoid cystic carcinoma also may show features of myoepithelial differentiation. Positive staining using antibodies for keratin, smooth muscle actin (Fig. 4-23), S-100 protein, and vimentin is commonly seen. In cases of tubular or solid growth pattern, the use of collagen type IV may be helpful to highlight the basal membrane material.

Differential Diagnosis

In small biopsy specimens, if the cylindromatous component is present, the main consideration in the differential diagnosis will be epithelial-myoepithelial carcinoma. In such cases, it is important to look carefully for the two rows of cells that are more commonly seen in adenoid cystic carcinoma. Because both of these tumors may share a similar immunohistochemical profile, an unequivocal diagnosis using limited biopsy material may not be possible, requiring complete surgical resection for proper classification. On the other hand, if the tumor shows the tubular or solid pattern, the main diagnostic consideration will be a conventional non–small cell carcinoma—namely, adenocarcinoma.

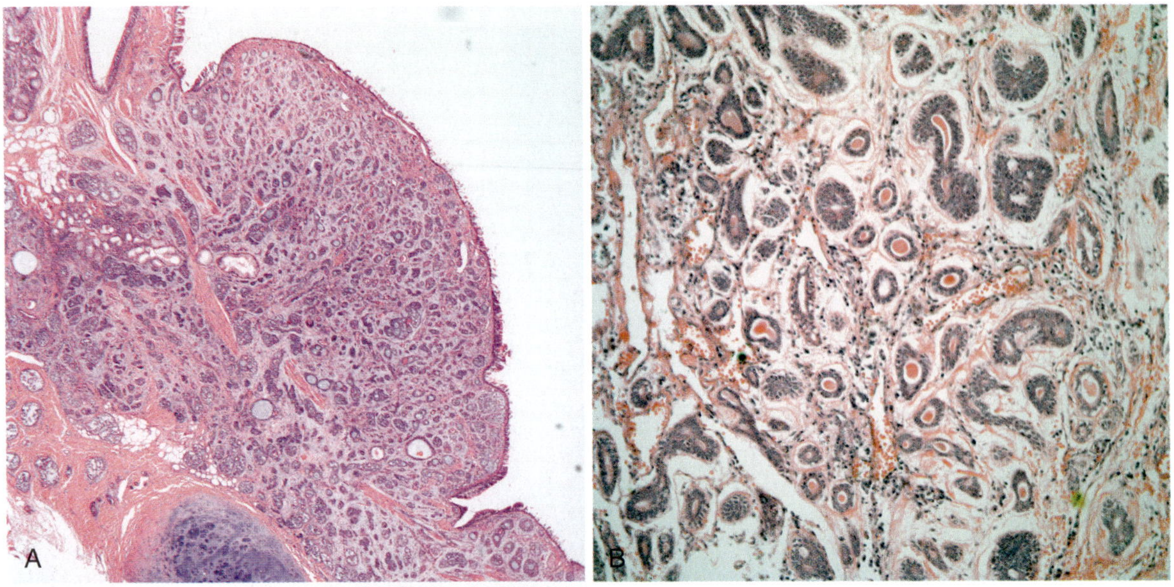

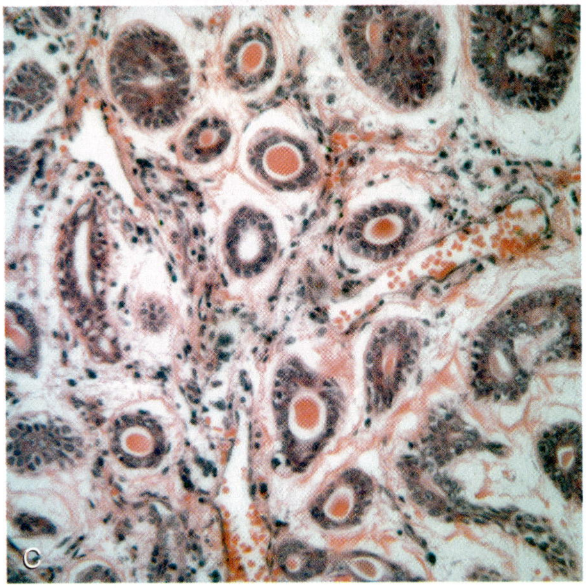

Figure 4-19 **A**, Low-power view of adenoid cystic carcinoma with a tubular growth pattern. **B**, Numerous glandular structures separated by thin fibroconnective tissue. **C**, Glandular areas composed of two rows of cells. Nuclear atypia and mitotic activity are absent.

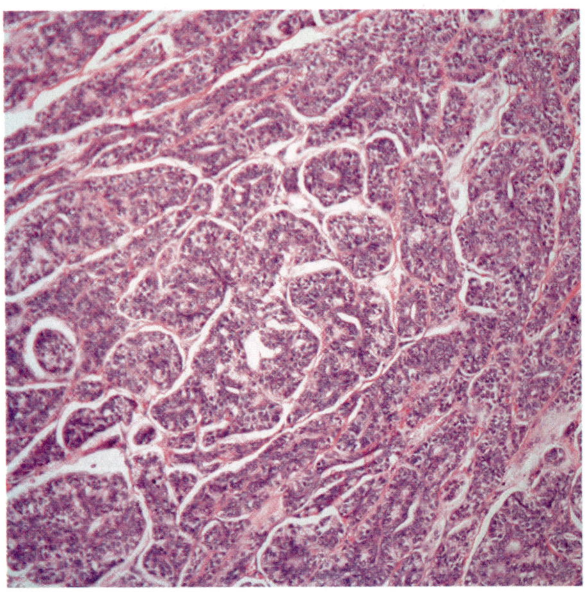

Figure 4-20 Adenoid cystic carcinoma. Tubular growth pattern with prominent solid component.

Clinical Behavior

Adenoid cystic carcinoma is a slow-growth tumor. Nevertheless, adenoid cystic carcinoma may behave aggressively, with widespread metastasis. The clinical stage at the time of diagnosis is very important in predicting clinical behavior.

ACINIC CELL CARCINOMA

Clinical Features

Acinic cell carcinoma also is known as Fechner's tumor, to honor the first clinician to describe this neoplasm in the lung.[19] It is an uncommon primary lung tumor that can manifest centrally or peripherally.[20–22] Most of the descriptions of these tumors have been isolated case reports. In a larger series,[20] the investigators found a higher prevalence in adults, with no predilection for either gender. In that report, a majority of tumors were

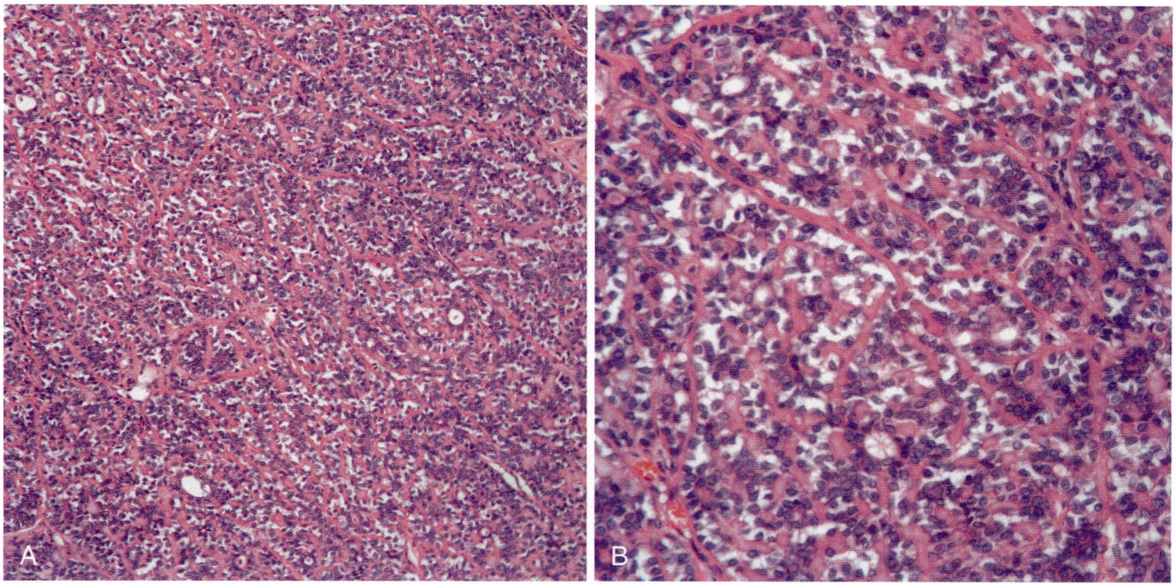

Figure 4-21 **A**, Low-power view of the solid component in an adenoid cystic carcinoma with tubular growth pattern. Note the presence of clear cells, small glandular structures, and myoepithelial cells separated by thin collagenous material. **B**, High-power view.

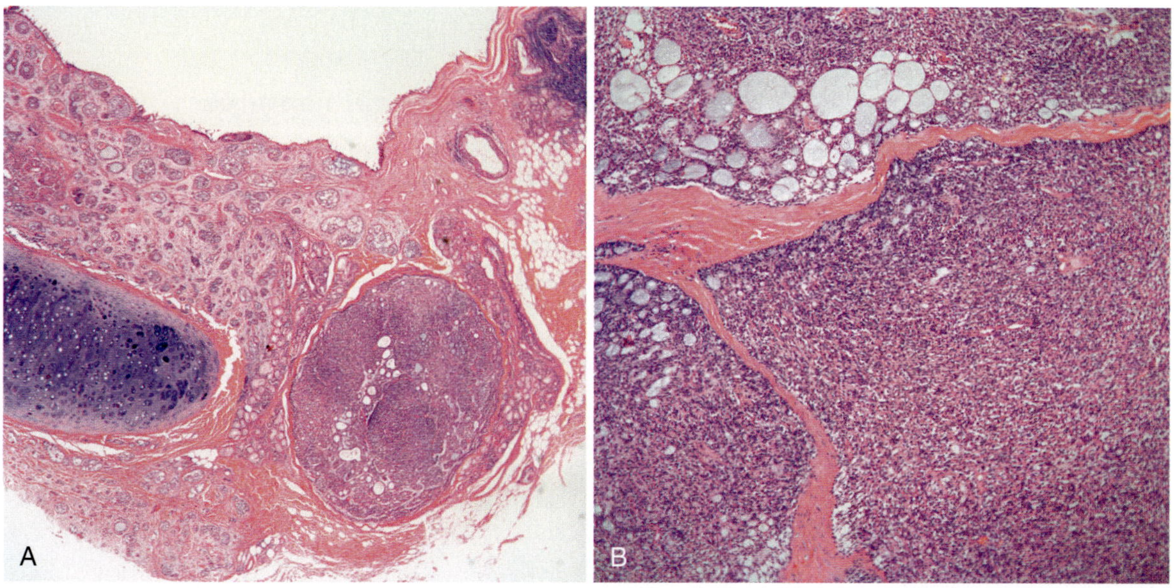

Figure 4-22 **A**, Low-power view of an adenoid cystic carcinoma showing tubular and solid growth patterns. **B**, Solid component of adenoid cystic carcinoma with only focal cystic areas.

located peripherally; accordingly, most of the patients were asymptomatic, and their tumors were discovered during routine radiographic examination. When these tumors arise in a central location, the patient will experience symptoms of obstruction, dyspnea, and cough.

Macroscopic Features

Acinic cell carcinomas in the lung are well-circumscribed tumors, which can range in size from 1 to 5 cm in greatest dimension. They are soft, with a homogeneous cut surface, without necrosis or hemorrhage.

Microscopic Features

The main histopathologic variants are acinar, oncocytic, and papillocystic. The *acinar* variant is composed of medium-sized cells with clear granular cytoplasm, displaying small nuclei toward the periphery of the cells (resembling a "signet ring cell"), and inconspicuous nucleoli (Fig. 4-24). Nuclear atypia and mitotic activity are

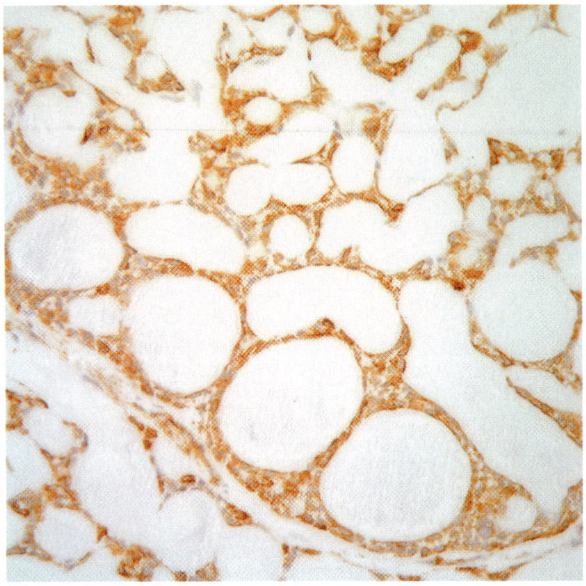

Figure 4-23 Smooth muscle actin showing a positive reaction in myopithelial cells.

uncommon. The neoplastic cells grow in cords or arranged in pseudoglandular formation, separated by fibrocollagen bands with an inflammatory infiltrate. In some areas, the pattern is observed to be more solid, with nests of tumor cells separated by a mild inflammatory infiltrate, whereas in other areas, the tumor cells float in alveolar spaces (Fig. 4-25). Necrosis and hemorrhage are absent. In the *oncocytic* growth pattern, the tumor has a more solid appearance (Fig. 4-26). The cells are of medium size with oncocytic cytoplasm and a central nucleus, and in some cells, nucleoli may be seen (Fig. 4-27). No mitotic activity or nuclear atypia is present in this growth pattern. In the *papillocystic* variant, the tumor may display areas of cystic structures lined by cells with acinar cell characteristics (Fig. 4-28), whereas in other areas the cystic component may be more prominent, with cystically dilated areas containing acellular material. The true nature of the acinar cell component becomes apparent at higher magnification (Fig. 4-29). In all three growth patterns, necrosis, hemorrhage, cellular atypia, and mitotic activity are rarely observed.

Histochemical and Immunohistochemical Features

The most useful histochemical stain is periodic acid–Schiff stain (PAS), which demonstrates the presence of glycogen in the tumor cells (Fig. 4-30). Mucicarmine may give focal positive staining for intracellular mucin. Immunohistochemical studies are not very helpful in the diagnosis of acinic cell carcinoma, because these tumors will stain with low-molecular-weight keratin (CAM 5.2) and epithelial membrane antigen (EMA). Some tumors have shown positive staining for α_1-antichymotrypsin and amylase (Fig. 4-31).

Ultrastructural Features

The role of electron microscopy in the diagnosis of acinic cell carcinomas cannot be overemphasized. The finding of dark, electron-dense granules or electron-lucent granules (immature zymogen granules) in the cytoplasm of the neoplastic cells is diagnostic for acinic cell carcinoma.

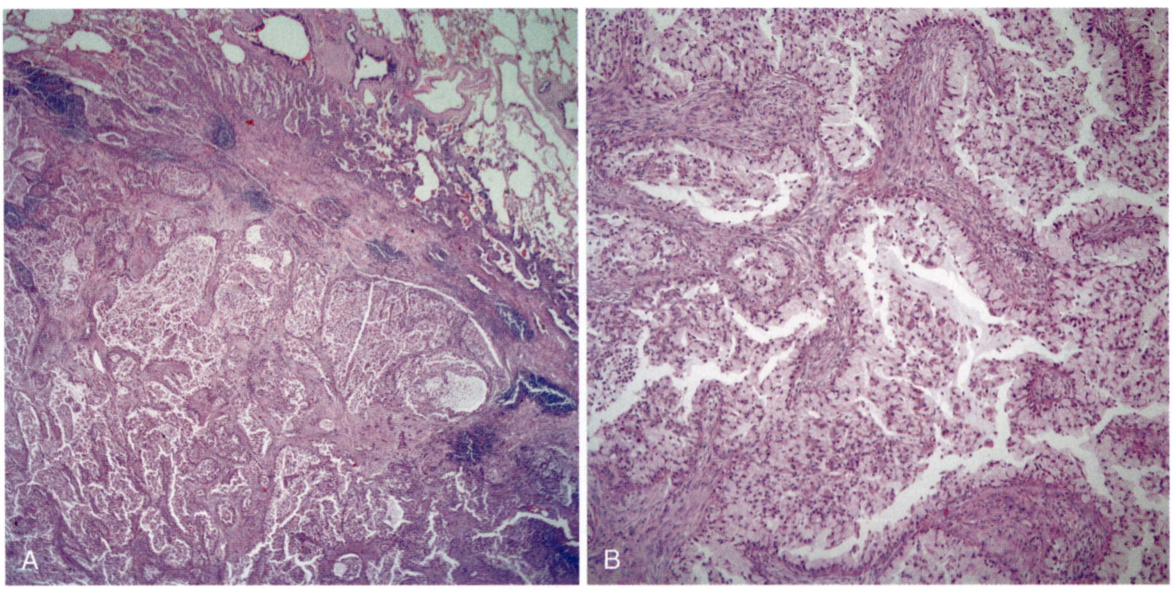

Figure 4-24 **A**, Low-power view of acinic cell carcinoma destroying lung parenchyma. **B**, Acinar growth pattern. Tumor cells are separated by thick bands of fibroconnective tissue with inflammatory reaction.

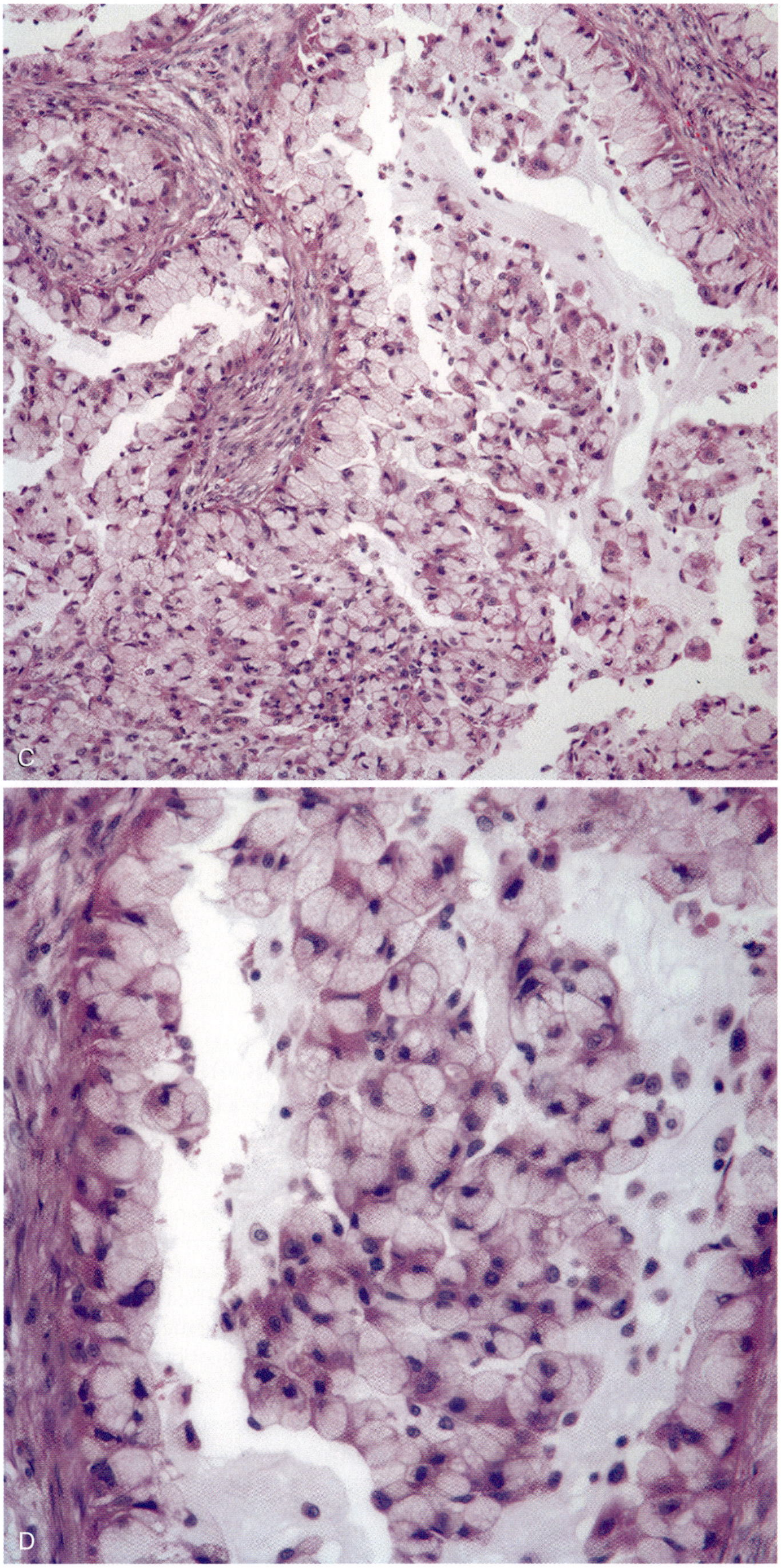

Figure 4-24—cont'd **C**, Tumor cells showing striking clear granular cytoplasm with nuclei displayed toward the periphery. **D**, High-power view showing clear cells with granular cytoplasm. Note the absence of nuclear pleomorphism or mitotic activity.

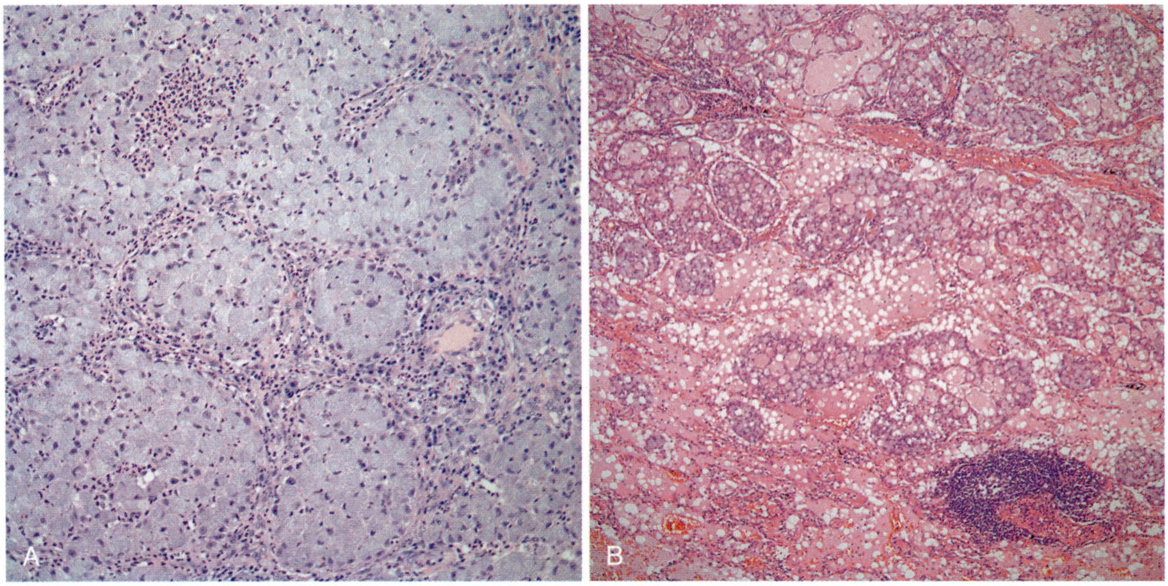

Figure 4-25 Acinic cell carcinoma, **A**, Islands of neoplastic cells with granular cytoplasm. **B**, Neoplastic cells filling alveolar spaces.

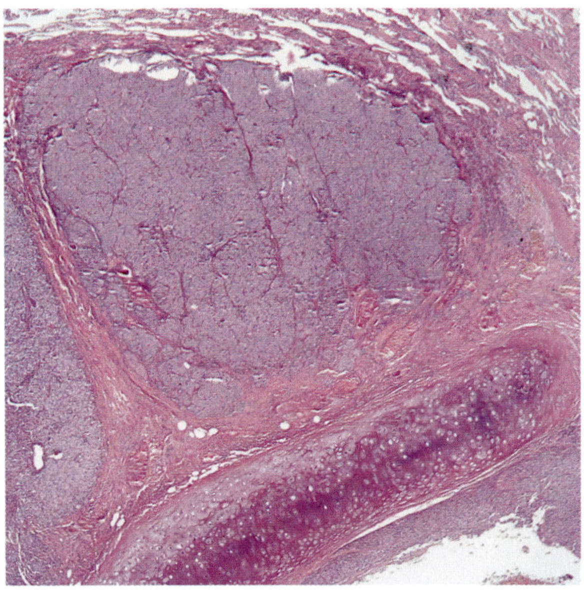

Figure 4-26 Acinic cell carcinoma showing a solid oncocytic cellular proliferation.

Differential Diagnosis

The scope of the differential diagnosis will depend primarily on the histologic growth pattern and cell type. When the tumor manifests prominent oncocytic features, the most important consideration in the differential diagnosis is oncocytic neuroendocrine carcinoma. In this setting, the use of immunohistochemical neuroendocrine markers such as chromogranin, synpatophysin, and CD56 may lead to the correct interpretation. When the tumor shows an acinar growth pattern with cells resembling signet ring cells, the most important diagnostic possibility is adenocarcinoma with signet ring cell features. In this setting, histochemical staining with mucicarmine will demonstrate the presence of intracellular mucin coupled with the presence of nuclear atypia, as well as mitotic activity, leading to a correct diagnosis.

Clinical Behavior

Acinic cell carcinomas usually are low-grade neoplasms. In some cases, however, the tumor may show aggressive behavior with widespread metastasis.

PLEOMORPHIC ADENOMA (MIXED TUMOR)

Clinical Features

Pleomorphic adenoma is an unusual primary tumor in the lung.[23–27] It appears to occur predominantly in adults, with a slight predilection for women. Patient age may range from 35 to 75 years. The tumor can occur in a central or peripheral location, and the signs and symptoms may be related to the anatomic distribution of the tumor. No predilection for any particular lung or lung segment has been documented.

Macroscopic Features

The endobronchial lesions may manifest as polypoid tumors, whereas those in the periphery of the lung may manifest as well-circumscribed tumors. The tumors may

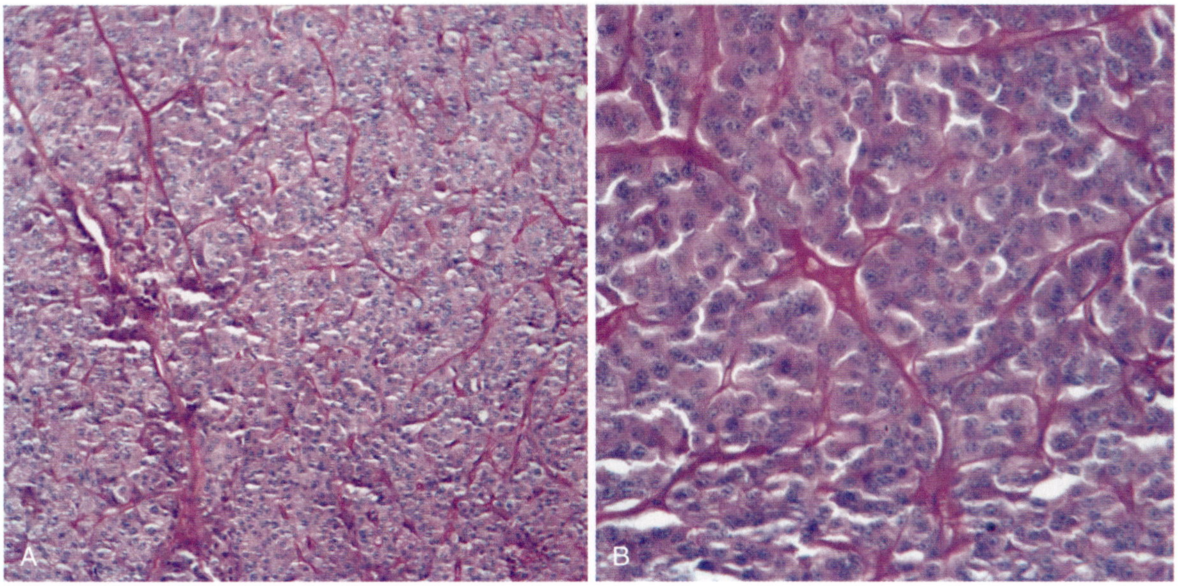

Figure 4-27 Acinic cell carcinoma, **A**, Oncocytic cells arranged in a nested pattern. **B**, High-power view showing absence of mitotic activity.

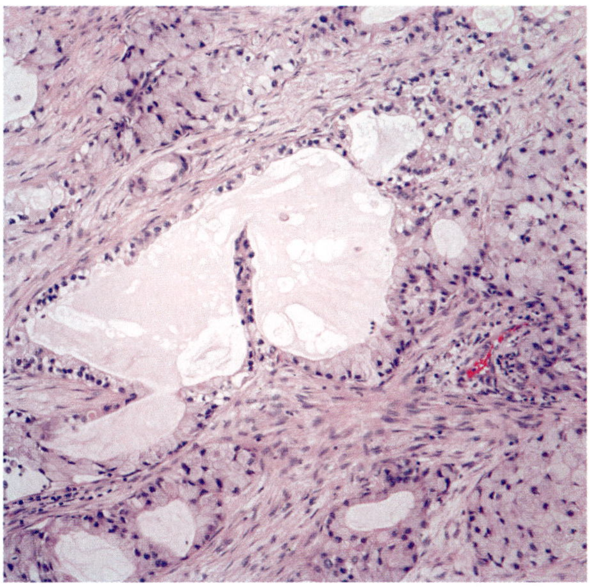

Figure 4-28 Acinic cell carcinoma. Cystic structures are mixed with solid areas.

range in size from 1 cm to more than 10 cm in diameter. Tumors in the central location are likely to be smaller, owing to their propensity to cause early symptoms.

Microscopic Features

Histologically, these tumors may be categorized as either conventional benign mixed tumors or, rarely, malignant mixed tumor (ex pleomorphic adenoma). By definition, pleomorphic adenomas are biphasic in composition—they may display both epithelial and mesenchymal areas (Fig. 4-32). The epithelial areas may show cystic or tubular structures, lined by a low cuboidal- or squamous cell–type epithelium, resembling adnexal elements (Fig. 4-33). In some cases, the epithelial component has a trabecular arrangement with a bland spindle cell–type mesenchymal component (Fig. 4-34). Alternatively, the epithelial component may show a solid myoepithelial proliferation composed of medium-sized cells with light eosinophilic cytoplasm, round nuclei, and inconspicuous nucleoli (Fig. 4-35). In some cases, the solid epithelial component may have a marked plasmacytoid appearance, with larger cells (Fig. 4-36). Mitotic activity and nuclear atypia are absent. The mesenchymal component most commonly is indicated by the presence of chondromyxoid stroma. Although mature cartilage is a rare finding, in some cases it may appear prominently, admixed with areas of keratinization or tubular or myoepithelial-type structures (Fig. 4-37).

In cases of malignant mixed tumor (ex pleomorphic adenoma), histologic features generally include areas of necrosis, hemorrhage, and vascular permeation by tumor cells. This tumor also is characterized by malignant spindle cell areas in which mitotic activity and cellular pleomorphism are common, along with remnants of glandular or tubular epithelial structures, which also may show atypical features (Fig. 4-38).

Immunohistochemical Features

The immunophenotype of mixed tumors is similar to that of other salivary gland–type tumors, displaying a myoepithelial differentiation. Tumor cells may show positive

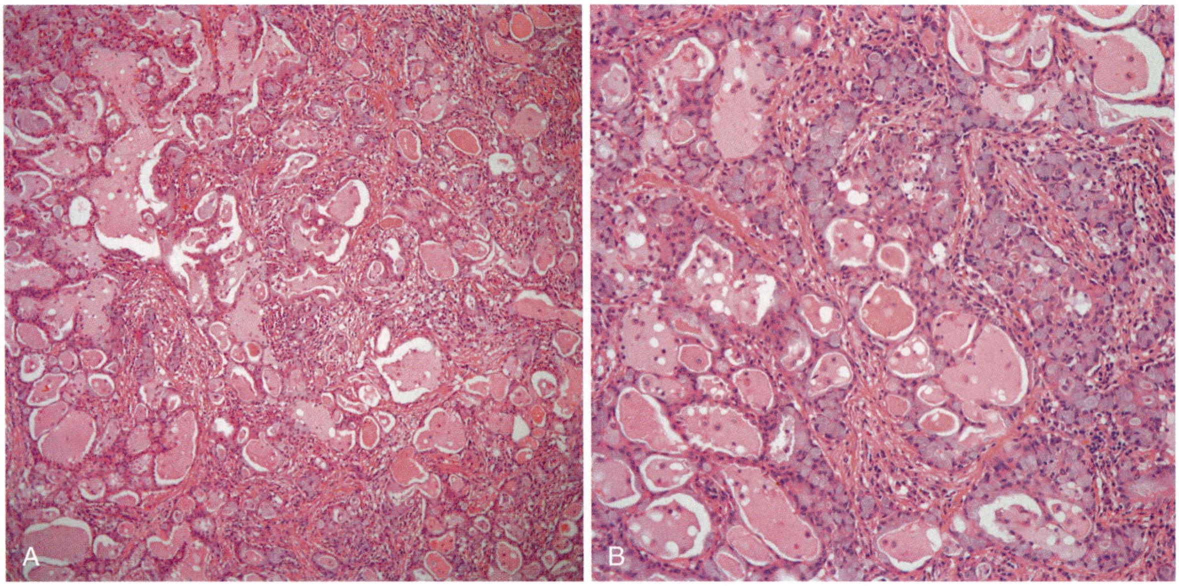

Figure 4-29 Acinic cell carcinoma. **A**, Prominent cystic growth pattern. **B**, Cystic growth pattern admixed with a more conventional acinar component.

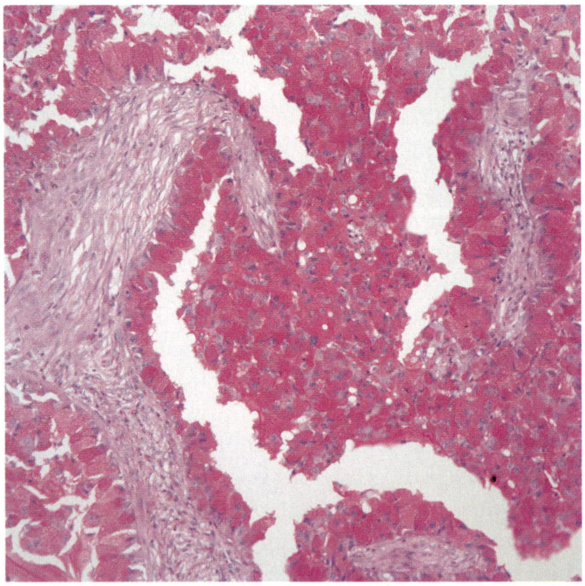

Figure 4-30 Acinic cell carcinoma. Strong positive reaction can be seen in tumor cells with periodic acid–Schiff (PAS) staining.

staining for low-molecular-weight keratin (i.e., CAM 5.2), smooth muscle actin, S-100 protein, and vimentin. In some tumors, staining for glial fibrillary acid protein (GFAP) also may be positive.

Differential Diagnosis

With small biopsy specimens, definitive diagnosis of mixed tumors may be very difficult. Considerations in the differential diagnosis will therefore depend largely on what the biopsy sample may show. Alternative diagnoses may range from another salivary gland–type tumor of the lung to a pure mesenchymal neoplasm. In cases with malignant histologic features identified in material from a complete surgical resection, the interpretation will depend on the identification of areas with a histologic pattern similar to that in benign mixed tumors. Otherwise, tumors may be classified as sarcomas or carcinosarcomas of the lung.

Clinical Behavior

For benign mixed tumors, complete surgical resection is curative. However, in tumors with malignant histologic features, clinical behavior is more aggressive and usually includes distant metastasis, which may require additional medical treatment.

EPITHELIAL-MYOEPITHELIAL CARCINOMA

Clinical Features

Epithelial-myoepithelial carcinoma is one of the most unusual salivary gland–type tumors of the lung.[28–33] The few reported cases have occurred in adults, and the tumors were centrally located. In keeping with this anatomic location, patients may present with obstructive symptoms, pneumonia, cough, dyspnea, or hemoptysis.

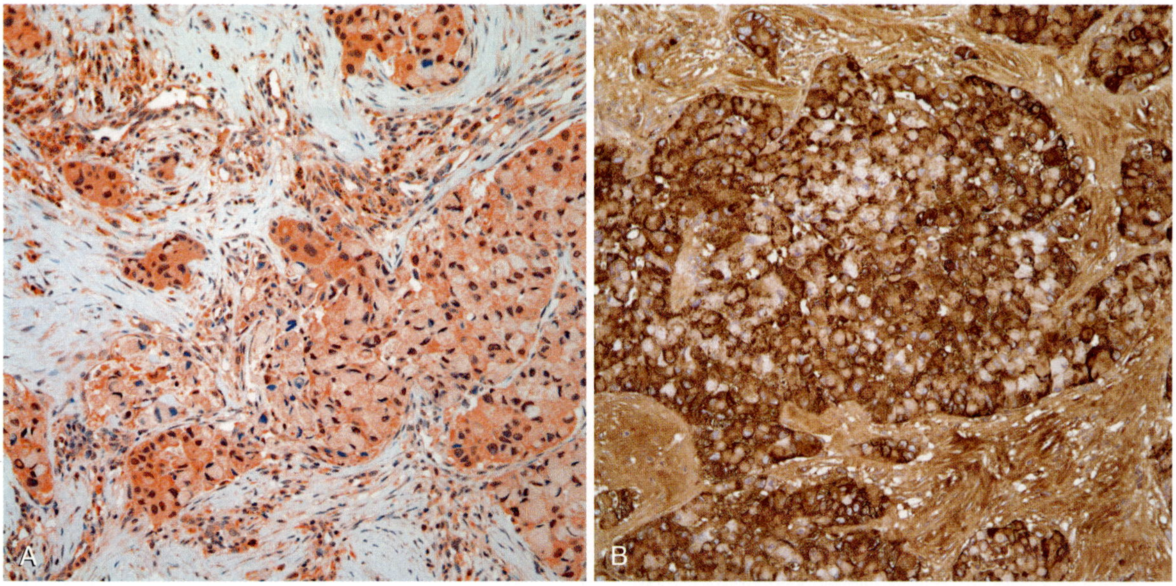

Figure 4-31 Acinic cell carcinoma. **A**, Immunohistochemical stain for amylase showing positive reaction in tumor cells. **B**, α_1-Antichimotrypsin showing strong positive reaction in tumor cells.

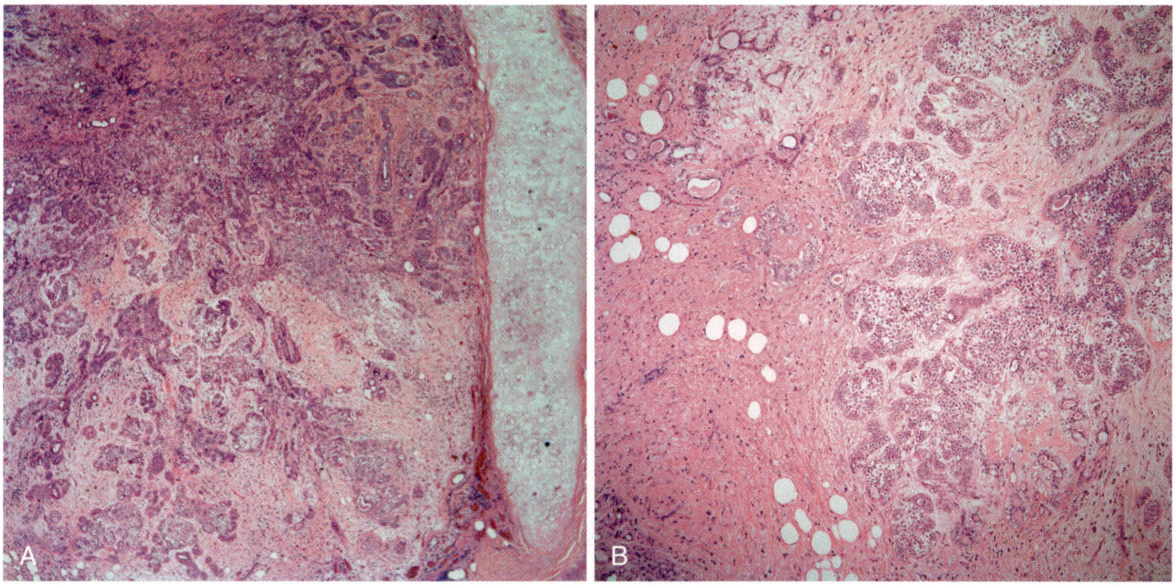

Figure 4-32 **A**, Low-power view of a mixed tumor. **B**, Mixed tumor showing areas of fibroconnective tissue, adipose tissue, and solid myoeithelial cells.

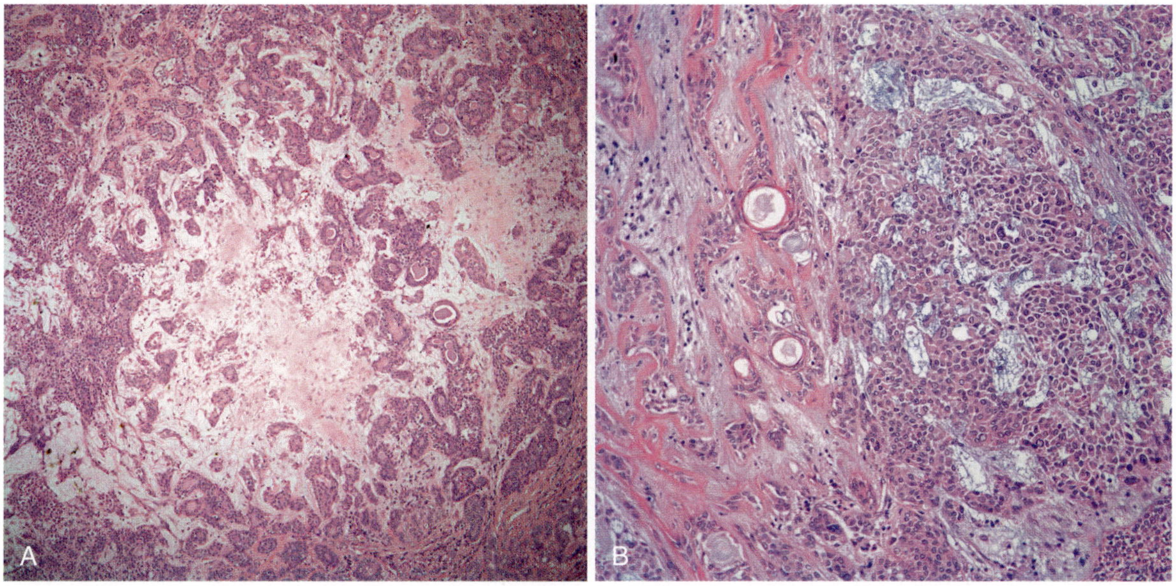

Figure 4-33 Mixed tumor. **A**, Myoepithelial cells embedded in fibrocollagenous tissue. **B**, Myoepithelial cells admixed with tubular adnexa–like structures.

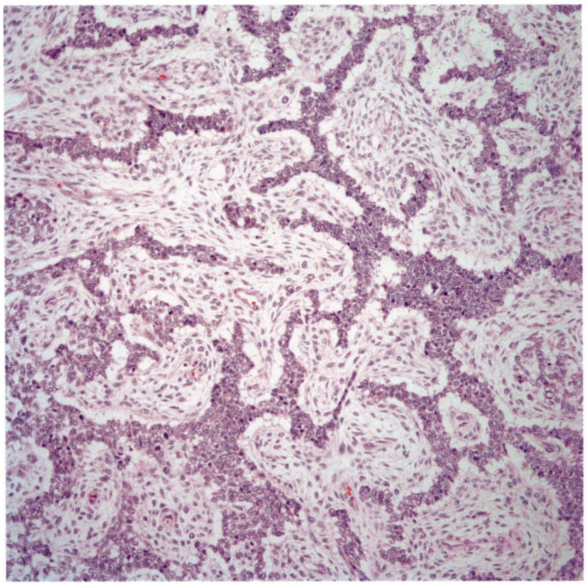

Figure 4-34 Mixed tumor showing myoepithelial cells arranged in a trabecular pattern and embedded in a bland spindle cell component.

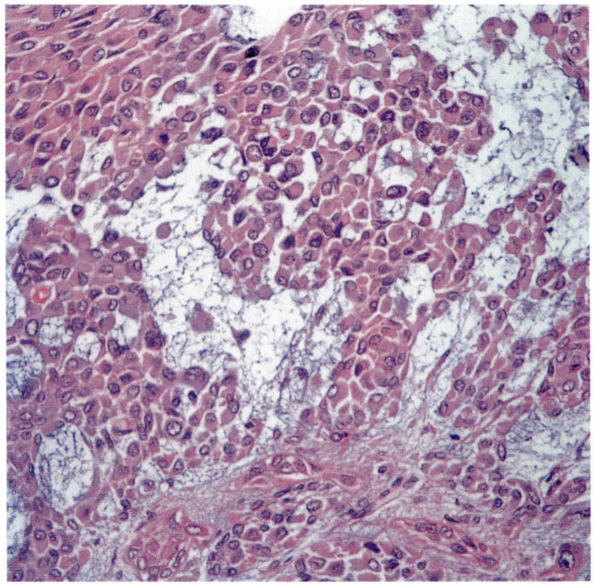

Figure 4-36 Mixed tumor. Solid myoepithelial component with prominent plasmacytoid appearance.

Macroscopic Features

The tumors appear to be well circumscribed, but not encapsulated, endobronchial lesions, ranging in size from 1 to 5 cm in greatest dimension. They may obstruct the airway lumen completely or partially.

Microscopic Features

The low-power view reveals a predominant glandular pattern, with glandular structures separated by thin fibroconnective tissue (Fig. 4-39). At higher magnification, the glandular component shows the characteristic dual cellular population of inner ductal epithelial cells surrounded by an outer layer of cells with clear cytoplasm (myoepithelial cells) (Fig. 4-40). In some areas the tumor has a more solid pattern, with only focal glandular differentiation (Fig. 4-41). Focal areas of squamous metaplasia and areas with sclerotic changes also may be seen (Fig. 4-42). The tumor does not show marked cellular atypia or increased mitotic activity. Areas of necrosis and hemorrhage are absent.

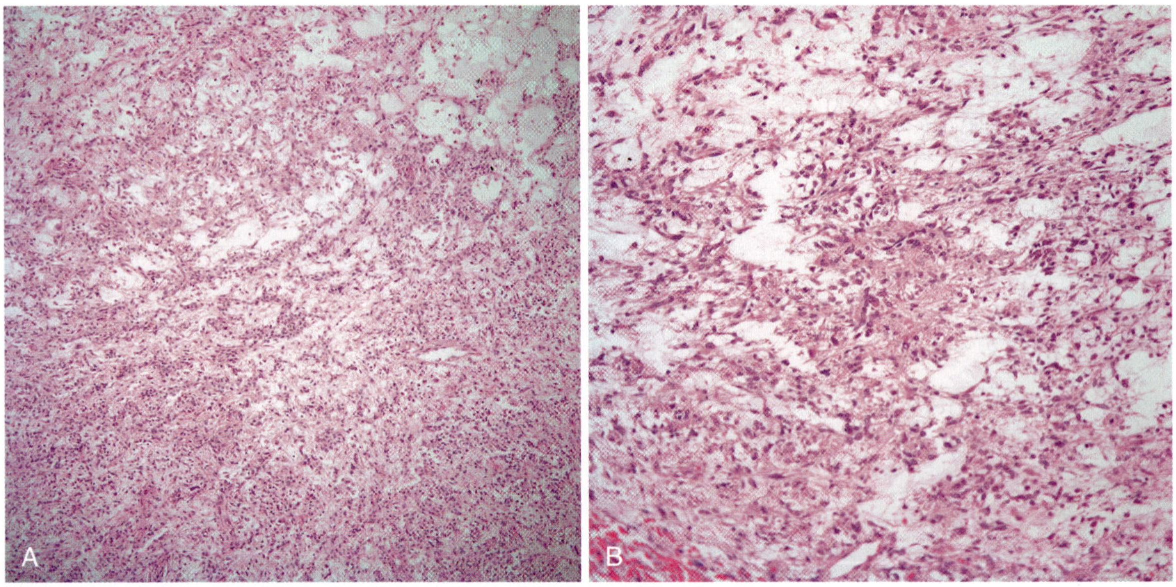

Figure 4-35 **A**, Mixed tumor with solid myoepithelial areas. **B**, High-power magnification of the solid myoepithelial component. Note the absence of nuclear atypia and mitotic activity.

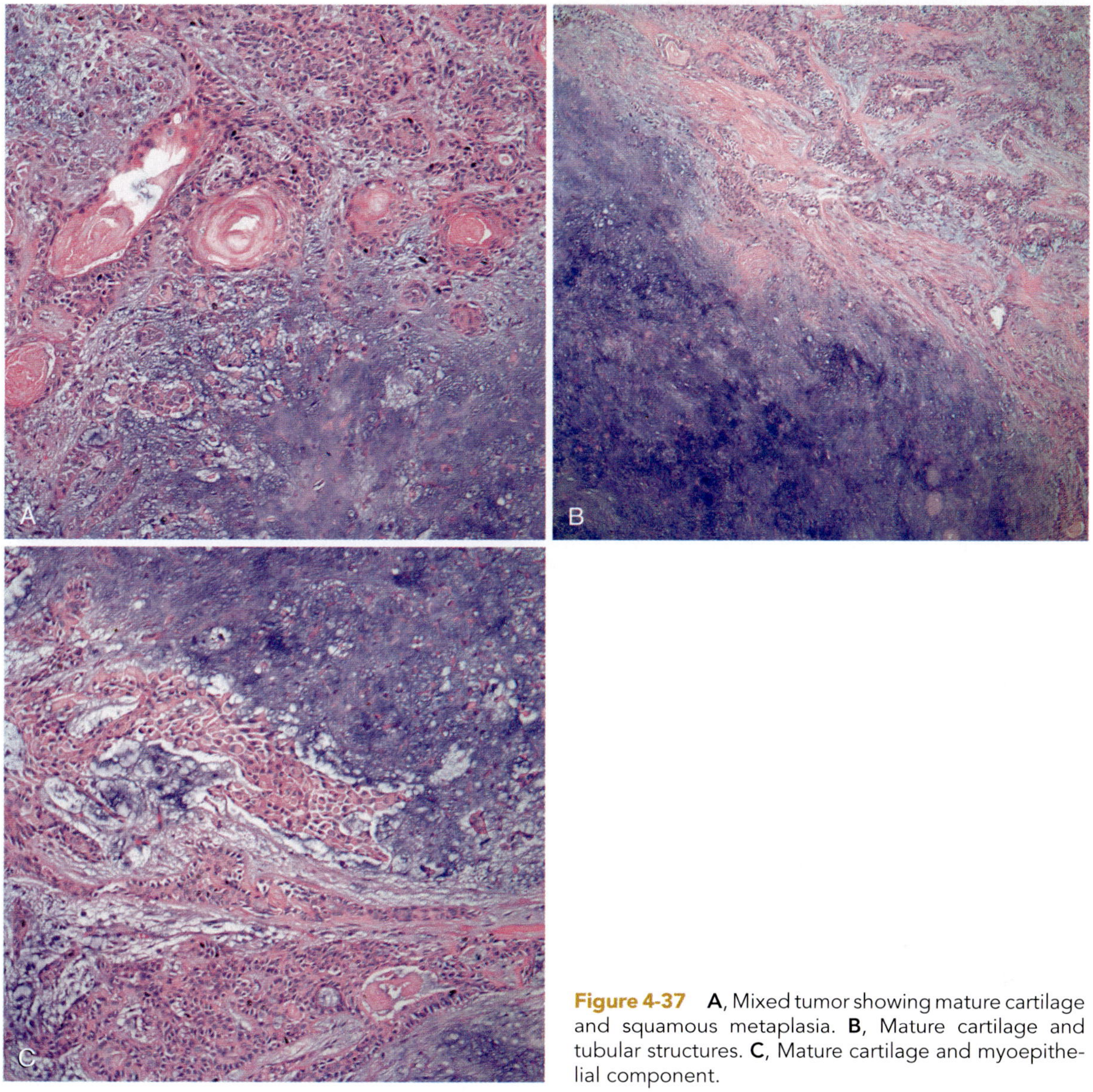

Figure 4-37 **A**, Mixed tumor showing mature cartilage and squamous metaplasia. **B**, Mature cartilage and tubular structures. **C**, Mature cartilage and myoepithelial component.

In some cases, a striking spindle cell component may be observed (Fig. 4-43).

Immunohistochemical Features

The tumor characteristically shows a dual cellular proliferation with positive staining for epithelial markers in the inner layer and for smooth muscle actin and S-100 protein in the outer layer. Focal weakly positive staining may be seen with CD117 and GFAP. Cases with positive staining for TTF-1 also have been reported.

Clinical Behavior

Because of the rarity of this tumor in the lung, assessing its malignant potential is difficult. Some evidence suggests, however, that the tumor may behave as a low-grade carcinoma with the potential to metastasize. Lymph node metastasis, although rare, is sometimes observed[33] (Fig. 4-44).

ONCOCYTOMAS

Oncocytomas occur very rarely in the lung, and only a few cases have been reported in the literature.[34-36] The histopathologic features described are similar to those of tumors occurring in the salivary glands. Because other tumors with similar characteristics occur more commonly in the lung, use of standard hematoxylin-eosin stains will not be sufficient for histopathologic diagnosis. Neuroendocrine carcinomas with oncocytic features or metastatic tumors with oncocytic features should be carefully ruled out by either immunohistochemical studies or clinical findings.

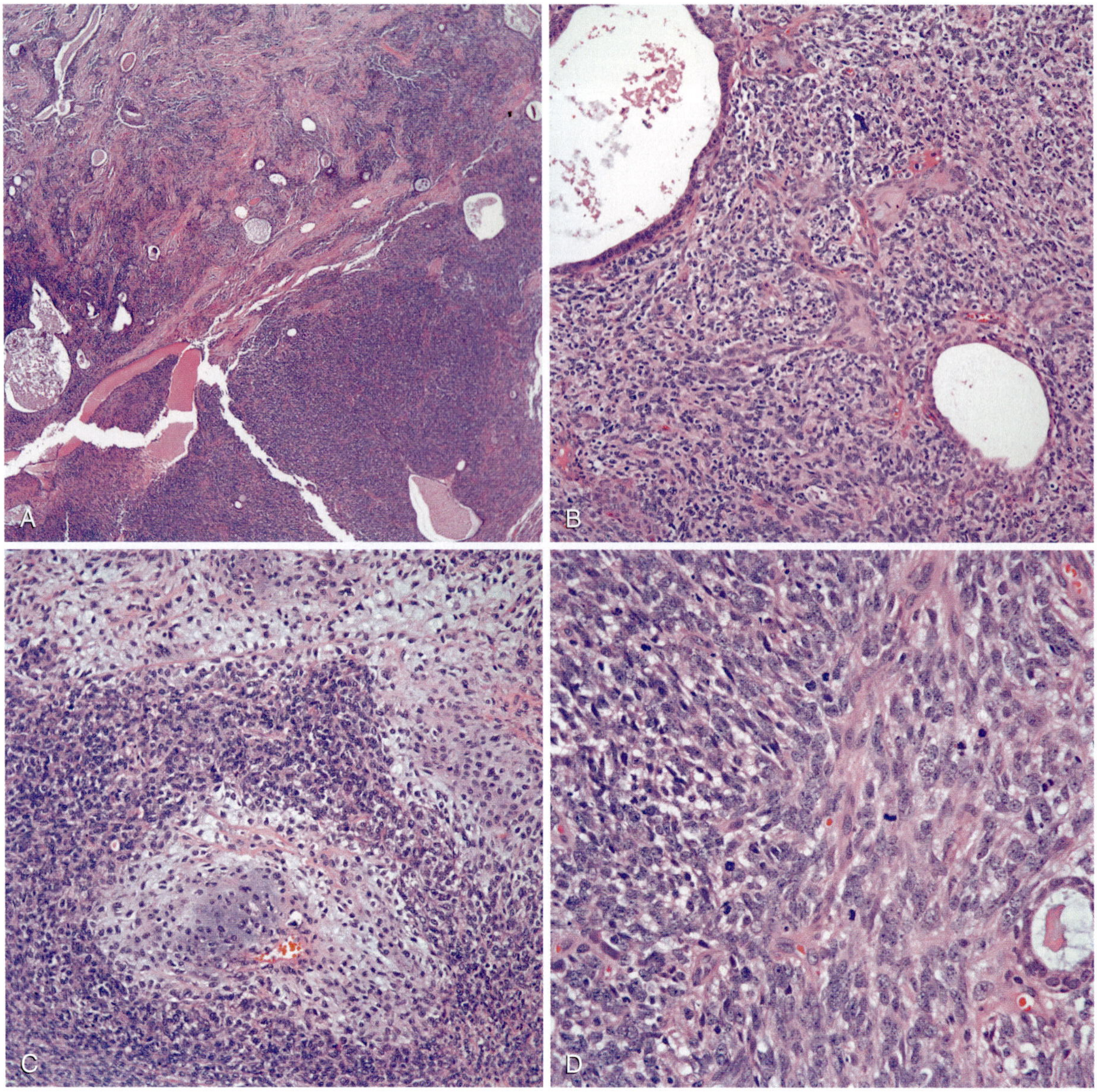

Figure 4-38 **A**, Malignant mixed tumor showing prominent solid areas. **B**, Prominent solid areas and residual cystic benign component. **C**, Solid component with residual benign chondroid component. **D**, Note the presence of nuclear atypia and mitotic activity in the solid spindle cell component.

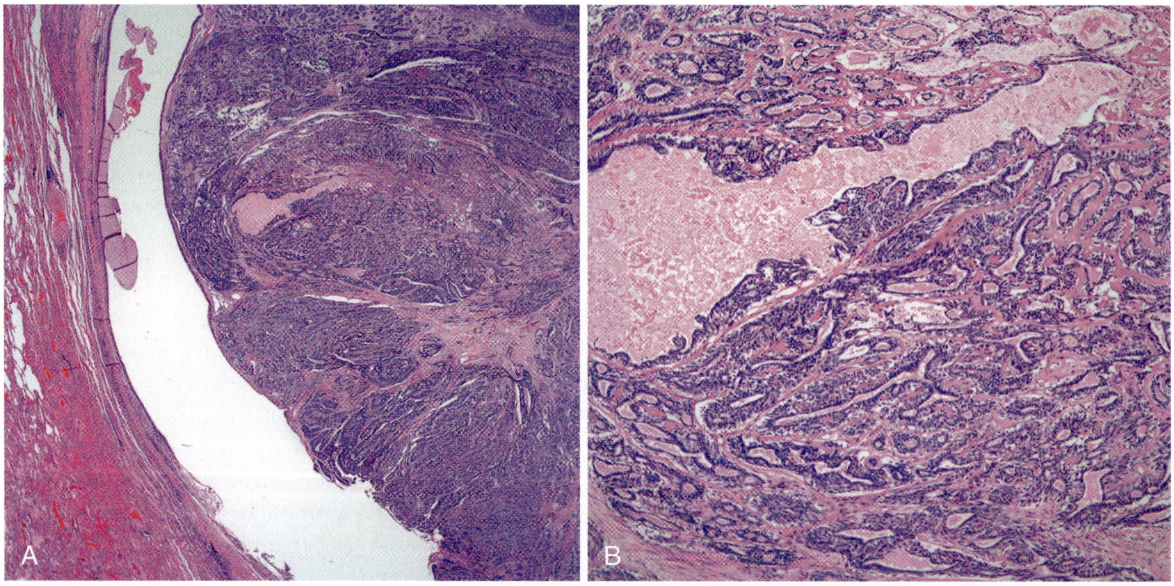

Figure 4-39 **A**, Low-power view of epithelial-myoepithelial carcinoma. **B**, Prominent glandular component of epithelial-myoepithelial carcinoma.

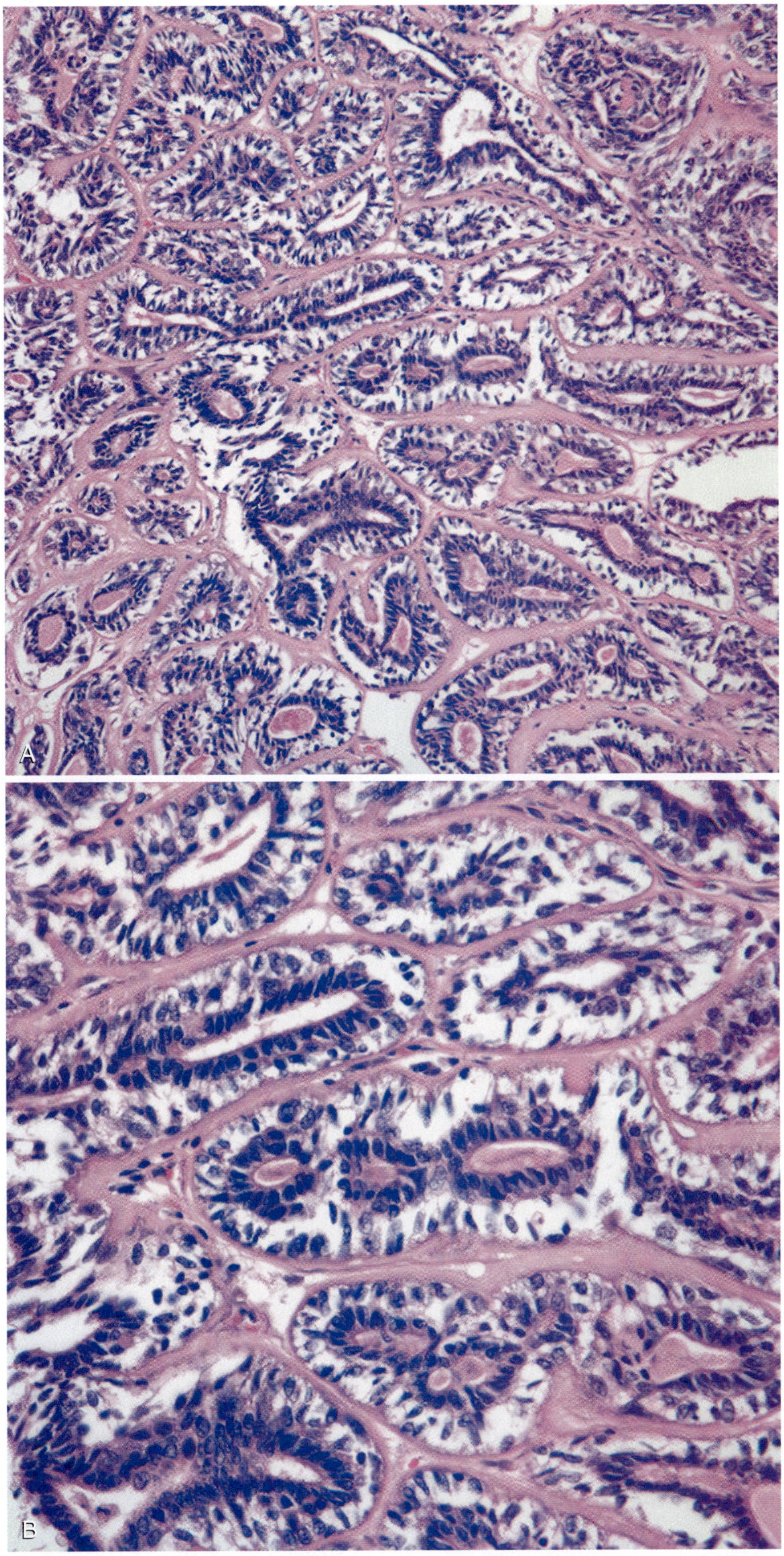

Figure 4-40 **A**, Epithelial-myoepithelial carcinoma showing the classic dual cellular proliferation. **B**, Glands composed of two cell populations, the inner epithelial component and the outer clear cell myoepithelial component.

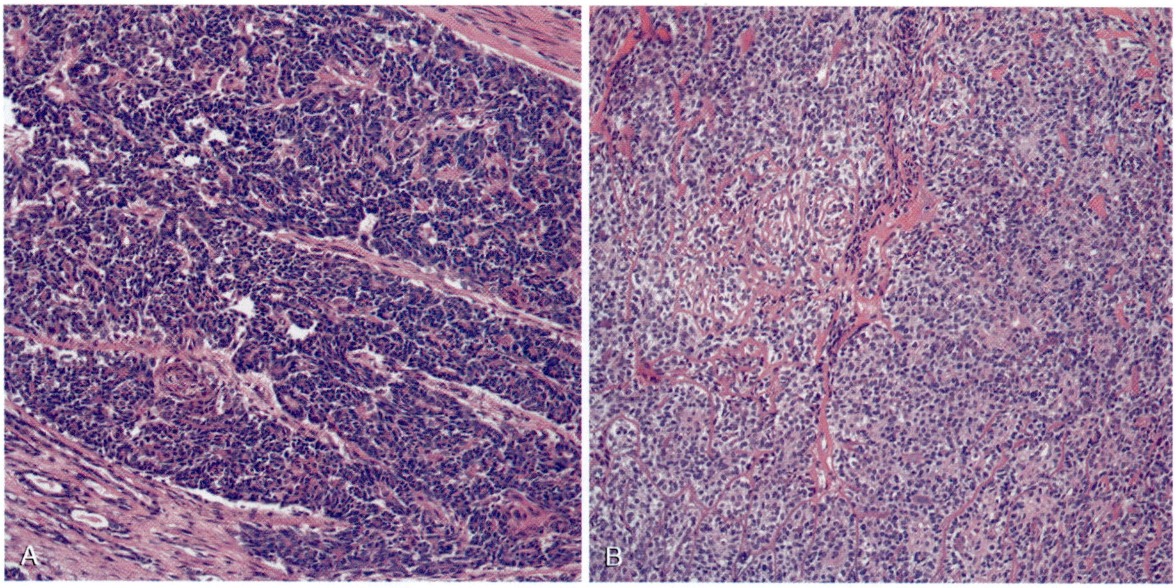

Figure 4-41 **A**, Epithelial-myoepithelial carcinoma showing a solid component. Small glandular structures are still visible. **B**, Solid component with presence of clear cells, separated by thin fibrocollagenous tissue.

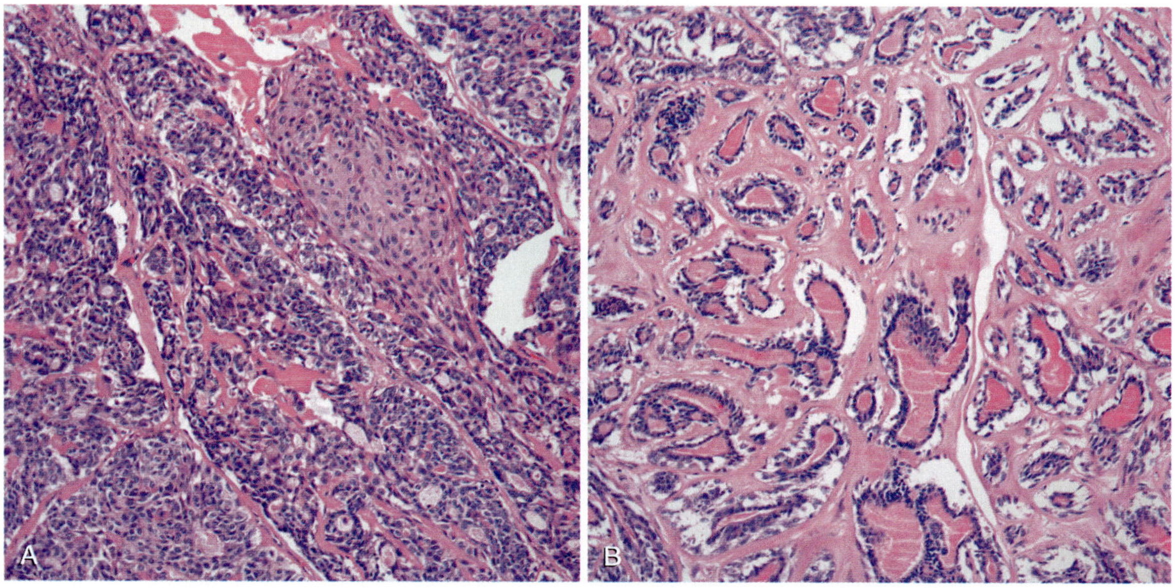

Figure 4-42 Epithelial-myoepithelial carcinoma. **A**, Solid component with focal areas of squamous metaplasia. **B**, Marked sclerotic changes.

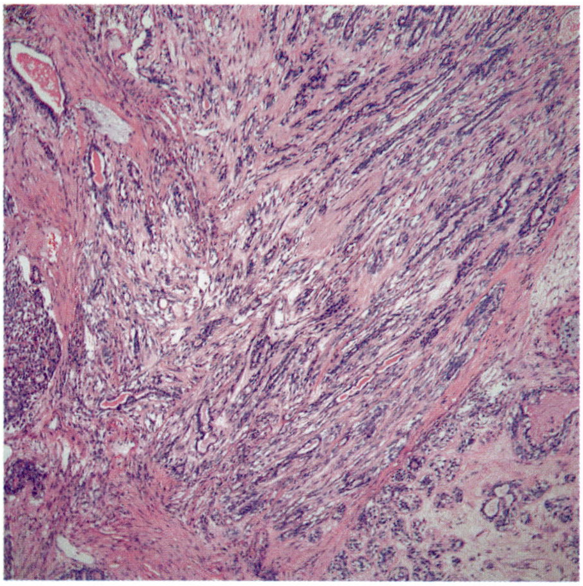

Figure 4-43 Epithelial-myoepithelial carcinoma with a prominent spindle cell component.

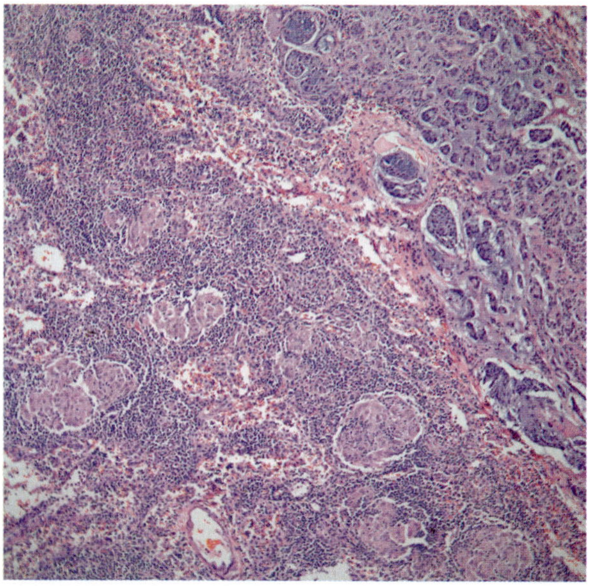

Figure 4-44 Lymph node showing metastatic epithelial-myoepithelial carcinoma.

REFERENCES

1. Moran CA. Primary salivary gland type tumors of the lung. *Semin Diagn Pathol.* 1995;12:106–122.
2. Dowling EA, Miller RE, Johnson IM, Collier FC. Mucoepidermoid tumors of the bronchi. *Surgery.* 1962;52:600–609.
3. Ozlu C, Christopherson WM, Allen JD. Mucoepidermoid tumors of the bronchi. *J Thorac Cardiovasc Surg.* 1961;42:24–31.
4. Axelson C, Burcharth F, Johansen A. Mucoepidermoid lung tumors. *J Thorac Cardiovasc Surg.* 1973;65:902–908.
5. Turnbull AD, Huvos AG, Goodner JT, Foote Jr FW. Mucoepidermoid tumors of the bronchial glands. *Cancer.* 1971;28:539–544.
6. Reichle FA, Rosemond GP. Mucoepidermoid tumors of the bronchus. *J Thorac Cardiovasc Surg.* 1966;51:443–448.
7. Klacsmann PG, Olson JL, Eggleston JC. Mucoepidermoid carcinoma of the bronchus. *Cancer.* 1979;43:1720–1733.
8. Barsky SH, Martin SE, Matthews M, Gazdar A, Costa JC. "Low grade" mucoepidermoid carcinoma of the bronchus with "high grade" biologic behavior. *Cancer.* 1983;51:1505–1509.
9. Seo IS, Warren J, Mirkin D, Weisman SJ, Grosfeld JL. Mucoepidermoid carcinoma of the bronchus in a 4-year-old child. *Cancer.* 1984;53:1600–1604.
10. Yousem SA, Hocholzer L. Mucoepidermoid tumors of the lung. *Cancer.* 1987;60:1346–1352.
11. Moran CA, Suster S, Koss MN. Primary adenoid cystic carcinoma of the lung: a clinicopathological and immunohistochemical study of 16 cases. *Cancer.* 1994;73:1390–1397.
12. Ishida T, Nishino T, Oka T, et al. Adenoid cystic carcinoma of the tracheobronchial tree: clinicopathology and immunohistochemistry. *J Surg Oncol.* 1989;41:52–59.
13. Heilbrunn AA, Crosby IK. Adenoid cystic carcinoma and mucoepidermoid carcinoma of the tracheobronchial tree. *Chest.* 1972;61:145–149.
14. Nomori H, Kaseda S, Kobayashi K, Ishihara T, Yanai N, Torikata C. Adenoid cystic carcinoma of the trachea and main stem bronchus: a clinical, histologic, and immunohistochemical study. *J Thorac Cardiovasc Surg.* 1988;96:271–277.
15. Inoue H, Iwashita A, Kanegae H, Higuchi K, Fujinaga Y, Matsumoto I. Peripheral pulmonary adenoid cystic carcinoma with substantial submucosal extension to the proximal bronchus. *Thorax.* 1991;46:147–148.
16. Conlan AA, Payne WS, Woolner LB, Sanderson DR. Adenoid cystic carcinomas (cylindroma) and mucoepidermoid carcinoma of the bronchus. *J Cardiothorac Surg.* 1978;76:369–377.
17. Markel SF, Abell MR, Haight L, French AJ. Neoplasms of bronchus commonly designated as adenomas. *Cancer.* 1964;17:590–604.
18. Payne WS, Ellis FH, Woolner LB, Moersch HJ. The surgical treatment of cylindroma (adenoid cystic carcinoma) and mucoepidermoid tumors of the bronchus. *J Thorac Cardiovasc Surg.* 1959;38:709–726.
19. Fechner RE, Bentnick BR, Askew Jr JB. Acinic cell tumor of the lung: a histologic and ultrastructural study. *Cancer.* 1972;29:501–508.
20. Moran CA, Suster S, Koss MN. Acinic cell carcinoma of the lung ("Fechner tumor"): a clinicopathologic, immunohistochemical, and ultrastructural study of five cases. *Am J Surg Pathol.* 1992;16:1039–1050.
21. Latz DR, Bubis JJ. Acinic cell tumor of the bronchus. *Cancer.* 1976;38:830–832.
22. Gharpure KJ, Desphande RK, Vishweshvara RN, et al. Acinic cell tumor of the bronchus (a case report). *Indian J Cancer.* 1985;22:152–156.
23. Davis PW, Briggs JC, Leal RME, Storring FK. Benign and malignant mixed tumours of the lung. *Thorax.* 1972;27:657–673.
24. Hayes MM, Van der Westhuizen NG, Forgie R. Malignant mixed tumors of the bronchus: a biphasic neoplasm of epithelial and myoepithelial cells. *Mod Pathol.* 1993;6:85–88.
25. Payne WS, Scier J, Woolner LB. Mixed tumors of the bronchus (salivary gland type). *J Thorac Cardiovasc Surg.* 1965;49:663–668.
26. Sakamoto H, Uda H, Tanaka T, Oda T, Morino H, Kikui M. Pleomorphic adenoma in the periphery of the lung: report of a case and review of the literature. *Arch Pathol Lab Med.* 1991;115:393–396.
27. Moran CA, Suster S, Askin FB, Koss MN. Benign and malignant salivary gland type tumors of the lung: clinicopathologic and immunohistochemical study of eight cases. *Cancer.* 1994;73:2481–2490.
28. Nistal M, García-Viera M, Martinez-García C, Paniagua R. Epithelial-myoepithelial tumor of the bronchus. *Am J Surg Pathol.* 1994;18:421–425.
29. Strickler JG, Hegstrom J, Thomas MJ, Yousem SA. Myoepithelioma of the lung. *Arch Pathol Lab Med.* 1987;111:1082–1086.
30. Tsuji N, Tateishi R, Ishiguro S, Terao T, Higashiyama M. Adenomyoepithelioma of the lung. *Am J Surg Pathol.* 1995;19:956–962.
31. Wilson RW, Moran CA. Epithelial-myoepithelial carcinoma of the lung: immunohistochemical and ultrastructural observations and review of the literature. *Hum Pathol.* 1997;28:631–635.
32. Chang T, Husain AN, Colby T, et al. Pneumocytic adenomyoepitheluioma: a distinct lung tumor with epithelial, myoepithelial, and pneumonic differentiation. *Am J Surg Pathol.* 2007;31:562–568.
33. Nguyen CV, Suster S, Moran CA. Pulmonary epithelial-myoepithelial carcinoma: a clinicopathological and immunohistochemical study of five cases. *Hum Pathol.* 2009;40(3):366–373.
34. Fechner RE, Bentnick BR. Ultrastructure of bronchial oncocytoma. *Cancer.* 1973;331:1451–1457.
35. Nielsen AL. Malignant bronchial oncocytoma: a case report and review of the literature. *Hum Pathol.* 1985;16:852–854.
36. Santos-Briz A, Jerrón J, Sastre R, Romero L, Valle A. Oncocytoma of the lung. *Cancer.* 1977;40:1330–1336.

5

Neuroendocrine Tumors of the Lung

Neuroendocrine carcinomas constitute an important group of primary neoplasms in the lung. Although the gamut of primary lung tumors that may show neuroendocrine differentiation is rather complex, involving tumors not only of epithelial but also of mesenchymal or neural origin, this chapter focuses mainly on epithelial tumors.

Neuroendocrine tumors are ubiquitous neoplasms that have been the subject of investigation for over a century. Although these low-grade tumors initially were described as neoplasms with a better prognosis than that for conventional carcinoma (carcinoid tumor), in time, different studies have conceptualized them as a family of neoplasms that may expand from an indolent and insignificant small lesion (so-called tumorlet), most often encountered by chance, to low-, intermediate-, and high-grade malignancies. To provide a better understanding of these tumors in terms of clinical course, behavior, and possible histogenesis, different studies including morphologic, immunohistochemical, and, more recently, molecular investigations, have attempted to classify this family of neoplasms; however, universal agreement is still lacking. Some reviews on the subject[1] either precede the most recent classification of lung tumors by the World Health Organization[2] (WHO) or have separated these tumors in the conventional three-way category system.[3] Although other studies have followed the WHO classification, those studies have stated the difficulty inherent in making these diagnoses using surgical biopsy specimens.[4]

The problem deepens owing to the fact that the designation given to some of these tumors may depend largely on the anatomic site in which they may appear. As an example, in the WHO classification for tumors of the pleura, lung, thymus, and heart,[2] tumors in the thymus are separated into low- and high-grade malignancy, whereas those in the lung are separated into a four-way category system.

HISTORICAL ASPECTS

Siegfried Oberndorfer[5] is credited for coining the term *carcinoid tumor* in 1907. In 1904, Bunting[6] from Johns Hopkins reported a case under the designation "multiple primary carcinomata" and made reference to other possible descriptions that dated back to the 18th century. Thus, it appears that this tumor may have been recognized well over a century ago. In 1914, Gossett and Masson[7] described similar tumors in the appendix and made an analogy with the previous description by Oberndorfer.[5] At the same time these tumors were being studied in the gastrointestinal tract, similar tumors in the respiratory tract, especially those occurring in the bronchial wall, were being reported as bronchial adenomas.[8,9] Gmelich and colleagues[10] identified the presence of Kulschitzky cells (K cells) in bronchioles and established the relationship of these cells and the occurrence of these neoplasms in the lung. Of interest, Hausman and Weimann[11] described a case with lymph node metastasis from a "pulmonary tumorlet." These investigators noted that such tumors have a low malignant potential. The so-called tumorlet measured 1.5 cm in greatest dimension and had spindle cell morphology, with lymph node metastasis, as noted. Azzopardi,[12] in a study of 100 cases of what he called "oat cell carcinoma," comprising 16 surgical cases and 84 cases from autopsy material, described positive structural features characteristic of this tumor that included streams, ribbons, rosettes, and ductules. As suggested by this definition and at least one of the illustrations presented in his review, some of the cases presented in this study may not represent oat cell carcinoma as it is defined today, corresponding instead to low- or intermediate-grade neuroendocrine carcinomas. A similar conclusion may be drawn from consideration of the 138 cases of oat cell carcinoma described by Yukato and associates,[13] in which some of those tumors, although neuroendocrine in nature, may not necessarily be of the oat cell type as it is defined today.

HISTOGENESIS, DIFFERENTIATION, MULTIDIRECTIONAL DIFFERENTIATION, DIVERGENT DIFFERENTIATION

Gould and colleagues[14] introduced the term *multidirectional differentiation* after observing the presence of neuroendocrine, mucosubstance-producing, and squamous cells in pulmonary carcinomas. These investigators also noted that certain tumors may share similar patterns of differentiation.[14] Further observations of interest in some cases included predominant features of squamous differentiation seen at electron microscopy.[14] Accordingly, the investigators designated those tumors as "neuroendocrine carcinomas with squamous differentiation." They also noted that some squamous and adenocarcinomas of the lung may show bound membrane and dense core granules at electron microscopy. Nevertheless, Gould[15] also warned about the possibility of cell populations that demonstrate similar or identical patterns of differentiation but which may not necessarily share identical or even closely related embryogenesis.

Earlier workers had documented the presence of non–small cell neoplasms that, histologically, looked like squamous cell carcinomas or adenocarcinomas and showed the presence of neurosecretory granules on ultrastructural studies. These neoplasms had been classified as atypical endocrine tumors. Such descriptions have raised concerns about the true significance of the many classification systems available for neuroendocrine tumors [16] To complicate matters further, some small cell carcinomas do not demonstrate immunohistochemical differentiation for neuroendocrine markers, nor are neurosecretory granules detected on ultrastructural studies; however, they do show the ultrastructural features of epithelial tumors. Regardless of the histologic subtype, all lung tumors have the potential to show neuroendocrine differentiation by immunohistochemistry or electron microscopy.

More recently, some investigators[17] have argued that the current revised classification of tumors by the WHO[2] in fact clearly defines each one of the neuroendocrine tumors of the lung. These workers have introduced the term *divergent differentiation*, stating that this concept applies to a subset of non–small cell carcinomas that are not considered morphologically neuroendocrine but that express neuroendocrine differentiation with neuroendocrine markers (so-called non–small cell carcinoma with neuroendocrine differentiation). In addition, Brambilla and colleagues[17] state that the so-called tumorlets do not differ in cellular components from the so-called typical carcinoid, and that these tumorlets also display divergent differentiation. Early reports of "metastatic tumorlets" are incorrect; such lesions represent the current so-called typical carcinoid.

CLASSIFICATIONS

Neuroendocrine lung neoplasms have been a subject of numerous classification systems. Many of them, although logical, fail to provide a practical approach; others, although practical, fail to properly define this complex group of tumors. This section reviews the most important past and present classification systems and evaluates their practical significance. The most important classification schema and diagnostic criteria are presented in Tables 5-1 and 5-2.

In 1977, Gould[18] introduced the terms *neuroendocrinoma* and *neuroendocrine carcinoma* by drawing an analogy between these tumors and the APUD (amine precursor uptake and decarboxylation) cell system neoplasms with respect to their aberrant secretory activities. Gould emphasized the numerous neoplasms that may belong to this APUD system, which is not limited to the respiratory tract or to a particular group of tumors—for example, carcinoid tumor. This investigator also elaborated on abandoning traditional terms such as *bronchial adenoma*, a term that does not convey the true nature of these neoplasms and yet is used to encompass a diverse group of tumoral conditions. This study highlights three important issues: First, the term *bronchopulmonary neuroendocrine tumor* is preferable to *bronchopulmonary carcinoid*; second, it is argued that "oat cell carcinomas" represent the malignant counterpart of carcinoid tumor; and third, the term *undifferentiated oat cell carcinoma* is in widespread use. In 1983, Gould and colleagues[19] presented a new classification system for neuroendocrine pulmonary neoplasms that included four categories instead of the conventional three. Their schema is as follows:

TABLE 5-1 HISTOPATHOLOGIC CLASSIFICATIONS OF NEUROENDOCRINE TUMORS OF THE LUNG

Authors	Tumor Designation	Equivalent (Conventional Classification)
Gould et al.[19]	Bronchopulmonary carcinoid	Conventional carcinoid
	Well-differentiated neuroendocrine carcinoma	Atypical carcinoid
	Neuroendocrine carcinoma of intermediate-size cells	Variant of small cell carcinoma
	Neuroendocrine carcinoma of small cell type	Small cell carcinoma
Paladugu et al.[21]	Kulchitzky cell carcinoma type I	Conventional carcinoid
	Kulchitzky cell carcinoma type II	Atypical carcinoid
	Kulchitzky cell carcinoma type III	Small cell carcinoma
Capella et al.[26]	Benign or low-grade malignant nonfunctioning well-differentiated tumor	Conventional carcinoid
	Low-grade malignant nonfunctioning well-differentiated carcinoma	Atypical carcinoid
	High-grade malignant functioning or nonfunctioning poorly differentiated carcinoma	Small, large, and intermediate cell
Travis et al.[28]	Typical carcinoid	Conventional carcinoid
	Atypical carcinoid	Atypical carcinoid
	Small cell carcinoma	Small cell carcinoma
	Large cell neuroendocrine carcinoma	
Huang et al.[30]	Well-differentiated neuroendocrine carcinoma	Conventional carcinoid
	Moderately differentiated neuroendocrine carcinoma	Atypical carcinoid
	Poorly differentiated neuroendocrine carcinoma	Atypical carcinoid with more mitosis
	Undifferentiated large cell neuroendocrine carcinoma	Large cell neuroendocrine carcinoma
	Undifferentiated small cell carcinoma	Small cell carcinoma
Moran and Suster[105]	Well-differentiated neuroendocrine carcinoma	Conventional carcinoid
	Moderately differentiated neuroendocrine carcinoma	Atypical carcinoid
	Poorly differentiated neuroendocrine carcinoma	Large cell and small cell neuroendocrine carcinoma

TABLE 5-2 CRITERIA FOR DIAGNOSIS OF NEUROENDOCRINE TUMORS OF THE LUNG ON COMPLETE SURGICAL RESECTION SPECIMEN

Tumor	Size	Mitotic Activity	Necrosis
Carcinoid tumorlet	<0.5 cm	None	None
Well-differentiated neuroendocrine carcinoma	>0.5 cm	<3 mitotic figures per 10 hpf	Minimal and focal
Moderately differentiated neuroendocrine carcinoma	>0.5 cm	>3 mitotic figures per 10 hpf	Comedo-like
Poorly differentiated neuroendocrine carcinoma			
Small cell carcinoma*		>10 mitotic figures per 10 hpf	Marked
Large cell neuroendocrine carcinoma†		>10 mitotic figures per 10 hpf	Marked

*On resected specimens. Criteria do not apply to biopsy specimens.
†On resected specimens. Diagnosis also requires positive histologic findings and immunohistochemical neuroendocrine markers.
hpf, high-power field.

Bronchopulmonary carcinoid: Typical histologic features, locally invasive, potential for recurrence, and distant metastasis. Bronchopulmonary carcinoid is separated from neuroendocrine carcinoma (see further on). The cases presented showed penetration of the bronchial wall and mediastinal soft tissue. In addition, six cases showed direct invasion into lymph nodes at the time of initial presentation.

Well-differentiated neuroendocrine carcinoma: Even though Gould and colleagues recognized that this designation may not be entirely satisfactory, this category is for tumors that retain a clearly organoid pattern, moderate cellular pleomorphism, mitosis, and "true" lymph node metastasis.

Neuroendocrine carcinoma of intermediate-size cells: This tumor type represents a variant of small cell neuroendocrine carcinoma; the cells are twice the size of "small cell" counterparts with prominent nucleoli and abundant mitotic figures. Of interest, the investigators noted that 7 of the 11 cases presented showed features of glandular or squamous differentiation.

Neuroendocrine carcinoma of small cell type: Typical "oat" cell carcinoma, abundant mitoses and inconspicuous nucleoli. The authors comment that not all tumors in this category are neuroendocrine and recommend the systematic use of immunohistochemistry to separate those tumors that are neuroendocrine from those which are not neuroendocrine.

In 1985, Warren and associates[20] presented a study of 81 cases of pulmonary neuroendocrine neoplasms assessing Gould's classification systems and determined their usefulness for the proper identification and treatment of patients with those neoplasms. Paladugu and colleagues[21] presented a new classification system for these neuroendocrine neoplasms, which they designated *bronchopulmonary Kulchitzky cell carcinomas* (KCCs), that reverted to a three-category schema. These investigators used the designations KCC-I, KCC-II, and KCC-III for typical carcinoid, atypical carcinoid, and small cell carcinoma, respectively. Of interest, they reported mortality rates of 1.7% for KCC-I and 27% for KCC-II. Histologically, the KCC-II tumors showed a mitotic activity level of 1 mitotic figure per high-power field. These workers concluded that their nomenclature is preferable to that of the Gould classification both because they consider the K cell to be the origin of these tumors and because it is simpler and less confusing. In 1972, however, Arrigoni and coworkers[22] had introduced the concept of "atypical carcinoid" by separating those tumors based on cellular atypia and mitotic activity with an average of 1 mitotic figure per 1 or 2 high-power fields, leaving a possibility of 5 to 10 mitotic figures per 10 high-power fields.

A point of interest is that in the Arrigoni,[22] Gould,[19] and Paladugu[21] classification systems, the number of mitotic figures per 10 high-power fields is subject to interpretation. On a background of that state of confusion, in 1982, Mills and associates[23] presented a study of 17 cases of atypical carcinoid tumors of the lung in which the mitotic count in those tumors ranged from 2 to 28 mitotic figures (mean, 14; median, 13) per 10 high-power fields. Also, Valli and colleagues[24] presented a study of 33 cases of atypical carcinoid tumors of the lung in which the mitotic activity ranged from 4 to 80 figures per 1.52 mm^2. Other reports[25] use the criterion of increased mitotic activity level with more than 1 mitotic figure per 1 or 2 high-power fields.

At that point, it was evident that the criterion used to separate carcinoid from atypical carcinoid by mitotic activity was less than ideal. In 1995, Capella and associates[26] revised the classification of neuroendocrine tumors of the lung, pancreas, and gut. Their reclassification follows:

- **Benign or low-grade malignant nonfunctioning well-differentiated tumor** as the equivalent for conventional carcinoid
- **Low-grade malignant nonfunctioning well-differentiated carcinoma** as the equivalent for atypical carcinoid
- **High-grade malignant functioning or nonfunctioning poorly differentiated carcinoma** as the equivalent for the large cell type and the small or intermediate cell type

The criterion separating typical from atypical carcinoid was established at no more than 3 mitotic figures per 10 high-power fields. These investigators added that if metastasis or gross invasion is present, tumors should be called "low-grade neuroendocrine carcinoma."

In 1991, Travis and coworkers[27] had presented a study of 35 cases of neuroendocrine carcinomas of the lung in which a proposed criteria was presented for large cell neuroendocrine carcinoma. In this study, previous criteria for other neuroendocrine carcinomas were followed, and the large cell carcinoma was presented as a tumor with a "neuroendocrine pattern," high mitotic activity with an average of 66 figures per 10 high-power fields, and prominent nucleoli. These workers suggested that the prognosis for large cell neuroendocrine carcinoma is between those of atypical carcinoid and small cell carcinoma. However, in 1998, Travis' group[28] presented a new study of neuroendocrine neoplasms in which their goals were to provide clear definitions for the four neuroendocrine tumors, and to modify the criteria for the diagnosis of carcinoid and atypical carcinoid. The "new" classification system placed large cell neuroendocrine carcinoma in the high-grade category of tumors, contrary to the investigators' previous study.[27] This new approach is as follows:

- **Conventional carcinoid tumor**: Restricted to no more than 1 mitotic figure per 10 high-power fields
- **Atypical carcinoid**: More than 2 but fewer than 10 mitotic figures per 10 high-power fields, or necrosis (often punctate)
- **Large cell neuroendocrine carcinoma**: Tumors with "neuroendocrine morphology," mitotic activity of more than 11 figures per 10 high-power fields, cytologic features of large cell carcinoma, and positive immunohistochemical staining for neuroendocrine markers
- **Small cell carcinoma**: Tumors with the cytology of small cell tumor cells (absent nucleoli), mitotic activity of more than 11 figures per 10 high-power fields, and frequent necrosis

This system is essentially repeated in the most recent version of the WHO Classification of Tumours of the Lung, Pleura, Thymus, and Heart.[2] Of note, however, it represents a classification for *resected* specimens. In a separate study on the reproducibility of the proposed classification of neuroendocrine lung tumors conducted by Travis and coworkers,[29] in which five experienced pulmonary pathologists participated in the evaluation of 40 surgically resected neuroendocrine tumors, unanimous agreement on classification was reached in only 55% of the cases. The most common disagreements were between large cell neuroendocrine carcinoma and small cell carcinoma. Finally, in 2002, Huang and associates[30] presented the most recent attempt to classify neuroendocrine tumors of the lung. These workers studied 234 cases, classified into five different categories. Their system essentially follows the Travis criteria[28] for the separation of carcinoid and atypical carcinoid (well- and moderately differentiated neuroendocrine carcinoma): The categories of large cell neuroendocrine carcinoma and small cell carcinoma are retained, with the prefix of "undifferentiated," with mitotic counts of more than 30 per 10 high-power fields. A new category is what the authors call "poorly differentiated neuroendocrine carcinoma," which is conceptualized as an atypical carcinoid with an increased mitotic count of more than 10 per 10 high-power fields.

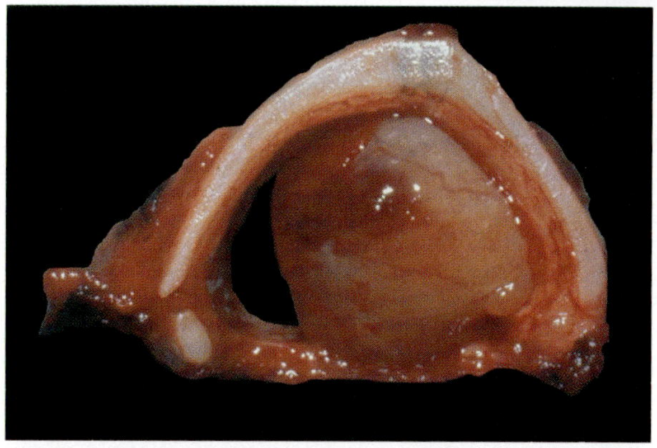

Figure 5-1 Gross illustration of an endobronchial well-differentiated neuroendocrine carcinoma obstructing the bronchial lumen.

GENERAL CLINICAL FEATURES

Neuroendocrine carcinomas of the lung may be associated with paraneoplastic syndromes including Cushing's syndrome, inappropriate secretion of antidiuretic hormone, and carcinoid syndrome. The last-named condition may be present in approximately 10% of patients whose tumor demonstrates a well-differentiated histologic pattern. In addition, depending on the location of the tumor, patients with carcinomas in the central location also may experience symptoms of pulmonary obstruction, dyspnea, cough, or chest pain. Patients with tumors in the periphery of the lung may be asymptomatic until the tumor reaches a larger size. Although neuroendocrine carcinomas may occur at any age, the tumors are more commonly encountered in the fifth to seventh decades of life. No gender predilection has been noted.

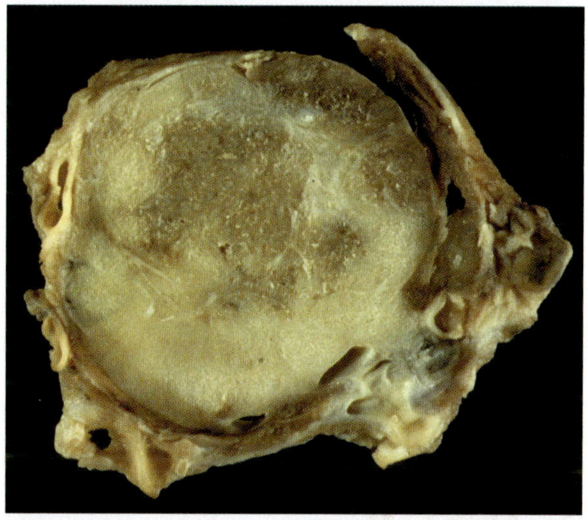

Figure 5-2 Gross specimen of an endobronchial well-differentiated neuroendocrine carcinoma, showing a rather homogeneous surface without necrosis or hemorrhage.

GENERAL MACROSCOPIC FEATURES

Those tumors occurring in the central location may manifest as polypoid tumors obstructing the lumen of the airway (Figs. 5-1 and 5-2). Tumor size may range from 1 cm to larger than 10 cm in diameter. These tumors are light brown, and the cut surface is tan and homogeneous in appearance. The presence of areas of necrosis or hemorrhage should alert the pathologist to the possibility of a higher grade (Fig. 5-3). In high-grade neuroendocrine carcinomas, it is common to encounter invasion into mediastinal structures at the time of diagnosis.

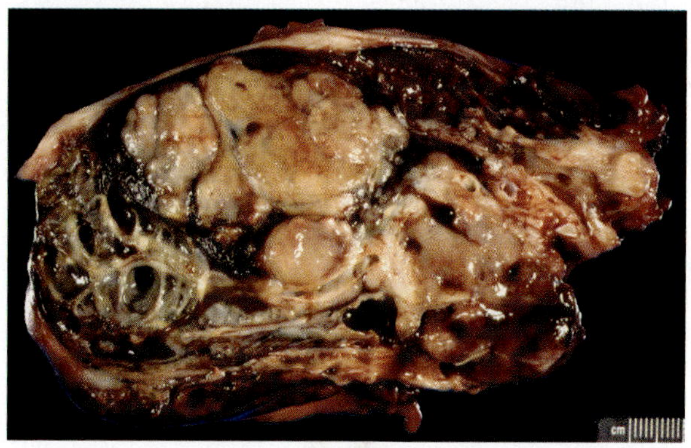

Figure 5-3 Gross specimen of a moderately differentiated neuroendcrine carcinoma. The large tumor mass shows areas of necrosis.

TUMORLET

The histopathologic features present in the so-called tumorlet are essentially the same as those in otherwise well-differentiated neuroendocrine carcinomas. As a matter of fact, the tumorlet may represent the true carcinoid tumor of the lung. However, the diagnosis of tumorlets is restricted to lesions no more than 0.5 cm in greatest dimension. Although this lesion more often is found incidentally in lung biopsy specimens, with the use of more sophisticated radiologic techniques, the diagnosis of tumorlet is becoming more common (Figs. 5-4 and 5-5).

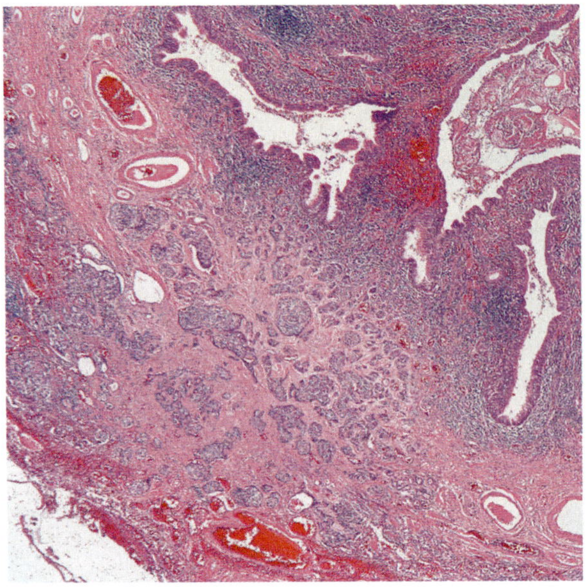

Figure 5-4 So-called tumorlet. The neuroendocrine tumor was less than 0.5 cm in greatest dimension.

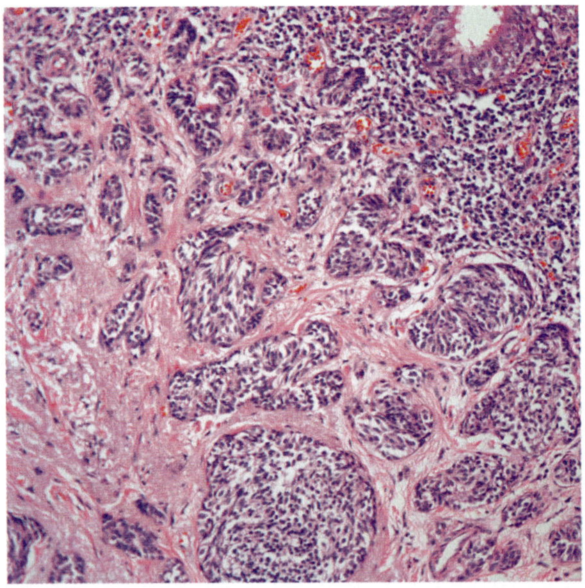

Figure 5-5 High-power view of a tumorlet showing histologic pattern similar to that of a well-differentiated neuroendocrine carcinoma.

WELL- AND MODERATELY DIFFERENTIATED NEUROENDOCRINE CARCINOMAS (CARCINOID AND ATYPICAL CARCINOID)

The current designation provided by the WHO[2] defines well- and moderately differentiated neuroendocrine carcinomas as having neuroendocrine morphology: organoid, trabecular, insular, palisading, ribbon, and rosette-like features. The difference between well- and moderately differentiated neuroendocrine carcinomas is that the former has fewer than 2 mitotic figures per 10 high-power fields, whereas the latter has 2 to 10 mitotic figures per 10 high-power fields. Clinically, both tumors may be associated with carcinoid syndrome[31] and show a spectrum of cell differentiation that includes spindle cells, oncocytic, and melanocytic features, among others.[32–37] Although the WHO still maintains the nomenclature of carcinoid and atypical carcinoid, some investigators believe that the most accurate designation for these neoplasms is that of neuroendocrine carcinoma, which conveys the true nature of these tumors.[22,38] This is the designation that is used in this section.

At low magnification, the tumor displays an organized growth pattern, which may show a nesting, solid, pseudoglandular, or trabecular arrangement composed of a rather homogeneous cellular proliferation characterized by small to medium-sized cells with moderate amounts of occasional cytoplasm, round to oval nuclei, and sometimes nucleoli (Figs. 5-6 to 5-10). Rosette formation may be readily identifiable (Fig. 5-11). The presence of necrosis in the form of comedo-like necrotic areas or hemorrhage, coupled with the presence of 2 or more mitotic figures per 10 high-power fields, is the criterion for classification as a moderately differentiated neuroendocrine carcinoma (Figs. 5-12 to 5-14).

Several histologic variants have been described for both well- and moderately differentiated neuroendocrine carcinomas.

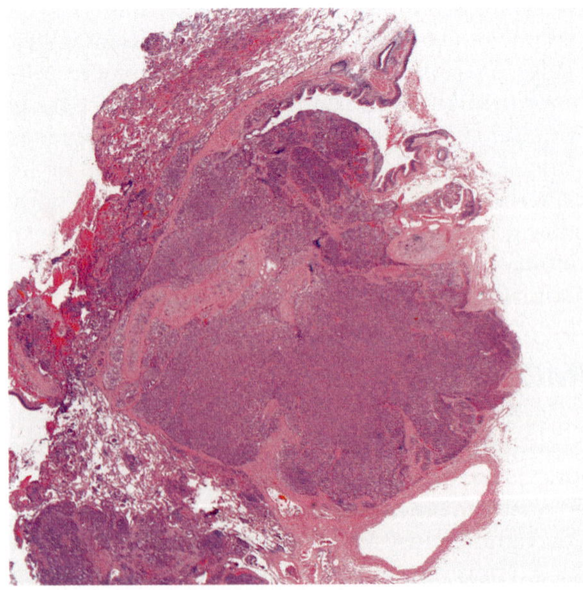

Figure 5-6 Low-power view of a well-differentiated neuroendocrine carcinoma.

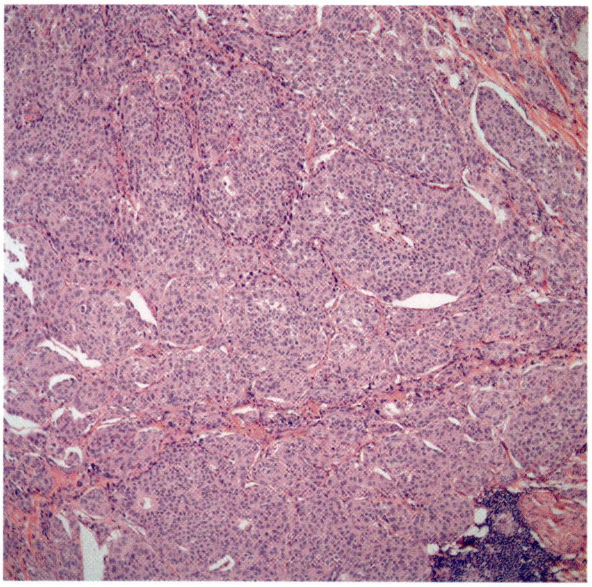

Figure 5-7 Classic nesting pattern in a well-differentiated neuroendocrine carcinoma.

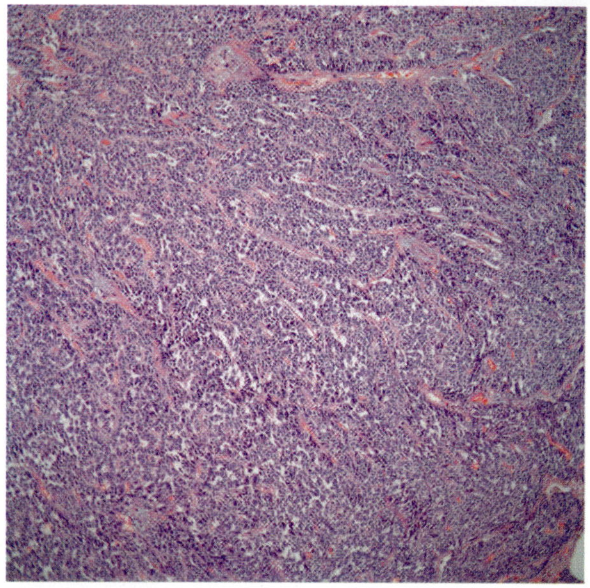

Figure 5-8 Trabecular arrangement in a well-differentiated neuroendocrine carcinoma.

Spindle cell neuroendocrine carcinoma: In this variant, although an organoid pattern may be present, the cell morphology is that of fusiform cells with inconspicuous nucleoli and finely dispersed chromatin (Fig. 5-15). In some cases the spindle cell proliferation may be associated with dilated blood vessels, imparting a hemangiopericytic pattern. However, this variant also may display nuclear atypia and increased mitotic activity (Figs. 5-16 and 5-17).

Oncocytic neuroendocrine carcinoma: The growth pattern of this neoplasm is essentially similar to

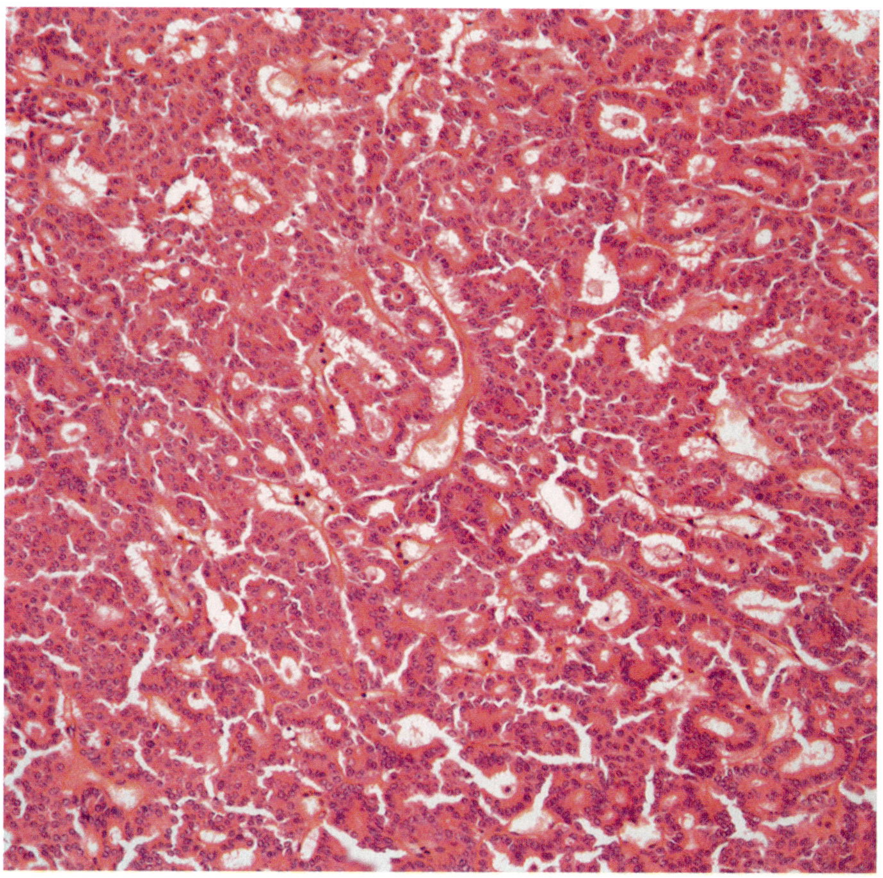

Figure 5-9 Glandular growth pattern in a well-differentiated neuroendocrine carcinoma.

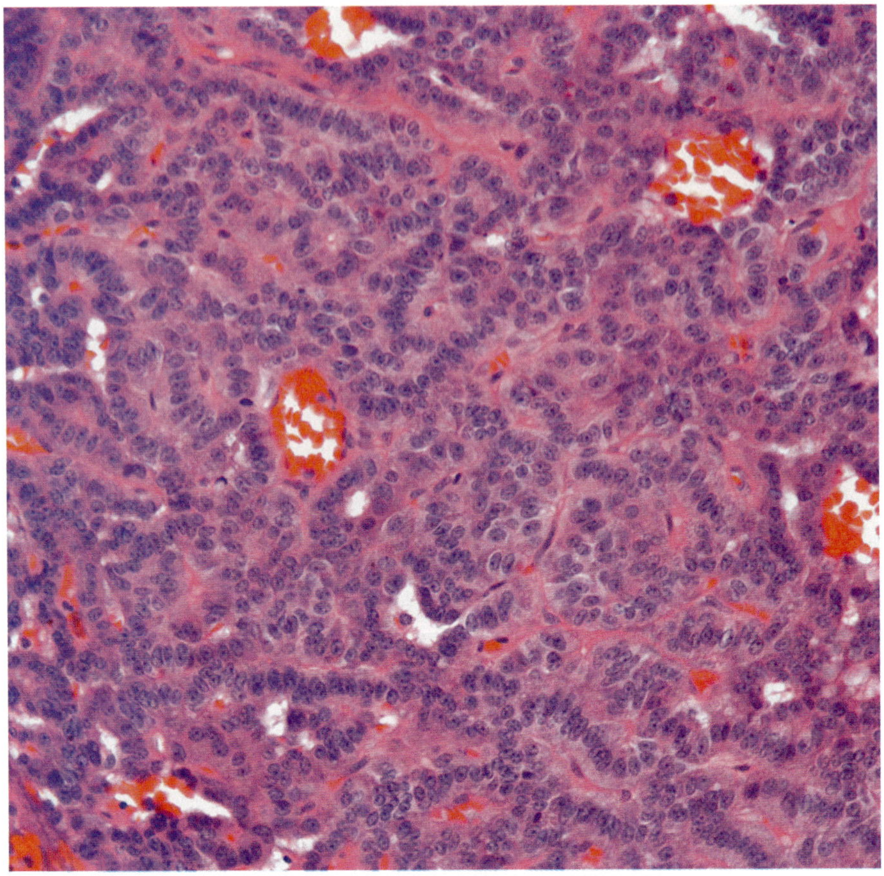

Figure 5-10 Organoid pattern in a well-differentiated neuroendocrine carcinoma.

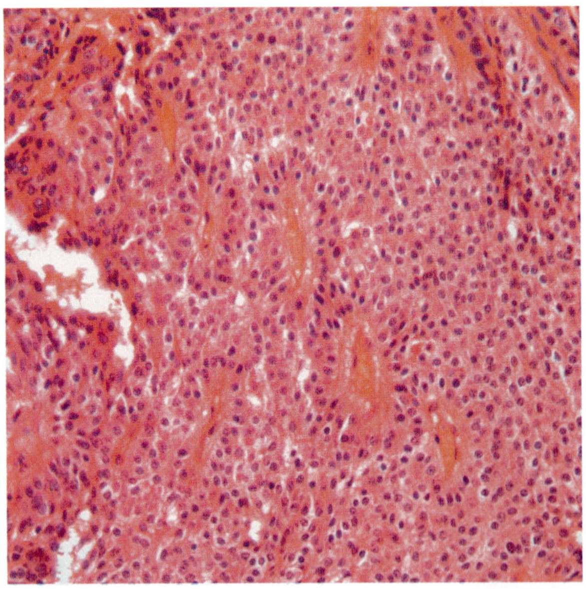

Figure 5-11 Rosette formation in a well-differentiated neuroendocrine carcinoma.

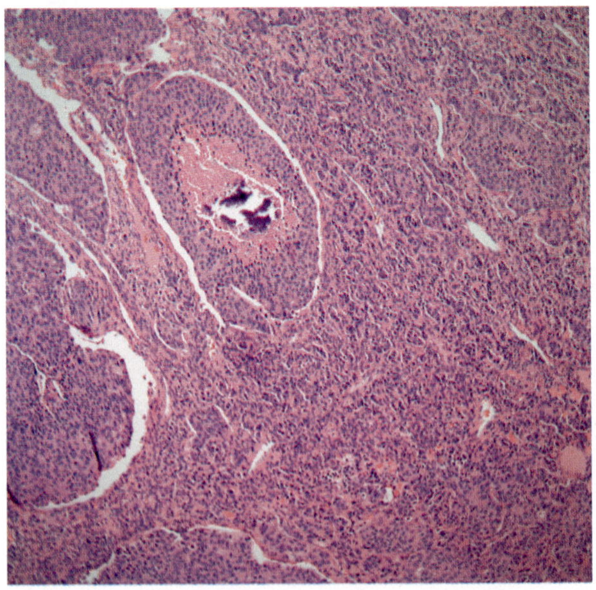

Figure 5-12 Moderately differentiated neuroendocrine carcinoma showing comedo-like necrosis and sheets of neoplastic cells.

that of the conventional cell type. The tumors may display a diffuse growth pattern or have a glandular appearance (Figs. 5-18 and 5-19). Cytologically, the cells are of medium size, with ample eosinophilic cytoplasm, round to oval nuclei, and sometimes prominent nucleoli. Clusters of oncocytic cells may be present among tumor cells (Figs. 5-20 and 5-21). This variant also may display features of moderately differentiated carcinoma, including increased mitotic activity (Fig. 5-22). Caution is in order, however, in

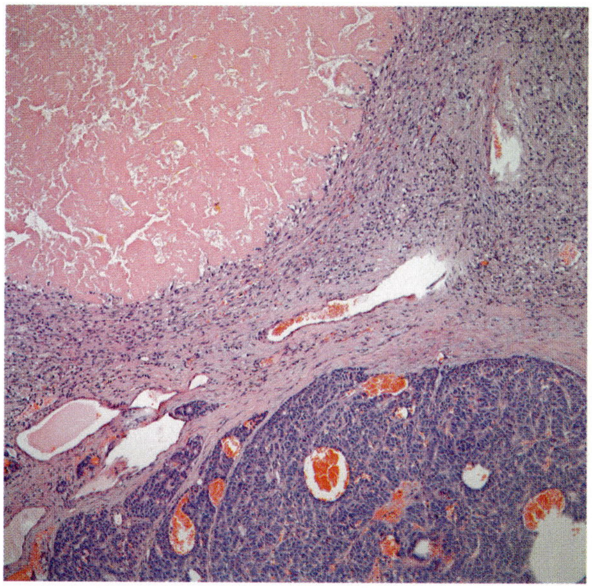

Figure 5-13 Moderately differentiated neuroendocrine carcinoma showing extensive areas of necrosis.

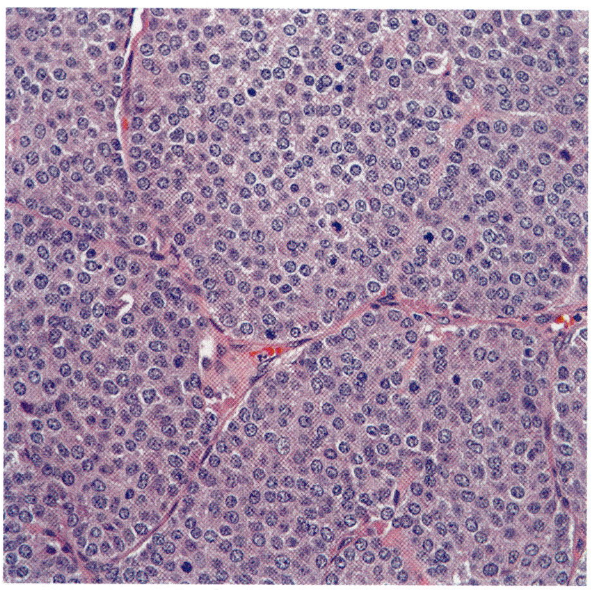

Figure 5-14 Moderately differentiated neuroendocrine carcinoma with increased mitotic activity.

assessing mitotic activity, because oncocytic tumors may display areas of nuclear atypia without mitotic activity.

Mucinous neuroendocrine carcinoma: This is a rare variant among primary neuroendocrine carcinomas of the lung. The presence of mucous material may be limited to the intraluminal component in some cases of glandular arrangement, or more rarely, the mucinous component may be intermixed with the neoplastic cellular proliferation (Fig. 5-23).

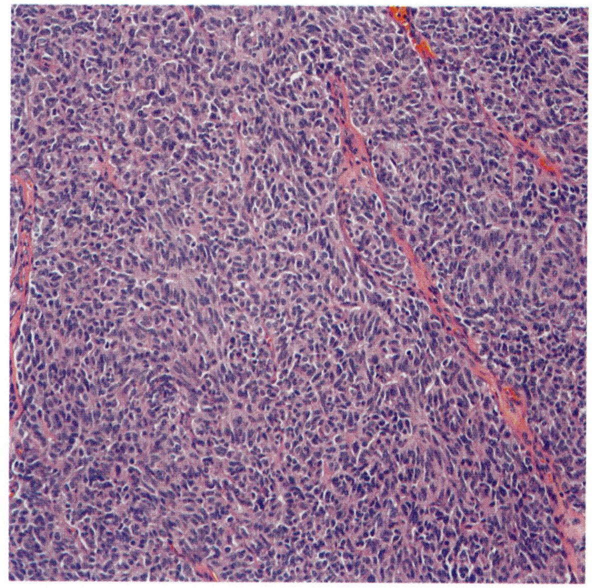

Figure 5-15 Well-differentiated neuroendocrine carcinoma with prominent spindle cell growth.

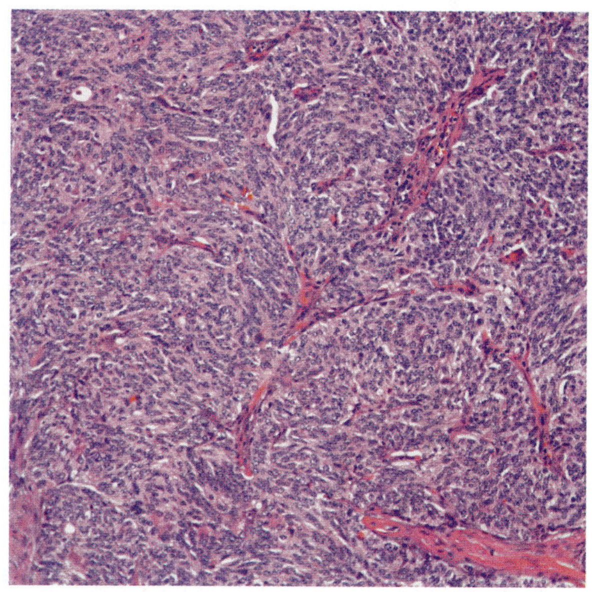

Figure 5-16 Moderately differentiated neuroendocrine carcinoma with prominent spindle cell growth and nuclear atypia.

Pigmented or melanocytic neuroendocrine carcinoma: The growth pattern of this variant is similar to that of the conventional type; however, melanin pigment may be present in cells (Fig. 5-24) or distributed along the fibroconnective tissue.

Clear cell neuroendocrine carcinoma: In this variant, the neoplastic cells are characterized by the presence of clear cytoplasm. This cytoplasmic feature may be seen in either spindle cell or conventional morphology (Fig. 5-25).

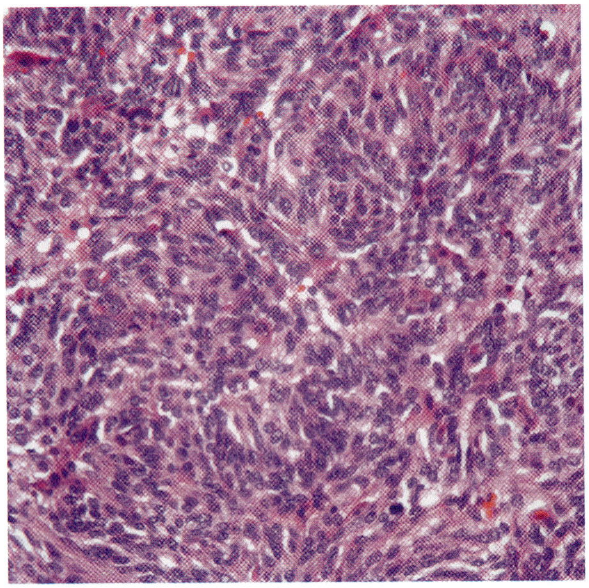

Figure 5-17 Moderately differentiated neuroendocrine carcinoma with spindle cell growth and increased mitotic activity.

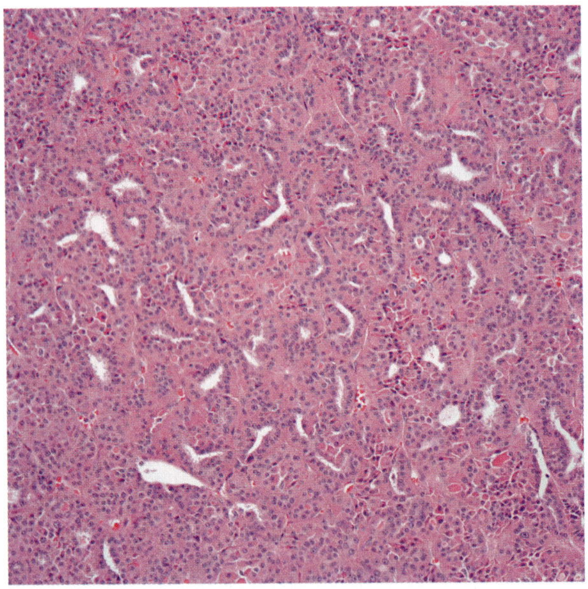

Figure 5-18 Well-differentiated neuroendocrine carcinoma with glandular and oncocytic features.

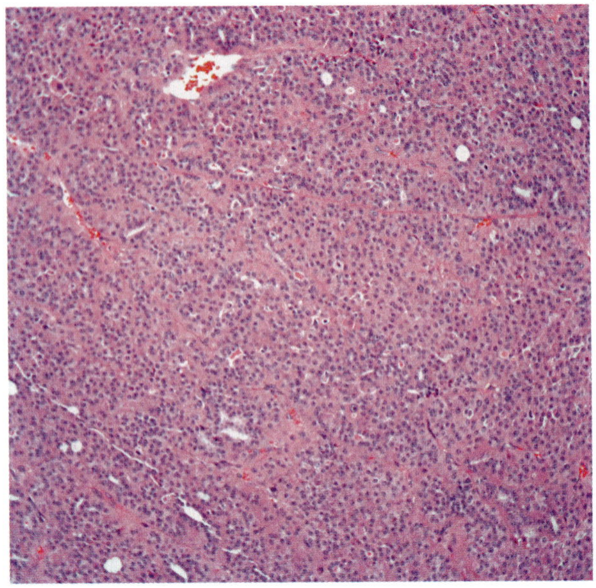

Figure 5-19 Well-differentiated neuroendocrine carcinoma with solid and oncocytic growth pattern.

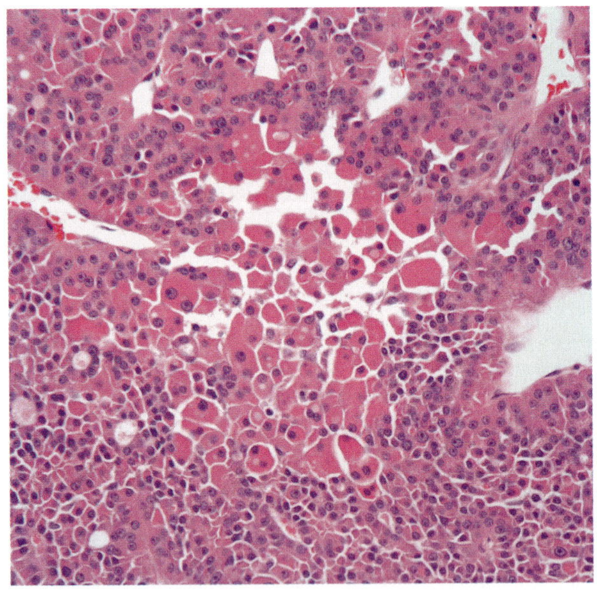

Figure 5-20 Well-differentiated neuroendocrine carcinoma with oncocytic growth pattern and clusters of so-called oncoblasts.

Angiectatic neuroendocrine carcinoma: This variant is characterized by the presence of large dilated spaces filled with blood, reminiscent of a vascular neoplasm. Closer inspection of the tumor cells, however, reveals the presence of areas of more conventional neuroendocrine morphology (Fig. 5-26).

Amyloid-like stroma: The morphology of these tumors is essentially the same as that of the conventional neuroendocrine tumor. However, the tumor cells are admixed with areas of hyalinization, imparting the appearance of an amyloid-like stroma. (Fig. 5-27).

Metaplastic bone formation: The growth pattern of this variant is the same as that of the conventional neuroendocrine tumor, in which well-formed bone is admixed with the neoplastic cellular proliferation (Fig. 5-28).

Immunohistochemical Features

Both well- and moderately differentiated neuroendocrine neoplasms show positive staining for neuroendocrine markers—namely, chromogranin, synaptophysin, and CD56. Thyroid transcription factor-1 also has been

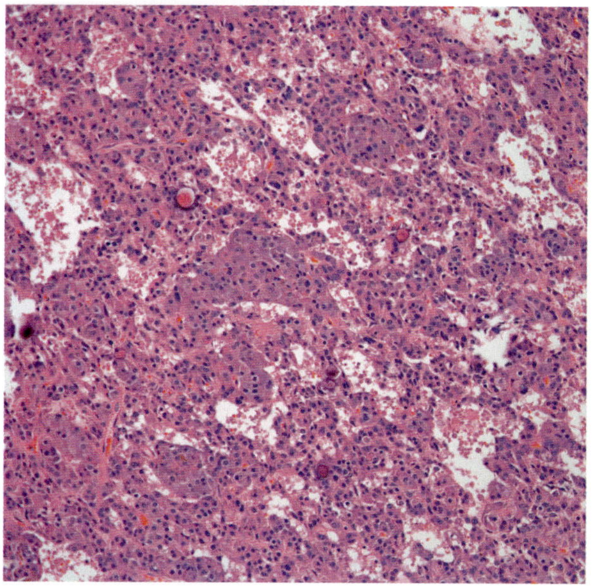

Figure 5-21 Moderately differentiated neuroendocrine carcinoma with disorganized oncocytic growth pattern.

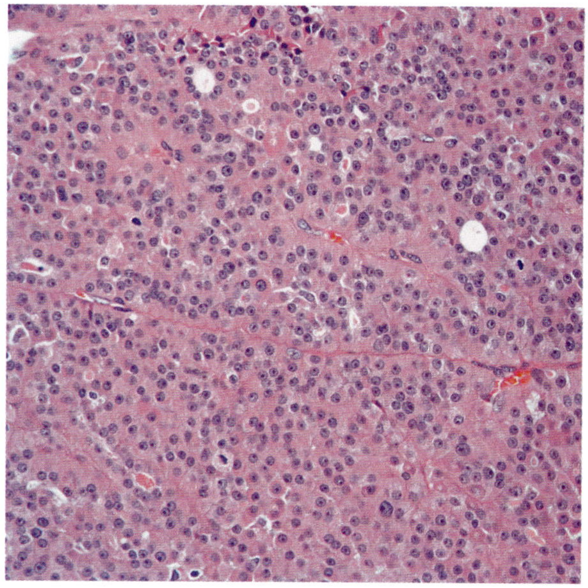

Figure 5-22 Moderately differentiated neuroendocrine carcinoma with oncocytic features. Note the presence of several mitotic figures.

shown to be helpful in the evaluation of neuroendocrine neoplasms of the lung.[39] Also, when proliferating markers such as Ki-67 are used to separate conventional and atypical carcinoids, a 4% cutoff was shown in one study to provide significant differences in 4-year overall survival rate.[40] This study used the classification of neuroendocrine neoplasms presented by the Arrigoni[22] and Warren[20] groups and was performed using resected specimens. The investigators demonstrated that with these tumors, accurate interpretation requires analysis of material from complete surgical resections, rather than biopsy specimens, in which labeling of proliferative markers may be deceiving.

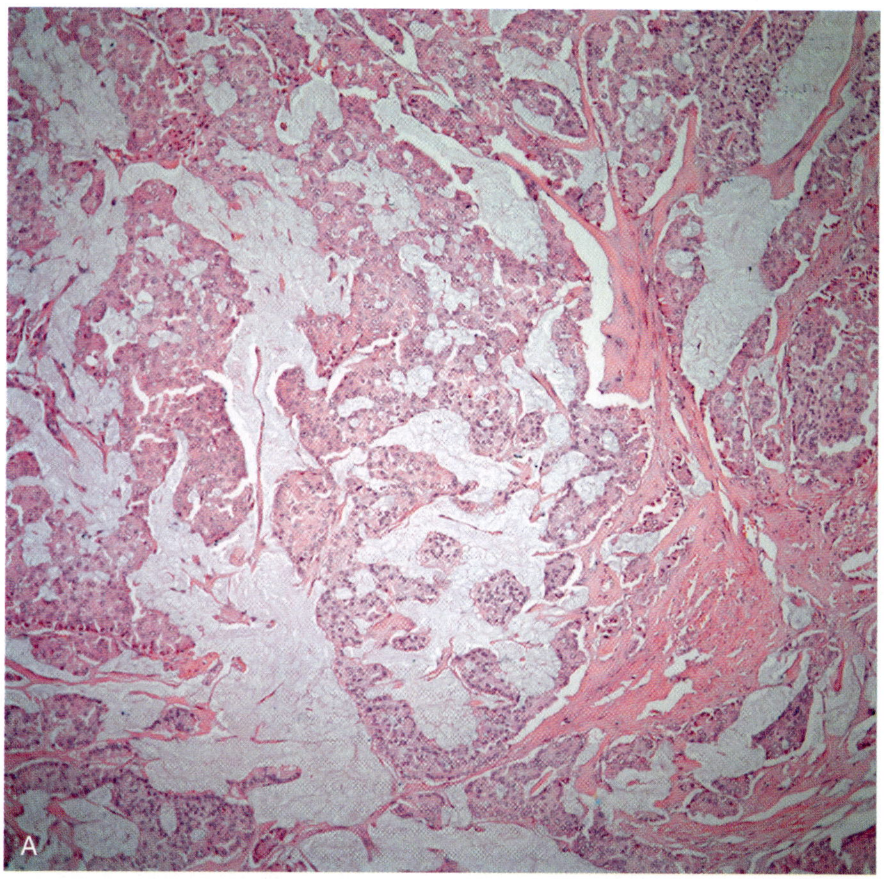

Figure 5-23 **A**, Well-differentiated neuroendocrine carcinoma with mucous stroma.

Continued

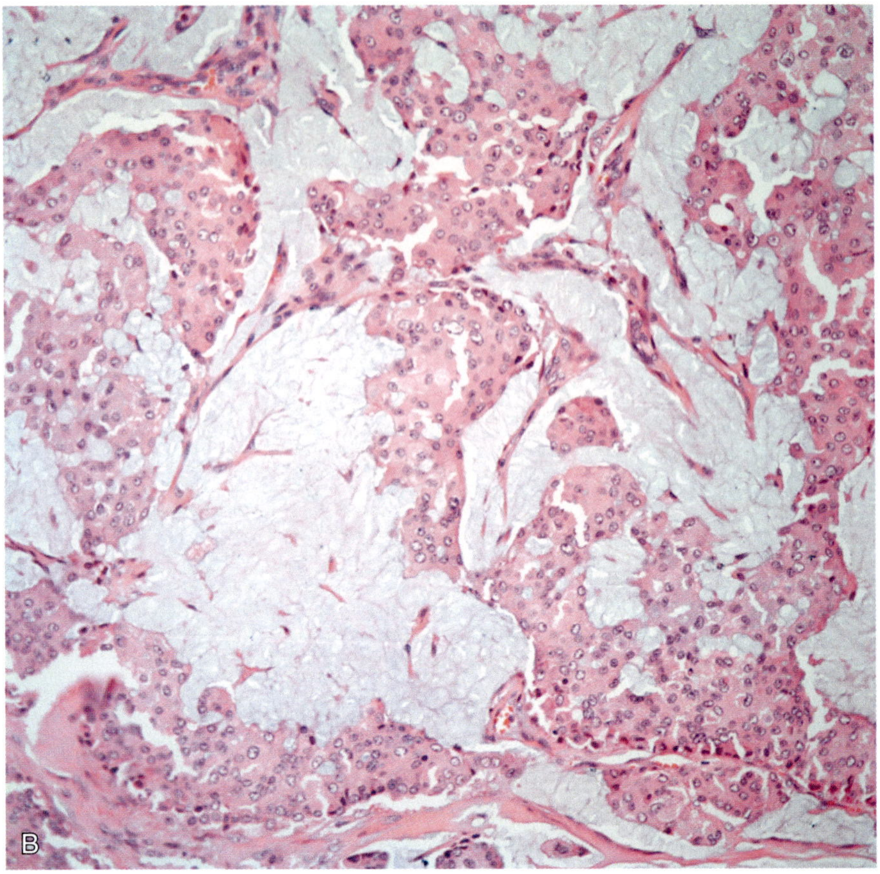

Figure 5-23—cont'd **B**, High-power view of the mucous component.

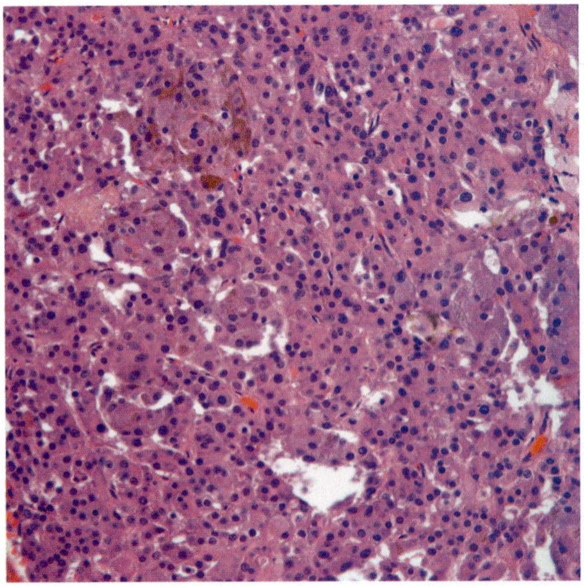

Figure 5-24 Well-differentiated neuroendocrine carcinoma with melanin pigment deposition.

Molecular Features

Well- and moderately differentiated tumors also have been the subject of more modern investigative techniques. In chromosomal studies, 11q deletions appear to be shared by both tumors.[41] Losses of 10q and 13q may also be responsible for the aggressive clinical behavior shown by some of these tumors.

Clinical Behavior

It is difficult to address patients' survival rates in a meaningful fashion, owing to the lack of real comparisons between previous and current schemas for the classification of these tumors. In 1984, Wilkins and associates,[42] using a schema most like that published by Arrigoni and colleagues, presented a study of 111 patients who underwent surgical resection for "bronchopulmonary carcinoid." Eleven of these patients had atypical carcinoid, and 45% died in a period of 33 months. The follow-up period for those who survived ranged from 16 to 48 months. Even though the investigators reported a survival rate of 82% for a 10-year period, supporting data are rather limited, and a clear-cut survival rate is not provided for the conventional carcinoid. A better-defined study of "typical carcinoid" is the one presented by Schreurs and coworkers[43] in a study of 93 patients over a period of 25 years. Although the histological criteria are not clearly mentioned in the presentation, Arrigoni's criterion for separating typical from atypical carcinoid probably was used. These workers reported a survival rate of 100% for

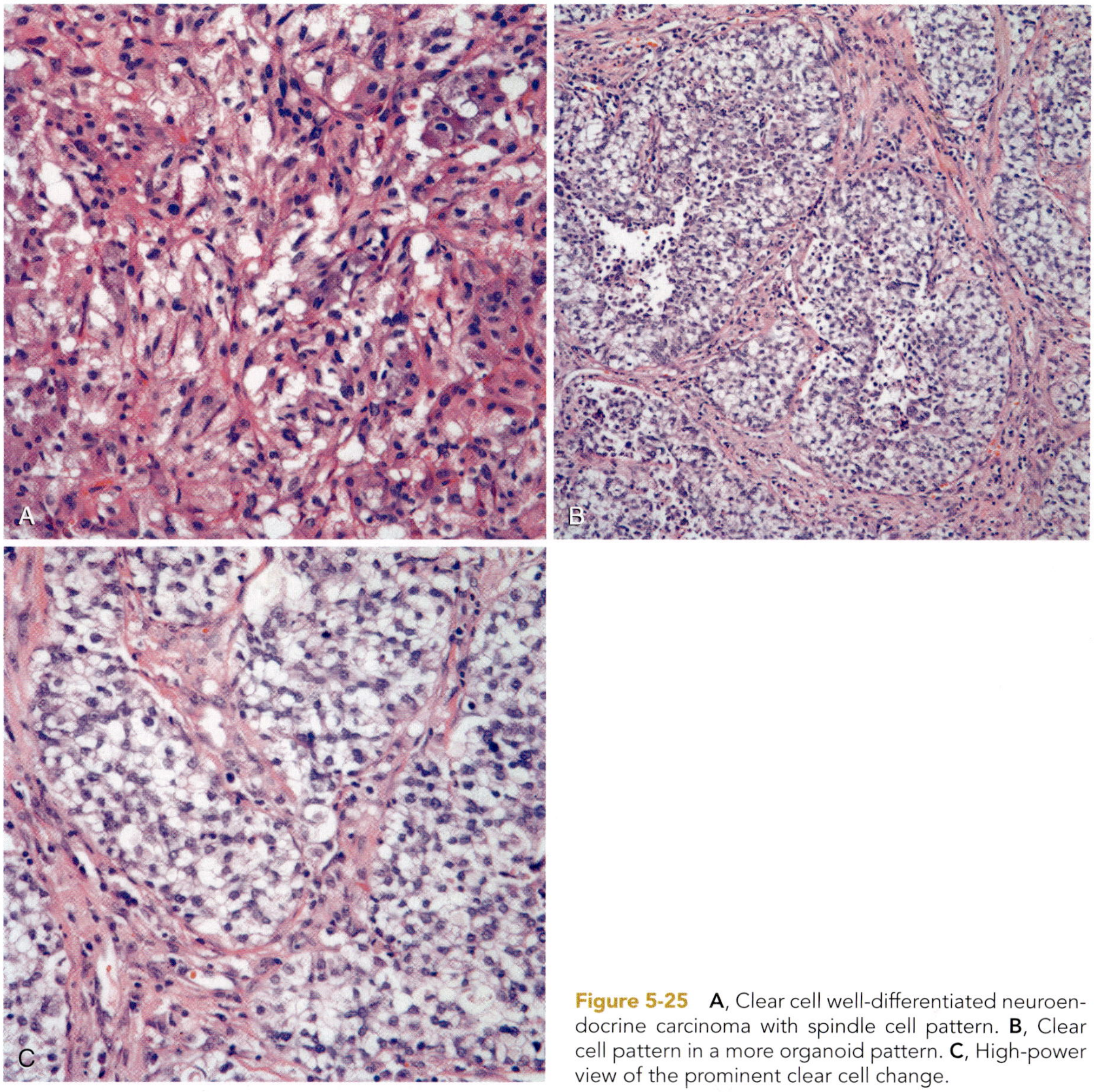

Figure 5-25 **A**, Clear cell well-differentiated neuroendocrine carcinoma with spindle cell pattern. **B**, Clear cell pattern in a more organoid pattern. **C**, High-power view of the prominent clear cell change.

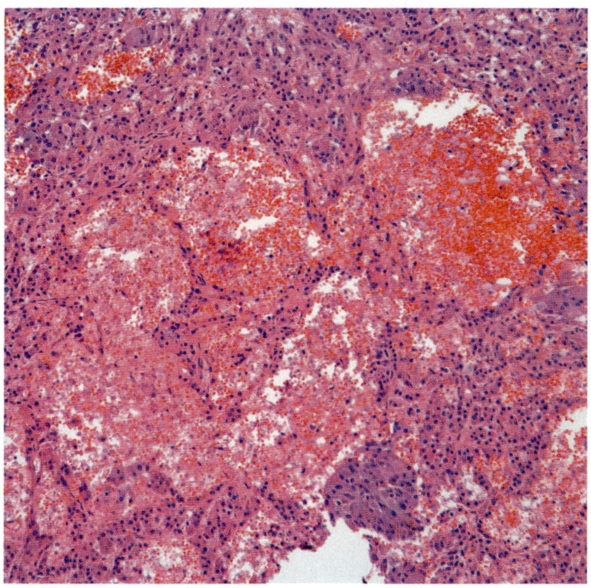

Figure 5-26 Well-differentiated neuroendocrine carcinoma with prominent angiectatic changes mimicking a vascular neoplasm.

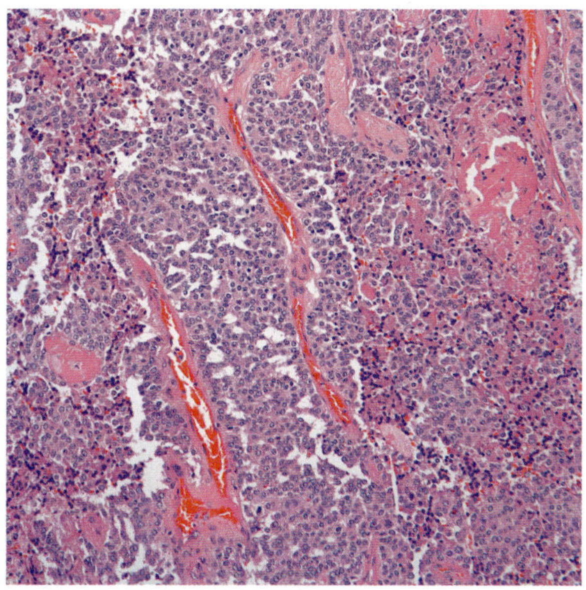

Figure 5-27 Well-differentiated neuroendocrine carcinoma with areas of hyalinization mimicking amyloid.

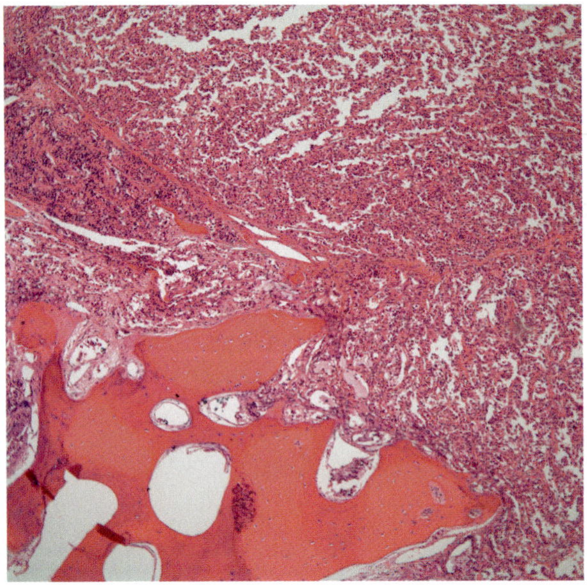

Figure 5-28 Well-differentiated neuroendocrine carcinoma with metaplastic bone formation.

86 patients at 5, 10, and 15 years after surgical treatment, with 7 dying of unrelated causes. The selection process for this study excluded patients with distant metastasis, however, suggesting that stage of the neoplasm at the time of diagnosis has an impact on the survival rate.

POORLY DIFFERENTIATED NEUROENDOCRINE CARCINOMA

Small Cell Carcinoma

Small cell carcinoma is defined by the WHO[2] as a malignant tumor with cells with scant cytoplasm and absent or inconspicuous nucleoli. Necrosis is extensive and mitotic count is high (60 mitotic figures per $2\,mm^2$). Obviously, such analysis can be accomplished accurately only in resected specimens and not in biopsy material. Nevertheless, in a study of 100 cases of small cell carcinoma,[44] the investigators claimed that in greater than 90% of the cases the diagnosis of small cell carcinoma can be established using small biopsy specimens. Most patients presenting with small cell carcinoma, however, have late-stage disease, precluding curative surgical resection, as has been noted in the literature.[45] Consequently, the surgical pathologist is provided with a small biopsy specimen in order to arrive at a definitive diagnosis.

The topic of small cell carcinoma has not been exempt from controversy. In 1985, Vollmer and colleagues[46] presented a study in which they addressed the issue of the subclassification of small cell carcinoma into oat cell type or intermediate type. However, in 1988, the Pathology Committee of the International Association for the Study of Lung Cancer recommended using the term *small cell carcinoma* for tumors previously designated as oat cell and intermediate subtypes.[47] Even terms such as *small cell neuroendocrine carcinoma*[48] may fall under scrutiny, because a proportion of these tumors may not show positive reaction to antibodies against neuroendocrine markers.

Macroscopic Features

Small cell carcinomas are usually in late stages at the time of diagnosis. The tumors are commonly central in location and large, with areas of necrosis (Fig. 5-29).

Microscopic Features

The tumor shows a dyscohesive cellular distribution composed of small cells with scant cytoplasm, round nuclei, and inconspicuous nucleoli. Single-cell necrosis or extensive areas of necrosis are common. In addition, the so-called Azzopardi phenomenon (denatured DNA around vessels imparting a bluish color or crush artifact–like image) is commonly observed in these tumors. The mitotic figure count in resected specimens or in open lung biopsies is more than 10 per 10 high-power fields (Fig. 5-30). Some areas show spindle cell morphology, with oval nuclei and inconspicuous nucleoli (Fig. 5-31). Of note, however, most of these features may be absent in a small transbronchial biopsy specimen, and the established criteria for diagnosis of small cell carcinoma may not be met in such material. Small biopsy specimens typically are characterized by the presence of crush artifact and few viable cells, with only occasional mitotic figures (Fig. 5-32).

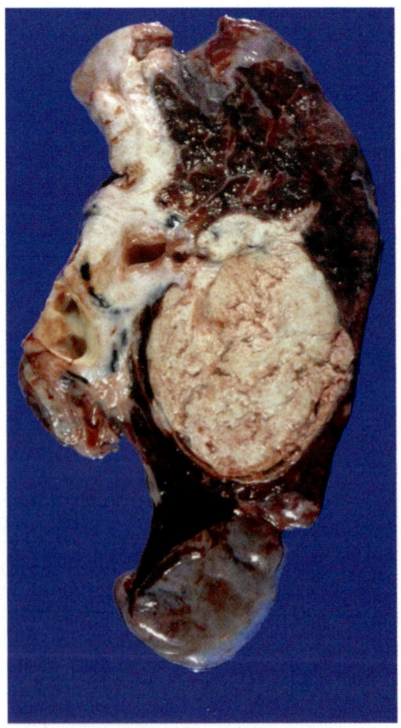

Figure 5-29 Gross specimen of a small cell carcinoma. The tumor is in a central location extending into lung parenchyma.

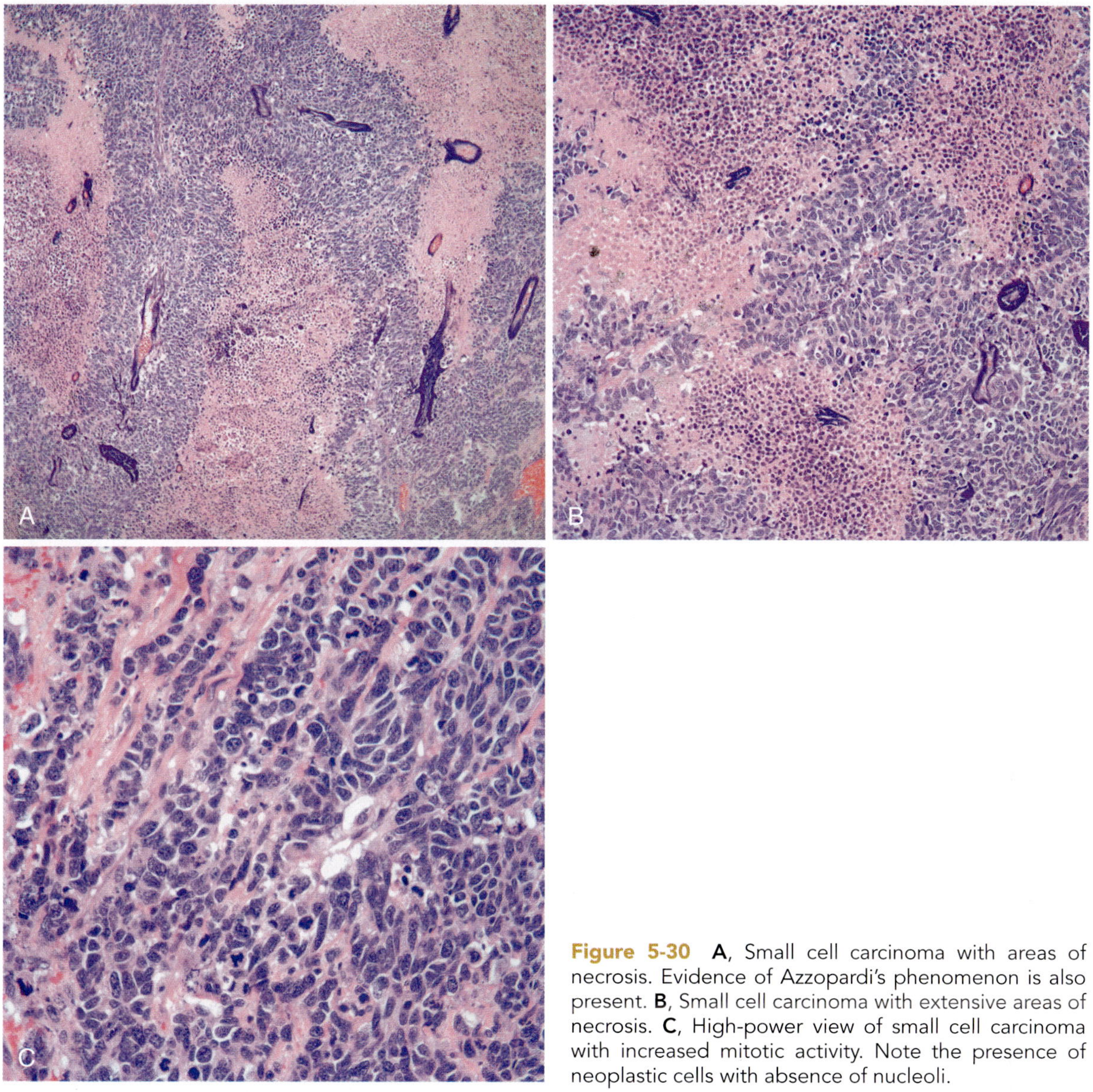

Figure 5-30 **A**, Small cell carcinoma with areas of necrosis. Evidence of Azzopardi's phenomenon is also present. **B**, Small cell carcinoma with extensive areas of necrosis. **C**, High-power view of small cell carcinoma with increased mitotic activity. Note the presence of neoplastic cells with absence of nucleoli.

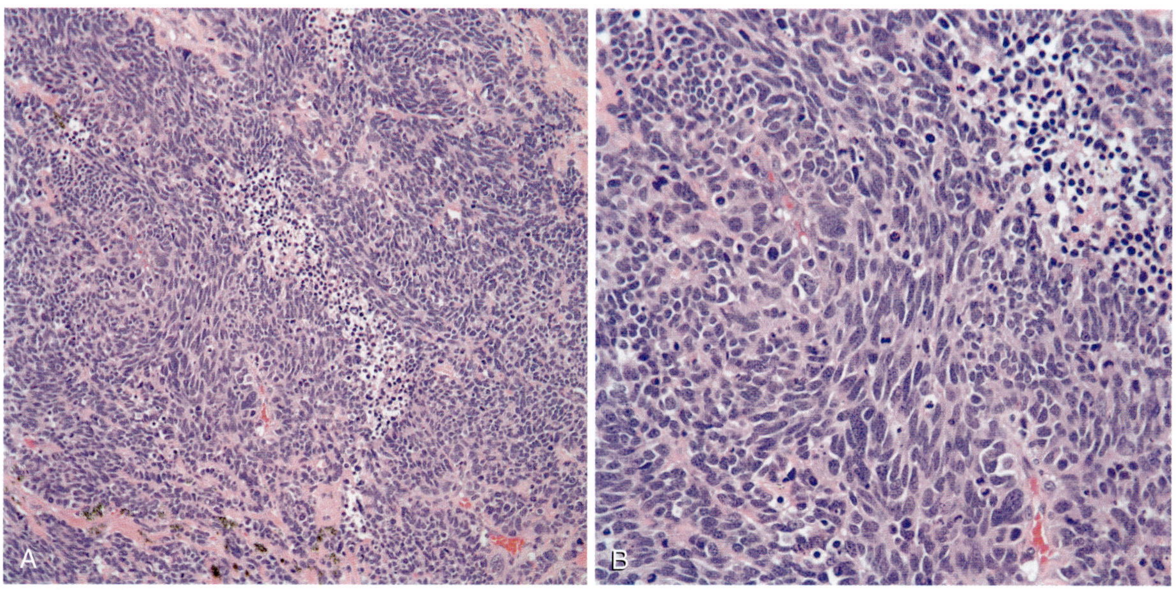

Figure 5-31 **A**, Small cell carcinoma with prominent spindle cell growth pattern. **B**, Small cell carcinoma with spindle cells and increased mitotic activity.

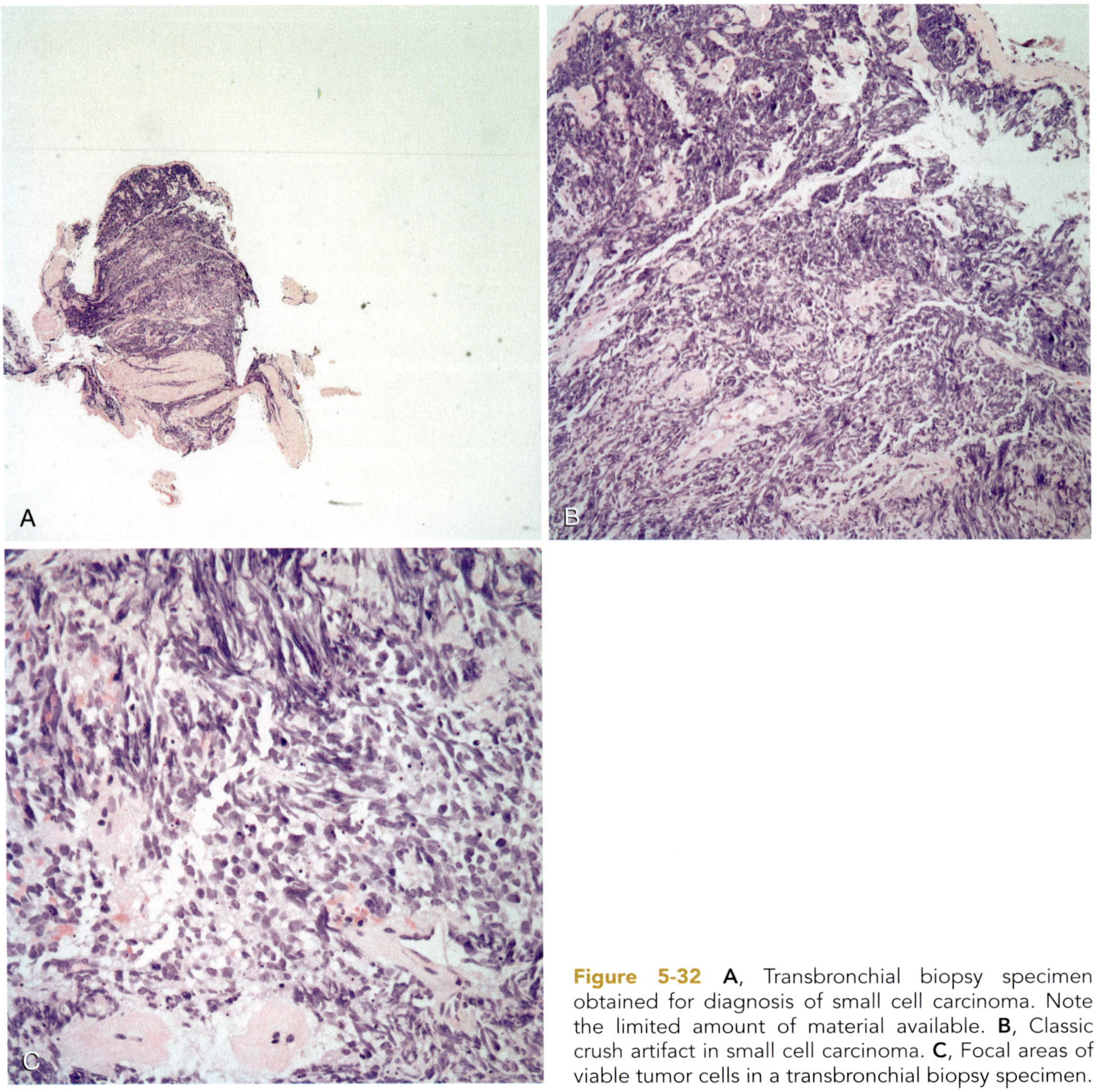

Figure 5-32 **A**, Transbronchial biopsy specimen obtained for diagnosis of small cell carcinoma. Note the limited amount of material available. **B**, Classic crush artifact in small cell carcinoma. **C**, Focal areas of viable tumor cells in a transbronchial biopsy specimen.

Immunohistochemical Features

In an immunohistochemical study of small cell carcinoma,[49] immunostaining for neuroendocrine markers such as chromogranin was positive in 60% of open lung biopsy specimens but only in 47% of transbronchial biopsy specimens, whereas synaptophysin staining showed 5% and 19% positivity, respectively. Nevertheless, most investigators concur that small cell carcinoma represents one end of the spectrum of neuroendocrine carcinomas of the lung. Also, in small, poorly preserved biopsy specimens in which the intensity of staining for neuroendocrine markers is marked, better-differentiated neuroendocrine tumors should be considered as an alternative diagnosis to small cell carcinoma.[50]

The impact of a diagnosis of small cell carcinoma cannot be overemphasized, because patients may undergo chemotherapy, radiation therapy, or both. It has been estimated in large studies that the long-term survival rate for patients with small cell carcinoma is approximately 10% at 2 years.[51]

Large Cell Neuroendocrine Carcinoma (Large Cell Carcinoma with Neuroendocrine Morphology, Large Cell Carcinoma with Neuroendocrine Differentiation)

By definition, large cell neuroendocrine carcinomas are poorly differentiated non–small cell carcinomas. According to the WHO classification,[2] the main feature distinguishing large cell neuroendocrine carcinoma from small cell carcinoma is the presence of prominent nucleoli in the former.

Macroscopic Features

Large cell neuroendocrine carcinomas are large neoplasms, usually in late stages at the time of diagnosis. The tumor may be in a central location, and it may manifest as a well-demarcated, solid, grayish mass, with or without apparent necrosis (Fig. 5-33).

Microscopic Features

Large cell neuroendocrine carcinomas will display a neuroendocrine morphology, including ribbons, rosettes, or nesting patterns combined with large zones of necrosis and a mitotic count higher than 11 mitotic figures per 2 mm^2 (average, 75 per mm^2) of viable tumor (Figs. 5-34 to 5-38). This latter definition applies to resected tumors only, so the diagnosis can hardly be accomplished using small biopsy specimens, in which viable tumor may not be adequate to evaluate for the so-called neuroendocrine pattern, or to permit a mitotic count of more than 11 mitotic figures.

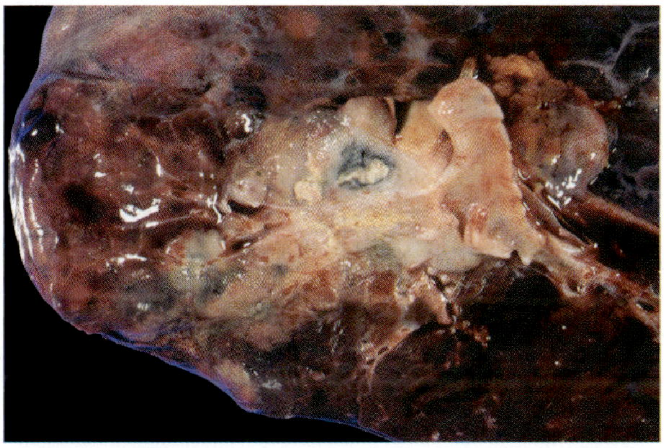

Figure 5-33 Gross specimen of a large cell neuroendocrine carcinoma in a central location extending into lung parenchyma.

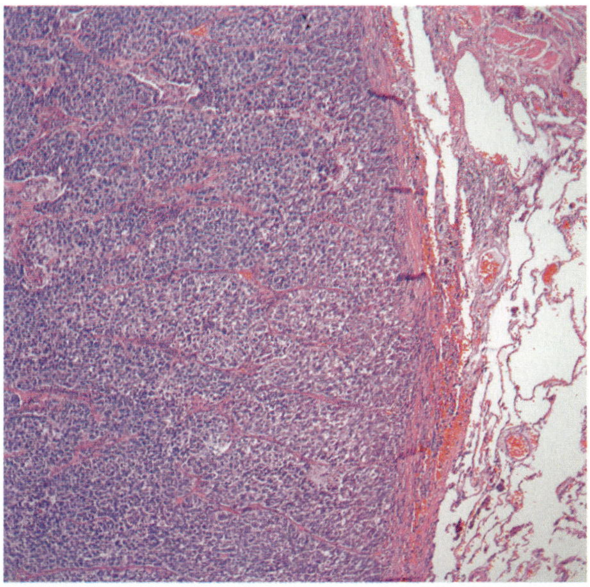

Figure 5-34 Large cell neuroendocrine carcinoma showing a nesting pattern.

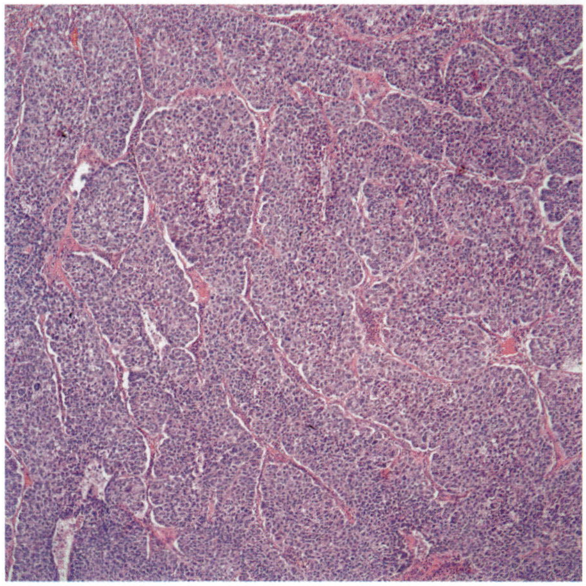

Figure 5-35 Large cell neuroendocrine carcinoma showing an organoid pattern of growth.

In 1988, Mooi and coworkers[52] described 11 primary lung carcinomas under the rubric of "non–small cell carcinoma with neuroendocrine features." These tumors had been diagnosed as either large cell carcinoma or squamous cell carcinoma, but they showed similarities to bronchial carcinoid and small cell carcinoma. In six of seven cases in which electron microscopy studies were available, the tumors showed dense core granules; all of the tumors showed positive staining for neuron-specific enolase (NSE). (Most of the antibodies that are available today for these studies may not have been available in 1988.) The investigators also stated that neuroendocrine features may be suspected from the light microscopic appearance. As suggested by some of the illustrations provided, some of those tumors, if not all, are similar to today's designation of large cell neuroendocrine carcinoma.

In 1997, Dresler and associates[53] analyzed 40 cases of large cell neuroendocrine carcinoma and concluded that large cell neuroendocrine carcinomas identified by histologic examination carry a poor prognosis. They also suggest that lesions previously categorized as large cell carcinoma with neuroendocrine features should be regarded as "large cell carcinoma with occult neuroendocrine differentiation." This latter suggestion specifically addresses an important issue: how to group tumors that have a "neuroendocrine pattern" yet fail to show immunoreactivity for neuroendocrine markers. According to currently accepted criteria, in order to make the diagnosis of large cell neuroendocrine carcinoma, "neuroendocrine morphology" and positive staining for at least one

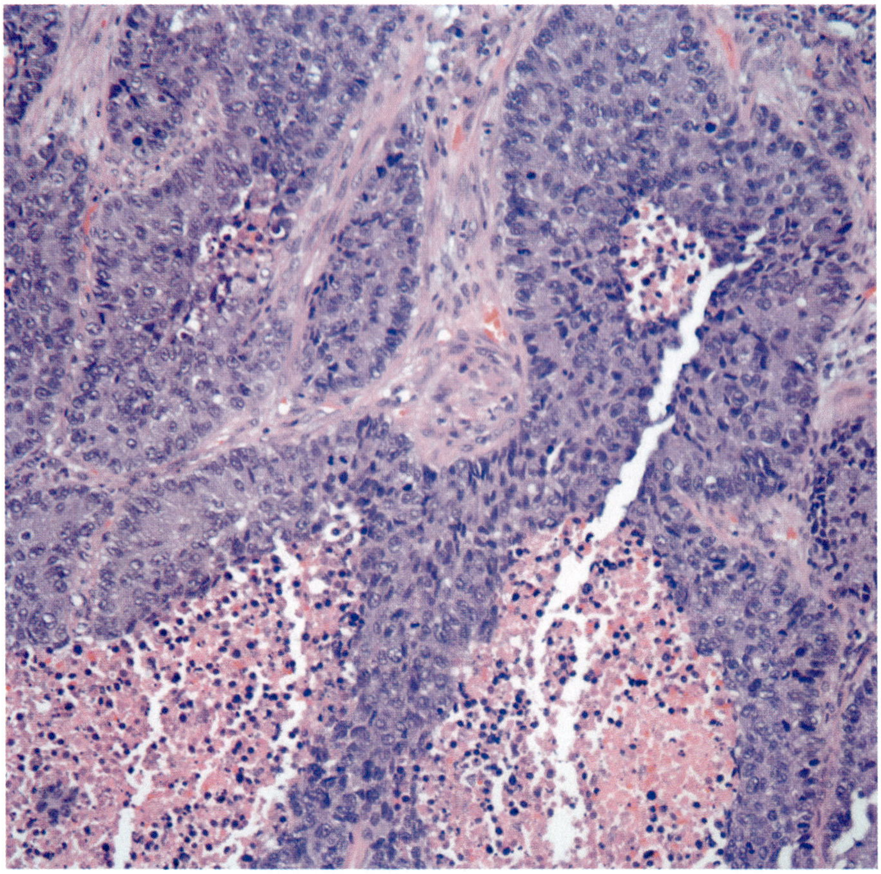

Figure 5-36 High-power view of a large cell neuroendocrine carcinoma showing extensive areas of necrosis.

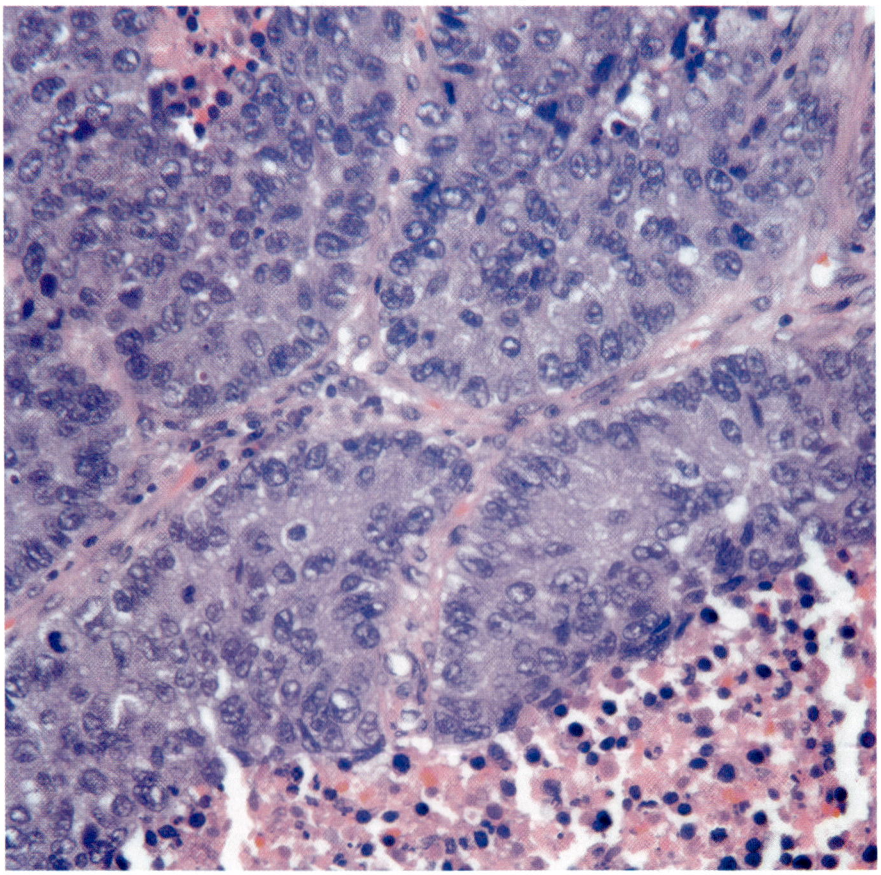

Figure 5-37 Large cell neuroendocrine carcinoma showing neoplastic cells with prominent nucleoli.

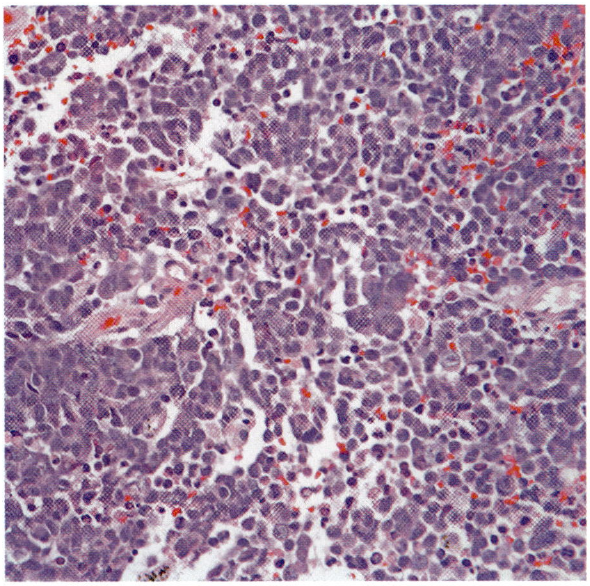

Figure 5-38 Large cell neuroendocrine carcinoma with a more disorganized growth pattern.

neuroendocrine marker are required.[2] This issue has become even more confusing because of the use of terms such as *small cell–like large cell neuroendocrine carcinoma* in some cytologic studies.[54]

Using the presence of nucleoli to separate small cell from non–small cell carcinoma may prove just as difficult as using cell size for their differentiation. Marchevsky and associates[55] evaluated 28 surgically resected high-grade pulmonary neuroendocrine carcinomas (16 small cell carcinomas and 12 large cell neuroendocrine carcinomas) by morphometric means. These workers recognized the presence of considerable overlap of nuclear features between these entities, which helped to separate only 9 of 28 cases studied, and suggested the use of more generic terminology such as "high-grade neuroendocrine carcinoma" or "grade III neuroendocrine carcinoma."

The topic of large cell neuroendocrine carcinoma has generated myriad publications attempting to clarify this confusing topic. For instance, in a study of 2070 large cell carcinomas, Iyoda and colleagues[56] divided them into four different categories: large cell neuroendocrine carcinoma, large cell carcinoma with neuroendocrine differentiation, large cell carcinoma with neuroendocrine morphology, and "classic" large cell carcinoma. In a multivariate analysis, the investigators grouped the first three entities into a single category, which they designated "large cell carcinoma with neuroendocrine features," separate from the "classic" large cell carcinoma. These workers concluded that tumors in this combined group are more aggressive. Tumors in which morphologic evidence of neuroendocrine change was absent were classified as "large cell carcinomas with neuroendocrine morphology." However, the multivariate analysis showed that the clinical behavior of these tumors was similar to that of tumors classified as "large cell neuroendocrine carcinoma" and "large cell carcinoma with neuroendocrine differentiation," as opposed to the "classic" large cell carcinoma. Nevertheless, their classification raises an important question: whether it is more important to determine neuroendocrine "differentiation" by immunohistochemical means, or whether a specific diagnosis is warranted for those tumors. Some other publications on this topic have lumped large cell neuroendocrine carcinomas and large cell carcinoma with neuroendocrine morphology under the same designation.[57] Unfortunately, in many recent publications on the subject, even as the investigators claimed to have used rigorous application of the WHO criteria,[2] their efforts have been concentrated on those tumors that fit the criteria of morphology and immunohistochemistry, leaving unanswered the question of what to do with tumors that may show the morphology but not the immunohistochemistry.[58–68] In other reports, it is very difficult to discern which cases were large cell neuroendocrine carcinoma, because the terminology used appears to be ambiguous.[69–72]

In some studies the use of more esoteric methods, such as chromosomal analysis and loss of heterozygosity (LOH) analysis, have been undertaken to separate tumors with features of large cell neuroendocrine carcinoma,[73] whereas in others the nomenclature used is not that assigned by the WHO classification system.[74] In some reports, these tumors have been correlated with pathologic stage; however, these tumors may manifest in different pathologic stages.[75] In some recent publications,[76,77] an emphasis has been on separation of large cell neuroendocrine carcinoma from small cell carcinoma by means of immunohistochemical and molecular studies. If the objective is to apply WHO criteria or any of the other schemas presented, such distinctions should not be a difficult task, because one neoplasm is small cell, and the other is non–small cell with prominent nucleoli. Furthermore, differentiating small cell from non–small cell carcinoma should not require immunohistochemical or molecular studies.

Alternatively, some reports have concentrated on non–small cell carcinomas with neuroendocrine differentiation or neuroendocrine morphology.[72,78–83] A study by Howe and associates[78] evaluated 439 cases of non–small cell carcinoma using immunohistochemical stains for neuroendocrine markers. The investigators reported that 36% of these tumors showed positive staining for at least one neuroendocrine marker and concluded that the presence of neuroendocrine differentiation in non–small cell carcinoma is of no prognostic significance, as also reported by other authors.[80] More recently, Ionescu and colleagues[83] arrived at similar conclusions after reviewing 609 cases of non–small cell carcinoma. In some cases, adenocarcinomas may show neuroendocrine differentiation. Some researchers have suggested that this is an important prognostic feature,[84] whereas others have taken a more circumspect approach.[85]

A few issues arise from critical analysis of the literature:

1. The diagnosis of large cell neuroendocrine carcinoma in most published series has been a diagnosis in retrospect after analysis for all large cell carcinomas.
2. Review of the cases included in a good number of publications, despite the "rigorous" application of the WHO criteria, suggests that some of the tumors included may not exactly belong in the category of "large cell neuroendocrine carcinoma."
3. The fact that resections have been evaluated speaks volumes to the issue that these tumors have already been initially treated as non–small cell carcinomas.
4. Although all investigators believe that these tumors are of high grade, they do not unanimously agree on the best method of treatment for patients diagnosed with large cell neuroendocrine carcinomas. Some workers have argued that large cell neuroendocrine carcinoma is potentially treatable with surgery,[64] whereas others advocate additional medical treatment.[86]
5. Some confusion remains regarding the use of terms such as *neuroendocrine differentiation* and *neuroendocrine morphology*.
6. Stage at presentation may still represent an important independent factor in the prognosis with these tumors.

Neuroendocrine morphology and differentiation can be summarized as follows:

Large cell neuroendocrine carcinoma refers to tumors with neuroendocrine pattern and positive staining for neuroendocrine markers—namely, chromogranin, synaptophysin, and CD56.

Large cell carcinoma with neuroendocrine features or morphology refers to tumors with neuroendocrine pattern but negative staining for neuroendocrine markers.

Large cell carcinoma with neuroendocrine differentiation refers to tumors with positive staining for neuroendocrine markers but absent neuroendocrine morphology.

Although any questions related to the issue of large cell carcinoma would be expected to be restricted to the concepts of neuroendocrine morphology or neuroendocrine differentiation, the WHO has identified yet another tumor that may prove even more confusing regarding the current classification, the so-called basaloid carcinoma of the lung.[87]

BASALOID CARCINOMA

Basaloid carcinoma initially was described as a new morphologic and phenotypical entity; however, close analysis of its histopathologic description reveals that in 19 of the 38 reported cases, the tumor showed areas of squamous cell carcinoma, adenocarcinoma, and large cell carcinoma, raising the possibility that at least one half of the tumors described may be grouped into one of those more specific categories. The WHO classification[2] recognizes that the distinction between large cell neuroendocrine carcinoma and basaloid carcinoma is difficult and often requires immunohistochemical studies. Furthermore, the WHO acknowledges that in 10% of cases of basaloid carcinoma, immunostaining for a neuroendocrine marker may be positive, thereby raising the possibility that "basaloid carcinoma" may represent a growth pattern, rather than a specific pathologic entity. Further studies on basaloid carcinoma have stressed the use of immunohistochemical studies—namely, immunostaining for cytokeratins 1, 5, 10, and 14 (34βE12)—to differentiate such tumors from large cell neuroendocrine carcinoma. However, Lyda and Weiss[88] reported an incidence of 5% positive staining for 34βE12 in neuroendocrine carcinomas.

Microscopic Features

Basaloid carcinoma typically appears as a well-defined tumor mass destroying lung parenchyma. As its name implies, the low-power view shows islands of tumor cells with palisading of the nuclei. The high-power view shows oval to spindle cells with elongated nuclei, and in some cells prominent nucleoli may be observed. Mitotic count in these tumors is high (Fig. 5-39).

CARCINOMAS WITH MIXED HISTOLOGIC PATTERN

In a small but well-represented number of cases, pulmonary carcinomas may show combined histologic patterns, particularly those of the small cell and non–small cell categories.[89–93] The general consensus is that these neoplasms display more aggressive clinical behavior than that typical of pure small cell carcinomas, leading to a lower survival rate. The possible association of small cell carcinoma and large cell neuroendocrine carcinoma, or large cell carcinoma with neuroendocrine differentiation, is an important topic that merits further investigation. It is debatable whether this distinction has a practical value in the treatment of patients, because both tumors are of high grade.

Molecular Biology

Genetic studies have been performed showing a gain of 3q in approximately 66% of small cell carcinomas and deletions of 10q, 16q, and 17p, which were less frequent in large cell neuroendocrine carcinomas than in small cell carcinomas.[94] Other studies have shown that gene expression profiling fails to distinguish small cell from large cell neuroendocrine carcinomas. This finding has prompted some investigators to suggest that both entities should be

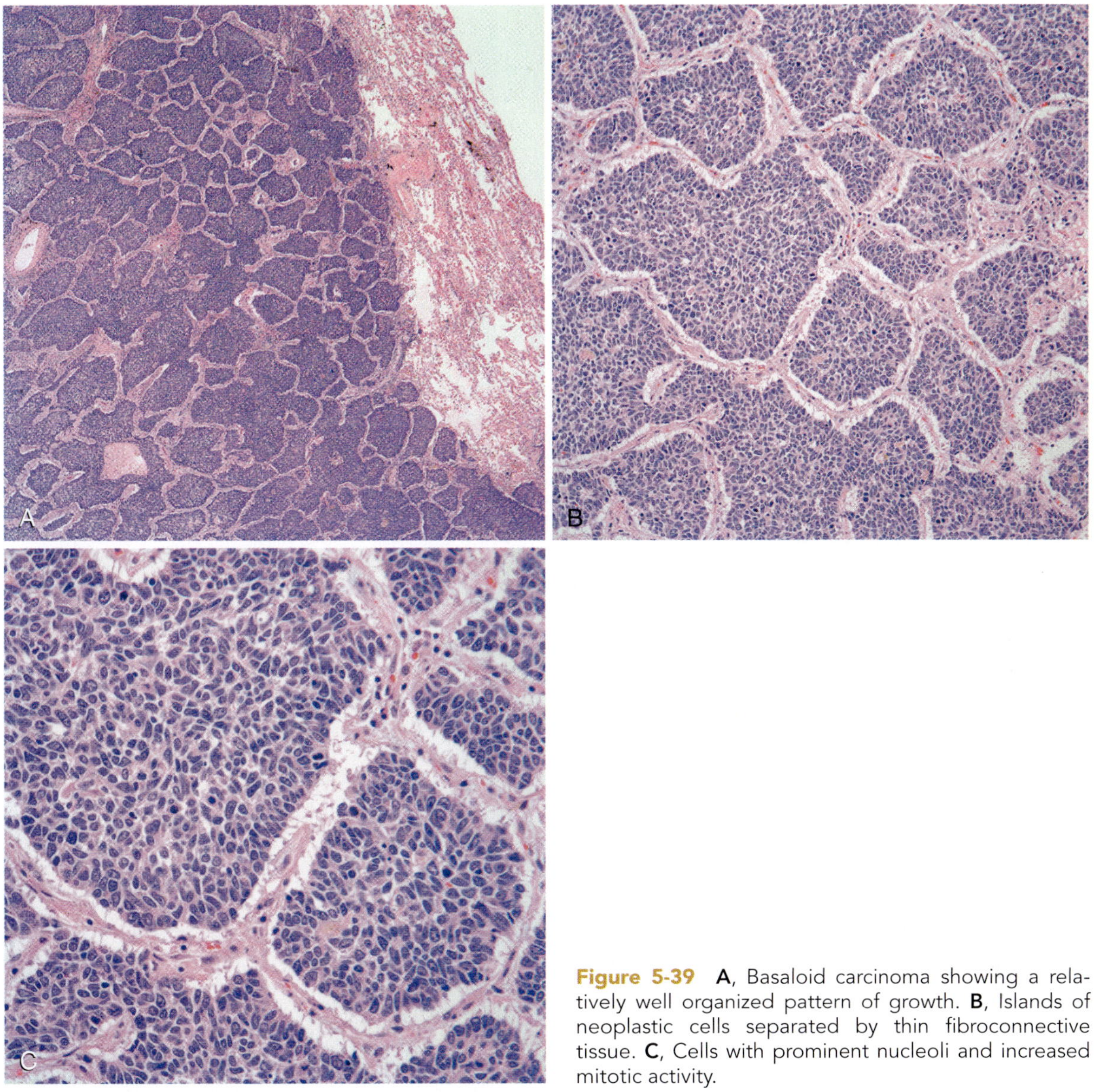

Figure 5-39 **A**, Basaloid carcinoma showing a relatively well organized pattern of growth. **B**, Islands of neoplastic cells separated by thin fibroconnective tissue. **C**, Cells with prominent nucleoli and increased mitotic activity.

grouped under the designation *high-grade neuroendocrine tumors*.[95] Other investigators have placed more emphasis on the spectrum of differentiation of neuroendocrine tumors: Studies of expression of gene products have found no evidence linking carcinoids and small cell carcinoma,[96,97] leading to the suggestion that small cell carcinomas are derived from epithelial cells, and that bronchial carcinoids are related to neural crest–derived tumors. It also appears that human p19ARF protein encoded by the beta transcript of the *p161NK4a* gene is more commonly lost in high-grade neuroendocrine carcinomas than in conventional non–small cell carcinomas.[98]

Analysis of p53, K-ras-2, and C-raf-1 by some workers has led to the suggestion that typical and atypical carcinoids are genetically distinct from high-grade neuroendocrine carcinomas.[99] It has been documented that loss of heterozygosity at 3p14.2-p21.3 is significantly more extensive in atypical carcinoids, whereas typical carcinoids are strongly positive for the cytoplasmic Fhit protein, similar to normal lung epithelia.[100] Of interest, the expression of Bcl-2 has been found to be involved in the pathogenesis of small cell carcinoma and carcinoid tumors of the lung.[101] Also, the expression of retinoblastoma protein (RB) in neuroendocrine tumors has disclosed the presence of the RB gene in patients with carcinoids and atypical carcinoids, whereas it is absent in patients with small cell and large cell neuroendocrine carcinoma.[102,103] More recently, it has been suggested that hASH-1 (human homologue of Mas1) is involved in the neuroendocrine differentiation of small and non–small cell carcinomas.[104]

Practical Approach

Based on current concepts and approaches, a practical classification system for neuroendocrine carcinomas may be conceptualized as follows[105]:

Surgical Resection Specimens

- Carcinoid—tumorlet (lesion less than 0.5 cm in greatest dimension)
- Well-differentiated neuroendocrine carcinoma—typical carcinoid (tumors with up to 3 mitotic figures per 10 high-power fields and absence of necrosis)
- Moderately differentiated neuroendocrine carcinoma—atypical carcinoid (tumors with 4 but fewer than 10 mitotic figures per 10 high-power fields and necrosis)
- High-grade neuroendocrine carcinoma:
  - Small cell carcinoma (with or without positive neuroendocrine markers; tumors with more than 10 mitotic figures per 10 high-power fields and necrosis)
  - Large cell neuroendocrine carcinoma—large cell carcinoma with positive neuroendocrine morphology and either positive or negative staining for neuroendocrine markers

Biopsy Specimens

- Neuroendocrine carcinoma—if the tumor is in the spectrum of well- or moderately differentiated neuroendocrine carcinoma (carcinoid or atypical carcinoid), and the tumor radiologically is larger than 5 mm in greatest diameter (specify the possibilities)
- Small cell carcinoma
- Squamous cell carcinoma
- Adenocarcinoma
- Non–small cell carcinoma

PULMONARY PARAGANGLIOMA

Although pulmonary paraganglioma is not part of the spectrum of neuroendocrine carcinomas, it is included in this chapter because it is part of the neuroendocrine family of tumors that may occur primarily in the lung. This neoplasm is exceedingly rare, and only a few well-described cases have been reported in the literature. The tumors appear to occur in adults, who may present with hypertension, increased serum norepinephrine, or Cushing's syndrome.[106–110]

Macroscopic Features

Tumor size ranges from less than 1 cm to more than 3 cm in greatest dimension. The tumors are endobronchial in location and may obstruct the bronchial lumen, producing symptoms of cough, wheezing, and dyspnea. The tumor may also appear at the periphery of the lung parenchyma.

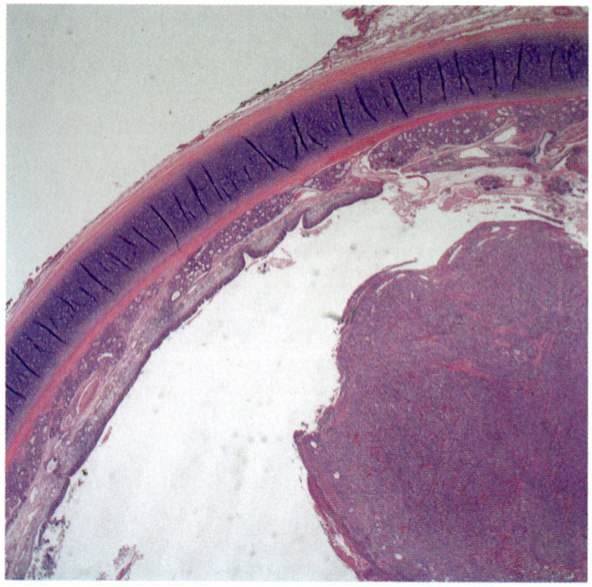

Figure 5-40 Bronchial paraganglioma.

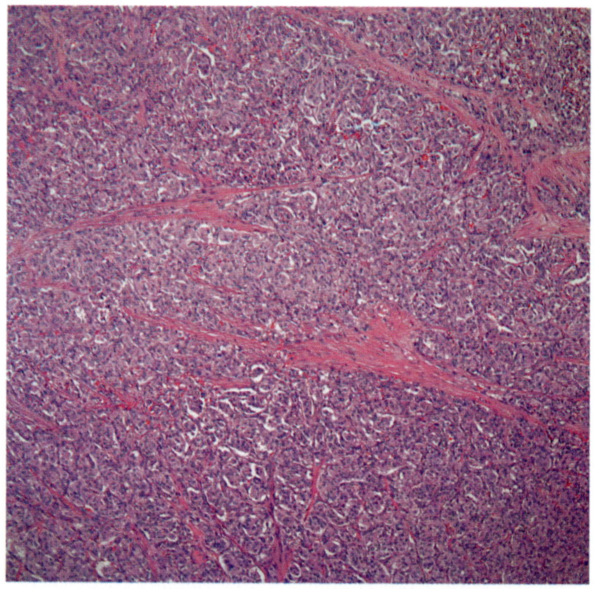

Figure 5-41 Paraganglioma with a well-organized nesting pattern—the so-called zellballen pattern.

Microscopic Features

At low magnification, the mass may appear as a polypoid tumor filling the bronchial lumen (Fig. 5-40). The classic low-power characteristic of paragangliomas is the so-called zellballen pattern (Fig. 5-41): The cells are arranged in a nesting pattern in which the nests are separated by thin fibroconnective tissue and ectatic blood vessels (Fig. 5-42). The tumor also may show oncocytic changes with a homogeneous cellular proliferation. On the high-power view, however, it is common to identify cells with macronuclei or bizarre nuclei with no mitotic activity (Fig. 5-43).[106–110] Also common is the presence of

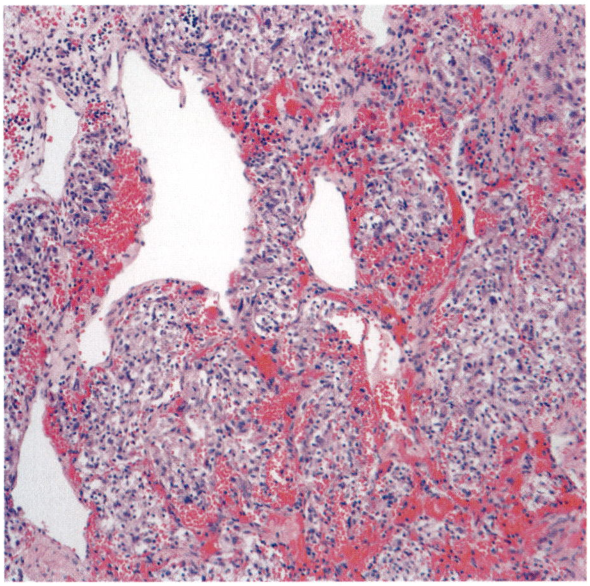

Figure 5-42 High-power view of paraganglioma showing nests of tumor cells and ectatic blood vessels.

large ectatic vessels or extensive areas of hyalinization (Fig. 5-44). In some cases, ganglion cells, represented by larger cells with esosinophilic cytoplasm, and prominent nucleoli, accompany the cellular proliferation. In other cases, the tumor may show spindle cell morphology (Fig. 5-45). In a few cases lymph node involvement has been reported.

Immunohistochemical Features

Like neuroendocrine carcinomas, paragangliomas react positively with neuroendocrine markers such as chromogranin, synaptophysin, or CD56. However, staining for keratin is negative in paragangliomas, whereas it is positive in neuroendocrine carcinomas. S-100 protein staining also is positive in sustentacular cells of paragangliomas.

Clinical Behavior

Surgical resection with close follow-up appears to be the treatment of choice, and in a majority of cases it is the only treatment.

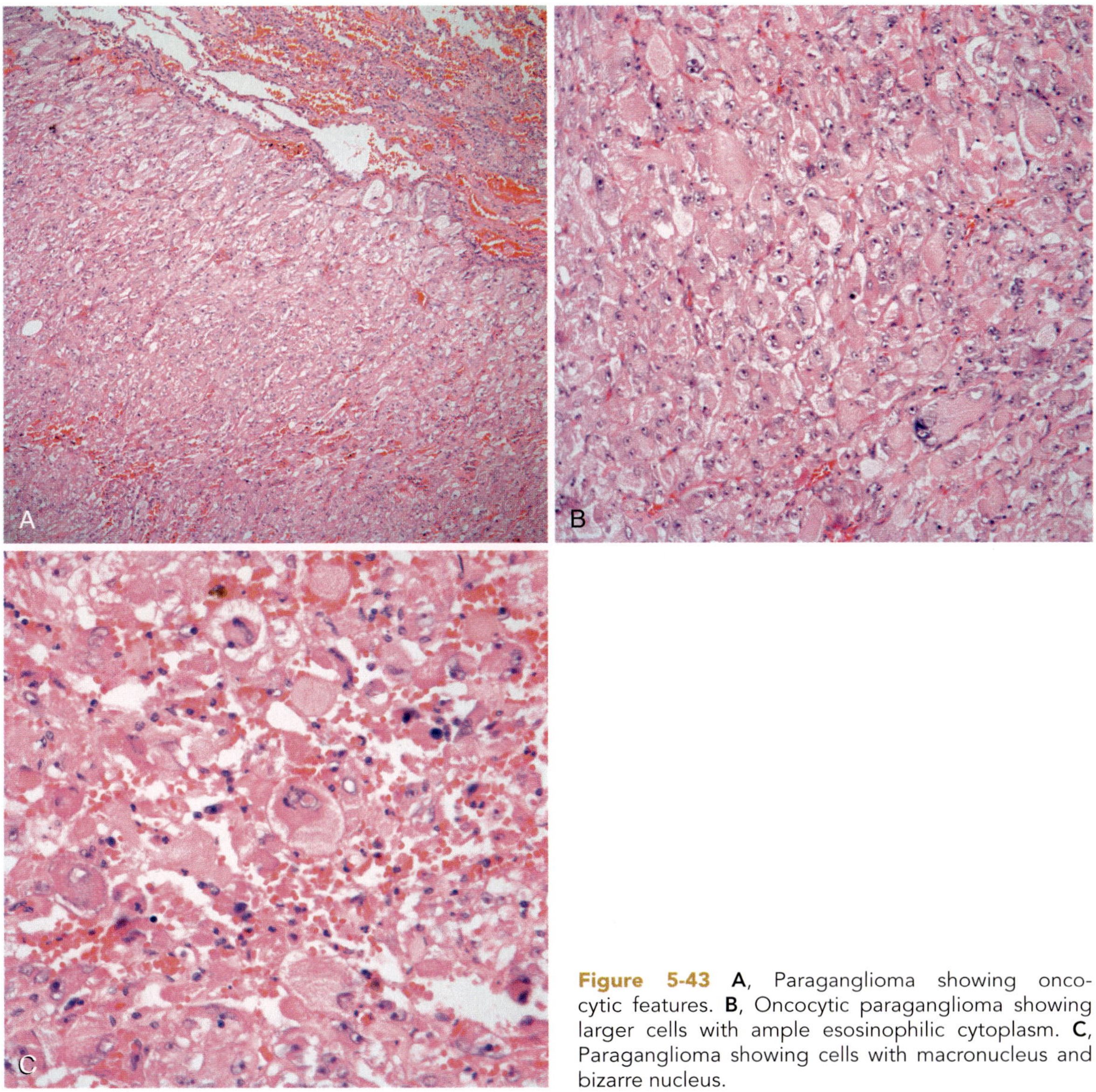

Figure 5-43 **A**, Paraganglioma showing oncocytic features. **B**, Oncocytic paraganglioma showing larger cells with ample esosinophilic cytoplasm. **C**, Paraganglioma showing cells with macronucleus and bizarre nucleus.

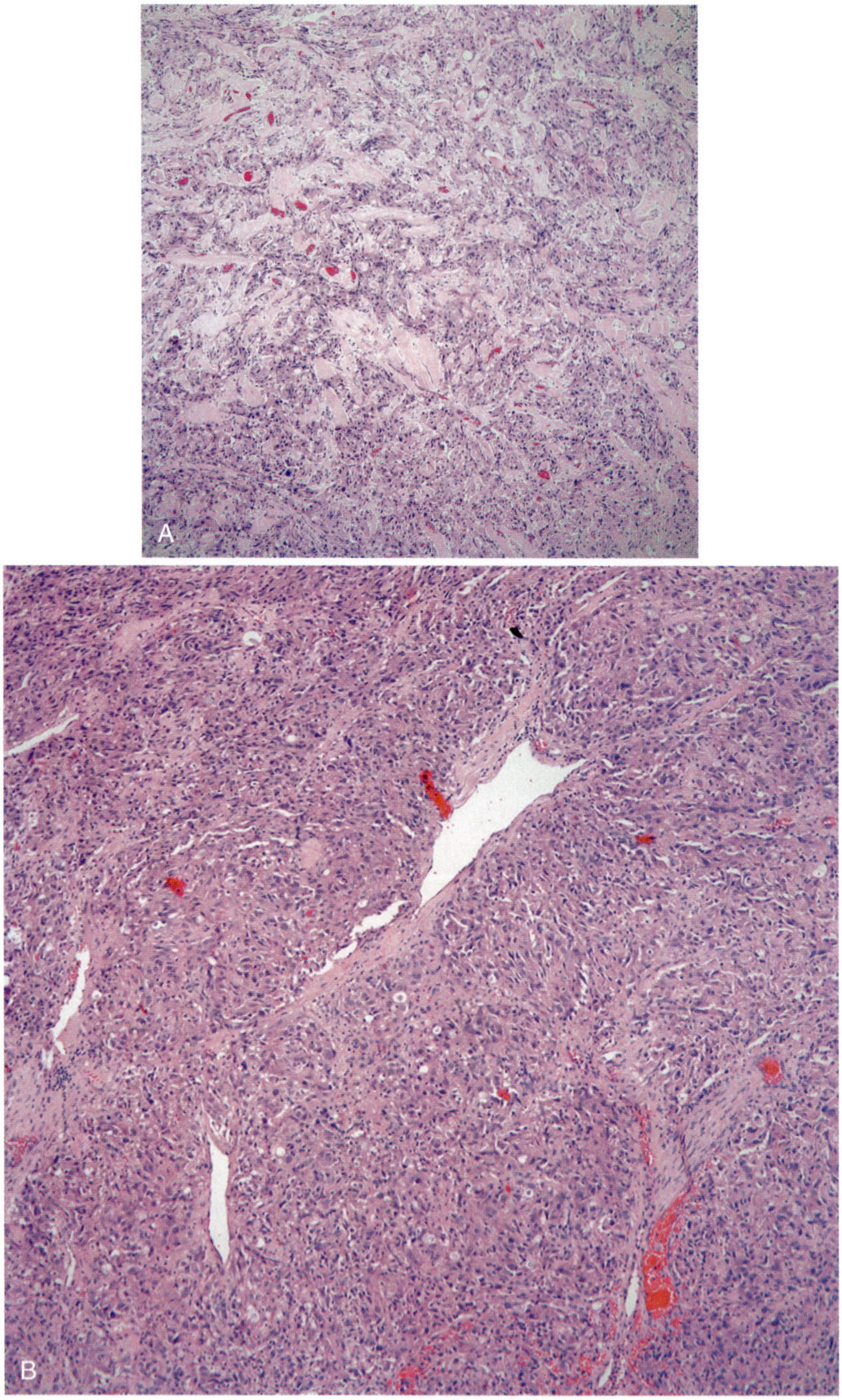

Figure 5-44 **A**, Paraganglioma with areas of hyalinization. **B**, Paraganglioma in which large ectatic vessels are evident.

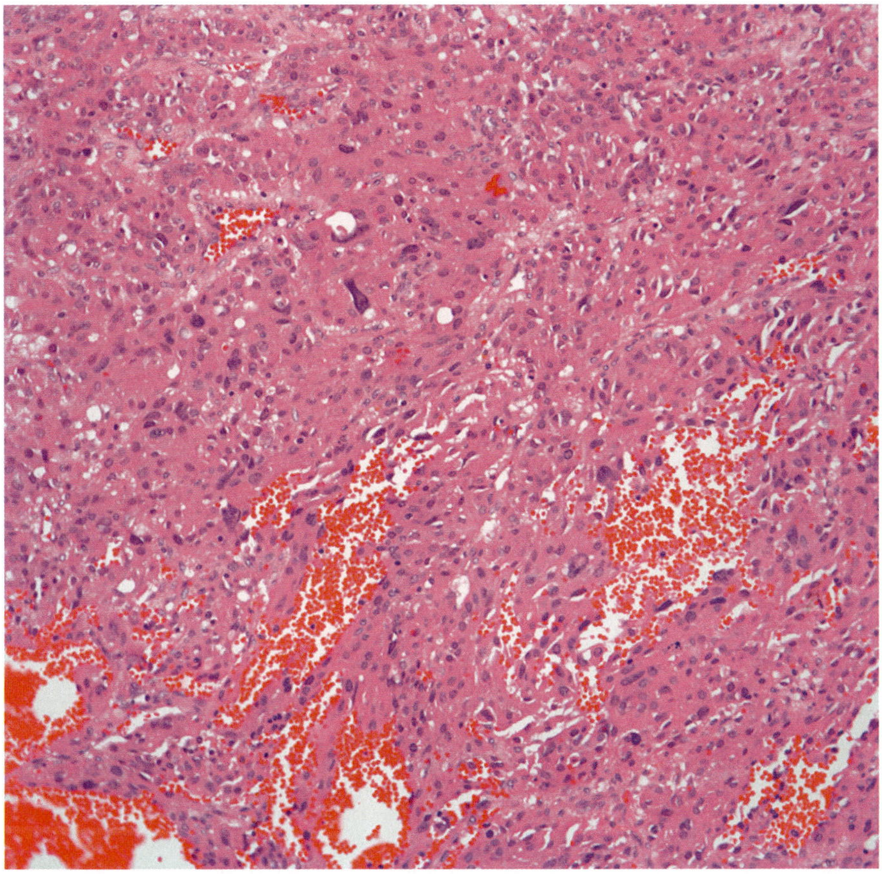

Figure 5-45 Paraganglioma with spindle cell growth pattern.

REFERENCES

1. Muller NL, Miller RR. Neuroendocrine carcinomas of the lung. *Semin Roentgenol.* 1990;25(1):96–104.
2. Beasley MB, Thunnissen FB, Hasleton PS, et al. Carcinoid tumor. In: Travis WD, Brambilla E, Müller-Hermelink HK, Harris CC, eds. *WHO Classification of Tumours: Tumours of the Lung, Pleura, Thymus and Heart*. Lyon, France: IARC Press; 2004.
3. Cerilli LA, Ritter J, Mills SE, Wick MR. Neuroendocrine neoplasms of the lung. *Am J Clin Pathol.* 2001;116(suppl 1):S65–S96.
4. Flieder DB. Neuroendocrine tumors of the lung: recent developments in histopathology. *Curr Opin Pulm Med.* 2002;8:275–280.
5. Oberndorfer S. Karzinoide Tumoren des Dunndarms. *Frankf Z Pathol.* 1907;425–432.
6. Bunting CH. Multiple primary carcinomata of the ileum. *Johns Hopkins Hosp Bull.* 1904;165(Dec.):389–394.
7. Gosset A, Masson P. Tumeurs endocrines de l'appendice. *Presse Med.* 1914;25:237–240.
8. Kinney FJ, Kovarik JL. Bone formation in bronchial adenoma. *Am J Clin Pathol.* 1965;44(1):52–56.
9. Heimburger IL, Kilman JW, Battersby JS. Peripheral bronchial adenomas. *J Thorac Cardiovasc Surg.* 1966;52(4):542–549.
10. Gmelich JT, Bensch KG, Liebow AA. Cells of Kultschitzky type in bronchioles and their relation to the origin of peripheral carcinoid tumor. *Lab Invest.* 1967;17(1):88–98.
11. Hausman DH, Weimann R. Pulmonary tumorlet with hilar lymph node metastasis. *Cancer.* 1967;20(9):1515–1519.
12. Azzopardi JG. Oat cell carcinoma of the bronchus. *J Pathol Bacteriol.* 1959;78(2):513–519.
13. Yutaka K, Ferguson TB, Bennett DE, Burford TH. Oat cell carcinoma of the lung. *Cancer.* 1969;23(3):517–524.
14. Gould VE, Memoli VA, Dardi LE. Multidirectional differentiation in human epithelial cancers. *J Submicrosc Cytol.* 1981;13(1):97–115.
15. Gould VE. Histogenesis and differentiation: a re-evaluation of these concepts as criteria for the classification of tumors. *Hum Pathol.* 1986;17(3):212–215.
16. Sheppard MN. Neuroendocrine differentiation in lung tumours. *Thorax.* 1991;46:843–850.
17. Brambilla E, Lantuejoul S, Sturm N. Divergent differentiation in neuroendocrine tumors. *Semin Diagn Pathol.* 2000;17(2):138–148.
18. Gould VE. Neuroendocrinomas and neuroendocrine carcinomas: APUD cell system neoplasms and their aberrant secretory activities. *Pathol Annu.* 1977;12:33–62.
19. Gould VE, Linnoila RI, Memoli VA, Warren WH. Neuroendocrine cells and neuroendocrine neoplasms of the lung. *Pathol Annu.* 1983;287–330.
20. Warren WH, Gould VE, Faber LP, Kittle CF, Memoli VA. Neuroendocrine neoplasms of the bronchopulmonary tract. *J Thorac Cardiovasc Surg.* 1985;89(6):819–825.
21. Paladugu RR, Benfield JR, Pak HY, Ross RK, Teplitz RL. Bronchopulmonary Kulchitzky cell carcinomas: a new classification scheme for typical and atypical carcinoids. *Cancer.* 1985;55(6):1303–1311.
22. Arrigoni MG, Woolner LB, Bernatz PE. Atypical carcinoid tumors of the lung. *J Thorac Cardiovasc Surg.* 1972;64(3):413–421.
23. Mills SE, Cooper PH, Walker AN, Kron IL. Atypical carcinoid tumor of the lung. *Am J Surg Pathol.* 1982;6(7):643–654.
24. Valli M, Fabris GA, Dewar A, Hornall D, Sheppard MN. Atypical carcinoid tumour of the lung: a study of 33 cases with prognostic features. *Histopathology.* 1994;24:363–369.

25. Grote TH, Macon WR, Davis B, Greco FA, Johnson DH. Atypical carcinoid of the lung: a distinct clinicopathologic entity. *Chest.* 1988;93(2):370–375.
26. Capella C, Heitz PU, Hofler H, Solcia E, Kloppel G. Revised classification of neuroendocrine tumours of the lung, pancreas and gut. *Virch Arch.* 1994;425:547–560.
27. Travis WD, Linnoila RI, Tsokos MG, et al. Neuroendocrine tumors of the lung with proposed criteria for large-cell neuroendocrine carcinoma. An ultrastructural, immunohistochemical, and flow cytometric study of 35 cases. *Am J Surg Pathol.* 1991;15(6):529–553.
28. Travis WD, Rush W, Flieder DB, et al. Survival analysis of 200 pulmonary neuroendocrine tumors with clarification of criteria for atypical carcinoid and its separation from typical carcinoid. *Am J Surg Pathol.* 1998;22(8):934–944.
29. Travis WD, Gal AA, Colby TV, Klimstra DS, Falk R, Koss MN. Reproducibility of neuroendocrine lung tumor classification. *Hum Pathol.* 1998;29:272–279.
30. Huang Q, Muzitansky A, Mark EJ. Pulmonary neuroendocrine carcinomas: a review of 234 cases and statistical analysis of 50 cases treated at one institution using a simple clinicopathologic classfication. *Arch Pathol Lab Med.* 2002;126:545–553.
31. Ricci C, Patrassi N, Massa R, Mineo C, Benedetti-Valentini F. Carcinoid syndrome in bronchial adenoma. *Am J Surg.* 1973;126(11):671–677.
32. Sklar JL, Churg A, Bensch KG. Oncocytic carcinoid tumor of the lung. *Am J Surg Pathol.* 1980;4(3):287–292.
33. Cebelin MS. Melanocytic bronchial carcinoid tumor. *Cancer.* 1980;46(8):1843–1848.
34. Wise WS, Bonder D, Aikawa M, Hsieh CL. Carcinoid tumor of lung with varied histology. *Am J Surg Pathol.* 1982;6(3):261–267.
35. Grazer R, Jacobs SB, Lucas P. Melanin-containing peripheral carcinoid of the lung. *Am J Surg Pathol.* 1982;6(1):73–78.
36. Gal AA, Koss MN, Hochholzer L, DeRose PB, Cohen C. Pigmented pulmonary carcinoid tumor. *Arch Pathol Lab Med.* 1993;117:832–836.
37. Tsutsumi Y, Yazaki K. Atypical carcinoid tumor of the lung, associated with giant-cell transformation in bone metastasis. *Acta Pathol Jpn.* 1990;40(8):609–615.
38. Memoli VA. Well-differentiated neuroendocrine carcinoma: a designation comes of age. *Chest.* 1991;10:892.
39. Sturm N, Rossi G, Lantuejoul S, et al. Expression of thyroid transcription factor-1 in the spectrum of neuroendocrine cell lung proliferations with special interest in carcinoids. *Hum Pathol.* 2002;33:175–182.
40. Costes V, Marty-Ane C, Picot MC, et al. Typical and atypical bronchopulmonary carcinoid tumors: a clinicopathologic and Ki-67-labeling study. *Hum Pathol.* 1995;26(7):740–745.
41. Walch AK, Zitzelsberger HF, Bauchinger M, et al. Typical and atypical carcinoid tumors of the lung are characterized by 11q deletions as detected by comparative genomic hybridization. *Am J Pathol.* 1998;153:1089–1098.
42. Wilkins EW, Grillo HC, Moncure AC, Scannell JG. Changing times in surgical management of bronchopulmonary carcinoid tumor. *Ann Thorac Surg.* 1984;38(4):339–344.
43. Schreurs JM, Westermann CJ, van den Bosch JM, Vanderschueren RG, Brutel de la Riviere A, Knaepen PJ. A twenty-five-year follow-up of ninety-three resected typical carcinoid tumors of the lung. *J Thorac Cardiovasc Surg.* 1992;104(5):1470–1475.
44. Nicholson S, Beasley MB, Brambilla E, et al. Small cell carcinomas (SCLC): a clinicopathologic study of 100 cases with surgical specimens. *Am J Surg Pathol.* 2002;26(9):1184–1197.
45. Zakowski MF. Pathology of small cell carcinoma of the lung. *Semin Oncol.* 2003;30(1):3–8.
46. Vollmer RT, Birch R, Ogden L, Crissman JD. Subclassification of small cell cancer of the lung: the Southern Cancer Study Group experience. *Hum Pathol.* 1985;16(3):247–252.
47. Hirsch FR, Matthews MJ, Aisner S, et al. Histopathologic classification of small cell lung cancer: changing concepts and terminology. *Cancer.* 1988;62(5):973–977.
48. Warren WH, Memoli VA, Jordan AG, Gould VE. Reevaluation of pulmonary neoplasms resected as small cell carcinomas. *Cancer.* 1990;65:1003–1010.
49. Guinee DG, Fishback NF, Koss MN, Abbondanzo SL, Travis WD. The spectrum of immunohistochemical staining of small-cell lung carcinoma in specimens from transbronchial and open lung biopsies. *Cancer.* 1994;102(4):406–414.
50. Warren WH, Gould VE. Differential diagnosis of small cell neuroendocrine carcinoma of the lung. *Chest Surg Clin N Am.* 1997;7(1):49–63.
51. Spiegelman D, Maurer LH, Ware JH, et al. Prognostic factors in small-cell carcinoma of the lung: an analysis of 1,521 patients. *J Clin Oncol.* 1989;7(3):344–354.
52. Mooi WJ, Dewar A, Springall D, Polak JM, Addis BJ. Non–small cell lung carcinomas with neuroendocrine features. A light microscopic, immunohistochemical and ultrastructural study of 11 cases. *Histopathology.* 1988;13:329–337.
53. Dresler CM, Ritter JH, Patterson GA, Ross E, Bailey MS, Wick MR. Clinical-pathological analysis of 40 patients with large cell neuroendocrine carcinoma of the lung. *Ann Thorac Surg.* 1997;63:180–185.
54. Yang YJ, Steele CT, Ou XL, Snyder KP, Kochman LJ. Diagnosis of high-grade pulmonary neuroendocrine carcinoma by fine-needle aspiration biopsy: nonsmall-cell or small-cell type? *Diagn Cytopathol.* 2001;25:292–300.
55. Marchevsky AM, Gal AA, Shah S, Koss MN. Morphometry confirms the presence of considerable nuclear size overlap between “small cells” and “large cells” in high-grade pulmonary neuroendocrine neoplasms. *Am J Clin Pathol.* 2001;116:466–472.
56. Iyoda A, Hiroshima K, Toyozaki T, Haga Y, Fujisawa T, Ohwada H. Clinical characterization of pulmonary large cell neuroendocrine carcinoma and large cell carcinoma with neuroendocrine morphology. *Cancer.* 2001;91:1992–2000.
57. Zacharias J, Nicholson AG, Ladas GP, Goldstraw P. Large cell neuroendocrine carcinoma and large cell carcinomas with neuroendocrine morphology of the lung: prognosis after complete resection and systematic nodal dissection. *Ann Thorac Surg.* 2003;75:348–352.
58. Takei H, Asamura H, Maeshima A, et al. Large cell neuroendocrine carcinoma of the lung: a clinicopathologic study of eighty-seven cases. *J Thorac Cardiovasc Surg.* 2002;124(2):285–292.
59. Mazieres J, Daste G, Molinier L, et al. Large cell neuroendocrine carcinoma of the lung: pathological study and clinical outcome of 18 resected cases. *Lung Cancer.* 2002;37:287–292.
60. Jung KJ, Lee KS, Han J, et al. Large cell neuroendocrine carcinoma of the lung: clinical, CT, and pathological findings in 11 patients. *J Thorac Imaging.* 2001;16:156–162.
61. Filosso PL, Ruffini E, Oliaro A, et al. Large-cell neuroendocrine carcinoma of the lung: a clinicopathologic study of eighteen cases and the efficacy of adjuvant treatment with octreotide. *J Thorac Cardiovasc Surg.* 2005;129(4):819–824.
62. Hage R, Seldenrijk K, Bruin PD, Swieten HV, Bosch JVD. Pulmonary large cell neuroendocrine carcinoma (LCNEC). *Eur J Cardiothorac Surg.* 2003;23:457–460.
63. Yamanishi M, Takeuchi S, Kurashina R, et al. High survival rate of 6 cases of pulmonary large cell neuroendocrine carcinoma formerly classified as small cell carcinoma. *J Nippon Med.* 2001;68:335–339.
64. Doddoli C, Barlesi F, Chetaille B, et al. Large cell neuroendocrine carcinoma of the lung: an aggressive disease potentially treatable with surgery. *Ann Thorac Surg.* 2004;77:1168–1172.
65. Paci M, Cavazza A, Annessi V, et al. Large cell neuroendocrine carcinoma of the lung: a 10-year clinicopathologic retrospective study. *Ann Thorac Surg.* 2004;77:1163–1167.

66. Jiang S-X, Kameya T, Shoji M, Dobashi Y, Shinada J, Yoshimura H. Neuroendocrine carcinoma of the lung: a histologic and immunohistochemical study of 22 cases. *Am J Surg Pathol.* 1998;22(5):526–537.
67. Skuladottir H, Hirsch FR, Hansen HH, Olsen JH. Pulmonary neuroendocrine tumors: incidence and prognosis of histological subtypes. A population-based study in Denmark. *Lung Cancer.* 2002;37(2):127–135.
68. Cooper WA, Thourani VH, Gal AA, Lee RB, Mansour KA, Miller JI. The surgical spectrum of pulmonary neuroendocrine neoplasms. *Chest.* 2001;119:14–18.
69. Veronesi G, Morandi U, Alloisio M, et al. Large cell neuroendocrine carcinoma of the lung: a retrospective analysis of 144 surgical cases. *Lung Cancer.* 2006;53:111–115.
70. Masuya D, Liu D, Ishikawa S, Yamamoto Y, Huang C-L, Yokomise H. Large cell carcinoma with neuroendocrine morphology of the lung. *Jpn J Thorac Cardiovasc Surg.* 2006;54:31–34.
71. Battafarano RJ, Fernandez FG, Ritter J, et al. Large cell neuroendocrine carcinoma: an aggressive form of non-small cell lung cancer. *J Thorac Cardiovasc Surg.* 2005;130:166–172.
72. Iyoda A, Hiroshima K, Baba M, Saitoh Y, Ohwada H, Fujisawa T. Pulmonary large cell carcinomas with neuroendocrine features are high-grade neuroendocrine tumors. *Ann Thorac Surg.* 2002;73:1049–1054.
73. Peng W-X, Sano T, Oyama T, Kawashima O, Nakajima T. Large cell neuroendocrine carcinoma of the lung: a comparison with large cell carcinoma with neuroendocrine morphology and small cell carcinoma. *Lung Cancer.* 2005;47:225–233.
74. Garcia-Yuste M, Matilla JM, Alvarez-Gago T, et al. Prognostic factors in neuroendocrine lung tumors: a Spanish Multicenter Study. Spanish Multicenter Study of Neuroendocrine Tumors of the Lung of the Spanish Society of Pneumonology and Thoracic Surgery (EMETNE-SEPAR). *Ann Thorac Surg.* 2000;70:258–263.
75. Iyoda A, Hiroshima K, Moriya Y, et al. Prognostic impact of large cell neuroendocrine histology in patients with pathologic stage Ia pulmonary non–small cell carcinoma. *J Thorac Cardiovasc Surg.* 2006;132:312–315.
76. Hiroshima K, Iyoda A, Shida T, et al. Dictinction of pulmonary large cell neuroendocrine carcinoma from small cell lung carcinoma: a morphological, immunohistochemical, and molecular analysis. *Mod Pathol.* 2006;19:1358–1368.
77. Nitadori J, Ishii G, Tsuta K, et al. Immunohistochemical differential diagnosis between large cell neuroendocrine carcinoma and small cell carcinoma by tissue microarray analysis with a large antibody panel. *Am J Clin Pathol.* 2006;125:682–692.
78. Howe MC, Chapman A, Kerr K, Dougal M, Anderson H, Hasleton PS. Neuroendocrine differentiation in non–small cell lung cancer and its relation to prognosis and therapy. *Histopathology.* 2004;46:195–201.
79. Carey FA, Save VE. Neuroendocrine differentiation in lung cancer. *J Pathology.* 1997;182:9–10.
80. Wertzel H, Grahmann PR, Bansbach S, Lange W, Hasse J, Bohm N. Results after surgery in undifferentiated large cell carcinoma of the lung: the role of neuroendocrine expression. *Eur J Cardiothorac Surg.* 1997;12:698–702.
81. Jensen SM, Gazdar AF, Cuttitta F, Russell EK, Linnoila I. A comparison of synaptophysin, chromogranin, and L-dopa decarboxylase as markers for neuroendocrine differentiation in lung cancer cell lines. *Cancer Res.* 1990;50:6068–6074.
82. Burnett HE, Zakhour HD, Walker C. Neuroendocrine and epithelial markers in diagnostic bronchial lung cancer biopsy specimens. *Eur J Cancer.* 1992;28A(4/5):853–855.
83. Ionescu D, Treaba D, Gilks CB, et al. Nonsmall cell lung carcinoma with neuroendocrine differentiation—an entity of no clinical or prognostic significance. *Am J Surg Pathol.* 2007;31(1):26–32.
84. Hiroshima K, Iyoda A, Shibuya K, et al. Prognostic significance of neuroendocrine differentiation in adenocarcinoma of the lung. *Ann Thorac Surg.* 2002;73:1732–1735.
85. Souhami RL. Neuroendocrine phenotype, chemosensitivity and prognosis in adenocarcinoma of the lung. *Ann Oncol.* 1991;2:323–324.
86. Iyoda A, Hiroshima K, Toyozaki T, et al. Adjuvant chemotherapy for large cell carcinoma with neuroendocrine features. *Cancer.* 2001;92:1108–1112.
87. Brambilla E, Moro D, Veale D, et al. Basal cell (basaloid) carcinoma of the lung: a new morphologic and phenotypic entity with separate prognostic significance. *Hum Pathol.* 1992;23(9):993–1003.
88. Lyda MH, Weiss LM. Immunoreactivity for epithelial and neuroendocrine antibodies are useful in the differential diagnosis of lung carcinomas. *Hum Pathol.* 2000;331:980–987.
89. McDowell EM, Trump BF. Pulmonary small cell carcinoma showing tripartite differentiation in individual cells. *Hum Pathol.* 1981;12(3):286–294.
90. Tsubota YT, Kawaguchi T, Hoso T, Nishino E, Travis WD. A combined small cell and spindle cell carcinoma of the lung: report of a unique case with immunohistochemical and ultrastructural studies. *Am J Surg Pathol.* 1992;16(11):1008–1115.
91. Adelstein DJ, Tomashefski JF, Snow NJ, Horrigan TP, Hines JD. Mixed small cell and non-small cell lung cancer. *Chest.* 1986;89(5):699–704.
92. Radice PA, Matthews MJ, Ihde DC, et al. The clinical behavior of "mixed" small cell/large cell bronchogenic carcinoma compared to "pure" small cell subtypes. *Cancer.* 1982;50(12):2894–2902.
93. Ruffini E, Rena O, Oliaro A, et al. Lung tumors with mixed histologic pattern. Clinico-pathologic characteristics and prognostic significance. *Eur J Cardiothorac Surg.* 2002;22:701–707.
94. Ullmann R, Petzmann S, Sharma A, Cagle PT, Popper HH. Chomosomal aberrations in a series of large-cell neuroendocrine carcinomas: unexpected divergence from small-cell carcinoma of the lung. *Hum Pathol.* 2001;32:1059–1063.
95. Jones MH, Virtanen C, Honjoh D, et al. Two prognostically significant subtypes of high-grade lung neuroendocrine tumours independent of small cell and large cell neuroendocrine carcinomas identified by gene expression profiles. *Lancet.* 2004;363:775–781.
96. Sampietro G, Tomasic G, Collini P, et al. Gene product immunophenotyping of neuroendocrine lung tumors. *App Immunohistochem Mol Morphol.* 2000;8(1):49–56.
97. Anbazhagan R, Tihan T, Bornman DM, et al. Classification of small cell lung cancer and pulmonary carcinoid by gene expression profiles. *Cancer Res.* 1999;59(10):5119–5122.
98. Gazzeri S, Valle VD, Chaussade L, Brambilla C, Larsen CJ, Brambilla E. The human p19ARF protein encoded by the beta transcript of the *p16INK4a* gene is frequently lost in small cell lung cancer. *Cancer Res.* 1998;58(17):3926–3931.
99. Przygodzki RM, Finkelstein SD, Langer JC, et al. Analysis of p53, K-ras-2, and C-raf-1 in pulmonary neuroendocrine tumors: correlation with histological tumors. *Am J Pathol.* 1996;148(5):1531–1541.
100. Kovatich A, Friedland DM, Druck T, et al. Molecular alteratons to human chromosome 3p loci in neuroendocrine lung tumors. *Cancer.* 1998;83:1109–1117.
101. Wang D-G, Johnston CF, Sloan JM, Buchanan KD. Expression of Bcl-2 in lung neuroendocrine tumours: comparison with p53. *J Pathol.* 1998;184:247–251.
102. Cagle PT, el-Naggar AK, Xu HJ, Xu SX, Benedict WF. Differential retinoblastoma protein expression in neuroendocrine tumors of the lung. Potential diagnostic implications. *Am J Pathol.* 1997;150:393–400.
103. Rusch VW, Klimstra DS, Venkatraman ES. Molecular markers help characterized neuroendocrine lung tumors. *Ann Thorac Surg.* 1996;62:798–810.

104. Ito T, Udaka N, Okudela K, Yazawa T, Kitamura H. Mechanisms of neuroendocrine differentiation in pulmonary neuroendocrine cells and small cell carcinoma. *Endocr Pathol.* 2003;14(2):133–139.
105. Moran CA, Suster S, Coppola D, Wick MR. Neuroendocrine carcinomas of the lung: a critical analysis. *Am J Clin Pathol.* 2009;131(2):206–221.
106. Shibahara J, Goto A, Niki T, Tanaka M, Nakajima J, Fukayama M. Primary pulmonary paraganglioma: report of a functioning case with immunohistochemical and ultrastructural study. *Am J Surg Pathol.* 2004;28(6):825–829.
107. Kee AR, Forrest CH, Brennan BA, Papadimitriou JM, Glancy RJ. Gangliocytic paraganglioma of the bronchus: a case report with follow-up and ultrastuctural assessment. *Am J Surg Pathol.* 2003;27:1380–1385.
108. Palau MA, Merino MJ, Quezado M. Corticotropin-producing pulmonary gangliocytic paraganglioma associated with Cushing's syndrome. *Hum Pathol.* 2006;37:623–626.
109. Aubertine CL, Flieder DB. Primary paraganglioma of the lung. *Ann Diagn Pathol.* 2004;8:237–241.
110. Dahir KM, Gonzales A, Revelo MP, Ahmed SR, Roberts JR, Blevins Jr LS. Ectopic adrenocorticotropic hormone hypersecretion due to a primary pulmonary paraganglioma. *Endocr Pract.* 2004;10:424–428.

6

Biphasic Tumors of the Lung

PULMONARY BLASTOMA
PLEUROPULMONARY BLASTOMA
PULMONARY CARCINOSARCOMA

Primary malignant biphasic tumors occurring in the lung parenchyma are rare, accounting for no more than 1% to 2% of all primary malignant tumors of the lung. The two most common neoplasms in this group are blastomas and carcinosarcomas. Not all pulmonary blastomas are biphasic, but because a majority are, the topic of pulmonary blastomas is covered in this chapter.

Pleuropulmonary blastomas also are included in this chapter. This tumor occurs predominantly in the pediatric population; however, the designation "blastoma" may cause it to be confused with blastoma in the adult.

The primary clinical and pathologic characteristics of these three neoplasms are summarized in Tables 6-1 and 6-2.

PULMONARY BLASTOMA

The group of tumors designated *pulmonary blastoma* probably represents less than 1% of all malignant primary lung neoplasms. Because of their rarity, these neoplasms often are addressed with similar tumors, such as pulmonary carcinosarcomas, in the category "biphasic tumors of the lung."[1] Pulmonary blastoma occasionally is confused with pleuropulmonary blastoma, a tumor that shares similar terminology but probably represents a different clinicopathologic entity.[2] As noted previously, not all pulmonary blastomas are biphasic tumors, and currently the World Health Organization (WHO) classifies the monophasic variant of pulmonary blastoma as "well-differentiated fetal adenocarcinoma." In this chapter, however, the term *blastoma* is used consistently.

Historical Aspects

In 1952, Barnard[3] described a tumor in a 40-year-old woman who had survived 10 years after a pneumonectomy for an intrapulmonary tumor. Histologically, the tumor was characterized by a mixture of carcinoma and sarcoma, which Barnard found to be similar to the embryomata of the kidney, so he designating it "embryoma of the lung." In 1961, Spencer[4] described three similar tumors that he termed *pulmonary blastoma*, noting that they resembled nephroblastomas found in the kidney. In addition, he suggested that such terminology would lend support to the theory of dual development of the lung from the laryngotracheal bud and pulmonary mesenchyma. This theory had already been presented by Waddell,[5] who suggested that the distal respiratory portion of the lung derives from the mesenchyma. However, other investigators disagreed with this view of lung histogenesis and supported the theory that the lung is formed from two germ cell layers. Many of these workers interpreted pulmonary blastoma as a form of carcinosarcoma that happened to resemble the fetal lung.[6,7] By the early 1970s, pulmonary blastoma had been reported only sporadically in the literature, with fewer than 20 cases mentioned.[8,9] All of the tumors occurred in adult patients and displayed the characteristic biphasic histologic features. Most of the cases had a fatal outcome, with variable range of survival. Nevertheless, there was still resistance to classifying pulmonary blastoma as a specific clinicopathologic condition, and on the basis of embryogenesis, some researchers still felt that it was a variant of carcinosarcoma.[10] To address this view, some studies were published suggesting that all of the epithelium-lined structures, including alveoli, are of endodermal origin, whereas pulmonary blastomas are composed of two distinct components: epithelial and mesenchymal.[11,12] Pulmonary blastomas have been described under a variety of names, including pulmonary endodermal tumor resembling fetal lung,[13,14] adenocarcinoma simulating fetal tubules in pseudoglandular stage,[15] and adenocarcinoma of the fetal lung type.[16]

Definition

In the most recent WHO classification of tumors of the lung, the definition of pulmonary blastoma was limited to tumors with a biphasic morphology—that is, tumors that show areas of well-differentiated fetal adenocarcinoma and primitive mesenchymal stroma.[17] *Fetal adenocarcinoma* (pulmonary blastoma, monophasic type) is defined as

TABLE 6-1 CLINICAL FEATURES OF PRIMARY BIPHASIC TUMORS

Characteristic	Monophasic Blastoma	Biphasic Blastoma	PPB	Carcinosarcoma
Age < 12 yr	Uncommon	Uncommon	Common	Uncommon
Smoking history	Common	Common	Negative	Common
Extrapulmonary involvement	Rare	Rare	Common	Rare
Cystic tumors	Rare	Rare	Common	Rare
Asymptomatic	Common	Rare	Rare	Rare
Prognosis	Better	Poor	Poor	Poor

PPB, pleuropulmonary blastoma.

TABLE 6-2 HISTOLOGIC CHARACTERISTICS OF BIPHASIC LUNG TUMORS

Histologic Feature	Monophasic Blastoma	Biphasic Blastoma	PPB	Carcinosarcoma
Malignant glands	Always	Always	Never	Common
Squamous cell carcinoma	Never	Never or very unusual	Never	Common
Undifferentiated large cell carcinoma	Never	Never	Never	Common
Morules	Common	Common	Never	Never
Sarcomatous component	Never	Always	Always	Always
Benign cystic component	Never	Never	Always	Never

PPB, pleuropulmonary blastoma.

a distinctive form of adenocarcinoma with histopathologic features resembling those of fetal lung tubules. However, the WHO investigators also added that some of these fetal adenocarcinomas may rarely show other subtypes of adenocarcinoma. This statement is a bit ambiguous, because a wide range of histologic features may be seen in otherwise nonfetal adenocarcinomas of the lung, leading to problems with the evaluation and classification of these tumors. In our own experience with many tumors similar to those reported in the literature, the monophasic variant of pulmonary blastoma has been associated with another neoplasm but displays a different histologic pattern.

As stated previously, both fetal adenocarcinoma and biphasic pulmonary blastoma are designated in this chapter as monophasic and biphasic blastomas, respectively, because the main characteristic of these tumors is the presence of a glandular proliferation that mimics pulmonary development in embryonic life between weeks 11 and 18. Use of this nomenclature is recommended to promote uniformity in the evaluation and classification of these tumors.

Clinical Features

Only a few series of pulmonary blastomas have been reported in the literature, and a majority of these reports discuss single, isolated cases, providing little meaningful clinical information.[18–21] Koss and associates[22] reported the largest series of pulmonary blastomas to date (including monophasic and biphasic tumors), analyzing data for 52 patients, and found that the great majority of these tumors occur in adults, with a mean and median age at diagnosis of 35 years. Two children younger than 10 years of age also were included in this group of patients, however. The occurrence of pulmonary blastomas in children is rare but has been recognized by other workers.[23–25] In Koss and coworkers' study, the tumors were more common among white patients than among African Americans, in a proportion of approximately 2:1, and no gender difference was noted. The most common clinical signs and symptoms were cough, hemoptysis, and chest pain; however, 21 of 52 patients (41%) were asymptomatic. Thirty-three of the 52 patients studied provided a history of tobacco use. In their series of six cases,[15] which was limited to monophasic blastomas (fetal adenocarcinoma), Kodama and colleagues found that the tumor occurs predominantly in men between the ages of 23 to 67 years, with clinical signs and symptoms similar to those reported by Koss's group.[22] In the five cases reported by Nakatani and coworkers,[14] all of the patients were women between the ages of 33 and 55 years with similar symptoms. Other investigators have observed similar clinical features in smaller series of cases.[16,26,27] On the basis of those studies, a reasonable conclusion is that pulmonary blastoma has the same clinical presentation as for other non–small cell carcinomas of the lung.

Macroscopic Features

Pulmonary blastomas are single pulmonary masses, well-circumscribed but not encapsulated. The cut surface may show a homogeneous or lobulated light tan surface. In some cases, the tumor also may appear as a dominant mass with adjacent nodules. The cut surface of the tumor also may show areas of hemorrhage or necrosis. Tumor size ranges from 1 cm to larger than 20 cm in greatest dimension. In Koss and coworkers' analysis,[22] only 36% of the tumors were less than 5 cm in size. A majority of tumors are found in the periphery of the lung (Fig. 6-1); however, a small percentage will be in an endobronchial location, with polypoid growth.

Microscopic Features

Monophasic Blastoma

As its name implies, the monophasic variant of pulmonary blastoma is composed exclusively of epithelial components and in many ways its appearance mimics the embryologic development of the lung during weeks 11 to 18 (Fig. 6-2). The tumor may be central (Fig. 6-3) or peripheral in location and usually appears to be well demarcated but not encapsulated (Fig. 6-4). The low-power

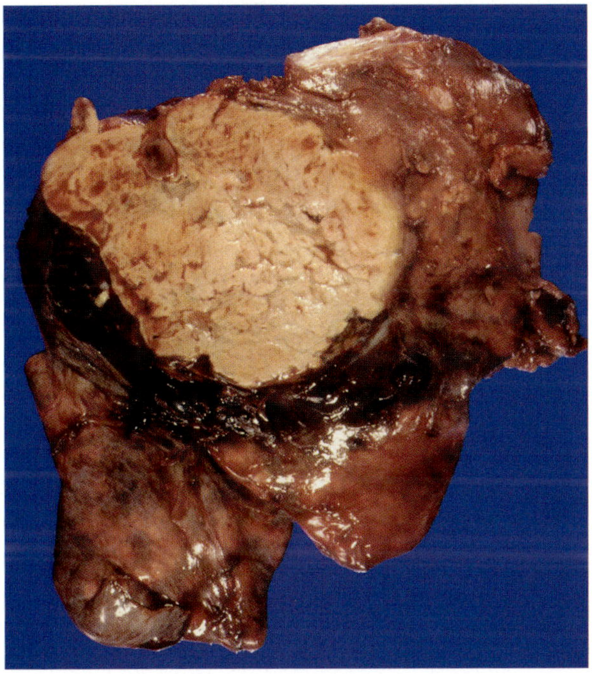

Figure 6-1 Well-demarcated pulmonary blastoma in the periphery of the lung parenchyma. The tumor cut surface is light tan with a homogeneous appearance.

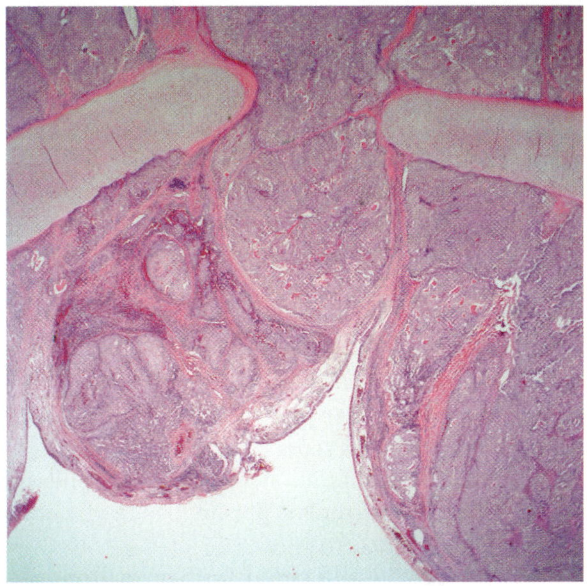

Figure 6-3 Low-power view of a centrally located monophasic pulmonary blastoma with polypoid growth.

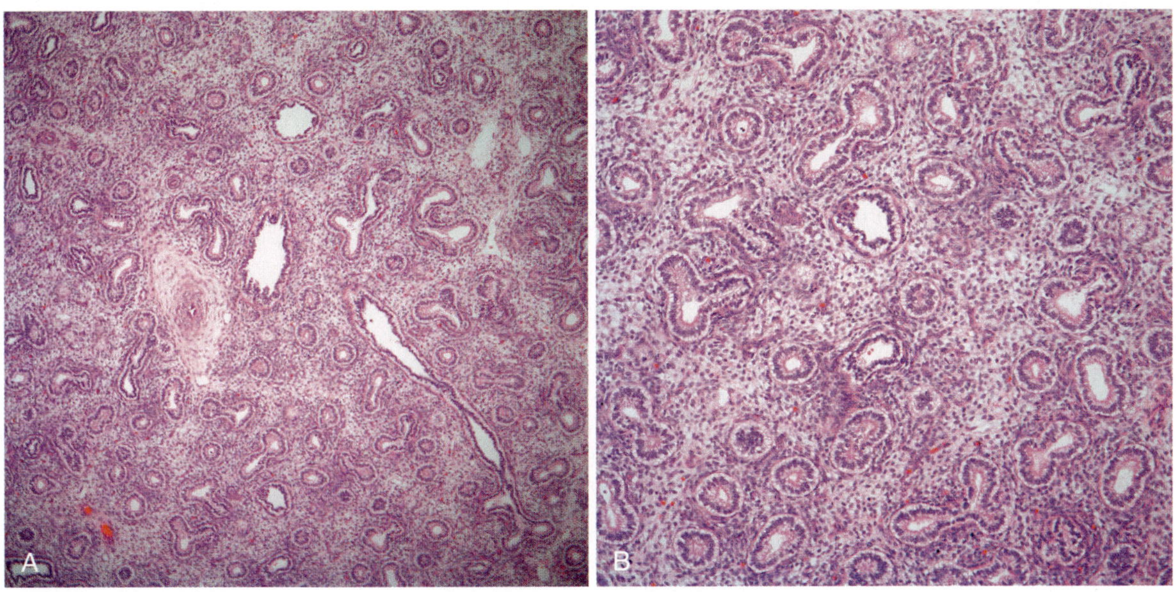

Figure 6-2 **A**, Low-power view of a section of fetal lung at approximately weeks 11 to 12. **B**, High-power view shows the classic glandular proliferation separated by stromal fibroblasts. Note the clearing of the cytoplasm.

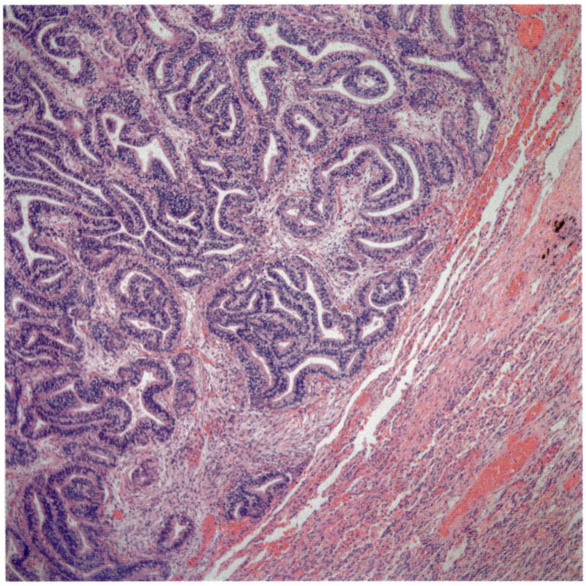

Figure 6-4 Monophasic pulmonary blastoma in the periphery of the lung parenchyma. Note the well-demarcated tumor destroying normal lung parenchyma.

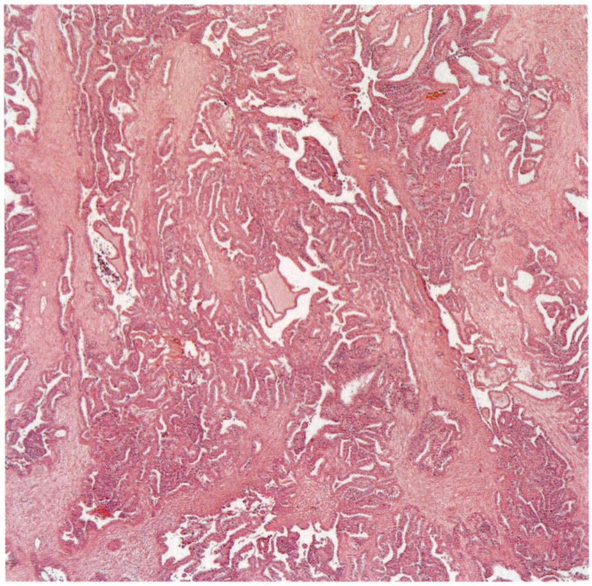

Figure 6-6 Monophasic pulmonary blastoma showing a glandular proliferation with pseudopapillary features. The bands of fibroconnective tissue are more prominent than in Figure 6-5.

view shows a malignant glandular neoplasm destroying normal lung architecture. Three growth patterns may be observed:

- Solid growth glandular pattern, with large lobules separated by thin fibrous septa (Fig. 6-5)
- Solid glandular proliferation with pseudopapillary features and more prominent fibrous bands of fibroconnective tissue (Fig. 6-6)
- Solid glandular proliferation with a cribriform-like pattern (Fig. 6-7)

These glands are of various sizes and shapes, and in many areas they are elongated, forming tubules with a minimal stromal component and resembling branching tubular structures (Fig. 6-8). The glandular elements are typical of two distinct types:

1. Columnar cells with clear cytoplasm, nuclei displayed toward the periphery, and relatively little atypia (Fig. 6-9)
2. Glandular elements lined by a single layer of cells, displaying various degrees of cytologic atypia (Fig. 6-10)

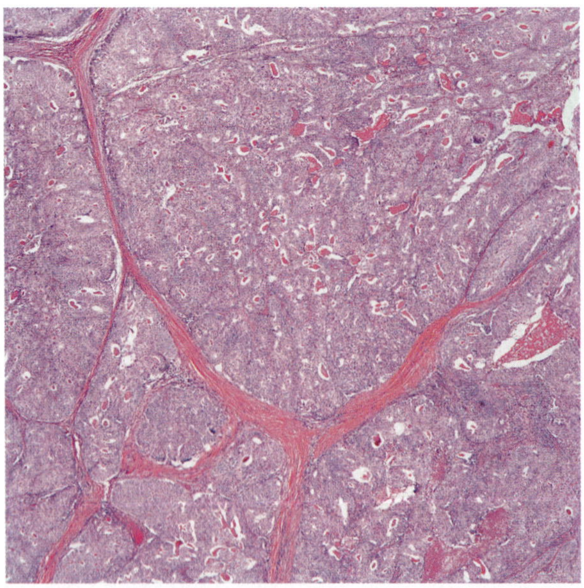

Figure 6-5 Monophasic pulmonary blastoma with a solid glandular pattern of growth. The tumor shows some lobulation separated by thin fibrous connective tissue.

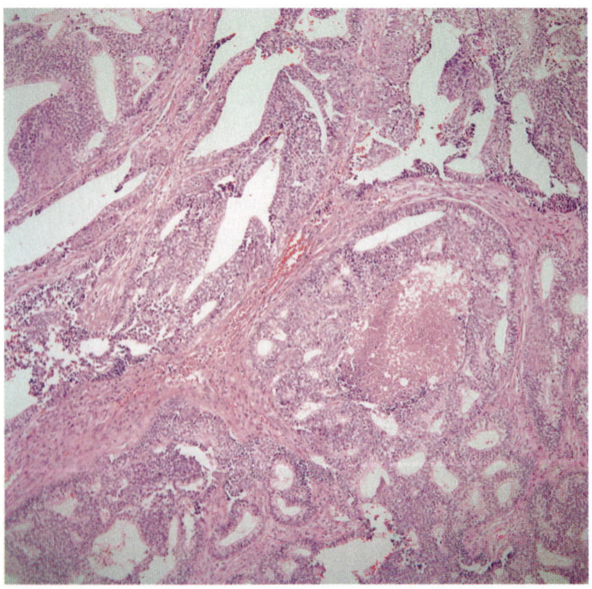

Figure 6-7 Monophasic pulmonary blastoma with a cribriform-like pattern.

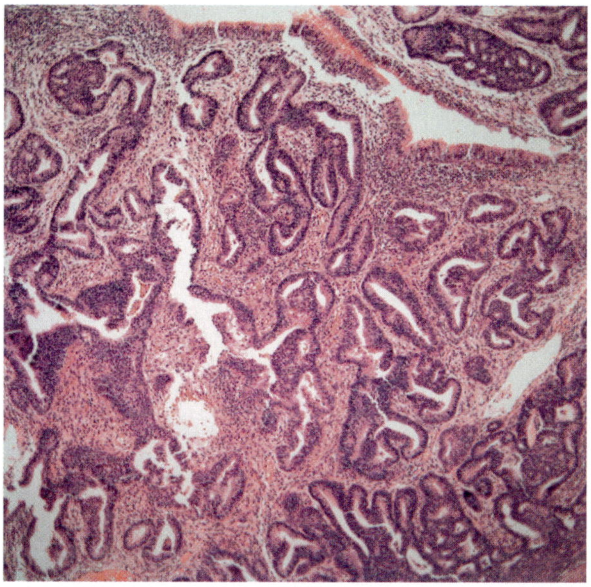

Figure 6-8 Monophasic pulmonary blastoma showing glands and tubular structures of different sizes.

Morules are identified in budding glandular structures; these can be rather inconspicuous (Fig. 6-11) or very prominent (Fig. 6-12), or they can fill the lumen of the glandular structures entirely (Fig. 6-13). These morules are small "squamoid-like" cellular aggregates, without significant cytologic atypia. Their presence has been observed in up to 85% of cases. Necrosis may be present in differing proportions ranging from focal in the form of comedo-like necrosis (Fig. 6-14) or extensive and admixed with glandular tumor structures (Fig. 6-15). Marked nuclear pleomorphism may be present, but it is not common and is absent in a majority of cases (Fig. 6-16). Monophasic pulmonary blastoma may show some unusual features, such as abundant foamy macrophages adjacent to tumor glands (Fig. 6-17), presence of cholesterol cleft granulomas (Fig. 6-18), metaplastic bone formation (Fig. 6-19), inflammatory changes of the fibroconnective tissue stroma (Fig. 6-20), or malignant glandular structures floating in alveolar spaces (Fig. 6-21).

Nakatani and colleagues[16] subdivided the monophasic blastomas (fetal adenocarcinoma) into two separate groups: low- and high-grade tumors. High-grade tumors were characterized by cells with prominent nucleoli, mitotic figures, and papillary infoldings. In at least two of the cases, however, a spindle cell component was recognized, which raises the possibility of a biphasic neoplasm from the outset. Of note, monophasic pulmonary blastomas may be associated with another type of malignancy. Cohen and associates[28] described a single

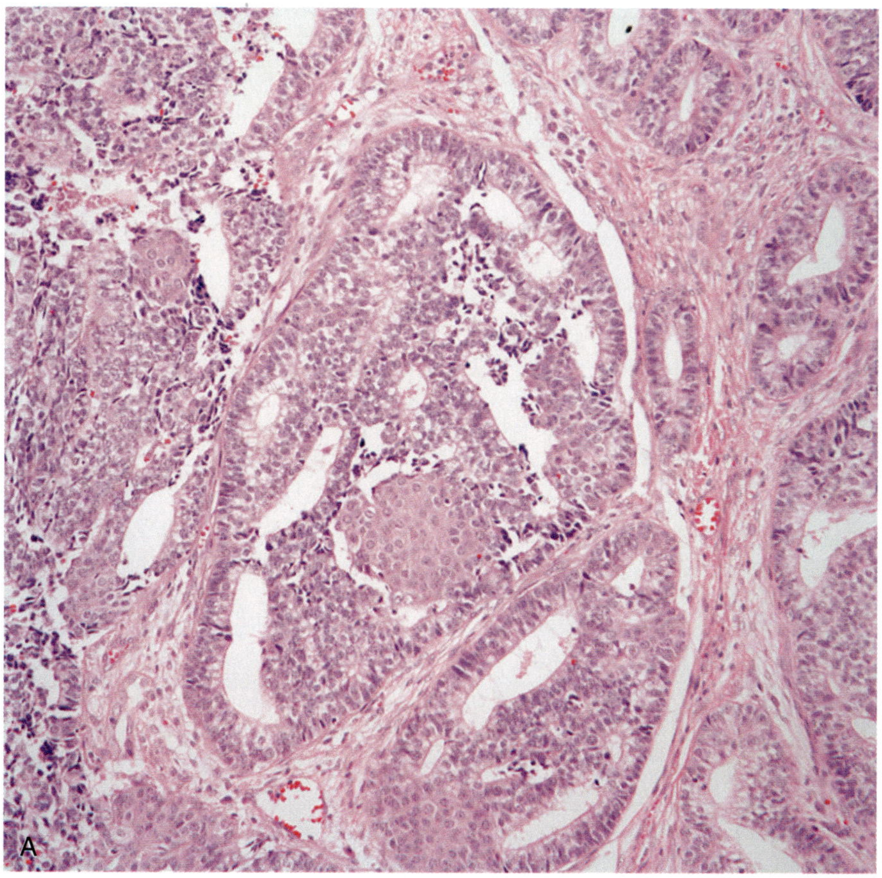

Figure 6-9 **A**, Low-power view of monophasic pulmonary blastoma composed of glandular structures lined by columnar-type epithelium.

Continued

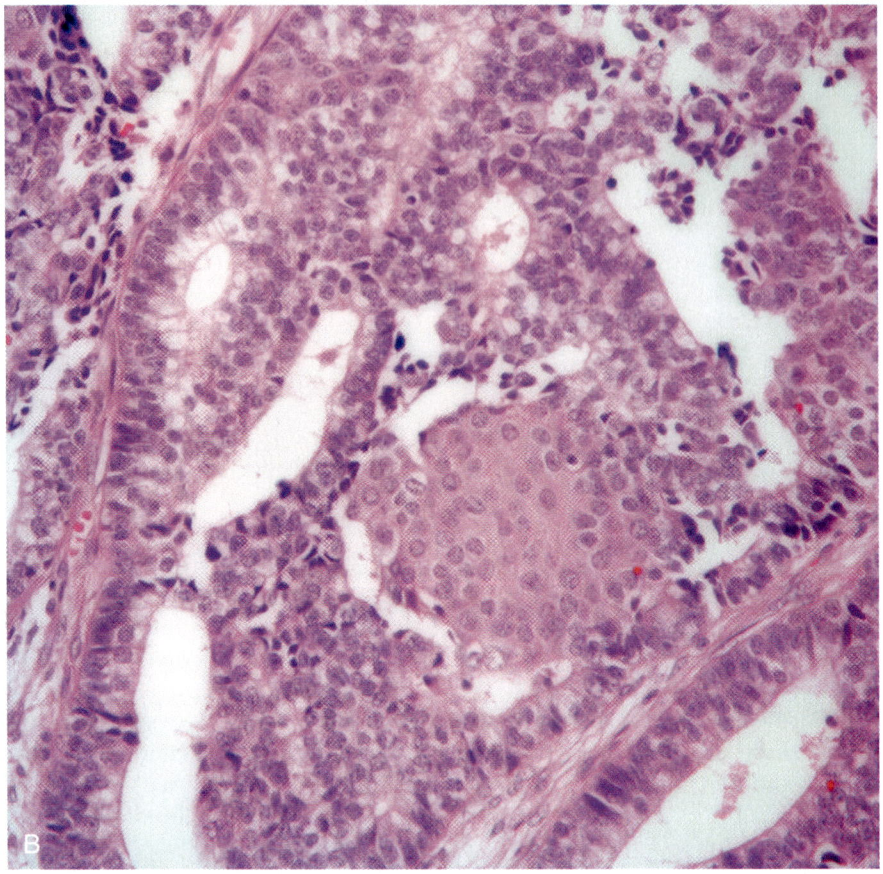

Figure 6-9—cont'd **B**, High-power view of the glandular structures with columnar epithelium and a squamous morule.

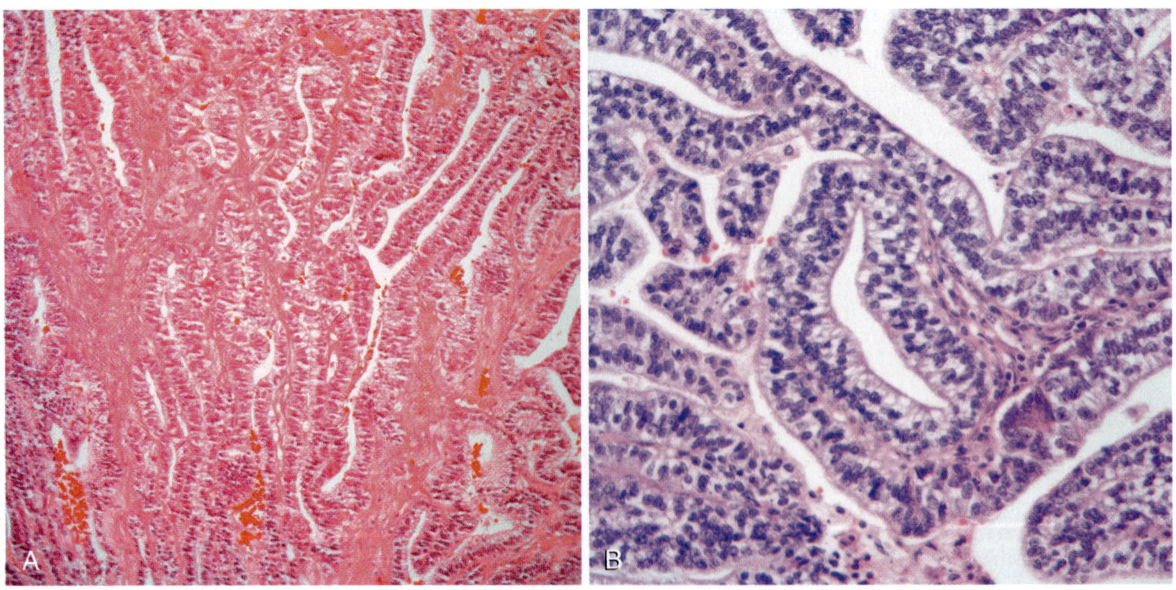

Figure 6-10 **A**, Low-power view of a monophasic pulmonary blastoma composed of glandular structures lined by a single row of cells. **B**, Higher-power view shows nuclear atypia and mitotic activity.

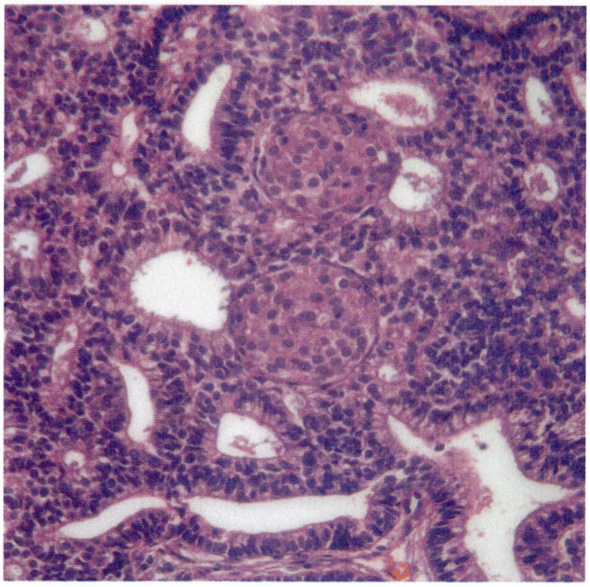

Figure 6-11 Monophasic pulmonary blastoma showing glandular structures with adjacent morules.

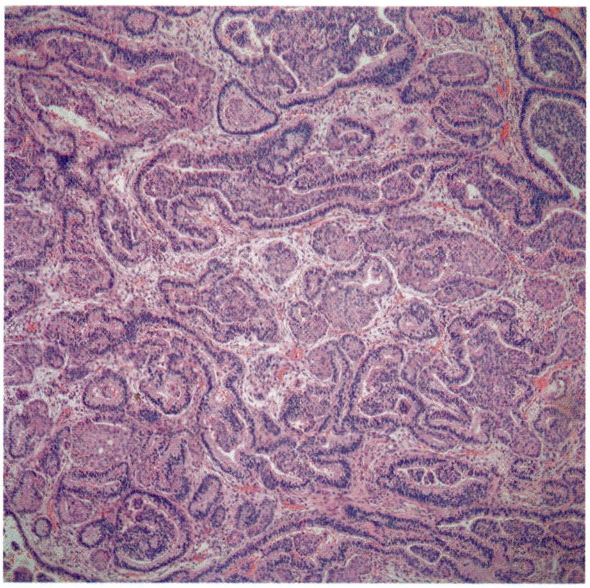

Figure 6-12 Monophasic pulmonary blastoma displaying numerous morules.

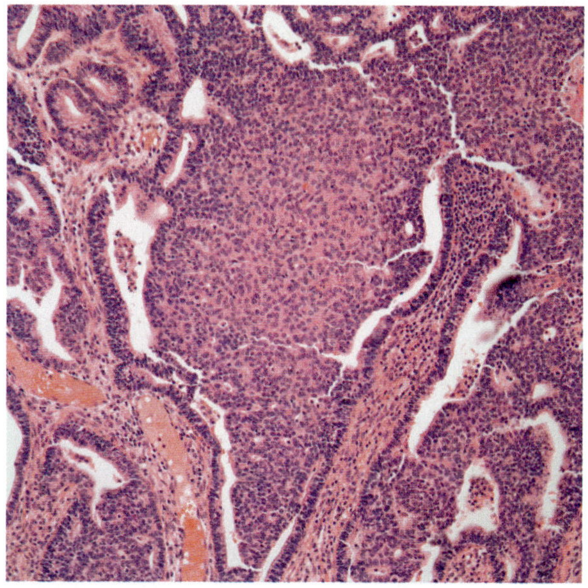

Figure 6-13 Large morules fill the glandular structures in this monophasic pulmonary blastoma.

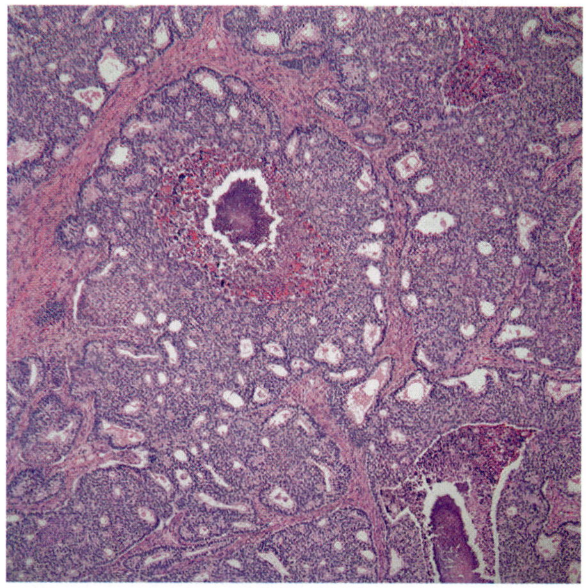

Figure 6-14 Monophasic pulmonary blastoma showing focal areas of necrosis, comedo-like type.

case in which the blastoma was associated with a melanoma, and in our own clinical experience, these tumors may be associated with hepatocellular differentiation (Fig. 6-22).

Biphasic Blastoma

At low magnification, biphasic blastomas will show a mixture of tubular epithelial structures separated by an immature spindle mesenchymal component. These components may be present in differing proportions (Fig. 6-23). The glandular component is similar to that in monophasic blastoma: tubular structures lined by pseudostratified, nonciliated columnar cells with typically clear cytoplasm. In this growth pattern, it often is possible to identify increased mitotic activity, necrosis, hemorrhage, and nuclear pleomorphism (Fig. 6-24). The stromal mesenchymal component is composed of an immature, monotonous proliferation of spindle cells that can be either fairly subtle or the predominant component of the tumor (Fig. 6-25). In addition, the mesenchymal component may vary in the spectrum of differentiation (Fig. 6-26). The presence of cartilage, bone, and skeletal muscle has been described in these cases[29] (Fig. 6-27).

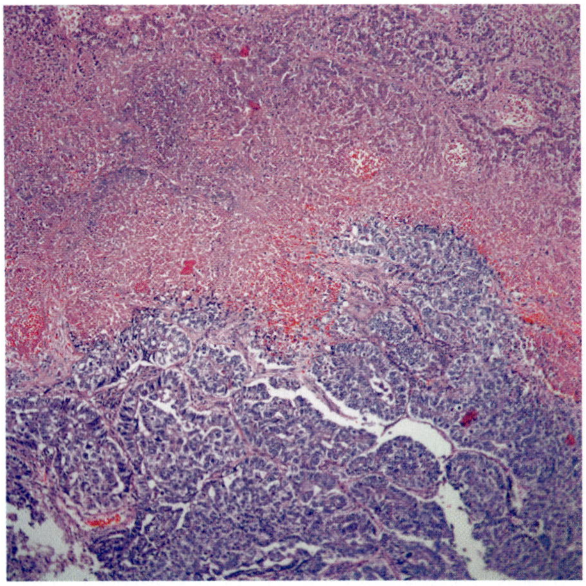

Figure 6-15 Monophasic pulmonary blastoma with areas of extensive necrosis.

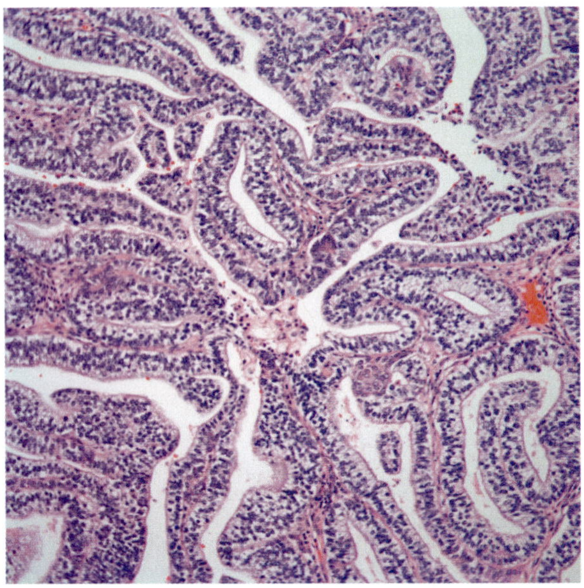

Figure 6-16 Monophasic pulmonary blastoma showing the typical endometrioid-like pattern. Nuclear atypia and pleomorphism are not marked in these tumors.

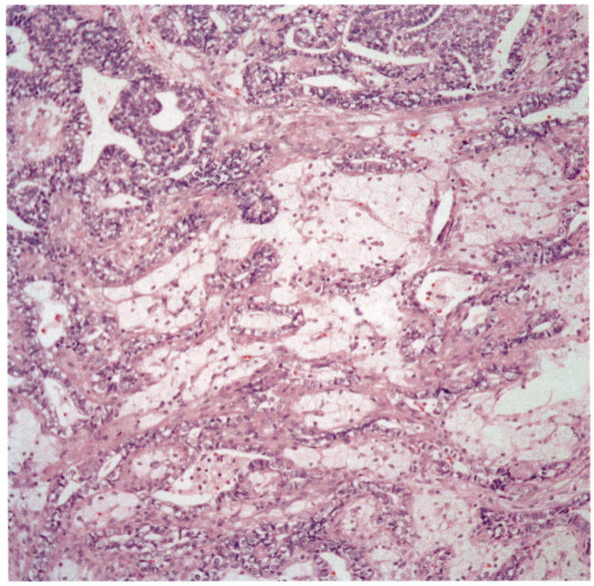

Figure 6-17 Monophasic pulmonary blastoma showing an extensive collection of foamy macrophages.

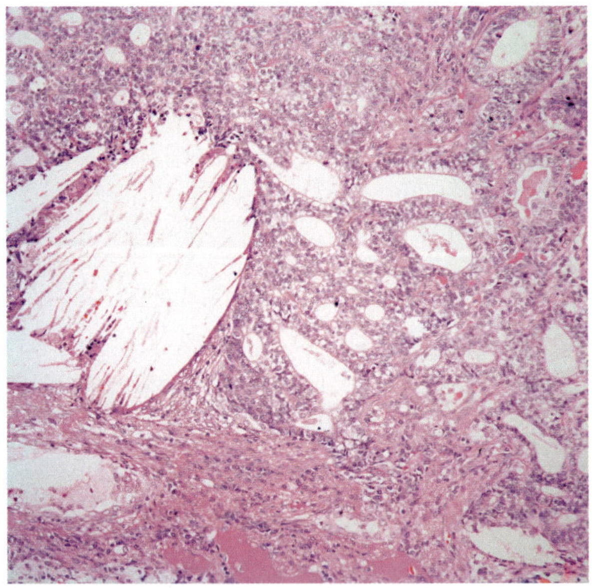

Figure 6-18 Monophasic pulmonary blastoma showing cholesterol cleft granulomas.

Some unusual cases show squamous cell carcinoma, and others display transition from blastic to more differentiated areas.[18,30]

Histochemical Features

The use of immunohistochemical stains may prove beneficial for evaluating monophasic blastomas, because such stains characteristically reveal the presence of intracellular glycogen, with periodic acid–Schiff (PAS) stain, and absence of intracellular mucin, with diastase–PAS stain and mucicarmine. In some cases, however, mucin may be present in intraluminal glandular structures. Similar features also are present in the epithelial component of biphasic neoplasms.

Immunohistochemical Features

The epithelial component of pulmonary blastomas shows positive staining for low-molecular-weight keratin (CAM5.2), epithelial membrane antigen (EMA), carcinoembryonic antigen (CEA), and thyroid transcription factor-1 (TTF-1).[14,16,22,31–34] The morular component of blastomas displays positive staining for neuroendocrine

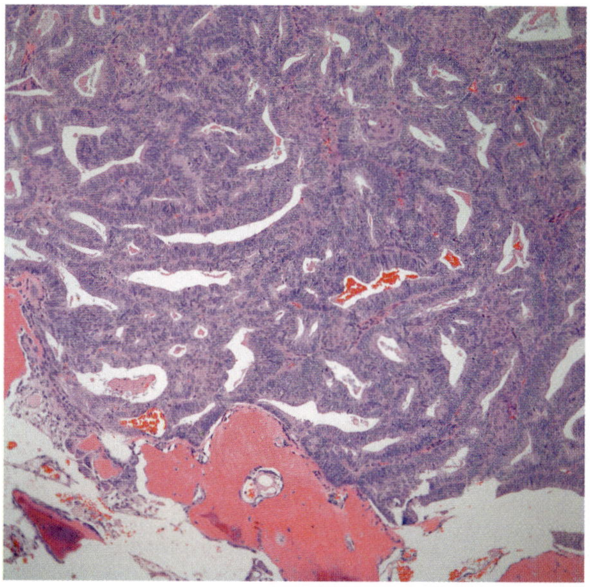

Figure 6-19 Monophasic pulmonary blastoma showing metaplastic bone formation.

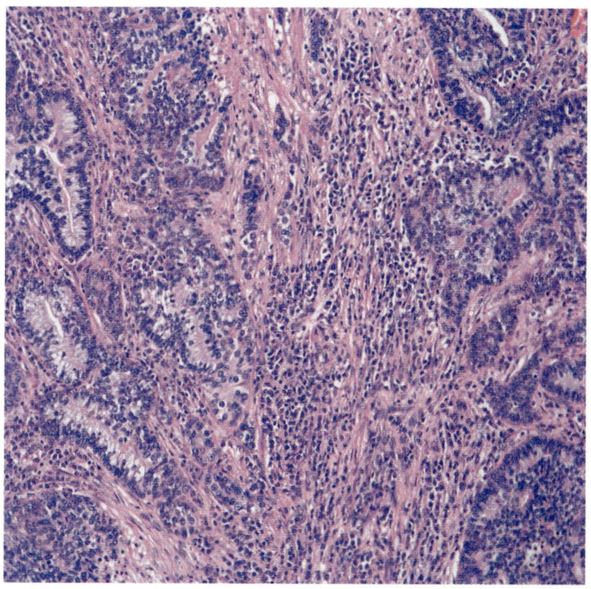

Figure 6-20 Monophasic pulmonary blastoma showing marked inflammatory reaction in fibroconnective tissue.

markers—namely, chromogranin and synaptophysin. Pacinda and associates[35] compared blastomas and carcinomas and found that both show positive staining for p53 and MDM2 protein, suggesting that they may have a similar pathogenesis.

Molecular Biology Features

Because of the rarity of these neoplasms, studies dealing with molecular changes have been limited. Bodner and Koss[36] analyzed mutations in the *p53* gene in 12 cases of monophasic and 9 cases of biphasic blastoma and found

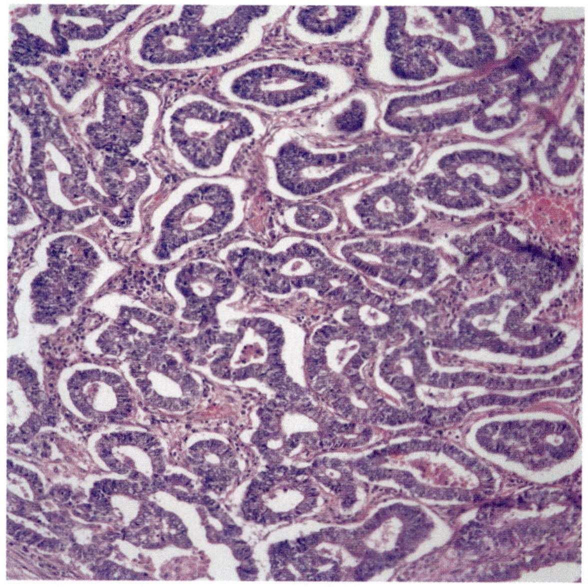

Figure 6-21 Tumor glandular structures floating in alveolar spaces in monophasic pulmonary blastoma.

that 5 of the 12 biphasic tumors (42%) had mutations in the *p53* gene, whereas none of the monophasic tumors did. Holst and colleagues[37] reported a similar experience, observing the presence of *p53* mutation by DNA genotyping in one of 7 cases of biphasic tumors, and no mutation in monophasic tumors. More recently, Nakatani and associates[38] studied the presence of B-catenin in pulmonary blastomas, identifying aberrant nuclear-cytoplasmic localization of B-catenin in both epithelial and mesenchymal components.

Differential Diagnosis

Because of the prominent glandular pattern, it is important to distinguish monophasic pulmonary blastoma from conventional adenocarcinoma, especially the so-called secretory endometrioid–like adenocarcinoma of the lung. Although this distinction may prove to be difficult in some cases, the presence of "morules" is a feature characteristic of pulmonary blastomas. The glandular proliferation also closely mimics the glandular development of the lung in embryonic weeks 11 to 18, displaying glands or tubular structures composed of cells with clear cytoplasm, displacement of the nuclei toward the base of the glands, and inconspicuous nucleoli. The use of histochemical stains such as PAS and mucicarmine may be effective, because the glands or tubular structures that compose pulmonary blastomas will fail to stain for intracellular mucin. In some cases, however, both of these histochemical stains may yield positive results in the lumen of the glandular structures. Immunohistochemical staining for neuroendocrine markers may be positive in the morular areas of pulmonary blastomas.

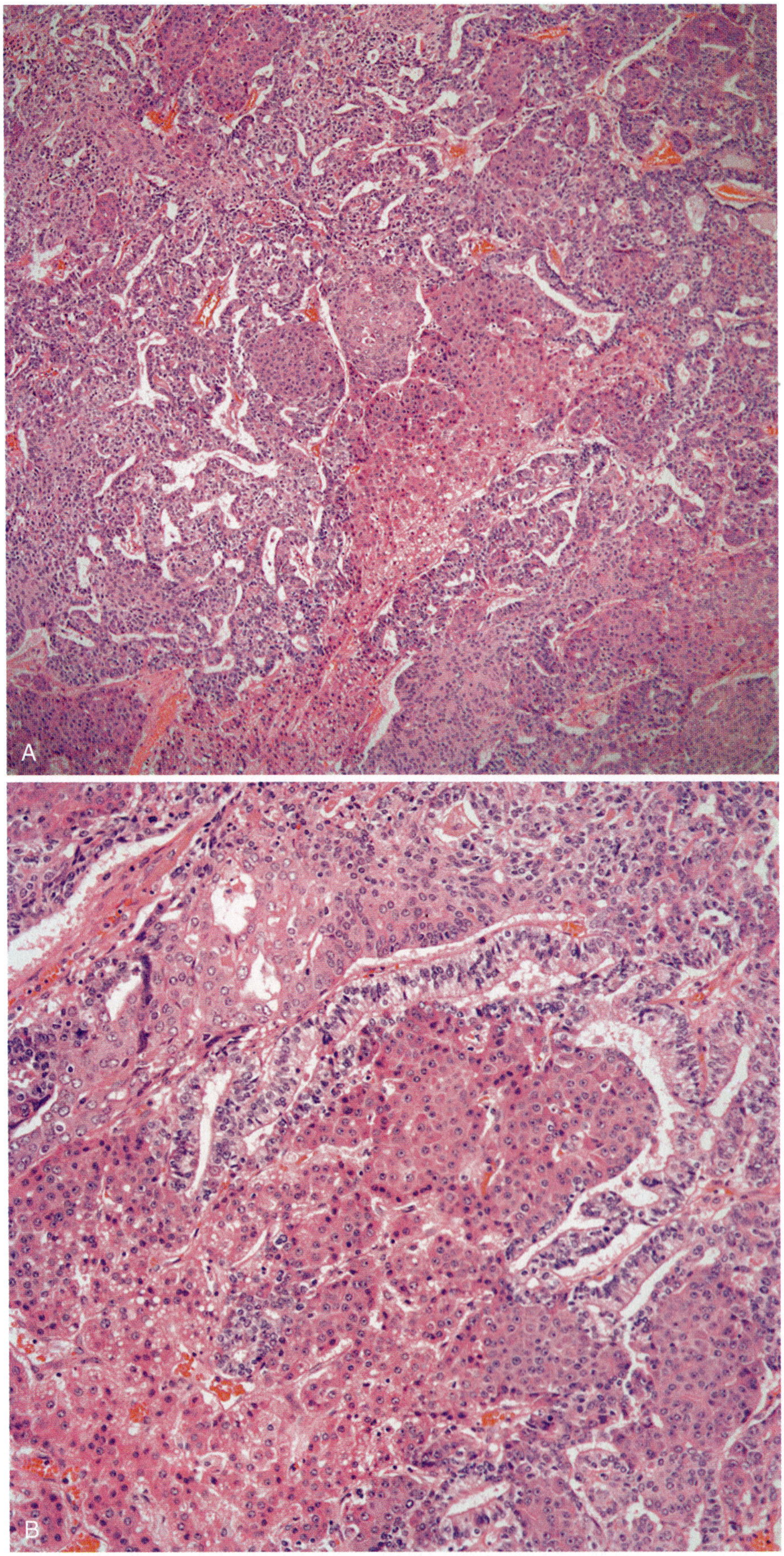

Figure 6-22 **A**, Low-power view of a monophasic pulmonary blastoma with hepatocellular differentiation. **B**, High-power view showing the two components as distinct entities.

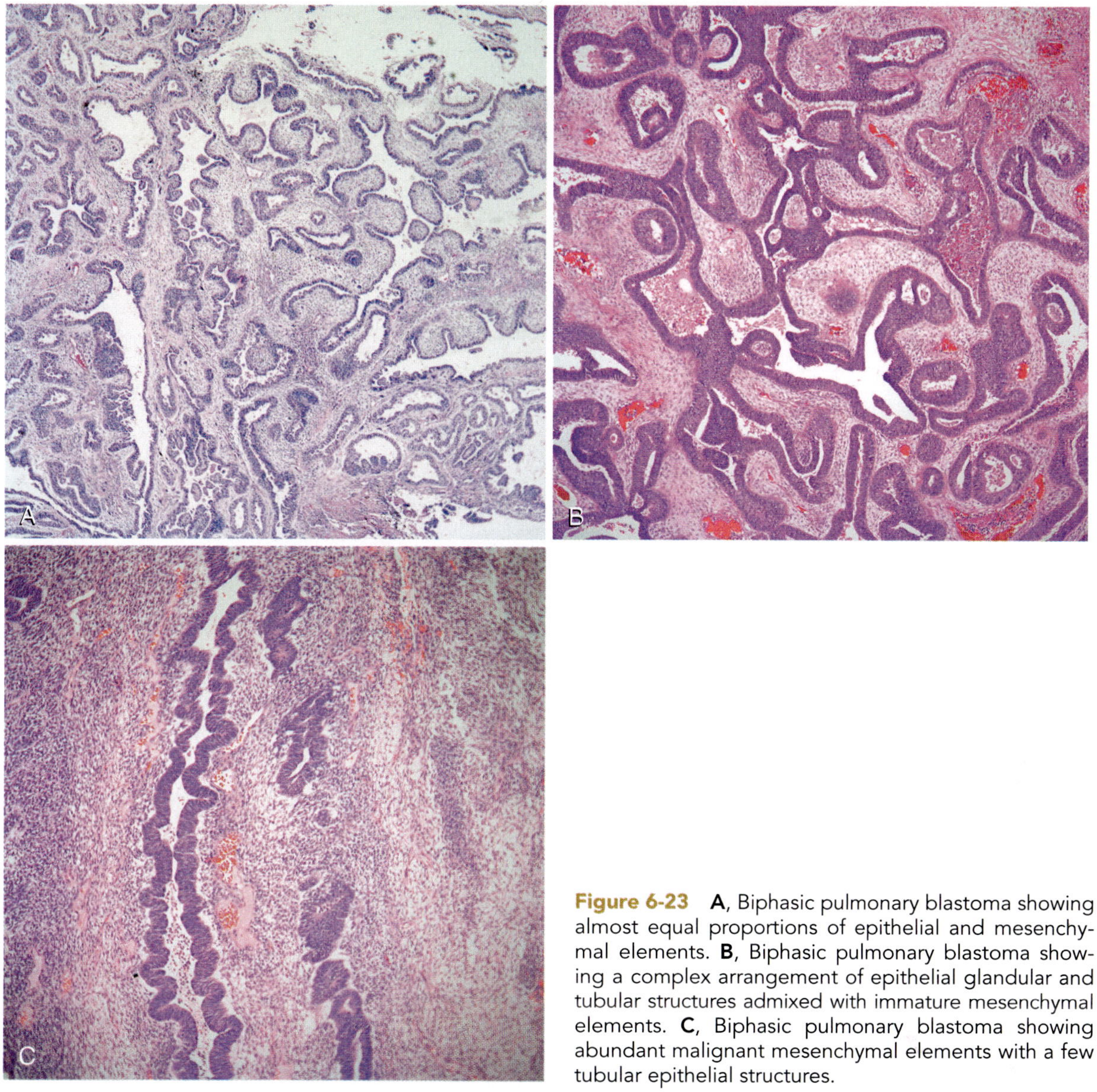

Figure 6-23 **A**, Biphasic pulmonary blastoma showing almost equal proportions of epithelial and mesenchymal elements. **B**, Biphasic pulmonary blastoma showing a complex arrangement of epithelial glandular and tubular structures admixed with immature mesenchymal elements. **C**, Biphasic pulmonary blastoma showing abundant malignant mesenchymal elements with a few tubular epithelial structures.

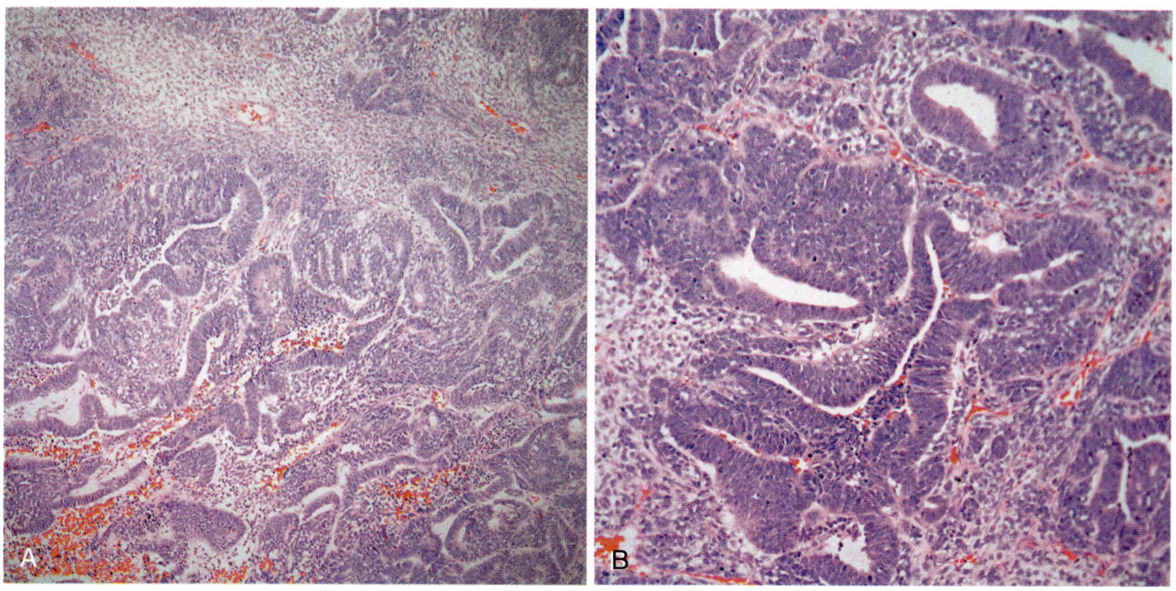

Figure 6-24 **A**, Low-power view of a biphasic pulmonary blastoma showing the classic epithelial component of tubular structures. **B**, High-power view of the epithelial component in a biphasic pulmonary blastoma showing a greater degree of cellular atypia and mitotic activity.

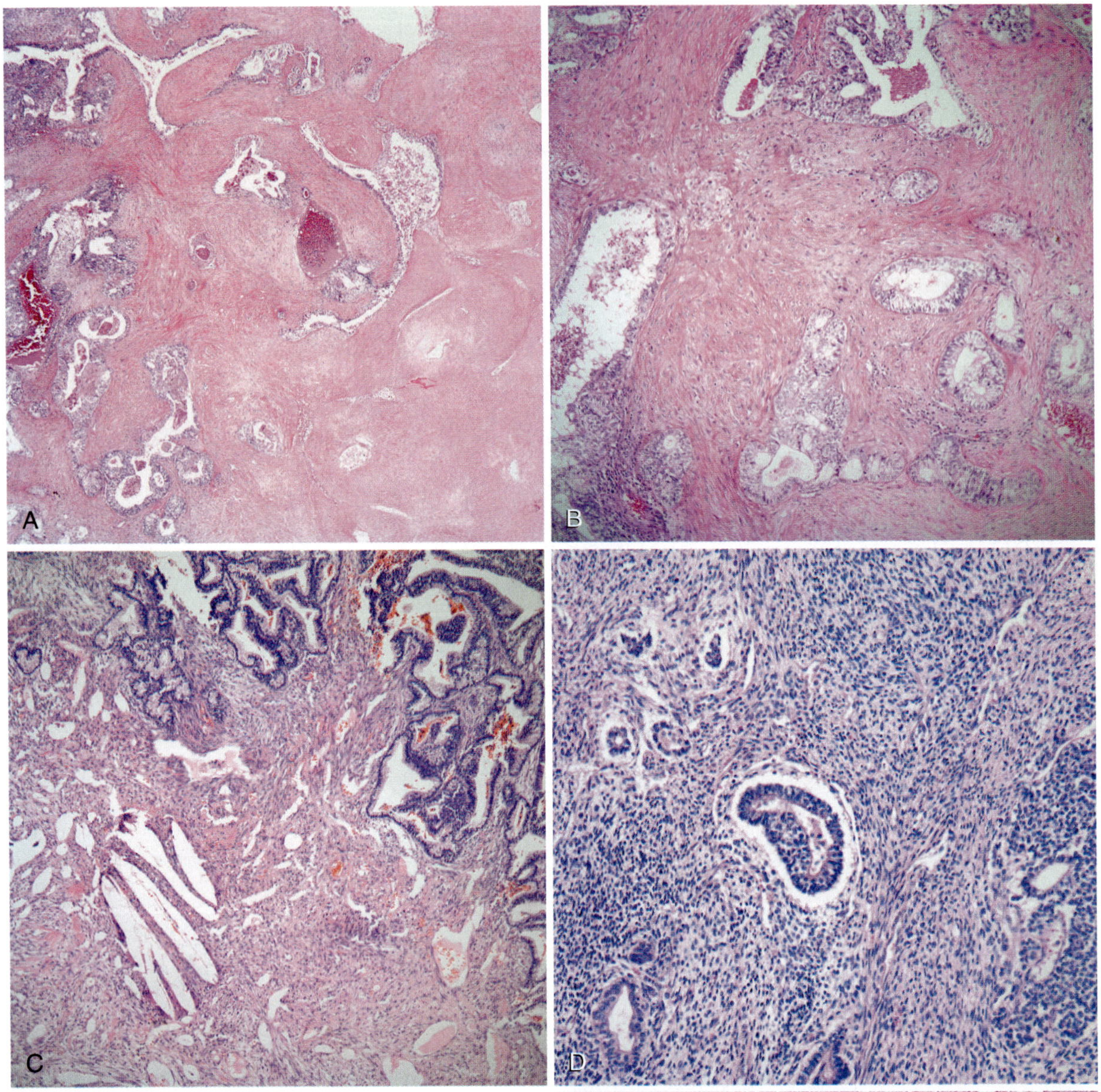

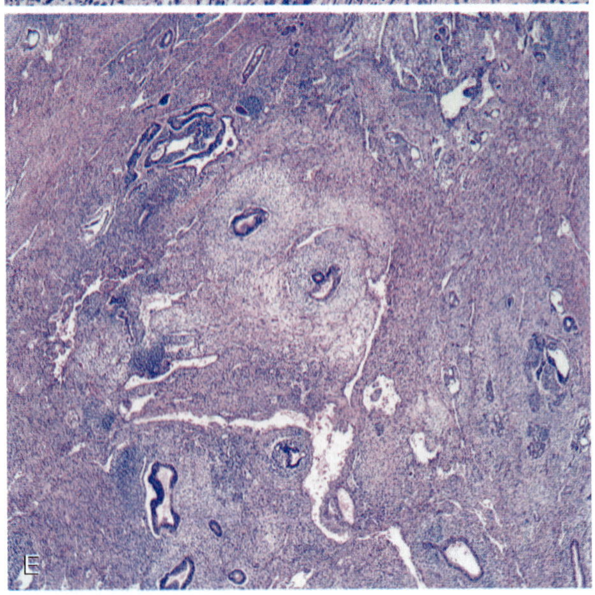

Figure 6-25 **A**, Biphasic pulmonary blastoma with extensive areas of a fibroma-like mesenchymal component. **B**, Biphasic pulmonary blastoma with a more pronounced mesenchymal spindle cell component. **C**, Biphasic pulmonary blastoma in which the mesenchymal spindle cell component predominates; a cholesterol clef granuloma also is present. **D**, Biphasic blastoma with predominance of the mesenchymal component. Note the presence of scattered epithelial glandular component. **E**, Low-power view of a biphasic blastoma in which the glandular component is negligible, so that the tumor may be mistaken for a benign process.

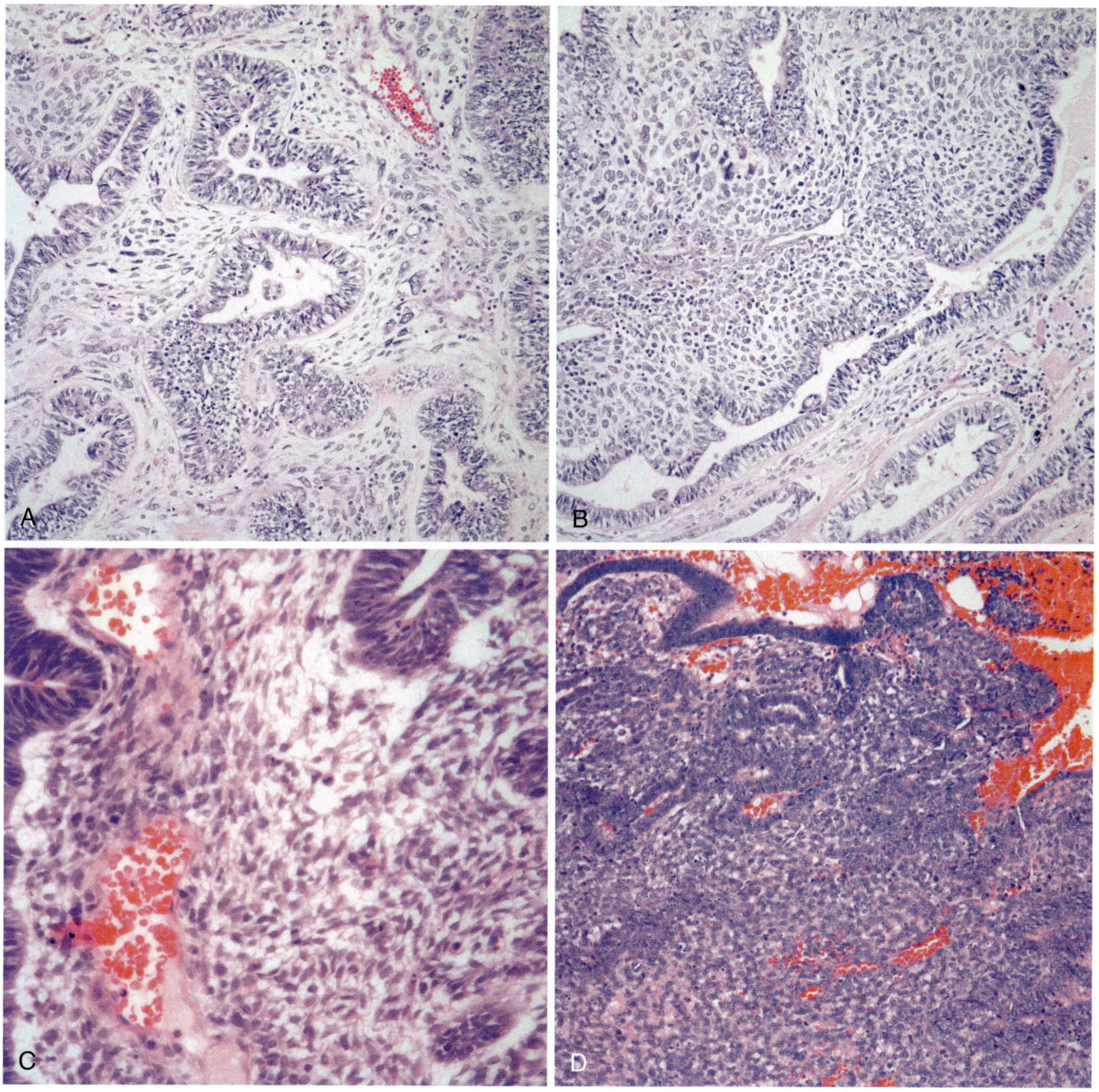

Figure 6-26 **A**, Low-power view of a biphasic blastoma in which the mesenchymal component shows a greater degree of atypia. **B**, Biphasic blastoma with a high-grade mesenchymal component. **C**, High-power view of the mesenchymal component showing nuclear atypia and mitotic activity. **D**, High-power view of an undifferentiated sarcomatous component. Note the presence of scattered glandular structures.

With biphasic tumors, the most important consideration in the differential diagnosis is carcinosarcoma, which will display light microscopic evidence of conventional carcinoma, adenocarcinoma, or squamous cell carcinoma associated with sarcoma of the conventional type. The correct diagnosis may necessitate a complete surgical resection, because the tumor in a small biopsy specimen may show only one of the components, either epithelial or mesenchymal.

Treatment and Prognosis

Although no specific and definitive treatment for pulmonary blastoma has emerged, the treatment of choice usually is complete surgical resection. Prognosis differs within the published series, and there appears to be a difference in survival rates, depending on the histologic type. In Kodama and colleagues' report of six cases of fetal adenocarcinoma, five of six patients died within a period of 34 months.[15] The size of the tumors in these patients ranged from 3 to 14 cm. In Nakatani and associates' series of five cases of "endodermal tumor resembling fetal lung," tumor size ranged from 2.2 to 5 cm, and four of the patients survived throughout the follow-up period of 24 to 108 months.[14] The fifth patient had a tumor size of 5 cm and died at 24 months after diagnosis. In Nakatani and associates' study of low- and high-grade tumors, grading appeared to correlate with survival;

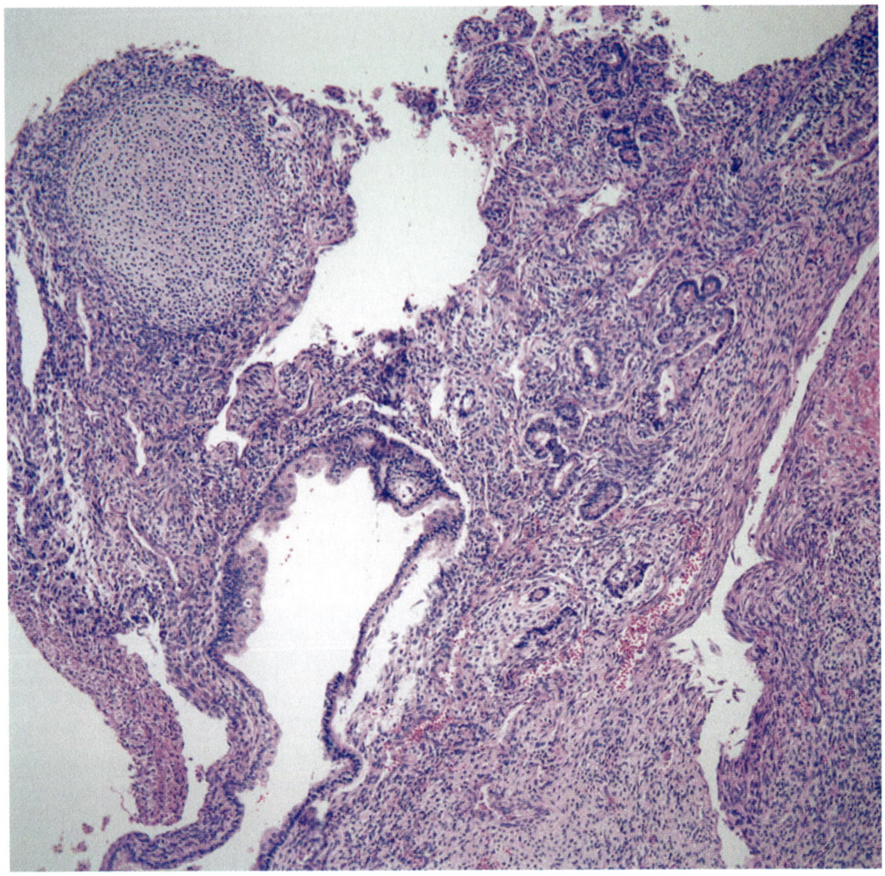

Figure 6-27 Biphasic pulmonary blastoma showing epithelial and mesenchymal components. Note the presence of cartilaginous differentiation.

tumors labeled as high-grade appeared to be more aggressive.[16] In their study of 52 pulmonary blastomas, Koss and coworkers found that in monophasic blastomas, the size of the tumor did not correlate with survival; however, the presence of lymphadenopathy, metastasis at initial presentation, tumor recurrence, and higher pathologic stage adversely affected survival.[22] This was also the case with biphasic tumors; however, a closer correlation was found between tumor size (larger than 5 cm in greatest dimension) and poor survival. In general, it appears that biphasic tumors behave more aggressively than monophasic tumors. More recently, Liman and associates[39] arrived at similar conclusions in a study addressing the survival rate for patients with biphasic pulmonary blastomas. Patients with smaller tumors fared better than those with large tumors.

PLEUROPULMONARY BLASTOMA

Primary pediatric intrapulmonary neoplasms are rare. In a study by Dishop and Kuruvilla[40] reviewing their 25-year experience at a large children's hospital, 14 (6.9 %) of 204 pediatric lung tumors could be classified as pleuropulmonary blastoma. The investigators concluded that pleuropulmonary blastoma and carcinoid tumor represent the most common malignant tumors in the pediatric age group. In another English language review of a 19-year experience, the investigators found 44 cases of intrapulmonary tumors and encountered only 3 cases of malignant neoplasms, one of which was classified as pleuropulmonary blastoma.[41]

Historical Aspects

Pleuropulmonary blastoma is a pediatric neoplasm; however, because the designation "blastoma" has been appended to this entity, some confusion between pleuropulmonary blastoma and conventional pulmonary blastoma in the adult has arisen. Before 1988, the terminology used for these neoplasms included the following: pulmonary blastoma (a true congenital neoplasm), pulmonary blastoma associated with cystic lesions, childhood pulmonary blastoma, pulmonary sarcoma arising in mesenchymal cystic hamartoma, mesenchymal cystic hamartoma, embryonal sarcoma, rhabdomyosarcoma arising in congenital cystic adenomatoid malformation, and sarcoma arising in bronchogenic cyst.[42–47] Manivel and coworkers[48] coined the term *pleuropulmonary blastoma* in their report of 11 pediatric tumors that involved not only the lung but also the pleura and mediastinum.

Definition

Pleuropulmonary blastoma was defined by Manivel and coworkers[48] as a tumor with primitive embryonic-like blastema and stroma with potential for sarcomatous differentiation and absence of an adenocarcinomatous component. This definition allows distinction of pleuropulmonary blastoma from the monophasic variant (fetal adenocarcinoma) and biphasic variants of conventional pulmonary blastoma, and also from pulmonary carcinosarcoma, owing to the absence of a malignant epithelial component. Some investigators, however, have considered pleuropulmonary blastoma to represent the pulmonary blastoma of childhood and have gone so far as to call it "the rightful pulmonary blastoma."[49] Whether or not this tumor is the true blastoma, in practice, pleuropulmonary blastoma and adult blastomas constitute two different histopathologic tumors that should not be confused with each other.

Clinical Features

Pleuropulmonary blastoma characteristically affects children younger than 15 years of age, but in rare instances it has been recorded in young adults.[50,51] Hill and coworkers[50] reported a case in a 36-year-old man who presented with a cystic and solid intrapulmonary mass; Zuker and colleagues[51] reported the case of a 19-year-old man with neurofibromatosis and pleuropulmonary blastoma. The tumor does not appear to have any gender predilection, affecting males and females approximately equally. Patients may present with clinical signs and symptoms of cough, fever, chest pain, lethargy, respiratory distress, anorexia, and weight loss.[46] Radiologically, partial or total opacification of the lung field and mediastinal shifting, pleural effusion, and hydropneumothorax have been observed.[48] Although the tumor usually manifests as a unilateral pulmonary mass, one case of bilateral cystic pleuropulmonary blastoma has been reported.[52] In addition, pleuropulmonary blastoma has been reported in association with other conditions, such as intestinal polyps and congenital cystic adenomatoid malformation.[53–55] Of note, however, congenital cystic adenomatoid malformation type 4 and pleuropulmonary blastoma type I may show similar features, making the distinction of these two conditions based on morphology alone very difficult.[55]

Macroscopic Features

The size and macroscopic characteristics of pleuropulmonary blastoma may vary according to specific histologic subtype. These tumors may attain a large size, and in a majority of cases tumor size appears to range from 5 cm to larger than 20 cm in greatest dimension. Some tumors may show a predominantly cystic nature, whereas others display a more homogeneous appearance, with soft, friable, gelatinous areas. A combination of both of these features may be visible in some tumors.[48,56–58] The cystic tumor may have a multilobate appearance with thin wall cysts.

Microscopic Features

Pleuropulmonary blastoma has been subdivided into three different histopathologic patterns.[59]

Pleuropulmonary blastoma type I is a tumor composed predominantly of cystic structures separated by thin, fibrous septa. Benign epithelium, in most cases a low cuboidal type, lines the cysts. Underneath the benign epithelium lies a more solid cellular proliferation, which may be composed of spindle or oval cells, depending on the differentiation of the tumor. In some cases, rhabdomyoblastic differentiation may be apparent, whereas in others, this differentiation becomes apparent only after immunostaining. A cambium-like layer similar to that seen in sarcoma botryoides may be present (Figs. 6-28 to 6-34).

Pleuropulmonary blastoma type II and type III may differ only in the amount of solid component. If the tumor displays mixed cystic and solid component, it should be classified as type II, whereas if it is predominantly solid, it should be classified as type III. Rhabdomyosarcomatous differentiation appears to be a common occurrence in these tumors, whereas areas of chondromyxoid change and well-formed hyaline cartilage may be seen in some cases (Figs. 6-35 to 6-40).

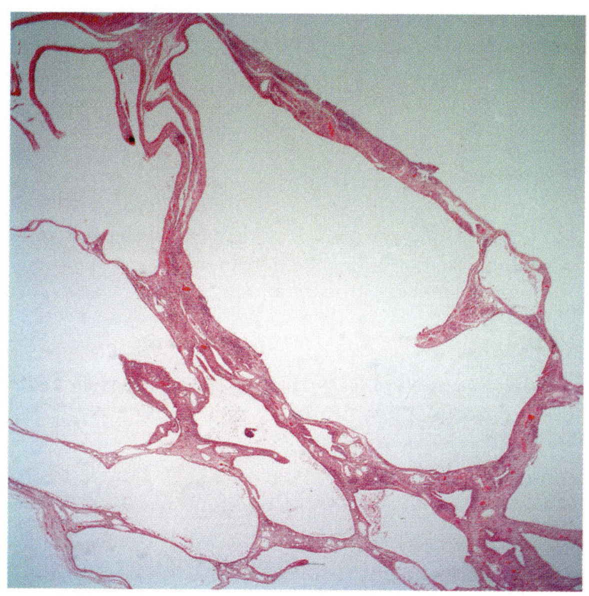

Figure 6-28 Low-power view of a type I pleuropulmonary blastoma. Note the cystic structures separated by minimal spindle cell elements.

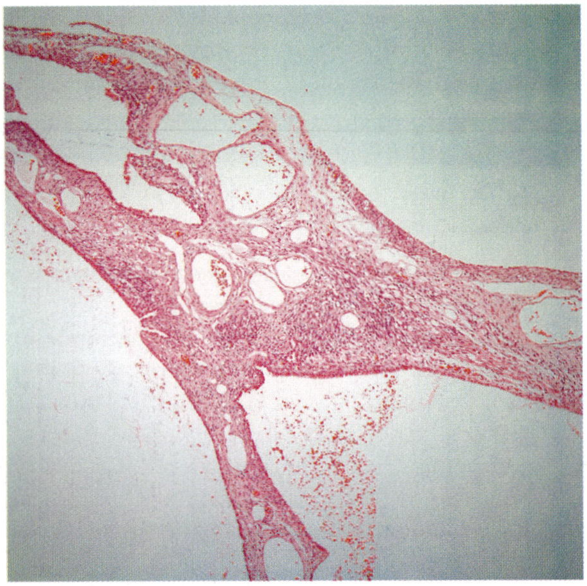

Figure 6-29 Intermediate-power view of a type I pleuropulmonary blastoma in which the spindle cell elements separating cystic structures are more apparent than in Figure 6-28.

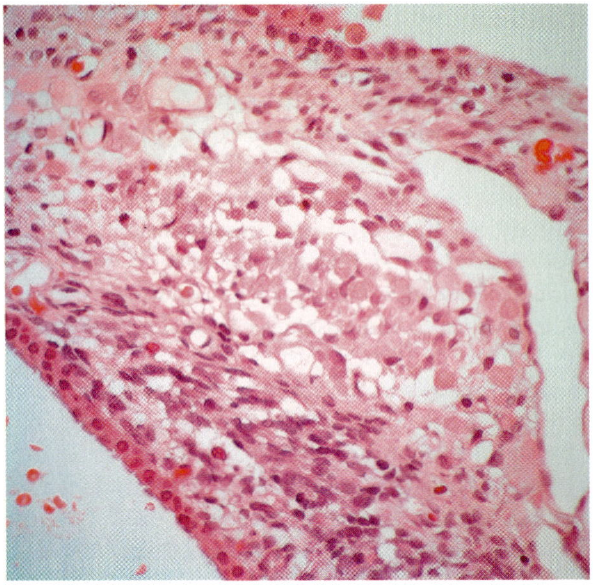

Figure 6-31 Closer view of the mesenchymal component of a type I pleuropulmonary blastoma showing rhabdomyoblastic differentiation.

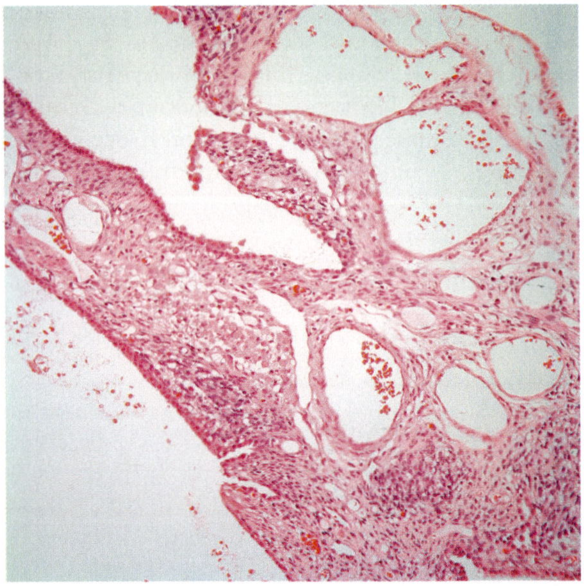

Figure 6-30 High-power view of a type I pleuropulmonary blastoma showing benign epithelium lining the cystic structures, with a mesenchymal component and other small cysts.

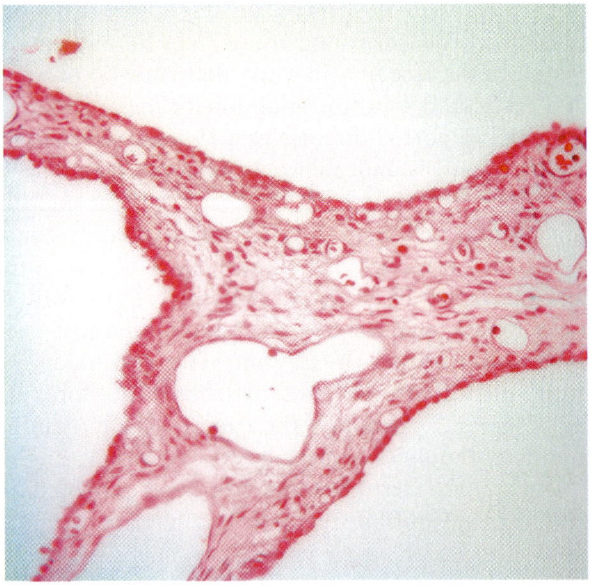

Figure 6-32 Closer view of the epithelial lining of the cystic structures composed of benign low cuboidal epithelium in a type I pleuropulmonary blastoma.

Immunohistochemical and Molecular Features

Immunohistochemical stains are used to define the type of sarcomatous component present in pleuropulmonary blastomas. Previous studies have documented positive staining for desmin, smooth muscle actin, vimentin, neuron-specific enolase, CD68, and other histiocytic markers. In the benign epithelium, positive staining for cytokeratin and epithelial membrane antigen is expected.

Owing to the rarity of pleuropulmonary blastoma, only a few cases have been analyzed by molecular studies. Some findings, however, appear to be relatively consistent; for instance, the presence of trisomies 8 and 2 has been documented in several studies.[60–64] In some of these studies, both anomalies have been detected in the same tumor. More recently, Kusafuka and associates[65] documented the presence of *p53* mutations in two of three cases of pleuropulmonary blastoma.

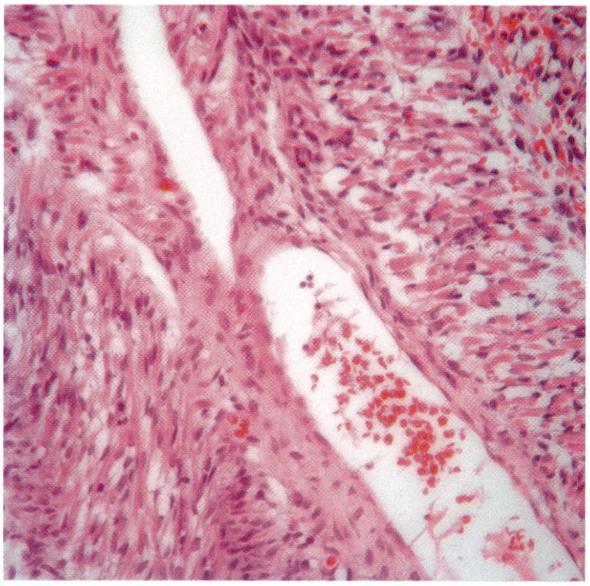

Figure 6-33 Pleuropulmonary blastoma type I showing multiple areas of skeletal muscle differentiation.

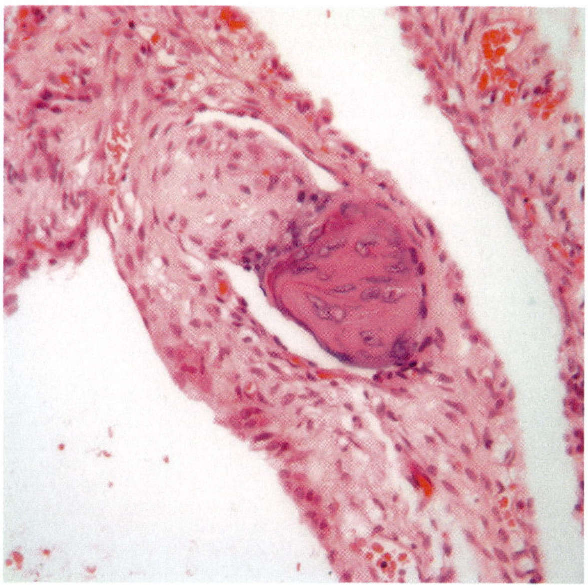

Figure 6-34 Pleuropulmonary blastoma type I showing metaplastic bone formation in the wall of a cyst.

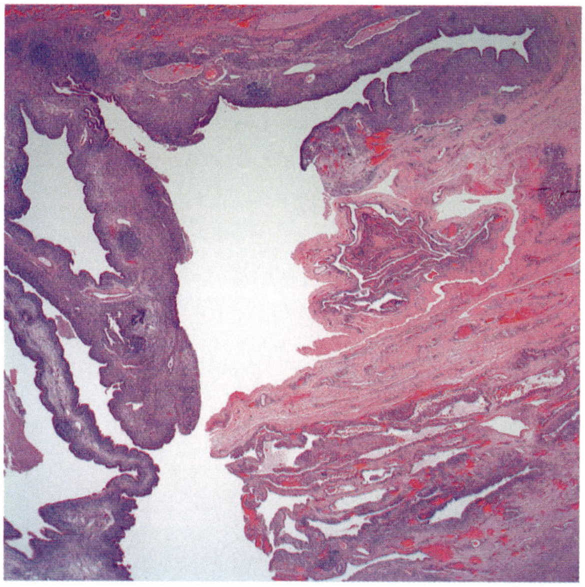

Figure 6-35 Low-power view of a type II pleuropulmonary blastoma. The spindle cell component is readily apparent.

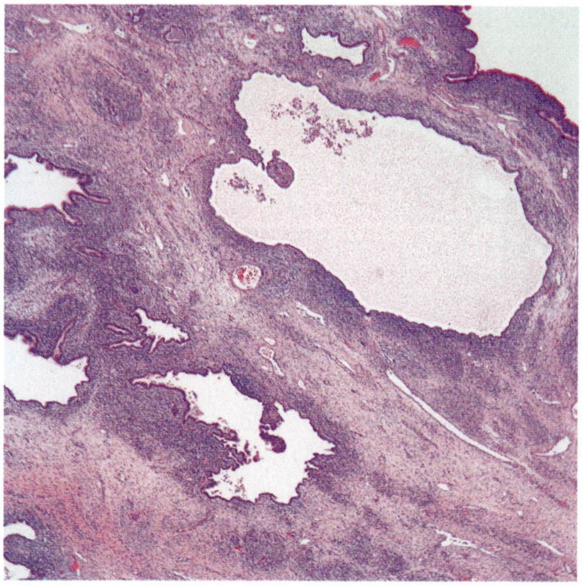

Figure 6-36 Pleuropulmonary blastoma type II with readily apparent cystic and mesenchymal components.

Treatment and Prognosis

The treatment and prognosis for pleuropulmonary blastoma are variable and will depend to some extent on histologic subtype. Priest and coworkers[59] documented a survival rate of 83% for type I and 42% for types II and III; however, the survival differences did not reach statistical significance. In a study of 11 cases, Indolfi and colleagues[66] stated that radical surgery should be the main goal of treatment, followed by chemotherapy and radiotherapy. Other workers have suggested that pleuropulmonary blastoma type II may respond to multimodal therapy.[67] The aggressive nature of pleuropulmonary blastoma types II and III also has been demonstrated by documentation of metastatic disease to the central nervous system.[68,69] More recently, Priest and coworkers[70] stated that a rigorous surveillance schedule for pleuropulmonary blastoma type I might detect early recurrences and may be an alternative to adjuvant chemotherapy. Some investigators have documented long-term survival.[71]

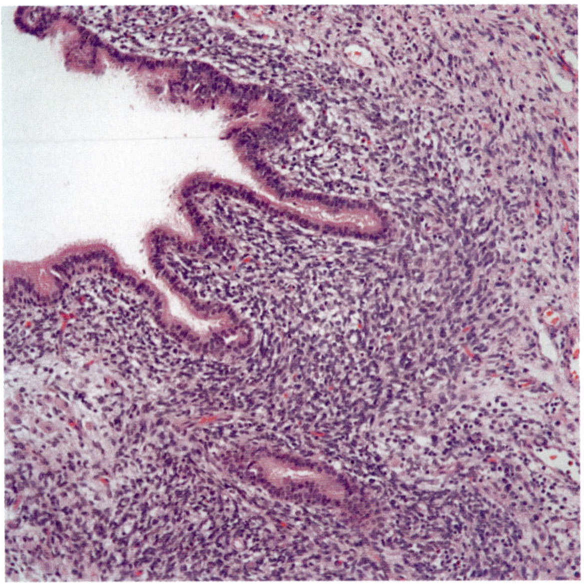

Figure 6-37 High-power view of a type II pleuropulmonary blastoma showing the malignant mesenchymal component associated with a cystic structure, lined by benign low columnar epithelium.

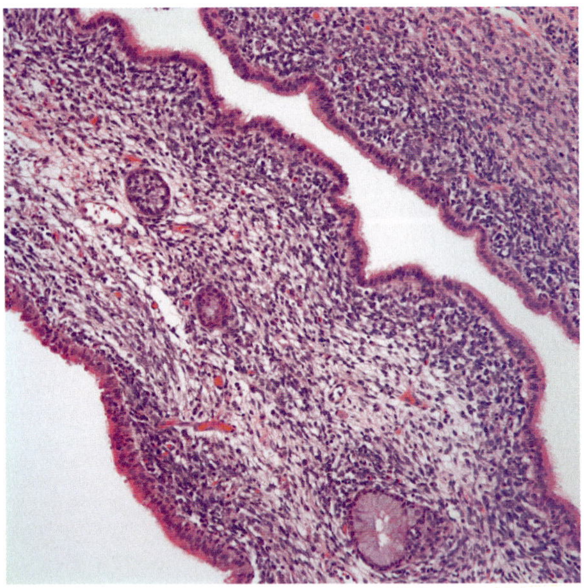

Figure 6-38 Pleuropulmonary blastoma type II. Benign glandular structures are entrapped in the wall of the cysts and admixed with the mesenchymal structures.

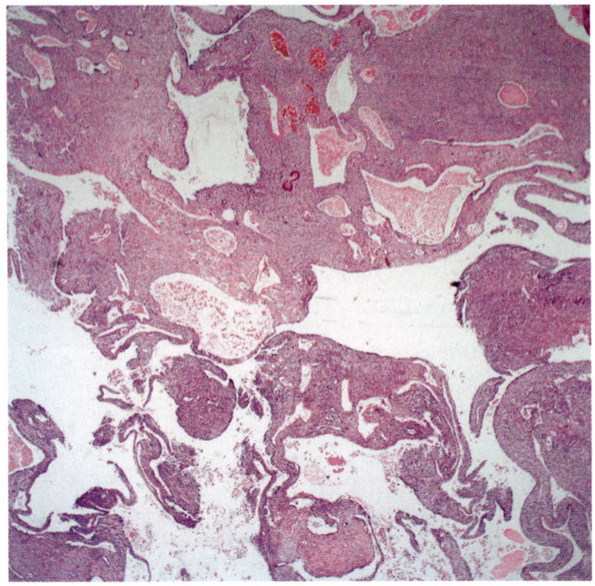

Figure 6-39 Low-power view of a type III pleuropulmonary blastoma with a predominant solid pattern.

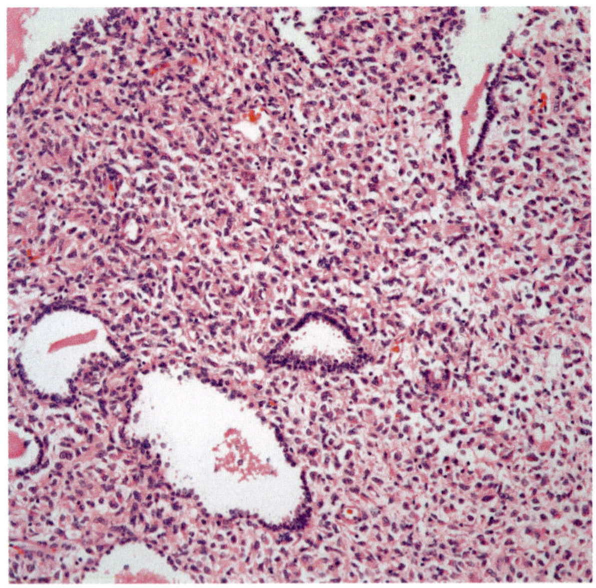

Figure 6-40 High-power view of the sarcomatous component of a type III pleuropulmonary blastoma with scattered epithelial benign cystic structures.

PULMONARY CARCINOSARCOMA

As with pulmonary blastoma, a majority of pulmonary carcinosarcomas have been classified as biphasic tumors of the lung. Histologically, however, carcinosarcomas do not share the same spectrum of differentiation as for pulmonary blastomas or pleuropulmonary blastomas. Therefore, it is very likely that carcinosarcomas represent a distinct clinicopathologic entity, and in this chapter, they are addressed separately from pulmonary blastomas and pleuropulmonary blastomas.

Historical Aspects

The classification of carcinosarcoma, and its existence as a separate clinicopathologic entity, have been debated for more than a century, ever since the initial description by Kika in 1908.[72] Many hypotheses have been presented, identifying carcinosarcoma as a dual type of tumor, collision tumor, combination tumor, composition tumor, or tumor derived from stem cells.[73] Most of those theories were presented in the early 20th century, and clear knowledge regarding tumor histogenesis in the original cases is not available today. It is clear, however, that all of these tumors show a biphasic cellular proliferation that on light microscopy resembles the histologic patterns of epithelial and sarcomatous neoplasms.

In 1938, Saphir and Vass[74] reviewed data for 153 reported carcinosarcomas from the literature, summarizing the contemporary theories regarding their origin. Of the 153 cases reported under that terminology, 7 cases were primary carcinosarcomas of the lung, and after careful analysis the investigators determined that at least 6 of those cases could not be classified as carcinosarcomas but probably represented carcinomas. These workers also stated that the carcinosarcomatous nature of those reported cases was questionable, except in 3 or 4 cases. In 1961, Moore[75] reported a case of carcinosarcoma of the lung, acknowledging the existence of 13 additional cases in the literature. Two different presentations for these tumors, central and peripheral, were outlined. Central tumors appear to show a pedunculated growth in an endobronchial location, whereas peripheral tumors appear to be more solid and larger. It appears that tumors in the peripheral location are more prone to local invasion and distant metastasis. A report from the Mayo Clinic[76] for the years 1915 to 1965 found 9 cases of carcinosarcoma of the lung, and also included a review of the existing literature. These cases mirrored those previously described in terms of presentation and histopathologic features. Critical review of these reports show that, in a majority of cases, the malignant epithelial component was that of squamous cell carcinoma, whereas the most common sarcomatous component was that of fibrosarcoma. These findings cast some doubt on the tumors' identification as carcinosarcoma, rather than spindle cell squamous cell carcinoma or sarcomatous carcinoma. In some cases, however, the epithelial component was that of adenocarcinoma. In addition, some workers have documented the spread of the tumor to regional lymph nodes, with both components present.[72,77] Although it is easy to dismiss cases in which the "sarcomatous" component was that of the fibrosarcoma type,[78] cases in which the sarcomatous component is of the heterologous type, such as malignant bone, cartilage, or striated muscle, are more problematic.[79–82] Nevertheless, some investigators explain the presence of malignant bone, cartilage, or muscle as reflecting divergent differentiation "committed" to mesenchymal tissues and prefer to categorize these tumors as biphasic sarcomatoid carcinomas.[83]

Definition

The conventional and classic definition of carcinosarcoma is a malignant tumor composed of carcinoma (e.g., squamous cell carcinoma, adenocarcinoma) and a malignant mesenchymal neoplasm such as osteosarcoma, chondrosarcoma, or rhabdomyosarcoma. In the most recent version of the WHO classification of lung tumors, however, carcinosarcomas are included in the family of sarcomatous carcinomas, and the WHO investigators state that carcinosarcomas belong to one of the following four groups of tumors that share similar histopathologic features and represent a "morphologic continuum": pulmonary blastoma, spindle cell carcinoma, pleomorphic carcinoma, and giant cell carcinoma. On the basis of that definition, these investigators do not appear to consider carcinosarcoma, or any of the other four tumors listed, to be specific clinicopathologic entities.

Clinical Features

In two of the largest series of primary carcinosarcomas of the lung published thus far,[84,85] the investigators found a male predominance, in a proportion as high as 7:1. The tumors also appear to be more common in adults, with a median age at diagnosis of 65 years. The clinical signs and symptoms will depend on the location of the tumor; patients with a centrally located tumor are most likely to experience early symptoms, because the tumor may obstruct a major airway. Central tumors have a propensity to grow in a polypoid fashion, to partly or almost completely obstruct the bronchial lumen. Thus, patients may present with cough, dyspnea, or hemoptysis. Patients with peripherally located tumors may not have symptoms until the tumor has attained a larger size and involves adjacent structures, such as the pleura. These patients are most likely to present with chest pain, weight loss, or obstructive pneumonia. An association between tobacco use and carcinosarcoma is likely.[84] Many patients do not present with any symptoms, and their tumors are discovered during a routine radiographic evaluation.[84]

Macroscopic Features

The macroscopic features of carcinosarcoma also may depend on the location of the tumor, because centrally located tumors may not attain a larger size, in contrast with those in the periphery of the lung. Tumor size may range from 2 cm to larger than 10 cm in greatest dimension. Areas of hemorrhage and necrosis are common. The tumors appear to be well circumscribed but not encapsulated, and the cut surface may be light brown and partly lobulated or homogeneous in appearance; a predominantly solid consistency is characteristic. In some cases in which heterologous differentiation is present, areas of cartilaginous change can be identified (Fig. 6-41). In their study of 66 patients with carcinosarcomas,[84] Koss and coworkers determined that central tumors are more common than peripheral tumors, and that the upper lobes are more commonly affected.

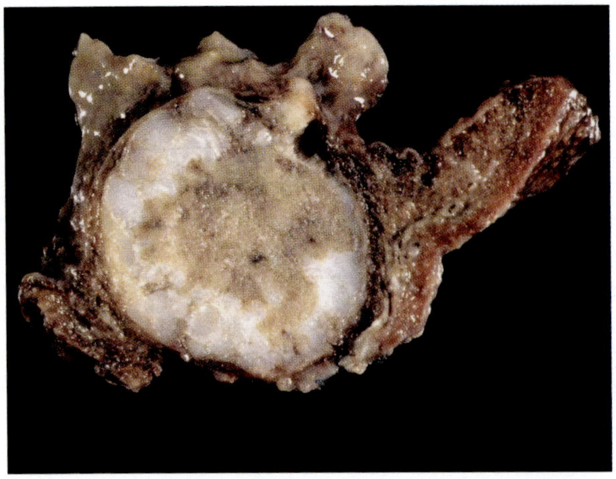

Figure 6-41 Carcinosarcoma showing a lobulated surface. The whitish areas represent cartilaginous differentiation.

Microscopic Features

This tumor may appear in a central location involving the main airway, or in the periphery of the lung as a well-circumscribed tumor mass (Fig. 6-42). The histopathologic features of this tumor are rather straightforward, with unequivocal areas of carcinoma and sarcoma (Figs. 6-43 to 6-53). The most common epithelial component in pulmonary carcinosarcoma is squamous cell carcinoma, and the second most common is adenocarcinoma, followed by adenosquamous carcinoma or large cell carcinoma. The histologic criteria for any of these carcinomas are essentially the same as the criteria described in Chapter 3. The sarcomatous component should be in the form of osteosarcoma, chondrosarcoma, or rhabdomyosarcoma, adhering to the same criteria as described for their counterparts in the soft tissues. The difference is that both components are intermingled, and although a predominance of one over the other may be seen, both should be clearly observed and differentiated in these carcinosarcomas. Extensive areas of hemorrhage or necrosis may be observed in some of these tumors, mainly those that reach a larger size.

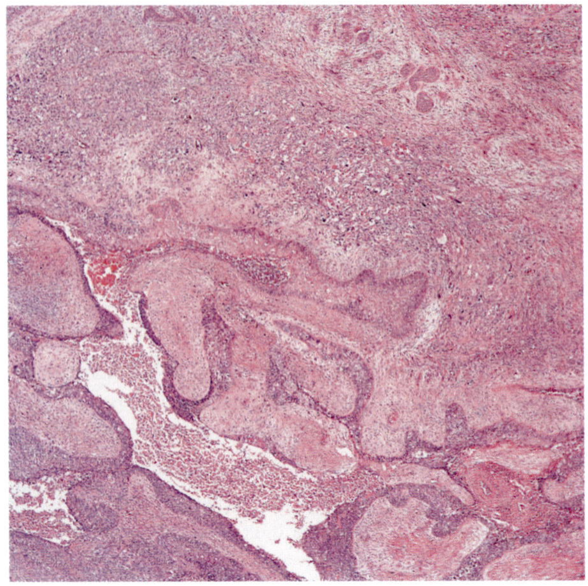

Figure 6-43 Carcinosarcoma of the lung. Areas of squamous cell carcinoma can be seen adjacent to areas of sarcoma.

Metastatic disease from carcinosarcomas has been documented not only in regional lymph nodes (Fig. 6-54) but also in kidney, bone, liver, spleen, and gastrointestinal tract. The histopathologic features of these metastatic tumors may include only epithelial components or only sarcomatous components, or both.

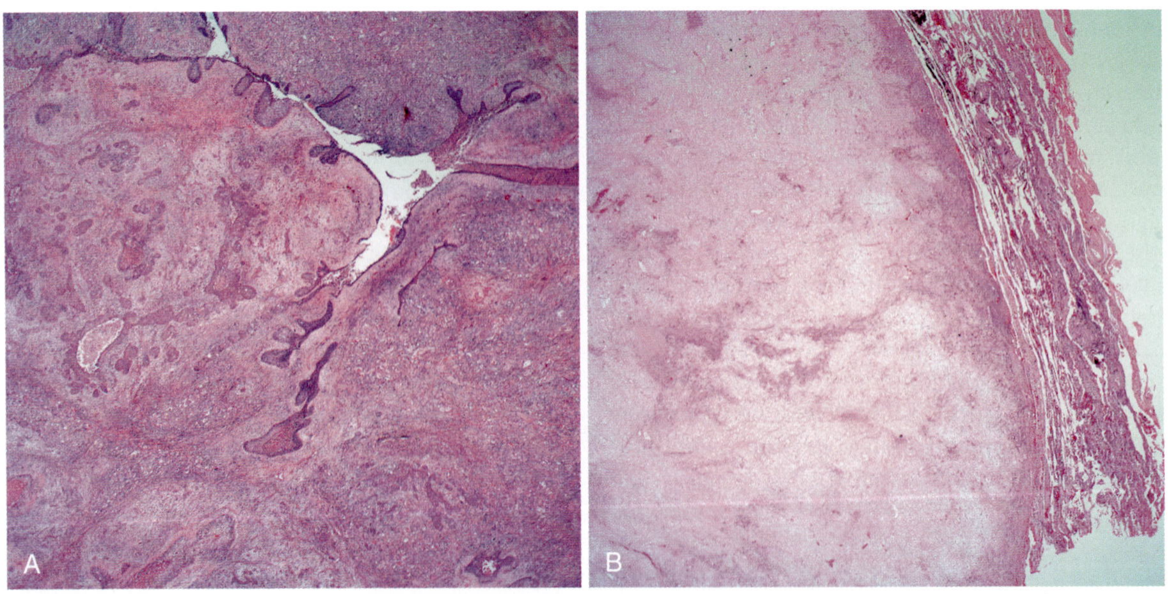

Figure 6-42 **A**, Carcinosarcoma of the lung obstructing the main airway. **B**, Peripheral carcinosarcoma manifesting as a well-circumscribed tumor mass.

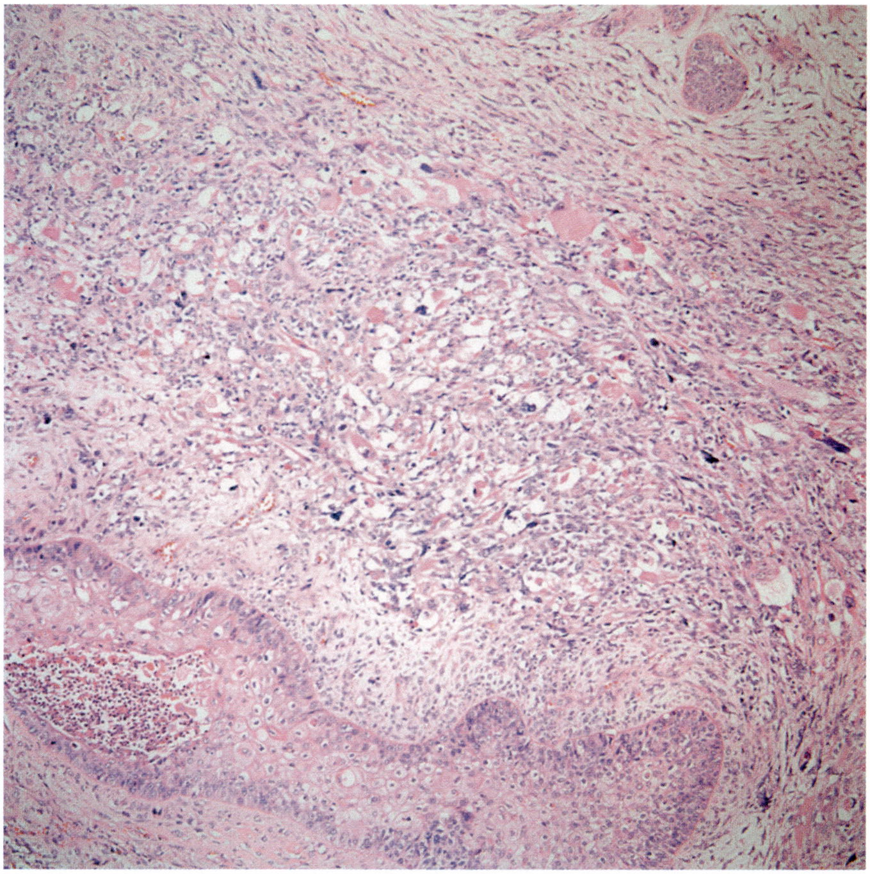

Figure 6-44 Higher magnification of a carcinosarcoma showing the contrast between the two neoplastic cellular populations (epithelial and mesenchymal).

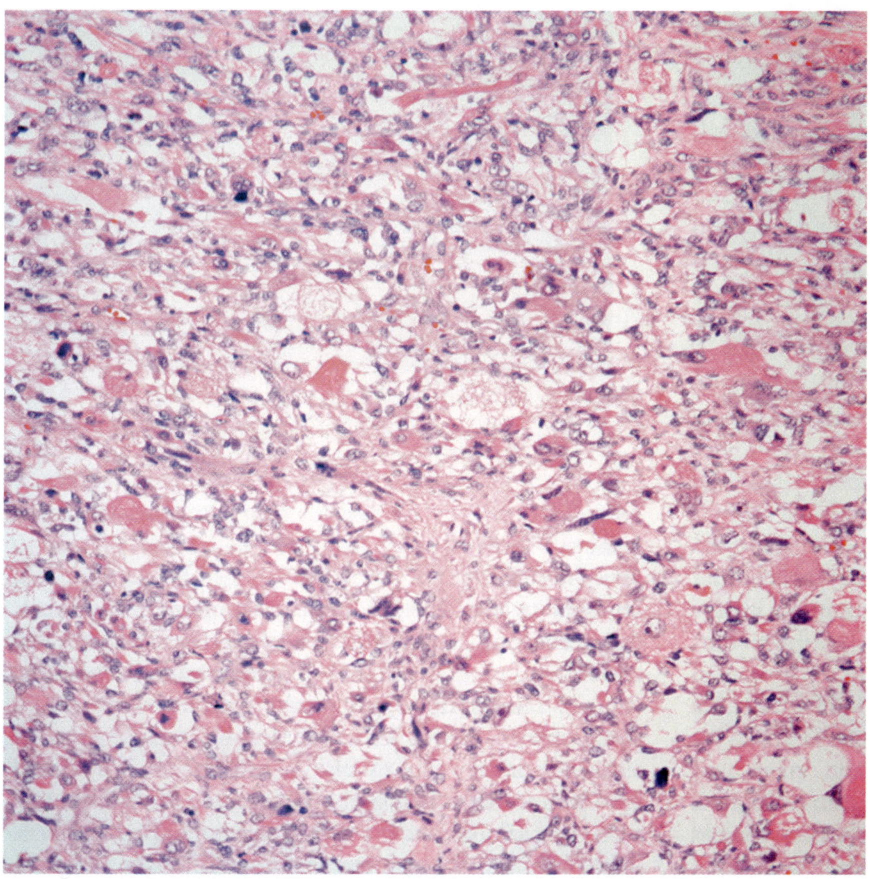

Figure 6-45 High-power magnification showing the rhabdomyosarcomatous differentiation in carcinosarcoma of the lung.

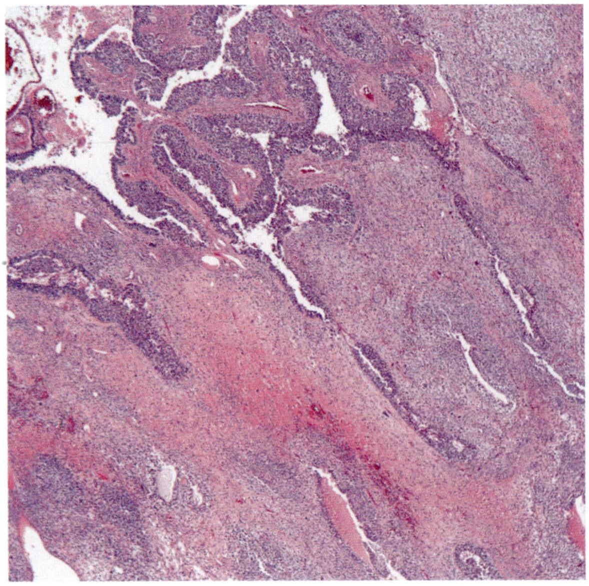

Figure 6-46 Carcinosarcoma of the lung. Areas of papillary carcinoma can be seen adjacent to areas of sarcoma.

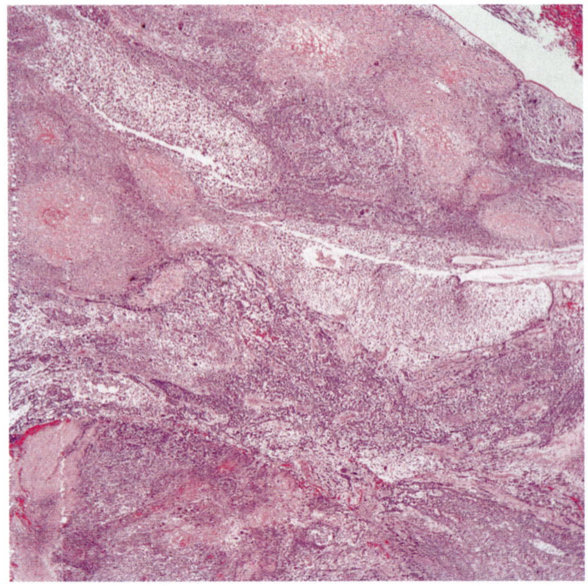

Figure 6-48 Low-power view of carcinosarcoma of the lung. Areas of keratinizing squamous cell carcinoma, undifferentiated sarcoma, and osteosarcoma can be seen.

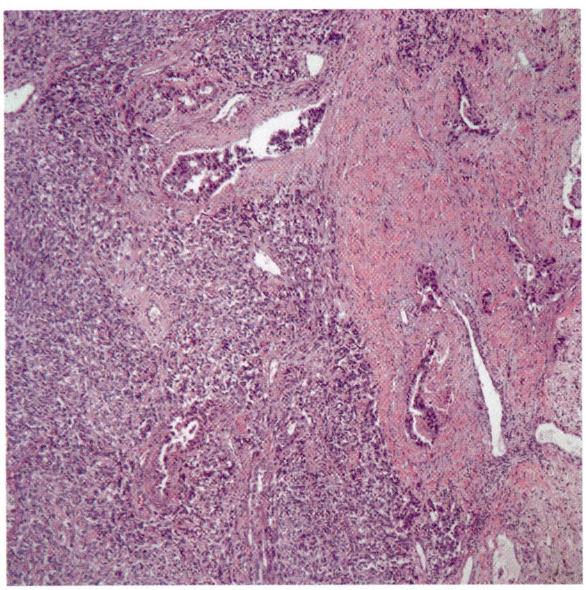

Figure 6-47 Carcinosarcoma of the lung showing an extensive sarcomatous component with areas of adenocarcinoma.

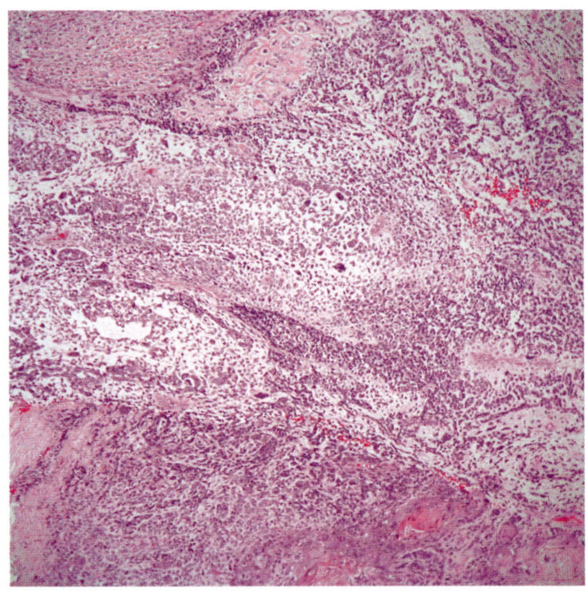

Figure 6-49 Closer view of carcinosarcoma of the lung showing the squamous cell carcinoma and osteosarcomatous component.

Immunohistochemical Features

Immunohistochemical studies may be helpful in determining the presence and amount of the different components within carcinosarcomas. The use of epithelial markers, including EMA and low- and high-molecular-weight cytokeratins, may prove to be beneficial in outlining the epithelial component. Keratin 5/6 and p63 may be useful in determining the presence of squamous cell carcinoma, whereas TTF-1 and CEA may be helpful in cases of adenocarcinoma. Muscle markers, including desmin, myoglobin, and Myo-D1, may be helpful in cases of rhabdomyosarcoma, and S-100 protein and Sox-2 in cases of chondrosarcoma. For diagnosis of osteosarcoma, however, it may be necessary to rely on the morphologic nature of the neoplasm. In this setting, immunohistochemical studies using collagen type IV may be useful when it is difficult to separate dense collagen and osteoid.[86,87] Even though these tumors may show a wide spectrum of positive staining using immunohistochemical markers, the diagnosis

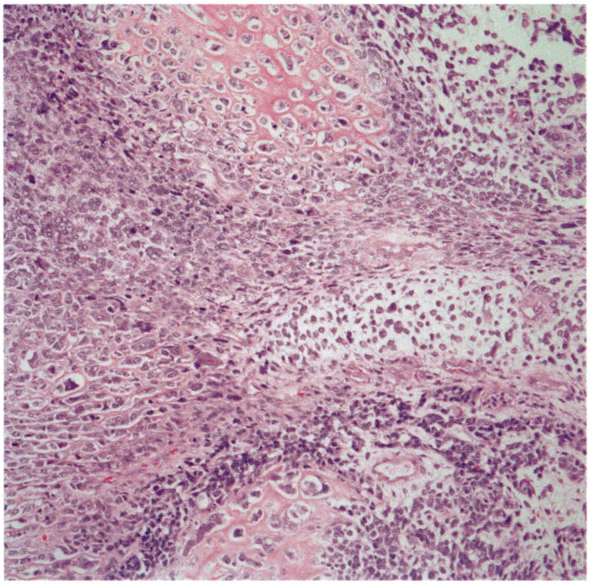

Figure 6-50 Higher-power view of carcinosarcoma of the lung. Areas of osteosarcoma can be seen.

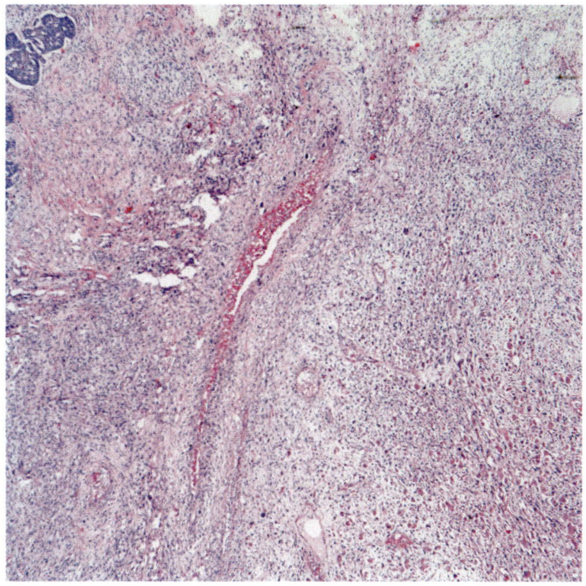

Figure 6-52 Carcinosarcoma of the lung in which the epithelial component is minimal.

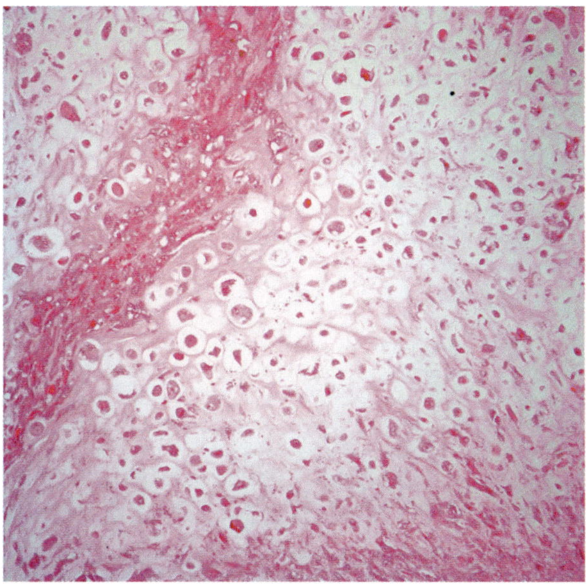

Figure 6-51 Carcinosarcoma of the lung with extensive areas of chondrosarcoma.

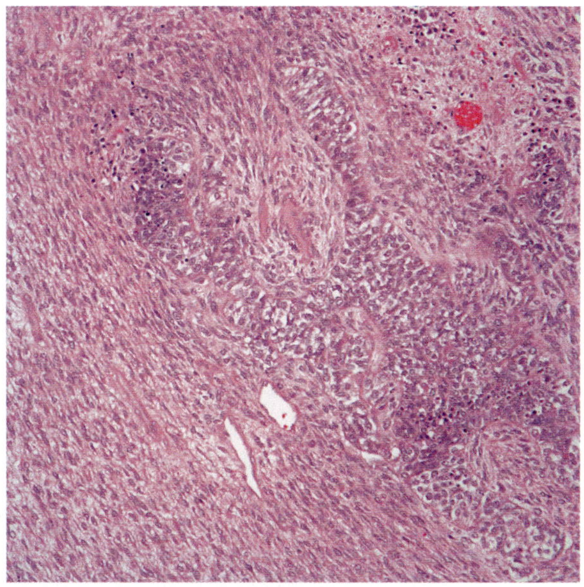

Figure 6-53 Carcinosarcoma of the lung in which the epithelial component is rather inconspicuous.

of carcinosarcoma is still made on morphologic grounds, because the two components of the tumor must be identified. Immunohistochemical markers should be used exclusively to demonstrate a specific characteristic of the tumor that may not be as obvious on morphologic evaluation. Of note, positive staining with either epithelial or mesenchymal markers does not imply that the heterologous component of the tumor is metaplastic in nature, as has been suggested by some authors.[88]

Differential Diagnosis

With a small biopsy specimen, the diagnosis of carcinosarcoma may prove to be very difficult to nearly impossible. Success will depend largely on the sample of the tissue obtained. Thus, the initial diagnosis in patients with this tumor may be either a malignant epithelial or malignant mesenchymal neoplasm. In the great majority of cases, the definitive diagnosis of carcinosarcoma is made from material obtained at complete surgical resection of the tumor.

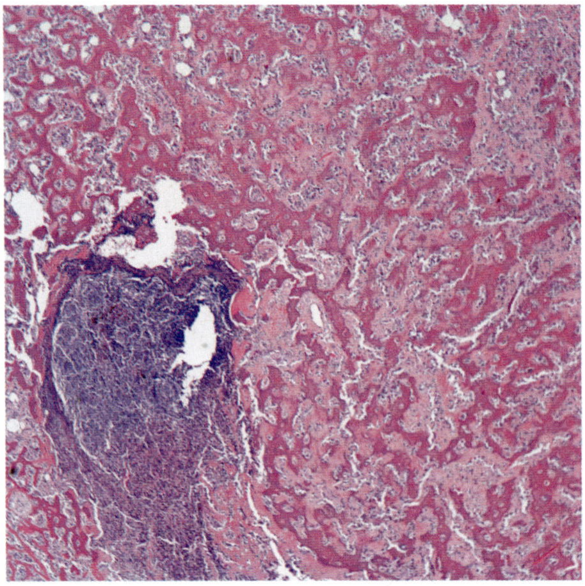

Figure 6-54 Osteosarcomatous component of a carcinosarcoma of the lung involving a regional lymph node.

Prognosis and Treatment

Although no specific treatment for carcinosarcoma has emerged, complete surgical resection appears to be the current treatment of choice. In a majority of cases, carcinosarcoma is difficult to diagnose from a small biopsy specimen; accordingly, most diagnoses are made after surgical resection of the tumor.

Gebauer[89] compared the prognosis for carcinosarcoma with that for other pulmonary sarcomas and concluded that patients with carcinosarcoma fare worse. Other workers have reported that the prognosis is comparable to that for other pulmonary carcinomas.[90] In the Mayo Clinic study by Davis and colleagues,[85] only 4 of 17 patients with carcinosarcoma survived follow-up periods ranging from 6 to 39 months, with a median survival of 1 year. Wick and associates[91] reported an overall 5-year survival rate for patients with sarcomatoid carcinomas (encompassing spindle cell carcinoma, carcinosarcoma, pulmonary blastoma, squamous cell carcinoma with pseudosarcomatous stroma, and pseudosarcoma) of approximately 20%. In Koss and coworkers' study of 66 patients, the overall survival rate for patients with carcinosarcoma was 21% at 5 years.[84] Although these results were similar to those of Wick's group,[91] the Koss investigators[84] stated that the histologic differences between carcinosarcoma and spindle cell carcinoma suggest that these tumors may be separate entities with similar behavior. This concept has been corroborated by other investigators,[92] who have found that tumors with heterologous components, such as osteosarcoma, chondrosarcoma, or rhabdomyosarcoma, may progress more rapidly, making the separation of the different components in a particular tumor very important and raising the possibility that carcinosarcoma may be a specific clinicopathologic entity.

REFERENCES

1. Berho M, Moran CA, Suster S. Malignant mixed epithelial/mesenchymal neoplasms of the lung. *Semin Diagn Pathol.* 1995;12(2):123–139.
2. Koss MN. Pulmonary blastomas. *Lung Cancer.* 1994;349–362.
3. Barnard WG. Embryoma of lung. *Thorax.* 1952;7:299–301.
4. Spencer H. Pulmonary blastoma. *J Pathol Bacteriol.* 1961;82:161–165.
5. Waddell WR. Organoid differentiation of the foetal lung: histologic study of the differentiation of mammalian foetal lung in utero and in transplants. *Arch Pathol.* 1949;47:227–247.
6. Souza RC, Peasly ED, Takaro T. Pulmonary blastomas—a distinct group of carcinosarcomas of the lung. *Ann Thorac Surg.* 1965;1:259–268.
7. Bauermeister DE, Jennings ER, Beland AH, Judson HA. Pulmonary blastoma—a form of carcinosarcoma. *Am J Clin Pathol.* 1966;46:322–329.
8. Chaudhuri MR, Eastham WN, Fredriksz PA. Pulmonary blastoma with diverse mesenchymal proliferation. *Thorax.* 1972;27:487–491.
9. Dixon DS, Breslow A. Pulmonary blastoma. *Am Rev Respir Dis.* 1973;108:968–971.
10. Roth JA, Elguezabal A. Pulmonary blastoma evolving into carcinosarcoma. A case study. *Am J Surg Pathol.* 1978;2:407–413.
11. Fung CH, Lo JW, Yonan TN, Milloy FJ, Hakami MM, Changus GW. Pulmonary blastoma. An ultrastructural study with a brief review of the literature and a discussion of pathogenesis. *Cancer.* 1977;39:153–163.
12. McCann MP, Fu YS, Kay S. Pulmonary blastoma. A light and electron microscopic study. *Cancer.* 1976;38:789–797.
13. Kradin RL, Young RH, Dickersin GR, Kirkham SE, Mark EJ. Pulmonary blastoma with argyrophil cells and lacking sarcomatous features (pulmonary endodermal tumor resembling fetal lung). *Am J Surg Pathol.* 1982;6:165–172.
14. Nakatani Y, Dickersin GR, Mark EJ. Pulmonary endodermal tumor resembling fetal lung: a clinicopathologic study of five cases with immunohistochemical and ultrastructural characterization. *Hum Pathol.* 1990;21:1097–1107.
15. Kodama T, Shimosato Y, Watanabe S, Koide T, Naruke T, Shimase J. Six cases of well-differentiated adenocarcinoma simulating fetal lung tubules in pseudoglandular stage. Comparison with pulmonary blastoma. *Am J Surg Pathol.* 1984;8:735–744.
16. Nakatani Y, Kitamura H, Inayama Y, et al. Pulmonary adenocarcinoma of the fetal lung type: a clinicopathologic study indicating differences in histology, epidemiology, and natural history of low-grade and high-grade forms. *Am J Surg Pathol.* 1998;22:399–411.
17. Travis WD, Brambilla E, Müller-Hermelink K, Harris CC. *Pathology and Genetics. Tumors of the Lung, Pleura, Thymus, and Heart.* World Health Organization (WHO). Lyon, France: IARC Press; 2004:40, 56.
18. Yazawa T, Ogata T, Kamma H, Shibagaki T, Iijima T, Horiguchi H. Pulmonary blastoma with a topographic transition from blastic to more differentiated areas. An immunohistochemical assessment of its embryonic nature using stage-specific embryonic antigens. *Virch Arch A Pathol Anat Histopathol.* 1991;419:513–518.
19. LeMense GP, Reed CE, Silvestri GA. Pulmonary blastoma: a rare lung malignancy. *Lung Cancer.* 1996;15:233–237.
20. Force S, Patterson GA. Clinical-pathologic conference in general thoracic surgery: pulmonary blastoma. *J Thorac Cardiovasc Surg.* 2003;126:1247–1250.
21. Kawano R, Hata E, Ikeda S, Yokota T. Pulmonary blastoma. *Jpn J Thorac Cardiovasc Surg.* 2005;53:611–614.
22. Koss MN, Hochholzer L, O'Leary T. Pulmonary blastomas. *Cancer.* 1991;67:2368–2381.
23. DiFurio MJ, Auerbach A, Kaplan KJ. Well-differentiated fetal adenocarcinoma: rare tumor in the pediatric population. *Pediatr Dev Pathol.* 2003;6:564–567.

24. Seballos R, Klein RL. Pulmonary blastomas in children: report of two cases and review of the literature. *J Pediatr Surg.* 1994;29:1553–1556.
25. Majid OA, Rajendran U, Baker LT. Pulmonary blastoma. *Ann Thorac Cardiovasc Surg.* 1998;4:47–52.
26. Robert J, Pache JC, Seium Y, de Perrot M, Spiliopoulos A. Pulmonary blastoma: report of five cases and identification of clinical features suggestive of the disease. *Eur J Cardiovasc Surg.* 2002;22:708–711.
27. Adluri RK, Boddu SR, Martin-Ucar A, Duffy JP, Beggs FD, Morgan WE. Pulmonary blastoma—a rare tumor with variable presentation. *Eur J Cardiovasc Surg.* 2006;29:236–239.
28. Cohen RE, Weaver MG, Montenegro HD, Abdul-Karim FW. Pulmonary blastoma with malignant melanoma component. *Arch Pathol Lab Med.* 1990;114:1076–1078.
29. Heckman CJ, Truong LD, Cagle PT, Font RL. Pulmonary blastoma with rhabdomyosarcomatous differentiation: an electron microscopic and immunohistochemical study. *Am J Surg Pathol.* 1988;12:35–40.
30. Olenick SJ, Fan CC, Ryoo JW. Mixed pulmonary blastoma and carcinosarcoma. *Histopathology.* 1994;25:171–174.
31. Addis BJ, Corrin B. Pulmonary blastoma, carcinosarcoma and spindle cell carcinoma: an immunohistochemical study of keratin intermediate filaments. *J Pathol.* 1985;147:291–301.
32. Berean K, Truong LD, Dudley Jr AW, Cagle PT. Immunohistochemical characterization of pulmonary blastoma. *Am J Clin Pathol.* 1988;89:773–777.
33. Garcia-Escudero A, Gonzalez-Campora R, Villar-Rodriguez JL, Lag-Asturano E. Thyroid transcription factor-1 expression in pulmonary blastoma. *Histopathology.* 2004;44:502–514.
34. Chejfec G, Cosnow I, Gould NS, Husain AN, Gould VE. Pulmonary blastoma with neuroendocrine differentiation in cell morules resembling neuroepithelial bodies. *Histopathology.* 1990;17:353–358.
35. Pacinda SJ, Ledet SC, Gondo MM, et al. *p53* and MDM2 immunostaining in pulmonary blastoma and bronchogenic carcinomas. *Hum Pathol.* 1996;27:542–546.
36. Bodner SM, Koss MN. Mutations in the *p53* gene in pulmonary blastomas: immunohistochemical and molecular studies. *Hum Pathol.* 1996;27:1117–1123.
37. Holst VA, Finkelstein S, Colby TV, Myers JL, Yousem SA. *p53* and *K-ras* mutational genotyping in pulmonary carcinosarcoma, spindle cell carcinoma, and pulmonary blastoma: implications for histogenesis. *Am J Surg Pathol.* 1997;21:801–811.
38. Nakatani Y, Miyagi Y, Takemura T, et al. Aberrant nuclear/cytoplasmic localization and gene mutation of B-catenin in classic pulmonary blastoma: beta-catenin immunostaining is useful for distinguishing between classic pulmonary blastoma and a blastomatoid variant of carcinosarcoma. *Am J Surg Pathol.* 2004;28:921–927.
39. Liman ST, Altinok T, Topcu S, et al. Survival of biphasic pulmonary blastoma. *Respir Med.* 2006;100:1174–1179.
40. Dishop MK, Kuruvilla S. Primary and metastatic lung tumors in the pediatric population: a review and 25-year experience at a large children's hospital. *Arch Pathol Lab Med.* 2008;132:1079–1103.
41. Papagiannopoulos K, Hughes S, Nicholson AG, Goldstraw P. Cystic lung lesions in the pediatric and adult population: surgical experience at the Brompton Hospital. *Ann Thorac Surg.* 2002;73:1594–1598.
42. Ashworth TG. Pulmonary blastoma, a true congenital neoplasm. *Histopathology.* 1983;7:585–594.
43. Holland-Moritz RM, Heyn RM. Pulmonary blastoma associated with cystic lesions in children. *Med Pedatr Oncol.* 1984;12:85–88.
44. Cohen M, Emms M, Kaschula ROC. Childhood pulmonary blastoma: a pleuropulmonary variant of the adult type pulmonary blastoma. *Pediatr Pathol.* 1991;11:737–749.
45. Fallon G, Schiller M, Kilman JW. Primary rhabdomyosarcoma of the bronchus. *Ann Thorac Surg.* 1971;9:179–182.
46. Weinberg AG, Currakino G, Moore GC, Votteler TP. Mesenchymal neoplasia and congenital pulmonary cysts. *Pediatr Pathol.* 1980;9:179–182.
47. Mark EJ. Mesenchymal cystic hamartoma of the lung. *N Engl J Med.* 1986;315:1255–1259.
48. Manivel JC, Priest JR, Watterson J, et al. Pleuropulmonary blastoma: the so-called pulmonary blastoma of childhood. *Cancer.* 1988;62:1516–1526.
49. Dehner LP. Pleuropulmonary blastoma is the pulmonary blastoma of childhood. *Semin Diagn Pathol.* 1994;11:144–151.
50. Hill DA, Sadeghi S, Schultz MZ, Burr JS, Dehner LP. Pleuropulmonary blastoma in an adult: an initial case report. *Cancer.* 1999;85:2368–2374.
51. Zuker NB, Dietl CA, Kenna S, Fischer EG, Gardner D. Unusual survival of an adult with pleuropulmonary blastoma and neurofibromatosis. *J Thorac Cardiovasc Surg.* 2007;134:541–542.
52. Picaud JC, Levrey H, Bouvier R, et al. Bilateral cystic pleuropulmonary blastoma in early infancy. *J Pediatr.* 2000;136:834–836.
53. Nur S, Badr R, Sandoval C, Brudniki A, Yeh A. Syndromic presentation of a pleuropulmonary blastoma associated with congenital cystic adenomatoid malformation. A case report. *J Pediatr Surg.* 2007;42:1772–1775.
54. Dosios T, Stinios J, Nicolaides P, Spyrakos S, Androulakakis E, Constantopoulos A. Pleuropulmonary blastoma in childhood. A malignant degeneration of pulmonary cysts. *Pediatr Surg Int.* 2004;20:863–865.
55. MacSweeny F, Papagiannopoulos K, Goldstraw P, Sheppard MN, Corrin B, Nicholson AG. An assessment of the expanded classification of congenital cystic adenomatoid malformation and their relationship to malignant transformation. *Am J Surg Pathol.* 2003;27:1139–1146.
56. Hachitanda Y, Aoyama C, Sato JK, Shimada H. Pleuropulmonary blastoma in childhood: a tumor of divergent differentiation. *Am J Surg Pathol.* 1993;17:382–391.
57. Herman TE, Siegel MJ. Neonatal pleuropulmonary blastoma, type I. *J Perinatol.* 2008;28:82–84.
58. Kukkady A, Upadhyay V, Pease PWB, Chan YF. Pleuropulmonary blastoma: four cases. *Pediatr Surg Int.* 2000;16:595–598.
59. Priest JR, McDermott MB, Bhatia S, Watterson J, Manivel JC, Dehner LP. Pleuropulmonary blastoma: a clinicopathological study of 50 cases. *Cancer.* 1997;80:147–161.
60. Hong B, Chen Z, Coffin CM, et al. Molecular cytogenetic analysis of pleuropulmonary blastoma. *Cancer Cytogenet.* 2003;142:65–69.
61. de Krijger RR, Claessen SM, van der Ham F, et al. Gain of chromosome 8q is a frequent finding in pleuropulmonary blastoma. *Mod Pathol.* 2007;20:1191–1199.
62. Sebire NJ, Rampling D, Malone M, Ramsay A. Gains of chromosome 8 in pleuropulmonary blastomas of childhood. *Pediatr Dev Pathol.* 2002;5:221–222.
63. Sciot R, Dal Cin P, Brock P, et al. Pleuropulmonary blastoma (pulmonary blastoma of childhood): genetic link with other embryonal malignancies? *Histopathology.* 1994;24:559–563.
64. Yang P, Hasegawa T, Hirose T, et al. Pleuropulmonary blastoma: fluorescence in situ hybridization analysis indicating trisomy 2. *Am J Surg Pathol.* 1997;21:854–859.
65. Kusafuka T, Kuroda S, Inoue M, et al. *p53* gene mutations in pleuropulmonary blastomas. *Pediatr Hematol Oncol.* 2002;19:117–128.
66. Indolfi P, Casale F, Carli M, et al. Pleuropulmonary blastoma: management and prognosis of 11 cases. *Cancer.* 2000;89:1396–1401.
67. Pinarli FG, Oguz A, Ceyda K, Memi L, Aylar P. Type II pleuropulmonary blastoma responsive to multimodal therapy. *Pediatr Hematol Oncol.* 2005;22:71–76.
68. Priest JR, Magnuson J, Williams GM, et al. Cerebral metastasis and other central nervous system complications of pleuropulmonary blastoma. *Pediatr Blood Cancer.* 2007;49:266–273.
69. Perdikogianni C, Stiakaki E, Danilatou V, Delides G, Kalmanti M. Pleuropulmonary blastoma: an aggressive intrathoracic neoplasm of childhood. *Pediatr Hematol Oncol.* 2001;18:259–266.

70. Priest JR, Hill DA, Williams GM, et al. Type I pleuropulmonary blastoma: a report from the International Pleuropulmonary Blastoma Registry. *J Clin Pathol.* 2006;24:4492–4498.
71. Romeo C, Impellizzeri P, Grosso M, Vitarelli E, Gentile C. Pleuropulmonary blastoma: long-term survival and literature review. *Med Pediatr Oncol.* 1999;33:372–376.
72. Kika G. *Gann.* 1908;2:84.
73. Kakos GS, Wiliams TE, Assor D, Vasko JS. Pulmonary carcinosarcoma: etiologic, therapeutic, and prognostic considerations. *J Thorac Cardiovasc Surg.* 1971;61:777–783.
74. Saphir O, Vass A. Carcinosarcoma. *Am J Cancer.* 1938;33(3):331–361.
75. Moore TC. Carcinosarcoma of the lung. *Surgery.* 1961;50(6):886–893.
76. Stackhouse EM, Harrison EG, Ellis FH. Primary mixed malignancies of lung: carcinosarcoma and blastoma. *J Thorac Cardiovasc Surg.* 1969;57:385–399.
77. Diaconita G. Bronchopulmonary carcinosarcoma. *Thorax.* 1975;30:682–686.
78. Heremans A, Verbeken E, Deneffe G, Demedts M. Carcinosarcoma of the lung: report of two cases and review of the literature. *Acta Clin Belg.* 1989;44:110–115.
79. Ludwigsen E. Endobronchial carcinosarcoma. *Virch Arch Path Anat Histol.* 1977;373:293–302.
80. Edwards CW, Saunders MA, Collins F. Mixed malignant tumour of the lung. *Thorax.* 1979;34:629–636.
81. Zimmerman KG, Sobonya RE, Payne CM. Histochemical and ultrastructural features of an unusual pulmonary carcinosarcoma. *Hum Pathol.* 1981;12:1046–1051.
82. Sarma DP, Deshotels SJ. Carcinosarcoma of the lung. *J Surg Oncol.* 1982;19:216–218.
83. Nappi O, Wick MR. Sarcomatoid neoplasms of the respiratory tract. *Semin Diagn Pathol.* 1993;10:137–147.
84. Koss MN, Hochholzer L, Frommelt RA. Carcinosarcomas of the lung: a clinicopathologic study of 66 patients. *Am J Surg Pathol.* 1999;23:1514–1526.
85. Davis MP, Eagan RT, Weiland LH, Pairolero PC. Carcinosarcoma of the lung: Mayo Clinic experience and response to chemotherapy. *Mayo Clin Proc.* 1984;59:598–603.
86. Cupples J, Wright J. An immunohistological comparison of primary carcinosarcoma and sarcoma. *Pathol Res Pract.* 1990;186:326–329.
87. Nappi O, Glasner SD, Swanson PE, Wick MR. Biphasic and monophasic sarcomatoid carcinomas of the lung. A reappraisal of "carcinosarcomas" and "spindle cell carcinomas. *Am J Clin Pathol.* 1994;102:331–340.
88. Rossi G, Cavazza A, Sturm N, et al. Pulmonary carcinomas with pleomorphic, sarcomatoid, or sarcomatous elements: a clinicopathologic and immunohistochemical study of 75 cases. *Am J Surg Pathol.* 2003;27:311–324.
89. Gebauer CHR. The operative prognosis of primary pulmonary sarcomas. *Scand J Thorac Cardiovasc Surg.* 1982;16:91–97.
90. Huwer H, Kalweit G, Straub U, Feindt P, Volkmer I, Gams E. Pulmonary carcinosarcoma: diagnostic problems and determinants of the prognosis. *Eur J Cardiothorac Surg.* 1996;10:403–407.
91. Wick MR, Ritter JH, Humphrey PA. Sarcomatoid carcinomas of the lung: a clinicopathologic review. *Am J Clin Pathol.* 1997;108:40–53.
92. Ishida T, Tateishi M, Kaneko S, et al. Carcinosarcoma and spindle cell carcinoma of the lung. *J Thorac Cardiovasc Surg.* 1990;100:844–852.

7

Mesenchymal Tumors of the Lung

Primary mesenchymal tumors of the lung, whether benign or malignant, are rare. Sarcomas with histopathologic features similar to those seen in soft tissues may arise in the bronchopulmonary region; thus, the histopathologic criteria for the diagnosis of pulmonary sarcomas or benign mesenchymal neoplasms are basically the same as those used when these tumors occur in more common locations, such as soft tissue or bone. Nevertheless, bronchopulmonary sarcomas are unusual tumors, accounting for no more than 1% of all the primary lung neoplasms. In 1954, Iverson[1] documented three cases of primary pulmonary sarcomas and noted that between 1900 and 1950, only 16 cases had been presented in the literature. In 1979, Eskenasy[2] reported 118 cases of primary lung sarcomas; however, close analysis showed that at least 68 of those cases, in today's nomenclature, would not be designated mesenchymal tumors. Included in this study were pediatric cases, which may account for the high volume of pulmonary sarcomas. Eskenasy[2] estimated a ratio of 1 sarcoma per every 30 to 35 cases, which appears to be fairly high, in view of the unusual occurrence of pulmonary sarcomas.

In a study from the Mayo Clinic encompassing a period of 28 years, Nascimiento and associates[3] encountered only 18 cases of primary pulmonary sarcomas in adult or young adult patients ranging in age from 22 to 77 years. Attanoos and coworkers[4] documented only 14 cases of primary sarcomas of the lung over a period of 30 years. These workers estimated that the incidence of primary sarcomas of the lung is in the range of 1 per every 550 bronchogenic carcinomas. Their study population ranged in age from 20 to 73 years, with a mean of 47 years. More recently, Keel and colleagues[5] documented 26 cases of primary pulmonary sarcoma in a similar population, in which patient age ranged from 18 to 75 years, with a mean of 48 years. In this study, no time frame was reported to permit determination of the frequency of these tumors; however, the evidence indicates that primary pulmonary sarcomas are relatively rare and account for less than 1% of all primary malignant neoplasms.

This chapter considers all mesenchymal neoplasms, whether they are benign or malignant, which are grouped according to their cell differentiation when known.

HAMARTOMA (BENIGN MESENCHYMOMA)

Hamartoma is the most common mesenchymal neoplasm in the lung. Debate continues over whether this tumor represents a hamartomatous lesion or a true neoplasm that should be termed *mesenchymoma*. Arguments in both camps are interesting and convincing, but both have concluded that the tumor is benign.[6–13] Two other lesions that are considered by some researchers to fall into the category of hamartoma are presented in this chapter under different designations: chondroma, defined as a mesenchymal neoplasm composed only of cartilage, and lipoma, as a similar lesion composed only of adipose tissue. The tumors that are designated here as hamartomas (or benign mesenchymomas) are composed of several tissue types.

Clinical Features

No predilection for either gender has been clearly documented for hamartomas, although in some series, male patients have predominated. Patient age may range from 17 to 77 years; however, the peak incidence is in the fifth and sixth decades of life. These tumors generally are intraparenchymal lesions and have been demonstrated to account for approximately 7% to 14% of all coin lesions. Central tumors also have been described but are rather uncommon and may account for approximately 10% of all lesions. The anatomic location of the tumor will determine symptomatology: When the tumor is intraparenchymal, patients may be completely asymptomatic, and the lesion usually is discovered during a routine chest radiographic examination. When the tumor is in a central location, patients may present with clinical signs and symptoms of bronchial obstruction including shortness of breath, cough, fever, and even weight loss. Although in the great majority of cases the tumor is a solitary mass, in some unusual cases multiple lesions may be noted on clinical presentation. The presence of intraparenchymal tumor in association with endobronchial tumor is even more unusual; nevertheless, such cases have been reported.

Macroscopic Features

Intraparenchymal lesions appear to be well circumscribed but not encapsulated and may be covered by a thin membranous tissue. On examination of the cut surface, the lesion appears to be slightly lobulated, with different-sized lobules apparent. The tumor is firm and whitish, with a mucoid or cartilaginous appearance. These lesions do not display areas of necrosis and hemorrhage. Tumor size may range from 1 cm to more than 10 cm in greatest dimension (Fig. 7-1).

Lesions that are in an endobronchial location are smaller than intraparenchymal tumors, at 1 to 3 cm in greatest dimension. The tumor is firm and white and may be attached to the bronchial wall.

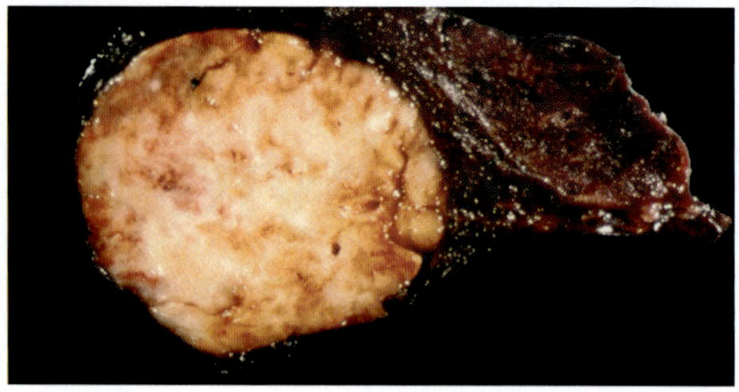

Figure 7-1 Large, well-circumscribed, predominantly cartilaginous hamartoma.

Histopathologic Features

Hamartomas are characterized by the presence of different types of tissues, including cartilage, adipose tissue, strands of smooth muscle, and invaginations of respiratory epithelium (Figs. 7-2 to 7-5). These tissues may appear in various proportions in different tumors, and to some extent this variability will depend on the size of the lesion. If the tumor is centrally located, the lesions may be composed predominantly of cartilage, with little adipose tissue, and covered by respiratory epithelium; however, the invagination of respiratory epithelium seen in intraparenchymal lesions may be absent. Cellular pleomorphism and nuclear atypia are not common, except in large lesions, in which some nuclear atypia of the cartilaginous component may be seen. In endobronchial lesions, it is possible to observe residual endobronchial glands admixed with cartilage or adipose tissue.

Treatment and Prognosis

The treatment of choice for these lesions is surgical resection, which may be accomplished by different techniques depending on the location and size of the tumor. These

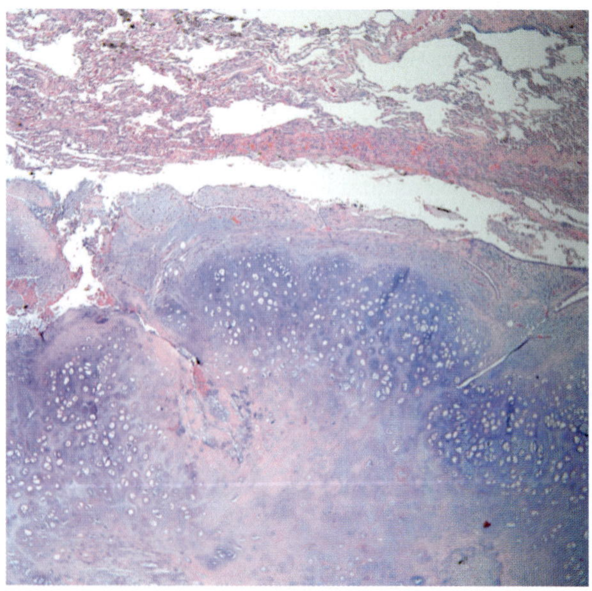

Figure 7-2 Pulmonary hamartoma. The tumor is well circumscribed and contains prominent mature cartilage.

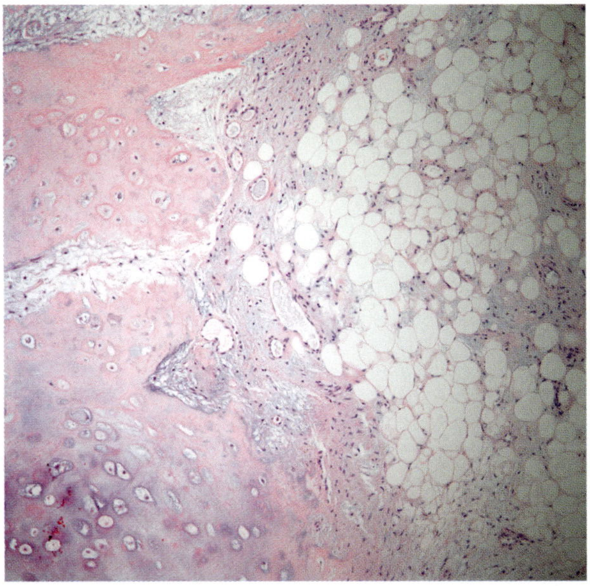

Figure 7-3 Pulmonary hamartoma showing a mixture of cartilage and adipose tissue.

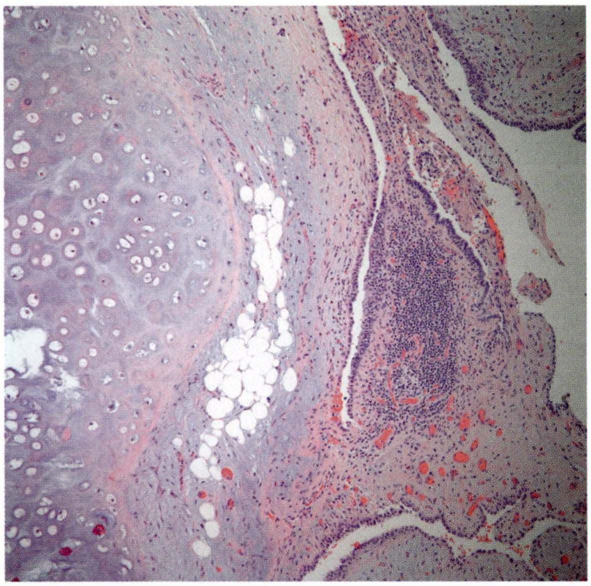

Figure 7-4 Pulmonary hamartoma. The typical epithelial invaginations are readily apparent.

lesions usually "shell out" easily, making them amenable to use of a more conservative surgical approach such as wedge resection. For larger or endobronchial tumors, the required surgical resection may be more extensive. These lesions are benign; therefore, complete surgical resection is curative. A few recurrences have been reported; these may be related to multicentricity.

TUMORS OF MUSCLE ORIGIN

Tumors of muscle origin constitute a family of both benign and malignant neoplasms including leiomyoma, leiomyosarcoma, and rhabdomyosarcoma.

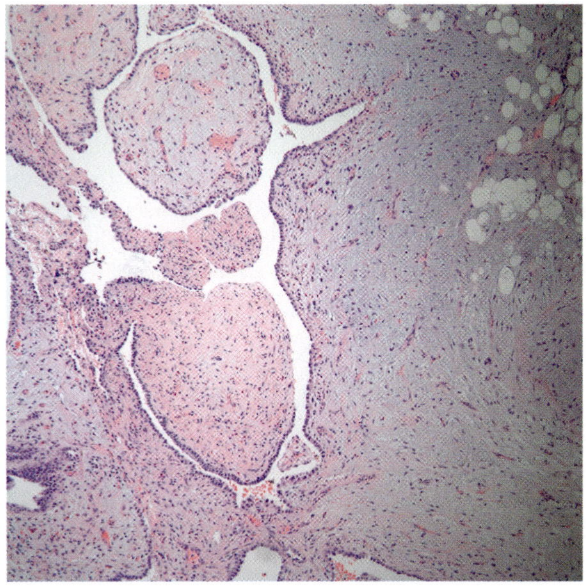

Figure 7-5 Pulmonary hamartoma with typical epithelial invaginations, myxoid areas, and adipose tissue.

Leiomyoma

Primary leiomyomas of the lung are rare; they are far less common than their malignant counterparts. In a majority of cases, leiomyomas are described in conjunction with other tumors of muscle origin, such as leiomyosarcomas, and they are thought to account for approximately 1% of all benign tumors of the lung. In earlier reports, the term *leiomyomatous hamartoma* has been used for these tumors when they appear to be multicentric.[14–17] Some researchers, however, have suggested that such neoplasms should not be considered to be primary lesions of the lung but should rather be regarded as metastatic tumors.

Horstmann and colleagues[18] documented a case of multiple pulmonary nodules in a 30-year-old pregnant woman that originally had been interpreted as leiomyomatous hamartomas and that underwent spontaneous regression during pregnancy and the postpartum period. The authors concluded that pulmonary fibroleiomyomatous hamartoma cannot be distinguished from the so-called benign metastasizing leiomyoma by clinical, radiologic, or histopathologic criteria, and that all of these tumors should be regarded as metastatic lesions from uterine tumors. Wolff and associates[19] documented nine cases (six in women and three in men) in which the patients had multiple pulmonary nodules that originated in the soft tissues or the uterus. The investigators concluded that the designation "fibroleiomyomatous hamartoma" should be abandoned.

Although the great majority of multiple pulmonary lesions occur in female patients, similar cases have been reported in male patients. In cases with multicentric tumors, however, no definitive explanation for the multicentricity of the tumor has been properly documented at the time of diagnosis and brief follow-up,[20] raising the possibility that in unusual circumstances, multicentric tumors may recur. In such cases, therefore, an appropriate clinical investigation should be undertaken in order to rule out the possibility of a metastatic tumor, from the uterus if the patient is female or from soft tissues if the patient is male. Primary leiomyomas in the lung do occur, but they are rare, and the vast majority of descriptions in the literature consist of single case reports or short series of cases.[21–42]

Clinical Features

This tumor appears to be more frequent in female patients, an observation that raises some concern about whether the possibility of uterine leiomyoma was adequately investigated in some of the reported cases. The tumor appears to affect patients of various ages, ranging from children younger than 10 years to adults older than 50 years of age. The highest incidence appears to be in adults, with an average age of 35 years.

Primary leiomyomas of the lung may occur in intraparenchymal or endobronchial locations. With central tumors, patients may present with clinical signs and symptoms of bronchial obstruction that may include cough, chest pain, shortness of breath, or hemoptysis. Other presenting manifestations may include atelectasis and obstructive pneumonia. Patients with intraparenchymal tumors may be completely asymptomatic; in such cases, the tumor usually is discovered on a routine chest radiograph.

Macroscopic Features

Leiomyomas may range in size from 1 cm to more than 10 cm in greatest dimension. However, in our experience these tumors are rarely longer than 5 cm. Intraparenchymal tumors are sharply circumscribed, but not encapsulated. They are of firm consistency and whitish and display a homogeneous-appearing cut surface (Fig. 7-6). Areas of hemorrhage or necrosis are not apparent. Centrally located tumors may appear to be pedunculated or attached to the wall of the bronchus, obliterating the lumen.

Histopathologic Features

These tumors appear as well-circumscribed masses obliterating normal lung parenchyma. Characteristically, they show a spindle cell proliferation arranged in fascicles that, in some areas, appear to intersect at 45-degree angles. The cellular proliferation is composed of fusiform cells with elongated nuclei, a moderate amount of eosinophilic cytoplasm, and inconspicuous nucleoli (Figs. 7-7 to 7-9). Intermixed with this spindle cell proliferation are areas showing entrapped structures resembling clefts that appear to be lined by respiratory epithelium. Centrally located tumors show morphologic features similar to those of tumors in an intraparenchymal location and usually are covered by a rim of respiratory epithelium. In either of these anatomic locations, the tumor may display focal areas of myxoid change. In general, leiomyomas of the lung do not show hemorrhage or necrosis, and within the cellular proliferation, nuclear atypia or mitotic activity are absent.

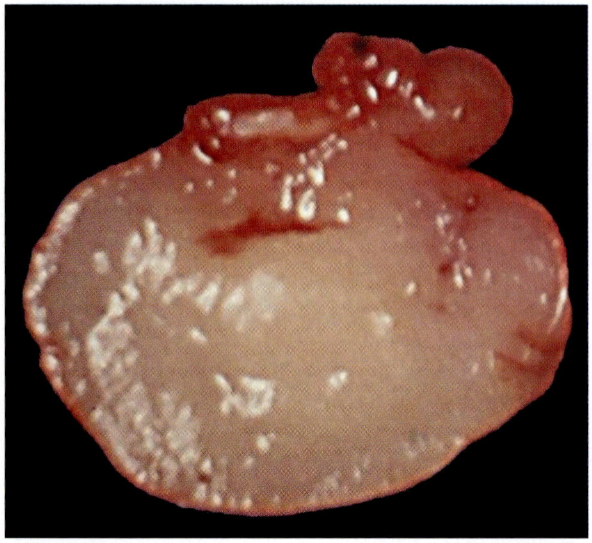

Figure 7-6 Pulmonary leiomyoma, gross specimen, with a smooth, glistening homogeneous-appearing surface.

Immunohistochemical Features

Although the diagnosis of leiomyoma usually is not challenging, in some cases immunohistochemical studies may aid in the diagnosis. Muscle markers, including muscle-specific actin, smooth muscle actin, and desmin, usually show positive staining in tumor cells. In some cases, keratin antibodies also may show positive staining.

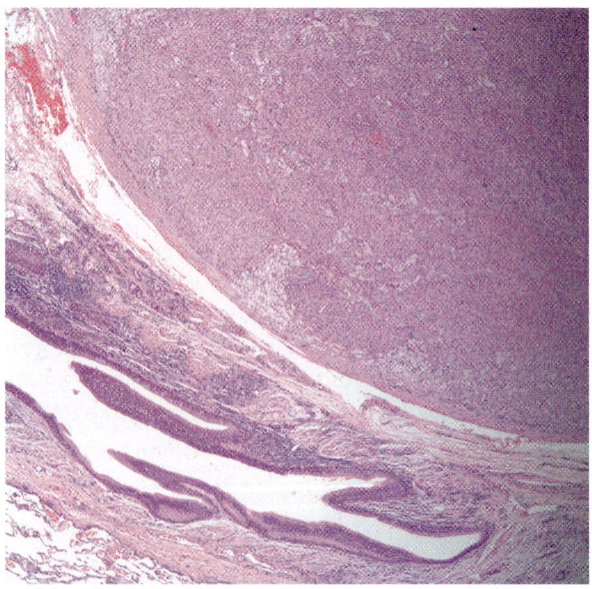

Figure 7-7 Low-power view of a pulmonary leiomyoma. The tumor was endobronchial in location.

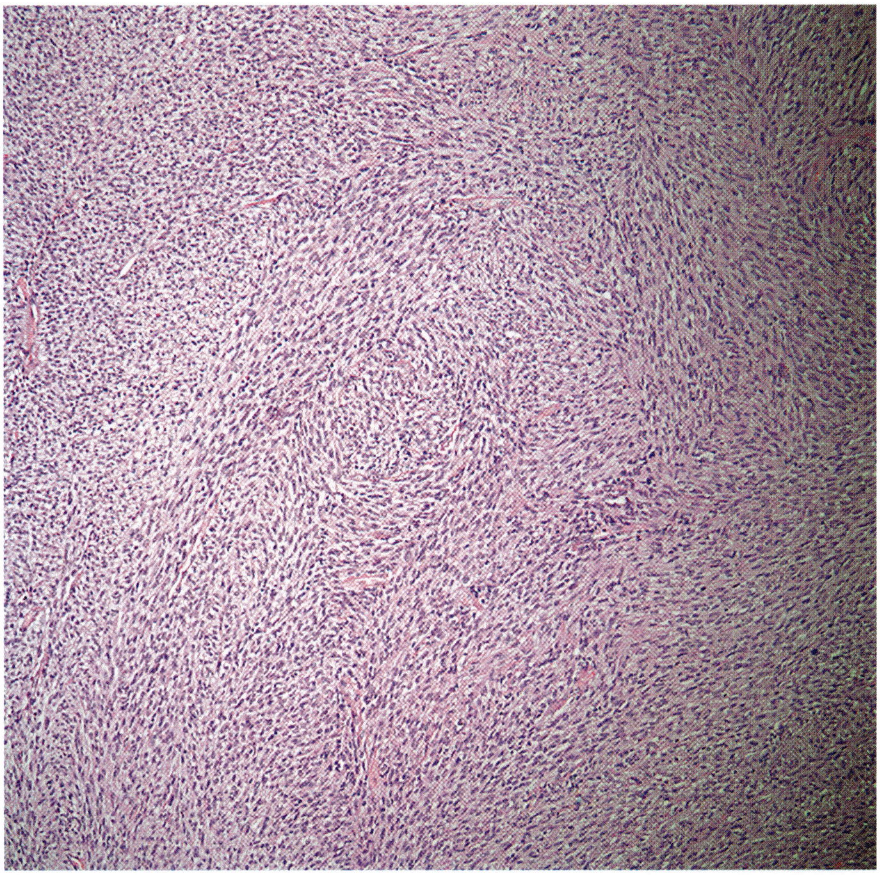

Figure 7-8 Intermediate-power view of a pulmonary leiomyoma showing a spindle cell proliferation. Necrosis and cellular pleomorphism are absent.

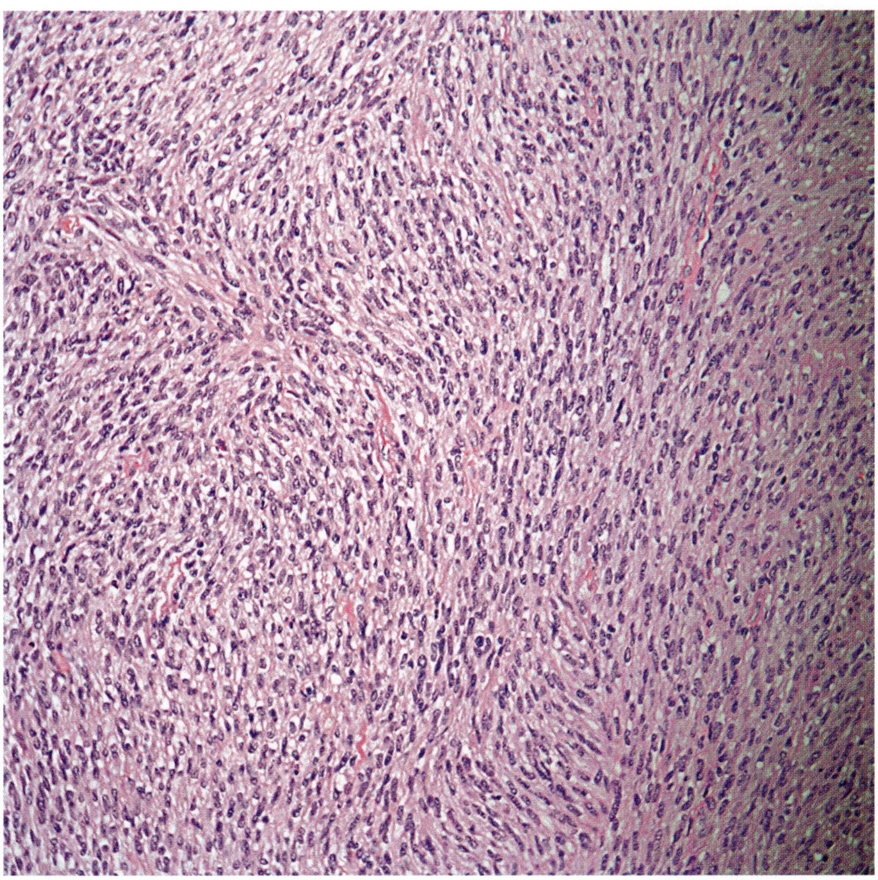

Figure 7-9 High-power view of a pulmonary leiomyoma showing absence of nuclear atypia and mitotic activity.

Differential Diagnosis

The most important consideration in the differential diagnosis is metastatic disease, either from a uterine leiomyoma (i.e., benign metastasizing leiomyoma) or from a leiomyosarcoma. In both of those instances, a good clinical history or physical examination will lead to the correct interpretation. Primary pulmonary leiomyosarcoma also should be considered, mainly in cases in which limited biopsy material is available for evaluation. Another important diagnostic possibility is primary benign neural tumor (schwannoma). In this setting, the use of other stains, including those for S-100 protein and neurofilament protein, may aid in arriving at a correct interpretation.

Treatment and Prognosis

The treatment of choice is complete surgical resection, which is curative. The surgical approach for these tumors may vary, depending on their location. Intraparenchymal tumors are more amenable to a conservative approach because these tumors “shell out” easily. Endobronchial tumors may be more challenging to resect conservatively, and in some cases, lobectomy or even pneumonectomy has been necessary.

Leiomyosarcoma

Primary leiomyosarcomas of the lung are rare; however, they are more common than their benign counterparts (leiomyomas). Essentially the same principles are applied to the diagnosis of these tumors; a careful clinical history and physical examination are necessary to rule out metastatic disease. The diagnostic criteria are similar to those for soft tissue leiomyosarcomas. Most of the information regarding pulmonary leiomyosarcomas has been presented as single case reports[21,43–61] or short series of cases,[31,62,63] with only a few larger series.[64,65] In some reported series, however, pulmonary leiomyosarcomas have been included in the general context of smooth muscle tumors[21,31] or with other sarcomas, such as fibrosarcomas.[64]

Clinical Features

Primary leiomyosarcomas in the lung are more common in adult patients; however, several cases occurring in children as young as newborns also have been described.[66–69] These tumors may appear as intraparenchymal masses or may arise in an endobronchial location. Clinical signs and symptoms may be related to the anatomic location of the tumor. Patients with tumors in a central location may present with symptoms of bronchial obstruction, including cough, shortness of breath, chest pain, and hemoptysis. Patients with peripheral tumors may present with more systemic complaints such as weight loss, or they may be completely asymptomatic, with the tumor discovered on a routine chest radiograph. Other presenting manifestations may include clubbing of the fingers, pleural effusion,[61] or Pancoast tumor.[49] A unique case of a renin-producing leiomyosarcoma has been reported.[70] On radiologic evaluation, no specific diagnostic hallmarks for leiomyosarcomas in the lung have been recognized.[71]

Macroscopic Features

Tumor size may range from 1 cm to more than 10 cm in greatest dimension. Intraparenchymal tumors appear to be well-demarcated masses that may be encapsulated or surrounded by a thin covering of fibroconnective tissue. The cut surface may appear a bit “whorly” and whitish, with a firm consistency (Fig. 7-10). Areas of hemorrhage and necrosis may be seen, and it is important to document such findings. Endobronchial tumors may manifest as pedunculated masses or may be firmly adherent to the bronchial wall. They are smaller than intraparenchymal tumors but may have the same gross features in terms of necrosis and hemorrhage.

Histopathologic Features

The morphologic features of primary leiomyosarcomas of the lung are similar to those seen in soft tissue tumors. The microscopic appearance is characterized by a spindle cellular proliferation arranged in broad fascicles of tumor cells that intersect at right angles, replacing normal lung parenchyma or protruding into the bronchial lumen. The cells have light eosinophilic cytoplasm, elongated “cigar-shaped”nuclei, and inconspicuous nucleoli. On the basis of their cytoarchitectural features, pulmonary leiomyosarcomas have been separated into three distinct histologic grades[65]:

- **Low-grade leiomyosarcomas:** Tumors are composed of a spindle cell proliferation, which on higher magnification shows mild cytologic atypia and a mitotic count of 1 to 3 mitotic figures per 10 high-power fields (Figs. 7-11 to 7-13). Cellular pleomorphism and hemorrhage and necrosis are absent.

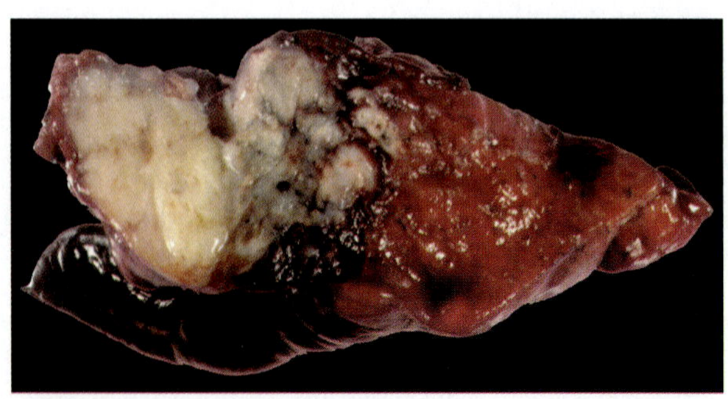

Figure 7-10 Pulmonary leiomyosarcoma, gross specimen, with focal areas of hemorrhage and necrosis.

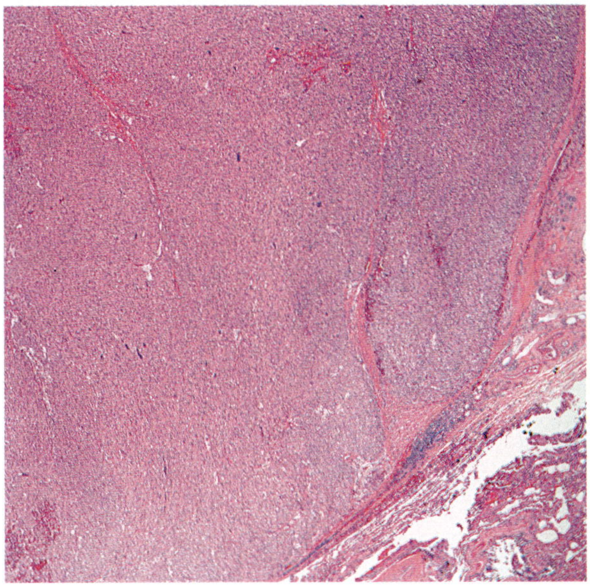

Figure 7-11 Low-grade pulmonary leiomyosarcoma. A spindle cell proliferation can be seen replacing lung parenchyma.

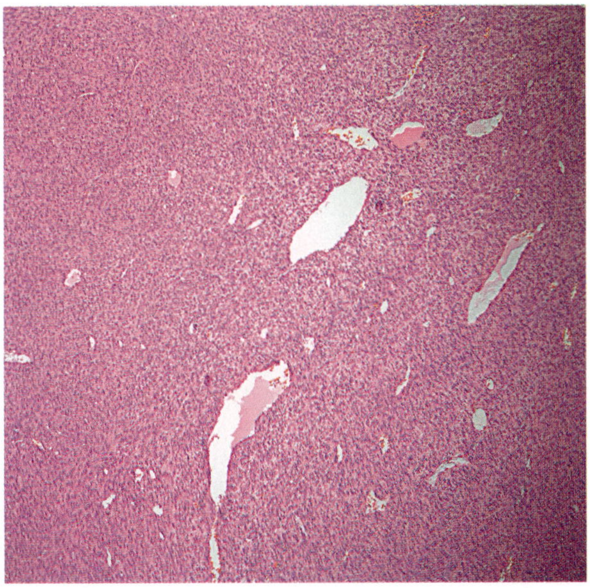

Figure 7-12 Low-grade pulmonary leiomyosarcoma with ectatic vessels.

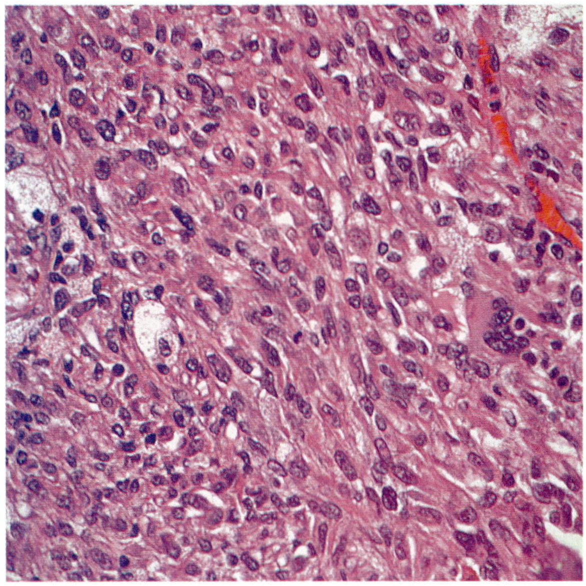

Figure 7-13 High-power view of a low-grade leiomyosarcoma showing mild nuclear atypia and scattered mitotic figures.

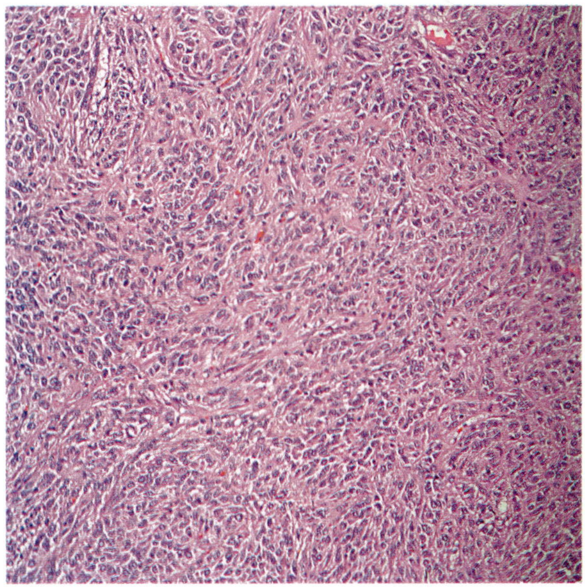

Figure 7-14 Intermediate-grade leiomyosarcoma with more obvious cellular atypia.

- **Intermediate-grade leiomyosarcoma:** The fascicular pattern of growth is preserved; however, the tumors show more prominent cellularity and increased mitotic activity in the range of 4 to 8 mitotic figures per 10 high-power fields (Figs. 7-14 to 7-16). Cytologic atypia is present but not marked, and occasionally, pleomorphic cells may be present. Necrosis and hemorrhage are absent.
- **High-grade leiomyosarcoma:** A more solid spindle cell proliferation is displayed, with areas still preserving the fascicular pattern of growth, which may acquire a storiform or hemangiopericytic pattern. Areas of necrosis or hemorrhage are readily identified. Degenerative changes, such as myxoid change and stromal hyalinization, can be seen. Cellular pleomorphism is marked, with larger cells that have prominent nucleoli; mitotic figures are easily identified and number more than 8 per 10 high-power fields (Figs. 7-17 to 7-21). In some cases, vascular invasion is identified.

Immunohistochemical Features

The tumor cells show positive staining for smooth muscle actin, desmin, and vimentin. As the tumor loses

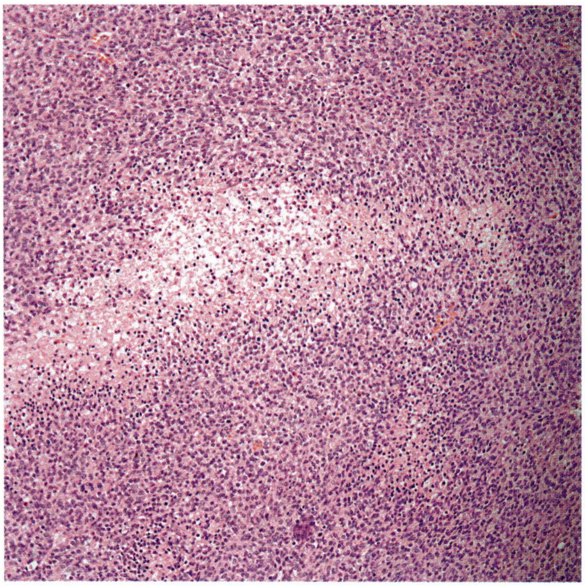

Figure 7-15 Intermediate-grade leiomyosarcoma showing a focal infarcted area.

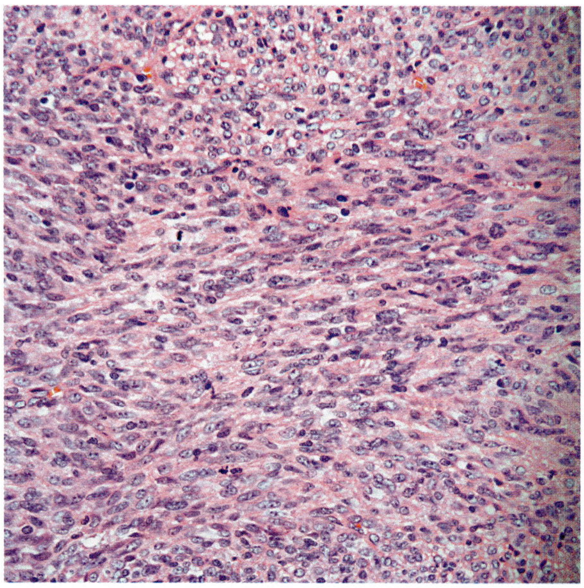

Figure 7-16 Intermediate-grade leiomyosarcoma with readily identifiable mitotic figures.

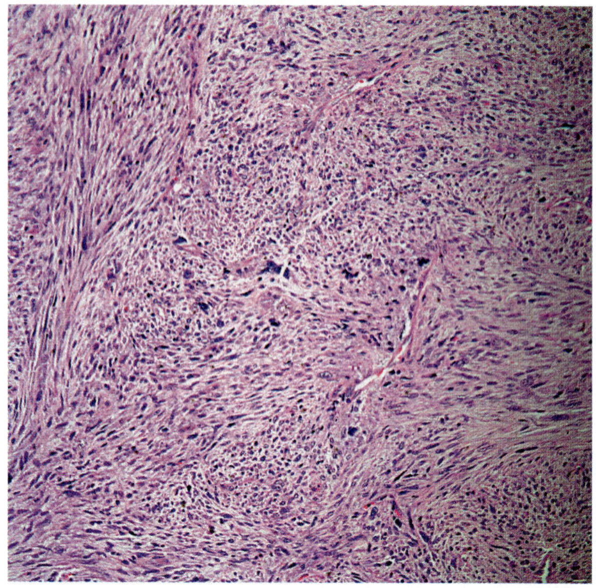

Figure 7-17 High-grade leiomyosarcoma with marked cellular atypia.

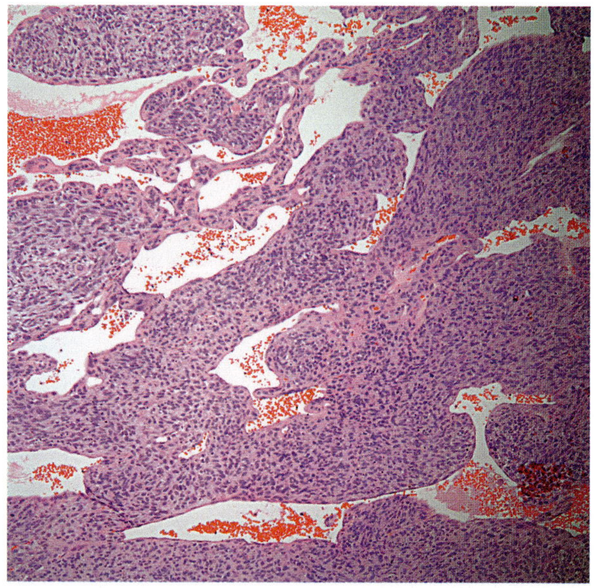

Figure 7-18 High-grade leiomyosarcoma with a hemangiopericytic pattern.

differentiation, however, variability in the staining pattern for these muscle markers may be noted. In high-grade tumors, the staining may be only focal, whereas in low-grade tumors, the staining may be stronger and diffuse. Leiomyosarcomas also may coexpress positive staining for keratin antibodies, so a wider than usual panel of immunohistochemical studies will be necessary to properly evaluate these neoplasms.

Molecular Studies

Schneider and associates[72] reported a case of a primary pulmonary leiomyosarcoma in a child. Karyotypic studies demonstrated consistent abnormalities of chromosomes 1, 5, 6, and 7; relative gain of chromosomes 2 and 11; and relative loss of chromosomes 9, 19, 20, and 22.

Differential Diagnosis

One of the most important considerations in the differential diagnosis is metastatic disease. The only way to distinguish between primary and metastatic disease is by careful analysis of findings on the clinical history and physical examination. On morphologic grounds, other spindle cell sarcomas may enter into the differential diagnosis, including monophasic synovial sarcoma, intrapulmonary solitary

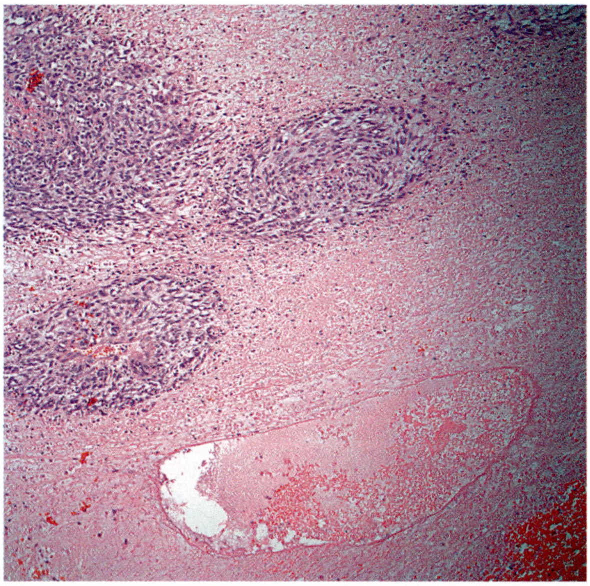

Figure 7-19 High-grade leiomyosarcoma with extensive areas of necrosis.

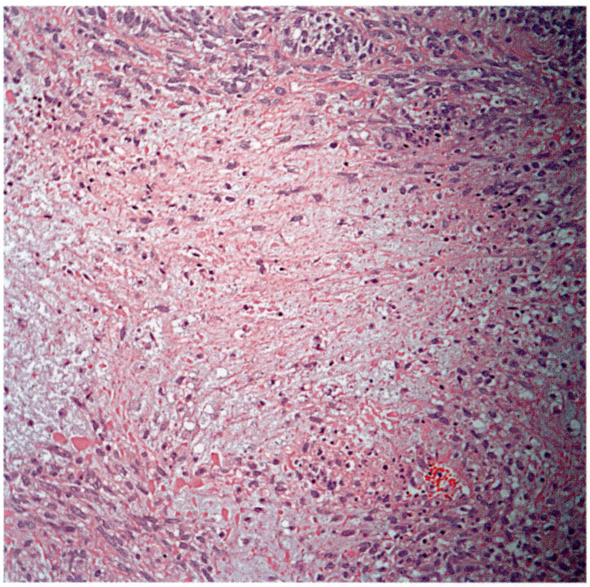

Figure 7-20 High-grade leiomyosarcoma showing myxoid changes.

fibrous tumor, and neurogenic sarcoma. In this setting, positive immunostaining for muscle markers (smooth muscle actin and desmin) and negative staining for S-100 protein and CD34 should indicate the correct interpretation. In high-grade tumors, pleomorphic carcinoma may enter into the differential diagnosis. Although pleomorphic carcinoma also may show focal staining for actin, it usually does not show positive staining for desmin and negative staining for keratin. In the same context, malignant melanoma also may be a consideration; the use of S-100 protein, HMB-45, and Melan A may be helpful in these cases.

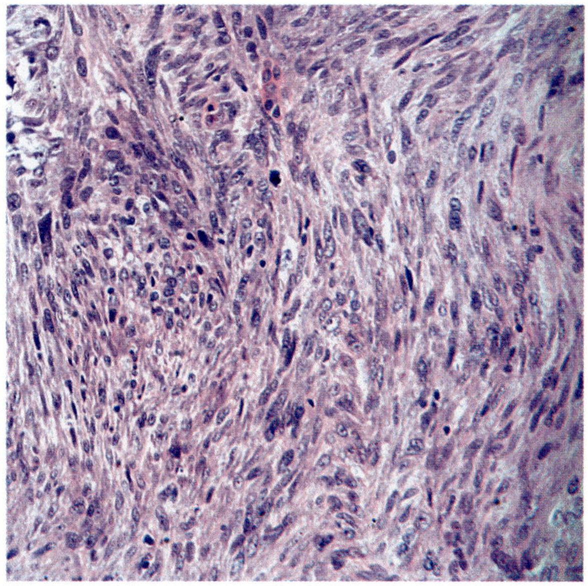

Figure 7-21 High-grade leiomyosarcoma showing mitotic figures and nuclear atypia.

Treatment and Prognosis

The initial treatment for patients with pulmonary leiomyosarcoma usually is surgical excision of the tumor. Once that is accomplished, the patient may be a candidate for adjuvant treatment (e.g., chemotherapy, immnotherapy, radiotherapy), depending on the clinical details of the case. Tumor size and degree of differentiation are important factors in determining prognosis. Tumors of low-grade malignancy may follow a more protracted course, whereas those of high-grade malignancy may exhibit more aggressive behavior. Widespread metastatic disease with spread to adjacent organs or viscera has been documented. In some cases of high histologic grade, fatal outcome within a 24-month period has been documented.[65]

Rhabdomyosarcoma

Primary pulmonary rhabdomyosarcomas are exceedingly rare in the adult population. Rhabdomyosarcoma may be encountered as a component of another neoplasm, such as carcinosarcoma; the tumor in its pure form is rare. Nevertheless, it has been described in adults as well as in children.[73–84] Some of the pediatric cases have been reported as cystic, raising the possibility that they may belong in the spectrum of pleuropulmonary blastomas.

Adult patients may present with clinical signs and symptoms of bronchial obstruction, including chest pain, shortness of breath, hemoptysis, and weight loss. These tumors may occur in a central or peripheral anatomic location, and tumor size may be more than 10 cm in greatest dimension.

Histopathologic Features

The tumors described in the adult population have been characterized by a closely packed spindle cell proliferation, arranged in fascicles and alternating with areas of discohesive cellular proliferation (Fig. 7-22). The spindle cell proliferation is arranged in a storiform pattern, and areas of necrosis and hemorrhage are readily identified (Figs. 7-23 and 7-24). At high magnification, the neoplastic cells can be seen to have moderate amounts of eosinophilic cytoplasm, oval nuclei, and, in some cells, prominent nucleoli (Figs. 7-25 to 7-27). Areas showing extensive pleomorphism with atypical mitotic figures are readily identified, as well as numerous rhabdomyoblasts (Fig. 7-28). Cross-striations are present in some cases, although they may be difficult to identify.

Immunohistochemical Features

The use of immunohistochemical studies, including staining for muscle markers, may aid in the diagnosis of rhabdomyosarcoma. Desmin, myoglobin, caldesmon, and myo-D are important markers that may show different staining patterns. The use of a wider panel of stains is important, however, because some tumors may show a stronger reaction with one or more of these markers. Rhabdomyosarcomas also may coexpress keratin positivity—hence the importance of expanding the panel of immunohistochemical studies performed.

Differential Diagnosis

Because of the rarity of primary rhabdomyosarcomas in the lung, considerations in the differential diagnosis should include other primary tumors of different histogenesis that may show the same pleomorphic features. The most important diagnostic consideration is pleomorphic carcinoma, an epithelial tumor that may show extensive areas of cellular pleomorphism, necrosis, hemorrhage, and spindle cell component. Pleomorphic carcinomas will not show positive staining for desmin, myoglobin, caldesmon, or myo-D, although they may show staining for smooth muscle actin. Another important diagnostic entity to consider is primary rhabdoid carcinoma of the lung. Rhabdoid carcinoma, as its name implies, usually shows a cellular proliferation that may closely resemble that of rhabdomyoblastic differentiation. Once again, staining for muscle markers—desmin, myoglobin, caldesmon, or myo-D—generally is negative in these tumors, whereas staining for keratin shows strong positive reaction in tumor

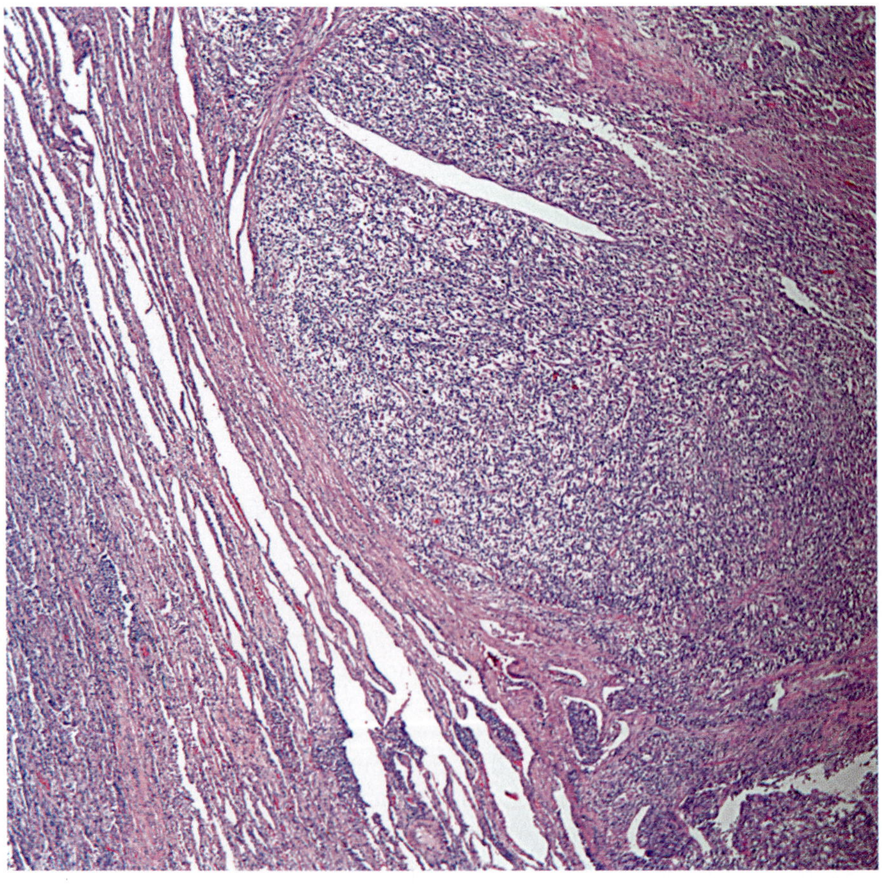

Figure 7-22 Low-power view of a pulmonary rhabdomyosarcoma. A pleomorphic spindle cell tumor can be seen replacing lung parenchyma.

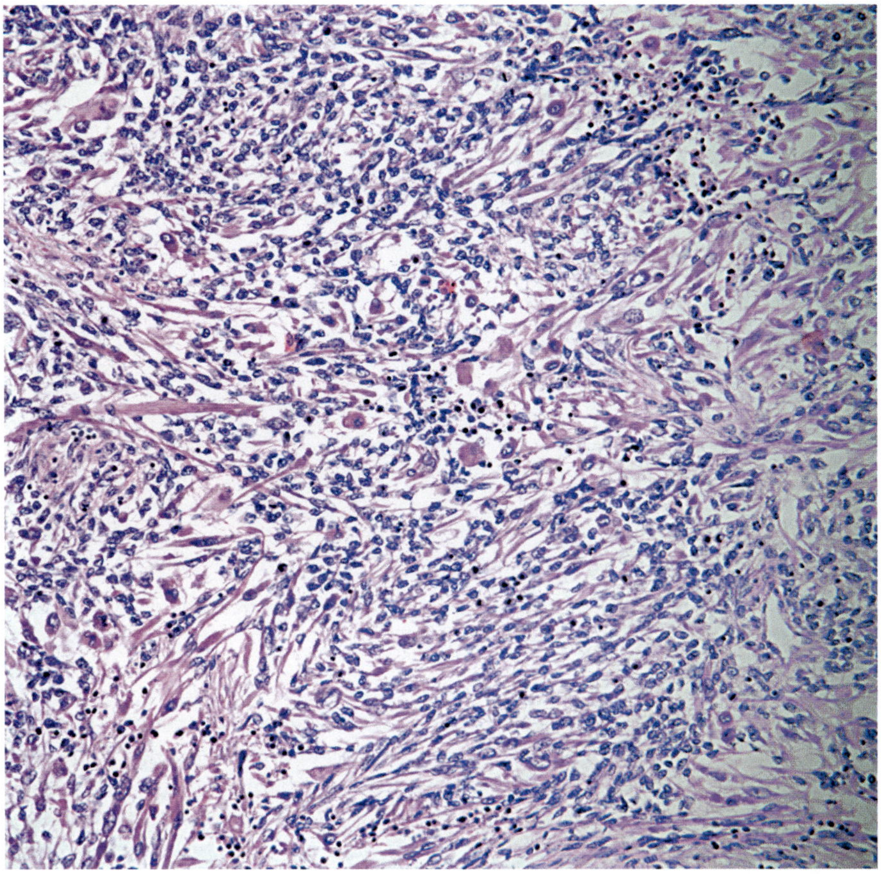

Figure 7-23 Rhabdomyosarcoma showing a mixture of spindle cells with numerous rhabdomyoblasts.

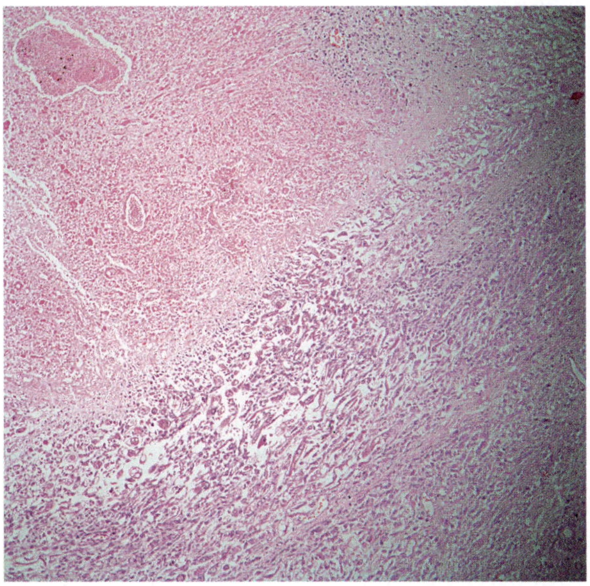

Figure 7-24 Rhabdomyosarcoma with extensive areas of necrosis.

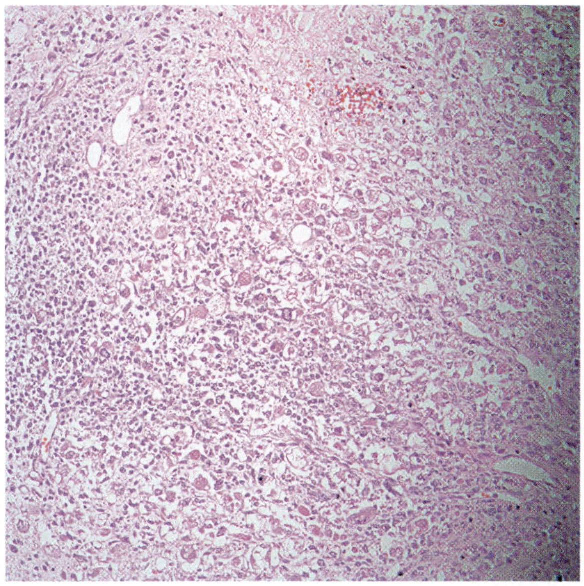

Figure 7-25 Rhabdomyosarcoma with degenerative areas and a spindle cell component.

cells. Because of the prominent spindle cell proliferation seen in pleomorphic rhabdomyosarcomas, other spindle cell sarcomas also should be considered in the differential diagnosis. In this setting, the use of a wider panel of antibodies should lead to a more accurate interpretation.

Treatment and Prognosis

The treatment for most primary rhabdomyosarcomas of the lung is complete surgical resection, followed by chemotherapy. In most of the published cases, the outcome

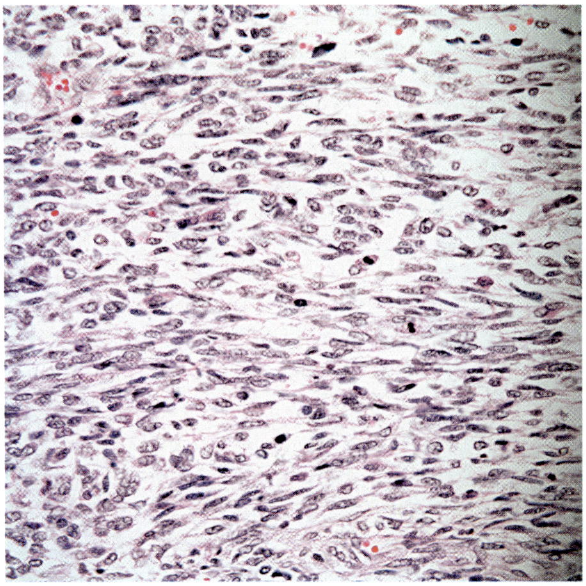

Figure 7-26 Rhabdomyosarcoma with a prominent spindle cell component. Note the presence of numerous mitotic figures.

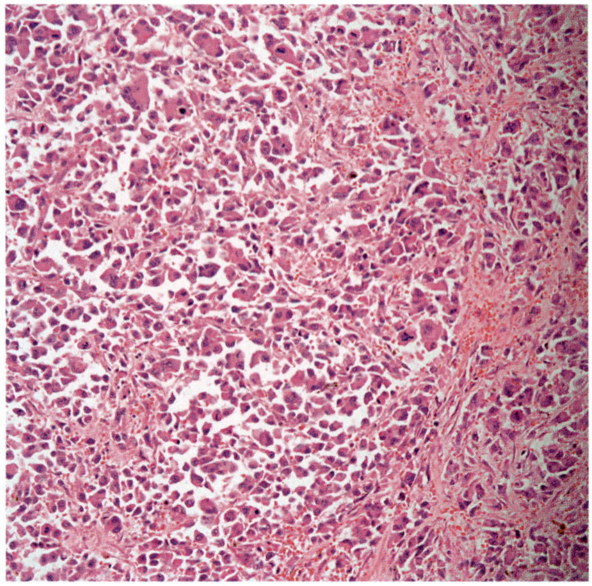

Figure 7-28 Rhabdomyosarcoma with marked cellular pleomorphism and mitotic activity.

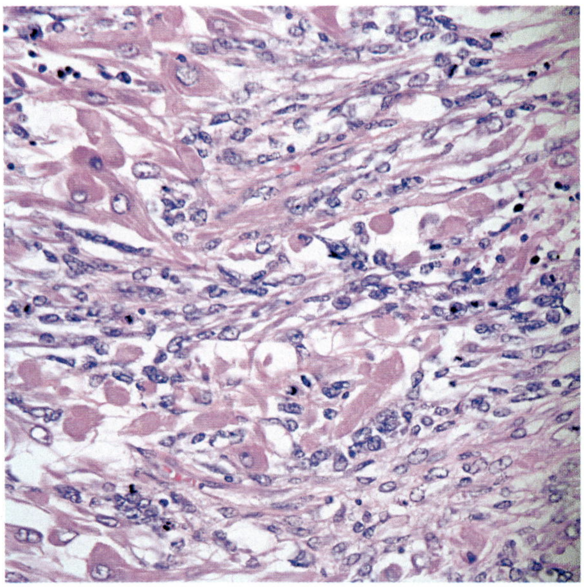

Figure 7-27 At higher magnification, the rhabdomyoblastic component is readily apparent in this rhabdomyosarcoma.

has been death, despite aggressive treatment, in as little as 24 months. Therefore, every effort should be made to obtain early diagnosis and accurate classification of these neoplasms.

TUMORS WITH PROMINENT FIBROBLASTIC COMPONENT

Tumors that show a prominent fibroblastic component are of varied histology and may include the entire spectrum of differentiation, ranging from benign to high-grade malignancy. Although these tumors are rarely encountered as primary lung neoplasms, it is important to include them as possibilities in the differential diagnosis for spindle cell tumors of the lung. Owing to advances in immunohistochemical studies and molecular techniques, some tumors that used to be classified as common, such as pulmonary fibrosarcoma, are now considered to be tumors of unusual occurrence. These changes have had a positive impact not only on diagnosis and classification of these rare tumors but also on the treatment of affected patients.

Some of the tumors that are discussed in this section also may be classified as biphasic tumors (adenofibromas), because they also may show some epithelial component in addition to the usual fibroblastic component; however, because of the prominence of their spindle cell fibroblastic component, they are included here. Similar claims can be made for hemangiopericytoma, which traditionally has been considered to be a vascular tumor; however, other lung tumors also may show a striking hemangiopericytic pattern, making this particular entity very difficult to diagnose as a primary lung tumor. It also shares immunohistochemical features with other tumors, especially with the intrapulmonary solitary fibrous tumor. Therefore, these tumors are grouped by histopathologic growth patterns, rather than similar histogenesis, which remains a matter of debate. The following tumors are discussed:

- Pulmonary adenofibroma
- Fibrosarcoma
- Intrapulmonary solitary fibrous tumor
- Hemangiopericytoma
- Monophasic synovial sarcoma

Pulmonary Adenofibroma

Pulmonary adenofibroma was described in 1993 as a glandular and spindle cell proliferation closely resembling adenofibromas of the genital tract and ovary.[85] The reporting investigators thought that these tumors might be benign hamartomatous lesions and alluded to at least two different cases in which different terminology might have been used for the same neoplasm.[86,87] In one of the previously described cases, the tumor was an incidental finding at autopsy and the stated diagnosis was fibroadenoma, owing to its close resemblance to similar tumors in the breast.[86] The other case belonged to a series of pulmonary hamartomas.[87] Therefore, it is possible that adenofibromas represent a variant of pulmonary hamartoma, without the presence of cartilage or adipose tissue.

Clinical Features

Adenofibromas occur in adults, who may be completely asymptomatic, with discovery of the pulmonary nodule made incidentally during a routine radiographic examination. The lesions often are described as intrapulmonary "coin" lesions.

Macroscopic and Histopathologic Findings

Pulmonary adenofibromas usually are rather small tumors that measure approximately 1 or 2 cm in greatest dimension. They are well-circumscribed, intraparenchymal lesions, not related to airways, with a firm to rubbery consistency. On histologic examination, the tumors display a spindle cell proliferation composed of oval cells embedded in a sclerotic background and arranged in a papillary growth pattern, reminiscent of those described in müllerian adenofibromas (Figs. 7-29 to 7-31). The spindle cells show elongated nuclei and scant cytoplasm. Myxoid changes and inflammatory infiltrate may be seen focally; cellular atypia and mitotic activity generally are absent. The tumor also shows complex, branching spaces lined by an epithelium that is surrounded by cuboidal or columnar cells. In some areas, gland-like spaces lined by tall columnar epithelium also may be seen (Figs. 7-32 and 7-33).

Immunohistochemical Features

Adenofibromas usually stain positively for vimentin, with positive staining for keratin and epithelial membrane antigen (EMA) in the epithelial lining. Staining for other antibodies including those for actin, desmin, S-100 protein, and CD34 is negative.

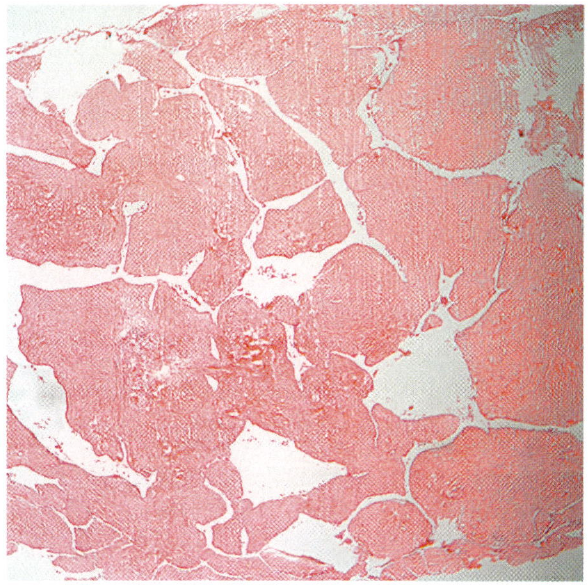

Figure 7-29 Pulmonary adenofibroma with a papillary-like pattern of growth.

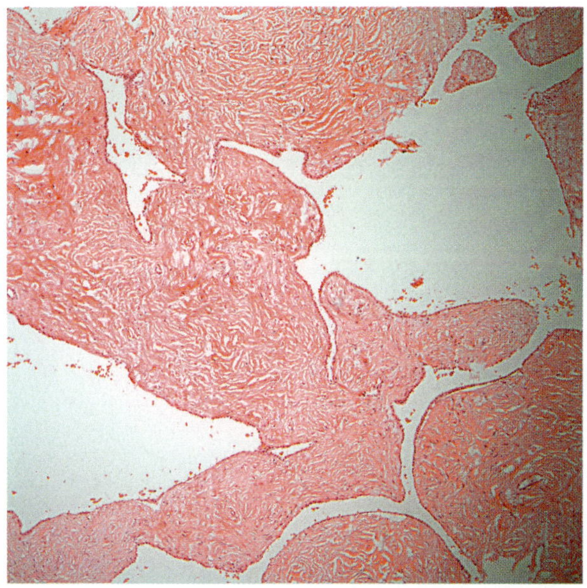

Figure 7-30 Pulmonary adenofibroma. Sclerotic areas lined by low cuboidal epithelium are visible.

Differential Diagnosis

Although the diagnosis of adenofibroma is straightforward, some malignant tumors that show a biphasic growth pattern may enter into the differential diagnosis, including pulmonary blastoma, carcinosarcoma, and biphasic synovial sarcoma. In these entities the spindle cell proliferation will show cellular atypia and mitotic activity, which generally is absent in pulmonary adenofibroma. In addition, negative staining for antibodies against keratin, EMA, S-100 protein, or Bcl-2 in the spindle cell component may provide valuable information in cases of synovial

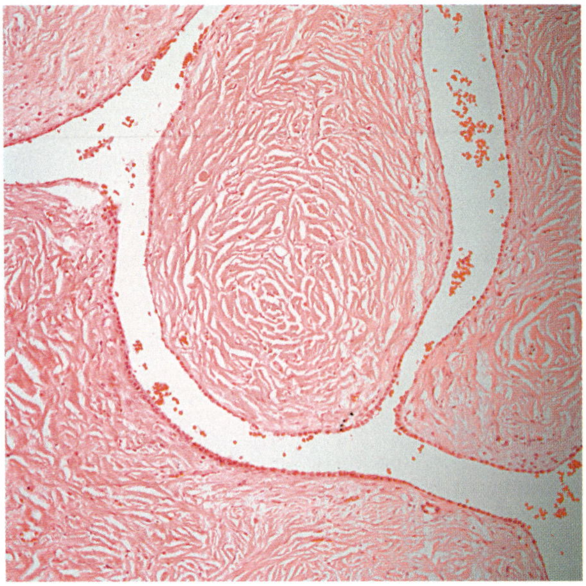

Figure 7-31 High-power view of a pulmonary adenofibroma showing marked sclerosis and a subtle spindle cell component of the stroma.

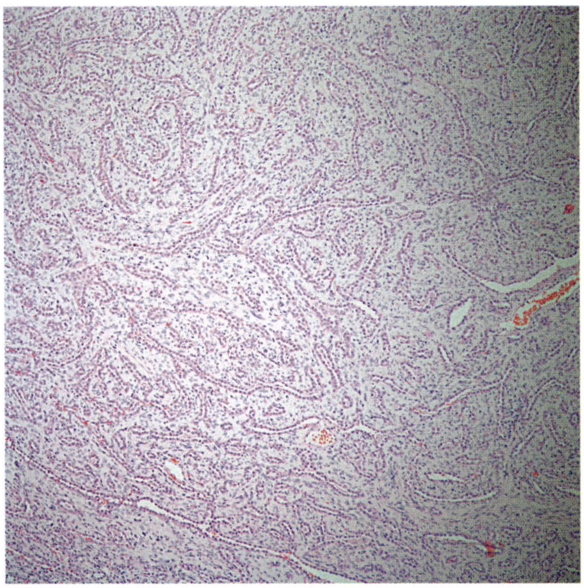

Figure 7-32 Pulmonary adenofibroma with a prominent glandular component.

sarcoma. Finally, the epithelial component of adenofibromas is benign and lacks atypia and mitotic activity, unlike that of blastoma or carcinosarcoma.

Treatment and Prognosis

Surgical resection by either tumor enucleation, wedge resection, or even lobectomy is the treatment of choice for adenofibromas. The clinical course of these tumors appears to be indolent; thus, complete surgical resection appears to be curative.

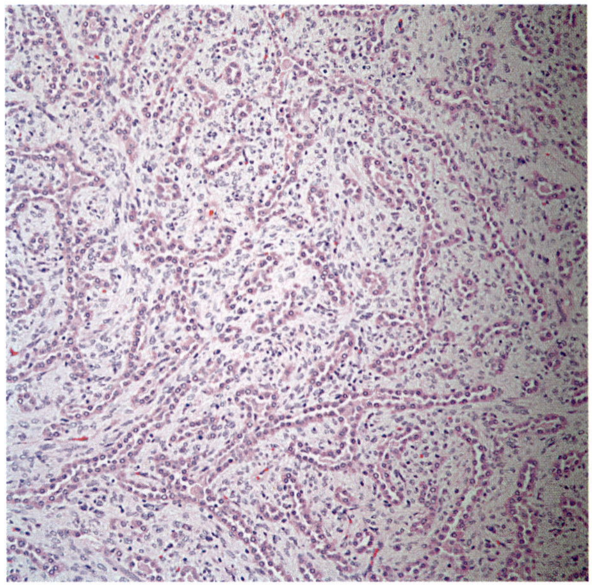

Figure 7-33 Pulmonary adenofibroma with glandular and stromal spindle cell components.

Fibrosarcoma

Fibrosarcomas represent a distinct tumor of rare occurrence, which in the past was claimed to be one of the most common sarcomas of the lung. With the use of immunohistochemical studies in current daily practice, however, it is possible that a good number of the cases previously reported as bronchopulmonary fibrosarcomas would now be classified as different neoplasms. In 1972, Guccion and Rossen[64] reported a study of 32 cases of primary pulmonary sarcomas in which they described 13 cases of bronchopulmonary fibrosarcoma and alluded to 48 previously reported cases. These tumors were separated by anatomic location into central and peripheral lesions; histologically, they appeared to range from low- to high-grade malignancy. The investigators noted similarities between fibrosarcomas with pleural involvement and what used to be called "localized fibrous mesothelioma" (currently classified as solitary fibrous tumors), citing their comparable behavior and metastatic potential. This analogy may have been the basis for the current term *intrapulmonary solitary fibrous tumor*.

Pettinato and colleagues[88] described five cases of bronchopulmonary fibrosarcoma, emphasizing the importance of separating this tumor from other sarcomas and linking it to the infantile fibrosarcoma of soft tissue. These workers also documented the indolent behavior displayed by some of these tumors and noted the possible difference in tumor behavior between pediatric and adult cases.

Clinical Features

Fibrosarcomas appear to affect people of all ages—they have been described in newborns, young children, adolescents, and older adults. No gender predilection has been recognized, nor any predilection for either lung or particular lung segment. Associated clinical signs and symptoms will depend largely on the anatomic location of the tumor and patient age at presentation. In young adults and in older persons with centrally located tumors, the clinical presentation may include shortness of breath, cough, chest pain, and hemoptysis, which are common findings in bronchial obstruction. Patients with peripheral tumors may be asymptomatic, and the tumor may be identified during a routine radiographic examination. Partial lung opacification may be seen on the chest film in some cases.

Macroscopic Features

The size of these tumors will depend on the anatomic location; tumors in a central location may be smaller than those in the periphery of the lung. In general, they have been described as ranging in size from 1 cm to more than 10 cm in greatest dimension. In a central location, the tumor may appear to obstruct the bronchial lumen and grow in a polypoid fashion, whereas intraparenchymal tumors may appear to be well circumscribed but not encapsulated. Regardless of their anatomic distribution, the tumors are firm to rubbery in consistency and whitish, and the cut surface may have a homogeneous, smooth appearance. Areas of necrosis or hemorrhage may be seen in high-grade tumors.

Histopathologic Features

The classic histopathologic description for fibrosarcoma is that of a spindle cell proliferation composed of elongated cells arranged in a herringbone-like pattern (Figs. 7-34 and 7-35). The spindle cells have scant cytoplasm, vesicular nuclei, granular chromatin, and inconspicuous nucleoli. The spindle cell proliferation is tightly packed, with little intercellular matrix (Fig. 7-36). Mitotic activity varies, with counts ranging from 2 or 3 (Fig. 7-37) to more than 10 mitotic figures per 10 high-power fields. Areas with extensive hyalinization, calcifications, and a discrete inflammatory infiltrate may be seen in some cases. Areas of necrosis are more common in high-grade tumors. Centrally located tumors are more likely to show features of low-grade histology, in contrast with the larger and more mitotically active peripheral tumors.

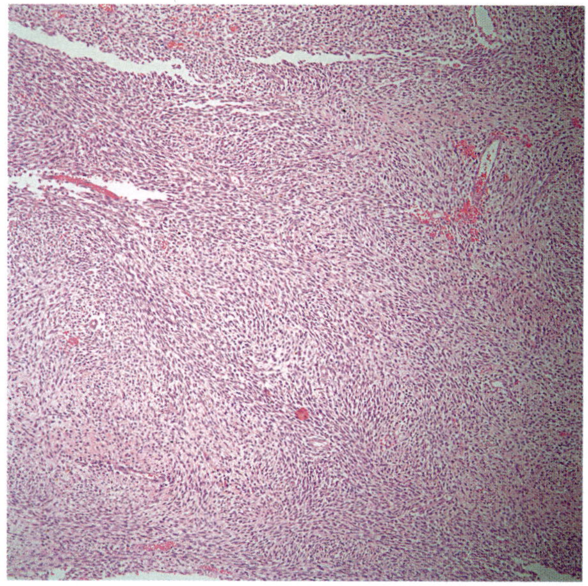

Figure 7-35 Pulmonary fibrosarcoma with a vague herringbone pattern.

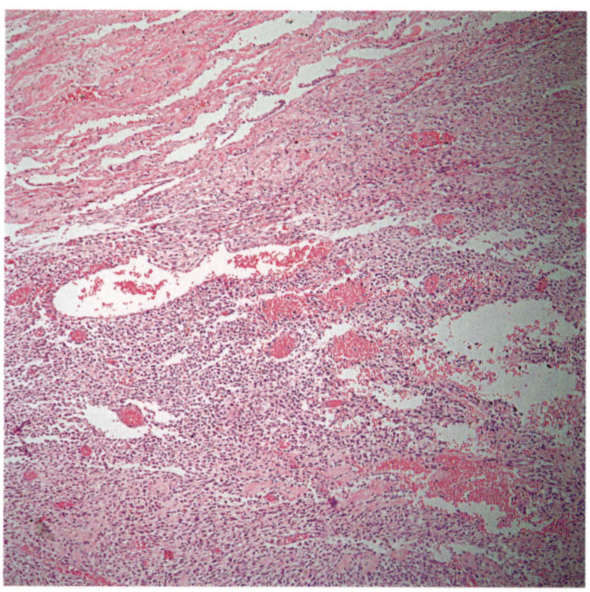

Figure 7-34 Low-power view of a pulmonary fibrosarcoma. Note the well-circumscribed tumor.

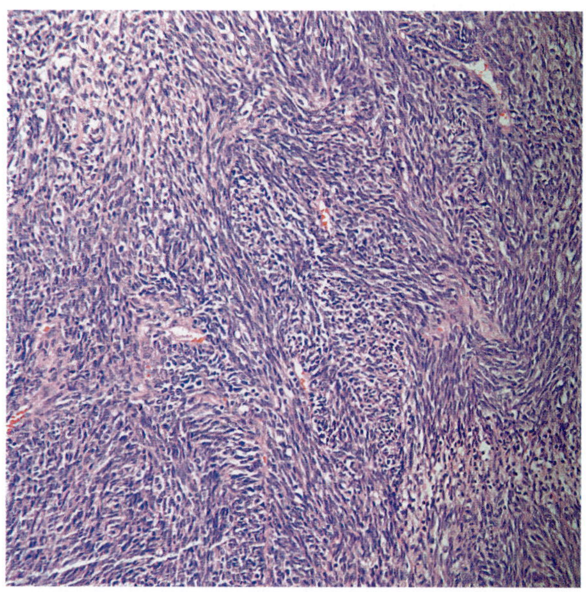

Figure 7-36 Pulmonary fibrosarcoma with an atypical spindle cell proliferation.

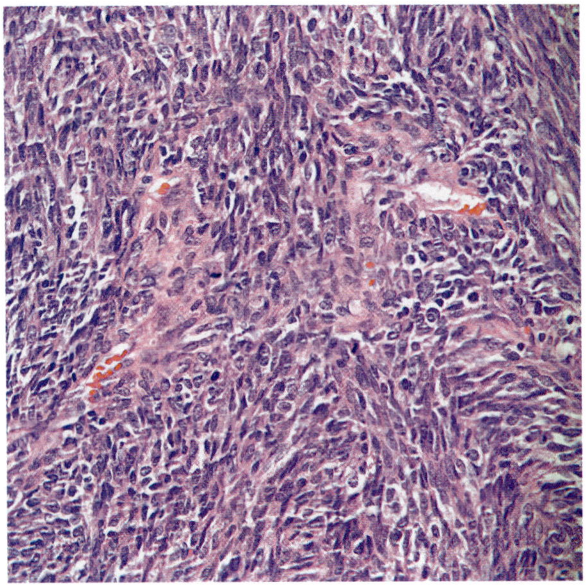

Figure 7-37 High-power view of a pulmonary fibrosarcoma showing nuclear atypia and mitotic figures.

Immunohistochemical Features

Because the histopathologic features described for bronchopulmonary fibrosarcoma also may be seen with intrapulmonary solitary fibrous tumor and synovial sarcoma, a battery of immunohistochemical staining procedures must be performed to accomplish proper histologic classification. The use of immunostains for keratin, EMA, CD34, Bcl-2, and vimentin is required. In cases of solitary fibrous tumor, CD34 and Bcl-2 may show positive staining, whereas keratin, EMA, and Bcl-2 may be of help in identifying synovial sarcoma. Vimentin will show positive staining in all of these tumors. When tumors of muscle origin enter into the differential diagnosis, the use of smooth muscle actin, desmin, or caldesmon may be of help. If immunohistochemical stains fail to identify the tumor with certainty, then molecular studies should be conducted, because synovial sarcomas are associated with a specific translocation that may aid in distinguishing them from fibrosarcoma. In essence, the diagnosis of fibrosarcoma in the lung has become one of exclusion.

Differential Diagnosis

As mentioned previously, the diagnosis of fibrosarcoma relies on distinguishing it from other tumors with similar histopathologic features, including monophasic synovial sarcoma, leiomyosarcoma, neurogenic sarcoma, and solitary fibrous tumor. The use of immunohistochemical studies is of great importance for accurate classification of these tumors.

Treatment and Prognosis

The treatment for fibrosarcoma is complete surgical resection, which may be followed by chemotherapy or radiation therapy, depending on the clinical circumstances. In the cases reported by Guccion and Rossen,[64] the tumors displayed aggressive clinical behavior, with development of metastatic disease within a period of 24 months. In the pediatric cases described by Pettinato and associates,[88] however, four of the children survived for periods ranging from 4 to 9 years. Accordingly, the investigators suggested that bronchopulmonary fibrosarcomas in children may carry a more favorable prognosis than that for tumors reported in adults.

Intrapulmonary Solitary Fibrous Tumor

Although solitary fibrous tumors of the pleura occur relatively frequently, their intrapulmonary counterparts are rather rare, and no sizable series of cases have been published thus far. A majority of the cases have been presented as individual case reports, and the histopathologic description has been that of a low-grade tumor with a low mitotic index. This observation raises the possibility that when this entity displays features of high-grade sarcoma, it may be classified as other than a "malignant" intrapulmonary solitary fibrous tumor.

Yousem and Flynn[89] are credited with the original description of these tumors in an intrapulmonary location. Their three cases represent the largest series reported to date, and the histopathologic features of these specimens resembled those of pleural solitary fibrous tumors. Subsequently, only a few additional case reports have been presented in the literature.[90–94]

Clinical Features

The tumor affects patients in various age groups, and although one pediatric case has been reported,[92] a majority of the cases appear to occur in adults. Patients may be completely asymptomatic, with the tumor identified during a routine radiographic examination, whereas others may present with nonspecific signs and symptoms such as cough, fatigue, and dyspnea. Hypoglycemia, a finding often encountered in pleural tumors, has not been reported in connection with intraparenchymal tumors. No predilection for gender, lung, or lung segment has been noted. On radiographic evaluation, some of these tumors have been described as "coin" lesions.

Macroscopic Features

The tumors appear to be well circumscribed, but not encapsulated, with no pleural involvement. Size may

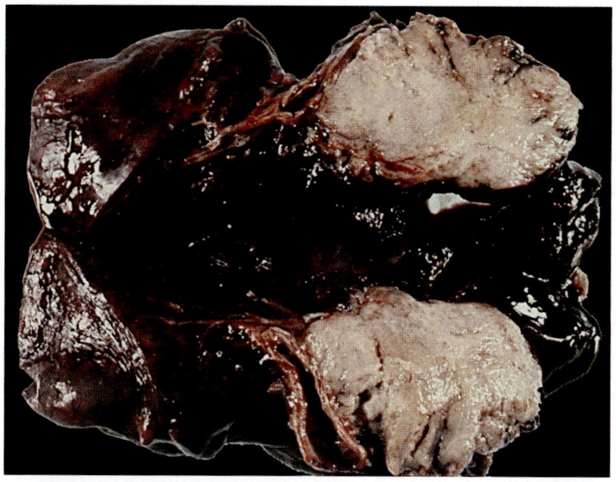

Figure 7-38 Intrapulmonary solitary fibrous tumor, gross specimen. The white tumor mass was firm in consistency and intraparenchymal in location. Note the viable airway.

range from 1 to 4 cm in greatest dimension. The tumors have been described as firm and white to gray in color, with a whorled appearance (Fig. 7-38). Areas of calcification may be seen. Focal areas of necrosis or hemorrhage have been observed in a few cases and may indicate a possibly higher-grade tumor.

Histopathologic Features

The basic histologic pattern in intraparenchymal tumors is the same as that described in pleural tumors. They may display hypo- and hypercellular areas with a spindle cell proliferation, which may adopt different histopathologic patterns, including the so-called patternless pattern and hemangiopericytic, neural, and angiofibromatous patterns. Areas of collagenization alternating with a spindle cell proliferation, composed of elongated, medium-sized cells with elongated nuclei and inconspicuous nucleoli in different proportions, are common features in these tumors (Figs. 7-39 to 7-44). The presence of different growth patterns within the same tumor is an indication that intrapulmonary solitary fibrous tumor may be the correct diagnosis. Although the histopathologic characteristics described in published cases have been similar to those of conventional solitary fibrous tumors with low or absent mitotic activity and absent necrosis and hemorrhage, numerous cases encountered in our own experience displayed the histopathologic features of malignant solitary fibrous tumors (unpublished data), including areas of increased mitotic activity (Figs. 7-45 and 7-46), necrosis, or hemorrhage. The spectrum of histopathologic features may be similar to that described for pleural tumors. An important feature of intrapulmonary solitary fibrous tumors is the presence of entrapped alveolar epithelium, which in some cases may mimic a biphasic lung neoplasm.

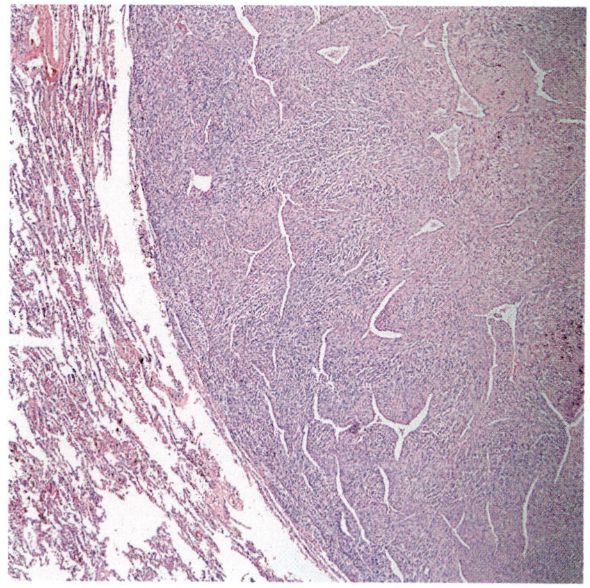

Figure 7-39 Low-power view of an intrapulmonary solitary fibrous tumor.

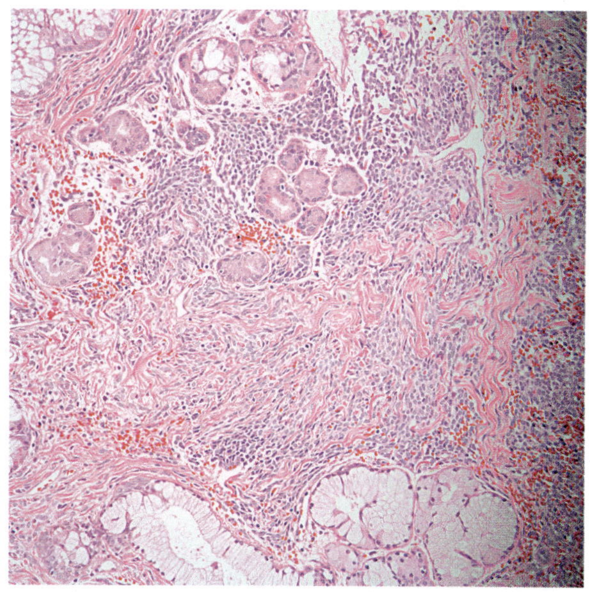

Figure 7-40 Intrapulmonary solitary fibrous tumor dissecting submucosal glands.

Immunohistochemical Features

Like their counterparts in the pleura, intrapulmonary solitary fibrous tumors will display positive staining for CD34 (Fig. 7-47), vimentin, and Bcl-2 (Fig. 7-48), whereas staining for keratin, actin, desmin, and S-100 protein is negative in the spindle cell component. In one of the reported cases,[93] the investigators performed genetic studies disclosing that the tumor was negative for *HMGA1* and *HMGA2* (high mobility group AT-hook 1 and 2) translocations.

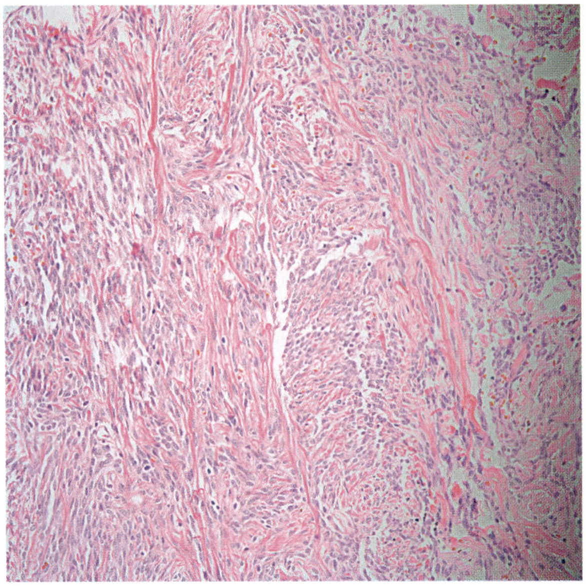

Figure 7-41 Intrapulmonary solitary fibrous tumor. A spindle cell proliferation is admixed with areas of prominent collagen deposition.

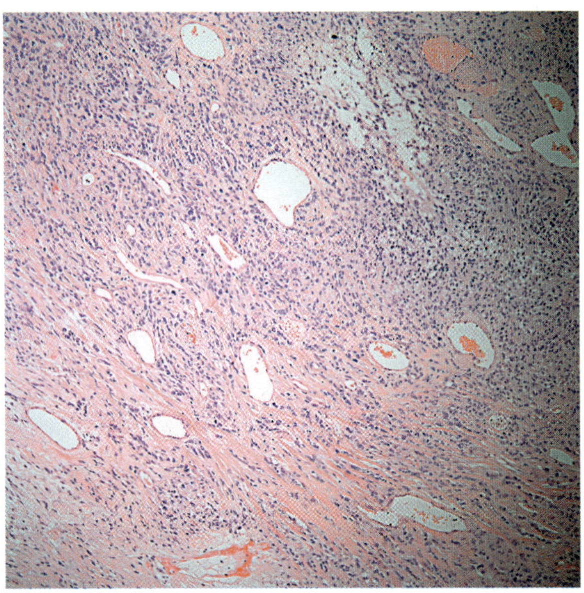

Figure 7-42 Intrapulmonary solitary fibrous tumor with a hemangiopericytic pattern.

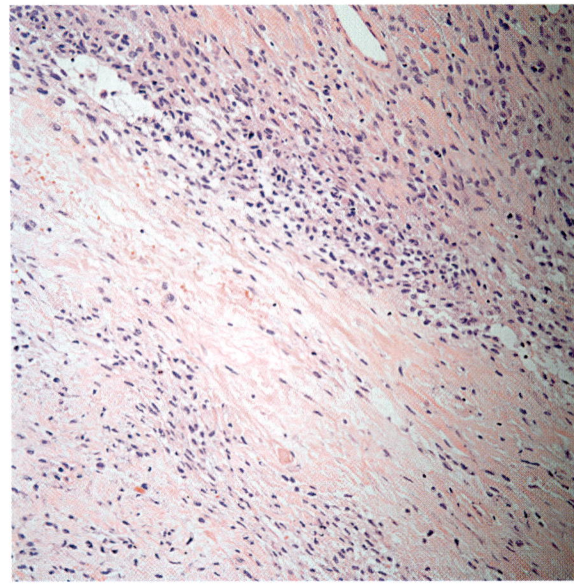

Figure 7-43 Intrapulmonary solitary fibrous tumor. Both hypo- and hypercellular areas are present.

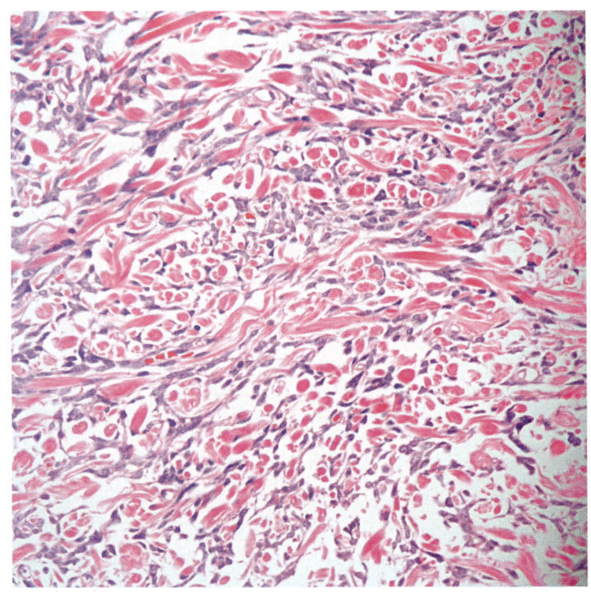

Figure 7-44 Intrapulmonary solitary fibrous tumor. The classic rope-like collagen is readily seen.

Differential Diagnosis

The most important consideration in the differential diagnosis is other spindle cell sarcomas—namely, fibrosarcoma and monophasic synovial sarcoma. Use of a panel of immunohistochemical stains may help with proper classification. It is vital to distinguish these tumors from other, higher-grade neoplasms, because the treatment for intrapulmonary solitary fibrous tumors is different from that for high-grade tumors. The presence of low mitotic activity, coupled with the positive staining pattern with use of CD34 and Bcl-2 and negative staining for epithelial markers including keratin and EMA, should lead to the correct interpretation.

Treatment and Prognosis

No large series with long follow-up have been presented, so the natural course of these tumors is unknown. In a majority of cases, the treatment has been complete surgical resection, with an uneventful postoperative course. The follow-up period has been short, however, and the histologic features described have been characteristic of benign or low-grade tumors with low mitotic activity.

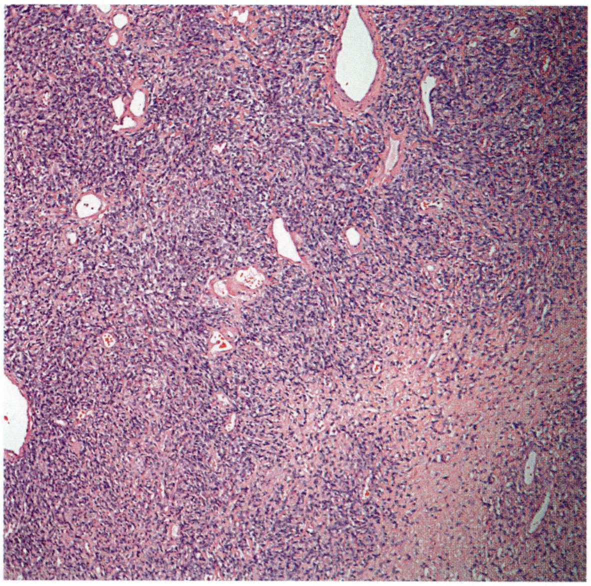

Figure 7-45 Intrapulmonary malignant solitary fibrous tumor. The hypercellular areas demonstrate marked cellular atypia.

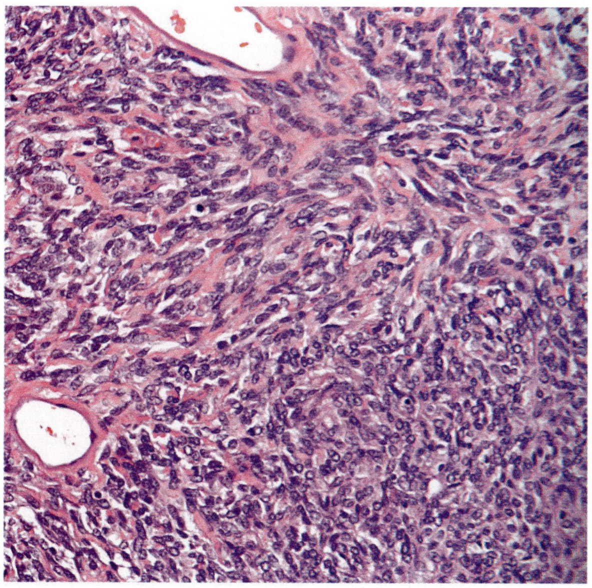

Figure 7-46 High-power view of an intrapulmonary malignant solitary fibrous tumor showing mitotic activity.

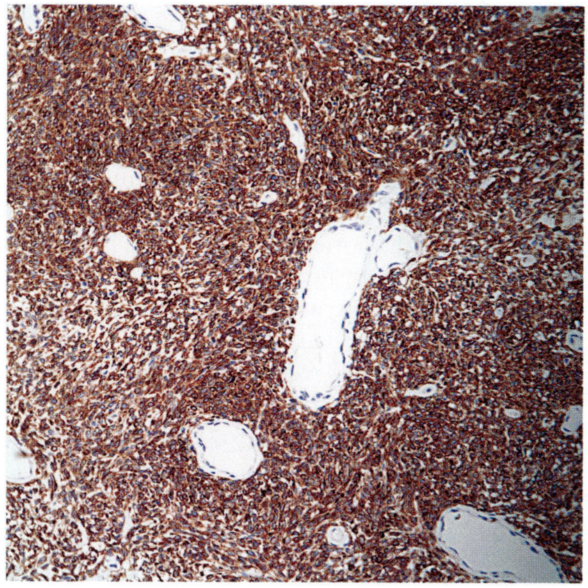

Figure 7-47 Solitary fibrous tumor. CD34 immunohistochemical staining produced a strong positive reaction in tumor cells.

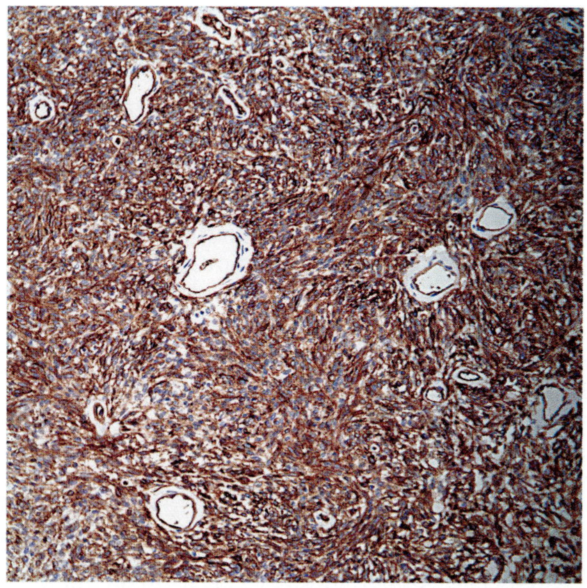

Figure 7-48 Solitary fibrous tumor. Bcl-2 immunohistochemical staining produced a strong positive reaction in tumor cells.

In cases in which the histologic pattern is similar to that of a high-grade sarcoma, surgical resection of the tumor may be followed by adjuvant treatment (e.g., chemotherapy, immunotherapy, radiotherapy).

Hemangiopericytoma

Whether hemangiopericytomas truly exist in the lung parenchyma has been a subject of controversy. Some investigators argue that many tumors may show a hemangiopericytic-like pattern of growth, and that in the lung, "hemangiopericytoma" may occur only as a growth pattern, rather than as a specific entity. The overlap of immunophenotype with that of other tumors, including the solitary fibrous tumor, which may show a hemangiopericytic growth pattern, has raised other issues regarding the validity of classifying hemangiopericytomas as a true clinicopathologic entity. Nevertheless, hemangiopericytomas have rarely been described as primary pulmonary neoplasms.[95,96]

In 1974, Meade and associates[95] reported 4 cases and analyzed the current literature, accumulating 24 additional cases of hemangiopericytoma that presumably had arisen in the lung parenchyma as a primary neoplasm. These investigators divided the hemangiopericytomas into benign and malignant tumors but also noted their lack of uniformity in appearance and growth. In 1987, Yousem and Hochholzer[96] reported the largest series of pulmonary hemangiopericytomas to date, describing 18 cases that were morphologically similar to soft tissue tumors. Although these workers separated the tumors into benign, undetermined, and malignant categories, they did not find any correlation between histologic pattern and clinical behavior except for the size of the tumor (>8 cm). To date, no large series of pulmonary hemangiopericytomas, detailing a longer follow-up period and additional immunohistochemical analysis, has been published to confirm or deny the existence of hemangiopericytoma in the lung. Nevertheless, the hemangiopericytic pattern commonly is seen as a growth pattern with several different tumors.

Clinical Features

Hemangiopericytomas have been described in young and older adults, without predilection for either lung or any lung segment. In the analysis of Meade and colleagues,[95] the tumor was reported more often in female patients, whereas Yousem and Hochholzer[96] did not find any gender predilection. The tumor appears to be more common among patients in the fifth decade of life, and patients may be completely asymptomatic or may present with nonspecific signs and symptoms such as cough, shortness of breath, and hemoptysis. Cases in which patients have presented with hypoglycemia or osteoarthropathy have been described[95,97]; these latter clinical manifestations also have been seen in association with solitary fibrous tumors. In contrast with previous studies, Yousem and Hochholzer[96] found that these tumors were more commonly seen in the periphery or midportion of the lung than in a central location. In only a few of their cases was the tumor centrally located.

Macroscopic Features

Hemangiopericytomas appear to occur in an endobronchial location, in the midlung field, or in the periphery of the lung. Tumor size may range from 1 cm to more than 10 cm in greatest dimension. The tumor usually is firm in consistency and appears to be well circumscribed but not encapsulated and light brown or tan, with or without areas of necrosis or hemorrhage. When the tumor is in an endobronchial location, it may show a polypoid growth pattern; cystic tumors also have been described.

Histopathologic Features

The histopathologic hallmark of hemangiopericytomas is a proliferation composed of oval to spindle cells growing around large, prominent, gaping, staghorn-like vessels with an attenuated endothelium, which may or may not contain red cells in their lumens (Figs. 7-49 and 7-50). The

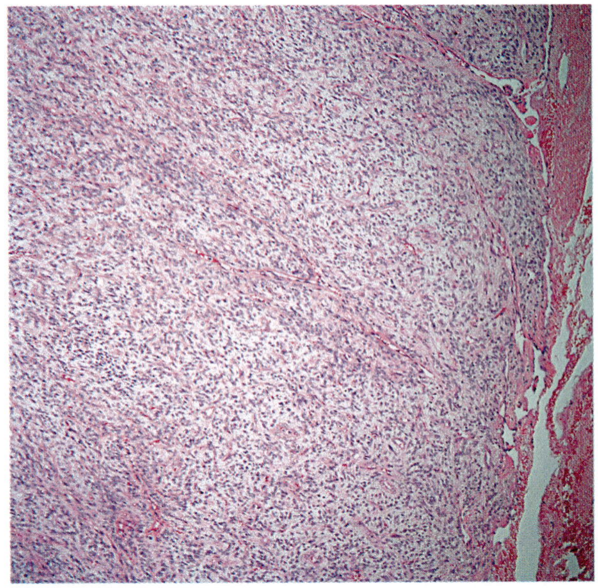

Figure 7-49 Low-power view of a hemangiopericytoma of the lung. Currently, this tumor may qualify as a solitary fibrous tumor.

cells have scant cytoplasm, oval nuclei, and inconspicuous nucleoli. Mitotic activity may vary, with counts ranging from none to more than 10 mitotic figures per 10 high-power fields (Fig. 7-51). Areas of hemorrhage and necrosis may be seen in some cases. The tumor usually appears to be fairly well circumscribed, but in some cases, tumor cells appear to infiltrate adjacent lung parenchyma.

Immunohistochemical Features

Because a hemangiopericytic pattern may be seen in many different tumors, it is important to perform a wide panel of immunohistochemical studies, which should include epithelial, muscle, neural, and vascular markers. Leiomyosarcomas may show areas of a hemangiopericytic pattern, and these tumors usually will demonstrate positive staining for muscle markers such as smooth muscle actin, desmin, or caldesmon. Synovial sarcoma, which also shows a hemangiopericytic pattern, demonstrates positive staining for keratin or EMA, or both, whereas neuronal tumors may show staining for S-100 protein or neurofilament protein. Some of the immunostains, however, may show reactivity when used with other tumors that also show a hemangiopericytic pattern. For instance, CD34 and Bcl-2 may stain positively in solitary fibrous tumors and synovial sarcomas, respectively. If the main distinction in the differential diagnosis is from synovial sarcoma, for example, an expected finding would be at least focal staining in tumor cells with keratin or EMA; in cases of solitary fibrous tumor, however, the issue is more complex, because both tumors share a similar immunophenotype. In this setting, careful evaluation of the morphology of the tumor may be more important. Solitary

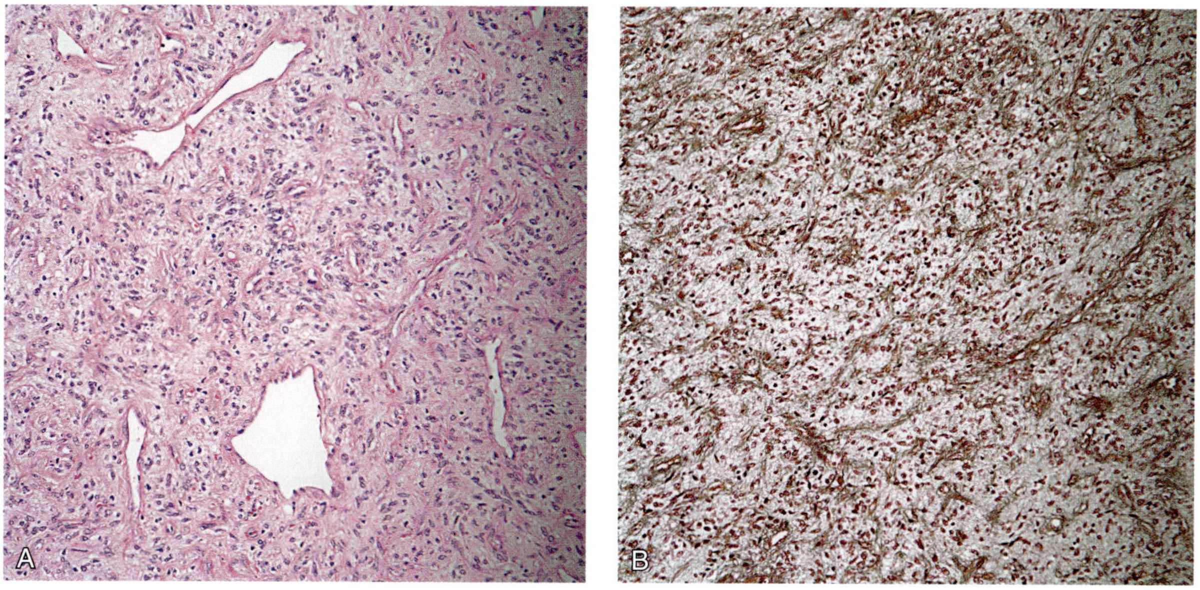

Figure 7-50 **A**, Hemangiopericytoma with ectatic vessels and spindle cell component. **B**, Reticulin staining highlights the presence of vessels and spindle cells.

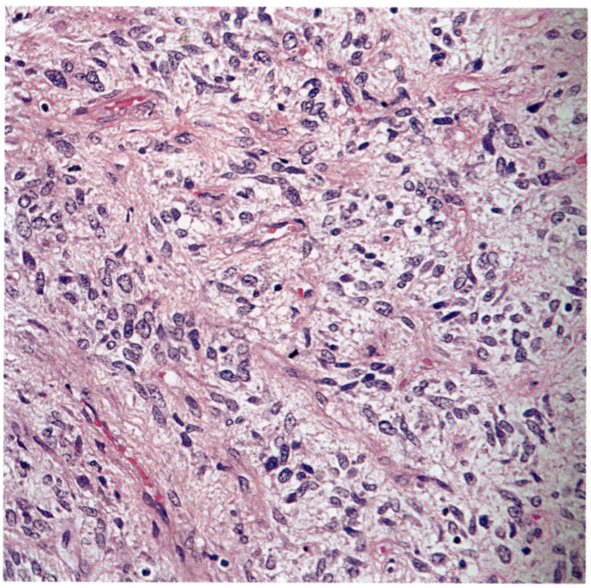

Figure 7-51 High-power view of a hemangiopericytoma showing scattered mitotic figures.

fibrous tumors usually show different patterns of growth within the same tumor, thus providing an important diagnostic feature.

Differential Diagnosis

The most important considerations in the differential diagnosis are solitary fibrous tumor, synovial sarcoma, and leiomyosarcoma. As indicated previously, a broad panel of immunohistochemical studies should be used to distinguish these tumors from one another. Also, when the possible diagnostic entities share a similar immunophenotype, a clear interpretation is very difficult. The current tendency is to label those tumors for which a designation of hemangiopericytoma versus solitary fibrous tumor is in question as the latter type.

Treatment and Prognosis

The largest series and reviews of pulmonary hemangiopericytoma have documented recurrences and metastatic disease in many patients. Accordingly, some researchers have suggested that all "hemangiopericytomas" are potentially malignant. Yousem and Hochholzer[96] were not able to identify with certainty any particular histopathologic feature to correlate with clinical behavior and further claimed that mitotic count was not reliable. Meade and colleagues[95] documented mortality rates of 32% to 50%, with higher rates in males than in females. The size of the tumor at the time of diagnosis appears to correlate with prognosis, and an arbitrary size of 8 cm or more has been mentioned as a cutoff size.

The treatment of choice is surgical resection, which may be followed by adjuvant medical therapy, depending on individual clinical circumstances, including the extent of disease at the time of diagnosis.

Monophasic Synovial Sarcoma

Primary intrathoracic sarcomas with features of synovial sarcomas of soft tissues are neoplasms of more recent description.[98,99] These tumors were first reported in an intrapulmonary location in 1995, in a series of 25 cases.[99] This original description constitutes the largest series to date of intrapulmonary monophasic synovial sarcomas.

Following this description, numerous case reports have been presented corroborating the diagnosis by means of immunohistochemistry or molecular biology techniques.[100–111] Other brief series of cases have expanded the anatomic distribution to include pleuropulmonary synovial sarcomas or have added molecular studies to the assessment protocol. Some studies, although they appear to present a larger number of cases, have emphasized gathering cases that may affect the pleura, lung, and mediastinum.[112–115] In one of these larger series, which reported 60 cases, it is very likely that some, if not a majority, of the cases reported as tumors of the lung may have been included in the initial description of the tumor, because both of these series came from the same institution.[99,115] Agreement appears to be unanimous that these tumors occur in the lung as well as in other thoracic locations. Only tumors occurring within the lung parenchyma are considered in the following discussion.

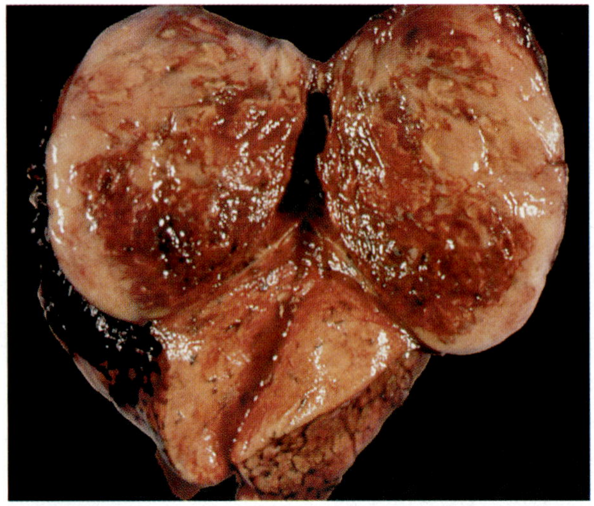

Figure 7-52 Intrapulmonary monophasic synovial sarcoma, gross specimen. Note the large intraparenchymal mass with focal areas of hemorrhage.

Clinical Features

The tumors affect a wide range of age groups, with reported cases in patients ranging from 16 to 77 years of age. The tumors affect both males and females, without any specific gender predilection. Clinical signs and symptoms typically are related to the anatomic distribution of the tumors. Patients with centrally located tumors may present with manifestations of bronchial obstruction, including shortness of breath, chest pain, cough, and hemoptysis; patients with peripheral tumors may be completely asymptomatic or may experience other nonspecific symptoms. In rare cases, patients may present with pneumothorax or may report a history of radiation therapy.[107,109]

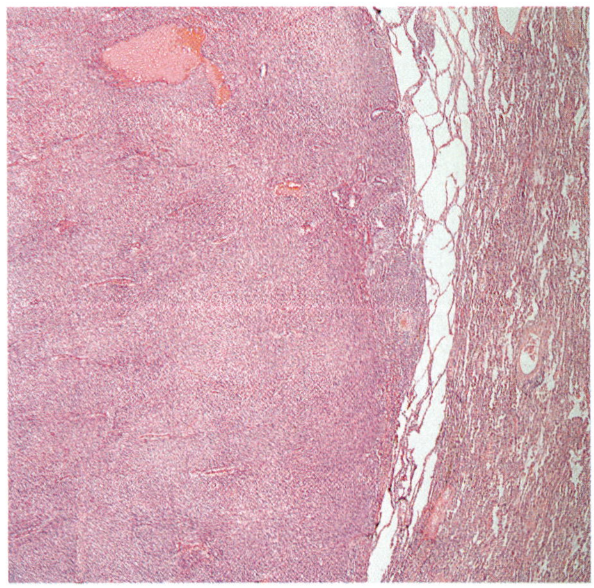

Figure 7-53 Low-power view of an intrapulmonary monophasic synovial sarcoma.

Macroscopic Features

As previously stated, the tumor may be centrally or peripherally situated in the lung. Size ranges from less than 1 cm to larger than 10 cm in greatest dimension. Monophasic synovial sarcomas usually are well circumscribed but not encapsulated and gray to tan in color. Necrosis, hemorrhage, and cystic changes may be seen in some cases (Fig. 7-52). The cut surface is smooth in appearance, with a rubbery to firm consistency. In some cases, the tumor appears to be infiltrative, with differing degrees of airway involvement.

Histopathologic Features

The low-power view shows a well-circumscribed tumor mass replacing normal lung architecture (Fig. 7-53). Higher magnification will reveal a spindle cell proliferation composed of plump, fusiform cells, with indistinct cytoplasm and oval nuclei (Figs. 7-54 to 7-56). The tumor characteristically consists of a relatively uniform, solid cell proliferation with minimal deposition of collagen. Some cases, however, may feature myxoid changes (Figs. 7-57 and 7-58) or epithelioid morphology composed of oval cells with indistinct borders and inconspicuous nucleoli. A prominent hemangiopericytic growth pattern with numerous ectatic branching vascular spaces may be seen in some tumors (Fig. 7-59). Neural-like palisading of tumor cells, reminiscent of peripheral nerve sheath tumors, also may be observed in some cases. Mitotic activity is variable, with counts ranging from 2 to more than 20 mitotic figures per 10 high-power fields. Areas of osteoid metaplasia, necrosis (Fig. 7-60), and hemorrhage may be seen. Entrapped alveolar epithelium may be present, mimicking the appearance of a biphasic tumor (Fig. 7-61).

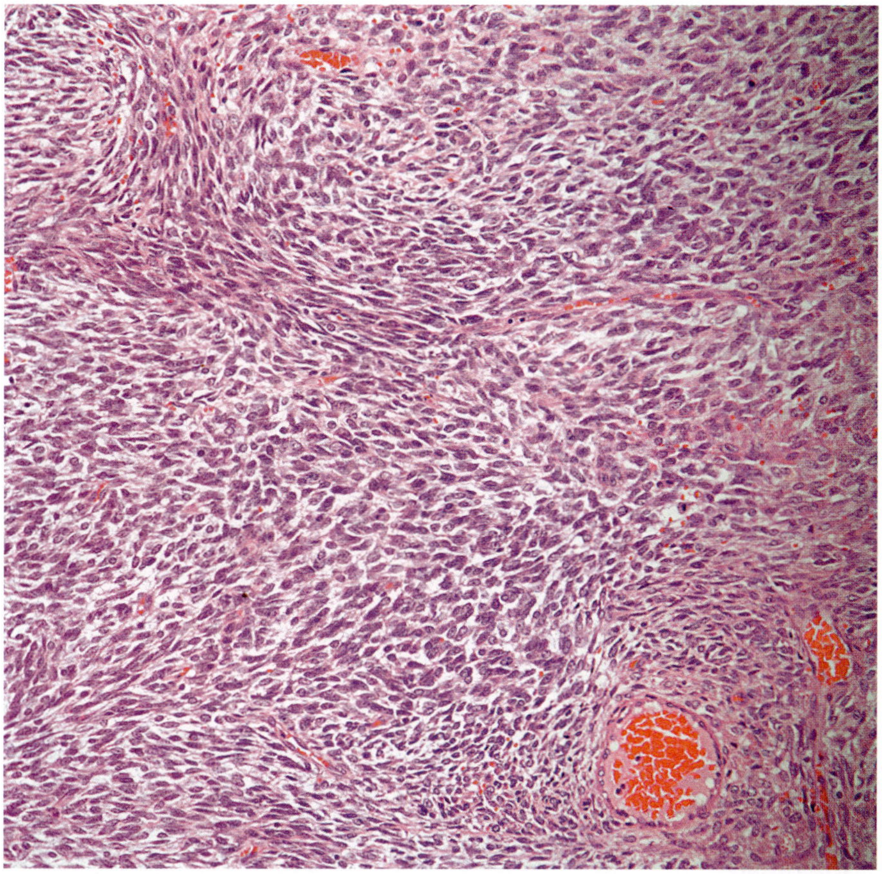

Figure 7-54 Intrapulmonary monophasic sarcoma with a prominent atypical spindle cell proliferation.

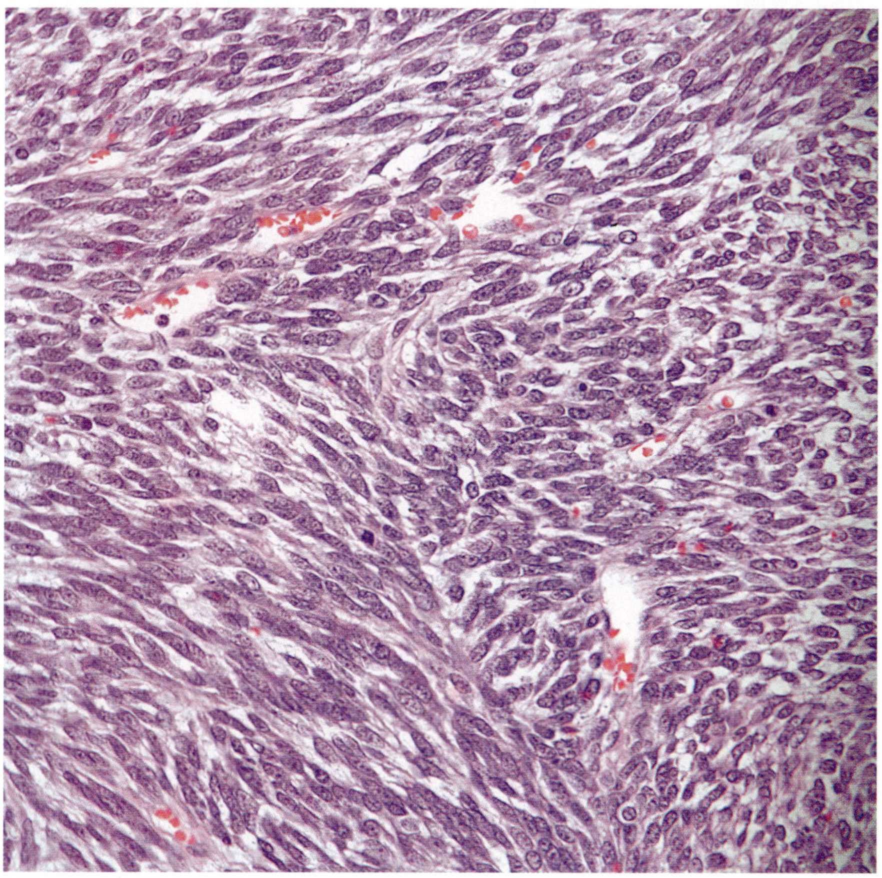

Figure 7-55 High-power view of an intrapulmonary monophasic synovial sarcoma showing mitotic activity.

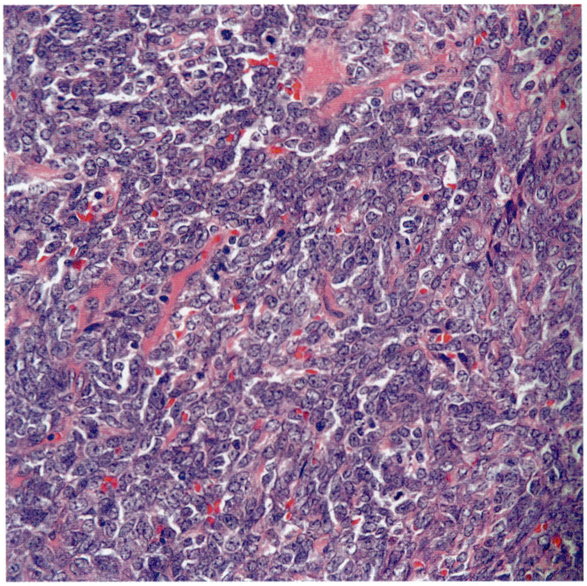

Figure 7-56 Intrapulmonary monophasic synovial sarcoma with epithelioid areas.

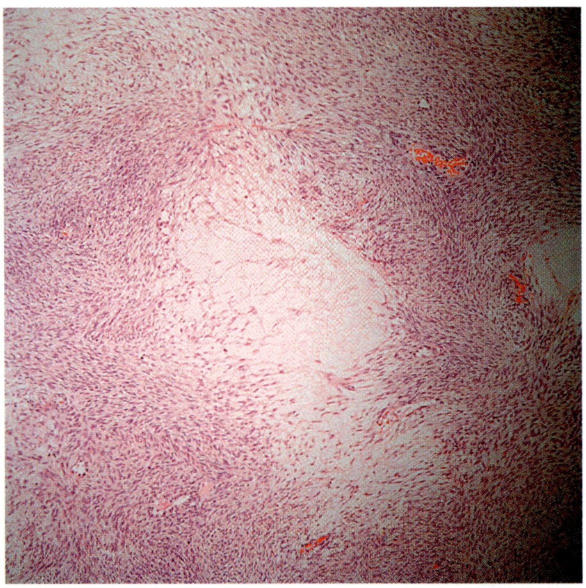

Figure 7-57 Intrapulmonary monophasic synovial sarcoma with focal myxoid areas.

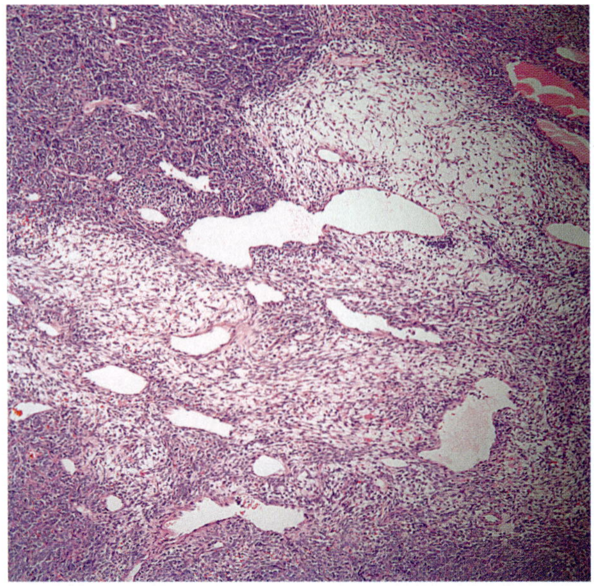

Figure 7-58 Intrapulmonary monophasic synovial sarcoma with extensive areas of myxoid change with ectatic blood vessels.

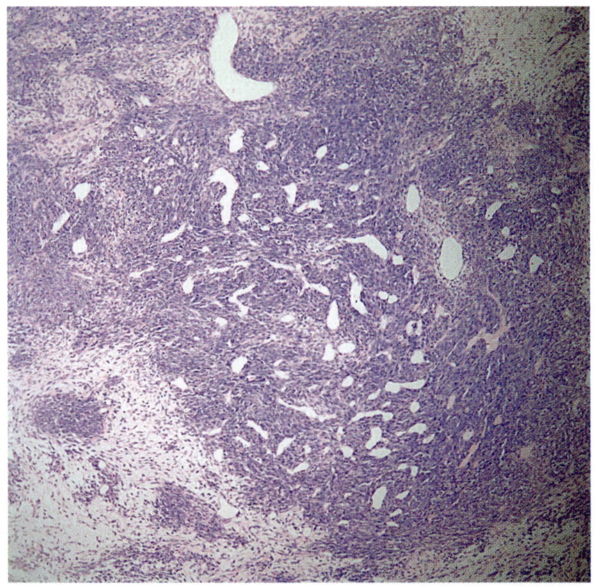

Figure 7-59 Intrapulmonary monophasic synovial sarcoma with a hemangiopericytic pattern.

Immunohistochemical Features and Molecular Biology

The hallmark of synovial sarcoma is positive staining for epithelial markers—namely, keratin and EMA. This positive staining may be focal, however, and although reactivity for both of these markers is positive in most cases, sometimes only one marker shows positive staining. Other markers also may help in the diagnosis of these tumors: Vimentin, Bcl-2, and CD99 have shown positive staining in tumor cells. Staining for smooth muscle actin, desmin, myoglobin, myo-D, CD31, and CD34 is negative in these tumors. Staining for S-100 protein may be focally positive in some cases.

Currently, the use of molecular techniques to detect the X;18 translocation is a standard approach to confirm the diagnosis of synovial sarcoma. This procedure may be helpful in approximately 90% of cases; in the remaining 10%, histopathologic analysis and immunohistochemical studies continue to be important assets in the evaluation of these tumors. Evaluation for *SYT-SSX* fusion genes also may be

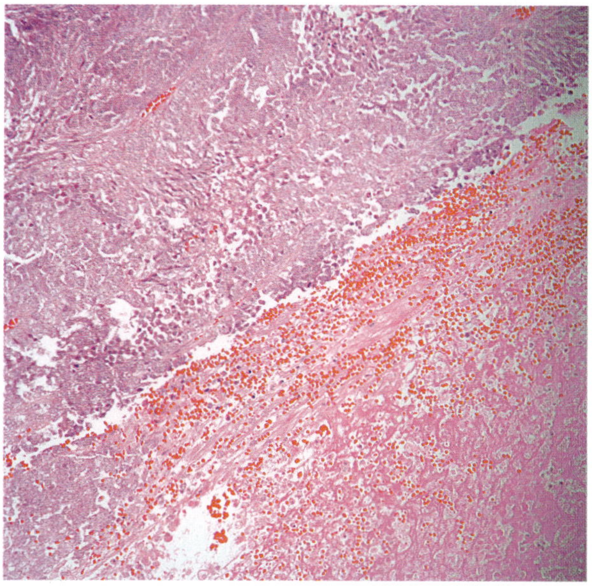

Figure 7-60 Intrapulmonary monophasic synovial sarcoma with extensive areas of necrosis.

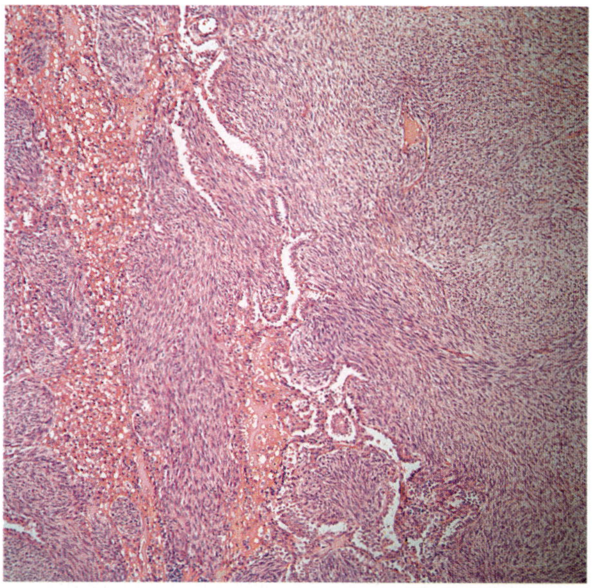

Figure 7-61 Intrapulmonary monophasic synovial sarcoma with entrapped alveolar epithelium. This appearance mimicks that of a biphasic tumor.

helpful, mainly for assessment of prognosis. Mezzelani and associates[116] conducted a study of 64 cases in which they evaluated fusion genes and suggested that *SYT-SSX1* fusion transcript appeared to be an independent prognostic factor associated with reduced metastasis-free survival, although not to a statistically significant degree. Boroumand and coworkers[117] reported a case of primary pulmonary synovial sarcoma for which an *SYT-SSX2* immunophenotype was established. The tumor, which demonstrated positive staining for CD117 (c-Kit), followed a rapidly progressive clinical course.

Treatment and Prognosis

The treatment for pulmonary synovial sarcoma is complete surgical resection of the tumor, accomplished by lobectomy or pneumonectomy. This may be followed by chemotherapy or radiation therapy, or both. The analysis for the fusion genes *SYT-SSX* usually is indicated if available, because of its implications for the behavior of this neoplasm. In the first series of cases reported,[99] follow-up data for periods ranging from 2 to 20 years were obtained: 6 patients died from the tumor; 8 patients were alive with disease, 4 patients were alive and well, and 4 patients had died of unrelated causes. Bégueret and colleagues[115] reported that at least one local recurrence developed in 36% of their patients, for whom the median survival was 44 months, and at least one distant metastasis occurred in 39%, for whom the median survival was 43 months. The investigators also determined 2- and 5-year disease-specific survival rates of 65% and 31%, respectively; the median disease-specific survival for the *SYT-SSX1* patient subset was 50 months, whereas for the *SYT-SSX2* patient subset it was 46 months.

MALIGNANT FIBROUS HISTIOCYTOMA

Although malignant fibrous histiocytoma has long been recognized as one of the most common sarcomas of soft tissues, it is rather rare as a primary lung neoplasm. A large proportion of soft tissue tumors will metastasize to the lung, however. The use of immunohistochemical studies in current practice has allowed for better characterization of many specimens of these tumors that otherwise would be classified as high-grade sarcoma.

In 1979, Bedrossian and associates[118] reported the first case of primary malignant fibrous histiocytoma in the lung, describing a 51-year-old man with an intrapulmonary neoplasm and no other history of tumor in the soft tissues. These investigators linked the histopathologic characteristics of this tumor to those of soft tissue tumors. By the mid-1980s, fewer than 25 additional cases had been described in the literature, and these were reported either as small series of cases or as individual case reports.[119–122] In 1987, Yousem and Hochholzer[123] described the largest series of primary malignant fibrous histiocytomas in the lung, consisting of 22 cases, and emphasized the importance of separating this entity from spindle cell carcinoma of the lung.

Clinical Features

Malignant fibrous histiocytoma appears to affect men and women equally, and although the tumor appears to be more common in adults in the fifth amd sixth decades of life, it also has been described in younger persons. In the series of cases presented by Yousem and Hochholzer,[123] patient age ranged from 18 to 80 years.

Clinical signs and symptoms will depend on the anatomic distribution of the tumor. Cough, weight loss, chest pain, shortness of breath, and hemoptysis are common but also may be seen with other types of tumors—namely, carcinomas. Some patients with primary malignant fibrous histiocytoma of the lung may be completely asymptomatic, and the tumor is discovered on a routine chest radiograph.

Macroscopic Features

The size of these tumors may range from 1 cm to more than 10 cm in greatest dimension. They may be central or peripheral in location, with ubiquitous distribution among the different pulmonary segments. The tumor mass is well circumscribed but not encapsulated and light tan, with or without areas of hemorrhage or necrosis (Fig. 7-62). In some tumors, it is possible to identify borders pushing into adjacent lung parenchyma. Extensive areas of necrosis also may be seen.

Histopathologic Features

The great majority of cases correspond to the pleomorphic type of malignant fibrous histiocytoma, which is characterized by a neoplastic spindle cell proliferation arranged in a storiform pattern with a cartwheel-like pattern around vessels. Admixed with this spindle cell proliferation are large pleomorphic cells with moderate amounts of cytoplasm, round to oval nuclei, and prominent nucleoli (Figs. 7-63 to 7-67). These larger cells also may be multinucleated, mimicking Reed-Sternberg cells seen in Hodgkin's lymphoma, or osteoclast-like. The tumor acquires a histiocytic-like cell proliferation with areas of more fibroblastic-type spindle cells. Mitotic

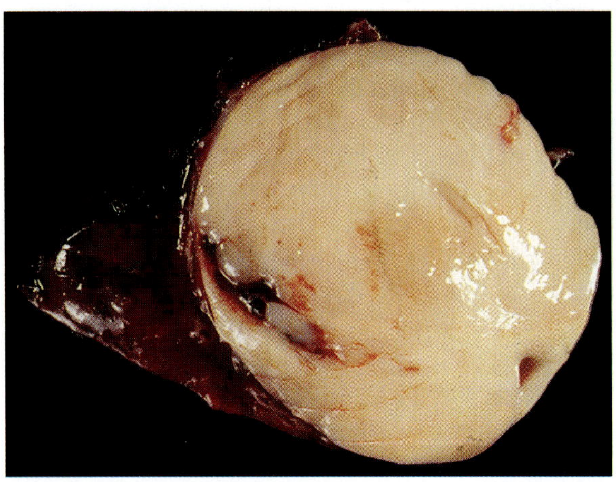

Figure 7-62 Intrapulmonary malignant fibrous histiocytoma, gross specimen. Note the large intraparenchymal tumor mass with focal areas of hemorrhage.

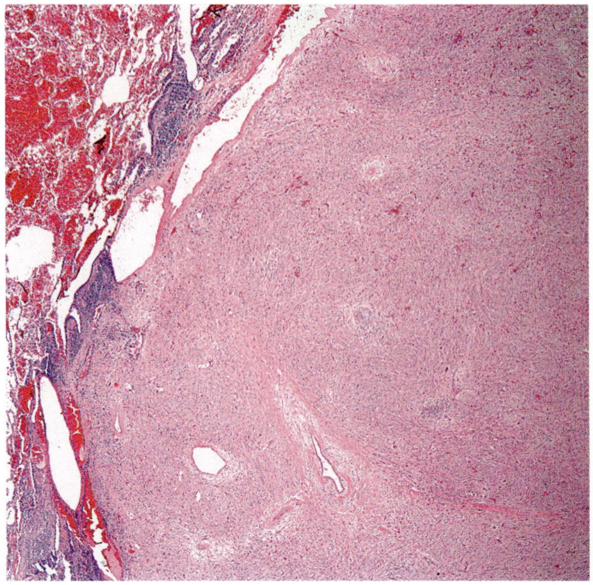

Figure 7-63 Low-power view of intrapulmonary malignant fibrous histiocytoma.

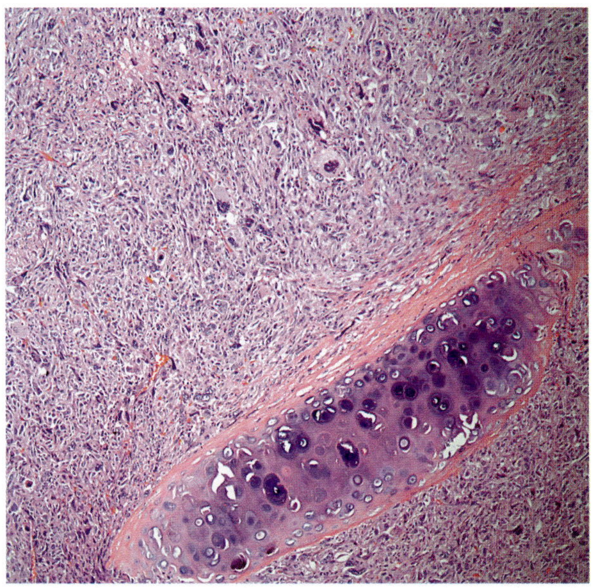

Figure 7-64 Intrapulmonary malignant fibrous histiocytoma with marked pleomorphism and destruction of the bronchial cartilage.

figures are readily identified, and areas of necrosis or hemorrhage can be seen in differing proportions. In some cases, myxoid and hemangiopericytic-like areas can be seen. An inflammatory infiltrate composed of plasma cells and lymphocytes also may be observed. Vascular invasion can be seen in approximately 50% of the cases of pulmonary malignant fibrous histiocytoma.

Immunohistochemical Features

Malignant fibrous histiocytoma characteristically shows positive staining for histiocytic markers, including CD68

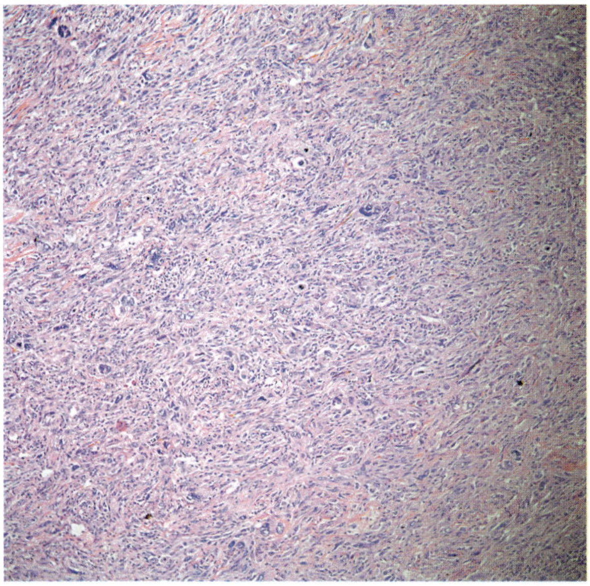

Figure 7-65 Intrapulmonary malignant fibrous histiocytoma composed of spindle cells arranged in a vaguely storiform pattern.

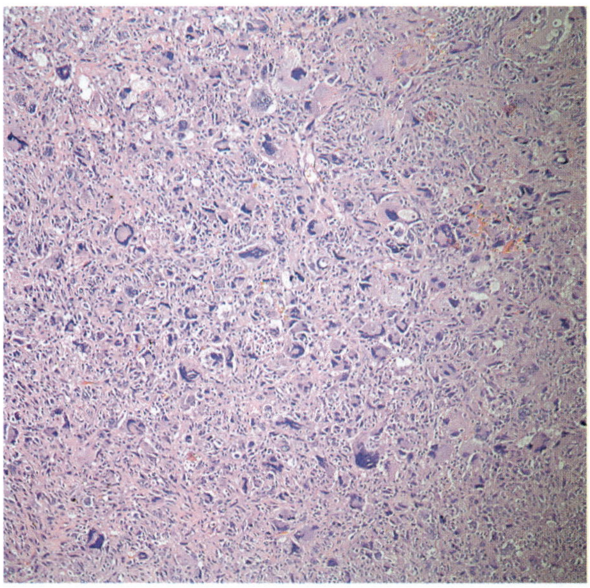

Figure 7-66 Malignant fibrous histiocytoma with prominent multinucleated giant cell component.

and α_1-antichymotrypsin, as well as vimentin. Staining for S-100 protein, desmin, actin, myoglobin, and caldesmon is negative, but in some cases, keratin staining may be positive. A wider than usual panel of immunostaining studies usually is performed to rule out another, more specific type of sarcoma.

Differential Diagnosis

The differential diagnosis for malignant fibrous histiocytoma in the lung encompasses other pleomorphic neoplasms, the most important being pleomorphic carcinoma,

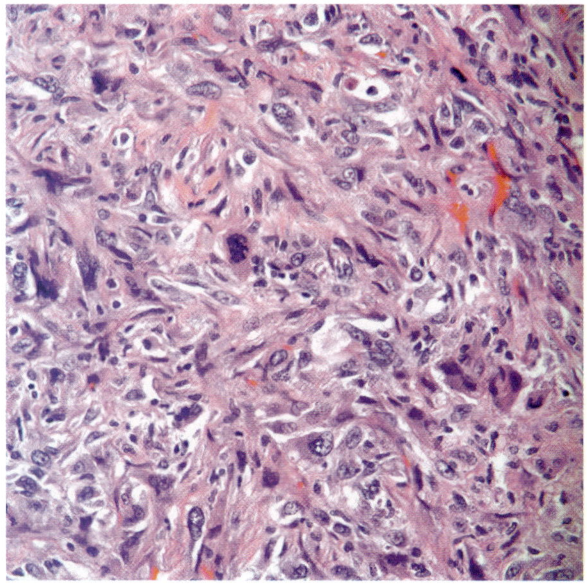

Figure 7-67 High-power view of a malignant fibrous histiocytoma showing atypical mitotic figures.

which is more common than and also is treated differently from malignant fibrous histiocytoma. In this setting, use of epithelial markers should be of help; in addition, it is possible to identify areas of more conventional squamous or adenocarcinoma in a majority of pleomorphic carcinomas. Another possibility to consider is pleomorphic rhabdomyosarcoma, which rarely can occur as a primary lung neoplasm. Rhabdomyosarcoma usually will display positive staining for muscle markers (desmin, myoglobin, myo-D) and a pattern of cross-striation on light microscopy. In diagnosing malignant fibrous histiocytoma, the most important task is to determine whether the tumor is primary or represents metastasis from a deep-seated neoplasm in soft tissues. A proper clinical history and complete physical examination are of the utmost importance in this setting.

Treatment and Prognosis

The treatment of pulmonary malignant fibrous histiocytoma is complete surgical resection followed by chemotherapy or radiation therapy, or both, depending on the individual circumstances. The clinical behavior of these tumors is aggressive, however, and metastatic disease is common. Although in some cases the course has not been rapidly progressive,[123] a majority of the patients have died within a period of 1 to 72 months.

BONE AND CARTILAGE TUMORS

Pulmonary neoplasms characterized by the presence of malignant cartilage or bone commonly are classified as biphasic or mixed epithelial and mesenchymal tumors of the lung. "Pure" neoplasms showing features of osteosarcoma or chondrosarcoma are exceedingly rare as primary malignant pulmonary neoplasms. As such, they represent a very small percentage of tumors occurring in the lung parenchyma. In terms of clinical or demographic characteristics, tumors in the lung do not resemble those in osseous areas: Tumors forming bone are classified as osteosarcoma, but the opposite is not true for cartilage-forming tumors in the lung, because they may represent benign conditions. The following tumors are discussed in this section:

- Osteosarcoma
- Chondroma
- Chondrosarcoma

Osteosarcoma

Osteosarcoma is exceedingly rare as a primary lung neoplasm, with fewer than 25 cases overall described in the literature.[124–135] The great majority of cases have been presented in the form of single case reports, and on the basis of clinical data, the anatomic distribution has been expanded to include more pleuropulmonary neoplasms. These tumors appear to be more common in older persons in the fifth to sixth decade of life. Patients may present with clinical signs and symptoms of cough, shortness of breath, chest pain, or hemoptysis or may be completely asymptomatic. Plain radiographs may not disclose osseous differentiation, and the tumor will appear as an intrapulmonary mass; thus, histologic examination is necessary for a definitive diagnosis. Although pulmonary osteosarcomas appear to affect older persons and not the younger patients with osseous osteosarcoma, it is essential to rule out the possibility of a primary osseous or soft tissue osteosarcoma. The lung is a well-recognized common site of metastases from osteosarcomas. One interesting clinical aspect of pulmonary osteosarcoma is the presence of normal levels of alkaline phosphatase, in contrast with the elevated levels seen in osteosarcomas of soft tissue and bone.

Macroscopic Features

The tumors have been described as firm, solid, "rock-hard" tumor masses of variable size, ranging from 4 cm to more than 20 cm in greatest dimension, with an average of 10 cm. They are well circumscribed, but not encapsulated, intraparenchymal masses. The cut surface may show solid bony areas or areas with cartilaginous change. Hemorrhage and necrosis are not common but may be present in some cases.

Histopathologic, Immunohistochemical, and Molecular Features

The diagnostic criteria for osteosarcoma in the lung are essentially the same as for osteosarcoma of bone. The tumor appears as a well-circumscribed mass obliterating normal lung parenchyma and displays a spindle cell proliferation composed of fusiform cells with scant cytoplasm and oval hyperchromatic nuclei admixed with osteoid and osteoclastic giant cells (Figs. 7-68 to 7-71). Nuclear atypia and mitotic activity are readily identified, but mitotic figures are not high in number. In some cases, extensive areas of cartilaginous differentiation also may be seen, leading to classification of some of these tumors as chondroblastic osteosarcomas.

The tumor characteristically demonstrates negative staining for epithelial, neural, vascular, and muscle markers. However, it may show positive staining for vimentin and

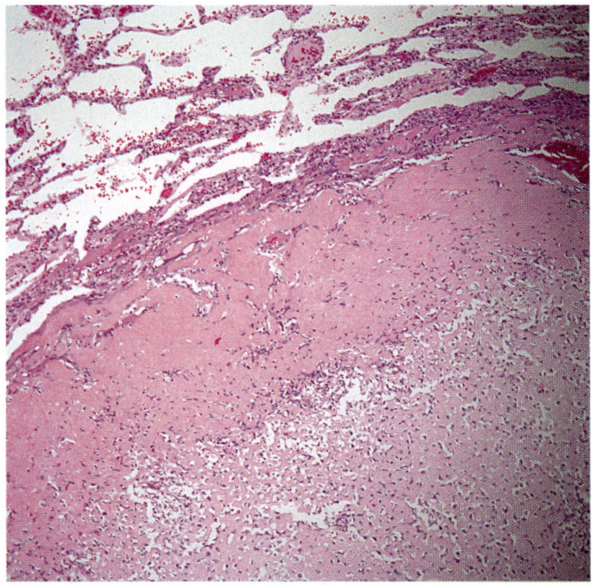

Figure 7-68 Low-power view of a primary osteosarcoma of the lung.

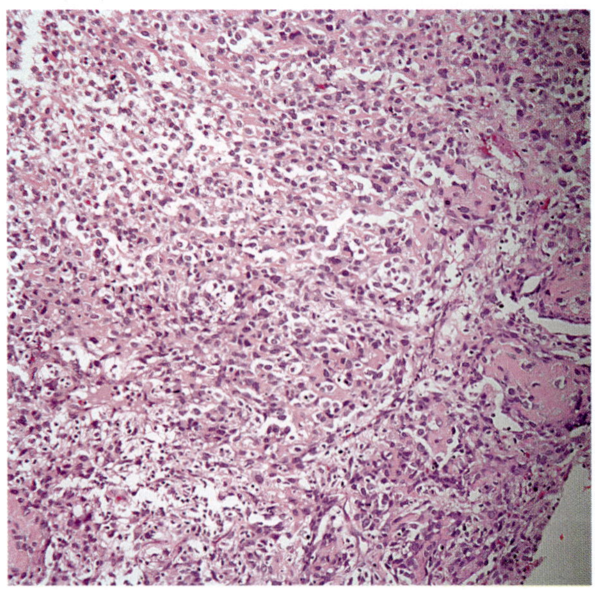

Figure 7-69 Osteosarcoma. Malignant spindle cells are admixed with focal areas of osteoid formation.

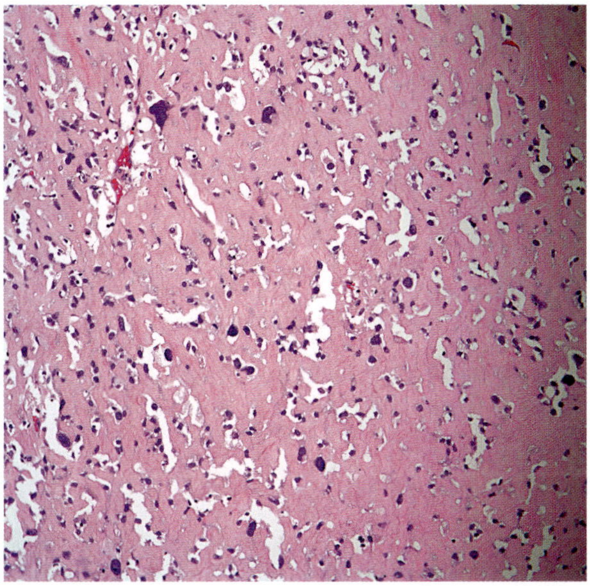

Figure 7-70 Pulmonary osteosarcoma with extensive areas of osteoid formation.

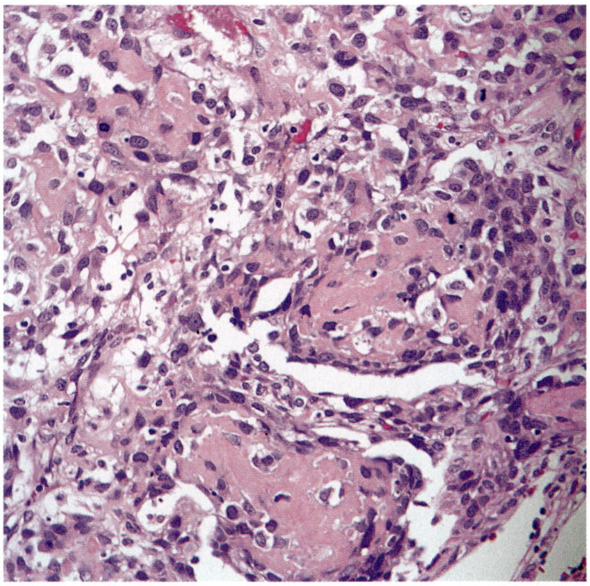

Figure 7-71 Pulmonary osteosarcoma showing osteoid formation and mitotic figures in the spindle cells.

for osteonectin, whereas osteopontin staining is negative. Using immunohistochemical and molecular techniques, Chapman and associates[129] studied a case of primary pulmonary osteosarcoma. The tumor cells demonstrated positive staining for Bcl-2 and cyclin D. Comparative genomic hybridization showed that genomic loss was more common than genomic gain, but no regions of high amplification were identified.

Differential Diagnosis

The most important consideration in the differential diagnosis is carcinosarcoma of the lung. In this setting, careful histologic evaluation for epithelial components is required. It is important to obtain a reasonable number of sections for histologic evaluation, because the epithelial component may be present in small percentages. Colby and coworkers[127] found that two of the cases initially thought to represent primary osteosarcomas were reclassified as carcinosarcomas, after careful evaluation and the use of immunohistochemical studies. Other primary tumors of the lung also may show bone formation, including synovial sarcoma and pleomorphic carcinomas. In these two conditions, however, the bone formation is that of metaplastic bone, rather than malignant osteoid. The use of immunohistochemical studies will lead to a more accurate interpretation in cases of an equivocal nature.

Treatment and Prognosis

In a majority of the reported cases, surgical resection has been the treatment of choice. This may be followed by adjuvant therapy (e.g., chemotherapy, radiation therapy, immunotherapy); however, no specific treatment for osteosarcomas of the lung has emerged. Distant metastases and recurrences have been documented. The clinical behavior of these tumors is aggressive, and in a majority of cases, the patients have not survived for longer than 12 months.

Chondroma

As mentioned previously, controversy remains over whether chondromas represent a specific benign tumoral condition, unrelated to the so-called hamartoma, or whether they are the same condition. Chondroma is presented here as a discrete clinical entity from a histopathologic perspective but not necessarily from a histogenetic perspective. The term *chondroma* has been used indiscriminately in the past for both tumoral conditions (hamartoma and chondroma) to denote a tumor that is composed exclusively of cartilage. Several cases have been described under the designation chondroma, and its unusual occurrence has been noted.

In 1977, Carney and colleagues[136] described an interesting association of gastric epithelioid leiomyosarcomas, functional paraganglioma, and pulmonary chondromas, which has since been known as Carney's triad. Carney[137] also commented on other cases in the literature with similar associations, noting the improbability of incidental occurrence of these tumors in young patients; he recommended that because at least two of these tumors are potentially lethal, careful evaluation of patients younger than 35 years should be undertaken. Additional reports of this triad also have been presented in the literature.[138,139] More recently, Rodriguez and associates[141] evaluated 42 patients with pulmonary cartilaginous tumors as a component of Carney's triad and concluded that these tumors are best designated as chondromas, because they differ histologically from cartilaginous hamartomas.

Macroscopic Features

The tumors appear to be well circumscribed and whitish, with a firm consistency, and the cut surface may have a smooth, mucoid, and lobulated appearance. Some tumors have been described as essentially mucoid or as displaying cystic changes. Tumor size varies but in general is approximately 3 cm in greatest dimension. In some cases, multiple tumors are apparent (Fig. 7-72).

Histopathologic Features

The histopathologic hallmark of chondromas is the presence of cartilage, which may be hyaline or myxoid in form. Under low magnification, a multilobate tumor with possible central degeneration or possible cystic changes is visible. Areas of calcification or ossification usually can be seen in the center or periphery of the lesion (Figs. 7-73 to 7-75). These tumors may be characterized by moderate cellularity, with some nuclear variability and binucleated cells. They lack mitotic activity or marked nuclear pleomorphism. Chondromas usually will not show the classic invagination of respiratory epithelium or the extensive adipose tissue content commonly observed in hamartomas.

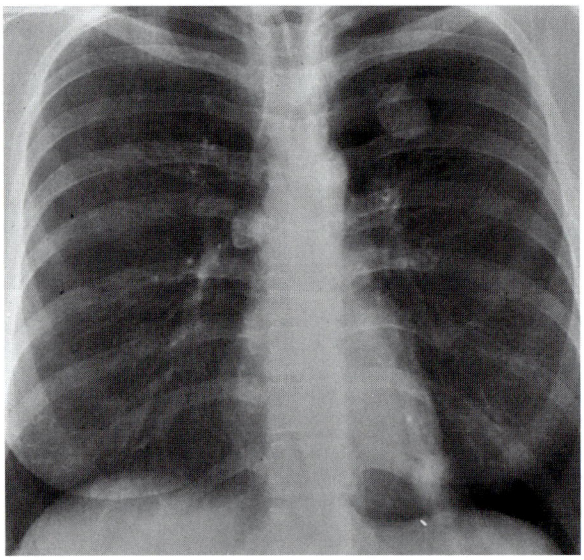

Figure 7-72 Chest radiograph showing chondromas of the lung.

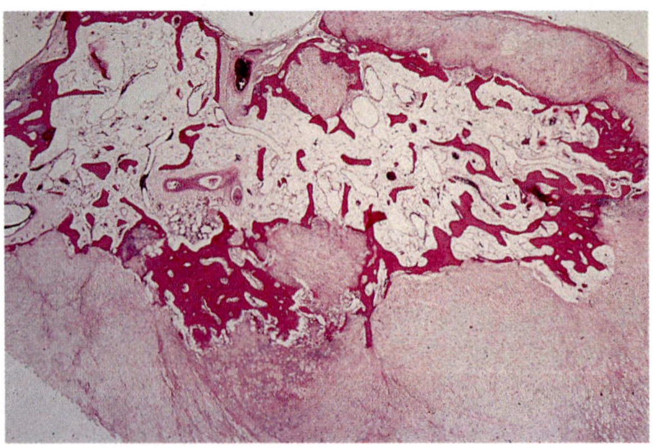

Figure 7-73 Pulmonary chondroma: mature bone and cartilage as seen at low magnification.

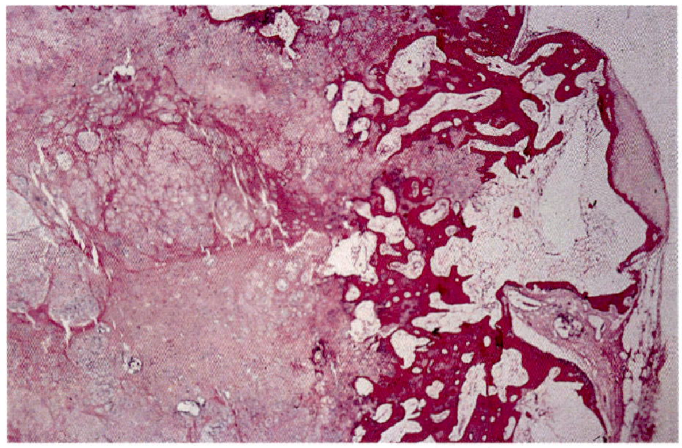

Figure 7-74 High-power view of a pulmonary chondroma showing predominantly mature bone and cartilage.

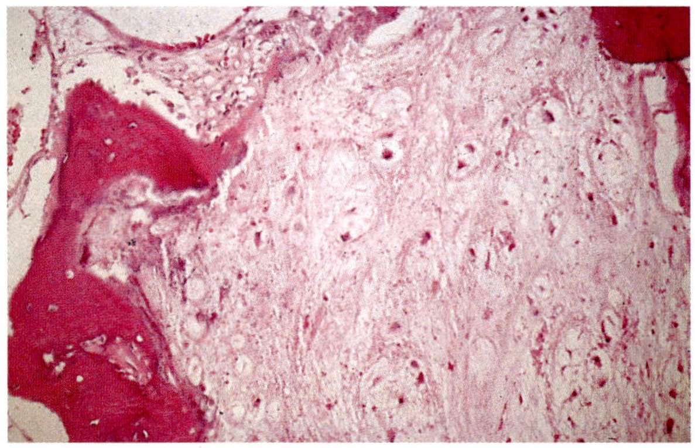

Figure 7-75 Pulmonary chondroma with focal chondroid atypia.

Differential Diagnosis

The most important consideration in the differential diagnosis is primary pulmonary chondrosarcoma. Chondromas in the lung also can be multifocal, giving the clinical impression of metastatic disease. In this setting, the absence of nuclear atypia and the overall qualities of the cartilage, coupled with negative clinical history for osseous neoplasms, will lead to the correct interpretation. When pulmonary hamartoma is suspected, histologic examination should show the presence of invaginations of respiratory epithelium or adipose tissue. The presence of pulmonary chondromas in a young patient should alert the clinician to the possibility of other tumors, especially those associated with Carney's triad.

Treatment and Prognosis

The treatment of choice is surgical resection. The methods used will depend on the individual clinical circumstances. Nevertheless, the tumor is benign, and complete surgical resection is curative.

Chondrosarcoma

Primary chondrosarcomas of the upper and lower respiratory tract are exceedingly rare.[142] The lung is a common site of metastatic disease from chondrosarcomas of bone origin; therefore, a careful analysis is essential before a diagnosis of primary pulmonary chondrosarcoma can be established. Only tumors occurring in the lower respiratory tract are addressed in the following discussion.

Numerous cases of primary chondrosarcomas of the lung have been described, mainly in the form of single case reports.[143–155] Some of these cases, however, may not represent true primaries. Although most researchers agree that these tumors are derived from bronchial cartilage, in general, pulmonary chondrosarcomas have been divided into tracheobronchial and pulmonary tumors. More essential to this discussion is separation of these neoplasms into primary and secondary tumors. Primary chondrosarcomas appear not to be related with any previous cartilaginous lesion and arise de novo. Secondary tumors are thought to arise from previous cartilaginous lesions, such as chondroma or hamartoma.

Clinical Features

Pulmonary chondrosarcomas occur in adults, and although the tumors have been described in various age groups, they may be more common among patients in the sixth and seventh decades of life. Clinical signs and symptoms may be related to the anatomic distribution of the tumor. Patients with centrally located tumors may present with shortness of breath, hemoptysis, cough, or other manifestations of bronchial obstruction. When the tumor is more distally located, patients may either present with similar manifestations or be asymptomatic.

Histopathologic Features

On gross examination, tumor size may range from 1 cm to more than 10 cm in greatest dimension. These tumors usually are irregular in shape but well circumscribed and white, with a firm consistency, and the cut surface may appear smooth and slightly lobulated (Fig. 7-76). Histologic examination reveals hyaline cartilage with numerous atypical chondrocytes, with two or more atypical nuclei (Figs. 7-77 and 7-78). Areas of myxoid change also may be seen in association with hyaline areas (Fig. 7-79). Hemorrhage, necrosis, and increased mitotic activity are not common in these tumors. Cases of dedifferentiated chondrosarcoma with a spindle cell component with cellular atypia and mitotic activity have been reported, however.[156] Tumors with a neoplastic cellular proliferation similar to that in myxoid chondrosarcomas (Figs. 7-80 and 7-81) and mesenchymal chondrosarcoma (Fig. 7-82) also have been described.[157]

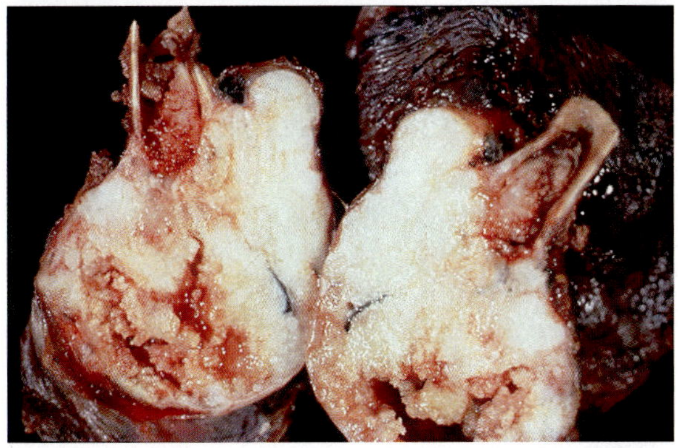

Figure 7-76 Primary chondrosarcoma of the lung, gross specimen. The large white tumor mass involves the main airway.

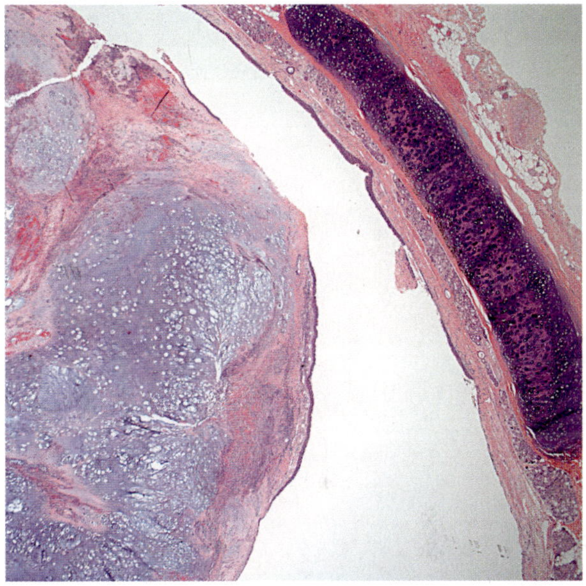

Figure 7-77 Low-power view of a primary chondrosarcoma of lung. Note the central location of the tumor.

Immunohistochemical Features

Although the diagnosis of chondrosarcoma should not pose a problem when the classic areas of hyaline cartilage are visible, the use of immunohistochemical studies may be helpful in cases of mesenchymal chondrosarcoma. In this setting, the use of S-100 protein and Sox-9 (Fig. 7-83) may help, because these markers appear to show positive staining not only in mesenchymal chondrosarcomas but also in conventional tumors.

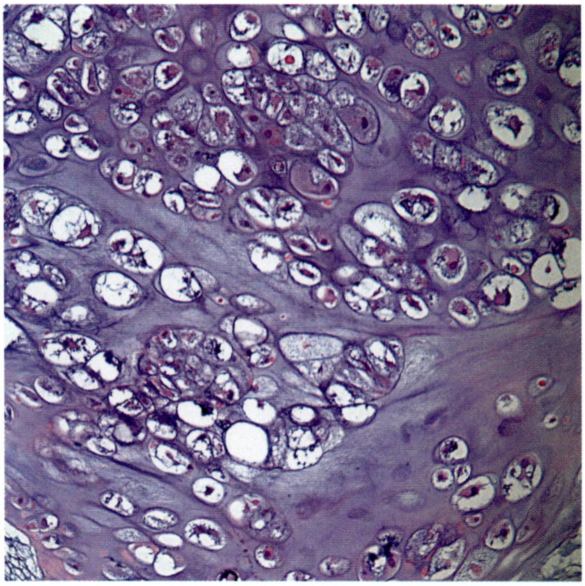

Figure 7-78 Low-grade chondrosarcoma of the lung with cartilaginous atypia.

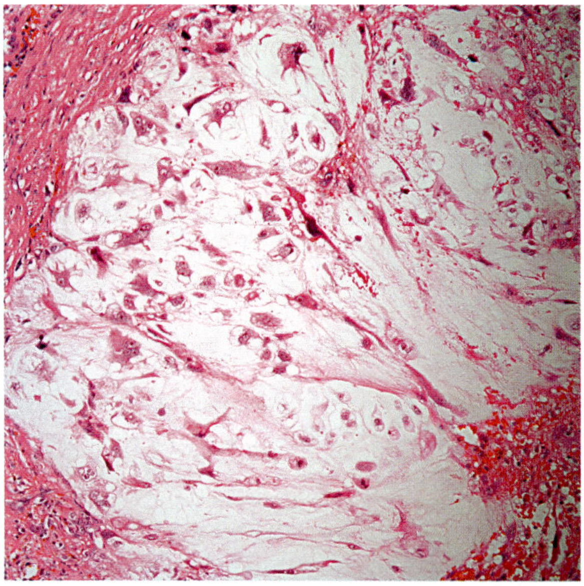

Figure 7-79 Myxoid changes in a primary chondrosarcoma of the lung.

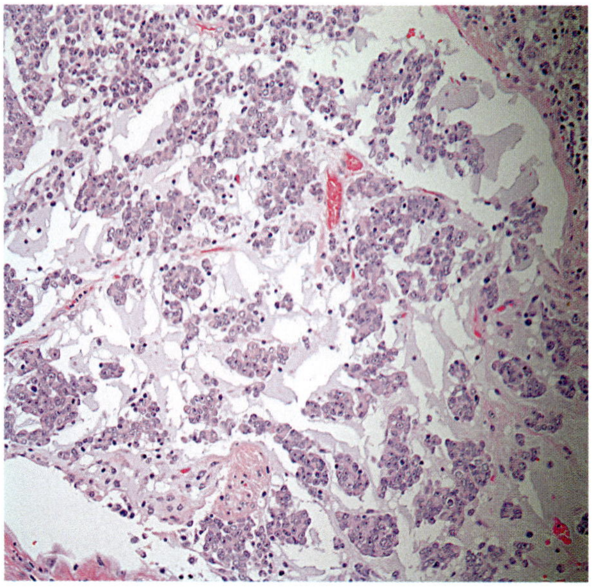

Figure 7-80 Primary myxoid chondrosarcoma of the lung. Extracellular pools of mucoid material are admixed with the neoplastic cellular proliferation.

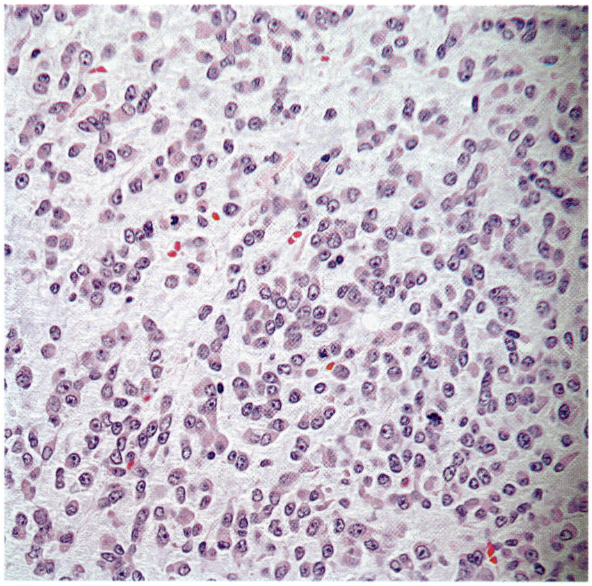

Figure 7-81 Primary pulmonary myxoid chondrosarcoma with cellular atypia and mitotic figures.

Differential Diagnosis

The most important consideration in the differential diagnosis is bronchial chondroma. With this neoplasm, the presence of binucleated or trinucleated atypical chondrocytes will point to the correct interpretation. Mesenchymal chondrosarcoma can be mistaken for a small cell carcinoma, and in such cases, use of keratin antibodies will make the correct diagnosis. In cases of dedifferentiated chondrosarcoma, it is important to identify both cartilaginous and spindle cell components. Metastatic chondrosarcoma to the lung must be ruled out by a complete clinical history.

Treatment and Prognosis

Surgical resection of the tumor is the treatment of choice. The effectiveness of radiation therapy or chemotherapy is still uncertain in tumors of lung origin. It has been suggested that tumors located centrally in the tracheobronchial area may be more amenable to complete surgical resection, leading to better long-term survival, whereas

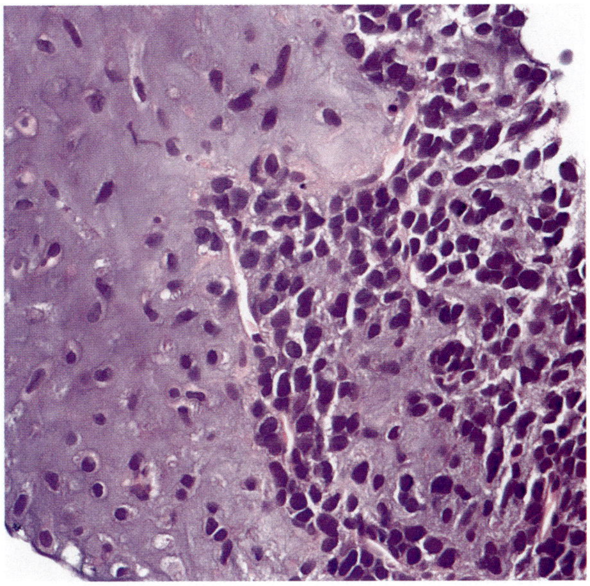

Figure 7-82 Primary mesenchymal chondrosarcoma of the lung.

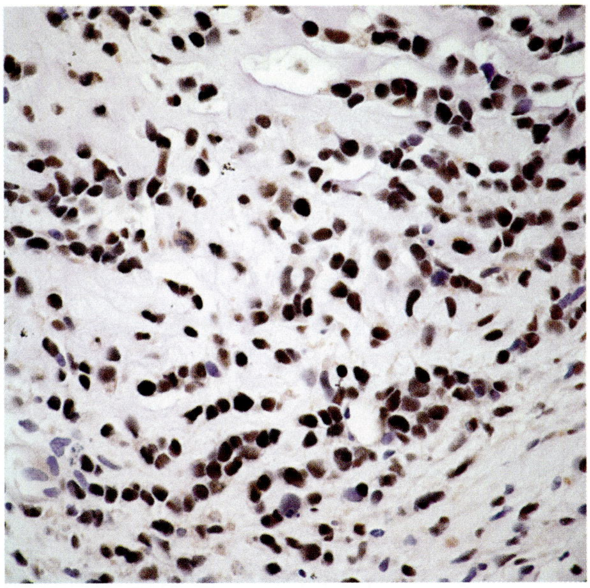

Figure 7-83 Sox-9 immunostaining is nuclear-positive in a mesenchymal chondrosarcoma of the lung.

those located more distally and in the lung parenchyma exhibit more aggressive behavior. Survival periods of more than 2 to 3 years have been observed; however, rapidly fatal outcomes in less than 12 months also have been reported.

ADIPOSE, MYXOID, AND FIBROMYXOID TUMORS

Adipose, myxoid, and fibromyxoid tumors constitute a heterogeneous group of neoplasms, consisting mostly of benign or low-grade tumors that occur rarely as primary lung neoplasms. Recognition of these tumors when they do occur is important, however, to avoid unnecessary procedures in patients who otherwise may be believed to have metastatic disease to the lung. Even though the histopathologic features of these tumors are similar to those of their counterparts in the soft tissues, obtaining a good clinical history is of utmost importance to proper classification of the tumor as a primary lung neoplasm. The following tumors are considered in this section:

- Lipoma
- Angiomyolipoma
- Liposarcoma
- Myxoma
- Aggressive angiomyxoma and malignant myxoid tumor
- Hyalinizing spindle cell tumor with giant cell rosettes

Lipoma

Primary adipose-forming tumors in the lung are exceedingly rare. However, the existence of lipomatous tumors in the lung, and more specifically in the bronchial area, has been documented numerous times in the literature, mainly in the form of individual case reports.[158–160] Although these tumors have been suggested to fall within the spectrum of hamartomas of the lung, their unique histopathologic features appear to be more akin to those of their soft tissue counterparts.

Clinical Features

The tumors predominantly affect adult men in the fifth and sixth decades of life, with a median age of 49 years. Because of the endobronchial location of the tumor, patients may present with clinical signs and symptoms of bronchial obstruction including cough, shortness of breath, and obstructive pneumonia. Some patients may be completely asymptomatic. One other feature that has been mentioned in association with these tumors is obesity.

Histopathologic Features

Tumor size may range from 1 cm to more than 5 cm in greatest diameter. The tumors are soft in consistency, yellowish, and well circumscribed, and they may appear as polypoid lesions obstructing the bronchial lumen (Fig. 7-84). On microscopic examination, the tumors are seen to be well circumscribed and composed of mature adipose tissue, with a surface lining of respiratory epithelium (Figs. 7-85 and 7-86). In some cases, myxoid areas and a spindle cell component may be present (Fig. 7-87). The tumor does not show atypical cells, hemorrhage, or necrosis.

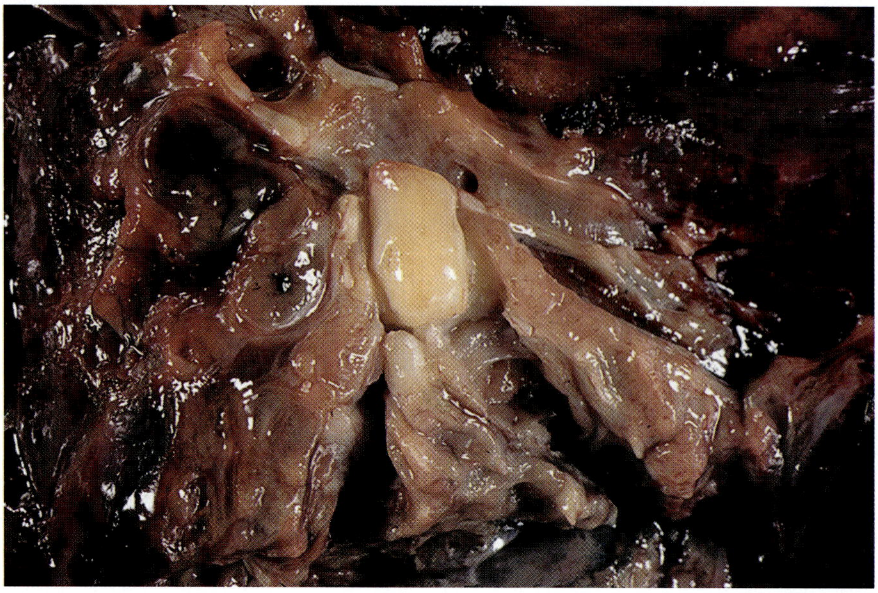

Figure 7-84 Bronchial lipoma, gross specimen. The yellowish tumor is well circumscribed.

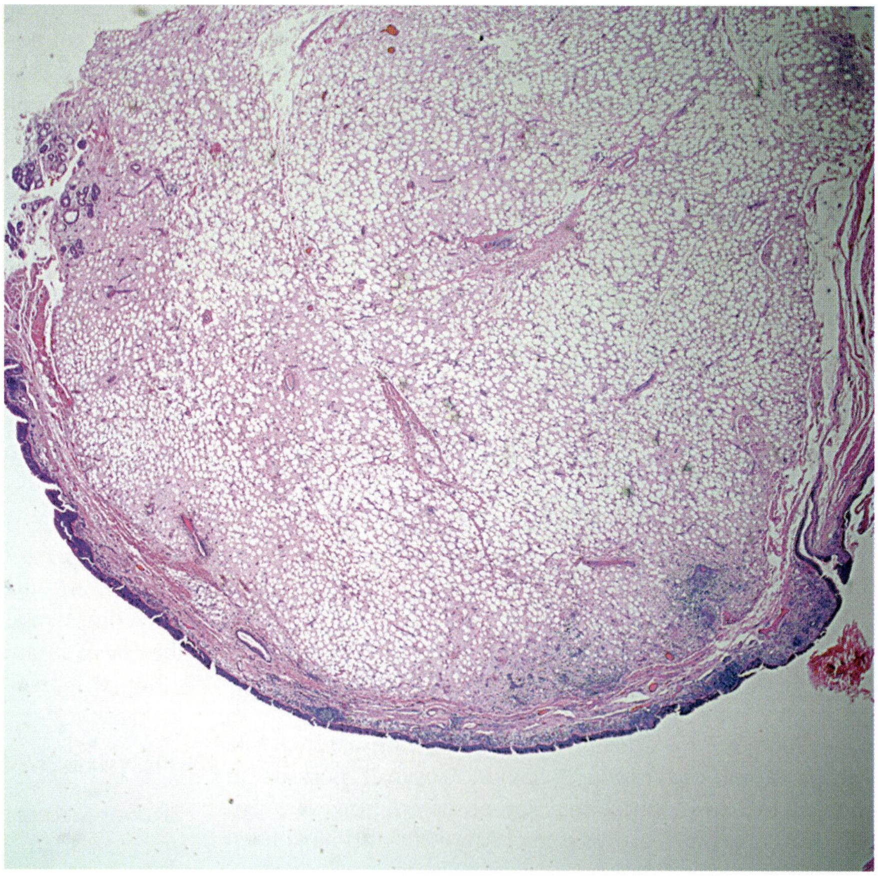

Figure 7-85 Low-power view of an endobronchial lipoma. Note that the tumor is composed mainly of mature adipose tissue.

Treatment and Prognosis

Surgical resection of the tumor is curative. Procedures that have been used range in extent from bronchotomy to lobectomy to pneumonectomy, depending on tumor location. Choice of surgical procedure is based on the specifics of the individual case.

Angiomyolipoma

Primary angiomyolipomas of the lung are exceedingly rare[161–166]; however, these tumors have been described in patients with and without a history of tuberous sclerosis. In some instances, the diagnosis is made at autopsy, whereas in others, the patient presents with an

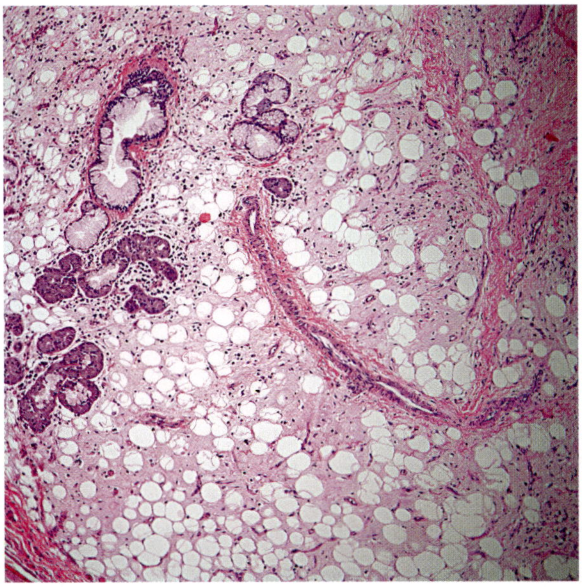

Figure 7-86 Endobronchial lipoma with sparing of the endobronchial glands.

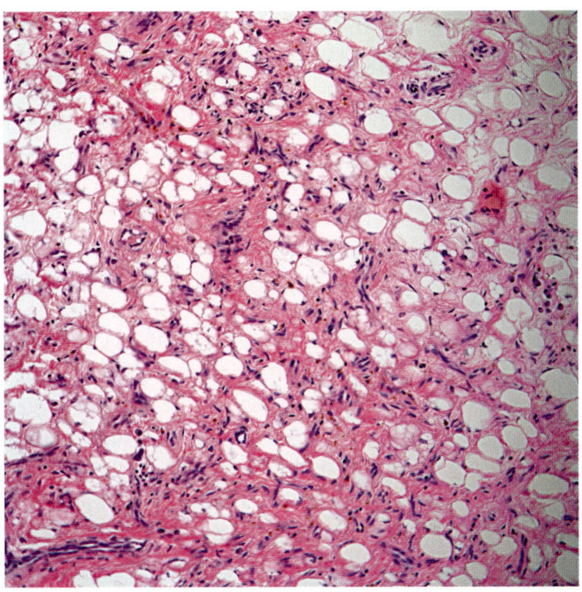

Figure 7-87 Endobronchial lipoma with a spindle cell component.

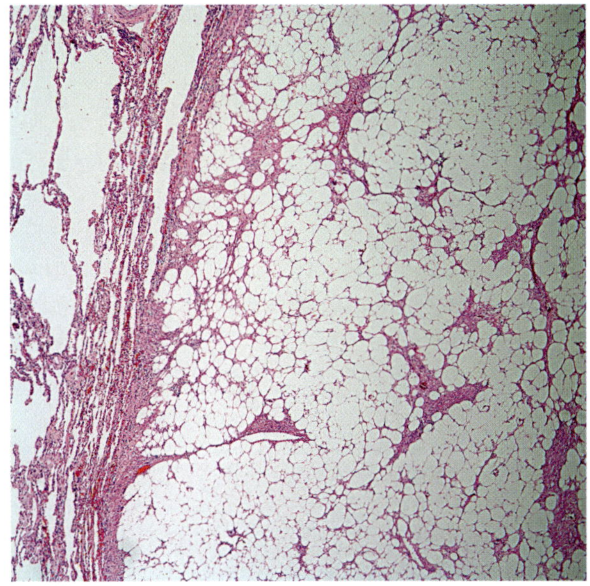

Figure 7-88 Low-power view of an intrapulmonary angiomyolipoma. Focal solid areas are present with abundant adipose tissue.

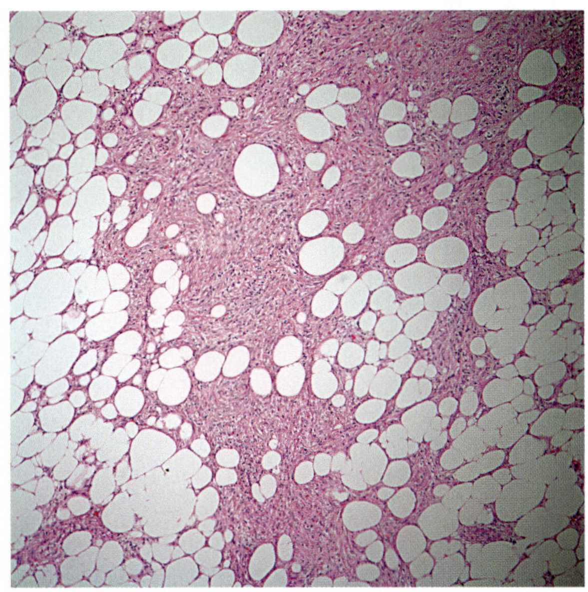

Figure 7-89 Pulmonary angiomyolioma. Solid areas composed of smooth muscle are present.

intrapulmonary mass. The tumor has been reported to affect the liver and lung simultaneously in some patients without a history of tuberous sclerosis.[163,166]

Histopathologic Features

On gross examination, the yellowish tumors appear to be well circumscribed, with a soft consistency, and are intraparenchymal in location. Tumor size may range from less than 1 cm to more than 3 cm in greatest dimension. Pulmonary angiomyolipomas show histopathologic features similar to those of the kidney tumors: abundant areas of mature adipose tissue, with solid areas of smooth muscle composed of spindle cells with light eosinophilic cytoplasm, oval nuclei, and inconspicuous nucleoli (Figs. 7-88 to 7-91). In some areas, cells with clear cytoplasm may be visible. Nuclear atypia and mitotic activity are not present. In addition to the adipose and muscle tissue, scattered vessels are distributed haphazardly. On immunohistochemical studies, the tumor may show positive staining for smooth muscle actin in the muscle areas, whereas S-100 protein may show positive staining in adipose tissue. HMB-45 staining can be either positive or negative in these tumors.

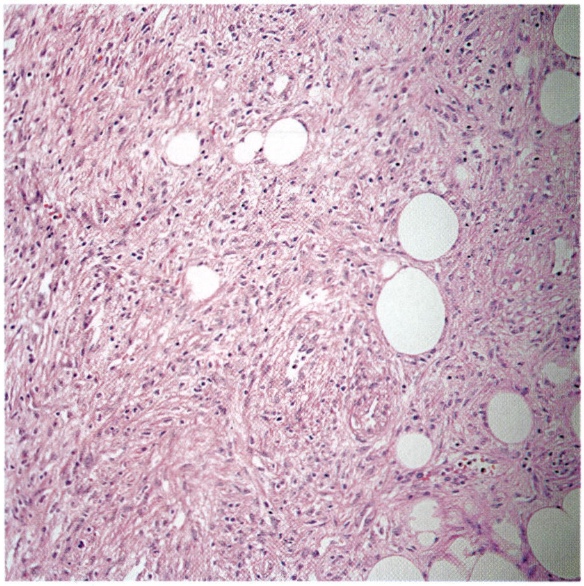

Figure 7-90 Pulmonary angiomyolipoma. Solid areas of smooth muscle are present with only focal adipose tissue.

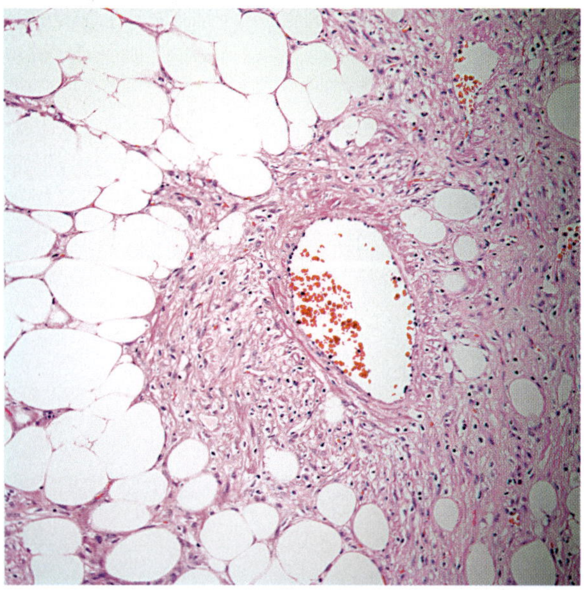

Figure 7-91 Pulmonary angiomyolipoma. Adipose tissue, smooth muscle, and ectatic vessels can be seen.

Treatment and Prognosis

Surgical resection is the treatment of choice and is curative. It is important to determine whether the patient has associated tuberous sclerosis, and to rule out the presence of other synchronous tumors elsewhere.

Liposarcoma

Primary liposarcomas of the lung have been reported sporadically in the literature.[167] As with other sarcomas, it is important to rule out the possibility of metastatic disease to the lung. Liposarcomas are known to metastasize to the lung and may show histopathologic growth patterns similar to those in soft tissues. Sawamura[167] reported a case of a 49-year-old woman who presented with a "coin lesion" in the lung. The patient died 6 months after surgical resection of the tumor, and at autopsy, no tumor was found outside of the lung.

An important point is that liposarcomas are more common in the mediastinum and in the chest wall; therefore, a primary tumor in those areas with extension into the lung parenchyma must be excluded. Some of the cases described have raised the possibility of a tumor originating from the pulmonary artery. The same histologic criteria used for tumors in the soft tissue are applicable for tumors in the lung parenchyma. It is imperative to obtain a proper sample, to ensure that a true lipomatous tumor is present, rather than a mixed epithelial-mesenchymal neoplasm. Because of the rarity of these tumors as primary lung neoplasms, it is difficult to determine a specific pattern of clinical behavior.

Myxoid Tumors

Myxoid tumors may range in behavior from benign to malignant, and a few reports expanding the histopathologic spectrum have been presented in the literature; however, these tumors occur only rarely. Matzuoka[169] and Huang[170] and their coworkers both have reported primary myxomas of the lung. In the case described by Matzuoka and colleagues,[169] the patient was an adult with a parenchymal tumor approximately 13 mm in diameter. The tumor described by Huang's group[170] appeared to have arisen from the pulmonary artery, and was larger at approximately 5 cm. Choi and associates[171] described a large intrapulmonary tumor in an adult patient that they classified as an aggressive angiomyxoma. Nicholson and coworkers[172] described two cases of a condition they termed *malignant myxoid endobronchial tumor*; however, they also noted that these tumors may represent the malignant component of a salivary gland–type tumor of the lung, which may be the so-called ex pleomorphic adenoma. Such cases may require additional study and complete sectioning to identify the presence of more conventional areas of salivary gland–type tumor of the lung.

Histopathologic Features

On macroscopic examination, these tumors may range in size from 1 cm to more than 5 cm in greatest dimension. They are soft in consistency and mucoid in appearance and have irregular borders; however, on gross inspection, it is difficult to determine which tumors correspond to which histologic category. The presence of hemorrhage or necrosis should raise the possibility of a more aggressive neoplasm. In tumors of the myxoma group, histopathologic features are similar to those of cardiac myxomas, including extensive areas of a myxoid stroma with the characteristic stellate cells, devoid of nuclear atypia or mitotic activity (Figs. 7-92 and 7-93). Aggressive angiomyxomas may show similar histopathologic features but also will display a vascular network or ectatic thick-walled vessels admixed with the myxoid component. Finally, "malignant myxoid tumors" may display features similar to those seen in myxoid chondrosarcoma or the malignant myxoid component of ex pleomorphic adenomas, including lobulation and a spindle cell component embedded in a myxoid background. The cellular proliferation generally shows nuclear atypia and mitotic activity. In some cases of malignant myxoid neoplasms (unpublished data), extensive sampling showed only myxoid areas with obvious malignant features. These findings suggest that these tumors may occur as primary lung neoplasms (Figs. 7-94 and 7-95).

Immunohistochemical studies may be helpful in ruling out more common epithelial, neuroendocrine, or mesenchymal neoplasms. Myxoid neoplasms usually demonstrate negative staining for CD34, CD31, keratin, muscle markers, and S-100 protein. Vimentin staining is positive, and CD34 will stain the vascular component of these lesions.

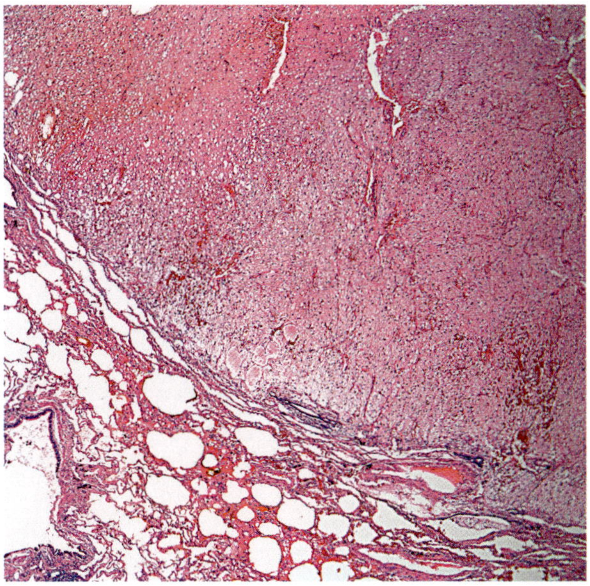

Figure 7-92 Low-power view of an intrapulmonary myxoma. The tumor is well circumscribed.

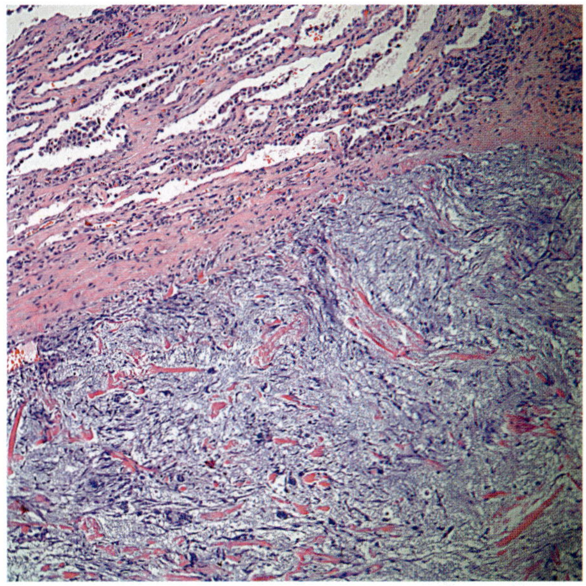

Figure 7-94 Primary myxoid sarcoma of the lung. Note the cellular atypia.

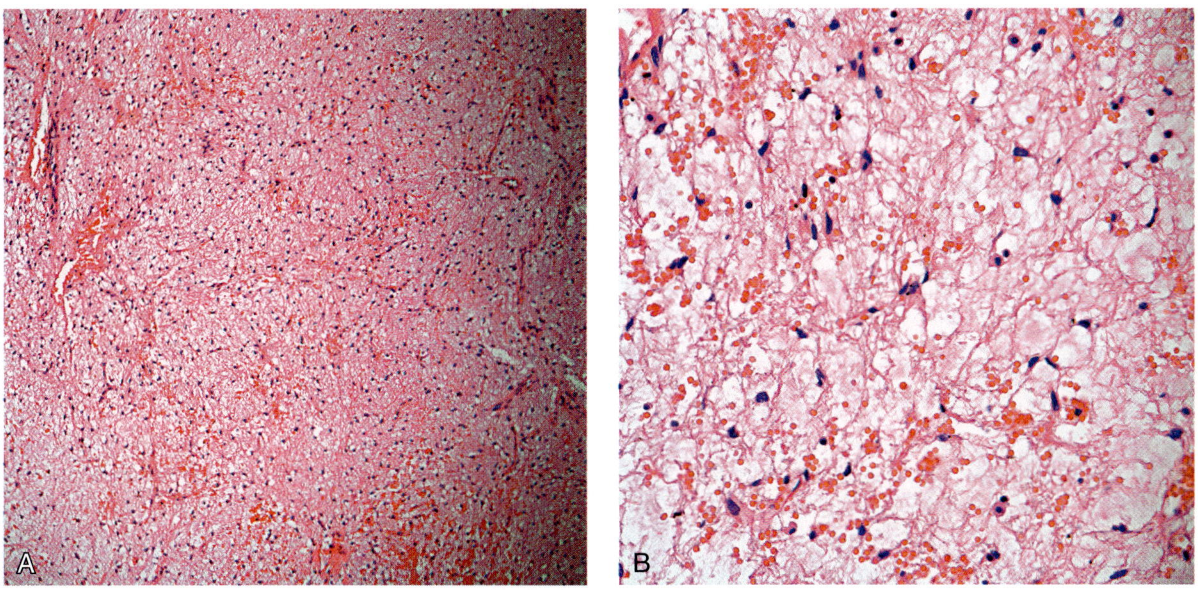

Figure 7-93 **A**, Intrapulmonary myxoma with marked myxoid changes and spindle cells. **B**, High-power view shows spindle cells without nuclear atypia.

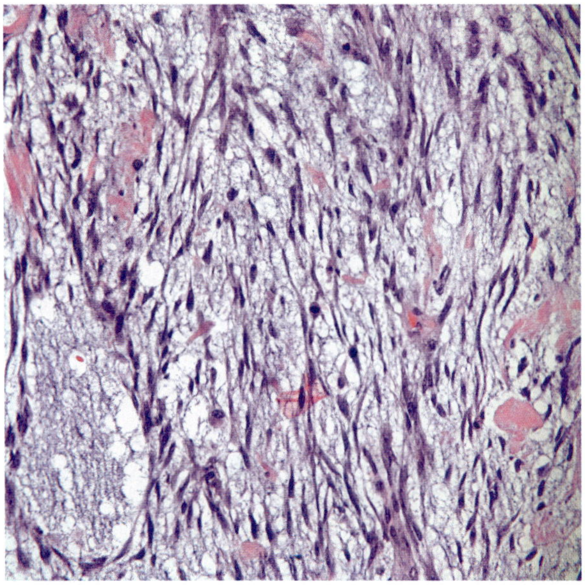

Figure 7-95 Primary myxoid sarcoma of the lung with nuclear atypia and mitotic activity.

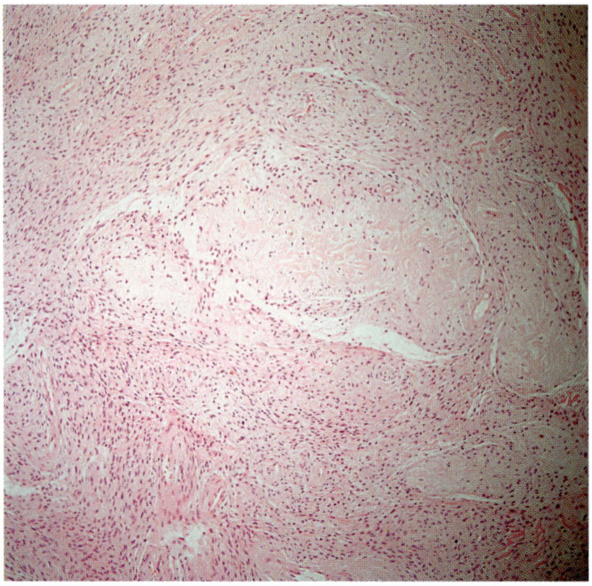

Figure 7-96 Hyalinizing spindle cell tumor with giant cell rosettes.

Treatment and Prognosis

The treatment of choice for myxomas and aggressive angiomyxomas is complete surgical resection, and it may be curative. In cases of malignant myxoid tumors, adjuvant treatment (chemotherapy, immunotherapy, or radiotherapy) may be required, depending on the individual circumstances.

Hyalinizing Spindle Cell Tumor with Giant Rosettes

This tumor, originally described in the soft tissues, occurs rarely, and it is even more rare as a primary lung neoplasm; only a few descriptions exist in the literature.[173,174] Magro and associates[174] first reported this lesion in a 20-year-old woman with multiple bilateral nodules. Although the investigators stated that the patient did not have a history of previous tumor, the presence of multiple bilateral pulmonary nodules highly suggests the possibility of metastatic disease to the lung. More recently, Kim and colleagues[173] described a 50-year-old woman who had a left lower mass approximately 7 cm in diameter and no other clinical history of previous tumor.

Histopathologic Features

The histopathologic features of this tumor are the same as those described for their soft tissue counterparts. The tumors display a spindle cell proliferation that may show myxoid or calcified areas. "Rosette-like" structures composed of collagen fibers, surrounded by spindle cells that impart the appearance of rosettes, are the identifying characteristic (Figs. 7-96 and 7-97). In some areas the tumor may also show a hemangiopericytic pattern, and scattered giant cells also may be present in the periphery. A bland overall cytologic appearance is characteristic, with no nuclear atypia or mitotic activity.

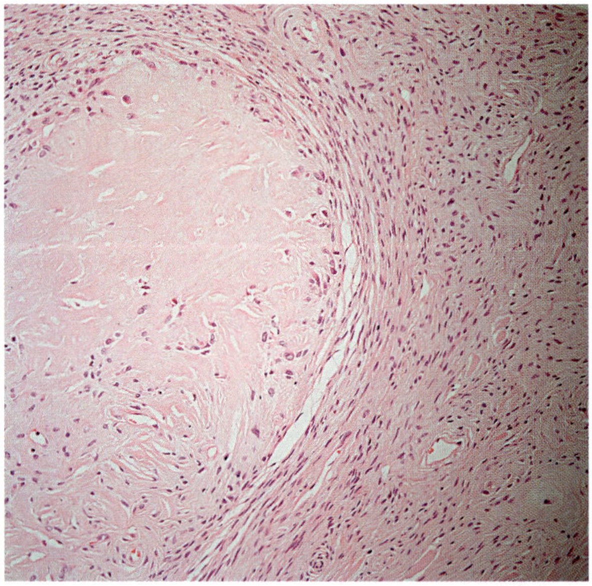

Figure 7-97 At higher magnification, this hyalinizing spindle cell tumor with giant cell rosettes shows lack of nuclear atypia and no mitotic activity.

Immunohistochemical studies are necessary to rule out other conditions that may present problems in the differential diagnosis. When intrapulmonary solitary fibrous tumor is suspected, the use of immunostains for CD34 and Bcl-2 may prove beneficial, because those stains give a negative reaction in the hyalinizing spindle cell tumor and a positive reaction in solitary fibrous tumors. Another condition that should be considered is adenofibroma; in this tumor, however, presence of an epithelial component should be an important clue to a correct diagnosis. Although vimentin staining is positive in hyalinizing spindle cell tumors, reaction to other immunostains, including those for muscle, neural, epithelial, and neuroendocrine markers, is negative.

Treatment and Prognosis

The treatment of choice is surgical resection of the tumor. Because of the rarity of this tumor in an intrapulmonary site, it is difficult to determine an unequivocal pattern of behavior; however, complete surgical resection may be curative.

NEUROGENIC TUMORS

The spectrum of tumors that show neural differentiation in the lung is just as extensive as that seen in the soft tissue, ranging from benign to malignant tumors. In unusual circumstances, the lung may show neuroglial heterotopias[175]; in this section, however, only tumoral conditions will be addressed.

Neural-derived tumors occurring primarily in the lung are exceedingly rare. In 1965, Bartley and Arean[176] described two cases, one malignant and one benign schwannoma, and reviewed the current literature of the time, noting that some of the previously reported diagnoses may not have been valid. In 1983, Roviaro and associates[177] reviewed the topic of primary pulmonary neurogenic tumors at a single institution over a period of 13 years and identified 4 cases in 1664 pulmonary neoplasms, drawing the conclusion that these tumors represent approximately 0.2% of all pulmonary neoplasms. These workers noted that the tumor in the lung was not associated with von Recklinghausen's disease; however, other investigators have documented the existence of primary neural tumors in the lung in patients with a history of neurofibromatosis.[178]

Schwannoma

Primary schwannomas of either benign or malignant histology, occurring primarily in the lung, have been described mainly in individual case reports.[179–186] Schwannomas appear to show an anatomic distribution similar to that for other, more common pulmonary tumors; they may be centrally located as an intrabronchial tumor or arise in the parenchyma of the lung as a peripheral tumor. Clinical signs and symptoms are related to anatomic location and may include shortness of breath, chest pain, or hemoptysis when the tumors are centrally located. Patients with peripheral tumors may present without any symptoms. Schwannomas have been described in patients of various age groups, ranging from young teenagers to adults older than 70 years of age.

Macroscopic Features

Schwannomas may appear as polypoid masses protruding and obliterating the bronchial lumen (Fig. 7-98) or may manifest as intraparenchymal tumors. They are well circumscribed but not encapsulated and surrounded by a thin membranous tissue and can range in size from 1 cm to more than 5 cm in greatest dimension. The cut surface of these tumors is smooth and homogeneous in appearance. When the histologic pattern is that of a malignant schwannoma, the tumor may show areas of necrosis or hemorrhage, features that should give the gross impression of a malignant neoplasm.

Histopathologic Features

Conventional schwannomas are characterized by a well-circumscribed tumor mass with a prominent spindle cell proliferation. The tumor may contain hypo- and hypercellular areas; however, it does not display nuclear atypia or mitotic activity (Figs. 7-99 to 7-101). Classic features of Antoni A and Antoni B can be seen in some tumors. In addition, some tumors have shown extensive areas of melanin pigment or the presence of psammoma bodies. These tumors characteristically show ectatic, thick-walled within the spindle cell proliferation. Malignant schwannomas also display a spindle cellular proliferation; however, the palisading of the nuclei characteristically seen in benign cases may not be present. Malignant schwannomas usually show areas of necrosis or hemorrhage, as well as nuclear atypia and mitotic activity (Figs. 7-102 to 7-104). In reported cases of malignant schwannoma, the histologic pattern has been that of an epithelioid schwannoma. Cases showing melanotic changes also have been described.

Immunohistochemical Features

Conventional schwannomas demonstrate a strong positive reaction for S-100 protein and negative staining for muscle, epithelial, and vascular markers. With malignant schwannomas, S-100 protein may not be as useful as in their benign counterparts, because the malignant tumors

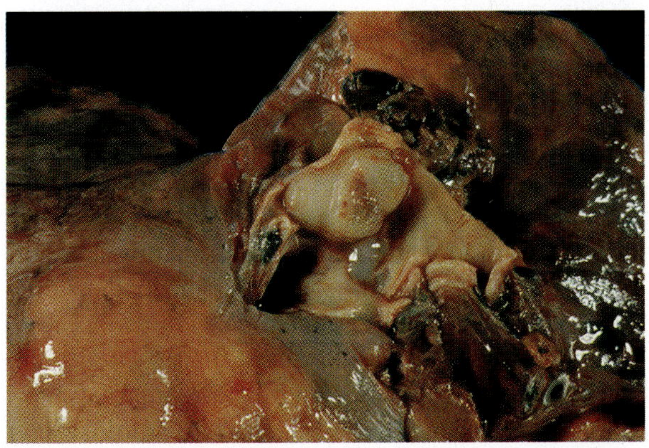

Figure 7-98 Pulmonary bronchial schwannoma, gross specimen. Note the attachment of the tumor to the bronchial wall.

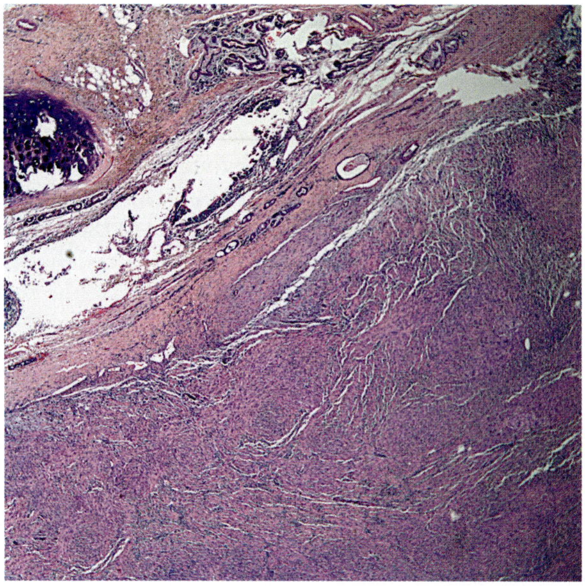

Figure 7-99 Low-power view of a bronchial schwannoma.

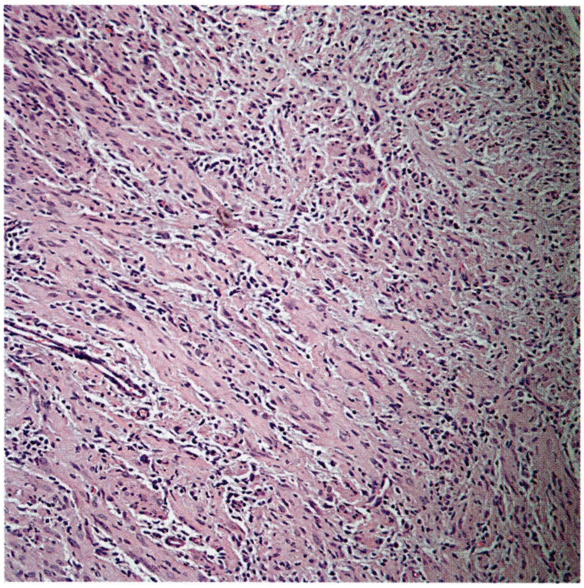

Figure 7-100 Bronchial schwannoma. A spindle cell proliferation is admixed with scattered inflammatory cells.

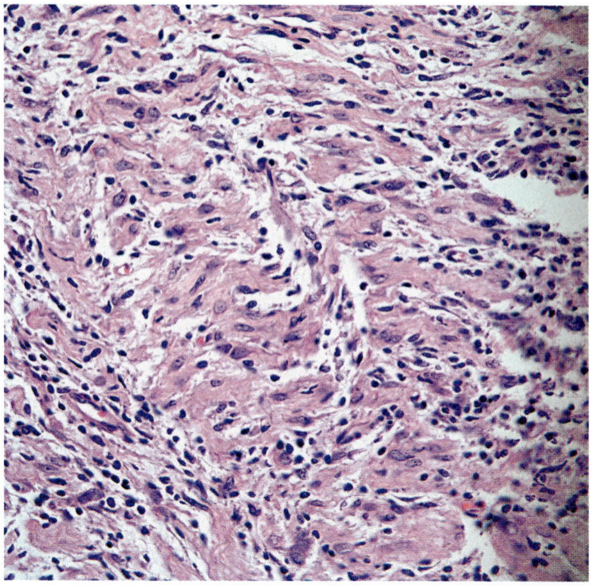

Figure 7-101 High-power view of the spindle cell proliferation in the bronchial schwannoma seen in Figure 7-100. Nuclear atypia and mitotic figures are lacking.

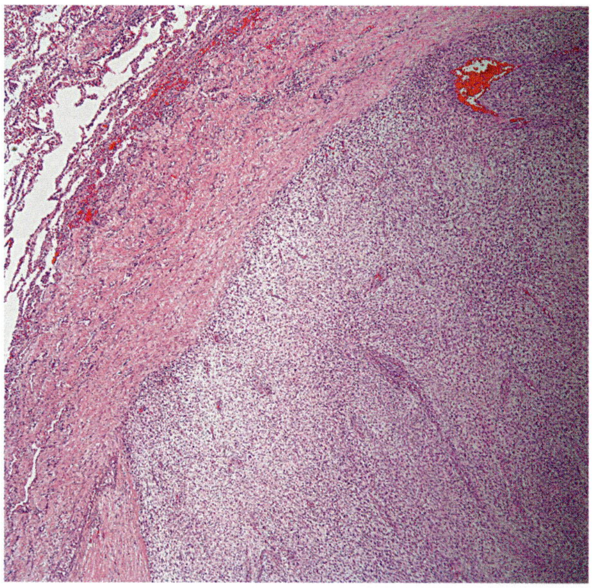

Figure 7-102 Malignant schwannoma of the lung. The well-demarcated tumor with spindle cell proliferation is seen destroying lung parenchyma.

may show negative staining for S-100 protein in a large proportion of cases, and positive reactions, when they occur, are not as strong as with the conventional schwannoma. Another marker that may show positive staining, but is not specific for schwannomas, is neurofilament protein.

Treatment and Prognosis

Surgical resection of the tumor is the treatment of choice and is curative for conventional schwannomas. With malignant schwannomas, however, adjuvant therapies may be required. Malignant schwannoma usually follows a rapidly progressive course with metastasis and eventual fatal outcome.

Neurofibroma and Ganglioneuroma

These tumors more commonly are encountered in the posterior mediastinum; on rare occasions, however, they have been described as either intrapulmonary or endobronchial tumors.[187–191] No definitive association has been made between these lung tumors and neurofibromatosis; however, this possibility needs to be explored clinically. The reported cases have been in adult patients, who may present with signs and symptoms of bronchial obstruction, including shortness of breath, chest pain, cough, and hemoptysis. Usually the tumors are single neoplasms;

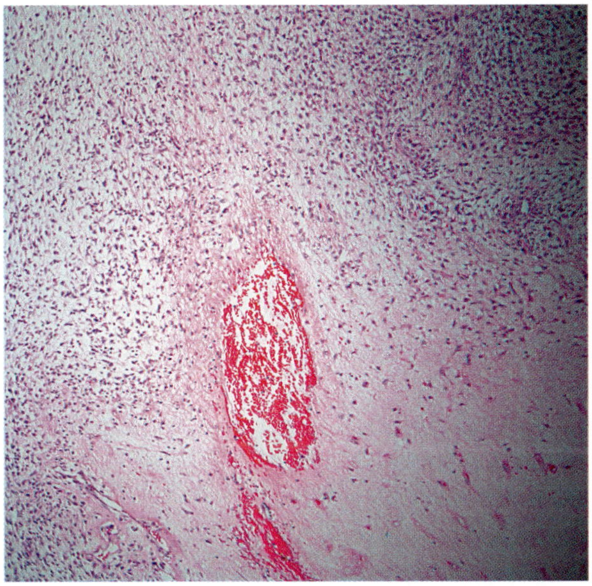

Figure 7-103 Malignant schwannoma of the lung. A thickened ectatic vessel and spindle cell proliferation are readily apparent.

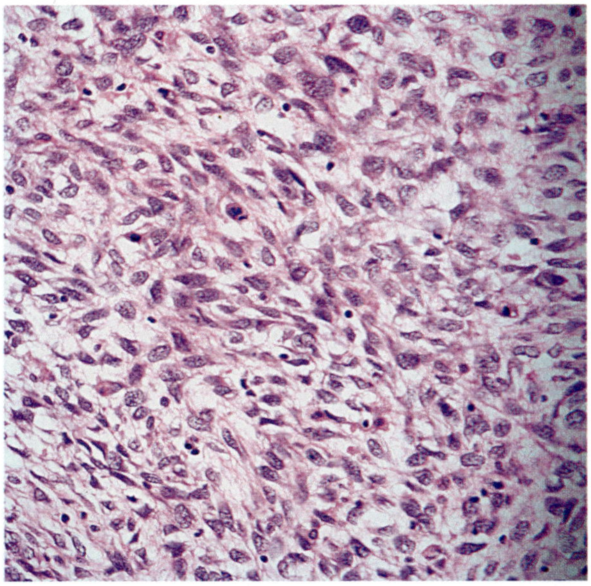

Figure 7-104 Malignant schwannoma of the lung. Microscopic features include an atypical spindle cell prolilferation with mitotic figures.

however, unusual cases of multiple pulmonary tumors have been described.[190]

Macroscopic Features

The tumors that are centrally located may grow as polypoid intraluminal tumors, with size ranging up to 3 cm in greatest dimension. The tumors are well circumscribed and sometimes encapsulated and are of soft consistency and gray-white in color; the cut surface has a homogeneous-appearing surface, without areas of hemorrhage or necrosis. Tumors that are intraparenchymal may reach a larger size of more than 5 cm in greatest dimension. They also are well circumscribed and may or may not be encapsulated.

Histopathologic Features

The tumors are characterized by a spindle cell proliferation embedded in a fibrocollagenous stroma. The spindle cells have scant eosinophilic cytoplasm and elongated nuclei. Nuclear atypia and mitotic activity are not features of these tumors (Figs. 7-105 to 7-107). In some cases, areas of myxoid change and more collagen deposition can be seen. In cases of ganglioneuroma, the spindle cellular proliferation is similar to that of neurofibromas,

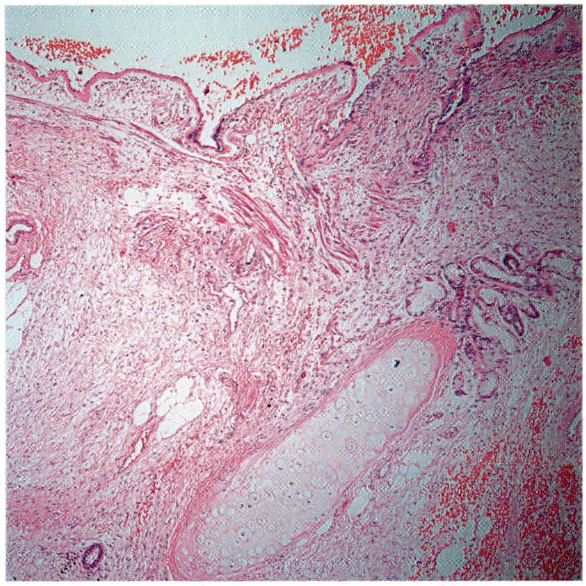

Figure 7-105 Low-power view of an endobronchial neurofibroma.

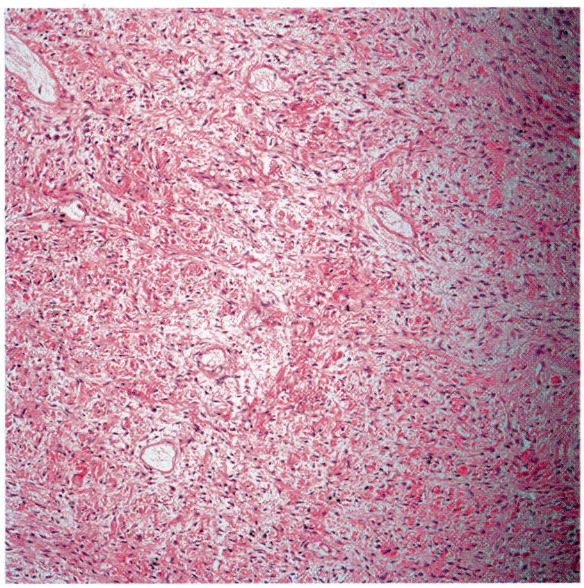

Figure 7-106 Neurofibroma. A bland spindle cell proliferation admixed with collagen is present.

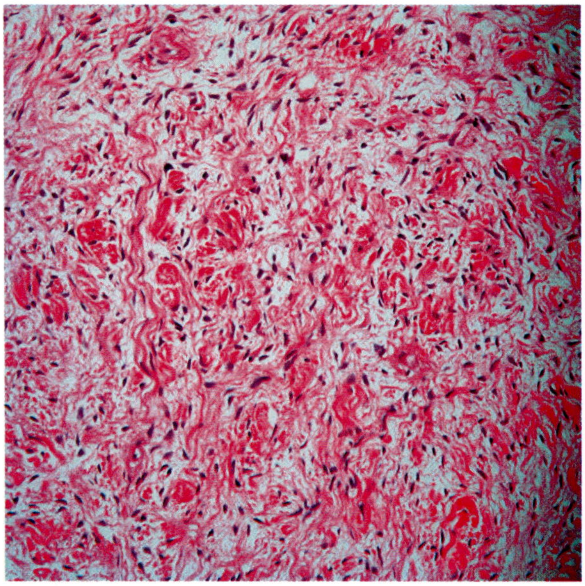

Figure 7-107 High-power view of an endobronchial neurofibroma lacking nuclear atypia and mitotic activity.

except that numerous ganglion cells are seen intermixed with the spindle cellular proliferation—hence the implication of ganglioneuroma. Immunohistochemical studies for detection of S-100 protein and neurofilament protein are positive in these tumors. Neu-N also may show positive staining in ganglion cells.

Differential Diagnosis

The most important consideration in the differential diagnosis is other benign spindle cell tumors of the lung, mainly leiomyomas or intrapulmonary solitary fibrous tumor. With both of these lesions, the use of immunohistochemistry aids in diagnosis; neurofibromas will show positive staining for S-100 protein or neurofilament protein and negative staining for muscle markers CD34 and Bcl-2, for which positive staining is seen in leiomyomas or solitary fibrous tumors, respectively.

Treatment and Prognosis

The treatment of choice is surgical resection by lobectomy or laser ablation. The specific procedure will be dictated by the clinical and radiologic presentation of the tumor. Complete surgical resection is curative in these patients.

Ependymoma

Ependymoma is unusual as a primary lung neoplasm. Crotty and coworkers[192] described a case of ependymoma in a 64-year-old woman who presented with a solitary lung nodule after being treated for a non–small cell carcinoma. The resected neoplasm was measured at 2 cm in diameter and was well circumscribed but not encapsulated. On histologic examination, the tumor was found to be composed of pleomorphic spindle cells with round to oval nuclei and prominent nucleoli, arranged in a subtle fascicular pattern with the presence of perivascular pseudorosettes. Other findings included increased mitotic activity and areas of necrosis. On immunohistochemical studies, the tumor cells showed positive staining for glial fibrillary acid protein, with less intense staining for vimentin, S-100 protein, and Leu-7.

Owing to the unusual occurrence of these tumors in the lung, it is difficult to assess clinical behavior and specific treatment.

Malignant Triton Tumor

Only a few cases of the unusual malignant "triton" tumor occurring in the lung parenchyma have been described.[193] By definition, triton tumors are characterized by the presence of malignant schwannoma and rhabdomyoblastic differentiation. The tumor has been described in children and adults with no history of neurofibromatosis. At presentation, clinical signs and symptoms may include shortness of breath, cough, and a large intrapulmonary mass. The tumors usually are larger than 5 cm in greatest dimension and have been described as soft in consistency with a gelatinous appearance. On histologic examination, like its soft tissue counterparts, the tumor is characterized by a spindle cell proliferation embedded in a loose or myxoid stroma replacing normal lung parenchyma. The spindle cell component may show marked cellular atypia characterized by bizarre cells and mitotic activity and may exhibit a fascicular growth pattern with subtle storiform growth and perivascular hyalinization of the vascular structures associated with the tumor. Merging with these neural areas are larger cells with eosinophilic cytoplasm and eccentric nuclei showing rhabdomyoblastic differentiation (Figs. 7-108 to 7-110).

Immunohistochemical studies using myoglobin and desmin will stain the rhabdomyoblastic component; the neural component may show at least focal positive staining for S-100 protein. The differential diagnosis for these tumors will depend on the material available for evaluation; however, malignant schwannoma and rhabdomyosarcoma are two distinct possibilities, owing to the two components present in these tumors. In addition, other primary or metastatic spindle cell sarcomas can be considered in the differential diagnosis. The use of immunohistochemical studies should lead to a correct interpretation.

Ganglioneuroblastoma

Ganglioneuroblastomas are exceedingly rare in the lung, and only a few cases have been described in the literature.[194,195] In appearance, these neoplasms resemble childhood tumors in the adrenal gland or posterior mediastinum. The cases described have been in patients

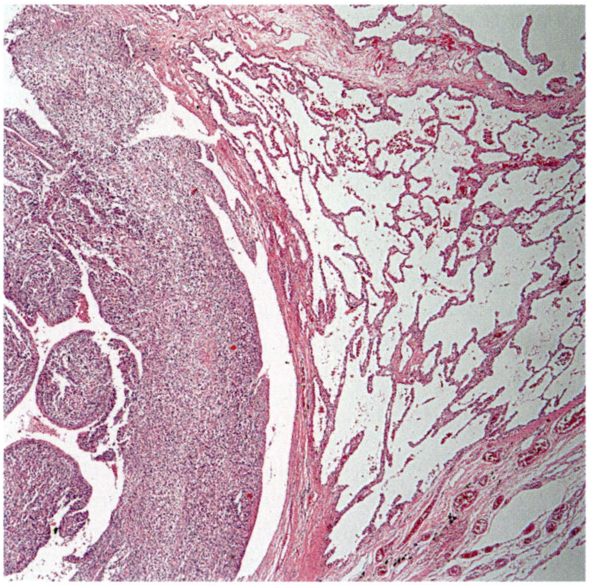

Figure 7-108 Low-power view of an intrapulmonary malignant triton tumor.

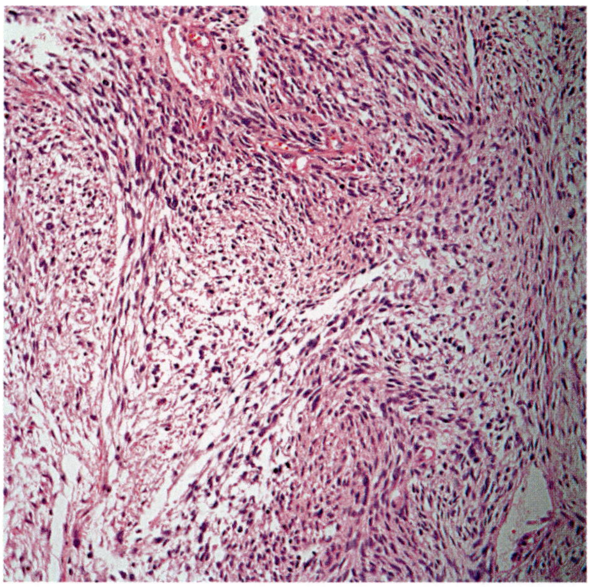

Figure 7-109 Intrapulmonary malignant triton tumor with a malignant spindle cellular proliferation.

between the ages of 20 and 47 years. Some of the patients presented with clinical signs and symptoms of cough, multiple endocrine neoplasia, gastric ulcers, and hypercalcemia; other patients have been asymptomatic.

Macroscopic Features

Ganglioneuroblastomas have been described as firm, well-circumscribed, tan to white, with a homogeneous surface, which can range in size up to 5 cm in diameter. The tumor may be located within the lung parenchyma without compromising bronchial structures, or may be seen in a peribronchial location, impinging on the bronchial lumen.

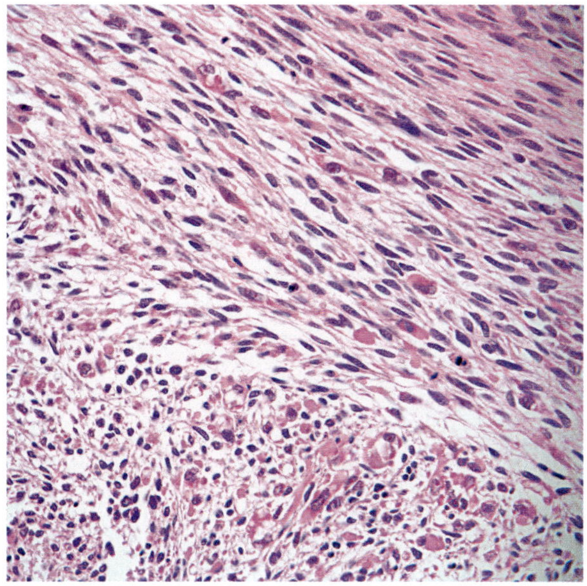

Figure 7-110 Intrapulmonary malignant triton tumor with rhabdomyoblastic differentiation.

Histopathologic Features

Ganglioneuroblastomas are characterized by the presence of a neoplastic cellular proliferation growing in sheets composed of rather small cells, with scant amounts of eosinophilic cytoplasm, round to oval nuclei, and in some cells, punctate nucleoli. Nuclear atypia and mitotic activity are present, along with areas of eosinophilic granular-like material characteristic of neurophil. The neoplastic cells appear to be connected to each other by thin cellular prolongations, and in some areas, rosettes also can be seen (Figs. 7-111 to 7-114). Areas of necrosis

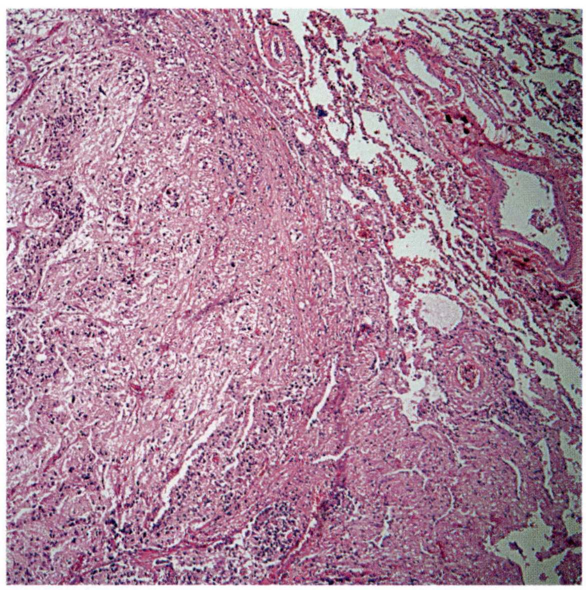

Figure 7-111 Low-power view of a primary pulmonary ganglioneuroblastoma. In this area of the tumor, neuroblastomatous differentiation is evident.

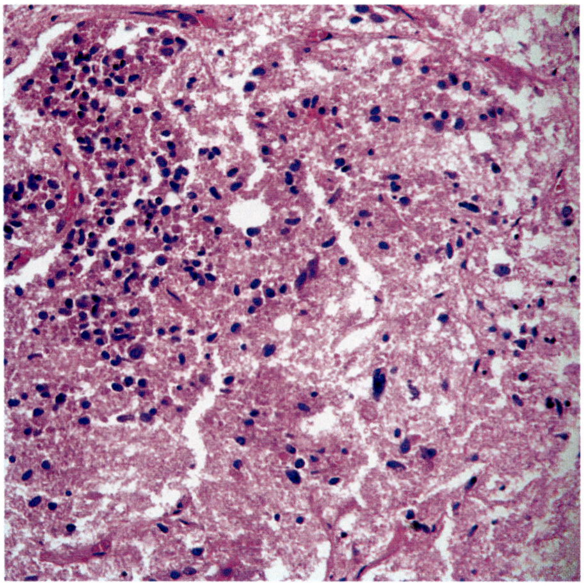

Figure 7-112 Higher-power view of the neuroblastomatous change in the tumor in Figure 7-111. Small cells are embedded in neuropil.

and cystic degeneration have been described. Admixed with this neoplastic cellular proliferation are larger cells with moderate amounts of eosinophilic cytoplasm, round to oval nuclei, and prominent nucleoli, representing ganglion differentiation. Immunohistochemical studies for neurofilament protein and S-100 protein may show focal staining in tumor cells, whereas Neu-N (for "neuronal nuclei") may show positive staining in the ganglion cells.

The differential diagnosis for ganglioneuroblastomas may pose some problems in cases in which limited biopsy tissue is available for evaluation. Other, more common primary lung neoplasms may be mistaken for ganglioneuroblastoma, including small cell carcinoma and small round blue cell tumor. In this setting, the use of immunohistochemical studies for epithelial or mesenchymal neoplasm should lead to a correct interpretation.

Treatment and Prognosis

The initial treatment is complete surgical resection of the tumor, which can be accomplished by lobectomy. It is difficult to assess whether patients with ganglioneuroblastomas will benefit from adjuvant therapy (e.g., chemotherapy, radiotherapy, immunotherapy), owing to the low frequency of this tumor. In at least two of the reported cases, the patient survived at least 1 year after initial diagnosis.

PULMONARY ARTERY SARCOMA

Any of the tumors described previously as occurring within the lung parenchyma or bronchial area also may originate from the wall of the pulmonary artery or vein.[196–207]

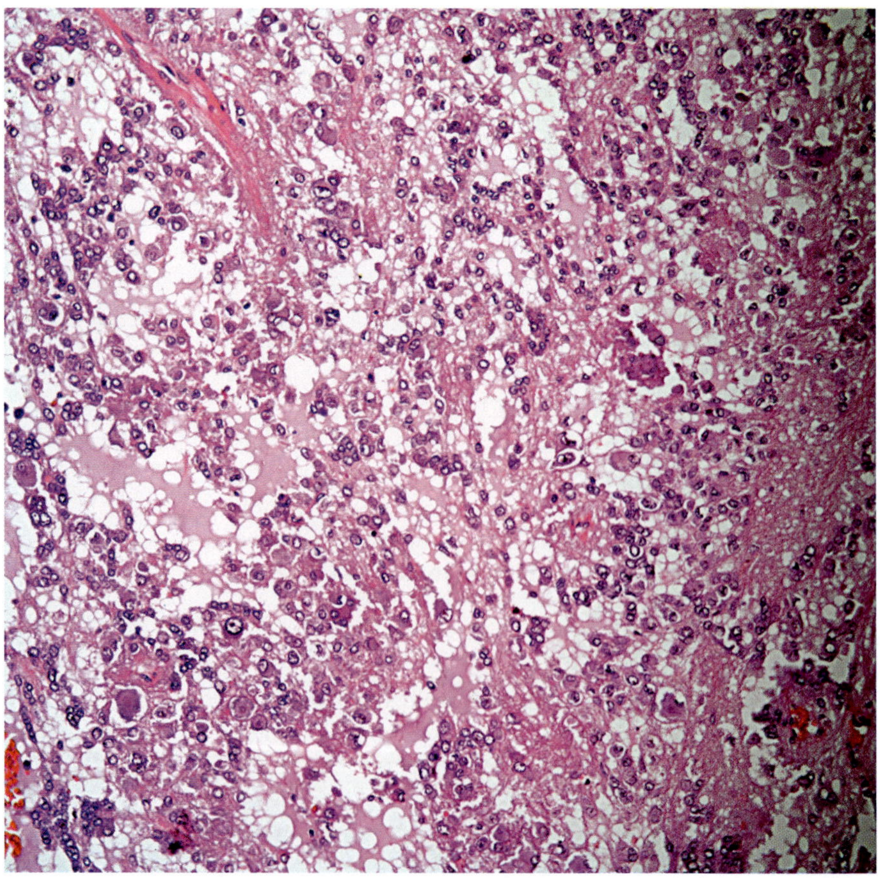

Figure 7-113 Primary ganglioneuroblastoma. Larger cells are seen admixed with scattered ganglion-like cells.

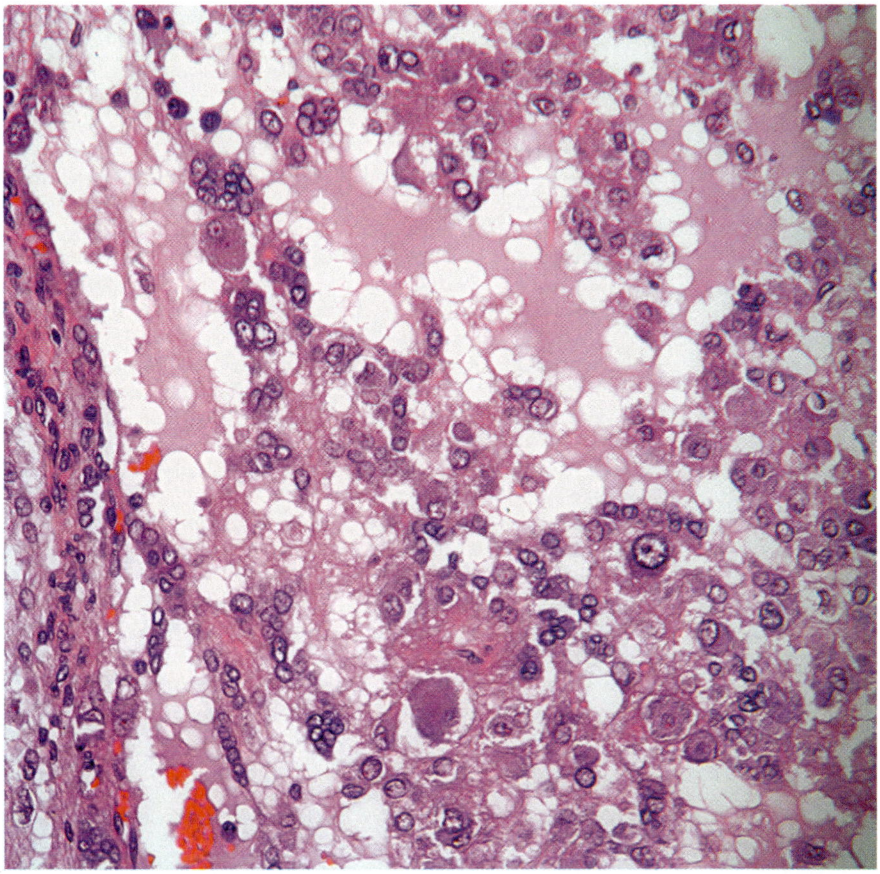

Figure 7-114 High-power view of a primary intrapulmonary ganglioneuroblastoma showing larger cells compatible with ganglion differentiation.

These tumors can be of vascular, muscle, osseous, or cartilaginous composition or may be of a more undifferentiated nature. For all tumors seen within the lumen of the pulmonary artery, it is essential to identify those with pulmonary artery origin because their treatment will differ. Because these tumors have been suggested to arise from pluripotent intimal cells, they also have been designated "intimal sarcoma." Most pulmonary artery sarcomas, however, probably arise from the pulmonary trunk.

In one of the largest series, Huo and associates[208] studied 12 cases (8 in men and 4 in women, between the ages of 34 and 69 years). In nine of those cases, the pulmonary trunk was involved, whereas in two cases, the tumor appeared to arise from the right pulmonary artery. The patients presented with variable clinical signs and symptoms including dyspnea, chest pain, cough, fatigue, and syncope. The initial diagnosis was not malignancy but rather pulmonary hypertension, pneumonia, asthma, or bronchitis.

On gross inspection, the tumor is seen to be attached to the pulmonary artery (Fig. 7-115), with or without extension along the vessel branches, possibly into the lung parenchyma. Histologic analysis may reveal the sarcoma to be a leiomyosarcoma, an angiosarcoma, or any other type of sarcoma. In the study by Huo's group,[208] eight cases showed distinct morphologic features that permitted more definitive classification: Two tumors were

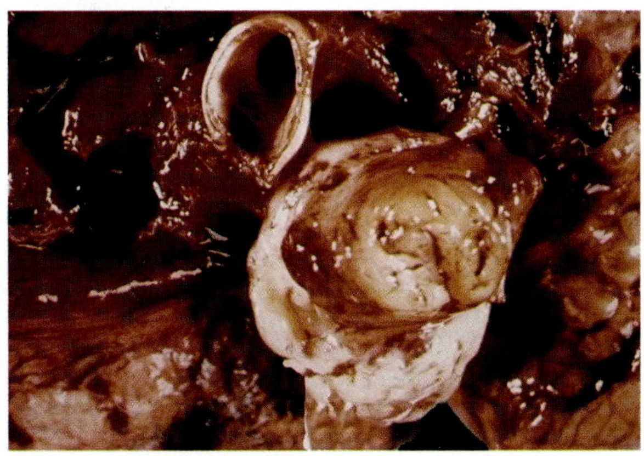

Figure 7-115 Pulmonary artery sarcoma, gross specimen. Note the tumor arising from the vessel. The airway is patent.

classified as rhabdomyosarcomas, four tumors as leiomyosarcomas, one osteosarcoma, and one as angiosarcoma. In four cases, no possible differentiation was noted, and those tumors were declared to be undifferentiated high-grade sarcomas. The use of immunohistochemical studies is important for proper classification of these tumors, and the use of vascular, neural, and muscle markers may help to obtain a definitive diagnosis.

The initial treatment is surgical and may be followed by chemotherapy or radiation therapy, or both, depending on the individual circumstances. The rate of intrathoracic metastases has been estimated to be approximately 50%, with a rate of distant metastasis of approximately 16%. The prognosis is still poor, however: Most of the patients in Huo and coworkers' study died of their disease within a period of 12 months.[208]

REFERENCES

1. Iverson L. Bronchopulmonary sarcoma. *J Thorac Surg*. 1954;27:130–148.
2. Eskenasy A. Primary lung sarcoma. A histopathologic study of 118 cases. *Morphol Embryol (Bucur)*. 1979;25:27–38.
3. Nascimiento AG, Unni KK, Bernatz PE. Sarcomas of the lung. *Mayo Clin Proc*. 1982;57:355–359.
4. Attanoos RL, Appleton MAC, Gibbs AR. Primary sarcomas of the lung: a clinicopathological and immunohistochemical study of 14 cases. *Histopathology*. 1996;29:29–36.
5. Keel SB, Bacha E, Mark EJ, Nielsen GP, Rosenberg AE. Primary pulmonary sarcoma: a clinicopathologic study of 26 cases. *Mod Pathol*. 1999;12:1124–1131.
6. Tomashefski JF. Benign endobronchial mesenchymal tumors: their relationship to parenchymal pulmonary hamartomas. *Am J Surg Pathol*. 1982;6:531–540.
7. Van den Bosch JM, Wagenaar S, Corrin B, Elbers JR, Knaepen PJ, Westermann CJ. Mesenchymoma of the lung (so called hamartoma): a review of 154 parenchymal and endobronchial cases. *Thorax*. 1987;42:790–793.
8. Bateson EM. So called hamartoma of the lung—a true neoplasm of fibrous connective tissue of the bronchi. *Cancer*. 1973;31:1458–1468.
9. Steele JD. The solitary pulmonary nodule. *J Thorac Cardiovasc Surg*. 1963;46:21–39.
10. Ray JF, Lawton BR, Magnin GE, et al. The coin lesion story: update 1976. Twenty years experience with early thoracotomy for 179 suspected malignant coin lesions. *Chest*. 1976;79:332–336.
11. Minasian H. Uncommon pulmonary hamartomas. *Thorax*. 1977;32:360–364.
12. Bateson EM. Cartilage-containing tumours of the lung (chondroma) and the mixed type (so called hamartoma): an unusual case of multiple tumours. *Thorax*. 1965;20:447–461.
13. Anderson MN. Multicentric hamartomas of the lung—report of a case with two additional lesions nine years after primary resection. *Ann Thorac Surg*. 1968;6:449–472.
14. Silverman J, Kay S. Multiple pulmonary leiomyomatous hamartomas: report of a case with ultrastructural examination. *Cancer*. 1976;38:1199–1204.
15. Burkhardt A, Otto HF, Kaukel E. Multiple pulmonary (hamartomatous?) leiomyomas. *Virchows Arch A Pathol Anat Histol*. 1981;394:133–141.
16. Kaplan C, Katoh A, Shamoto M, et al. Multiple leiomyomas of the lung: benign or malignant? *Am Rev Respir Dis*. 1973;108:656–659.
17. Martin E. Leiomyomatous lung lesions: a proposed classification. *AJR Am J Roentgenol*. 1983;141:269–272.
18. Horstmann JP, Pietra G, Harman JA, Cole NG, Grinspan S. Spontaneous regression of pulmonary leiomyomas during pregnancy. *Cancer*. 1977;39:314–321.
19. Wolff M, Kaye G, Silva F. Pulmonary metastases (with admixed epithelial elements) from smooth muscle tumors: report of nine cases, including three males. *Am J Surg Pathol*. 1979;3:325–342.
20. Nistal M, Hardisson D, Riestra ML. Multiple pulmonary leiomyomatous hamartomas associated with bronchogenic cyst in a man. *Arch Pathol Lab Med*. 2003;127:194–196.
21. Yellin A, Roseman Y, Lieberman Y. Review of smooth muscle tumours of the lower respiratory tract. *Br J Dis Chest*. 1984;78:337–351.
22. Lajos TZ, Meckstroth CV. Pedunculated leiomyoma of the lung: report of a case. *Chest*. 1967;52:114–116.
23. Van Way CW, McCraken RL, Carlisle BB. Leiomyoma of the lower respiratory tract. *Ann Thorac Surg*. 1968;6:273–276.
24. Sweet R. Pulmonary leiomyoma. *AJR Am J Roentgenol*. 1969;107:823–826.
25. Inberg MV, Sutinen S, Tala E. Leiomyoma of the lung and intercostal space: report of four cases. *Scand J Thorac Cardiovasc Surg*. 1969;3:52–58.
26. Sabbagh AH, O'Hare JE, Fritz JM. Pulmonary leiomyoma. *Ariz Med*. 1974;5:359–360.
27. Orlowski TM, Stasiak K, Kolodziej J. Leiomyoma of the lung. *J Thorac Cardiovasc Surg*. 1978;76:257–261.
28. Yamada H, Katoh O, Yamaguchi T, Natsuaki M, Itoh T. Intrabronchial leiomyoma treated by localized resection via bronchoscopy and bronchoplasty. *Chest*. 1987;91:283–285.
29. White SH, Ibrahim NBN, Forrester-Wood CP, Jeyasingham K. Leiomyomas of the lower respiratory tract. *Thorax*. 1985;40:306–311.
30. Vera-Román JM, Sobonya RE, Gomez-Garcia JL, Sanz-Bondia JR, Paris-Romeu F. Leiomyoma of the lung. Literature review and case report. *Cancer*. 1983;52:936–941.
31. Gal AA, Brooks JJ, Pietra GG. Leiomyomatous neoplasms of the lung: a clinical, histologic, and immunohistochemical study. *Mod Pathol*. 1989;2:209–216.
32. Defore Jr WW, Miller JI. Leiomyoma of the lung: a case report. *J Miss State Med Assoc*. 1981;22(3):49–50.
33. Ogawa J, Inoue H, Koide S, Kawada S, Shohtsu A, Osamura Y. Leiomyoma of the lung—report of a case. *Tokai J Exp Clin Med*. 1983;8:129–133.
34. Mathur RM, Sen G, Yadav KS. Endobronchial leiomyoma. *Indian J Cancer*. 1993;30:16–19.
35. Kim KH, Suh JS, Han WS. Leiomyoma of the bronchus treated by endoscopic resection. *Ann Thorac Surg*. 1993;56:1164–1166.
36. Ayabe H, Tsuji H, Tagawa Y, Tomita M, Tsuda N, Chen J. Endobronchial leiomyoma: report of a case treated by bronchoplasty and a review of the literature. *Surg Today*. 1995;25:1057–1060.
37. Ozçelik U, Kotiloğlu E, Göçmen A, Senocak ME, Kiper N. Endobronchial leiomyoma: a case report. *Thorax*. 1995;50:101–102.
38. Gotti G, Haid MM, Paladini P, Di Bisceglie M, Volterrani L, Sforza V. Pedunculated pulmonary leiomyoma with large cyst formation. *Ann Thorac Surg*. 1993;56:1178–1180.
39. Paik HC, Lee DY, Bae KM. Pulmonary leiomyoma: a case report. *Yonsei Med J*. 1993;34:381–385.
40. Lee CH, Juang YC, Hsueh C. Leiomyoma of the bronchus: report of a case successfully treated by Nd-YAG laser via fiberoptic bronchoscope. *J Formos Med Assoc*. 1990;89:1012–1014.
41. Karnak I, Akcoren Z, Senocak ME. Endobronchial leiomyoma in children. *Eur J Pediatr Surg*. 2000;10:136–139.
42. Bilgin S, Yilmaz A, Okur E, Düzgün S, Tahaoğlu C, Akkaya E. Primary endobronchial leiomyoma: a case report. *Tuberk Toraks*. 2004;52:272–274.
43. Zuricalday CG, Lor F, Turner CG. Primary pedunculated leiomyosarcoma of the lung. *Thorax*. 1982;37:153–154.
44. Wang NS, Seemayer TA, Ahmed MN, Morin J. Pulmonary leiomyosarcoma associated with an arteriovenous fistula. *Arch Pathol*. 1974;98:100–105.
45. Wick MR, Scheithauer BW, Piehler JM, Pairolero PC. Primary pulmonary leiomyosarcomas: a light and electron microscopic study. *Arch Pathol Lab Med*. 1982;106:510–514.
46. Capewell M, Webb JN, Crompton GK. Primary leiomyosarcoma of the lung presenting with a persistent pneumothorax. *Thorax*. 1986;41:649–650.
47. Schanher PW. Primary pulmonary leiomyosarcoma: case report and review of literature. *Ann Surg*. 1975;181:20–21.
48. Guillan RA, Wilen CJW, Zelman S. Primary leiomyosarcoma of the lung. *Chest*. 1969;56:452–454.

49. Shoji F, Yoshino I, Takeshita M, Sumiyoshi S, Sueishi K, Maehara Y. Pulmonary leiomyosarcoma presenting as a Pancoast tumor. *Pathol Res Pract*. 2007;203:745–748.
50. Shimono T, Yuasa H, Yuasa U, et al. Pulmonary leiomyosarcoma extending into left atrium or pulmonary trunk: complete resection with cardiopulmonary bypass. *J Thorac Cardiovasc Surg*. 1998;115:460–461.
51. Patel S, Jindrak KF, Anandarao N. Primary pedunculated leiomyosarcoma of the lung. *N Y State J Med*. 1991;91:29–31.
52. Gil RL, Albrechtsson U, Jakobsson B. Pulmonary leiomyosarcoma appearing as a cyst. Report of one case and review of the literature. *Thorac Cardiovasc Surg*. 1985;33:250–252.
53. Stark P, Frood L. Primary leiomyosarcoma of the lung originating in an emphysematous bulla. *Rofo*. 1989;151:738–739.
54. McNamara JJ, Paulson DL, Kingsley WB, Salinas-Izaquirre SF, Urschel Jr HC. Primary leiomyosarcoma of the lung. *J Thorac Cardiovasc Surg*. 1969;57:635–641.
55. Kulpati DD, Kamath RK, Singhal VS, Saha MM. Primary leiomyosarcoma of lung. *Indian J Chest Dis Allied Sci*. 1981;23(3):148–150.
56. Pedersen VM, Schulze S, Madsen KH, Krogdahl AS. Primary pulmonary leiomyosarcoma. *Scand J Thorac Cardiovasc Surg*. 1984;18:251–254.
57. Carlson DH, Hanelin J. Leiomyosarcoma of the thorax. *J Can Assoc Radiol*. 1978;29:221–224.
58. Dowell AR. Primary pulmonary leiomyosarcoma: report of two cases and review of the literature. *Ann Thorac Surg*. 1974;17:384–394.
59. Chaudhuri MR. Primary leiomyosarcoma of the lung. *Br J Dis Chest*. 1973;67:75–80.
60. Koizumi N, Fukuda T, Ohnishi Y, et al. Pulmonary myxoid leiomyosarcoma. *Pathol Int*. 1995;45:879–884.
61. Passamonte PM, Luger AM. Primary pulmonary leiomyosarcoma with digital clubbing and pleural effusion. Case report. *Mo Med*. 1984;667–668.
62. Morgan PGM, Ball J. Pulmonary leiomyosarcomas. *Br J Dis Chest*. 1980;74:245–252.
63. Ramanathan T. Primary leiomyosarcoma of the lung. *Thorax*. 1974;29:482–489.
64. Guccion JG, Rosen SH. Bronchopulmonary leiomyosarcoma and fibrosarcoma: a study of 32 cases and review of the literature. *Cancer*. 1972;30:836–847.
65. Moran CA, Suster S, Abbondanzo SL, Koss MN. Primary leiomyosarcomas of the lung: a clinicopathologic and immunohistochemical study of 18 cases. *Mod Pathol*. 1997;10:121–128.
66. Jimenez JF, Uthman EO, Townsend JW, Gloster ES, Seibert JJ. Primary bronchopulmonary leiomyosarcoma in childhood. *Arch Pathol Lab Med*. 1986;110:348–351.
67. Ownby D, Lyon G, Spock A. Primary leiomyosarcoma of the lung in chilhood. *Am J Dis Child*. 1976;130:1132–1133.
68. Takeda F, Yamagiwa I, Ohizumi H, Shiono S. Leiomyosarcoma of the main bronchus in a girl: a long-time survivor with multiple lung metastases. *Pediatr Pneumonol*. 2004;37:368–374.
69. Lai DS, Lue KH, Su JM, Chang H. Primary bronchopulmonary leiomyosarcoma of the left main bronchus in a child presenting with wheezing and atelectasis of the left lung. *Pediatr Pneumonol*. 2002;33:318–321.
70. Kawai K, Fukamizu A, Kawakami Y, et al. A case of renin producing leiomyosarcoma originating in the lung. *Endocrinol Jpn*. 1991;38:603–609.
71. Fitoz S, Atasoy C, Kizilkaya E, Başekim C, Karsli F. Radiologic findings in primary pulmonary leiomyosarcoma. *J Thorac Imaging*. 2000;15:151–152.
72. Schneider BF, Lovell MA, Golden WL. Cytogenetic abnormalities in primary bronchopulmonary leiomyosarcoma of childhood. *Cancer Genet Cytogenet*. 1998;105:145–150.
73. Przgodzki RM, Moran CA, Suster S, Koss MN. Primary pulmonary rhabdomyosarcomas: a clinicopathologic and immunohistochemical study of three cases. *Mod Pathol*. 1995;8:658–661.
74. Avagnina A, Elsner B, De Marco L, Bracco AN, Nazar J, Pavlovsky H. Pulmonary rhabdomyosarcoma with isolated small bowel metastasis. A report of a case with immunohistochemical and ultrastructural studies. *Cancer*. 1984;53:1948.
75. Bleisch VR, Kraus FT. Polypoid sarcoma of the pulmonary trunk. *Cancer*. 1980;46:314.
76. Conquest HF, Thornton JL, Massie JR, Coxe 3rd JW. Primary pulmonary rhabdomyosarcoma. *Ann Surg*. 1965;161:688.
77. Gondon LZ, Boss H. Primary rhabdomyosarcoma of lung. *Cancer*. 1955;8:588.
78. Forbes GB. Rhabdomyosarcoma of bronchus. *J Pathol*. 1955;70:427.
79. Drennan JM, McCormack RJM. Primary rhabdomyosarcoma of the lung. *J Pathol*. 1960;79:147.
80. Lee SH, Rengachary SS, Paramesh J. Primary pulmonary rhabdomyosarcoma. *Hum Pathol*. 1981;12:92.
81. Fallon G, Schiller M, Kilman JW. Primary rhabdomyosarcoma of the bronchus. *Ann Thorac Surg*. 1971;12:650.
82. Murphy JJ, Blair GK, Fraser GC, et al. Rhabdomyosarcoma arising within congenital pulmonary cysts. *J Pediatr Surg*. 1992;27:1364.
83. Ueda K, Gruppo R, Unger F, Martin L, Bove K. Rhabdomyosarcoma arising in congenital cystic adenomatoid malformation. *Cancer*. 1977;40:383.
84. Allan BT, Day DL, Dehner LP. Primary pulmonary rhabdomyosarcomas of the lung in children. *Cancer*. 1987;59:1005–1011.
85. Suster S, Moran CA. Pulmonary adenofibroma: report of two cases of an unusual type of hamartomatous lesion of the lung. *Histopathology*. 1993;23:547–551.
86. Scarff RW, Gowar FJS. Fibroadenoma of the lung. *J Pathol Bacteriol*. 1944;56:257–259.
87. Butler CH, Kleinerman J. Pulmonary hamartoma. *Arch Pathol*. 1969;88:584–592.
88. Pettinato G, Manivel JC, Saldana MJ, Peyser J, Dehner LP. Primary bronchopulmonary fibrosarcoma of chilhoood and adolescence: reassessment of a low grade malignancy. Clinicopathologic study of five cases and review of the literature. *Hum Pathol*. 1989;20:463–471.
89. Yousem SA, Flynn SD. Intrapulmonary localized fibrous tumor: intraparenchymal so-called localized fibrous mesothelioma. *Am J Clin Pathol*. 1988;89:365–369.
90. Aufiero TX, McGary SA, Campbell DB, Phillips PP. Intrapulmonary benign fibrous tumor of the pleura. *J Thorac Cardiovasc Surg*. 1995;110:549–551.
91. Caruso RA, LaSpada F, Gaeta M, Minutoli I, Inferrera C. Report of an intrapulmonary solitary fibrous tumor: fine-needle aspiration cytologic findings, clinicopathological, and immunohistochemical features. *Diagn Cytopathol*. 1996;14:64–67.
92. Kanamori Y, Hashizume K, Sugiyama M, et al. Intrapulmonary solitary fibrous tumor in an eight-year-old male. *Pediatr Pulmonol*. 2005;40:261–264.
93. Sagawa M, Ueda Y, Matsubara F, et al. Intrapulmonary solitary fibrous tumor diagnosed by immunohistochemical and genetic approaches: report of a case. *Surg Today*. 2007;37:423–425.
94. Sakurai H, Tanaka W, Kaji M, Yamazaki K, Suemasu K. Intrapulmonary localized fibrous tumor of the lung: a very unusual presentation. *Ann Thorac Surg*. 2008;86:1360–1362.
95. Meade JB, Whitwell F, Bickford BJ, Waddington JK. Primary haemangiopericytoma of lung. *Thorax*. 1974;29:1–15.
96. Yousem SA, Hochholzer L. Primary pulmonary hemangiopericytoma. *Cancer*. 1987;59:549–555.
97. Paullada JJ, Lisci-Garmilla A, Gonzáles-Angulo A, et al. Hemangiopericytoma associated with hypoglycemia. Metabolic and electron microscopic studies of a case. *Am J Med*. 1968;44:990–994.
98. Suster S, Moran CA. Primary synovial sarcoma of the mediastinum: a clinicopathologic, immunohistochemical, and ultrastrutural study of 15 cases. *Am J Surg Pathol*. 2005;29:569–578.

99. Zeren H, Moran CA, Suster S, Fishback NF, Koss MN. Primary pulmonary sarcomas with features of monophasic synovial sarcoma: a clinicopathological, immunohistochemical, and ultrastructural study of 25 cases. *Hum Pathol.* 1995;26:474–480.
100. Kaplan MA, Goodman MD, Satish J, et al. Primary pulmonary sarcoma with morphologic features of monophasic synovial sarcoma and chromosome translocation t(X;18). *Am J Clin Pathol.* 1996;105:195–199.
101. Noguera R, Navarro S, Cremades A, et al. Translocation (X;18) in a biphasic synovial sarcoma with morphologic features of neural differentiation. *Diagn Mol Pathol.* 1998;7:16–23.
102. Hisaoka M, Hashimoto H, Iwamasa T, Ishikawa K, Aoki T. Primary synovial sarcoma of the lung: report of two cases confirmed by molecular detection of *SYT-SSX* fusion gene transcripts. *Histopathology.* 1999;34:205–210.
103. Roberts CA, Seemayer TA, Neff JR, Alonso A, Nelson M, Bridge JA. Translocation (X;18) in primary synovial sarcoma of the lung. *Cancer Genet Cytogenet.* 1996;88:49–52.
104. Terasaki H, Niki T, Hasegawa T, et al. Primary synovial sarcoma of the lung: a case report confirmed by molecular detection of *SYT-SSX* fusion gene transcripts. *Jpn J Clin Oncol.* 2001;31:212–216.
105. Mikami Y, Nakajima M, Hashimoto H, Kuwabara K, Sasao Y, Manabe T. Primary poorly differentiated monophasic synovial sarcoma of the lung. A case report with immunohistochemical and genetic studies. *Pathol Res Pract.* 2003;199:827–833.
106. Niwa H, Masuda S, Kobayashi C, Oda Y. Pulmonary synovial sarcoma with polypoid endobronchial growth: a case report, immunohistochemical and cytogenetic study. *Pathol Int.* 2004;54:611–615.
107. Deraedt K, Debiec-Rychter M, Sciot R. Radiation-associated synovial sarcoma of the lung following radiotherapy for pulmonary metastasis of Wilms' tumour. *Histopathology.* 2006;48:463–477.
108. Watanabe R, Kamiyoshihara M, Kaira K, Motegi A, Takise A. Spontaneous expectoration of primary pulmonary synovial sarcoma. *J Thorac Oncol.* 2006;1:1025–1026.
109. Esaka EJ, Celebrezze JU, Golde SH, Chiossi G, Thomas RL. Pulmonary synovial sarcoma presenting as pneumothorax during pregnancy. *Obstet Gynecol.* 2008;111:555–558.
110. Jiang J, Zhou J, Ding W. Primary pulmonary synovial sarcoma, a rare primary neoplasm: two case reports and review of the current literature. *Respirology.* 2008;13:748–750.
111. Banerjee D, Gorse SJ, Cotter M, Johnson RC. Sonographic and pathologic features of metastatic synovial sarcoma of the lung presenting as breast neoplasm. *Breast J.* 2004;10:372.
112. Essary LR, Vargas SO, Fletcher CD. Primary pleuropulmonary synovial sarcoma: reappraisal of a recently described anatomic subset. *Cancer.* 2002;94:459–469.
113. Okamoto S, Hisaoka M, Daa T, Hatakeyama K, Iwamasa T, Hashimoto H. Primary pulmonary synovial sarcoma: a clinicopathologic, immunohistochemical, and molecular study of 11 cases. *Hum Pathol.* 2004;35:850–856.
114. Bégueret H, Galateau-Salle F, Guillou L, et al. Primary intrathoracic synovial sarcoma: a clinicopathologic study fo 40 t(X;18)-positive cases from the French Sarcoma Group and the Mesopath Group. *Am J Surg Pathol.* 2005;29:339–346.
115. Hartel PH, Fanburg-Smith JC, Frazier A, et al. Primary pulmonary and mediastinal synovial sarcoma: a clinicopathologic study of 60 cases and comparison with five prior series. *Mod Pathol.* 2007;20:760–769.
116. Mezzelani A, Mariani L, Tamborini E, et al. *SYT-SSX* fusion genes and prognosis in synovial sarcoma. *Br J Cancer.* 2001;85:1535–1539.
117. Boroumand N, Raja V, Jones DV, Haque AK. *SYT-SSX2* variant of primary pulmonary synovial sarcoma with focal expression of CD117 (c-kit) protein and poor clinical outcome. *Arch Pathol Lab Med.* 2003;127:e201–e204.
118. Bedrossian CWM, Verani R, Unger K, Salman J. Pulmonary malignant fibrous histiocytoma: light and electron microscopic studies of one case. *Chest.* 1979;75:186–189.
119. Sajjad SM, Begin LR, Dail DH, Lukeman JM. Fibrous histiocytoma of lung—a clinicopathological study of two cases. *Histopathology.* 1981;5:325–334.
120. Kern WH, Hughes RK, Meyer BW, Harley DP. Malignant fibrous histiocytoma of the lung. *Cancer.* 1979;44:1793–1801.
121. McDonnel T, Kyriakos M, Roper C, Mazoujjian G. Malignant fibrous histiocytoma of the lung. *Cancer.* 1988;61:137–145.
122. Lee JT, Shelburne JD, Linder J. Primary malignant fibrous histiocytoma of the lung: a clinicopathologic and ultrastructural study of five cases. *Cancer.* 1984;53:1124–1130.
123. Yousem SA, Hochholzer L. Malignant fibrous histiocytoma of the lung. *Cancer.* 1987;60:2532–2541.
124. Nosanchuk JS, Weatherbee L. Primary osteogenic sarcoma in lung: report of a case. *J Thorac Cardiovasc Surg.* 1969;58:242–247.
125. Bhalla M, Thompson BG, Harley R, McLoud TC. Primary extraosseous pulmonary osteogenic sarcoma: CT findings. *J Comput Assist Tomogr.* 1992;16:974–976.
126. Loose JH, el-Naggar AK, Ro JY, Huang WL, McMurtrey MJ, Ayala AG. Primary osteosarcoma of the lung. Report of two cases and review of the literature. *J Thorac Cardiovasc Surg.* 1990;100:867–873.
127. Colby TV, Bilbao JE, Battifora H, Uni K. Primary osteosarcoma of the lung: a reappraisal following immunohistologic study. *Arch Pathol Lab Med.* 1989;113:1147–1150.
128. Connolly JP, McGuyer CA, Sageman WS, Bailey H. Intrathoracic osteosarcoma diagnosed by CT scan and pleural biopsy. *Chest.* 1991;100:265–267.
129. Chapman AD, Pritchard SC, Yap WW, et al. Primary pulmonary osteosarcoma: case report and molecular analysis. *Cancer.* 2001;91:779–784.
130. Matono R, Maruyama R, Ide S, et al. Extraskeletal osteosarcoma of the pleura: a case report. *Gen Thorac Cardiovasc Surg.* 2008;56:180–182.
131. Yamazaki K, Okabayashi K, Hamatake D, et al. Primary osteosarcoma of the lung: a case report. *Ann Thorac Cardiovasc Surg.* 2006;12:126–128.
132. Magishi K, Yoshida H, Izumi Y, Ishikawa N, Kubota H. Primary osteosarcoma of the lung: report of a case. *Surg Today.* 2004;34:150–152.
133. Niimi R, Matsumine A, Kusuzaki K, et al. Primary osteosarcoma of the lung: a case report and review of the literature. *Mod Oncol.* 2008;25:251–255.
134. Stark P, Smith DC, Watkins GE, Chun KE. Primary intrathoracic extraosseous osteogenic sarcoma: report of three cases. *Radiology.* 1990;174:725–726.
135. Reingold IM, Amromin GD. Extraosseous osteosarcoma of the lung. *Cancer.* 1971;28:491–498.
136. Carney JA, Sheps S, Go V, Gorden H. The triad of gastric leiomyosarcoma, functioning extra-adrenal paraganglioma and pulmonary chondroma. *N Engl J Med.* 1977;296:1517–1518.
137. Carney JA. The triad of gastric epithelioid leiomyosarcoma, fuctioning extra-adrenal paraganglioma, and pulmonary chondroma. *Cancer.* 1979;43:374–382.
138. Mesina MS, Sampson MG, Nelson S. Carney's triad: role of transthoracic needle biopsy. *Am Rev Respir Dis.* 1983;126:311–313.
139. Tisell LE, Angervall L, Dahl I, Merck C, Zachrisson BF. Recurrent and metastasizing gastric leiomyoblastoma (epithelioid leiomyosarcoma) associated with multiple pulmonary chondro-hamartomas: long survival of a patient treated with repeated operations. *Cancer.* 1978;41:259–265.
140. Bini A, Grazia M, Petrella F, Chittolini M. Multiple chondromatous hamartomas of the lung. *Interact Cardiovasc Thorac Surg.* 2002;1:78–80.

141. Rodriguez FJ, Aubry MC, Tazelaar HD, Slezak J, Carney JA. Pulmonary chondroma: a tumor associated with Carney's triad and different from pulmonary hamartoma. *Am J Surg Pathol.* 2007;31:1844–1853.
142. Moran CA, Suster S, Carter D. Laryngeal chondrosarcomas. *Arch Pathol Lab Med.* 1992;117:914–917.
143. Daniels AC, Conner GH, Strauss FH. Primary chondrosarcoma of the tracheobronchial tree. *Arch Pathol.* 1967;84:615–624.
144. Rees GM. Primary chondrosarcoma of lung. *Thorax.* 1970;25:366–371.
145. Morgan AD, Salama FD. Primary chondrosarcoma of the lung. Case report and review of the literature. *J Thorac Cardiovasc Surg.* 1972;64:460–466.
146. Sun CCJ, Kroll M, Miller JE. Primary chondrosarcoma of the lung. *Cancer.* 1982;50:1864–1866.
147. Yellin A, Schwartz L, Hersho E, Lieberman Y. Chondrosarcoma of the bronchus. Report of a case with resection and review of the literature. *Chest.* 1983;84:224–226.
148. Morgenroth A, Pfeuffer HP, Viereck HJ, Heine WD. Primary chondrosarcoma of the left inferior lobar bronchus. *Respiration.* 1989;56:241–244.
149. Jazy FK, Cormier WJ, Panke TW, Shehata WM, Amongero FJ. Primary chondrosarcoma of the lung. A report of two cases. *Clin Oncol.* 1984;10:273–279.
150. Azimullah PC, Teengs JP, Boerma EJ. Chondrosarcoma of the lobar bronchus with prolonged postoperative survival. *Eur Respir J.* 1984;7:1537–1538.
151. Hayashi T, Tsuda N, Iseki M, Kishikawa M, Shinozaki T, Hasumoto M. Primary chondrosarcoma of the lung. A clinicopathologic study. *Cancer.* 1993;72:69–74.
152. Parker LA, Molina PL, Bignault AG, Fidler ME. Primary pulmonary chondrosarcoma mimicking bronchogenic cyst on CT and MRI. *Clin Imaging.* 1996;20:181–183.
153. Watanabe A, Ito M, Nomura F, Saka H, Sakai S, Shimokata K. Primary chondrosarcoma of the lung—a case report with immunohistochemical study. *Jpn J Med.* 1990;29:616–619.
154. Alkotob LM, Miller R, Mehta AC. Primary endobronchial chondrosarcoma. *J Bronchol.* 2001;8:110–111.
155. Shah ND, Diwanji SR. Primary chondrosarcoma of the lung with cutaneous and skeletal metastases. *Singapore Med J.* 2007;48:e196–e199.
156. Steurer S, Huber M, Lintner F. Dedifferentiated chondrosarcoma of the lung: case report and review of the literature. *Clin Lung Cancer.* 2007;8:439–442.
157. Huang HY, Hsieh MJ, Chen WJ, Ko SF, Yang BY, Huang SC. Primary mesenchymal chondrosarcoma of the lung. *Ann Thorac Surg.* 2002;73:1960–1962.
158. Moran CA, Suster S, Koss MN. Endobronchial lipomas: a clinicopathological study of four cases. *Mod Pathol.* 1992;7:212–214.
159. Matsuba K, Saito T, Ando K, Shirakusa T. Atypical lipoma of the lung. *Thorax.* 1991;46:685.
160. Schraufnagel DE, Morin JE, Wang NS. Endobronchial lipoma. *Chest.* 1979;75:97–99.
161. Guinee Jr DG, Thornberry DS, Azumi N, Przygodzki RM, Koss MN, Travis WD. Unique pulmonary presentation of an angiomyolipoma. Analysis of clinical, radiographic, and histopathologic features. *Am J Surg Pathol.* 1995;19:476–480.
162. Wu K, Tazelaar HD. Pulmonary angiomyolipoma and multifocal micronodular pneumocyte hyperplasia associated with tuberous sclerosis. *Hum Pathol.* 1999;30:1266–1268.
163. Saito M, Tsukamoto T, Takahashi T, Sai K, Fujii H, Nagashima K. Multifocal angiomyolipoma affecting the liver and lung without tuberous sclerosis. *J Clin Pathol.* 2004;57:221–224.
164. Ito M, Sugamura Y, Ikari H, Sekine I. Angiomyolipoma of the lung. *Arch Pathol Lab Med.* 1998;122:1023–1025.
165. Marcheix B, Brouchet L, Lamarche Y, et al. Pulmonary angiomyolipoma. *Ann Thorac Surg.* 2006;82:1504–1506.
166. Garcia TR, Maestre J. Angiomyolipoma of the liver and lung: a case explained by the presence of perivascular epithelioid cells. *Pathol Res Pract.* 2002;198:363–367.
167. Sawamura K, Hashimoto T, Nanjo S, et al. Primary liposarcoma of the lung: report of a case. *J Surg Oncol.* 1982;19:243–246.
168. Nicolas M, Moran CA, Suster S. Pulmonary metastases from liposarcoma: a clinicopathological and immunohistochemical study of 24 cases. *Am J Clin Pathol.* 2005;47:219–220.
169. Matzuoka H, Takata Y, Maeda S. Primary pulmonary myxoma. *Ann Thorac Surg.* 2005;79:329–330.
170. Huang SC, Lee ML, Chen SJ, Wu MZ, Chang CI. Pulmonary artery myxoma as a rare cause of dyspnea for a young female patient. *J Thorac Cardiovasc Surg.* 2006;131:1179–1180.
171. Choi YD, Kim JH, Nam JH, Choi C, Na KJ, Song SY. Aggressive angiomyxoma of the lung. *J Clin Pathol.* 2008;61:962–964.
172. Nicholson AG, Baandrup U, Florio R, Sheppard MN, Fisher C. Malignant myxoid endobronchial tumour: report of two cases with a unique histological pattern. *Histopathology.* 1999;35:313–318.
173. Kim L, Yoon YH, Choi SJ, et al. Hyalinizing spindle cell tumor with giant rosettes arising in the lung: report of a case with FUS-CREB3L2 fusion transcripts. *Pathol Int.* 2007;57:153–157.
174. Magro C, Fraggetta F, Manusia M. Hyalinizing spindle cell tumor with giant rosettes: a previously undescribed lesion of the lung. *Am J Surg Pathol.* 1998;22:1431–1433.
175. Kershisnik MM, Kaplan C, Craven CM, Carey JC, Townsend JJ, Knisely AS. Intrapulmonary neuroglial heterotopia. *Arch Pathol Lab Med.* 1992;116:1043–1046.
176. Bartley TD, Arean VM. Intrapulmonary neurogenic tumors. *J Thorac Cardiovasc Surg.* 1965;50:114–123.
177. Roviaro G, Montorsi M, Varoli F, Binda R, Cecchetto A. Primary pulmonary tumors of neurogenic origin. *Thorax.* 1983;38:942–945.
178. Unger PD, Geller SA, Anderson PJ. Pulmonary lesions in a patient with neurofibromatosis. *Arch Pathol Lab Med.* 1984;108:654–657.
179. Malik SK, Behera D, Kalra S, Dhaliwal RS, Banerjee CK. Intrabronchial schwannoma. A case report. *Scand J Thorac Cardiovasc Surg.* 1987;21:281–282.
180. Bosch X, Ramirez J, Font J, et al. Primary intrapulmonary benign schwannoma. A case with ultrastructural and immunohistochemical confirmation. *Eur Respir J.* 1990;3:234–237.
181. Ashkan K, Casey ATH. Pulmonary apex schwannoma. *J Neurol Neurosurg Psychiatry.* 1997;63:719.
182. Simansky DA, Aviel-Ronen S, Reder I, Paley M, Refaely Y, Yellin A. Psammomatous melanotic schwannoma: presentation of a rare primary lung tumor. *Ann Thorac Surg.* 2000;70:671–672.
183. Drowlands D, Edwards C, Collins F. Malignant melanotic schwannoma of the bronchus. *J Clin Pathol.* 1987;40:1449–1455.
184. Uchiyama M, Shimoyama Y, Usami N, et al. Primary pulmonary malignant schwannoma with extension to the tracheal carina. *J Thorac Cardiovasc Surg.* 2007;133:265–267.
185. Kitamura H, Kitamura H. Primary epithelioid malignant schwannoma of the lung. *Pathol Int.* 1994;44:317–324.
186. Togashi K, Hirahara H, Sugawara M, Oguma F. Primary malignant schwannoma of the lung. *Jpn J Thorac Cardiovasc Surg.* 2003;51:692–695.
187. Suzuki H, Sekine Y, Motohashi S, et al. Endobronchial neurogenic tumors treated by transbronchial electrical snaring and Nd-YAG laser abrasion: report of three cases. *Surg Today.* 2005;35:243–246.
188. Mahapatro RC, Bhavthankar AG, Kolhatkar MK. Neurofibroma of lung. *J Indian Med Assoc.* 1976;67:182–184.
189. Batori M, Lazzaro M, Lonardo MT, et al. A rare case of pulmonary neurofibroma: clinical and diagnostic evaluation and surgical treatment. *Eur Rev Med Pharmacol Sci.* 1999;3:155–157.
190. Charalambos Z, Dountsis A, Dahabreh J. Multiple bilateral recurrent neurofibromas of the lungs. *Eur J Cardiothorac Surg.* 2003;24:826.

191. Markaki S, Edwards C. Intrapulmonary ganglioneuroma: a case report. *Arch Anat Cytol Path*. 1987;35:183–184.
192. Crotty TB, Hooker RP, Swensen SJ, Scheithauer BW, Myers JL. Primary malignant ependymoma of the lung. *Mayo Clin Proc*. 1992;67:373–378.
193. Moran CA, Suster S, Koss MN. Primary malignant "triton" tumor of the lung. *Histopathology*. 1997;30:140–144.
194. Cooney TP. Primary pulmonary ganglioneuroblastoma in an adult: maturation, involution and the immune response. *Histopathology*. 1981;5:451–463.
195. Hochholzer L, Moran CA, Koss MN. Primary pulmonary ganglioneuroblastoma: a clinicopathologic and immunohistochemical study of two cases. *Ann Diagn Pathol*. 1998;2(3):154–158.
196. Balduin R, Drigo R, Schiraldi C, Carraro R. Ante mortem diagnosis of primary leiomyosarcoma of the pulmonary artery. *Respiration*. 1986;49:307–310.
197. Kimura I, Kiuchi H, Sakamoto Y, Yamamoto K, Dohi Y, Takahama M. Primary osteogenic sarcoma of pulmonary artery. *Jpn J Med*. 1990;29:32–37.
198. Berney CR, Roche B, Kurt AM, Spiliopoulos A, Mégevand R. Leiomyosarcoma of the pulmonary hilar vessels. *Thorac Cardiovasc Surg*. 1991;40:48–51.
199. Goldblum JR, Rice TW. Epithelioid angiosarcoma of the pulmonary artery. *Hum Pathol*. 1995;26:1275–1277.
200. Baker PB, Goodwin RA. Pulmonary artery sarcomas: a review and report of a case. *Arch Pathol Lab Med*. 1985;109:35–39.
201. Robaish AA, Lien DC, Slatnik J, Nguyen GK. Sarcoma of the pulmonary artery trunk: report of a case complicated with hemopericardium and cardiac tamponade. *Can J Cardiol*. 1995; 11:707–709.
202. Thijs LG, Kroon TAJ, van Leeuwen TM. Leiomyosarcoma of the pulmonary trunk associated with pericardial effusion. *Thorax*. 1974;29:490–492.
203. Nerlich A, Permanetter W, Ludwig B, Remberger K. Primary leiomyosarcoma of the truncus pulmonalis: report of a case with typical features and unusual metastases. *Pathol Respir Pract*. 1990;186:296–299.
204. Pain JA, Sayer RE. Primary leiomyosarcoma of the pulmonary artery. *Eur J Respir Dis*. 1984;65:139–145.
205. Faul JL, Wahl T, Ihnken K, Berry GJ, Doyle RL, Whyte RI. Superior vena cava syndrome caused by pulmonary artery sarcoma. *J Thorac Cardiovasc Surg*. 1999;118:749–750.
206. Okuno T, Matsuda K, Ueyama K, et al. Leiomyosarcoma of the pulmonary vein. *Pathol Int*. 2000;50:839–846.
207. Huo L, Lai S, Gladish G, Czerniak BA, Moran CA. Pulmonary artery angiosarcoma: a clinicopathologic and radiological correlation. *Ann Diagn Pathol*. 2005;9:209–214.
208. Huo L, Moran CA, Fuller GN, Gladish G, Suster S. Pulmonary artery sarcoma: a clinicopathologic and immunohistochemical study of 12 cases. *Am J Clin Pathol*. 2006;125:419–424.

8

Vascular Tumors of the Lung

Primary vascular tumors of the lung are rare and represent a small percentage of primary lung neoplasms. They may be benign or malignant; however, no association with any specific factors has been found. Vascular tumors can be classified as follows:

Benign Vascular Tumors

- Angiolymphoid hyperplasia with eosinophilia (epithelioid hemangioma)
- Capillary hemangiomatosis
- Hemangioma
- Lymphangioma

Malignant Vascular Tumors

- Angiosarcoma
- Epithelioid hemangioendothelioma
- Kaposi sarcoma

The most important clinical and immunohistochemical features are summarized in Table 8-1.

ANGIOLYMPHOID HYPERPLASIA WITH EOSINOPHILIA

Angiolymphoid hyperplasia with eosinophilia (ALHE), or epithelioid hemangioma, is an unusual lesion that has only recently been described as a primary pulmonary tumor.[1] Before this designation, considerable controversy had existed regarding the classification of similar lesions described by other names—for example, Kimura's disease, epithelioid hemangioma, angioreticuloma of the heart, atypical vascular proliferation of large vessels, and hemangioendothelioma of bone. Some researchers have attempted to unify these terms under a single clinicopathologic entity[2]; for the most part, however, such attempts have failed, and currently it is accepted that Kimura's disease and ALHE represent two different conditions.[3–22] Nevertheless, an important point is that regardless of their specific name, both of these conditions primarily affect anatomic sites other than the lung, including subcutaneous tissue, salivary glands, the orbit, and lymph nodes. Both conditions also have an unknown etiology, and thus far, not a single case of aggressive behavior has been reported for either lesion. Thus, ALHE in the lung is likely to follow a clinical course similar to that observed for benign lesions reported outside of the thoracic cavity.

Clinical Features

The only two reported cases of pulmonary ALHE were in a man and a woman 27 and 60 years of age, respectively. A history of asthma and a pulmonary mass was recorded for one patient; the second patient presented with a history of cough and dyspnea and radiographic evidence of a pulmonary mass. Neither patient had any evidence of nodal or soft tissue disease.

Macroscopic Features

Both patients underwent resection of the pulmonary mass. The tumors were well circumscribed but not encapsulated, of soft consistency, grayish, and the cut surface is partly cystic. Tumor size ranged from 2 to 3 cm in greatest dimension. Hemorrhage and necrosis were not described in either lesion.

TABLE 8-1 MOST COMMON CLINICAL AND IMMUNOHISTOCHEMICAL FEATURES OF VASCULAR TUMORS OF THE LUNG

Tumor	Presentation	Histopathologic Features	Positive Immunohistochemical Staining
Angiolymphoid hyperplasia with eosinophilia	Tumor nodule	Eosinophils, lymphoid hyperplasia, endothelial hyperplasia	CD31, CD34, factor VIII
Hemangioma	Tumor nodule	Capillary, cavernous Lack of atypia or mitosis	CD31, CD34, factor VIII
Capillary hemangiomatosis	Diffuse	Widespread presence of small interstitial capillaries containing red cells	CD31, CD34, factor VIII
Lymphangioma	Tumor nodule, diffuse	Abnormal proliferation and dilatation of pulmonary lymphatics	CD31, CD34 (weak), D2-40 in lymphatics
Angiosarcoma	Multiple nodules	Cellular atypia, mitosis, necrosis/ hemorrhage	CD31, CD34, factor VIII
Epithelioid hemangioendothelioma	Multiple nodules	Nodules in different stages of development—sclerotic, myxoid Calcified Rarely, mitotic figures	CD31, CD34, factor VIII
Kaposi sarcoma	Multiple nodules	Spindle cells with vascular slits; hyaline droplets, mitotic figures	CD31, CD34

Histopathologic Features

At low magnification, the ALHE process was seen as a well-circumscribed tumor replacing normal lung parenchyma with extensive areas of eosinophilic infiltrate, medium-sized vessel proliferation, and aggregates of lymphoid nodules (Figs. 8-1 to 8-3). Higher magnification revealed a proliferation of small-caliber vessels with hyperplastic endothelial lining and extensive deposition of eosinophils (Figs. 8-4 and 8-5). In some areas the process involved larger-caliber vessels (Fig. 8-6), and more discrete involvement of the airway was seen (Fig. 8-7). The epithelioid component showed medium-sized cells with large nuclei and eosinophilic cytoplasm. Some cells displayed prominent cytoplasmic vacuoles. In focal areas, the alveoli were filled with eosinophils, mimicking the histologic picture in an eosinophilic pneumonia (Fig. 8-8).

Immunohistochemical Features

Although the identification of the two reported cases of ALHE was accomplished using hematoxylin-eosin–stained sections, immunohistochemical studies may help in distinguishing ALHE from other, more common

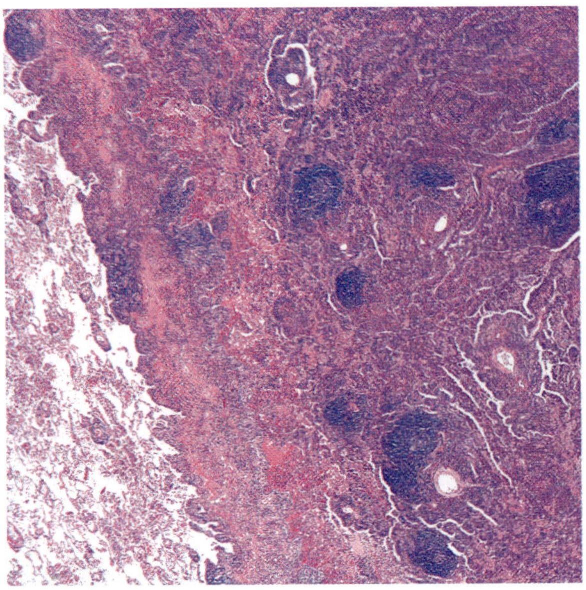

Figure 8-1 Angiolymphoid hyperplasia with eosinophilia. Low-power view shows a well-circumscribed tumor nodule replacing normal lung architecture.

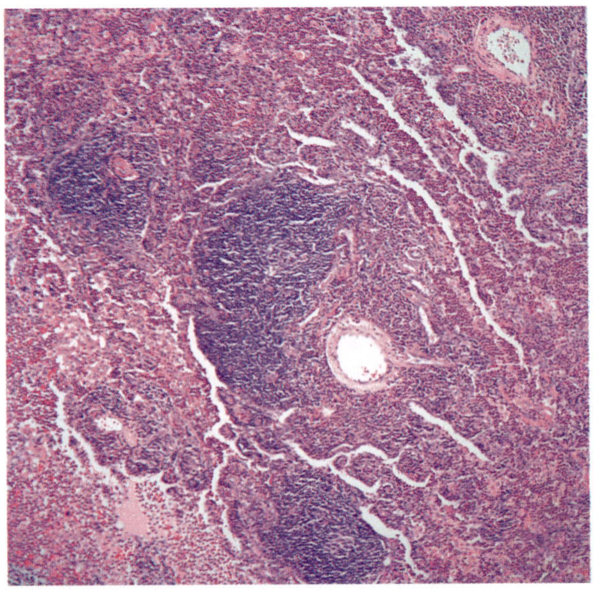

Figure 8-2 Angiolymphoid hyperplasia with eosinophilia. Focal lymphoid hyperplasia and extensive vascular proliferation are present.

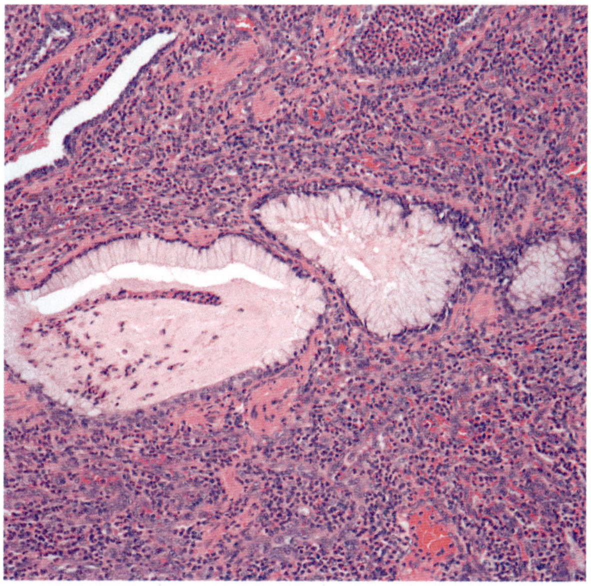

Figure 8-3 Angiolymphoid hyperplasia with eosinophilia. The process is seen surrounding normal endobronchial glands.

pulmonary conditions that may behave more aggressively. CD31, CD34, and factor VIII will help in identifying vessels; lymphoid markers, including leukocyte common antigen (LCA) and B and T cell markers such as L-26 and UCHL-1, may show the dual lymphoid population of these lesions. Keratin antibodies also may stain entrapped alveolar tissue.

Differential Diagnosis

Several conditions should be considered in the differential diagnosis for ALHE, ranging from benign inflammatory and infectious diseases to malignant lymphoproliferative disorders. Eosinophilic pneumonia may be confused with ALHE in small biopsy specimens, owing to the extensive presence of eosinophils; however, the clinical finding of a pulmonary nodule or mass would be unusual for eosinophilic pneumonia, which is a more diffuse process. Infectious conditions caused by parasites or fungal organisms may be associated with similar findings of a pulmonary mass with eosinophilia; in such cases, however, the identification of the causative organisms by light microscopy or tissue cultures will lead to the correct interpretation. Because of the presence of the lymphocytic component, ALHE also may be confused with a low-grade lymphoma, which can manifest as a pulmonary mass. In cases of pulmonary lymphoma, however, the lymphocytic proliferation will show clonality on immunohistochemical studies, rather than the polymorphous component of ALHE.

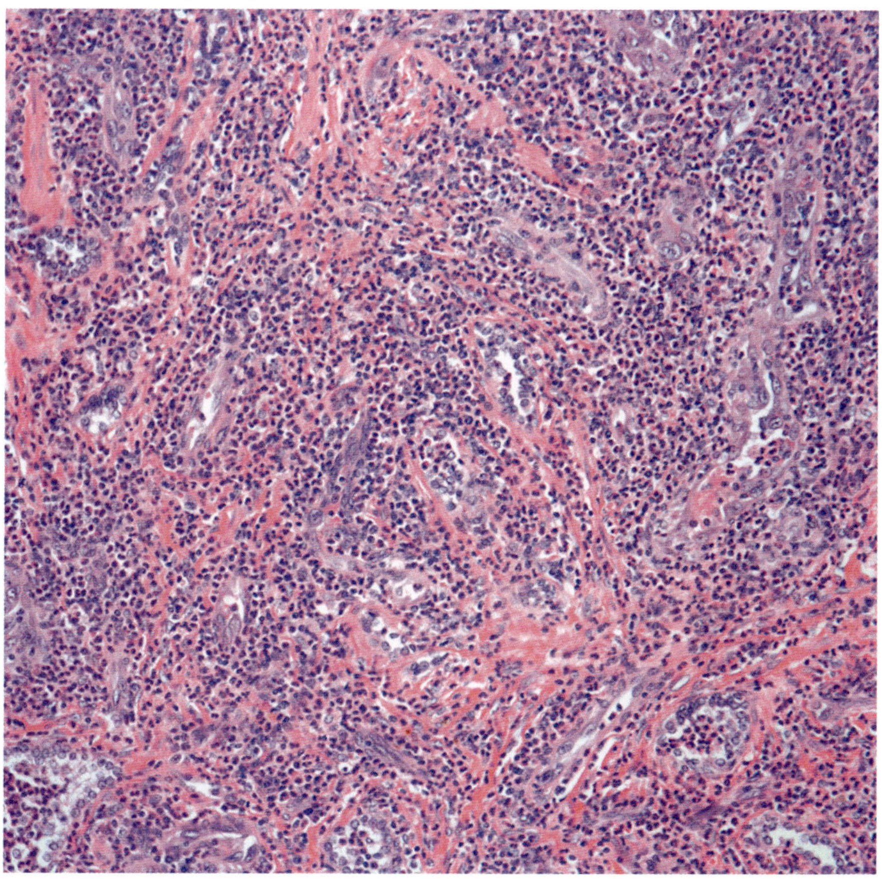

Figure 8-4 Angiolymphoid hyperplasia with eosinophilia. Note the extensive vascular proliferation with hyperplastic changes.

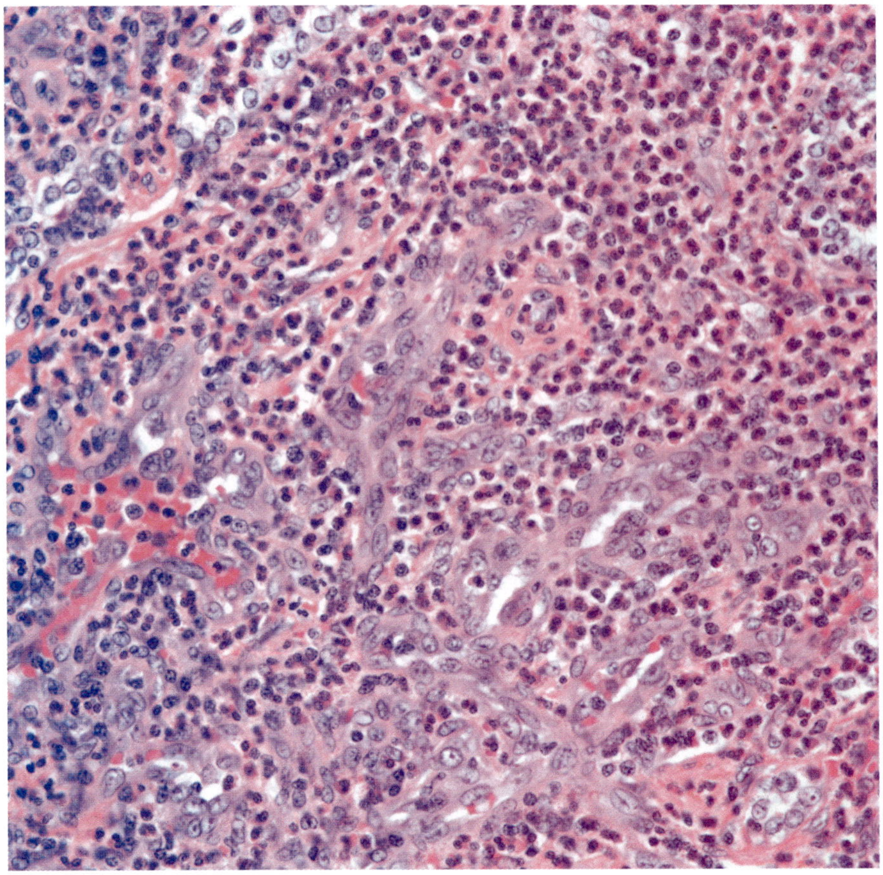

Figure 8-5 Angiolymphoid hyperplasia with eosinophilia. Endothelial hyperplasia with prominent eosinophilic inflammatory component is present.

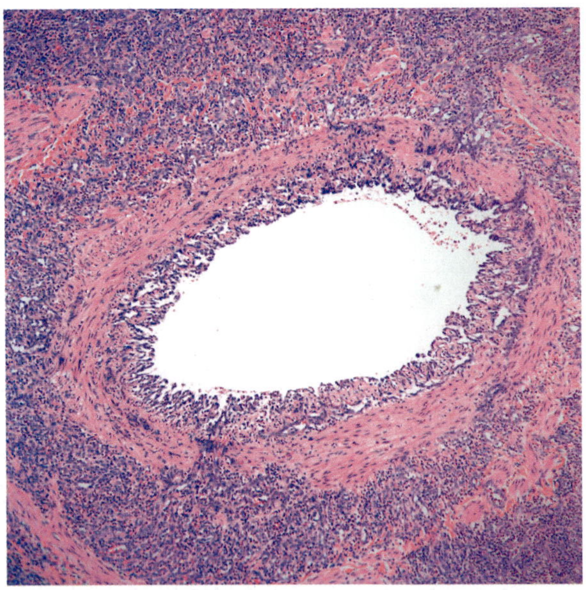

Figure 8-6 Angiolymphoid hyperplasia with eosinophilia with involvement of a large vessel.

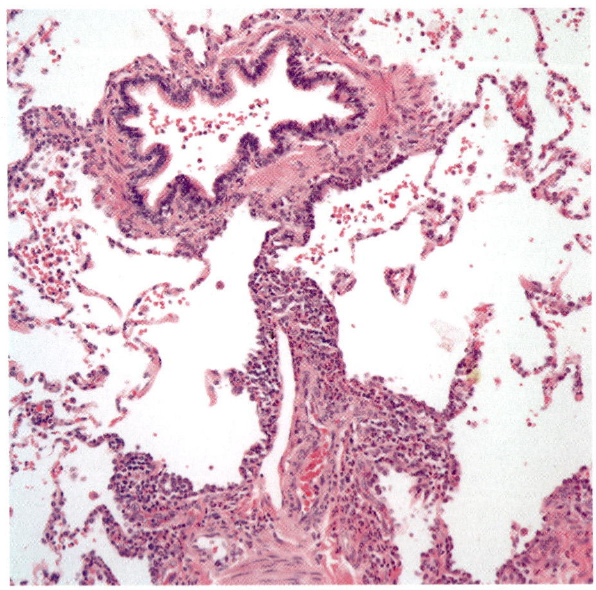

Figure 8-7 More discrete involvement by angiolymphoid hyperplasia with eosinophilia near the airway.

Treatment and Prognosis

Surgical resection is the treatment of choice and is curative in these lesions. The behavior of similar lesions outside of the thoracic cavity has been described as benign.

CAPILLARY HEMANGIOMATOSIS

Capillary hemangiomatosis is a rare vascular lesion characterized by proliferation of capillary channels. The lesion appears to occur at any age, without any gender predilec-

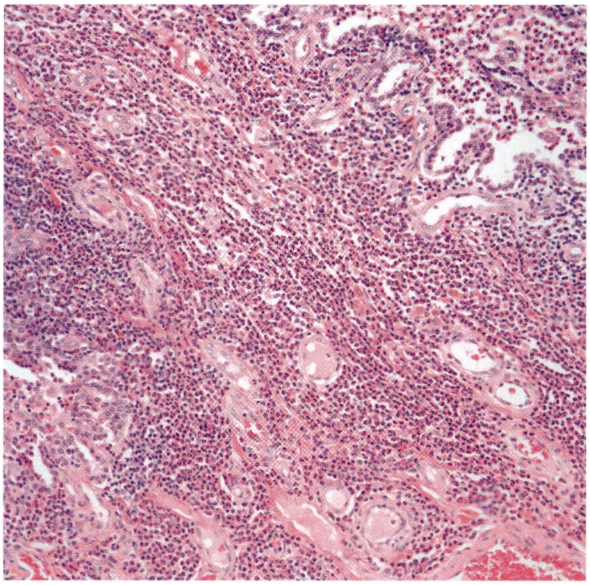

Figure 8-8 Angiolymphoid hyperplasia with eosinophilia. The extensive intra-alveolar deposition of eosinophils resembles that in eosinophilic pneumonia.

tion, and in many instances it is diagnosed at autopsy after the patient has died from the disease.

Historical Aspects

The first description of this lesion was made by "Wagenvoort" and colleagues,[23] who in 1978 described a 71-year-old woman who presented with a 3-week history of respiratory infection and dyspnea. Over a period of 5 months, the patient's clinical condition deteriorated, eventuating in death. Autopsy findings included the presence of heavy and firm lungs with a nodular cut surface. On histologic examination, atypical capillary-like channels were seen to be distributed in the fibrous septa and interstitium, around the bronchi, and in the pulmonary blood vessels, particularly the veins. The patient also had a cavernous-type hemangioma in the spleen that did not resemble the lesion in the lungs. Almost simultaneously, Rowen and associates[24] described three children between the ages of 4 and 7 years in whom autopsy revealed the presence of what was described as "pulmonary hemangiomatosis." These investigators concluded that the presence of a combination of diffuse interstitial infiltration and bloody pleural effusion in a child is pathognomonic for capillary hemangiomatosis. Histologic features include cavernous-type and capillary changes. Although in most cases the diagnosis of capillary hemangiomatosis has been made at autopsy, Wagenaar and coworkers[25] described the case of a 12-year-old girl in whom recurrent severe hemoptysis required a left pneumonectomy. The histopathologic findings indicated capillary hemangiomatosis. Of interest, the clinical picture was favorable at the 36-month follow-up evaluation, suggesting that if the diagnosis of pulmonary capillary hemangiomatosis is made early, aggressive treatment may prevent a fatal outcome.

Clinical Features

Capillary hemangiomatosis can affect children and adults of all ages, without predilection for either gender. Most cases, however, are diagnosed during the third and fourth decades of life. Langleben and colleagues[26] described capillary hemangiomatosis in three siblings who had died of pulmonary hypertension. The investigators concluded that capillary hemangiomatosis may have an autosomal recessive inheritance pattern. Similarly, Oviedo and coworkers[27] described two cases of congenital pulmonary capillary hemangiomatosis in which the affected neonates had other anomalies, including renal and bladder agenesis and hypertrophic cardiomyopathy. Although pulmonary hypertension is a common clinical finding in pulmonary capillary hemangiomatosis regardless of the age of the patient,[28] other findings may suggest different entities, such as interstitial lung disease.[29,30]

Clinical signs and symptoms of capillary hemangiomatosis may include cough, hemoptysis, respiratory distress, and chest pain.[31] More recently, Havlik and associates[32] retrospectively studied autopsy findings in a series of 140 patients and noted the presence of pulmonary capillary hemangiomatosis–like foci in approximately 5.7% of the cases. These workers concluded that these findings were incidental, and because none of the patients had a known history of pulmonary hypertension, the hemangiomatosis-like foci were not thought to contribute to the clinical outcome. In some unusual cases, capillary hemangiomatosis may arise in patients with hereditary hemorrhagic telangiectasia.[33]

Macroscopic Features

Two patterns are recognized by which capillary hemangiomatosis may compromise the lung parenchyma. The *diffuse* pattern is characterized by a congested lung parenchyma with areas of consolidation and multicystic sponge-like areas, which may be more conspicuous in the lower lobes (Fig. 8-9). In other cases, the cut surface of the lung parenchyma has been described as liver-like. The *multifocal* pattern is characterized by multiple, patchy, reddish-brown and white areas of consolidation.[34] The lung parenchyma can be affected in differing proportions; reported cases have ranged from 10% involvement to extensive diffuse involvement with the entire lung parenchyma described as deeply congested[35,36] (Figs. 8-10 to 8-12).

Microscopic Features

The histopathologic features of capillary hemangiomatosis echo the gross appearance in terms of pulmonary involvement, which can be diffuse or patchy and may be

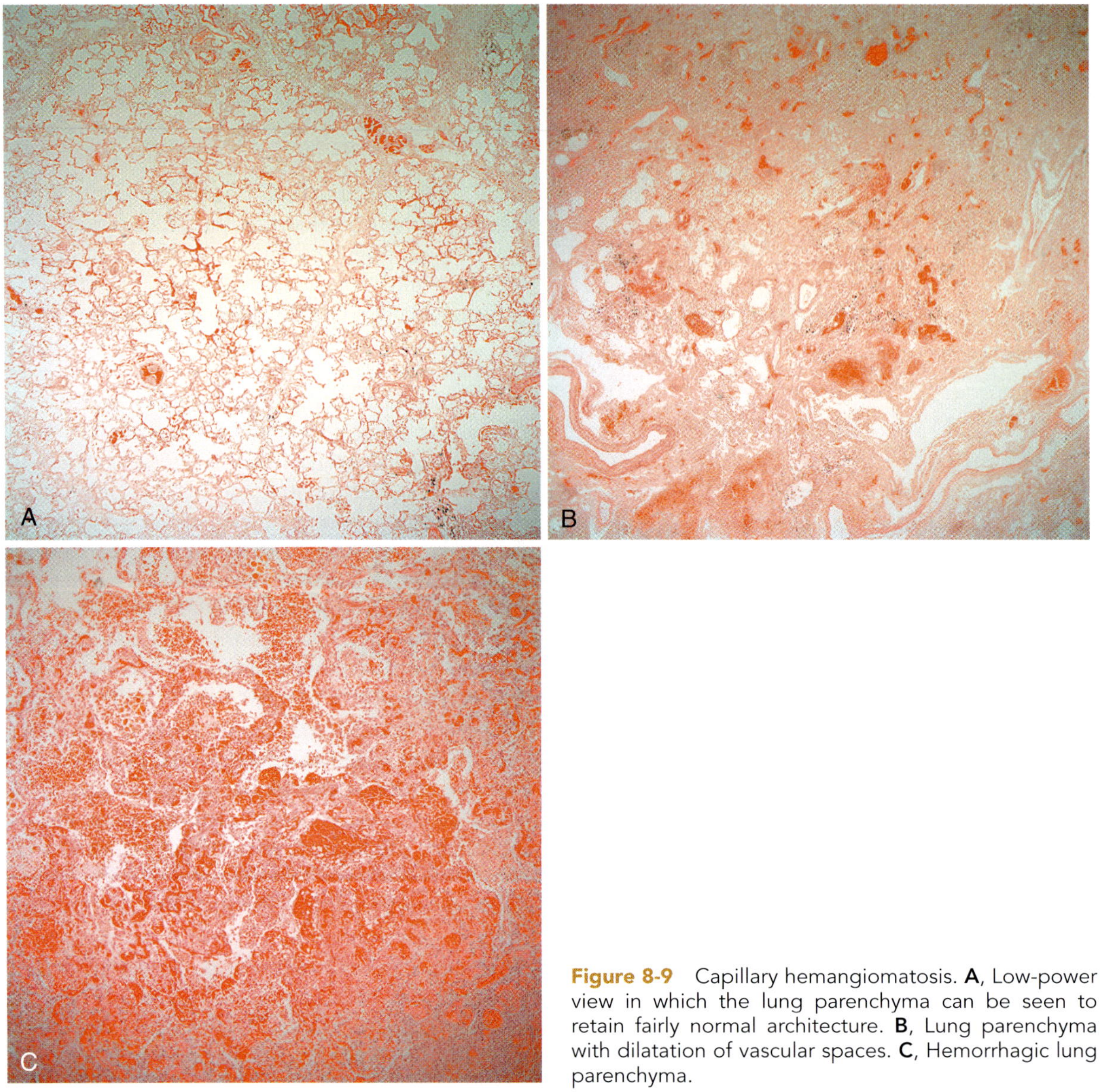

Figure 8-9 Capillary hemangiomatosis. **A**, Low-power view in which the lung parenchyma can be seen to retain fairly normal architecture. **B**, Lung parenchyma with dilatation of vascular spaces. **C**, Hemorrhagic lung parenchyma.

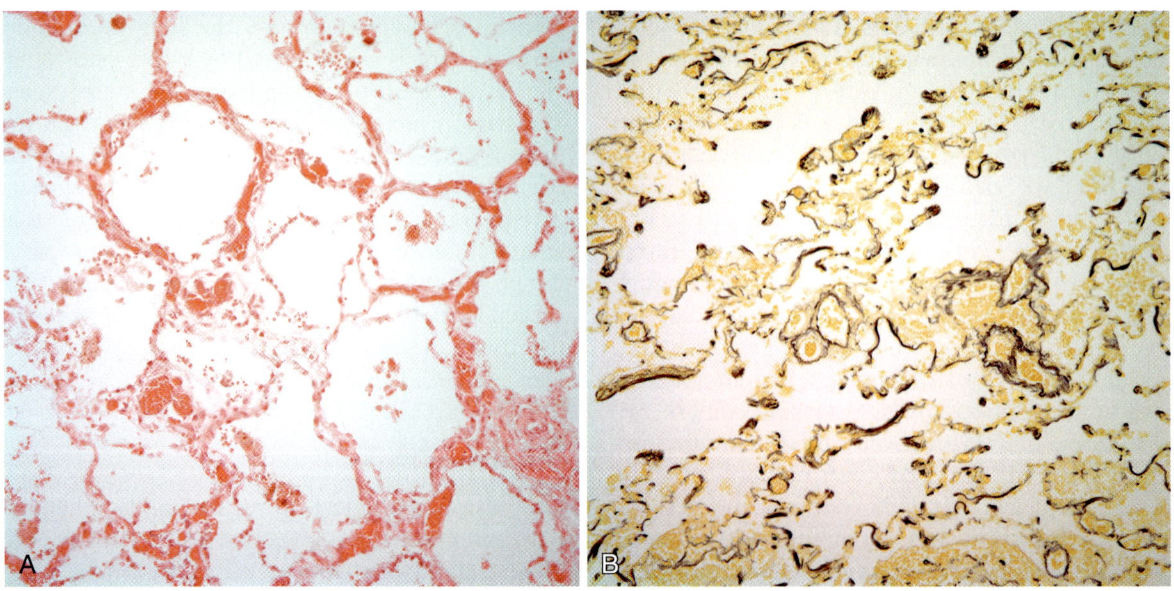

Figure 8-10 **A**, Capillary hemangiomatosis showing a proliferation of dilated capillaries in the interstitium filled with blood. **B**, Elastic stain reveals the vascular proliferation.

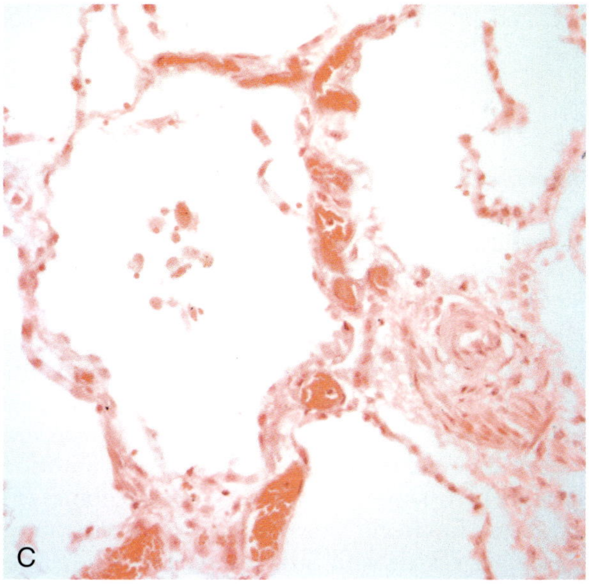

Figure 8-10—cont'd C, At higher magnification, the capillary proliferation is seen to follow the outlines of the alveoli.

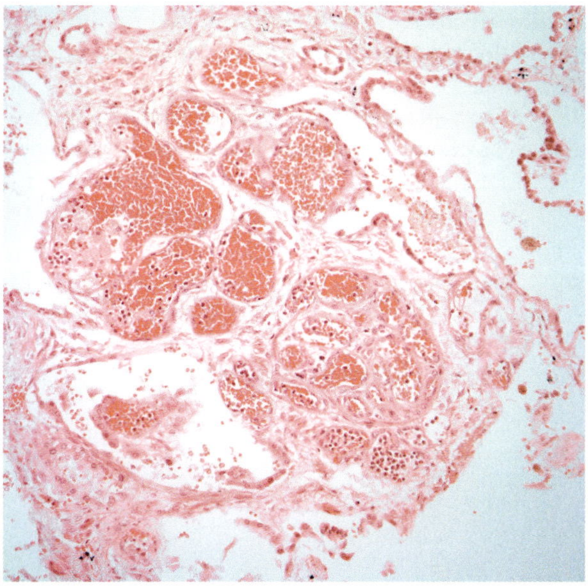

Figure 8-11 Capillary hemangiomatosis with obvious areas of vascular proliferation.

characterized by expansion of the pulmonary congestion into the interstitium. Higher magnification reveals a proliferation of small capillaries distributed along the interstitium and infiltrating into the bronchovascular bundle. The capillary proliferation does not display cytologic atypia, although mitotic figures may be seen occasionally. It may extend transmurally into larger vessels and bronchi, resulting in the narrowing of their lumens. Adjacent pulmonary vasculature also may show features of hypertrophy. One of the most reliable histologic features of capillary hemangiomatosis is the presence of double capillaries (or more) along both sides of the alveolar wall. In advanced cases, however, extensive sheets or nodules of capillaries may be seen.[30]

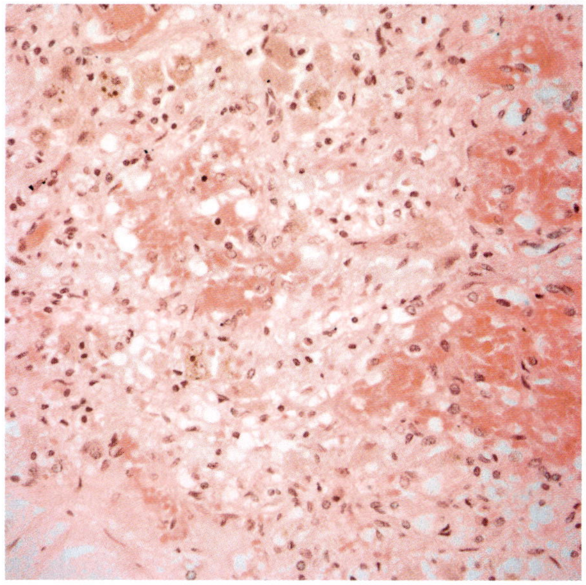

Figure 8-12 Lung parenchyma showing capillary proliferation admixed with histiocytes.

Differential Diagnosis

In small transbronchial biopsy specimens, an accurate diagnosis of capillary hemangiomatosis may prove difficult to obtain, because the lung parenchyma may not be represented. An open lung biopsy may be necessary; however, the benefits of this procedure must be weighed against the possible complications, including hemorrhage. When the histologic findings include pools of blood and areas of fibrosis, capillary hemangiomatosis may be mistaken for conventional cavernous hemangioma. Pulmonary interstitial disease should be considered in cases in which the lung parenchyma shows an inflammatory infiltrate without the capillary proliferation. Pulmonary veno-occlusive disease also may be considered in the differential diagnosis. Both capillary hemangiomatosis and veno-occlusive disease display extensive vascular obstruction; in capillary hemangiomatosis, however, the process originates from the capillaries, whereas in veno-occlusive disease the process originates from pulmonary venules and small veins.[37] Some researchers[38] have suggested that capillary hemangiomatosis may be an angioproliferative process secondary to postcapillary obstruction, rather than a separate disease.

Treatment and Prognosis

The treatment of capillary hemangiomatosis is surgical resection of affected lung tissue; however, this may prove to be a radical procedure owing to the extensive nature of the process in the lung parenchyma. Because patients often present with pulmonary hypertension and severe hemoptysis, the outcome may be fatal if the condition is not diagnosed and treated promptly. Successful treatment with pneumonectomy has been reported. In addition, some success with treatment with recombinant interferon alfa-2a has been documented.[39]

HEMANGIOMA

Primary pulmonary hemangiomas are exceedingly rare benign vascular tumors.[40–58] They have been described in both pediatric and adult patients, without any predilection for either gender or for any specific anatomic area.

Patients may present with a variety of nonspecific clinical signs and symptoms, including fever and pneumonia. More specific manifestations related to the location of the tumor have included hemoptysis, dyspnea, and hemopneumothorax. A case of pulmonary hemangioma in a child with partial trisomy D has been reported. The initial radiologic evaluation may reveal a solitary pulmonary mass or multiple pulmonary nodules. A case of giant cell hemangioma and a case of concurrent hemangiomas of the liver and lung have been described.

Macroscopic Features

As noted, hemangiomas may manifest either as a single intrapulmonary mass or as multiple pulmonary nodules. The tumor may range in size from 1 cm to greater than 3 cm in greatest dimension and often appears as a cystic mass with a glistening surface. On examination of the cut surface, thin-walled cysts of different sizes, which are filled with blood, may be observed (Fig. 8-13). In some cases the tumor may appear to be encapsulated, and less frequently, it has been reported to manifest as a pseudocyst. Hemangioma also may manifest as a bronchial tumor, and in unusual cases it may grow in a polypoid fashion.

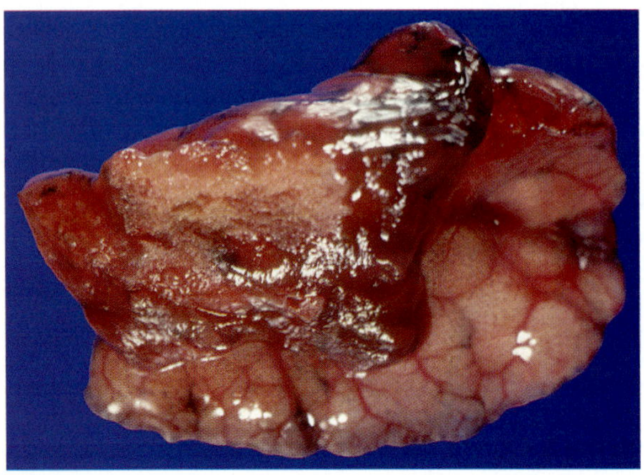

Figure 8-13 Pulmonary hemangioma, gross specimen. Note the focal sponge-like features and areas of hemorrhage are evident.

Microscopic Features

Pulmonary hemangiomas are histologically similar to those arising in more common locations, such as the skin or superficial soft tissues, and like other hemangiomas, they occur in two histologic patterns, cavernous and capillary. *Cavernous* hemangiomas are characterized by dilated, cyst-like structures filled with blood, thin walls, and adjacent inflammatory reaction in a background of fibroconnective tissue, which can display thickened, dilated vasculature (Figs. 8-14 and 8-15). The cellular proliferation does not show cytologic atypia, although mitotic figures rarely may be present. *Capillary* hemangiomas (Figs. 8-16 and 8-17) are characterized by the proliferation of small-caliber vessels with little intervening stromal reaction. The vessels may show hyperplastic changes, and occasionally, mitotic figures may be observed. When the tumor grows in a polypoid fashion in the bronchial wall, the surface may show inflammatory changes similar to those described in pyogenic granulomas of the skin. In both histologic patterns, the tumor replaces normal lung parenchyma.

The correct diagnosis can be made without the use of immunohistochemical stains. However, hemangiomas demonstrate positive staining for vascular markers such as factor VIII, CD34, and CD31 in the vascular proliferation.

Differential Diagnosis

The diagnosis of pulmonary hemangioma is rather straightforward. However, in areas in which a cavernous

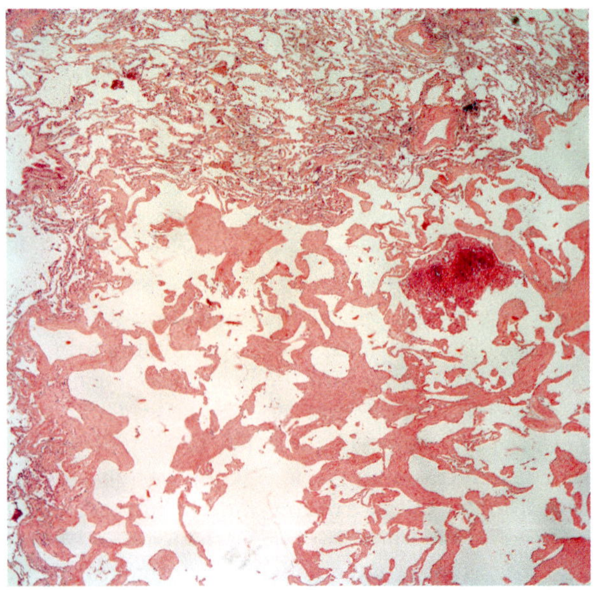

Figure 8-14 Low-power view of a pulmonary cavernous hemangioma.

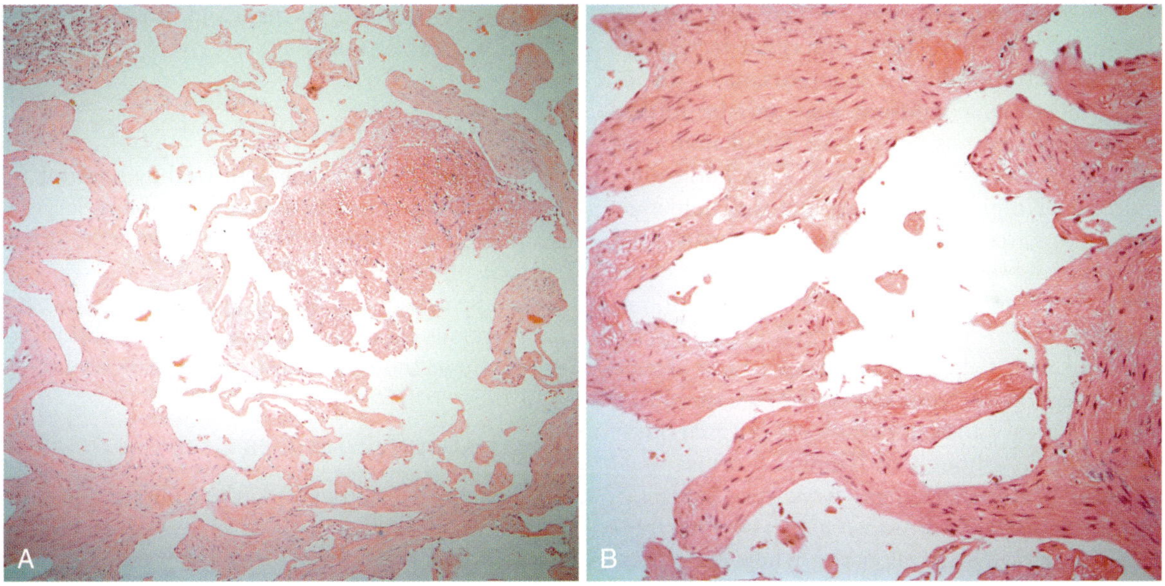

Figure 8-15 **A**, Pulmonary cavernous hemangioma with dilated, thick-walled vessels. **B**, Higher-power view of the dilated vascular spaces.

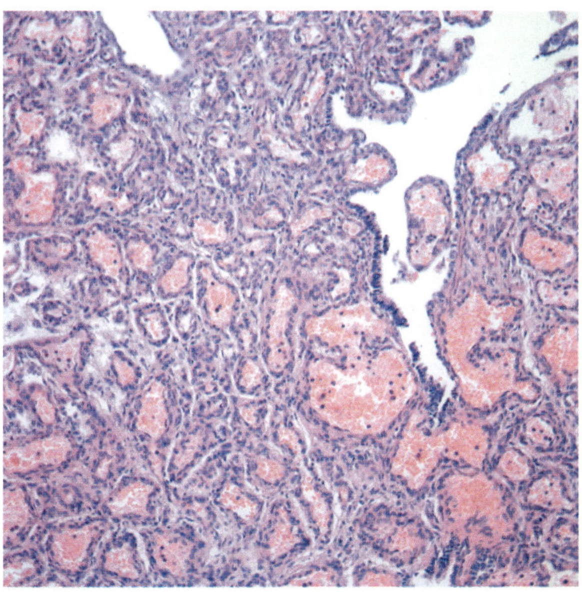

Figure 8-16 Pulmonary capillary hemangioma with extensive dilated capillary proliferation. Note the remaining normal respiratory epithelium.

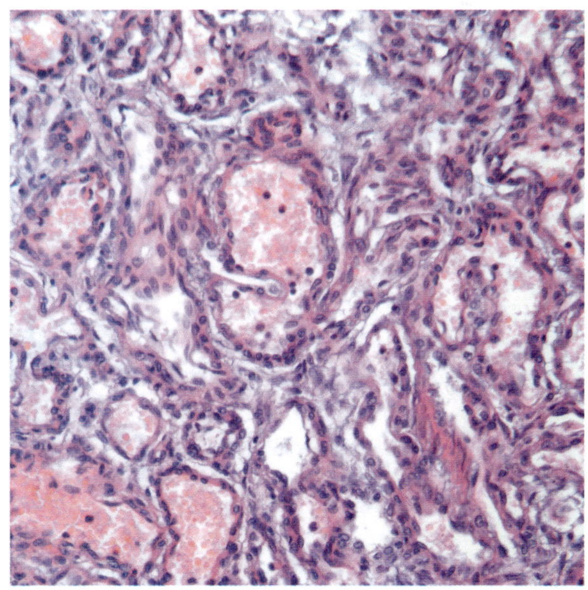

Figure 8-17 Pulmonary capillary hemangioma. Higher-power view of the capillary proliferation reveals absence of cellular atypia.

hemangioma shows dilated vascular spaces filled with blood, the tumor may resemble the so-called sclerosing hemangioma (pneumocytoma). In this setting, the positive staining for vascular markers will lead to the correct interpretation, because negative staining for those markers is characteristic of sclerosing hemangiomas. One possible consideration in the differential diagnosis for capillary hemangioma is angiolymphoid hyperplasia with eosinophilia. However, this clinical entity is characterized by the presence of lymphoid hyperplasia and eosinophilia, which generally are absent in capillary hemangioma.

Prognosis and Treatment

Hemangiomas are benign tumors that are cured by complete surgical resection, which can be accomplished by lobectomy, wedge resection, or sleeve resection. When the tumors are multiple, the procedure may be more extensive.

LYMPHANGIOMA

By definition, pulmonary lymphangioma is the abnormal proliferation of lymphatics within pulmonary parenchyma. This process may be the result of congenital errors of lymphatic development, which can lead to several conditions that have been described by various names in the literature. Thus, it is important to distinguish among the many conditions that may be related to lymphatic abnormalities, including lymphangiomas, lymphangiectasis, lymphangiomatosis, lymphatic dysplasia syndrome, lymphangioleiomyomatosis, hemangiolymphangioma, generalized lymphangiomatosis, and diffuse pulmonary lymphangiomatosis.[59–62] Because of the diverse nature of these conditions, proper correlation of clinical findings and histopathologic findings is imperative. For this reason, Faul and associates[59] have argued that the classification of lymphatic disorders should be based on both clinical and histopathologic criteria. Some of these conditions, although of lymphatic origin, may follow a clinical course that ranges from very benign to more aggressive. Some conditions, such as lymphangiectasis, may affect primarily neonates, wherease others, including lymphangioleiomyomatosis, are more common in young female patients. Still other conditions, such as lymphatic dysplasia syndrome, may constitute entirely different clinicopathologic entities. Some of these conditions may affect other extrathoracic areas, in addition to the lung parenchyma. The focus here is on the benign tumoral condition referred to as *lymphangioma*, although this particular tumor also has been referred to as "lymphangiomyoma" in the literature. Also, some of the previously reported cases of lymphangiomyoma or lymphangioma may represent different conditions, such as lymphangioleiomyomatosis or alveolar adenoma.[63,64]

Two different patterns of lung parenchyma involvement have been described: solitary pulmonary mass and diffuse pulmonary involvement.[60,61,65–73] Lymphangiomas may involve other mediastinal structures, including the pericardium, in addition to the lung and pleura.[60,61,64,74] Tazeelar and colleagues[60] coined the term *diffuse pulmonary lymphangiomatosis* in their description of nine cases, including those in children and young adults. Clinical signs and symptoms reported in these patients varied and included cough, shortness of breath, asthma, chylous effusions, and evidence of restriction on pulmonary function tests. The investigators determined that this condition was a separate entity from previously described lymphatic lesions. In seven of the patients, however, the process was not limited to the lung but also involved the mediastinum. Therefore, when the process is more diffuse in the lung parenchyma, it also is highly likely to extend outside the lung, or even outside the thoracic cavity. Nevertheless, these workers[60] clearly defined *lymphangiomatosis* as a process in which the number of complex anastomosing lymphatic channels is increased, in contrast with *lymphangiectasis*, in which the existing lymphatic channels are dilated.

When the process involves a solitary lung mass, some patients may be asymptomatic, whereas others experience symptoms of lung obstruction. Both presentations have been described in both male and female patients and in children as well as in adults.

Macroscopic Features

The solitary lesion is characterized by a tumor mass that destroys lung parenchyma and may be as large as 10 cm in greatest dimension. The gross tumor has a glistening surface, but the cut surface reveals a cystic configuration. The cystic structures may contain yellowish or serosanguineous fluid. When the process is diffuse, the lung parenchyma may have a honeycomb appearance.

Microscopic Features

Under low magnification, the solitary mass does not appear to be a well-defined process replacing the lung parenchyma but rather is seen as a proliferation of ectatic lymphatic channels, of differing sizes, that merge with the normal alveolar parenchyma. Higher-power examination of these lymphatic channels reveals an endothelial lining that does not exhibit cellular atypia or mitotic activity (Figs. 8-18 to 8-21). Acellular fluid, without blood, is present within the lumens of the lymphatic channels. However, when the tumor also displays a component of hemangioma (hemangiolymphangioma), some of the lumens may contain hemorrhagic fluid. When the process is more diffuse, it replaces extensive areas of normal alveolar lung parenchyma, displaying many cystically dilated spaces and taking on a honeycomb- or sponge-like appearance. In both presentations, it is possible to identify a smooth muscle component of variable proportion relative to overall composition. Adjacent

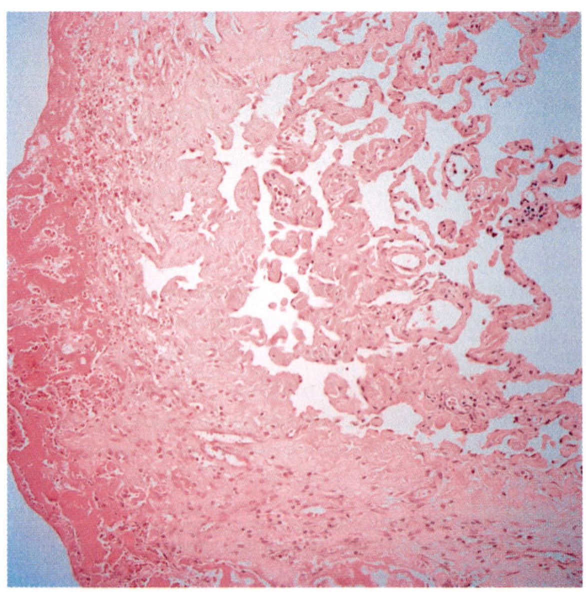

Figure 8-18 Pulmonary lymphangioma with involvement of pleura and lung parenchyma.

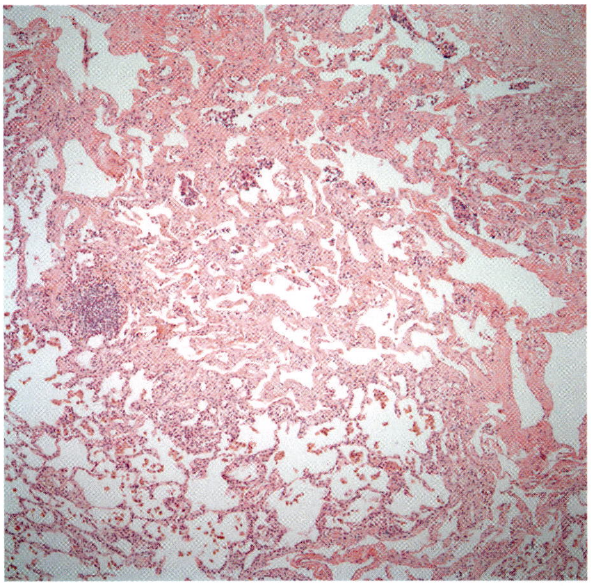

Figure 8-19 Pulmonary lymphangioma involving lung parenchyma in a subpleural pattern.

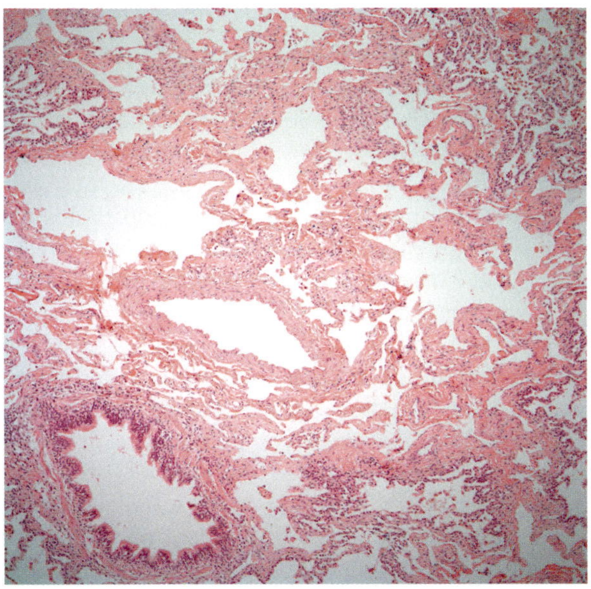

Figure 8-20 Pulmonary lymphangioma involving areas near other vascular structures and airway.

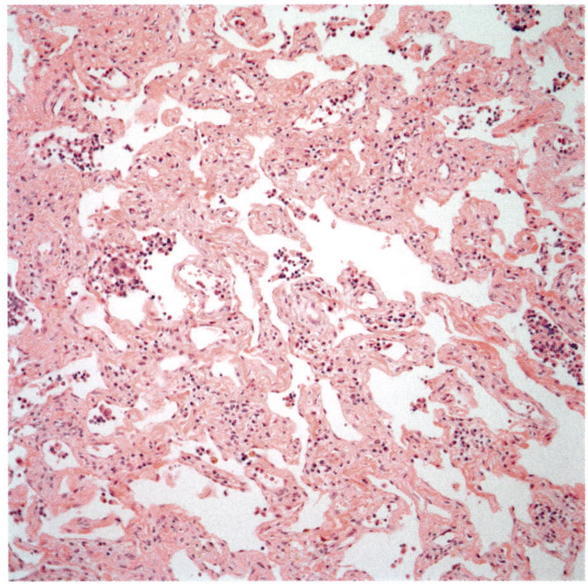

Figure 8-21 Pulmonary lymphangioma. Note tumor replacing extensive areas of normal lung parenchyma.

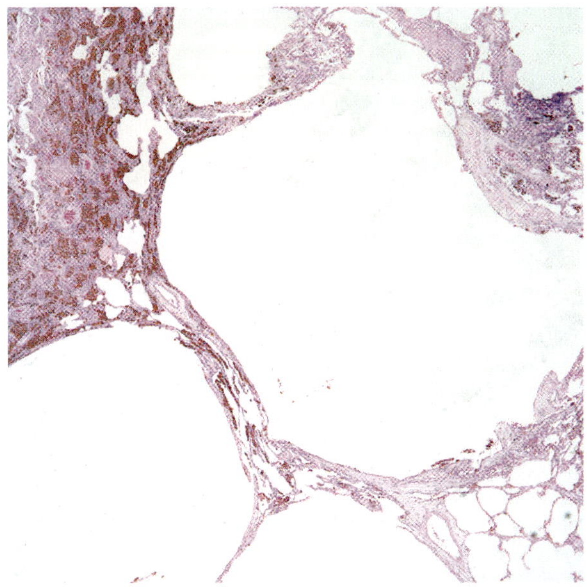

Figure 8-22 Pulmonary lymphangioma showing dilated lymphatics. Note the presence of iron-pigmented macrophages in the lung parenchyma.

lung parenchyma may show iron-filled or foamy macrophages, with little inflammatory reaction of the interstitium (Figs. 8-22 to 8-24). Areas of frank hemorrhage and necrosis are not common in lymphangiomas.

Immunohistochemical Features

Immunohistochemical studies may be useful in cases in which the diagnosis is not readily apparent. Staining for CD34, CD31, and factor VIII may give a weakly positive reaction in the endothelial lining. More recently, some investigators have claimed that D2-40 is a reliable marker for lymphoendothelium.[62] Lymphangiomas also may show positive staining for smooth muscle actin and desmin in the smooth muscle component. A majority of cases show negative staining for HMB-45 and estrogen and progesterone receptors, with only a single reported case documenting progesterone receptor positivity.[60]

Differential Diagnosis

Although the diagnosis of lymphangioma does not usually pose a problem, some conditions warrant specific consideration in the differential diagnosis. For a solitary lung

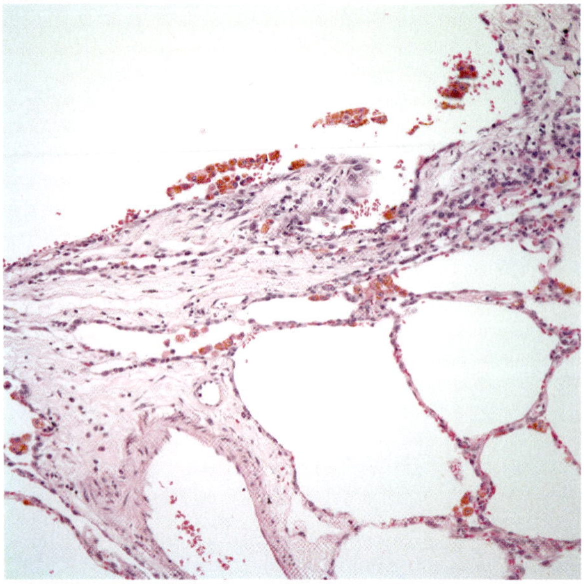

Figure 8-23 Dilated lymphatics contrasted with normal alveoli.

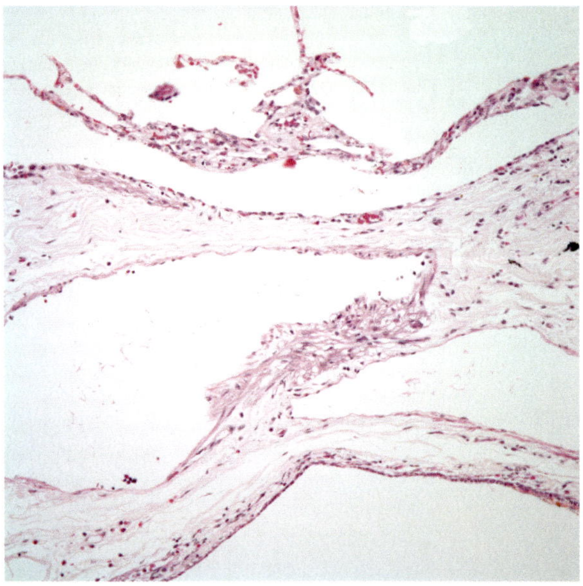

Figure 8-24 Dilated lymphatics with one showing focal muscle proliferation.

mass, the so-called alveolar adenoma and hemangioma may be considered. Alveolar adenomas should not demonstrate positive staining with vascular markers, whereas hemangioma should display abundant blood in the vascular lumens. When the process is diffuse, the most important differential diagnostic consideration is lymphangioleiomyomatosis. In this setting, clinical information (occurrence in a young female patient), findings on immunohistochemical studies (HMB-45 positivity), and the histologic distribution (diffuse) of the process are important clues to an accurate diagnosis.

Prognosis and Treatment

The treatment of choice for lymphangioma is surgical resection of the tumor. This procedure may range in extent from a wedge resection to a pneumonectomy, according to the particular circumstances. Although the prognosis with localized lymphangioma is good, a diffuse process involving mediastinal areas may be more difficult to manage.

ANGIOSARCOMA

Primary angiosarcomas of the lung are exceedingly rare. In a study of rare pulmonary tumors of the lung at a major institution in the years 1980 to 1990, Miller and Allen[75] encountered only 2 cases in a series of more than 10,000 pulmonary tumors and estimated the occurrence of this malignancy to be approximately 0.02%. Differentiation of primary from metastatic angiosarcoma in the lung can be quite difficult, however, because the clinical, radiologic, and histopathologic features of each are similar. In a study by Pate and Ryu[76] of 15 patients with angiosarcoma of the lung, all of the patients were diagnosed with metastatic disease to the lung, and in 12 of these cases the diagnosis was made ante mortem. The most common radiographic feature was presence of multiple pulmonary nodules; the most common clinical manifestation was hemoptysis. The designation of some cases as primary pulmonary tumors has been debated, either because they did not display all of the histopathologic features of angiosarcoma or because available clinical information was inadequate to rule out a possible extrapulmonary origin. Nevertheless, some well-documented cases of primary angiosarcomas of the lung have been reported, and in other instances the diagnosis has been made with confidence because no other site of malignancy was encountered.[77–84]

In cases reported as primary angiosarcoma of the lung, clinical presentation has varied, with tumors occurring in both young and older adults. In many instances, multiple bilateral pulmonary nodules are evident on radiographic examination, making the distinction from metastatic disease an impossible task. A history of environmental exposure, irradiation, or farming has been reported in some patients; presenting clinical signs and symptoms may include shortness of breath, hemoptysis, or frank pulmonary hemorrhage. In some unusual cases, the pulmonary angiosarcoma has been associated with other malignancies of different histologic type.[78] Complete physical and radiologic evaluation will be required to determine the primary site, owing to the difficulty in distinguishing primary from metastatic angiosarcoma.

Macroscopic Features

Although a majority of cases will manifest with multiple pulmonary nodules of various sizes distributed haphazardly throughout the lung parenchyma, presentation as a

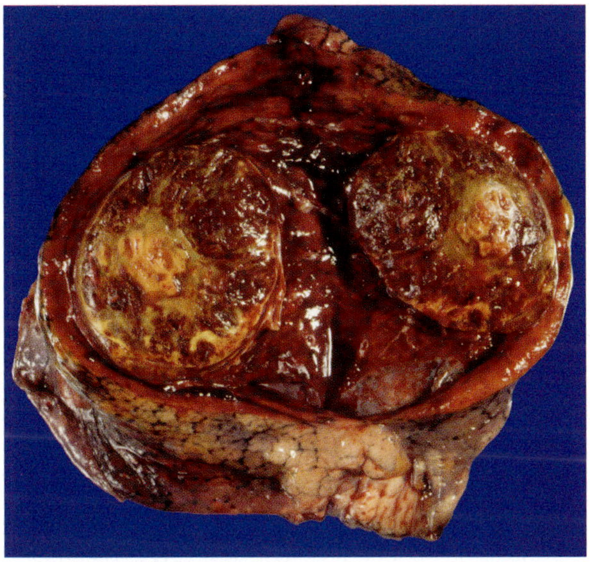

Figure 8-25 Angiosarcoma, gross specimen. Note the extensive areas of hemorrhage and focal necrosis.

single pulmonary mass has been reported[79,82] (Fig. 8-25). The tumors appear hemorrhagic and ill-defined, and can reach more than 5 cm in greatest dimension.

Histopathologic Features

The histopathologic features of pulmonary angiosarcoma are similar to those described for soft tissue angiosarcomas. The low-power view may show areas of hemorrhage, with a prominent vascular proliferation with cells arranged in cords (Fig. 8-26). In some cases, areas of a more solid epithelioid cellular proliferation also may be observed. Higher magnification will reveal an atypical vascular proliferation of anastomosing channels composed of plump, hyperchromatic endothelial cells (Fig. 8-27). Intravascular papillary tufts and areas of fibrin thrombi also may be present. In the solid areas, the cellular proliferation is composed of medium-sized cells with mild to moderate amounts of eosinophilic cytoplasm, round to oval nuclei, and inconspicuous nucleoli. Mitotic figures are readily identified. In some cases, this solid cellular proliferation may be composed of spindle cells (Fig. 8-28) with vascular slits resembling those in Kaposi sarcoma. Focal areas of hemorrhage and necrosis may be present (Figs. 8-29 to 8-32). The neoplastic pattern may mimic that of papillary tumors; however, these papillary tufts are composed of cells lining areas of fibroconnective tissue. In other areas it is possible to observe plump cells resembling the so-called hobnail cells seen in other epithelial tumors. Although pulmonary angiosarcomas are not encapsulated, extensive areas of fibroconnective tissue occasionally may be present in the periphery of the tumor.

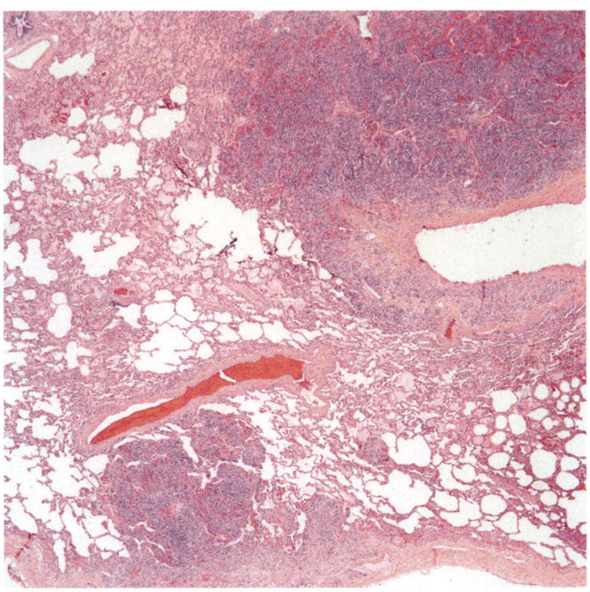

Figure 8-26 Low-power view of an angiosarcoma showing two distinct nodules in the lung parenchyma.

Immunohistochemical Features

The use of immunohistochemical markers may aid in distinguishing angiosarcoma from other malignant neoplasms. Angiosarcomas display positive staining for factor VIII, CD34, and CD31. In some instances, however, angiosarcomas may show focal staining in tumor cells for epithelial markers including pan-keratin and epithelial membrane antigen (EMA). Therefore, it is important to correlate the morphologic findings with the immunohistochemical results.

Differential Diagnosis

Because angiosarcomas may manifest as multiple pulmonary nodules, the possibility of metastatic disease from tumors outside of the thoracic cavity needs to be considered. In this setting, epithelial tumors such as carcinoma or melanoma enter into the differential diagnosis. Immunohistochemical studies using different types of keratins, CEA, and other carcinomatous epitopes may be useful in this aspect of the diagnostic investigation. Immunostaining for S-100 protein, HMB-45, and Melan A should help in distinguishing melanoma from angiosarcoma.

Of the other primary pulmonary neoplasms that may manifest in similar fashion, the most important is epithelioid hemangioendothelioma. A common clinical presentation for this tumor is one of multiple pulmonary nodules; however, the histologic features of epithelioid hemangioendothelioma—namely, the presence of a myxoid or "chondroid-like" stroma and the lack of pleomorphism—will distinguish it from angiosarcoma. On immunohistochemical studies, both tumors share the same immunophenotype of vascular differentiation. In cases in which angiosarcomas are formed by spindle cells,

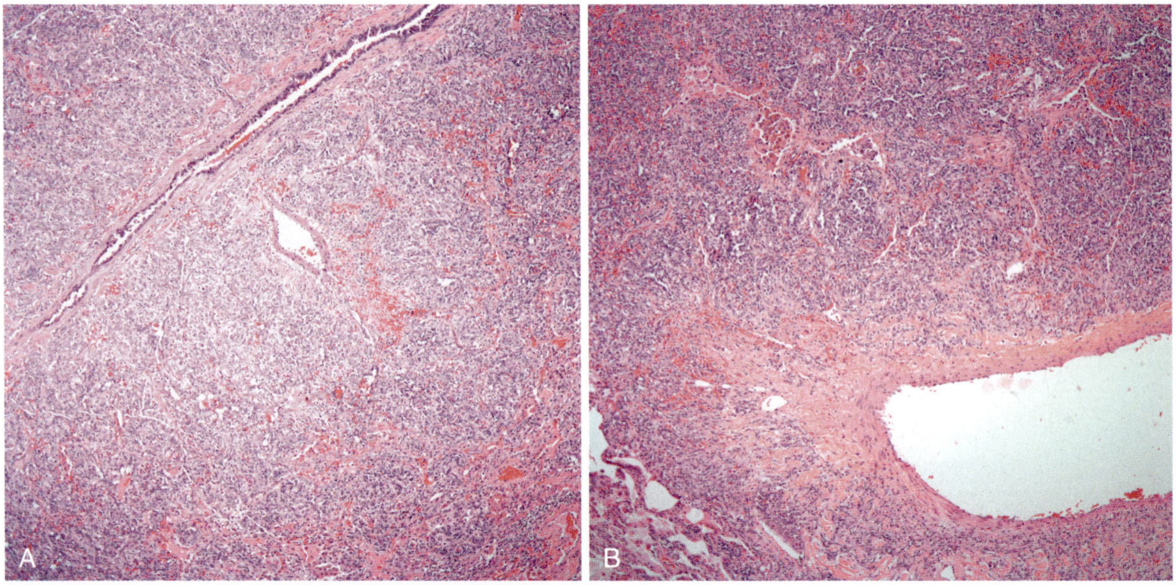

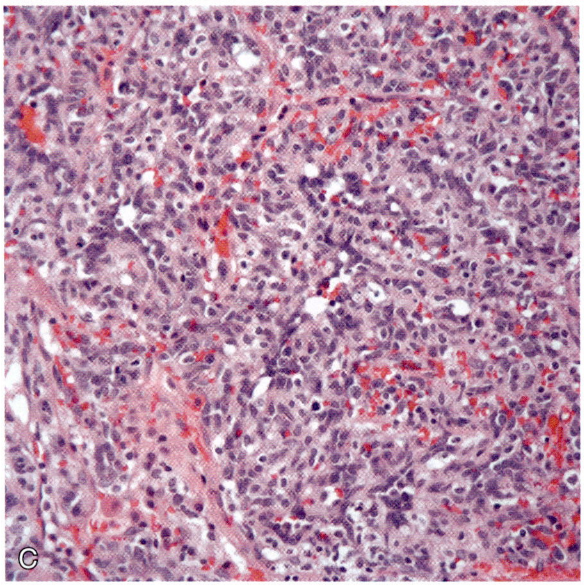

Figure 8-27 **A**, Angiosarcoma with solid appearance. Note compression of an airway structure. **B**, Angiosarcoma with prominent angiotropism. **C**, At higher magnification, vascular spaces with cellular atypia and mitotic figures are evident.

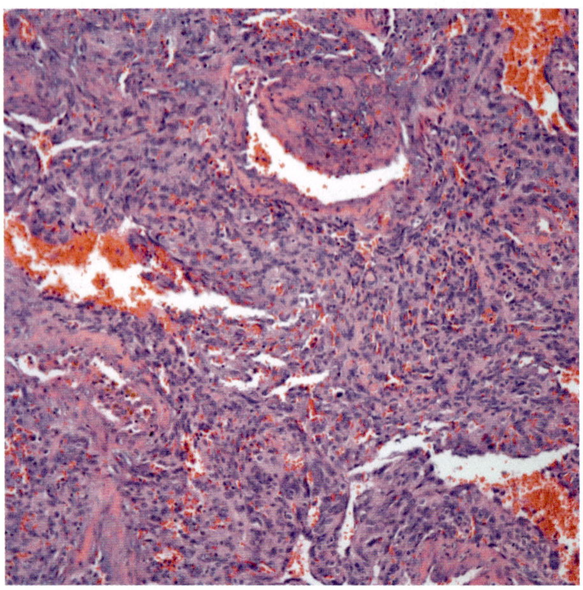

Figure 8-28 Angiosarcoma with spindle cell growth pattern.

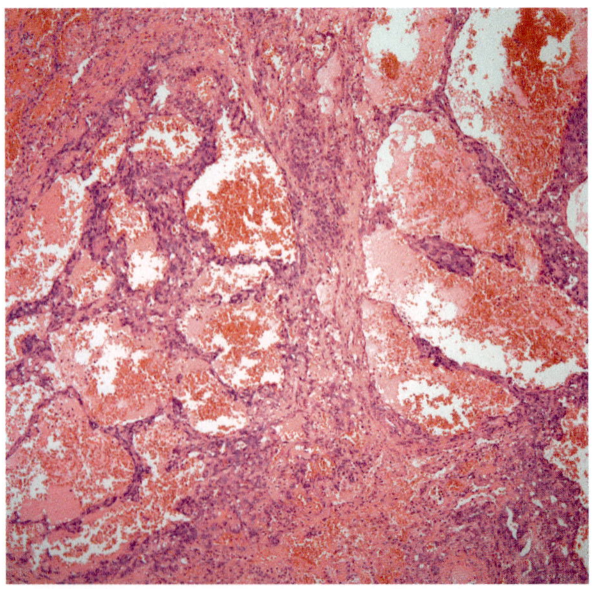

Figure 8-29 Low-power view of an angiosarcoma with large pools of blood.

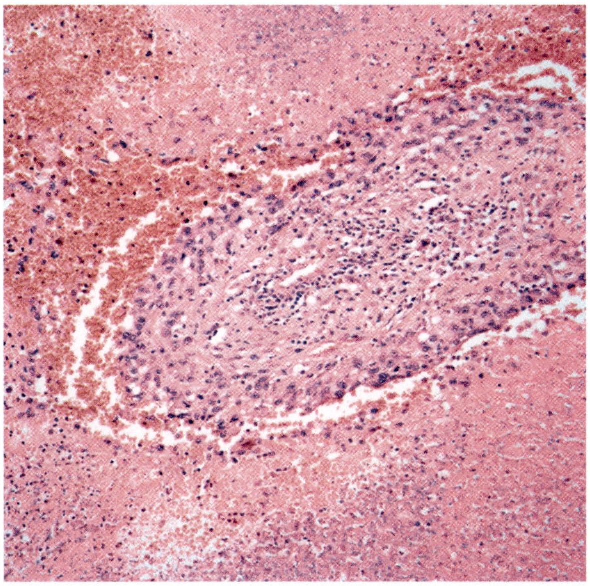

Figure 8-30 Angiosarcoma with areas of hemorrhage.

the tumor may resemble Kaposi sarcoma. The presence of other, more conventional areas of angiosarcoma and the use of immunohistochemical studies will lead to the correct interpretation, however.

Prognosis and Treatment

The prognosis for angiosarcoma is poor, and patients eventually die of their disease with metastatic spread. Different therapeutic modalities have been used, including surgery, chemotherapy, and radiation therapy, alone and in combination. In a case described by Kojima and coworkers,[82] a patient was treated with a combination of chemotherapy and immunotherapy with recombinant interleukin-2. The 1-year follow-up evaluation showed no evidence of recurrence.

EPITHELIOID HEMANGIOENDOTHELIOMA

Epithelioid hemangioendothelioma is rare but is more common by far than angiosarcoma in the lung. Because both of these tumors have similar clinical presentations, some cases that were reported as angiosarcomas may in fact have been epithelioid hemangioendothelioma. Nevertheless, epithelioid hemangioendothelioma is a tumor of ubiquitous distribution and may be seen more commonly in other anatomic sites, including soft tissue, liver, and bone.

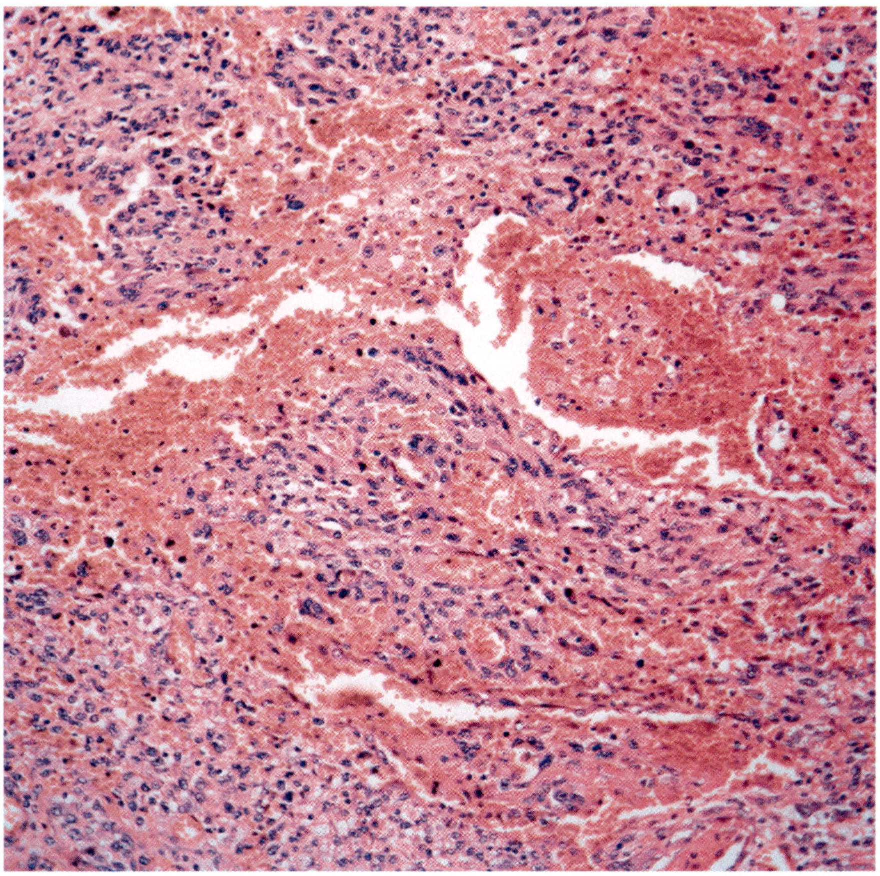

Figure 8-31 Angiosarcoma with spindle cell features and extravasated blood.

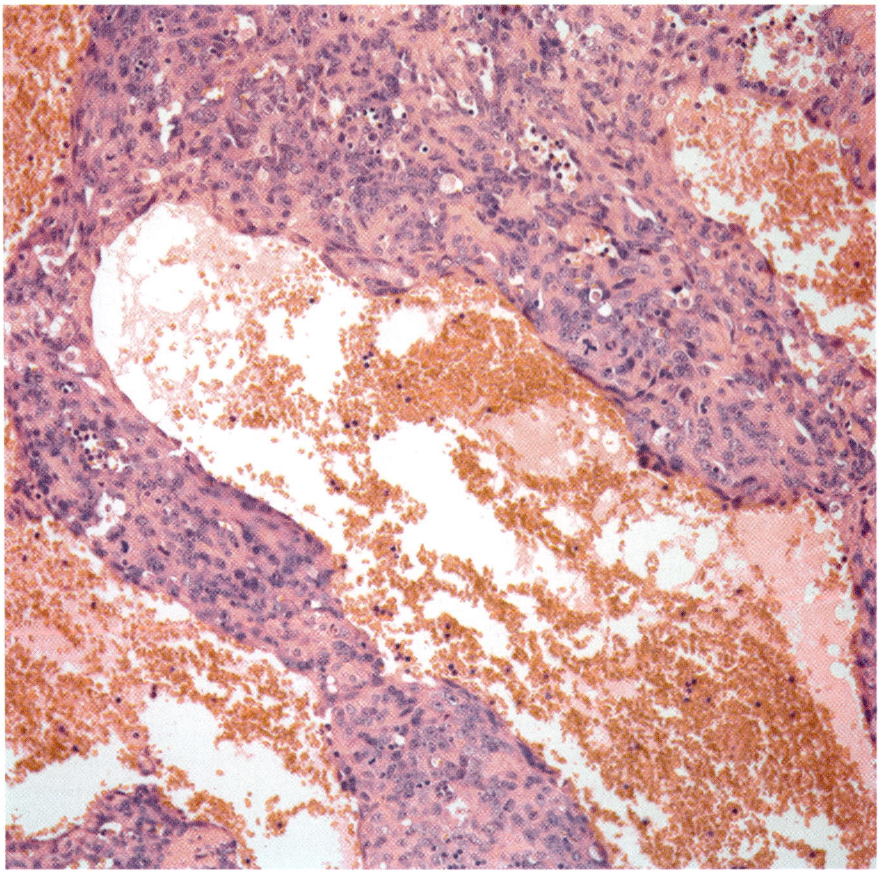

Figure 8-32 Close-up view of an angiosarcoma showing prominent cellular atypia and atypical mitotic figures.

Historical Aspects

In 1960, Smith and associates[85] described the case of a 53-year-old woman who presented with chronic fatigue and a long-standing radiographic abnormality of bilateral calcified densities in the lungs. The initial impression, despite the "chondromatous character" of the lesion, was one of metastatic carcinoma. Over the 11-year history recorded for this patient, however, no other malignancy had been demonstrated. Thus, the investigators designated this particular tumor as a primary chondrosarcoma of the lung.

In 1973, Farinacci and colleagues[86] described a 28-year-old woman whose radiographic films revealed numerous opacities in both lungs. The histologic interpretation in this case was "multifocal pulmonary lesions of possible decidual origin" (so-called pulmonary deciduosis). Both of those cases, in retrospect, can be identified as epithelioid hemangioendothelioma of the lung. It was not until 1975, when Dail and Liebow[87] presented a series of 20 cases in abstract form at the American Association of Pathologists and Bacteriologists, that this new entity was recognized under the designation "intravascular bronchioloalveolar tumor (IVBAT)," which the study authors described as a bronchioloalveolar tumor with a peculiar propensity for hyalinization. At least two thirds of the reported cases were in females.

Following this presentation, Corrin and coworkers[88] reported three additional cases in which the tumors were studied by ultrastructural means. The cells displayed features suggestive of smooth muscle, myofibroblasts, and endothelial differentiation. Accordingly, these workers suggested a vascular origin from precursor mesenchymal cells for this clinical entity. Although the histogenesis of IVBAT was still in question, some investigators recorded lymphatic involvement,[89] whereas others added the designation "sclerosing" to IVBAT (i.e., IVSBAT) to denote the histopathologic features of this tumor.[90] Ferrer-Roca,[90] who reported a case with ultrastructural findings, suggested a pneumocytic origin for this tumor. Meanwhile, several additional reports of IVBAT appeared in the literature.[91–93] Even though the designation IVBAT persisted, some workers suggested a probable vascular origin[94,95] and proposed names such as "sclerosing interstitial vascular tumor" and "sclerosing angiogenic tumor."

In 1982, Weiss and Enzinger[96] presented a series of 41 cases of a vascular tumor that often had been mistaken for carcinoma, which they designated "epithelioid hemangioendothelioma." These workers studied six of the cases using immunohistochemical techniques; in all six cases, the tumor demonstrated positive staining for factor VIII. The clinical course was between that typical for hemangioma and that observed for angiosarcoma—hence the proposed designation epithelioid hemangioendothelioma. In addition, the investigators described their experience with a few cases of similar histologic character in the liver and in the lung. They recommended use of the terms *benign* and *malignant* when possible but also acknowledged that they had not been able to predict prognosis on the basis of histologic findings in all cases.

Despite the accumulated experience with this tumor, in 1983 Dail and associates[97] reported their experience with 20 cases in the lung under the designation of intravascular, bronchiolar, and alveolar tumor (IVBAT), even though they acknowledged the endothelial origin of the tumor. In a more comprehensive review, Weiss and colleagues[98] analyzed the ubiquitous distribution of this neoplasm by comparing similar tumors in soft tissue, liver, lung, and bone. Other researchers,[99–101] however, were of the opinion that IVBAT represents a pulmonary angiosarcoma with a variable clinical course. Use of the designation IVBAT continues in the literature,[102,103] although the more appropriate term *epithelioid hemangioendothelioma*[104] currently is accepted as correct.

Clinical Features

Because of the rarity of epithelioid hemangioendothelioma, many case reports have described rather unusual associations or presentations. Some of these reported features include younger age at diagnosis, alveolar hemorrhage with pleural effusion, multiple site involvement, metastatic spread, and unusual association with other tumors.[105–110]

In the series of 20 cases reported by Dail and coworkers,[97] women comprised 80% of the cases, and patient age ranged from 12 to 61 years, with a sizable percentage of the cases diagnosed in persons younger than 40 years of age. Nine of the patients described were asymptomatic, whereas others presented with nonspecific symptoms including cough, dyspnea, and pleuritic pain. The investigators also documented that most of their patients presented with bilateral lung disease.

In the series of 21 patients presented by Kitaichi and colleagues,[111] similar findings were reported: The age distribution ranged from 14 to 64 years, female patients outnumbered the males (13 females and 8 males), and 15 patients presented with bilateral pulmonary disease, whereas only 6 had unilateral lung disease. These workers found that male patients are more likely to present with overt symptomatology (50%). Bagan and associates[112] reviewed the existing literature and noted that in most series the tumor was more common in women, with an age range of 7 to 72 years.

Macroscopic Features

Epithelioid hemangioendothelioma is characterized by the presence of multiple nodules replacing normal lung parenchyma. The nodules may range in size from a few millimeters to 2 or 3 cm in diameter, and their consistency may range from calcified to soft, with a somewhat mucoid appearance. The nodules are distributed haphazardly in the lung parenchyma and may involve the pleural surface.

Histopathologic Features

Low-power magnification reveals the presence of several nodules replacing normal lung architecture (Fig. 8-33). These nodules display different stages of development; some show areas of calcification and ossification, while others show a characteristic chondromyxoid background, and still others may show a predominant solid cellular proliferation (Figs. 8-34 to 8-38). Polypoid nodules are

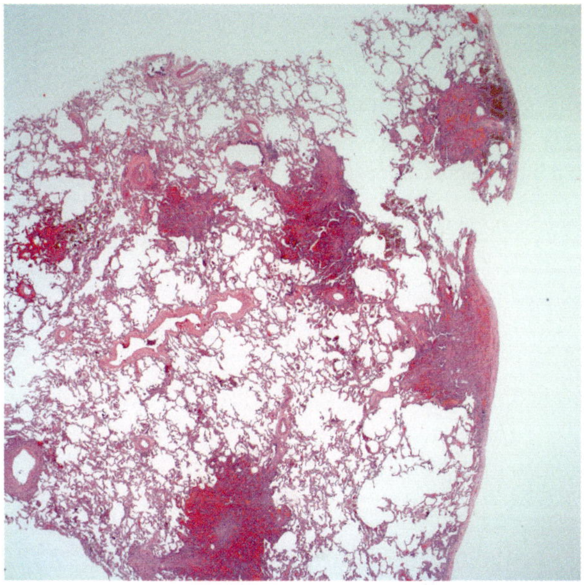

Figure 8-33 Epithelioid hemangioendothelioma with several intrapulmonary nodules.

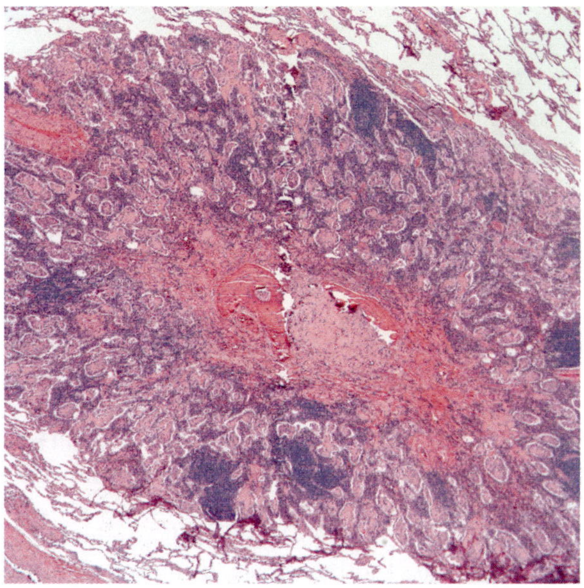

Figure 8-34 Epithelioid hemangioendothelioma with central ossification.

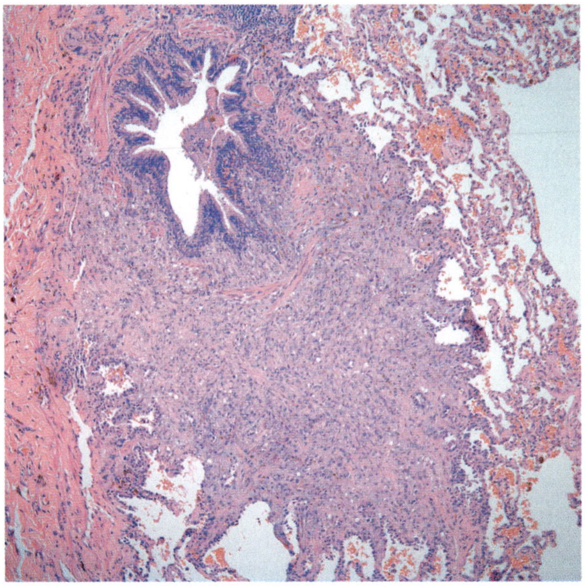

Figure 8-35 Epithelioid hemangioendothelioma. A nodule with a high degree of cellularity can be seen.

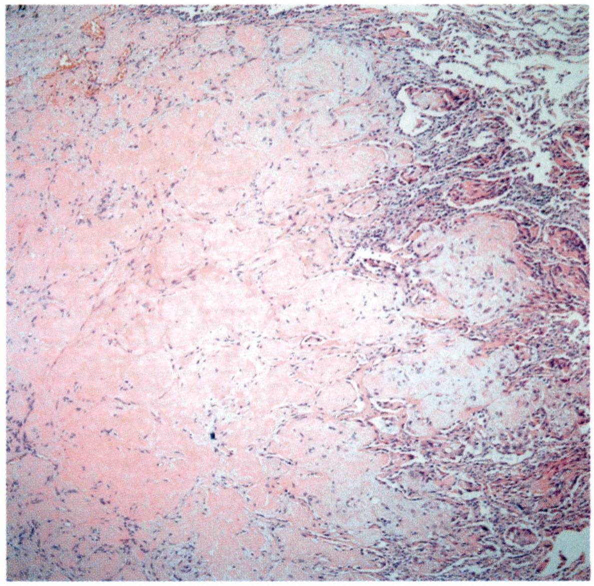

Figure 8-37 Epithelioid hemangioendothelioma. A nodule with more extensive hyalinization can be seen.

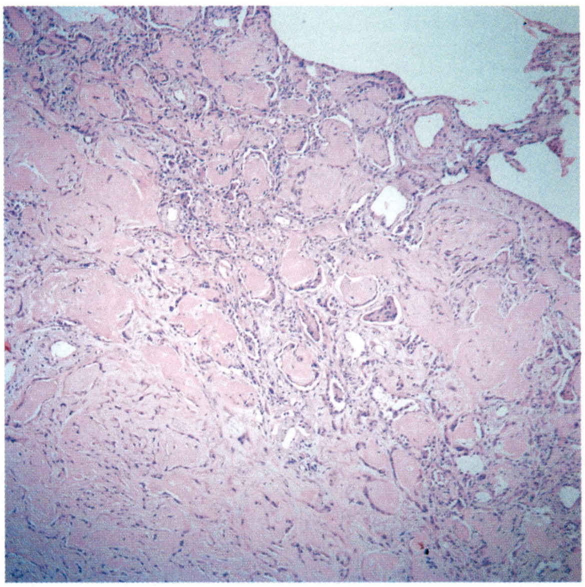

Figure 8-36 Epithelioid hemangioendothelioma. The typical chondroid stroma associated with epithelioid cells can be seen.

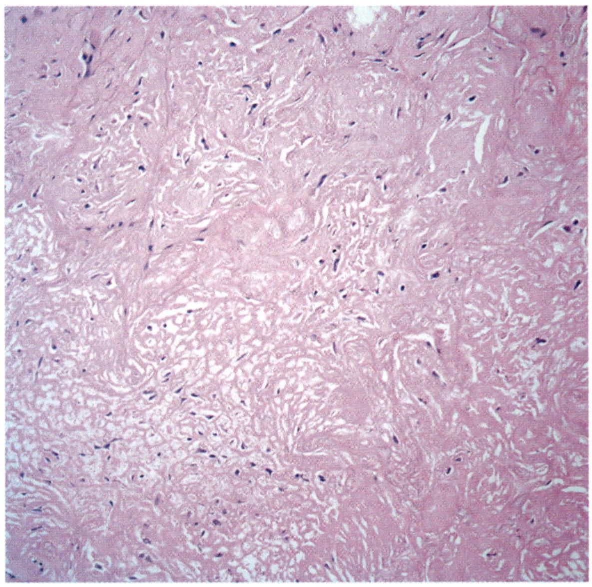

Figure 8-38 Epithelioid hemangioendothelioma with extreme hyalinization with only scant cellular elements.

arranged within alveolar spaces or are seen infiltrating into interstitial areas. At higher magnification, the tumor cells are seen to be arranged in small nests or cords within the myxoid background. The cytologic features include a cellular proliferation composed of medium-sized cells with light eosinophilic to pinkish cytoplasm, small nuclei, and inconspicuous nucleoli. In some areas, the cells are arranged in cords with their nuclei displayed toward the periphery, mimicking signet ring cell carcinoma cells or rhabdoid cells. In other areas, features suggestive of lumen formation, with red cells in the lumens, can be identified. Sometimes the neoplastic cells are admixed with prominent inflammatory infiltrate, and the tumor exhibits an intra-alveolar spreading pattern (Figs. 8-39 to 8-44). Although necrosis may be seen in a few cases, mitotic activity and cellular pleomorphism are lacking.

Immunohistochemical Features

Immunohistochemical vascular markers may be helpful in diagnosing epithelioid hemangioendothelioma. The use of CD31, CD34, and factor VIII may be helpful when a metastatic tumor of epithelial origin is being considered. Ohori and coworkers[113] studied the presence of estrogen

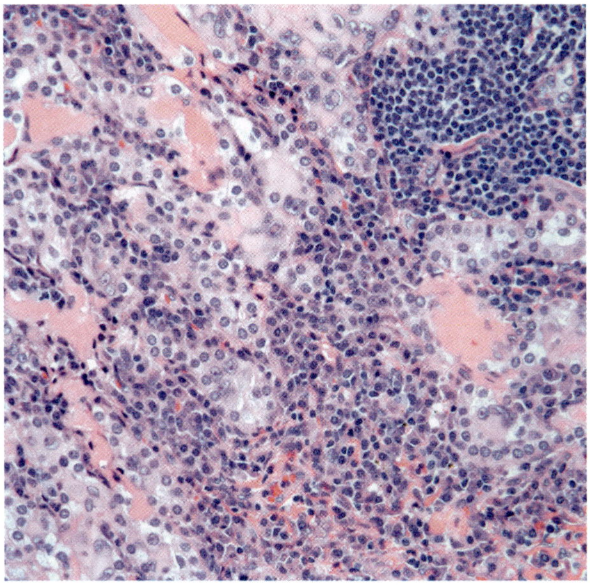

Figure 8-39 Epithelioid hemangioendothelioma with a prominent inflammatory process composed mainly of plasma cells.

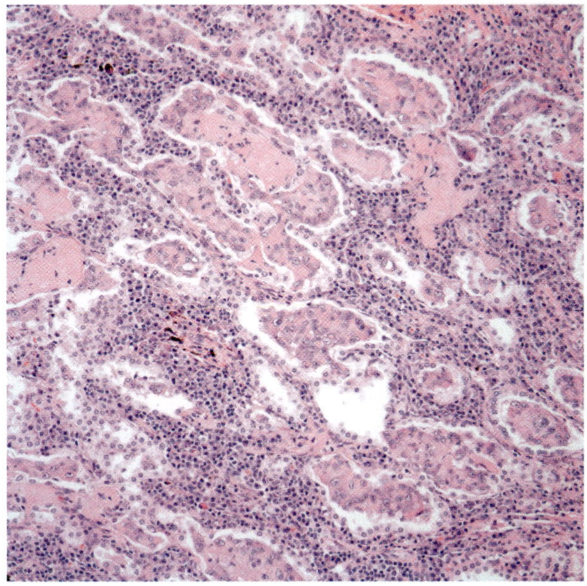

Figure 8-40 Epithelioid hemangioendothelioma with intra-alveolar spread.

and progesterone receptors in epithelioid hemangioendothelioma, among other conditions, and found positive staining for 17β-estradiol in one of the five cases studied. Kumazawa and associates[114] also reported the expression of glucocorticoid receptors.

Differential Diagnosis

Because of the unilateral or bilateral involvement of the lungs, metastatic carcinoma usually is considered in the differential diagnosis. In some cases, the histopathologic features also may mimic those of adenocarcinoma.[115]

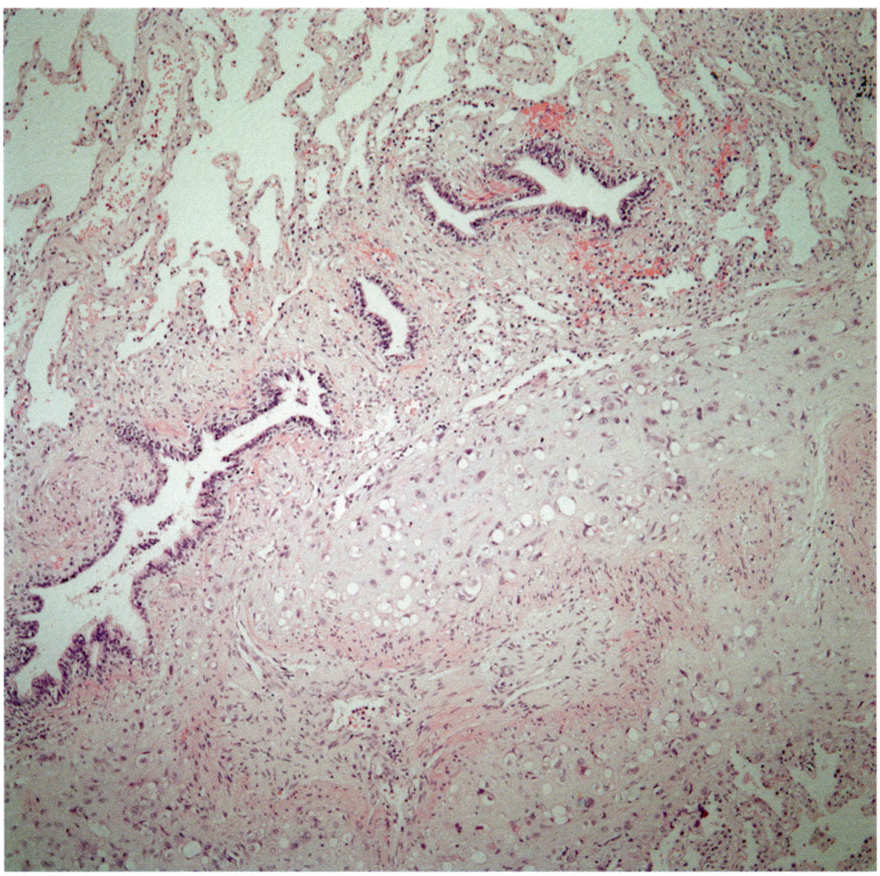

Figure 8-41 Epithelioid hemangioendothelioma with peribronchial spread resembling almost-normal bronchial cartilage.

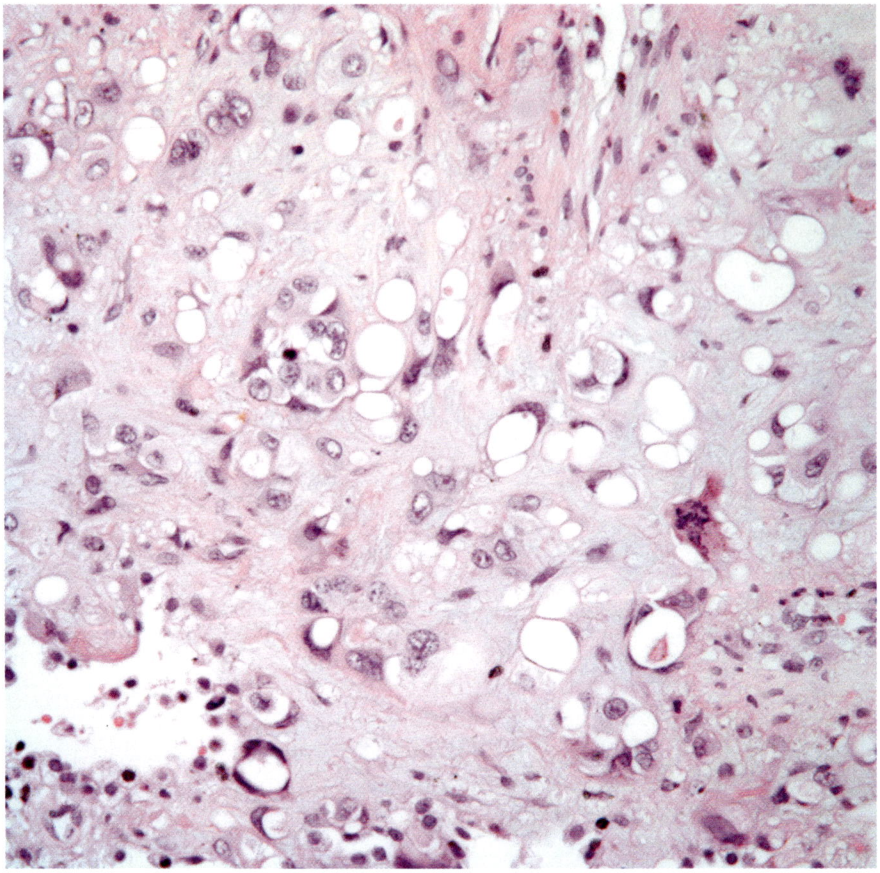

Figure 8-42 Epithelioid hemangioendothelioma with areas closely resembling signet ring cells.

Metastatic carcinoma is unlikely, however, in younger patients, who may be otherwise asymptomatic. The use of immunohistochemical markers CD31, CD34, and factor VIII in histopathologic analysis should lead to the correct interpretation. Angiosarcoma may share the immunohistochemical profile of positive vascular markers and the clinical presentation of pulmonary nodules, however. With epithelioid hemangioendothelioma, careful histologic examination of the tumor nodules should reveal a chondromyxoid background and possibly calcification or ossification, which would be unusual for angiosarcoma. In addition, compared with

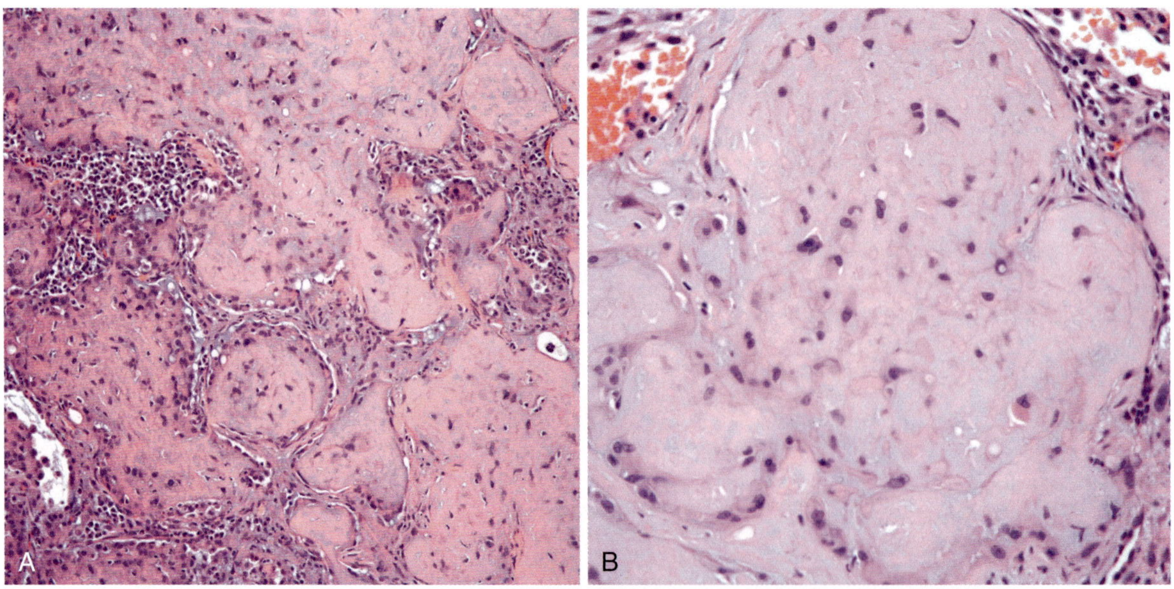

Figure 8-43 **A**, Epithelioid hemangioendothelioma with prominent chondroid stroma. **B**, Higher-power view showing epithelioid cells with absence of nuclear atypia or mitotic activity.

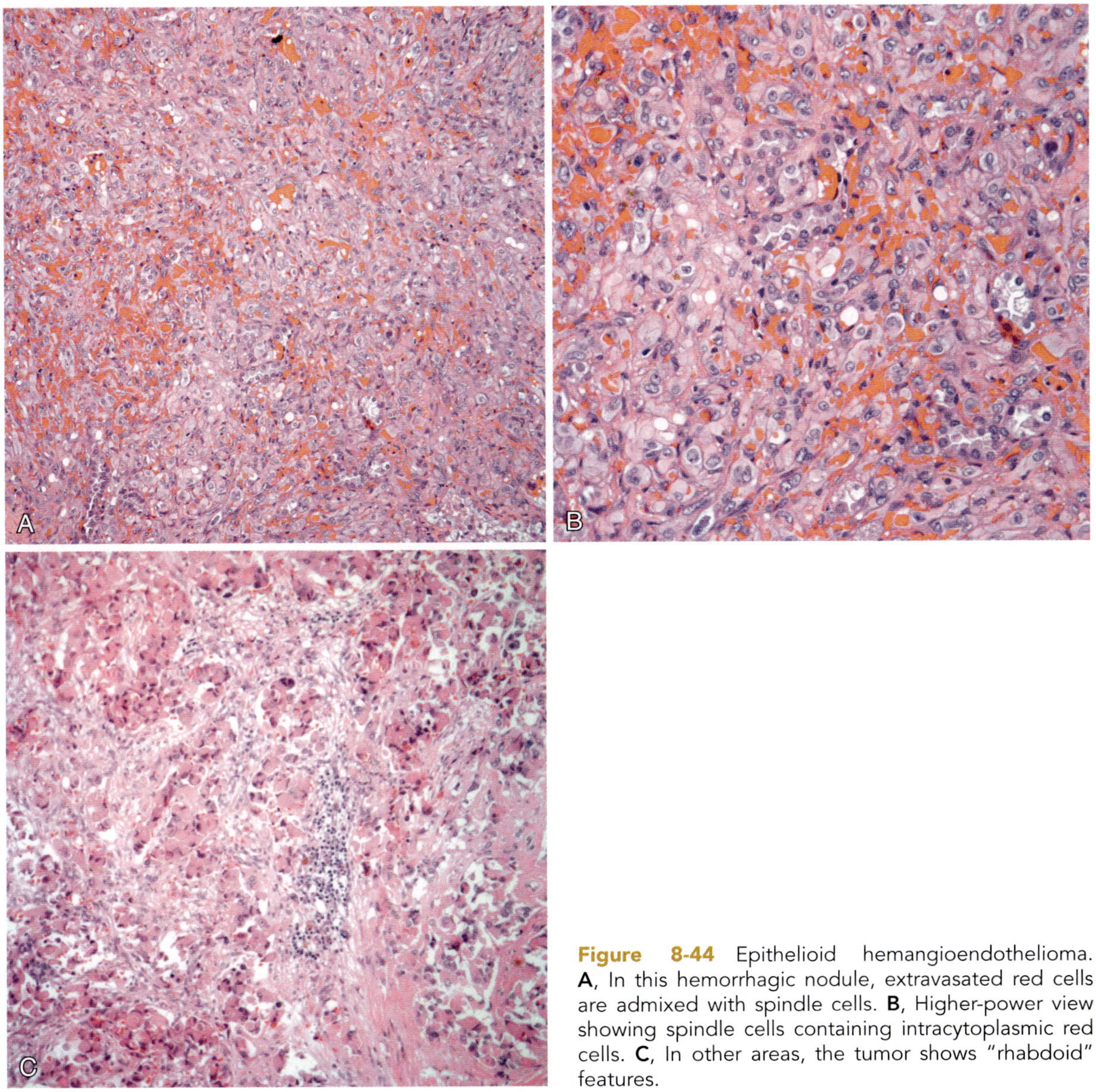

Figure 8-44 Epithelioid hemangioendothelioma. **A**, In this hemorrhagic nodule, extravasated red cells are admixed with spindle cells. **B**, Higher-power view showing spindle cells containing intracytoplasmic red cells. **C**, In other areas, the tumor shows "rhabdoid" features.

epithelioid hemangioendotheliomas, angiosarcomas display more mitotic activity and cellular atypia.

Prognosis and Treatment

No specific treatment for epithelioid hemangioendothelioma is available. Surgery may be beneficial in cases in which the nodules are not numerous.[116] The use of radiation therapy or chemotherapy has been attempted in some patients. Some investigators have suggested a possible role for steroid treatment in cases in which the tumor cells have shown reactivity for glucocorticoids,[114] whereas others have documented improvement in patients treated with bevacizumab.[117] Spontaneous regression of these tumors has also been observed in some patients.[111] The clinical behavior of epithelioid hemangioendothelioma is rather unpredictable. In some patients the course is aggressive, with a fatal outcome within 1 year, while in other patients the course may be more protracted, with one patient surviving for as long as 16 years.[118–120] The prognosis may be worsened by such factors as extensive intravascular, interstitial, and pleural spread[97] and the presence of liver nodules, hemorrhagic manifestations (hemoptysis), or pleural effusion.[112]

KAPOSI SARCOMA

Kaposi sarcoma is a malignant vascular neoplasm of unusual occurrence. Before the AIDS (acquired immunodeficiency syndrome) epidemic, the tumor most frequently was seen in the skin and soft tissues of older persons, usually on the lower extremities. Currently, Kaposi sarcoma most commonly affects patients infected with HIV. It still occurs more often as a skin and soft tissue tumor, rather than a visceral neoplasm.

Primary Kaposi sarcoma of the lung is exceedingly rare. Before the AIDS epidemic, some cases were documented in patients with various types of immunosuppression,[121] and a few cases occurred in patients who apparently were not immunocompromised.[122] Antman and colleagues[113] documented primary Kaposi sarcoma of the lung in a patient who appeared to be immunocompetent. The patient, a 32-year-old man, presented with clinical signs and symptoms of shortness of breath, hemoptysis, and syncope. Radiographic studies showed bilateral pulmonary infiltrates, and on biopsy, the findings were those characteristic of Kaposi sarcoma. The patient received chemotherapy, but no clinical response was obtained, and he died 3 months after initial diagnosis. Postmortem examination revealed metastatic lesions in the occipital lobe and liver. This case occurred after the AIDS epidemic had been recognized; therefore, the patient was properly evaluated for immune status. More recently, Martinez and associates[123] reported the case of a 49-year-old man with idiopathic pulmonary fibrosis and HIV-negative serostatus who underwent bilateral lung transplantation; bilateral pulmonary nodules developed within 6 months. The histopathologic findings were consistent with Kaposi sarcoma. The incidence of this neoplasm in transplant recipients is approximately 6%,[123] but Kaposi sarcoma is extremely rare as a pulmonary tumor. Of note, the spread of Kaposi sarcoma to the lung is not limited to patients with AIDS, because it also has been reported in HIV-negative patients.[124]

Since the AIDS epidemic became well known, the great majority of cases of primary pulmonary Kaposi sarcoma have been associated with that particular syndrome. In a report from Nash and Fligiel,[125] two patients who presented with hemoptysis and pulmonary hemorrhage, respectively, but no evidence of systemic Kaposi sarcoma, were diagnosed on lung biopsy with pulmonary Kaposi sarcoma. Bach and coworkers[126] described a patient with persistent pyrexia and no cutaneous lesions. Sadaghdar and Eden[127] reported the case of a patient presenting with fulminant respiratory failure who experienced relapse of his respiratory failure after treatment with chemotherapy. Joshi and associates[128] reported the case of a 51-year-old man presenting with shortness of breath, dry cough, and generalized fatigue. Chest radiographic imaging revealed multiple bilateral pulmonary nodules that on histologic evaluation were found to be consistent with Kaposi sarcoma.

Although in a majority of cases the clinical presentation was one of multiple pulmonary nodules, unusual cases of a solitary pulmonary nodule also have been described. Roux and colleagues[129] reported the case of a 35-year-old man who presented with cough, dyspnea, and hemoptysis and no history of cutaneous lesions. Chest radiograph revealed an irregular solitary nodule that on histopathologic evaluation showed features consistent with Kaposi sarcoma.

Pulmonary involvement by Kaposi sarcoma in patients with AIDS, originating most likely in the skin, does not occur as frequently as might be expected. Nash and Fligiel[130] evaluated the lungs of 17 men who had died from AIDS complications and found that the lung was involved in 6 cases. Similarly, Meduri and associates[131] documented the extensive parenchymal and pleural involvement by Kaposi sarcoma at autopsy in 11 patients who died with AIDS. Over a 4-year period, Garay and coworkers[132] evaluated 318 cases of AIDS-associated Kaposi sarcoma and identified 19 patients with pulmonary involvement. In a French study, Fouret and colleagues[133] identified nine cases of pulmonary Kaposi sarcoma among 84 patients with AIDS, all of whom had a history of cutaneous Kaposi sarcoma. In a large retrospective study of 140 HIV-positive patients, Mitchel and coworkers[134] encountered 39 patients (21%) with cutaneous Kaposi sarcoma. Of those 39, 19 had endobronchial lesions consistent with Kaposi sarcoma. Eight of those 19 had lesions limited to the endobronchial area, whereas 11 had extensive involvement. These investigators concluded that endobronchial lesions are relatively common in patients with cutaneous Kaposi sarcoma. Miller and associates[135] documented similar findings in a study of 361 HIV-positive patients, of whom 29 (8%) had tracheobronchial lesions. In contrast with the Western experience, in a study of HIV-related Kaposi sarcoma in African patients, Pozniak and colleagues[136] documented 47 patients with epidemic Kaposi sarcoma and stated that pulmonary involvement by this tumor is common but that coexisting pulmonary infections were uncommon.

Some studies have been more specific, exploring pulmonary involvement by Kaposi sarcoma in women and children.[137,138] Haramati and Wong[136] identified seven women with AIDS and cutaneous Kaposi sarcoma in whom the tumor caused diffuse lung disease. Theron and coworkers[137] documented the cases of six HIV-positive children between the ages of 18 months and 10 years, all of whom had lymphadenopathy. It was unclear whether these patients' pulmonary Kaposi sarcoma represented a primary disease or an extension from another primary site; however, this report highlights the ubiquitous distribution of the pulmonary lesion. This neoplasm also is associated with human herpesvirus (KSHV), as demonstrated by analyses of lung biopsy tissue and bronchial lavage fluid. Howard and associates[139] described the presence of a KSHV DNA sequence in lavage fluid obtained from HIV-infected patients with pulmonary involvement by Kaposi sarcoma, noting that this finding correlates with the clinical diagnosis of the tumor. Tamm and colleagues[140] studied the presence of human herpesvirus 8 (HHV8) in 100 consecutive bronchoalveolar lavage (BAL) fluid samples using a nested polymerase chain reaction (PCR) assay. These workers concluded that the detection of HHV8 DNA in BAL fluid is restricted to patients with Kaposi sarcoma, and that this finding is highly sensitive and specific for detection of pulmonary involvement by Kaposi sarcoma.

Macroscopic Features

A majority of reports of primary and metastatic pulmonary Kaposi sarcoma have documented bilateral pulmonary nodules. It appears, however, that pulmonary Kaposi sarcoma may manifest in two different patterns. In the first pattern, the tumor is limited to the endobronchial area; in the second, extensive involvement of the lung parenchyma is characteristic. Most cases will display both patterns, but extensive lung parenchymal involvement without endobronchial involvement,[141] or the reverse of this presentation, has been reported. The pulmonary nodules vary in size, ranging from only a few millimeters to more than 3 cm in diameter. These nodules can involve not only the lung parenchyma but also the pleural surface. The macroscopic appearance is that of a small reddish nodule that may or may not be hemorrhagic.

Histopathologic Features

The low-power view reveals that the lung parenchyma has been replaced by nodules of different sizes, which may show prominent hemorrhagic changes. These nodules may be interspersed with areas of normal lung parenchyma and may be situated in a subpleural or pleural location. Higher-power examination of the nodules shows a prominent spindle cell proliferation composed of elongated cells with fusiform nuclei and inconspicuous nucleoli. The spindle cell proliferation displays characteristic vascular slits, which may contain numerous red blood cells or hemosiderin. In addition, areas of hyaline droplets intermixed with red cells and spindle cells may be visible. Mitotic figures are readily identifiable, but tumor necrosis is not common and, when present, is not marked (Figs. 8-45 to 8-50). In some areas, ectatic large vessels or airway structures may be seen surrounded by the spindle cell proliferation. Some investigators have stated that the lymphatic distribution of Kaposi sarcoma in lung is a hallmark finding in open lung biopsy specimens.[142] Tumor cells may show positive staining for vascular markers including CD31, CD34, and factor VIII.[128]

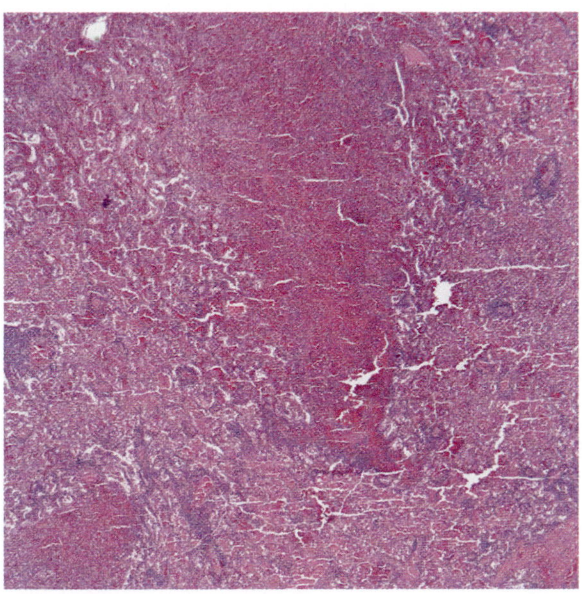

Figure 8-45 Low-power view of a Kaposi sarcoma in the lung with extensive areas of hemorrhage and subtle changes suggestive of nodule formation.

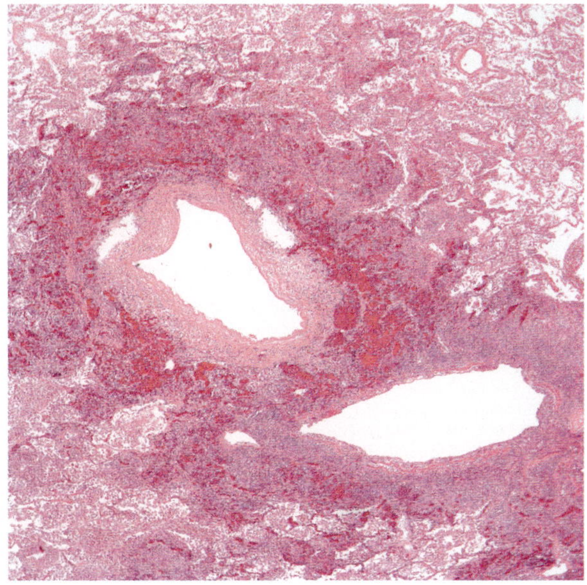

Figure 8-46 Low-power view of a Kaposi sarcoma showing prominent vascular tropism.

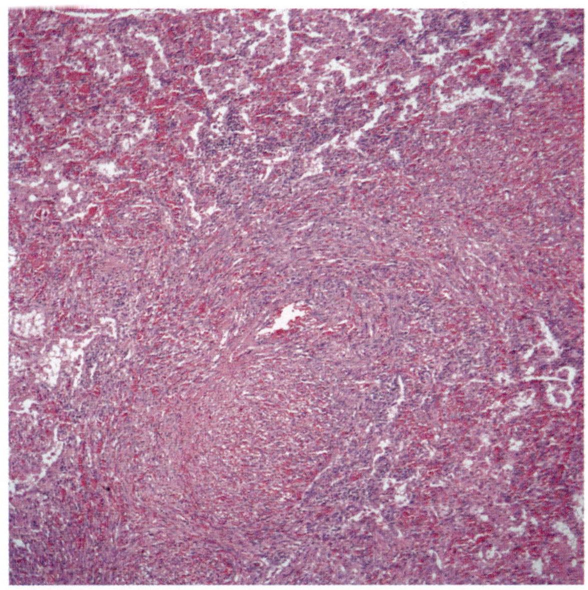

Figure 8-47 Kaposi sarcoma. This nodule in the lung parenchyma is composed of spindle cells with extravasated red cells.

Prognosis and Treatment

The prognosis for patients with Kaposi sarcoma may be affected by multiple factors including HIV serostatus, clinical presentation, and extent of the lesion at the time of diagnosis. In all reported cases, the outcome

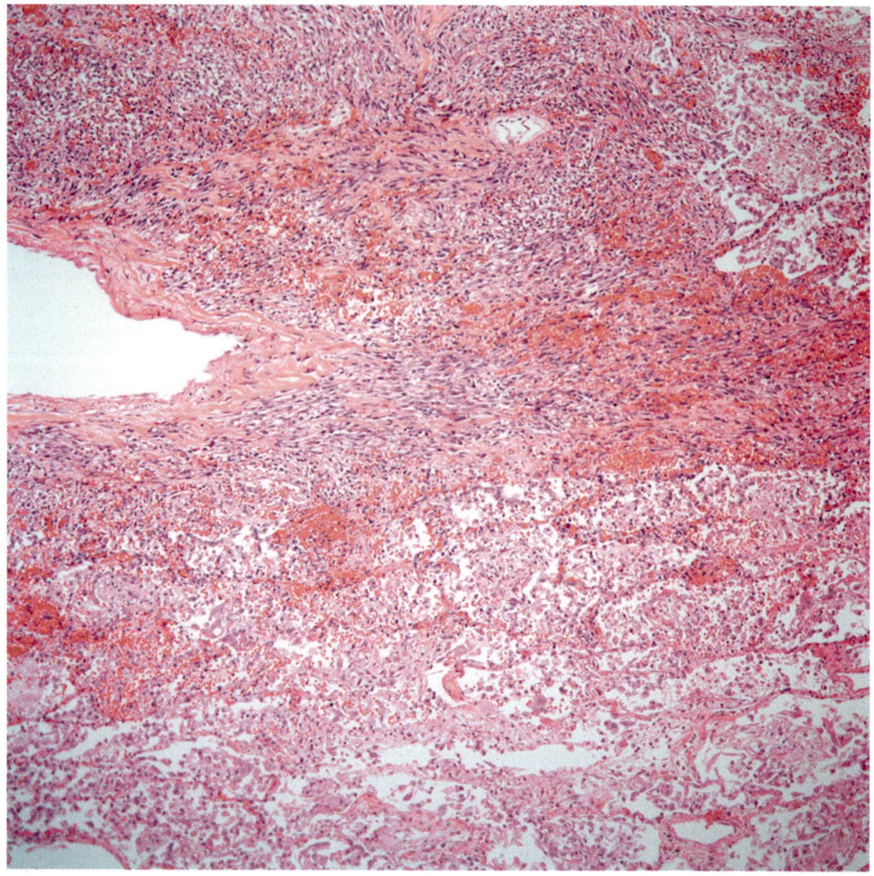

Figure 8-48 Kaposi sarcoma composed of spindle cells around a large vessel. Note the normal lung parenchyma with collections of macrophages.

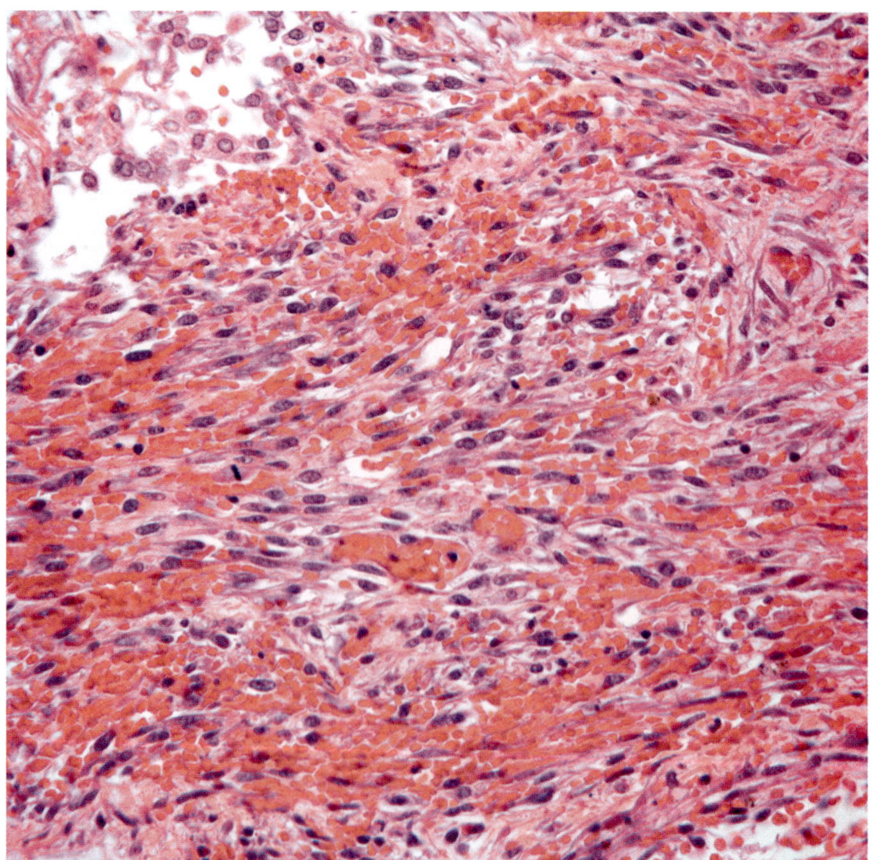

Figure 8-49 Kaposi sarcoma with prominent spindle cell proliferation and the classic vascular slits filled with red cells.

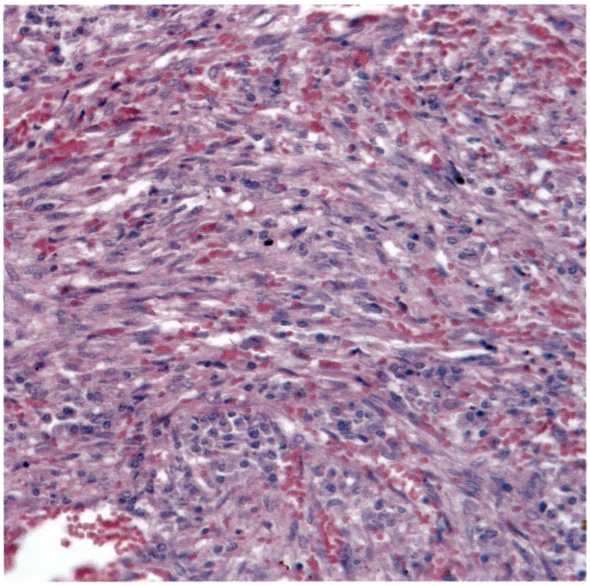

Figure 8-50 Kaposi sarcoma. At higher magnification, some of the spindle cells are seen to contain hyaline intracytoplasmic globules.

was death of the patient, but an important point in this context is that in a majority of the cases, the pulmonary lesions of Kaposi sarcoma are associated with AIDS. The tumor usually metastasizes within and outside of the thoracic cavity. Some investigators have claimed a response to irradiation[143] or chemotherapy.[144] However, Kaplan and associates[145] reported that the median survival in patients with this lesion was only 2 months, and that Kaposi sarcoma generally is a late manifestation of AIDS.

REFERENCES

1. Moran CA, Suster S. Angiolymphoid hyperplasia with eosinophilia (epithelioid hemangioma) of the lung: a clinicopathologic and immunohistochemical study of two cases. *Am J Clin Pathol.* 2005;123:762–765.
2. Rosai J, Gold J, Landy R. The histiocytoid hemangiomas: a unifying concept embracing several previously described entities of skin, soft tissue, large vessels, bone and heart. *Hum Pathol.* 1979;10:707–730.
3. Suster S. Nodal angiolymphoid hyperplasia with eosinophilia. *Am J Clin Pathol.* 1987;88:236–239.
4. Fetsch JF, Weiss SW. Observations concerning the pathogenesis of epithelioid hemangioma (angiolymphoid hyperplasia). *Mod Pathol.* 1991;4:449–455.
5. Konishi N, Tamura T, Kawai C, Shirai T. IgE associated nephropathy in a patient with subcutaneous eosinophilic lymphoid granuloma (Kimura's disease). *Virchows Arch A Pathol Anat Histol.* 1981;392:127–134.
6. Moesner J, Pallesen R, Sorensen B. Angiolymphoid hyperplasia with eosinophilia (Kimura's disease): a case with dermal lesions in the knee region and a popliteal arteriovenous fistula. *Arch Dermatol.* 1981;117:650–653.
7. Saxe N, Kahn LB. Angiolymphoid hyperplasia with eosinophilia. Report of three cases. *S Afr Med J.* 1977;52:454–457.
8. Fernandez LA, Olsen TG, Barwick KW, Sanders M, Kaliszewski C, Inagami T. Renin in angiolymphoid hyperplasia with eosinophilia. Its possible effect on vascular proliferation. *Arch Pathol Lab Med.* 1986;110:1131–1135.
9. Reed RJ, Terazakis N. Subcutaneous angioblastic lymphoid hyperplasia with eosinophilia (Kimura's disease). *Cancer.* 1972;29:489–497.
10. Olsen TG, Helwig EB. Angiolymphoid hyperplasia with eosinophilia: a clinicopathologic study of 116 patients. *J Am Acad Dermatol.* 1985;12:781–796.
11. Chan JKC, Hui PK, Ng CS, Yuen NW, Kung IT, Gwi E. Epithelioid hemangioma (angiolymphoid hyperplasia with eosinophilia) and Kimura's disease in Chinese. *Histopathology.* 1989;15:557–574.
12. Chun SI, Ji HG. Kimura's disease and angiolymphoid hyperplasia with eosinophilia: clinical and histopathologic differences. *J Am Acad Dermatol.* 1992;27:954–958.
13. Kempf W, Haeffner AC, Zepter K, et al. Angiolymphoid hyperplasia with eosinophilia: evidence for a T-cell lymphoproliferative origin. *Hum Pathol.* 2002;23:1023–1029.
14. Hidayat AA, Font RL, Zimmermann LE. Angiolymphoid hyperplasia with eosinophilia (Kimura's disease) of the orbit and ocular adnexa. *Am J Ophthalmol.* 1983;96:176–189.
15. Kuo TT, Hsueh S, Su IJ, Gonzalez-Crussi F, Chen JS. Histiocytoid hemangioma of the heart with peripheral eosinophilia. *Cancer.* 1985;55:2854–2861.
16. Googe PB, Harris NL, Mihm MC. Kimura's disease and angiolymphoid hyperplasia with eosinophilia: two distinct histopathologic entities. *J Cutan Pathol.* 1987;14:263–271
17. Urabe A, Tsuneyoshi M, Enjoji M. Epithelioid hemangioma versus Kimura's disease: a comparative clinicopathologic study. *Am J Surg Pathol.* 1987;11:758–766.
18. Kuo TT, Shih LY, Chan HL. Kimura's disease: involvement of regional lymph nodes and distinction from angiolymphoid hyperplasia with eosinophilia. *Am J Surg Pathol.* 1988;12:843–854.
19. Hui PK, Chan JK, Ng CS, Kung IT, Gwi E. Lymphadenopathy of Kimura's disease. *Am J Surg Pathol.* 1989;13:177–186.
20. Hosaka N, Minato T, Yoshida S, et al. Kimura's disease with unusual eosinophilic epithelioid granulomatous reaction: a finding possibly related to eosinophil apoptosis. *Hum Pathol.* 2002;33:561–564.
21. Chen H, Thompson LD, Aguilera NS, Abbondanzo SL. Kimura's disease: a clinicopathologic study of 21 cases. *Am J Surg Pathol.* 2004;28:505–513.
22. Cooper PH. Is histiocytoid hemangioma a specific pathologic entity?. *Am J Surg Pathol.* 1988;12:815–817.
23. Wagenvoort CA, Beetstra A, Spijker J. Capillary haemangiomatosis of the lungs. *Histopathology.* 1978;2:401–406.
24. Rowen M, Thompson JR, Williamson RA, Wood BJ. Diffuse pulmonary hemangiomatosis. *Radiology.* 1978;127:445–451.
25. Wagenaar SS, Mulder JJS, Wagenvoort CA, van de Bosch JM. Pulmonary capillary hemangiomatosis diagnosed during life. *Histopathology.* 1989;14:212–214.
26. Langleben D, Heneghan JM, Batten AP, et al. Familial pulmonary capillary hemangiomatosis resulting in primary pulmonary hypertension. *Ann Intern Med.* 1988;109:106–109.
27. Oviedo A, Abramson LP, Worthington R, Dainauskas JR, Crawford SE. Congenital pulmonary capillary hemangiomatosis: report of two cases and review of the literature. *Pediatr Pulmonol.* 2003;36:253–256.
28. Ishii H, Yanagimoto K, Iwabuchi K, et al. Two different manifestations of the effect of apoptosis on pulmonary capillary hemangiomatosis; localized and diffuse lesions. *Histopathology.* 2003;43:300–308.
29. Vevaina JR, Mark EJ. Thoracic hemangiomatosis masquerading as interstitial lung disease. *Chest.* 1988;93:657–659.
30. Eltorky MA, Headley AS, Winer-Muram H, Garrett Jr HE, Griffin JP. Pulmonary capillary hemangiomatosis: a clinicopathologic review. *Ann Thorac Surg.* 1994;57:772–776.
31. Lawler LP, Askin FB. Pulmonary capillary hemangiomatosis: multidetector row CT findings and clinicopathologic correlation. *J Thorac Imaging.* 2005;20:61–63.

32. Havlik DM, Massie LW, Williams WL, Crooks LA. Pulmonary capillary hemangiomatosis–like foci: an autopsy study of 8 cases. *Am J Clin Pathol.* 2000;113:655–662.
33. Varnholt H, Kradin R. Pulmonary capillary hemangiomatosis arising in hereditary hemorrhagic telangiectasia. *Hum Pathol.* 2004;35:266–268.
34. Erbersdobler A, Niendorf A. Multifocal distribution of pulmonary capillary haemangiomatosis. *Histopathology.* 2002;40:88–91.
35. Ishii H, Iwabuchi K, Kameya T, Koshino H. Pulmonary capillary hemangiomatosis. *Histopathology.* 1996;29:275–278.
36. Whitaker JS, Pickering CAC. Pulmonary capillary haemangiomatosis. *Diagn Histopathol.* 1983;6:77–84.
37. Frazier AA, Franks TJ, Mohammed TLH, Ozbudak IH, Galvin JR. From the Archives of the AFIP: Pulmonary veno-occlusive disease and pulmonary capillary hemangiomatosis. *Radiographics.* 2007;27:867–882.
38. Lantuejoul S, Sheppard MN, Corrin B, et al. Pulmonary veno-occlusive disease and pulmonary capillary hemangiomatosis. A clinicopathologic study of 35 cases. *Am J Surg Pathol.* 2006;30:850–857.
39. White CW, Sondheimer HM, Crouch EC, Wilson H, Fan LL. Treatment of pulmonary hemangiomatosis with recombinant interferon alfa-2a. *N Engl J Med.* 1989;320:1197–1200.
40. Brill PW, Symchych P, Winchester P. Capillary hemangioma of the lung. *Radiology.* 1977;124:184, 224.
41. Bowyer JJ, Sheppard M. Capillary haemangioma presenting as a lung pseudocyst. *Arch Dis Childhood.* 1990;65:1162–1164.
42. Galliani CA, Beatty JF, Grosfeld JL. Cavernous hemangioma of the lung in an infant. *Pediatr Pathol.* 1992;12:105–111.
43. Forsee JH, Mahon HW, James LA. Cavernous hemangioma of the lung. *Ann Surg.* 1950;131:418–423.
44. Davis MM, Bugaieski EM, Heifetz SA. Pathological case of the month. *Arch Pediatr Adolesc Med.* 1996;150:1309–1310.
45. Paul KP, Borner C, Muller KM, Vogt-Moykopf I. Capillary hemangioma of the right main bronchus treated with sleeve resection in infancy. *Am Rev Respir Dis.* 1991;143:876–879.
46. Wodenhouse GE. Hemangioma of the lung. *J Thorac Surg.* 1948;17:408–415.
47. Iwasaki M, Kobayashi H, Nomoto T, Arai T, Kondoh T. Primary racemose hemangioma of the bronchial artery. *Intern Med.* 2001;40:650–653.
48. Abrahams NA, Colby TV, Pearl R, Chipps BE, Juris AL, Leslie KO. Pulmonary hemangiomas of infancy and childhood: report of two cases and review of the literature. *Pediatr Dev Pathol.* 2002;5:283–292.
49. Harding JR, Williams J, Seal RM. Pedunculated capillary hemangioma of the bronchus. *Br J Dis Chest.* 1978;72:336–342.
50. Kayser K, Zink S, Link B, et al. Endobronchial juvenile hemangioma—a case report of a neonate including immunohistochemical monitoring and nuclear, cellular, and vascular morphometry. *Virchows Arch.* 2001;438:192–197.
51. Sirmali M, Demirag F, Aydin E, Karasu S, Kaya S. A pulmonary cavernous hemangioma causing massive hemoptysis. *Ann Thorac Surg.* 2003;76:1275–1276.
52. Kobayashi A, Ohno S, Bando M, Oshikawa K, Sugiyama Y. Cavernous hemangioma of lungs and liver in an asymptomatic girl. *Respiration.* 2003;70:647–650.
53. Fine SW, Whitney KD. Multiple cavernous hemangiomas of the lung: a case report and review of the literature. *Arch Pathol Lab Med.* 2004;128:1439–1441.
54. Fugo K, Matsuno Y, Okamoto K, et al. Solitary capillary hemangioma of the lung: report of 2 resected cases detected by high-resolution CT. *Am J Surg Pathol.* 2006;30:750–753.
55. Maeda R, Isowa N, Sumitomo S, Matsuoka K. Pulmonary cavernous hemangioma. *Gen Thorac Cardiovasc Surg.* 2007;55:177–179.
56. Quijano G, Drut R. Multiple congenital infantile hemangiomas of the lung in partial trisomy D. *J Clin Pathol.* 2007;60:943–945.
57. Capizzani TR, Patel H, Hines MH, Mott RT, Petty JK. A unique case of a giant congenital pulmonary hemangioma in a newborn. *J Pediatr Surg.* 2008;43:574–578.
58. Bhaskar J, Sharma A. Spontaneous hemo-pneumothorax as a result of venous hemangioma. *Tex Heart Inst J.* 2006;33:91–92.
59. Faul JL, Berry GJ, Colby TV, et al. Thoracic lymphangiomas, lymphangiectasis, lymphangiomatosis, and lymphatic dysplasia syndrome. *Am J Respir Crit Care Med.* 2000;161:1037–1046.
60. Tazelaar HD, Kerr D, Yousem SA, Saldana MJ, Langston C, Colby TV. Diffuse pulmonary lymphangiomatosis. *Hum Pathol.* 1993;24:1313–1322.
61. Marom EM, Moran CA, Munden RF. Generalized lymphangiomatosis. *AJR Am J Roentgenol.* 2004;182:1068.
62. Copeland J, Muller KM, Muller AM. Pulmonary haemangiolymphangioma—a new entity of pulmonary vascular tumours? *Histopathology.* 2008;52:527–529.
63. Bush JK, McLean RL, Sieker HO. Diffuse lung disease due to lymphangiomyoma. *Am J Med.* 1969;46:645–654.
64. Wada A, Tateishi R, Terazawa T, Matsuda M, Hattori S. Lymphangioma of the lung. *Arch Pathol.* 1974;98:211–213.
65. Drut R, Mosca HH. Intrapulmonary cystic lymphangioma. *Pediatr Pulmonol.* 1996;22:204–206.
66. Limmer S, Krokowski M, Kujath P. Pulmonary lymphangioma. *Ann Thorac Surg.* 2008;85:336–339.
67. Lee CH, Kim YD, Kim K, et al. Intrapulonary cystic lymphangioma in a 2-month-old infant. *J Korean Med Sci.* 2004;19:458–461.
68. Nagayasu T, Hayashi T, Ashizawa K, et al. A case of solitary pulmonary lymphangioma. *J Clin Pathol.* 2003;56:396–398.
69. Takahara T, Morisaki Y, Torigoe T, et al. Intrapulmonary cystic lymphangioma: report of a case. *Surg Today.* 1998;28:1310–1312.
70. Hamada K, Ishii Y, Nakaya M, Sawabata N, Fukuda K, Suzuki H. Solitary lympangioma of the lung. *Histopathology.* 1995;27:482–483.
71. Wilson C, Askin FB, Heitmiller RF. Solitary pulmonary lymphangioma. *Ann Thorac Surg.* 2001;71:1337–1338.
72. Kim WS, Lee KS, Kim I, et al. Cystic intrapulmonary lymphangioma: HRCT findings. *Pediatr Radiol.* 1995;25:206–207.
73. Milovic I, Oluic D. Lymphangioma of the lung associated with respiratory distress in a neonate. *Pediatr Radiol.* 1992;22:156.
74. Carlson KC, Parnassus WN, Klatt EC. Thoracic lymphangiomatosis. *Arch Pathol Lab Med.* 1987;111:475–477.
75. Miller DL, Allen MS. Rare pulmonary tumors. *Mayo Clin Proc.* 1993;68:492–498.
76. Patel AM, Ryu JH. Angiosarcoma in the lung. *Chest.* 1993;103:1531–1535.
77. Spragg RG, Wolf PL, Haghighi P, Abraham JL, Astarita RW. Angiosarcoma of the lung with fatal pulmonary hemorrhage. *Am J Med.* 1983;74:1072–1076.
78. Ott RA, Eugene J, Kollin J, Kanas RJ, Conston DE, Chi JC. Primary pulmonary angiosarcoma associated with multiple synchronous neoplasms. *J Surg Oncol.* 1987;35:269–276.
79. Palvio DHB, Paulsen SM, Henneberg EW. Primary angiosarcoma of the lung presenting as intractable hemoptysis. *Thorac Cardiovasc Surg.* 1987;35:105–107.
80. Sheppard MN, Hansell DM, Du Bois RM, Nicholson AG. Primary epithelioid angiosarcoma of the lung presenting as pulmonary hemorrhage. *Hum Pathol.* 1997;27:383–385.
81. Pandit SA, Fiedler PN, Westcott JL. Primary angiosarcoma of the lung. *Ann Diagn Pathol.* 2005;9:302–304.
82. Kojima K, Okamoto I, Ushijima S, et al. Successful treatment of primary pulmonary angiosarcoma. *Chest.* 2003;124:2397–2400.
83. Segal S, Lenchner GS, Cichelli AV, Promisloff RA, Hofman WI, Baiocchi GA. Angiosarcoma presenting as diffuse alveolar damage. *Chest.* 1988;94:214–216.
84. Yousem SA. Angiosarcoma presenting in the lung. *Arch Pathol Lab Med.* 1986;110:112–115.
85. Smith EA, Cohen RV, Peale AR. Primary chondrosarcoma of the lung. *Ann Intern Med.* 1960;53:838–846.

86. Farinacci CJ, Blauw AS, Jennings EM. Multifocal pulmonary lesions of possible decidual origin (so-called pulmonary deciduosis). *Am J Clin Pathol*. 1973;59:508–514.
87. Dail D, Liebow AA. Intravascular brochiololoalveolar tumor [abstract]. *Am J Pathol*. 1975;78:6a, 7a.
88. Corrin B, Manners B, Millard M, Weaver L. Histogenesis of the so-called "intravascular bronchioloalveolar tumours." *J Pathol*. 1979;128:163–167.
89. Wenisch HJC, Lulay M. Lymphogenous spread of an intravascular bronchioloalveolar tumor. *Virchows Arch A Path Anat Histol*. 1980;387:117–123.
90. Ferrer-Roca O. Intravascular and sclerosing bronchio-alveolar tumor. *Am J Surg Pathol*. 1980;4:375–381.
91. Sherman JL, Rykwalder PJ, Tashkin DP. Intravascular bronchioloalveolar tumor. *Am Rev Respir Dis*. 1981;123:468–470.
92. Marsh K, Kenyon WE, Earis JE, Pearson MG. Intravascular bronchioloalveolar tumor. *Thorax*. 1982;37:474–475.
93. Emery RW, Fox AL, Raab DE. Intravascular bronchioloalveolar tumour. *Thorax*. 1982;37:472–473.
94. Azumi N, Churg A. Intravascular and sclerosing bronchioloalveolar tumor: a pulmonary sarcoma of probable vascular origin. *Am J Surg Pathol*. 1981;5:587–596.
95. Weldon-Linne CM, Victor TA, Christ ML, Fry WA. Angiogenic nature of the "intravascular bronchioloalveolar tumor" of the lung. *Arch Pathol Lab Med*. 1981;105:174–179.
96. Weiss SW, Enzinger FM. Epithelioid hemangioendothelioma: a vascular tumor often mistaken for a carcinoma. *Cancer*. 1982;50:970–981.
97. Dail DH, Liebow AA, Gmelich JT, et al. Intravascular, bronchiolar, and alveolar tumor of the lung (IVBAT). An analysis of twenty cases of a peculiar sclerosing endothelial tumor. *Cancer*. 1983;51:452–464.
98. Weiss SW, Ishak KG, Dail DH, Sweet DE, Enzinger FM. Epithelioid hemangioendothelioma and related lesions. *Semin Diagn Pathol*. 1986;3:259–287.
99. Eggleston JC. The intravascular bronchioloalveolar tumor and the sclerosing hemangioma of the lung: misnomers of pulmonary neoplasia. *Semin Diagn Pathol*. 1985;2:270–280.
100. Bhagavan BS, Dorfman HD, Murthy MSN, Eggleston JC. Intravascular bronchioloalveolar tumor (IVBAT): a low-grade sclerosing epithelioid angiosarcoma of lung. *Am J Surg Pathol*. 1982;6:41–52.
101. Corrin B, Harrison WJ, Wright DH. The so-called intravascular bronchioloalveolar tumor of lung (low grade sclerosing angiosarcoma): presentation with exptrapulmonary deposits. *Diagn Histopathol*. 1983;6:229–237.
102. Sicilian L, Warson F, Carrington CB, Hayes J, Gaensler EA. Intravascular bronchioloalveolar tumor (IV-BAT). *Respiration*. 1983;44:387–394.
103. Sweeny WB, Vesoulis Z, Blaum LC. Intravascular bronchioloalveolar tumor: a distinctive surgical and pathological entity. *Ann Thorac Surg*. 1986;42:702–704.
104. Yousem SA, Hochholzer L. Unusual thoracic manifestations of epithelioid hemangioendothelioma. *Arch Pathol Lab Med*. 1987;111:459–463.
105. Rock MJ, Kaufman RA, Lobe TE, Hensley SD, Moss ML. Epithelioid hemangioendothelioma of the lung (intravascular bronchioloalveolar tumor) in a young girl. *Pediatr Pulmonol*. 1991;11:181–186.
106. Struhar D, Sorkin P, Greif J, Marmor S, Geller E. Alveolar haemorrhage with pleural effusion as a manifestation of epithelioid haemangioendothelioma. *Eur Respir J*. 1992;5:592–593.
107. Bollinger BK, Laskin WB, Knight CB. Epithelioid hemangioendothelioma with multiple site involvement. *Cancer*. 1994;73:610–615.
108. Van Kasteren ME, van der Wurff AA, Palmen FM, Dolman A, Miseré JF. Epithelioid haemangioendothelioma of the lung: clinical and pathological pitfalls. *Eur Respir J*. 1995;8:1616–1619.
109. Briens E, Caulet-Maugendre S, Desrues B, et al. Alveolar haemorrhage revealing epithelioid haemangioendothelioma. *Respir Med*. 1997;91:111–114.
110. Bralet MP, Terris B, Vilgrain V, et al. Epithelioid hemangioendothelioma, multiple focal nodular hyperplasias, and cavernous hemangiomas of the liver. *Arch Pathol Lab Med*. 1999;123:846–849.
111. Kitaichi M, Nagai S, Nishimura K, et al. Pulmonary epithelioid haemangioendothelioma in 21 patients including three with partial spontaneous regression. *Eur Respir J*. 1998;12:89–96.
112. Bagan P, Hassan M, Le Pimpec Barthes F, et al. Prognostic factors and surgical indications of pulmonary epithelioid hemangioendothelioma: a review of the literature. *Ann Thorac Surg*. 2006;82:2010–2013.
113. Ohori NP, Yousem SA, Alpan ES, Colby TV. Estrogen and progesterone receptors in lymphangioleiomyomatosis, epithelioid hemangioendothelioma, and sclerosing hemangioma of the lung. *Am J Clin Pathol*. 1991;96:529–535.
114. Kumazawa Y, Maeda K, Ito M, et al. Expression of glucocorticoid receptor and 11β hydroxysteroid dehydrogenase in a case of pulmonary epithelioid hemangioendothelioma. *J Clin Pathol*. 2002;55:61–64.
115. Hristova EN, Krishnamurthy S, Ro J, Ayala AG. Pulmonary epithelioid hemangioendothelioma with prominent signet ring cell features mimicking metastatic adenocarcinoma. *Ann Diagn Pathol*. 2003;7:160–164.
116. Schattenberg T, Pfannschmidt J, Herpel E, Schnabel PA, Mechtersheimer G, Dienemann H. Bilateral surgical resection in pulmonary epithelioid hemangioendothelioma. *Thorac Cardiovasc Surg*. 2007;55:199–210.
117. Belmont L, Zemoura L, Couderc LJ. Pulmonary epithelioid haemangioendothelioma and bevacizumab. *J Thorac Oncol*. 2008;3:557–558.
118. Saleiro S, Barbosa M, Souto Moura C, Almeida J, Ferreira S. Epithelioid hemangioendothelioma—a rare pulmonary tumor. *Rev Port Pneumol*. 2008;3:421–425.
119. Ledson MJ, Convery R, Carty A, Evans CC. Epithelioid haemangioendothelioma. *Thorax*. 1999;54:560–561.
120. Corrin B, Dewar A, Simpson CGB. Epithelioid hemangioendothelioma of the lung. *Ultrastruct Pathol*. 1996;20:345–347.
121. Mesmin F, Gomez H, Behar C, Caulet T. Lymphoblastic leukemia and Kaposi's sarcoma. *Pediatr Radiol*. 1979;8:185–187.
122. Antman KH, Nadler L, Mark EJ, Montella DL, Kirkpatrick P, Halpern J. Primary Kaposi's sarcoma of the lung in an immunocompetent 32-year-old heterosexual white man. *Cancer*. 1984;54:1696–1698.
123. Martinez S, McAdams HP, Youens KE. Kaposi sarcoma after bilateral lung transplantation. *J Thorac Imaging*. 2008;23:50–53.
124. Coll J, Pedro-Botet J, Pallas JO, Gimenez-Arnau AM, Barranco C. Classic Kaposi's sarcoma with pulmonary involvement in an HIV-negative woman. *Clin Exp Dermatol*. 1995;20:410–412.
125. Nash G, Fligiel S. Kaposi's sarcoma presenting as pulmonary disease in the acquired immunodeficiency syndrome: diagnosis by lung biopsy. *Hum Pathol*. 1984;15:999–1001.
126. Bach MC, Bagwell SP, Fanning JP. Primary pulmonary Kaposi's sarcoma in the acquired immunodeficiency syndrome: a cause of persistent pyrexia. *Am J Med*. 1988;85:274.
127. Sadaghdar H, Eden E. Pulmonary Kaposi's sarcoma presenting as fulminant respiratory failure. *Chest*. 1991;100:858–860.
128. Joshi M, Markelova N, Palacio D, Schapira RM. A patient with HIV, dyspnea, and multiple pulmonary nodules. *Chest*. 2006;130:1924–1928.
129. Roux FJ, Bancal C, Dombret MC, et al. Pulmonary Kaposi's sarcoma revealed by a solitary nodule in a patient with acquired immunodeficiency syndrome. *Am J Respir Crit Care Med*. 1994;149:1041–1043.
130. Nash G, Fligiel S. Pathologic features of the lung in the acquired immune deficiency syndrome (AIDS): an autopsy study of seventeen homosexual males. *Am J Clin Pathol*. 1984;81:6–12.

131. Meduri GU, Stover DE, Lee M. Pulmonary Kaposi's sarcoma in the acquired immune deficiency syndrome. Clinical, radiographic, and pathololgic manifestations. *Am J Med*. 1986;81:11–18.
132. Garay SM, Belenko M, Fazzini E, Schinella R. Pulmonary manifestations of Kaposi's sarcoma. *Chest*. 1987;91:39–43.
133. Fouret PJ, Touboul JL, Mayaud CM, Akoun GM, Roland J. Pulmonary Kaposi's sarcoma in patients with acquired immune deficiency syndrome: a clinicopathological study. *Thorax*. 1987;42:262–268.
134. Mitchell DM, McCarthy M, Flemming J, Moss FM. Bronchopulmonary Kaposi's sarcoma in patients with AIDS. *Thorax*. 1992;47:726–729.
135. Miller RF, Tomlinson MC, Cottrill CP, Donald JJ, Spittle MF, Semple SJ. Bronchopulmonary Kaposi's sarcoma in patients with AIDS. *Thorax*. 1992;47:721–725.
136. Pozniak AL, Latif AS, Neill P, Houston S, Chen K, Robertson V. Pulmonary Kaposi's sarcoma in Africa. *Thorax*. 1992;47:730–733.
137. Haramati LB, Wong J. Intrathracic Kaposi's sarcoma in women with AIDS. *Chest*. 2000;117:410–414.
138. Theron S, Andronikou S, Du Plessis JD, et al. Pulmonary Kaposi sarcoma in six children. *Pediatr Radiol*. 2007;37:1224–1229.
139. Howard M, Brink N, Miller R, Tedder R. Association of human herpes virus with pulmonary Kaposi's sarcoma. *Lancet*. 1995;346:712.
140. Tamm M, Reichenberger F, McGandy CE, et al. Diagnosis of pulmonary Kaposi's sarcoma by detection of human herpes virus 8 in bronchoalveolar lavage. *Am J Respir Crit Care Med*. 1998;157:458–463.
141. Gruden JF, Huang L, Webb WR, Gamsu G, Hopewell PC, Sides DM. AIDS-related Kaposi sarcoma of the lung: radiographic findings and staging system with bronchoscopic correlation. *Radiology*. 1995;195:545–552.
142. Purdy LJ, Colby TV, Yousem SA, Battifora H. Pulmonary Kaposi's sarcoma: premortem histologic diagnosis. *Am J Surg Pathol*. 1986;10:301–311.
143. Nobler MP. Pulmonary irradiation for Kaposi's sarcoma in AIDS. *Am J Clin Oncol*. 1985;8:441–444.
144. Gill PS, Akil B, Colletti P, et al. Pulmonary Kaposi's sarcoma: clinical findings and results of therapy. *Am J Med*. 1989;87:57–61.
145. Kaplan LD, Hopewell PC, Jaffe H, Goodman PC, Bottles K, Volberding PA. Kaposi's sarcoma involving the lung in patients with the acquired immunodeficiency syndrome. *J Acquir Immune Defic Syndr*. 1988;1:23–30.

9

Lung Tumors Derived from Presumed Ectopic Tissues

Tumors derived from presumed ectopic tissue constitute a family of tumors that are rarely encountered as primary intrapulmonary neoplasms. This is a diverse group in terms of not only histology and presentation but also clinical behavior. Nevertheless, the diagnostic criteria are essentially the same as those for such tumors occurring in the usual anatomic site. In view of their rarity as primary lung neoplasms, it is important to rule out a possible metastatic lesion before a definitive diagnosis of primary pulmonary neoplasm is rendered. Thus, careful clinicopathologic correlation, including information from appropriate radiologic investigations, is essential in the evaluation and diagnosis of these tumors.

The tumors and conditions described in this chapter, which by themselves have no particular clinical or histologic associations, can be categorized as follows:

- Glomangioma/glomangiosarcoma
- Melanoma
- Meningioma/meningothelial-like nodules/diffuse meningotheliomatosis
- Teratoma
- Thymoma

The most important clinical and immunohistochemical features are presented in Tables 9-1 and 9-2, respectively.

GLOMANGIOMA AND GLOMANGIOSARCOMA

Of glomangioma and glomangiosarcoma, the former is by far the more common. Glomangiomas occur more often in the nail bed and in superficial and deep soft tissues but also have been described in a more ubiquitous distribution that includes the gastrointestinal and gynecologic systems and the head and neck.[1–6] The tumors are assumed to originate from the glomus body, which is a specialized arteriovenous anastomosis made up of Suquet-Hoyer canals and is more commonly seen in the deep dermis and subungual area. Over the years, considerable debate has arisen regarding whether glomangioma represents a true tumor or a hyperplasia. Of note, however, the existence of glomangiosarcoma, an entity with aggressive clinical behavior, indicates that glomangioma may be a true neoplasm as well.

Although glomus tumors occurring in the respiratory system have been reported, they are exceedingly rare. The trachea is the most common location, and although most of the reported cases are of the benign type (glomangioma), cases of glomangiosarcoma also have been described.[7–10] This chapter focuses only on tumors of the lower respiratory tract, occurring in the bronchus and lung.

Primary pulmonary or bronchial glomangiomas and glomangiosarcomas are, for the most part, reported as curiosities or in small series of cases.[11–18] Tang and coworkers[11] are given credit for the first description of a glomangioma in the lung. This case was in a 67-year-old woman in whom radiographic evaluation revealed a mass in the left lung, suggesting a possible diagnosis of glomus tumor. The patient had two distinct intrapulmonary nodules, indicating the possibility of multicentric disease. Mackay and associates[12] described a 19-year-old patient with a coin lesion in the lung. A more detailed history disclosed that the patient also had a soft tissue tumor with similar histologic features; therefore, in this case, it is most likely that the lesion in the lung represented metastatic disease from an extrapulmonary origin.

Alt and colleagues[13] reported the case of a 34-year-old asymptomatic man with a coin lesion in the lung. These workers proposed that the term *glomus tumor* be reserved

TABLE 9-1 COMMON CLINICAL FEATURES

Tumor	Age Group	Anatomic Site	Prognosis
Glomangioma	Young and older adults	Central or peripheral location	Good
Glomangiosarcoma	Young and older adults	Central or peripheral location	Aggressive behavior
Melanoma	Young and older adults	Central or peripheral location	Variable aggressiveness
Meningioma	Young and older adults	Intraparenchymal	Good
Meningothelial-like nodule	Any age	Intraparenchymal	Good
Diffuse meningotheliomatosis	Young and older adults	Intraparenchymal	Good
Teratoma	Any age	Central or peripheral location	
Mature			Good
Malignant component			Aggressive behavior
Thymoma	Young and older adults	Intraparenchymal	Good

TABLE 9-2 IMMUNOHISTOCHEMICAL STAINS*

Tumor	Actin	Vimentin	S-100	EMA	Keratin	LCA	TdT	CEA	CD34
Glomangioma/glomangiosarcoma	+	+	−	−	−	−	−	−	±
Melanoma	−	+	+	−	−	−	−	±	−
Meningioma	−	+	±	+	±	−	−	−	±
Thymoma	−	±	−	±	+	+	+	−	−

*The immunohistochemical results for a teratoma will vary depending on the tissues present.

−, negative; +, positive; CEA, carcinoembryonic antigen; EMA, epithelial membrane antigen; LCA, leukocyte common antibody; S-100, S-100 protein; TdT, terminal deoxynucleotidyl transferase.

for those tumors composed of endothelium-lined vascular spaces surrounded by smooth muscle. Koss and associates[14] reported two additional cases of intrapulmonary glomangiomas in two asymptomatic patients who were 40 and 51 years of age, respectively. Gaertner and coworkers[15] collected five cases; in one of these, however, the tumor originated in the mediastinum, and one case was that of a glomangiosarcoma. The three patients with glomangiomas were adults, and the intrapulmonary lesion was discovered incidentally during follow-up for different reasons. The patient diagnosed with glomangiosarcoma appeared to have tumor-related signs and symptoms, such as hemoptysis. More recently, three additional reports of glomangiomas have been presented,[16–18] and in contrast with previous cases in which the tumor occurred in the lung parenchyma, the tumors were located within the bronchus, obstructing the lumen.

Clinical Features

No specific clinical features can be assigned to glomangioma or glomangiosarcoma. In the reported cases many patients have been asymptomatic, and the tumor was discovered during either a routine radiographic evaluation or an investigation for a different problem. When these tumors occur in a central location, however, the patient is more likely to present with some symptomatology related to bronchial obstruction—namely, cough, chest pain, or hemoptysis. Because glomangiomas are very unusual tumors, the clinical impression tends to be that of a different, more common bronchial neoplasm. Glomangiomas can occur in young adults or in older patients, between the ages of approximately 20 to 65 years, and have been described in both men and women and in white, black, and Asian patients.

Macroscopic Features

Glomangiomas may manifest as either central or peripheral tumors. In a majority of the cases, the tumor arises within the lung proper. These neoplasms may appear as well-circumscribed tumor nodules that range in size from 1 to 6 cm in greatest dimension. In a few cases, two separate nodules have been described. The tumors are of soft consistency and tan in color, with a smooth, homogeneous-appearing surface. In a few cases, "encapsulated" tumor nodules with dilated spaces seen on the cut surface have been described. Glomangiomas characteristically do not show areas of necrosis or hemorrhage. By contrast, glomangiosarcomas tend to be larger tumors with areas of hemorrhage or necrosis.

Microscopic Features

The spectrum of histopathologic features is broader for glomangiomas occurring in the soft tissue than for those observed in the lung, which tend to be of the solid mucohyaline type. The low-power view is that of a well-demarcated tumor nodule surrounded by normal lung parenchyma (Fig. 9-1). Even at low magnification, the tumor is characterized by a fairly homogeneous cellular proliferation in which tumor cells are admixed with ectatic vascular spaces (Fig. 9-2). Those arising in a central location will show partial obstruction of the bronchial lumen, with histopathologic features similar to those of tumors arising within the lung parenchyma. Higher magnification reveals a homogeneous cellular proliferation composed of medium-sized cells, with round to oval nuclei, clear to lightly eosinophilic cytoplasm, and ectatic vascular spaces (Figs. 9-3 to 9-8). The cellular proliferation

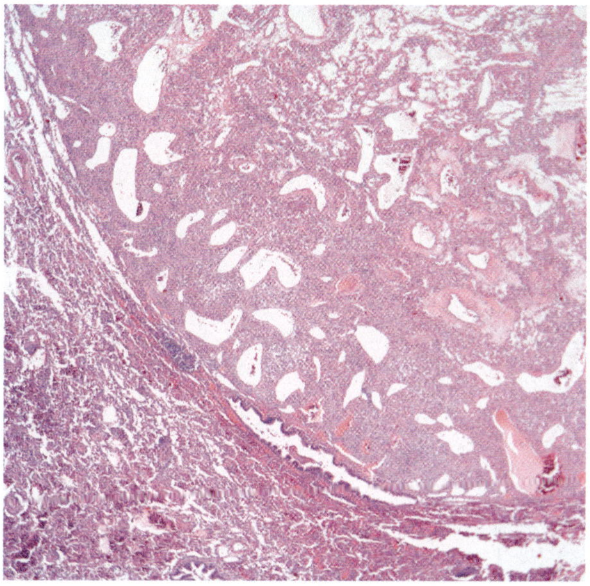

Figure 9-1 Low-power view of an intrapulmonary glomus tumor. The tumor is well circumscribed, but not encapsulated.

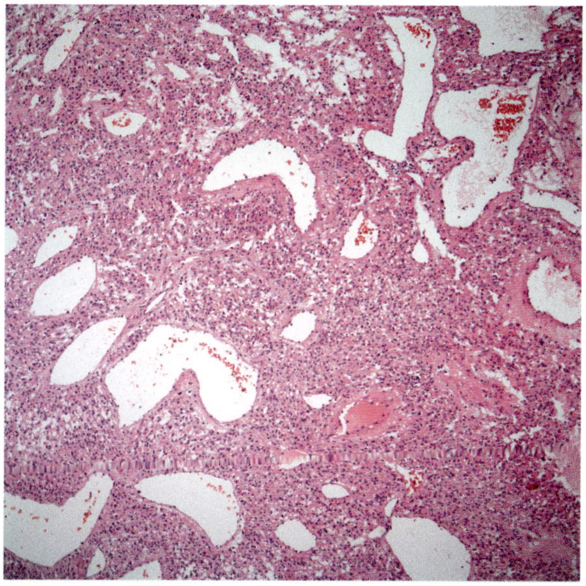

Figure 9-2 Intrapulmonary glomus tumor. Solid areas are combined with prominent ectatic vessels.

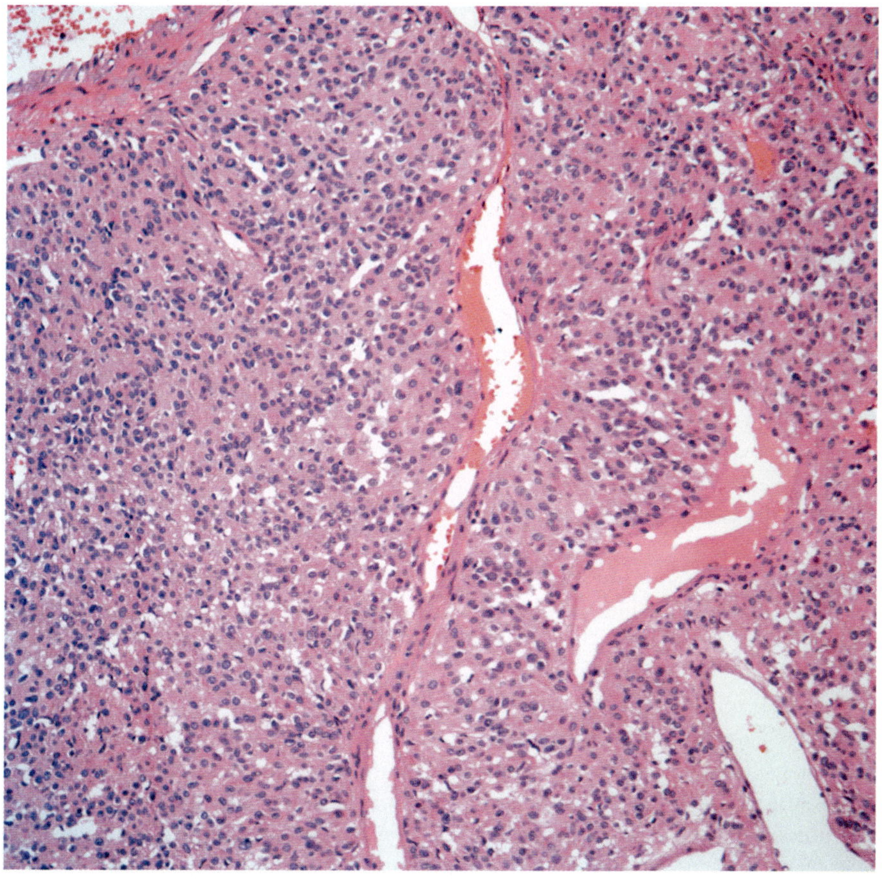

Figure 9-3 Glomus tumor showing solid areas.

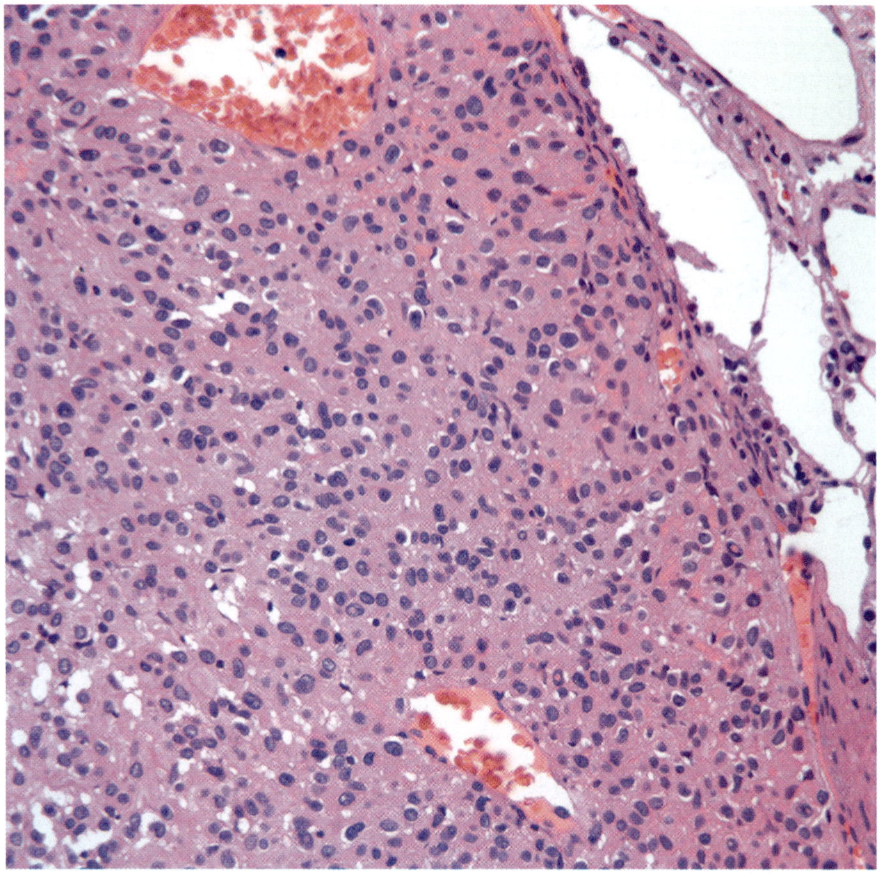

Figure 9-4 Glomus tumor with solid areas composed of cells with oncocytic features.

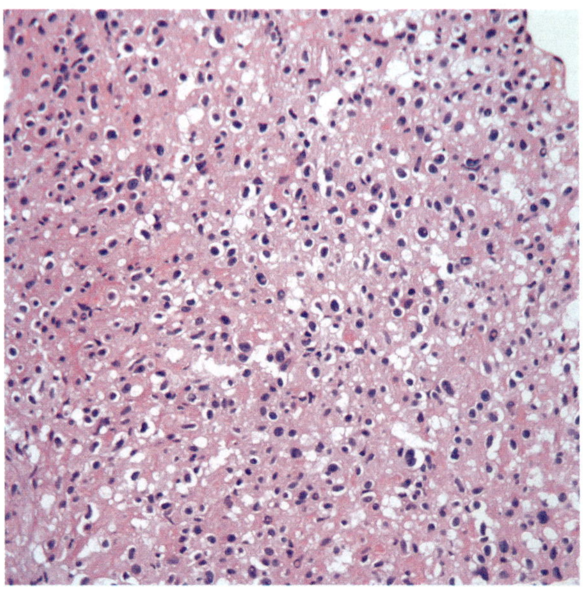

Figure 9-5 Glomus tumor composed of cells with light esosinophilic or clear cytoplasm.

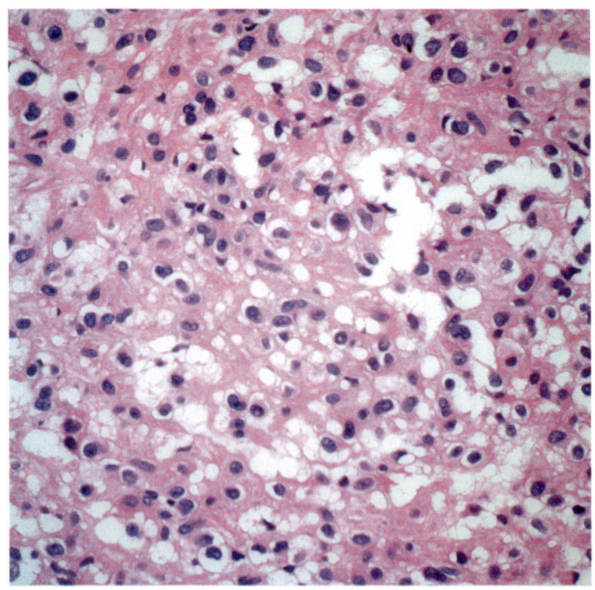

Figure 9-6 High-power view of a glomus tumor showing cells with clear cytoplasm. Note the absence of nuclear atypia and mitotic activity.

is characterized by clear cytoplasm, giving a “fried egg” appearance, whereas the vascular spaces show perivascular hyalinization (Figs. 9-9 to 9-11). Glomangiomas characteristically do not display evidence of necrosis or mitotic activity.

Glomangiosarcoma will display areas reminiscent of glomangiomas; at low magnification, however, it is possible to observe areas of necrosis, which may not necessarily be extensive. The higher-power view reveals areas of nuclear atypia and mitotic activity (Figs. 9-12 to 9-14).

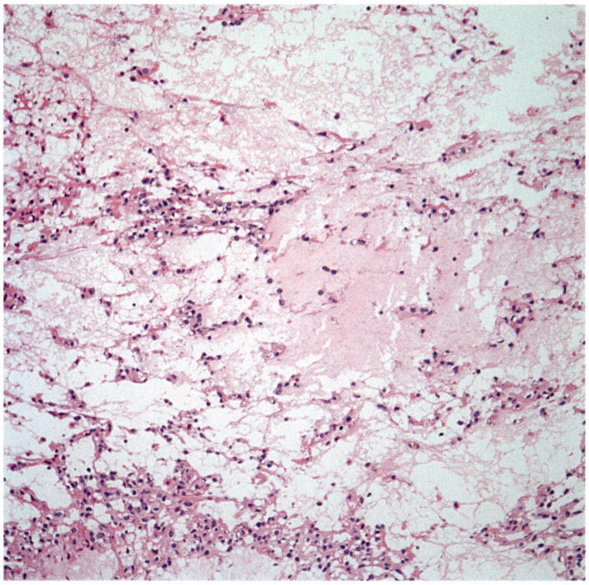

Figure 9-7 Glomus tumor with abundant mucoid material, with cords of tumor cells.

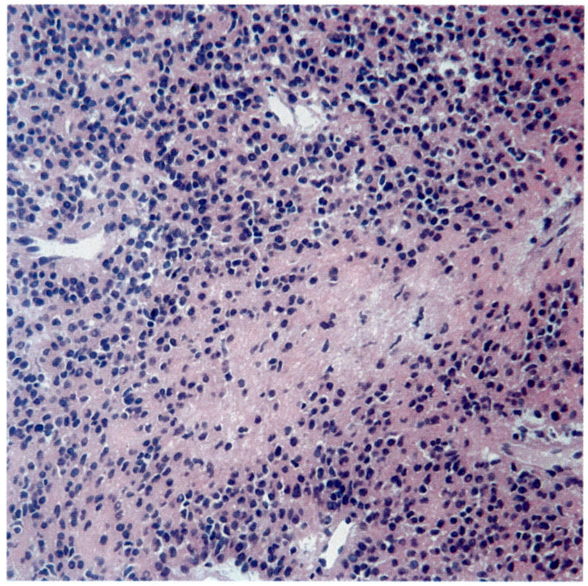

Figure 9-8 Glomus tumor with solid areas and neural-like features.

Areas demonstrating transition from conventional glomangioma to glomangiosarcoma may be observed and are helpful in arriving at a correct interpretation (Fig. 9-15).

Immunohistochemical Features

The most consistent finding on immunohistochemical studies is positive staining for vimentin and muscle-specific actin (Fig. 9-16). Glomangiomas may show positive staining for other markers as well, including smooth muscle actin, desmin, neuron-specific enolase, and Leu-7. These tumors characteristically show negative staining for keratins, epithelial membrane antigen (EMA), myoglobin, chromogranin, S-100 protein, and HMB-45. Although in some cases of intrapulmonary glomangiomas, the tumors have displayed negative staining for CD34,[14] Hatori and coworkers[19] reported a study of six cases of glomus tumor (subungual in location) in which positive staining for CD34 was observed in vascular endothelial cells and tumor cells.

Differential Diagnosis

The differential diagnosis for glomangiomas in the lung may be challenging, owing to their rarity as primary lung

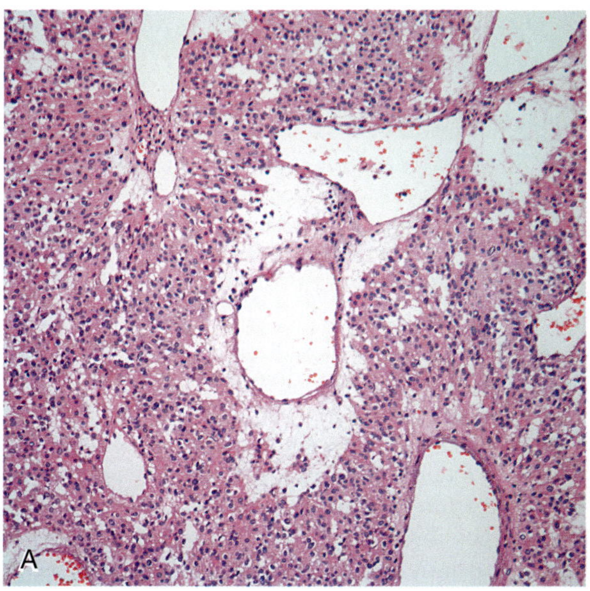

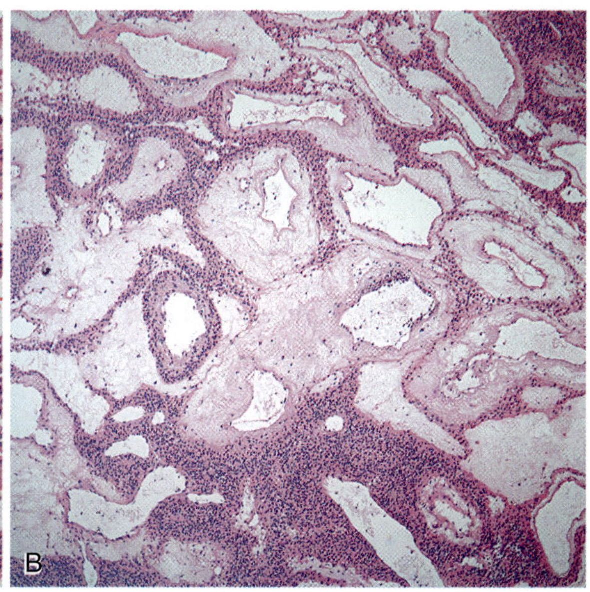

Figure 9-9 **A**, Glomus tumor with prominent dilated vessels. Note the edematous perivascular areas. **B**, Markedly edematous perivascular areas.

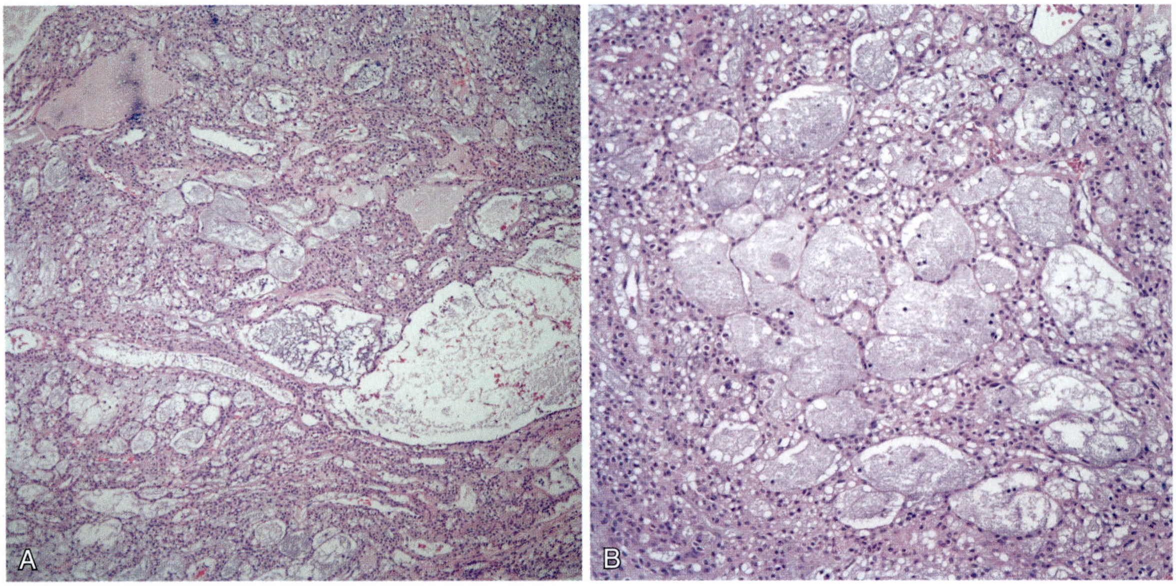

Figure 9-10 **A**, Glomus tumor with solid areas combined with cystic-like spaces filled with mucoid material. **B**, This growth pattern resembles that of a salivary gland tumor.

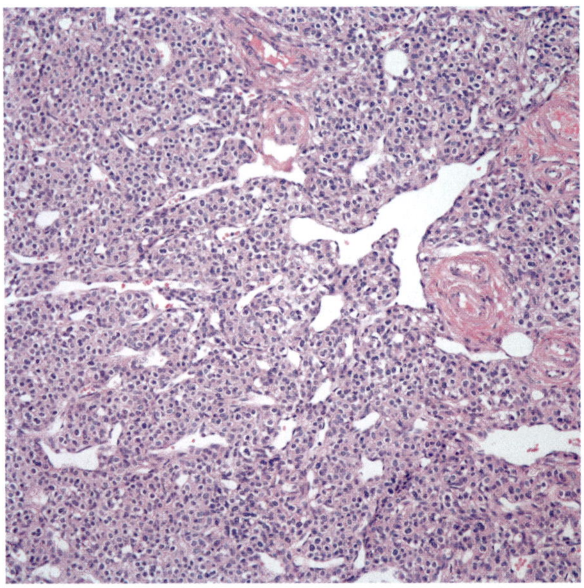

Figure 9-11 Glomus tumor with a prominent hemangiopericytic growth pattern.

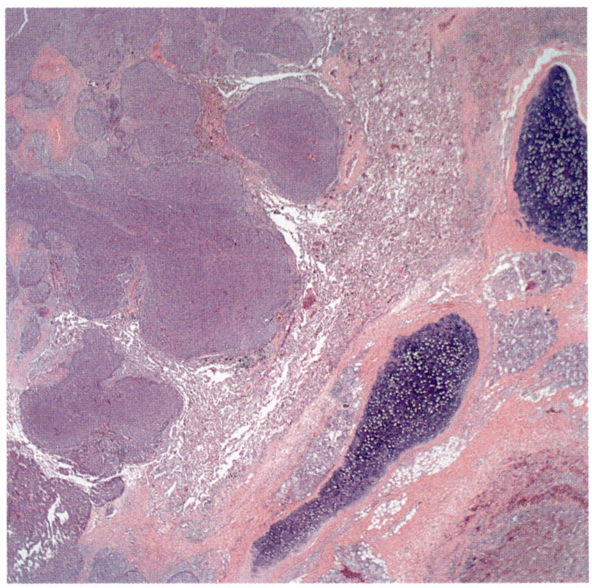

Figure 9-12 Low-power view of a pulmonary glomangiosarcoma showing a disorganized growth pattern.

neoplasms. Tumors that may have some macroscopic and histopathologic features in common include clear cell "sugar" tumor and well-differentiated neuroendocrine carcinoma (carcinoid tumor). Histologic findings in both of these entities may include dilated vascular spaces, lack of mitotic activity and necrosis, and a cellular proliferation composed of medium-sized cells with clear or lightly eosinophilic cytoplasm. The use of immunohistochemical studies, especially that showing positive staining of tumor cells for muscle-specific actin, will lead to the correct interpretation, because sugar tumors and neuroendocrine carcinomas demonstrate negative reactivity for muscle markers. Sugar tumors also may show positive staining for CD34, S-100 protein, and HMB-45, whereas neuroendocrine carcinomas will show positive staining for keratin, EMA, and neuroendocrine markers such as chromogranin or synaptophysin. In cases of glomangiosarcoma, the main issue will be the identification of more conventional areas of glomangioma and positive staining for muscle-specific actin. Leiomyosarcoma is a valid differential diagnostic possibility, however, because this tumor may have a similar immunophenotype. In this clinical scenario, the identification of more conventional areas of glomangioma is crucial to arriving at a more specific diagnosis.

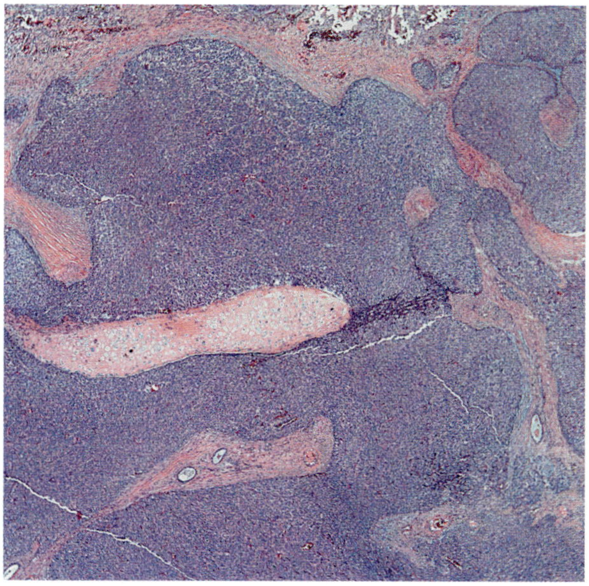

Figure 9-13 Intrapulmonary glomangiosarcoma. Lobules of tumor cells and extensive fibrocollagenous stroma can be seen.

Treatment and Prognosis

With glomangioma, complete surgical resection of the tumor is curative. Either wedge resection or lobectomy may be performed, depending on the clinical and radiologic findings. With glomangiosarcoma, surgical resection followed by chemotherapy appears to be a reasonable approach; however, because the rate of occurrence in the lung is exceedingly low, cumulative information is insufficient to determine the exact nature of these tumors. Nevertheless, it is likely that they follow an aggressive course, with widespread metastasis.

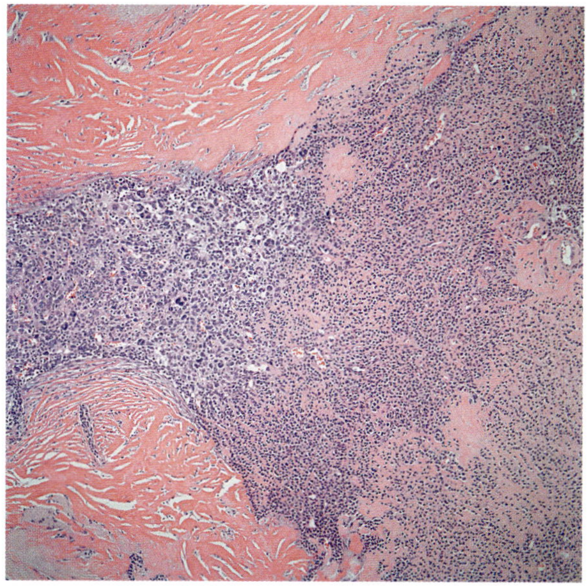

Figure 9-15 Areas of transition from glomangioma to glomangiosarcoma.

MELANOMA

Primary melanomas of the lung are rare, and the criteria for diagnosis as primary lung neoplasms are rather controversial. The lung is not an unusual site for metastatic disease from melanomas, however. In a study of 324 patients with malignant melanoma over a follow-up period of 24 months from diagnosis, Gromet and colleagues[20] found that the thorax was the initial site of relapse in 13 patients, 12 of whom were asymptomatic. The investigators concluded that the thorax is a common site for relapse, and

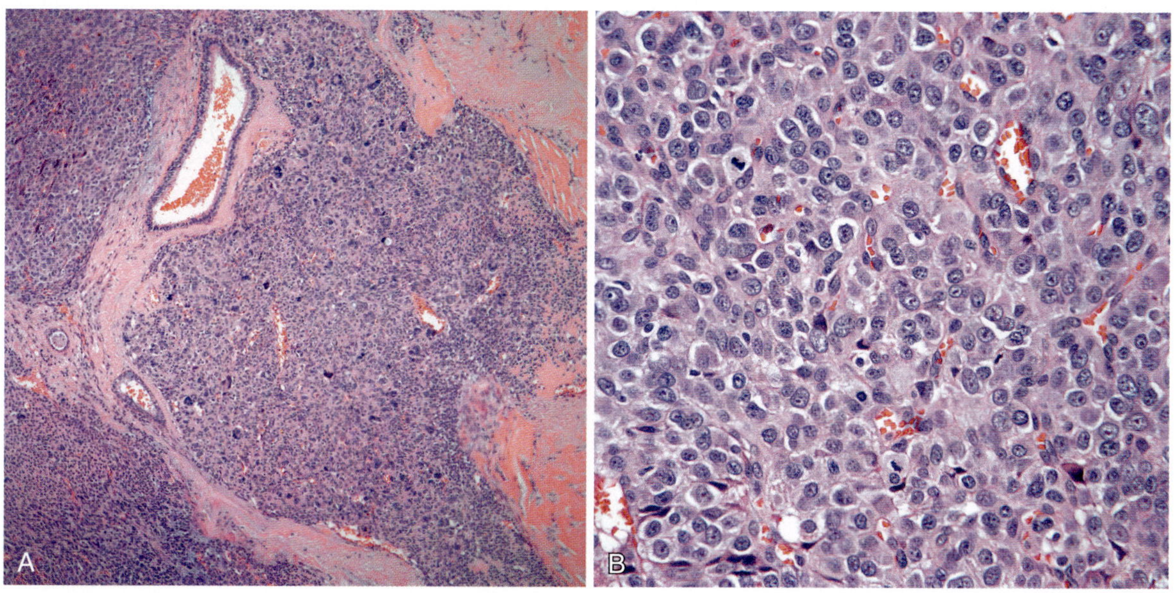

Figure 9-14 **A**, Glomangiosarcoma with prominent cellular atypia. **B**, Mitotic figures are readily identified.

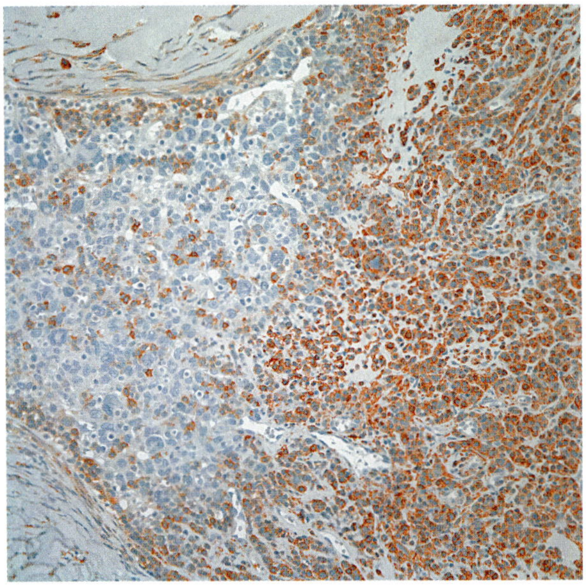

Figure 9-16 Immunohistochemical staining for smooth muscle actin produces a strong positive reaction to tumor cells in an area of transition between glomangioma and glomangiosarcoma.

that early detection of resectable metastases correlates with longer survival. Panagopoulos and Murray[21] evaluated 30 patients with metastatic melanoma of unknown primary origin and determined that 5 patients (16%) presented with lung metastases. These findings suggest that it is essential to obtain a detailed history, especially concerning previous cutaneous tumors, before any attempt at making the diagnosis of a primary pulmonary malignant melanoma.

The existence of primary melanomas of the lung is well known; however, most of the literature consists of case reports.[22–48] Some of the older reports do not present enough clinical, radiologic, or histologic information for proper definition of the entities described as primary lung tumors, whereas others cite a history of cutaneous tumor.[22–25] It is possible that the first description of primary melanoma in the lung was reported by Reid and Metha.[26] Although these investigators presented two cases, one of the tumors was a tracheal melanoma. The other, described as "bronchial melanoma," was diagnosed in a 60-year-old woman who was found at bronchoscopy to have a mass in the posterior basal bronchus. The patient had no previous history of tumor and was treated with pneumonectomy. No other malignancy was found.

Most of the historically accepted criteria for the diagnosis of primary pulmonary melanoma were originally presented by Jensen and Egedorf,[49] as follows: (1) no history of cutaneous lesion; (2) no history of ocular tumor; (3) single tumor in the lung; (4) morphology of the lung tumor compatible with primary neoplasm; (5) no spread of melanoma in other organs at the time of diagnosis; and (6) autopsy proven. Allen and Drash[28] reiterated the diagnostic criteria for melanomas in other areas and suggested that for a confident diagnosis of melanoma as a primary lung neoplasm, three additional findings should be documented: (1) junctional change with "dropping off" or "nesting" of malignant cells just beneath the bronchial epithelium; (2) invasion of the bronchial epithelium in an area in which the bronchial epithelium is not ulcerated; and (3) obvious melanoma beneath the epithelium. In numerous reports, the likelihood that the neoplasm was in fact a primary pulmonary melanoma has been diminished, because a previous cutaneous melanoma may have undergone spontaneous regression. Thus, the diagnosis of primary malignant melanoma of the lung is very difficult, if not impossible, to make convincingly.

In one of the largest series of primary lung melanomas, Wilson and Moran[50] noted that not all of the diagnostic criteria will necessarily be met in a single case. In this study, the incidence of primary malignant melanoma of the lung was assessed at 0.01% over a period of 45 years. Even though the eight cases described mirrored previous case reports to some extent, not all of the parameters were identified in each individual case. For instance, one of the strongest criteria for the diagnosis of pulmonary melanoma is the presence of in situ melanoma; however, some metastatic melanomas to the lung will display histopathologic features of in situ melanoma, despite manifesting as a single pulmonary mass.[51]

When the clinical and histologic criteria for the diagnosis of pulmonary melanoma are examined in more detail, it is apparent that some of the 1967 criteria may not necessarily apply in current practice. For instance, the use of autopsy to confirm the diagnosis is less relevant today than it may have been some years ago, because it is now possible to evaluate a patient for an occult tumor in the eye or elsewhere. It also is possible to evaluate the possibility of widespread metatatic disease at the time of diagnosis. More recently, in a study of 15 patients presenting with lung melanomas who had no history of melanoma, de Wilt and colleagues[52] analyzed the findings on which a diagnosis of metastatic or primary lung neoplasm was based. As acknowledged by the investigators, this group of patients may represent approximately 5% of those in whom the primary site is unknown. Eleven of the 15 patients presented with a single tumor, and in 7 cases, the diagnosis of primary pulmonary melanoma was very likely. These workers concluded that the distinction between primary and metastatic melanoma of the lung is best accomplished on the basis of clinical behavior (pattern of spread), rather than on histopathologic criteria. De Wilt and co-investigators,[52] like Wilson and Moran,[50] were not able to apply the entire set of criteria to any individual case. They argued that although the dilemma over primary and metastatic disease is of considerable interest, it may be irrelevant to the optimal management of these patients, and recommended that each case be evaluated on an individual basis.

Clinical Features

The clinical signs and symptoms of primary melanomas of the lung are nonspecific and are similar to those of primary lung carcinomas: cough, dyspnea, fever, chest pain, hemoptysis, and other signs of bronchial obstruction. Bronchoscopic findings may suggest melanoma if the lesion is pigmented; however, such pigmentation is not always present. The tumor does not have any predilection for a particular gender and usually is diagnosed in adult patients with a mean age of 51 years. Past or present cutaneous or ocular tumor must be excluded by history or physical and radiologic evaluations.

Macroscopic Features

The presence of a single tumor has been proposed as an important parameter for diagnosis; however, it should be kept in mind that a single tumor may also occur in metastatic disease. These tumors appear well defined, with or without obvious pigment (Fig. 9-17). The cut surface may be tan in color with a homogeneous surface, with or without areas of hemorrhage or necrosis. Tumor size may range from 1 cm to larger than 5 cm in greatest dimension, and the presentation may be one of polypoid bronchial lesions partially obstructing the lumen or as an intraparenchymal mass.

Microscopic Features

The spectrum of histopathologic features is similar to that seen in melanomas of the skin. The tumor may show in situ changes of the bronchial epithelium in many cases, but not in all (Figs. 9-18 to 9-20). These in situ changes may mimic those of carcinomas. Underneath the bronchial epithelium, the tumor may grow in an organoid, nested, diffuse, or spindle cell pattern (Figs. 9-21 to 9-26). The neoplastic cellular proliferation may be composed of medium-sized cells with moderate amounts of eosinophilic cytoplasm, round to oval nuclei, prominent nucleoli, and easily identified mitotic activity. The cellular proliferation may be composed of rather smaller cells with round nuclei and inconspicuous nucleoli, mimicking the growth pattern of a small cell carcinoma. In spindle cell melanomas, the tumor may be composed of fusiform cells with elongated nuclei and inconspicuous nucleoli. Pseudonuclear inclusion and mitotic activity can be easily identified. Areas of necrosis or hemorrhage may be observed, regardless of the growth pattern. Melanin pigment is present in a majority of cases; less commonly, however, it may appear only in focal areas.

Immunohistochemical Features

Immunohistochemical stains may be of great value in the diagnosis of pulmonary melanoma. Since these tumors

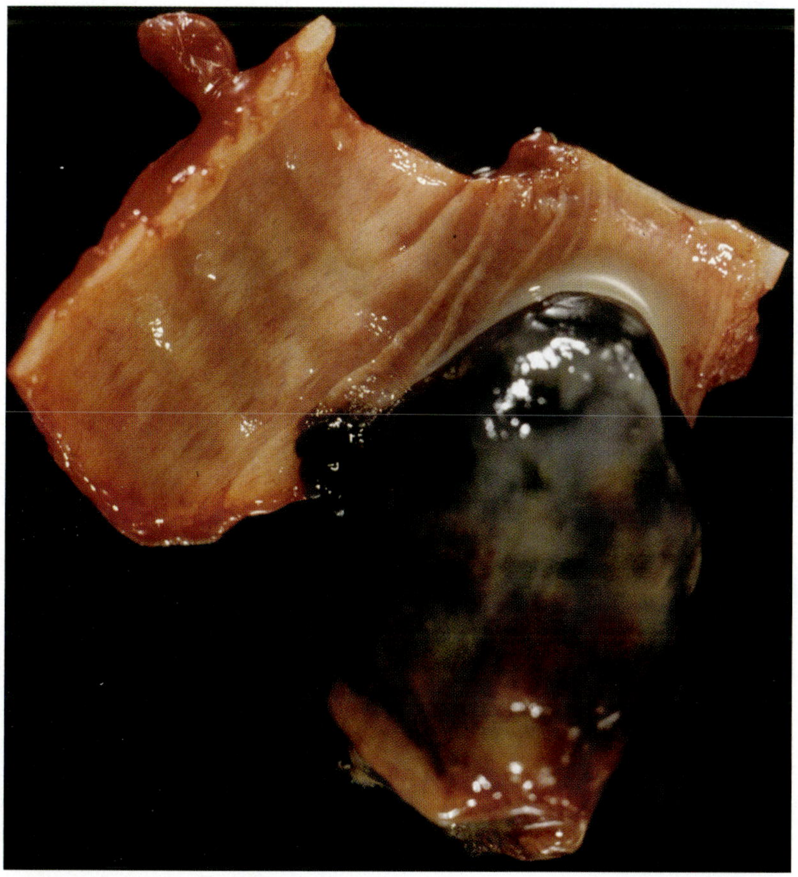

Figure 9-17 Bronchial melanoma, gross specimen. The tumor mass is the prominent pigmented lesion.

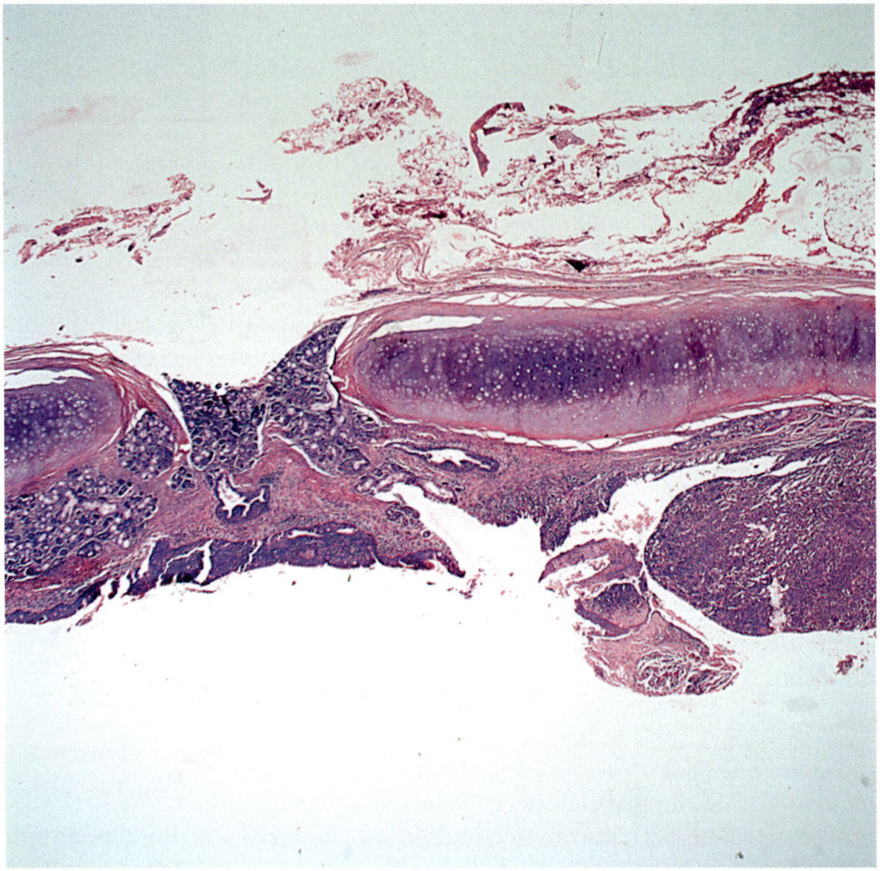

Figure 9-18 Bronchial melanoma with areas of transition between normal epithelium to in situ melanoma.

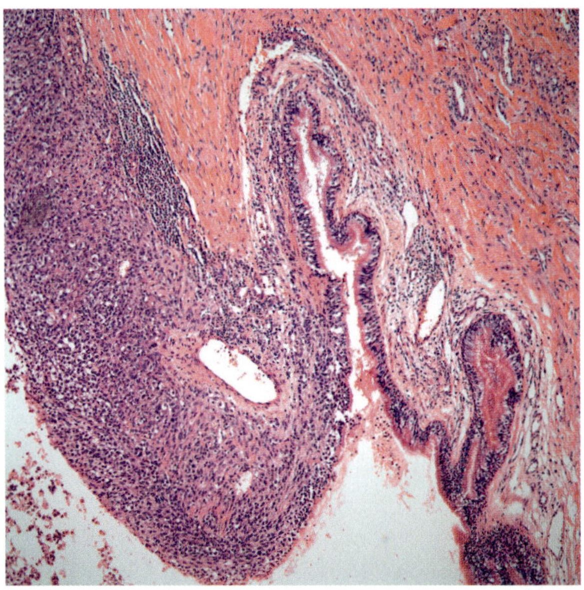

Figure 9-19 Bronchial melanoma showing areas of transition between normal epithelium and in situ changes of melanoma.

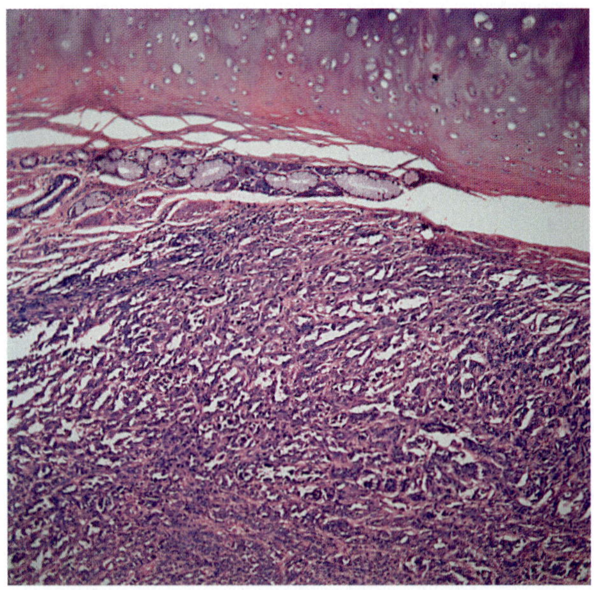

Figure 9-20 Bronchial melanoma. Full-thickness involvement of the bronchial mucosa can be seen. Note the presence of a few endobronchial glands and bronchial cartilage.

are very unusual as primary lung neoplasms, and since melanomas may also share some immonophenotypic features with lung carcinomas, it is important to perform a panel of immunohistochemical stains that may allow for a proper designation of these tumors. Melanomas react positively with S-100 protein, HMB-45, and Melan A; thus, these stains should be part of the panel. They may also be positive for carcinoembryonic antigen (CEA),[50] and some spindle cell melanomas may be negative for HMB-45.[53] Therefore, it is important to add other

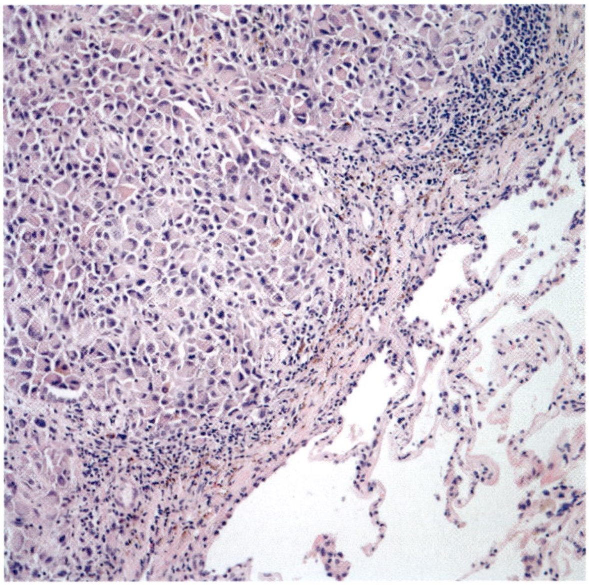

Figure 9-21 Pulmonary melanoma with prominent rhabdoid features.

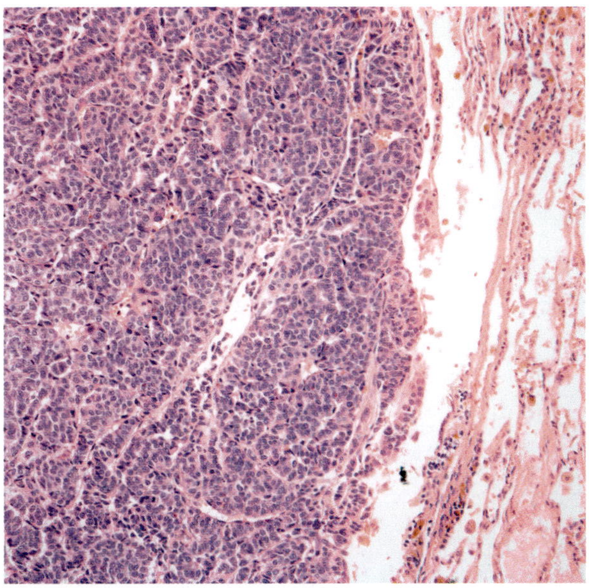

Figure 9-22 Pulmonary melanoma with a nested pattern, mimicking neuroendocrine carcinoma.

putative epithelial markers, such as keratins and EMA, to the panel.

Differential Diagnosis

Any attempt at a differential diagnosis is rather impractical because melanoma can mimic any primary tumor in the lung, including carcinomas that do not show the conventional squamous or adenocarcinomatous features. The histopathologic picture observed in some pleomorphic or sarcomatoid carcinomas of the lung is readily applicable to certain cases of melanoma. Some neuroendocrine tumors also may share histopathologic features with

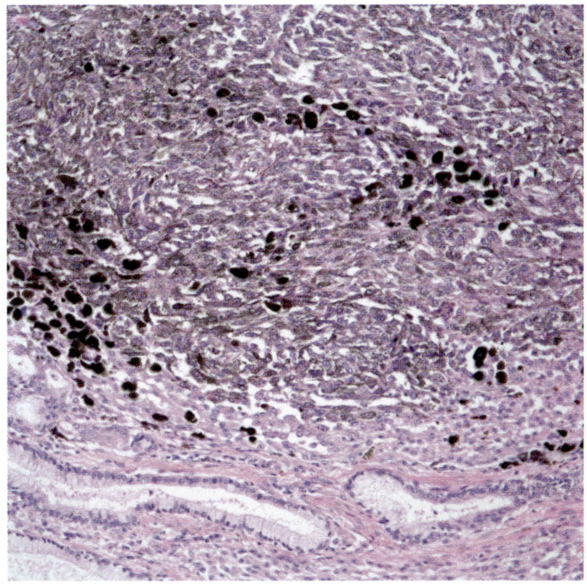

Figure 9-23 Pulmonary melanoma with prominent pigmented areas.

melanoma, including the presence of melanin pigment. Therefore, an immunohistochemical panel is essential in cases in which a nonepithelial malignancy is strongly suspected. A thorough clinical and radiologic evaluation is necessary to make the distinction between primary and metastatic disease.

Treatment and Prognosis

The treatment of choice for primary melanomas of the lung is complete surgical resection, and the prognosis is variable. Some tumors behave aggressively, whereas others exhibit a protracted course. In the series of 8 patients reported by Wilson and Moran,[50] five patients died of their disease between 4 and 32 months after initial diagnosis; two patients were alive with metastasis between 4 and 30 months after initial diagnosis; and one patient was alive without evidence of metastatic disease at 108 months after initial diagnosis. In the cases described by de Wilt and associates,[52] the 5-year survival rate was 42%, and the investigators concluded that resection in patients with pulmonary melanoma without a known primary can result in long-term survival.

MENINGIOMA

Meningiomas occur predominantly in the central nervous system; however, they also commonly occur in ectopic locations such as the scalp, orbital fossa, maxillary antrum, and frontal sinus.[54] When pulmonary meningiomas manifest in conjunction with a central nervous system tumor with otherwise "benign" histology, they have been regarded by some investigators as

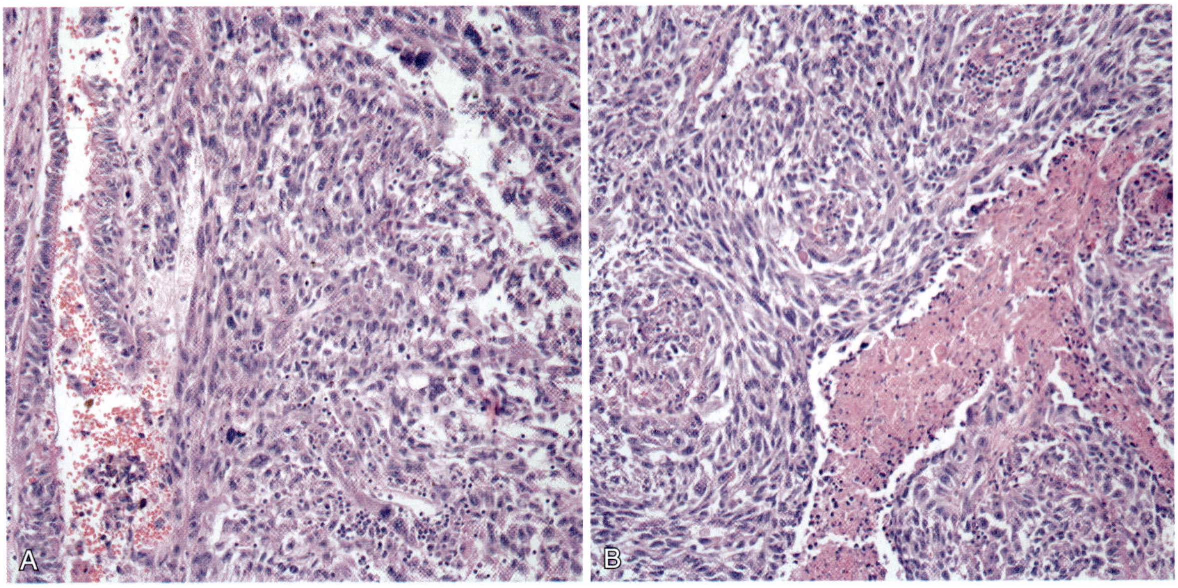

Figure 9-24 **A**, Pulmonary spindle cell melanoma. Note the remnants of respiratory epithelium. **B**, Spindle cell melanoma with focal areas of necrosis and prominent cellular atypia.

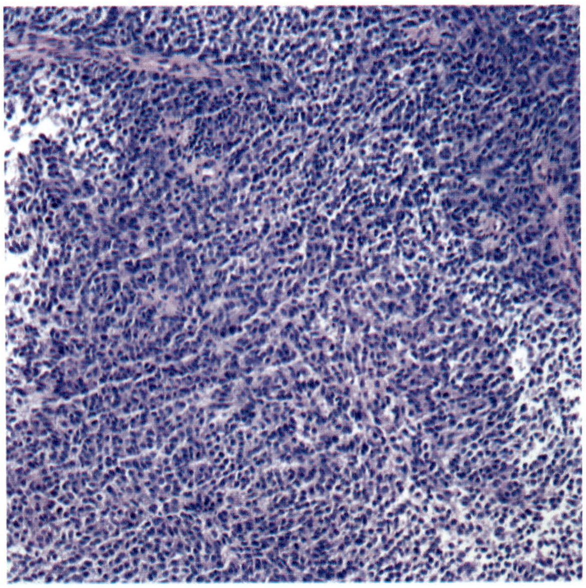

Figure 9-25 Pulmonary melanoma (so-called small cell type), mimicking a small cell carcinoma.

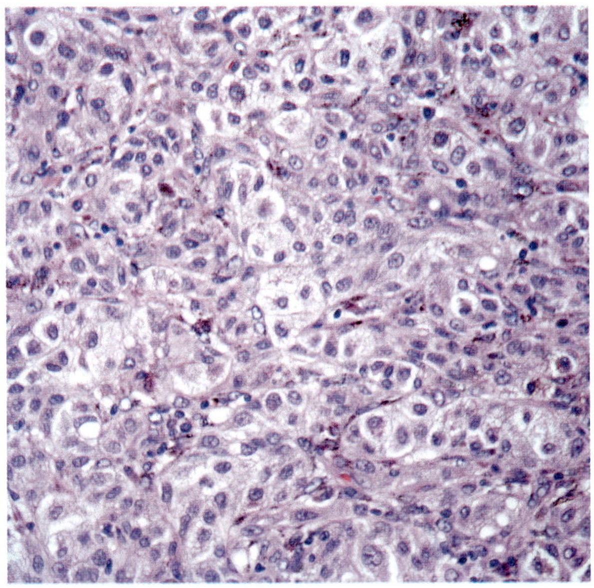

Figure 9-26 Pulmonary melanoma with clear cell features.

"benign metastasizing meningioma"[55] or as late metastasis in patients with a previous history of central nervous system tumors.[56] Metastases detected up to 19 years later have been reported in some patients.[56] In 1960, Hoye and colleagues[57] suggested a set of four diagnostic criteria for extracranial meningiomas: (1) direct extension from an intracranial tumor; (2) extracranial growth from arachnoid cell rests along cranial nerve sheaths; (3) proliferation of ectopic embryonic rests of arachnoid cells; and (4) extracranial metastases from intracranial tumors. The appearance of meningiomas in the lung may be best explained by the proliferation of ectopic embryonic rests of arachnoid cells.

The occurrence of ectopic primary pulmonary meningiomas is well documented. Because they are rare, most of the literature consists of case reports. Kemnitz and colleagues[58] are given credit for the first description of a primary pulmonary meningioma, in a 59-year-old woman. Since then, numerous case reports describing similar findings have been presented.[59-69] Based on these cases, patients tend to be adults and are predominantly female. A majority of tumors were discovered incidentally during routine physical examination. Related symptoms were recorded in only a few cases. In the only large series published, the study authors reported 10 cases of primary pulmonary meningioma.[70] Their findings are similar to those from previous reported cases. The patients were adults between the ages of 30 and 72 years (mean, 51 years), and their tumors were discovered incidentally. Only one patient in this series had symptoms (cough) related to the intrapulmonary tumor. The female predominance previously reported was not apparent in this study. Although the investigators[70] argued that the occurrence of intrapulmonary meningiomas remains speculative, they acknowledged that meningothelial-like nodules arising in the lung were a possible and more logical origin for pulmonary meningiomas. Associated meningothelial-like nodules were not found in any of the 10 cases of pulmonary meningioma in this series; however, in some more recent cases this association has been reported.[71,72] An explanation still needs to be provided for the origin of the meningothelial-like nodules themselves, however, indicating that the theory concerning ectopic embryonic rests may have some merit. Although the great majority of intrapulmonary meningiomas are benign, malignant intrapulmonary meningiomas have been reported.[73,74]

The diagnosis of malignancy can be problematic. Prayson and Farver[73] assigned a malignant classification to one case on the basis of histologic features, including nuclear pleomorphism and increased mitotic activity (15 mitotic figures per 10 high-power fields). In a case described by van der Meij,[74] however, it appears that the authors designated the tumor as malignant based on invasiveness (tumor invaded pleura, esophagus, intrapulmonary vessels, hilar lymph nodes, and peribronchial fat) and destruction of bronchial cartilage, rather than the histologic features of the meningioma, which showed 0 to 1 mitotic figures per square millimeter. Both features should be taken into account in order to accurately predict behavior.

Macroscopic Features

Pulmonary meningiomas are well-circumscribed tumors and often are found in a subpleural location. They are solid and whitish in color with a homogeneous-appearing cut surface (Fig. 9-27). Areas of necrosis and hemorrhage are not common, except in cases in which malignant features are present. Tumor size ranges from 1 cm to larger than 5 cm; in a majority of cases, however, average sizes range between 3 and 4 cm.

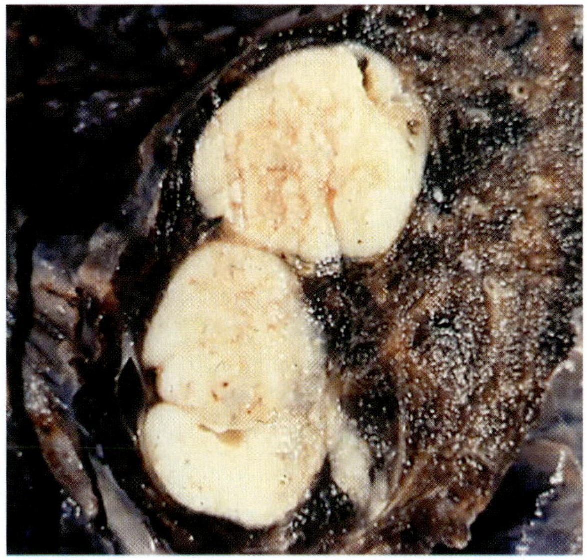

Figure 9-27 Pulmonary meningioma, gross specimen. The tumor mass is well circumscribed but not encapsulated. The cut surface has a homogeneous appearance.

Histologic Features

Intrapulmonary meningiomas display features similar to those in the central nervous system (Figs. 9-28 to 9-37). Transitional meningiomas are well circumscribed, but not encapsulated, and are surrounded by normal lung parenchyma. The cellular proliferation is composed of plump, slightly spindle-shaped cells arranged in lobules or whorls and interspersed with collagenized vascular structures. At high magnification, the cells have indistinct borders, pale eosinophilic cytoplasm, round to oval nuclei, and inconspicuous nucleoli. Psammoma bodies may be present toward the periphery of the tumor, but they may be completely absent in some cases. Areas resembling microcystic meningioma or clusters of xanthoma cells may be seen focally. Cellular atypia, if present, may be only focal, and mitotic activity is absent. Fibrous meningiomas are characterized by a spindle cell proliferation composed of fusiform cells with indistinct cell borders, pale eosinophilic cytoplasm, elongated nucleus, and inconspicuous nucleoli. More conventional areas of transitional meningiomas may be present in the periphery of these tumors. Mitotic activity is absent, as it is in transitional meningiomas. More recently, Rowsell and colleagues[75] described an intrapulmonary meningioma characterized by cords and fascicles of spindle cells, and epithelioid cells surrounded by abundant mucoid stroma. The investigators diagnosed this case as chordoid meningioma. In one case described as malignant meningioma, the tumor displayed more cytological atypia and increased mitotic activity,[73] whereas another showed an infiltrative growth pattern without increased mitotic activity.

Immunohistochemical Features

The two immunohistochemical stains that will aid in the diagnosis of meningiomas most consistently are vimentin and EMA. Some other stains that have been reported to give as weakly or focally positive reaction in intrapulmonary meningiomas include CD34, S-100 protein, keratin, and progesterone receptor. However, in all cases in which such staining has been reported to be positive, staining for vimentin and EMA also has been positive. Therefore,

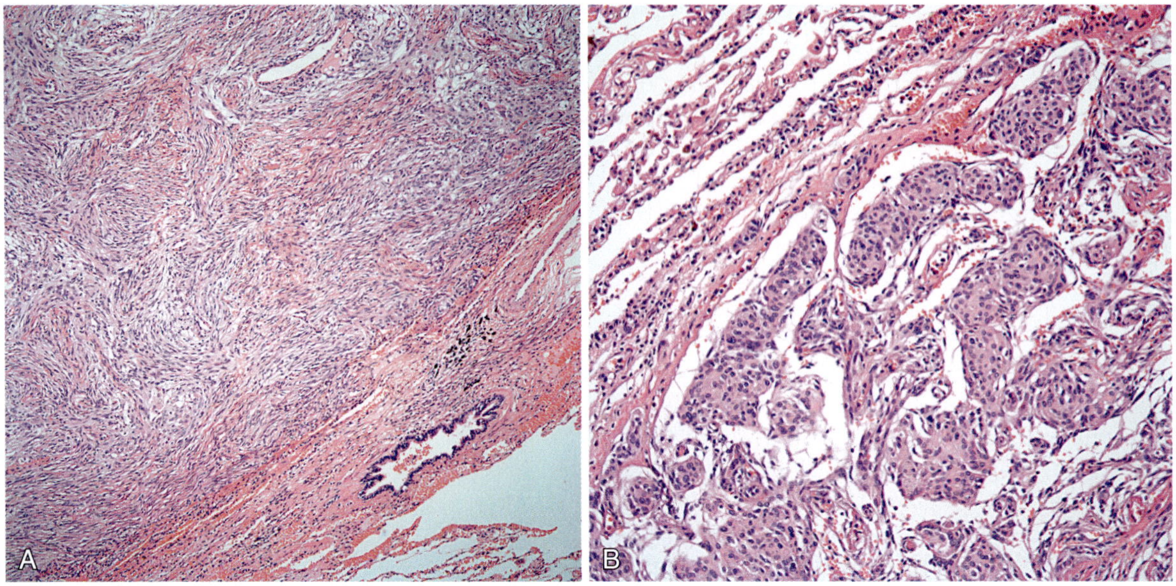

Figure 9-28 **A**, Intrapulmonary fibrous meningioma. **B**, Intrapulmonary transitional meningioma. Both tumors are well circumscribed but not encapsulated.

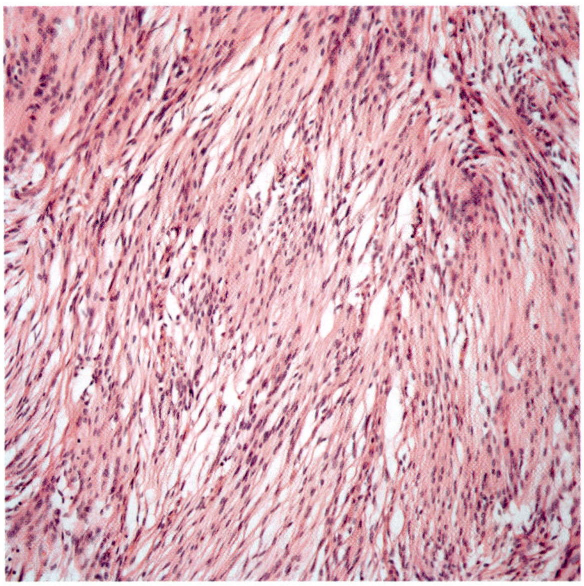

Figure 9-29 Fibrous meningioma with prominent spindle cell proliferation, mimicking a fibroblastic tumor.

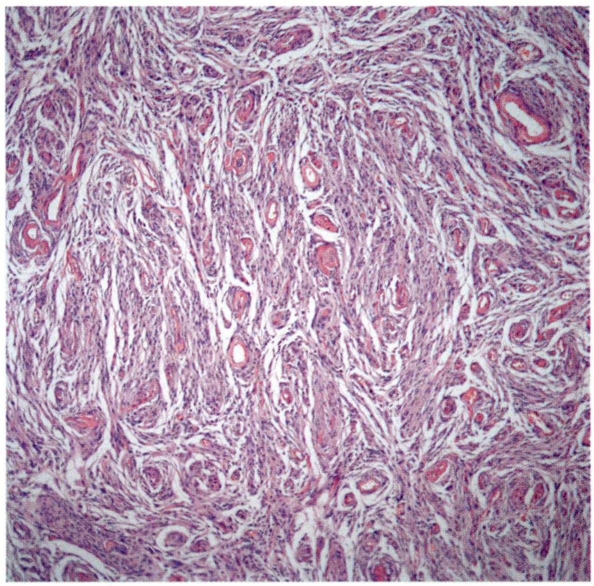

Figure 9-30 Fibrous meningioma with prominent ectatic vessels interspersed with the spindle cell proliferation.

careful evaluation of the histopathologic features of the tumor and the respective immunohistochemical profile is essential.

Differential Diagnosis

The most important consideration in the differential diagnosis is metastasis from a cranial meningioma. Once this possibility has been ruled out, a few other specific clinical entities may warrant consideration as indicated by the histopathologic features of the meningioma. Intrapulmonary spindle cell thymoma may rarely manifest as an intrapulmonary tumor. In this setting, the presence of psammoma bodies and whorling of cells would be unusual features for thymoma. Thymomas also would have a strong positive reaction on staining for keratin and either weak or negative staining for EMA. In cases of fibrous meningioma, inflammatory pseudotumor also may enter into the differential diagnosis. The absence of plasma cells or a more meaningful inflammatory component would be an unusual finding for inflammatory pseudotumor. Intrapulmonary fibrous tumor also may be considered; however, solitary fibrous tumors will display more characteristic histopathologic features and are likely

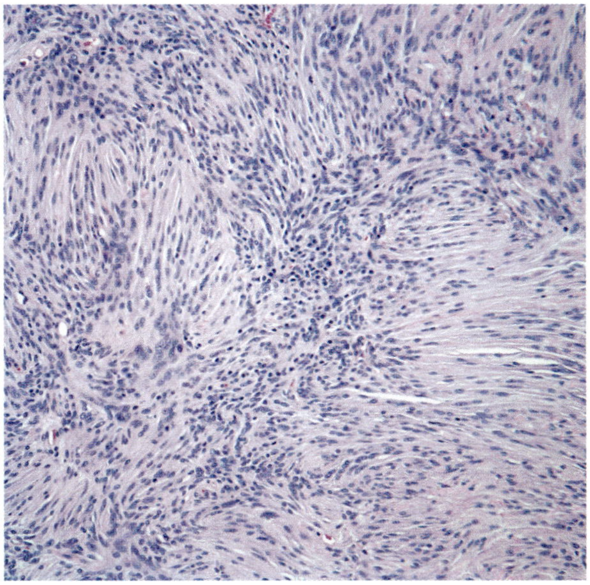

Figure 9-31 Intrapulmonary fibrous meningioma with prominent spindle cell proliferation, showing neural features.

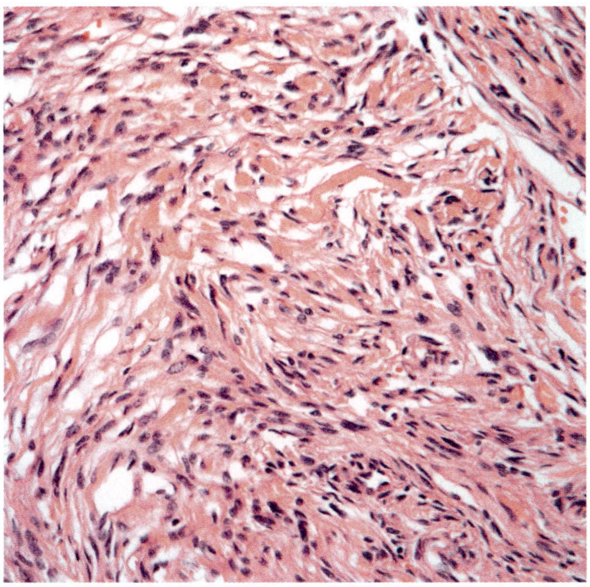

Figure 9-32 Fibrous meningioma with features mimicking those of an intrapulmonary solitary fibrous tumor.

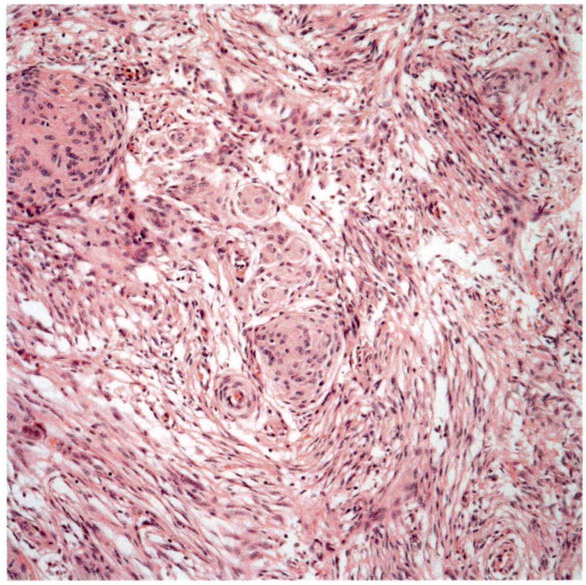

Figure 9-33 Fibrous meningioma with focal areas of transitional meningioma.

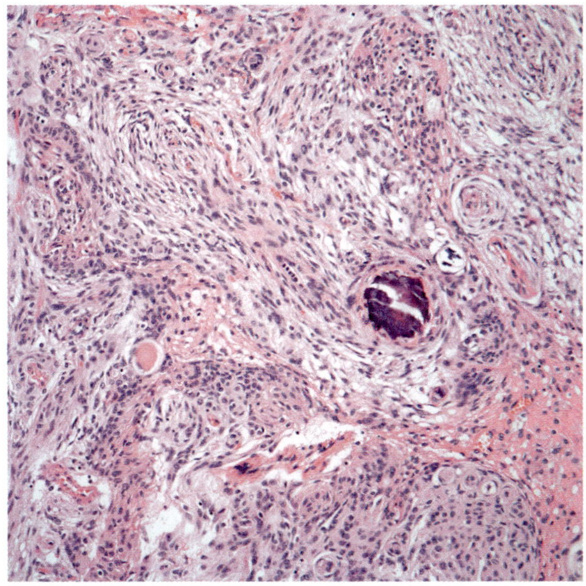

Figure 9-34 Intrapulmonary meningioma with fibrous and transitional areas and focal calcification.

to demonstrate positive staining for CD34 and negative staining for EMA.

Treatment and Prognosis

The treatment of choice for intrapulmonary meningioma is complete surgical resection. In a majority of cases, the tumor has manifested indolent clinical behavior. The available data are too limited to permit determination of the optimal treatment for cases that follow a more aggressive course, or for cases that are deemed malignant from the beginning.

MENINGOTHELIAL-LIKE NODULES AND DIFFUSE PULMONARY MENINGOTHELIOMATOSIS

These small tumor nodules have been reported in the lung for more than 50 years; however, they previously were believed to be chemodectomas.[76–83] Although the designation of "chemodectomas of the lung" was essentially reserved for lesions found incidentally in autopsy material, in several reports, the patients presented with "coin

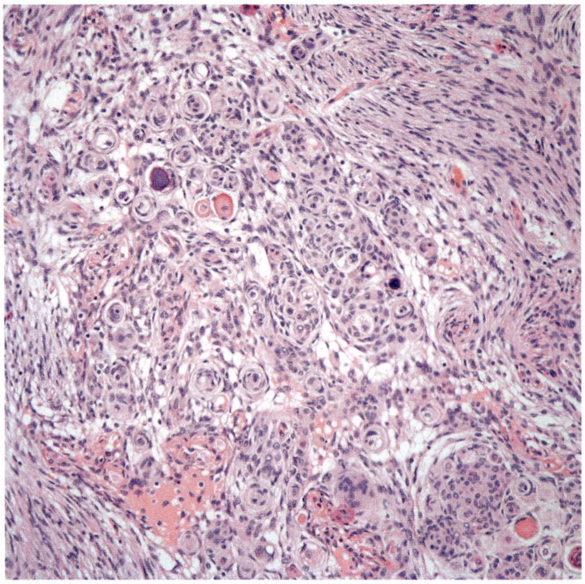

Figure 9-35 Intrapulmonary meningioma with predominant transitional features.

lesions" that were ultimately diagnosed as chemodectomas. Some investigators considered that these lesions were induced by pulmonary thromboemboli,[84,85] whereas others studying similar tumors in the head and neck theorized that they were caused by prolonged and severe hypoxia.[86] These chemodectomas were diagnosed on autopsy, however, and their discovery was incidental and unrelated to the main pathology for which the lungs were evaluated. Although a majority of cases featured single nodules, there are several others in which numerous nodules were reported in the lung parenchyma. Zak and Chabes[87] reported three autopsy cases in which multiple lung lesions were present, which the authors classified as "pulmonary chemodectomatosis." No detailed description as to the number and distribution of these nodules was provided.

In 1975, Kuhn and Askin[88] evaluated several tumors from one patient under electron microscopy. Histologically, the tumors were similar to minute chemodectomas of lung. The authors concluded that these lesions had little resemblance to paragangliomas, and were more similar to meningiomas. Churg and Warnock recorded similar findings[89] in a study of 26 cases using electron microscopy. These workers concluded that these so-called minute chemodectomas are not related to paragangliomas, and their findings suggested that meningeal arachnoid cells might be present. More recently, Gaffey and associates[90] studied 23 of these tumors using electron microscopy and immunohistochemistry, and concluded that a more accurate term for these lesions would be "meningothelial-like nodule." The investigators found that these lesions are more common in women, and that the majority are discovered during autopsy. The occur-

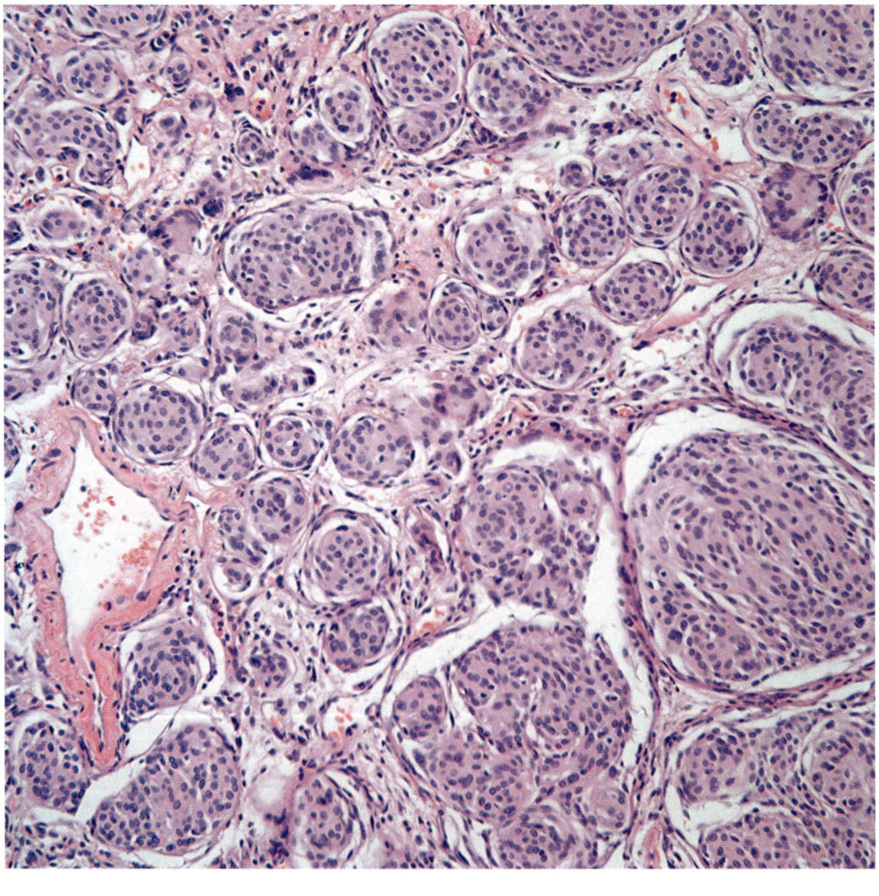

Figure 9-36 Intrapulmonary meningioma with "whorling."

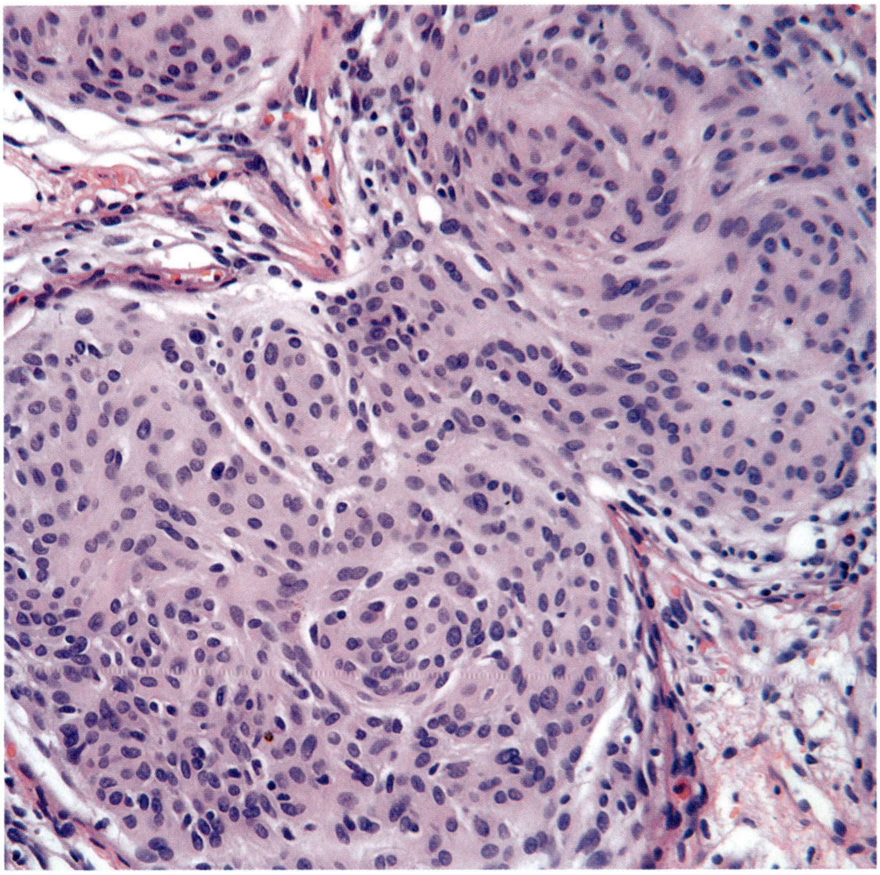

Figure 9-37 High-power view of an intrapulmonary meningioma showing lack of nuclear atypia or mitotic activity.

rence was estimated at approximately 1 in every 60 autopsies. No particular association to any specific disease was determined. The tumor nodules varied in size from 1 to 3 mm, and were found in pleural or parenchymal locations. These clinical findings, especially the wide spectrum of patient ages (range, 12 to 91 years) and predominance in females, mirror those reported previously in the literature.

Recently, a new entity termed *pulmonary meningotheliomatosis* has been described.[91] The reported series consisted of five patients who presented with bilateral diffuse pulmonary involvement. Female patients predominated (four women and one man), and the age range was 54 to 75 years. Some patients presented with dyspnea and shortness of breath, leading to open lung biopsy for diagnosis. In three of the patients, a history of previous malignancy was noted, and follow-up for possible metastatic disease was ongoing. The lesions matched the description of those reported as meningothelial-like nodules, except that the patients were symptomatic, had bilateral lung disease with clinical evidence of restrictive lung disease, and displayed evidence of diffuse reticulonodular pulmonary infiltrates on radiologic examination. Other cases involving multiple pulmonary nodules similar to meningothelial-like nodules have been reported, however. Ionescu and associates[92] published a series of 35 cases in which they documented the existence of multiple bilateral nodules in 3 of the patients. Kukoki and Sellawi[93,94] also have documented cases in which imaging revealed multiple bilateral pulmonary nodules.

Histopathologic Features

The low-power view shows small aggregates or interstitial nodules distributed in a subpleural or parenchymal location. These nodules range in size from 1 to 3 mm in greatest dimension. The high-power view reveals a proliferation of oval to spindle cells with moderate amounts of eosinophilic cytoplasm, indistinct cell borders, and oval nuclei with finely dispersed chromatin and inconspicuous nucleoli. In some areas, a "whorling" arrangement of tumor cells may be apparent, whereas in others the cells may show pseudonuclear inclusions. The nodules do not show evidence of mitotic activity, prominent cellular atypia, necrosis, or hemorrhage (Fig. 9-38); however, many may be located near ectatic blood vessels. Adjacent lung parenchyma may show areas of hemosiderin-laden macrophages or may demonstrate a histologic picture that is completely within normal limits. Either single or multiple nodules may be seen within the lung parenchyma.

In meningotheliomatosis, these nodules are more obvious, and depending on the number of sections available for study, it may be possible to identify multiple nodules distributed along the lung parenchyma (Fig. 9-39).

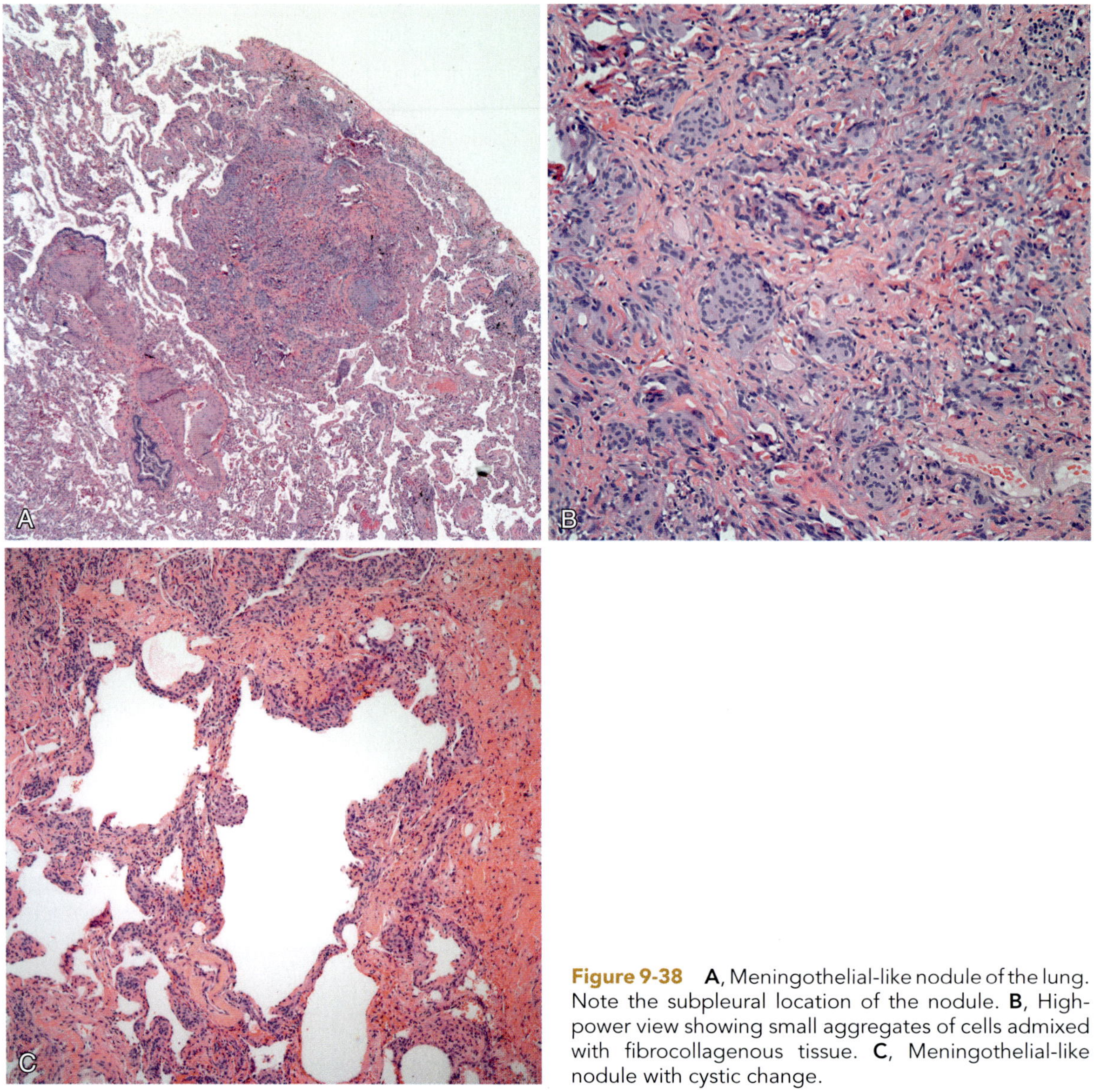

Figure 9-38 **A**, Meningothelial-like nodule of the lung. Note the subpleural location of the nodule. **B**, High-power view showing small aggregates of cells admixed with fibrocollagenous tissue. **C**, Meningothelial-like nodule with cystic change.

Immunohistochemical and Molecular Biology Features

The immunohistochemical findings in meningothelial-like nodules and meningotheliomatosis are similar to those described for pulmonary meningiomas. The nodules are most consistently positive for vimentin and EMA. Tumor cells are negative for keratins, muscle-specific actin, smooth muscle actin, chromogranin, synaptophysin, and CD34.

At the molecular level, Niho and coworkers[95] demonstrated monoclonal expansion by the X-chromosome–linked human androgen receptor gene assay (HUMARA) in 7 of the 11 cases studied and concluded that meningothelial-like nodules may be reactive proliferations. Ionescu and associates[92] published a comparative study of intracranial meningiomas and pulmonary meningothelial-like nodules in which mutational analysis was used to demonstrate loss-of-heterozygosity alterations at different chromosomal loci in both lesions. The investigators concluded that these conditions are unrelated, and that the lung lesions may represent a reactive process.

Differential Diagnosis

On histopathologic examination, meningothelial nodules may be confused with carcinoid tumorlets. The histologic features of carcinoid tumorlets are similar to those of neuroendocrine tumors, however; their main feature is an organoid, nested pattern, in which the cells react with epithelial markers such as keratins, and also with neuroendocrine markers such as chromogranin and synaptophysin. Metastatic disease, most likely from a neuroendocrine tumor such as paraganglioma,

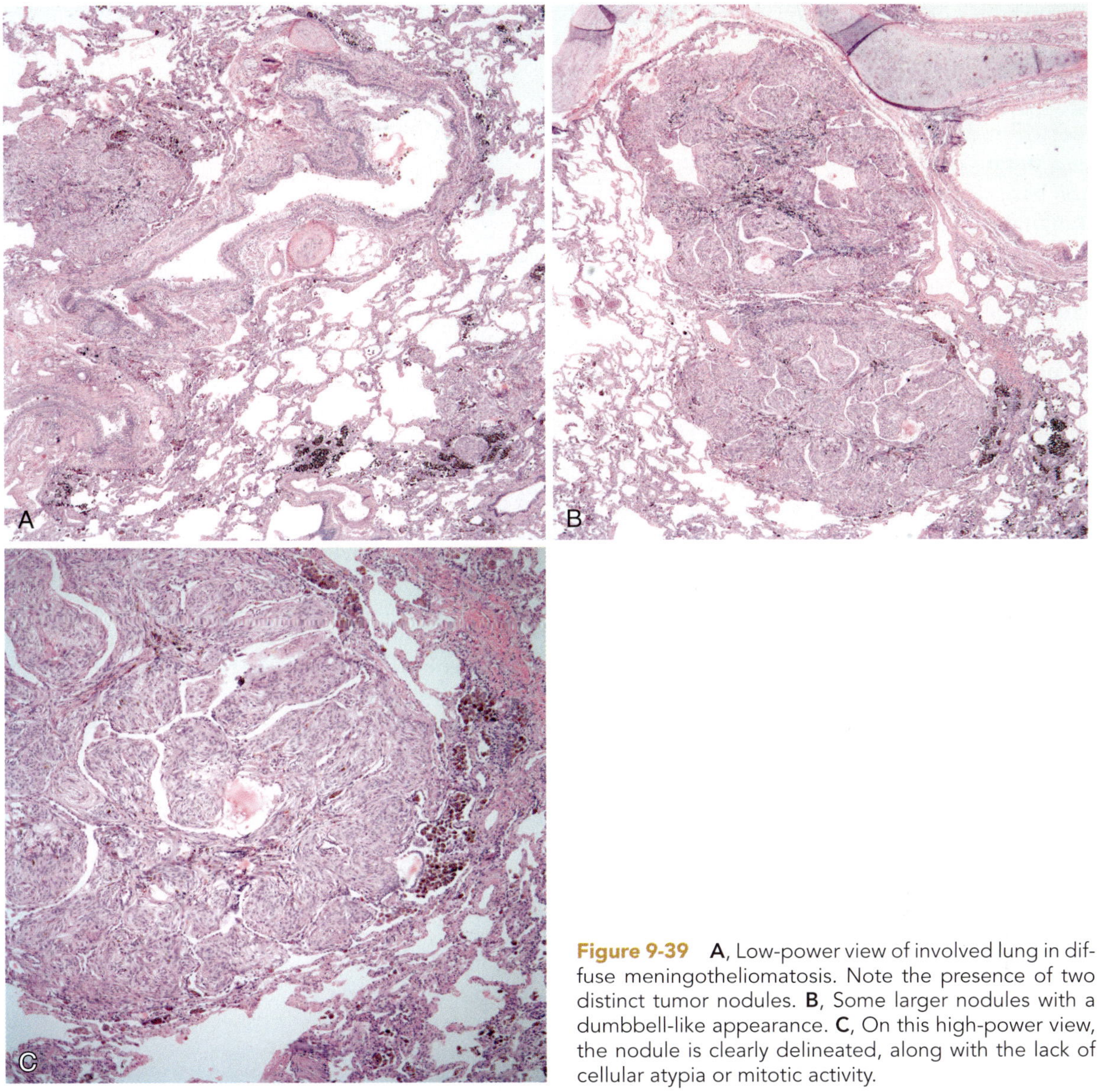

Figure 9-39 **A**, Low-power view of involved lung in diffuse meningotheliomatosis. Note the presence of two distinct tumor nodules. **B**, Some larger nodules with a dumbbell-like appearance. **C**, On this high-power view, the nodule is clearly delineated, along with the lack of cellular atypia or mitotic activity.

is another possibility in the differential diagnosis. The use of appropriate immunohistochemical studies using epithelial and neuroendocrine markers will lead to the correct interpretation.

Treatment and Prognosis

These tumors are benign, and complete surgical resection is curative. In approximately 65% of the reported cases, the diagnosis is based on findings in autopsy material, whereas in the remaining 35%, it derives from analysis of surgical resected material unrelated to these lesions. As new modalities and techniques in diagnostic imaging emerge, however, it is very likely that sampling of these tumor nodules may become a routine part of diagnostic surgical pathology practice.

TERATOMA

Intrapulmonary germ cell tumors are exceedingly rare. Germ cell tumors occur more often along the midline and in the thorax, and they are far more common in the anterior mediastinum. Of the tumors within this family, teratomas are most likely to occur in an intrapulmonary location; nevertheless, caution is warranted in making a definitive diagnosis of primary intrapulmonary teratoma. Germ cell tumors of testicular or ovarian origin may metastasize to the lung, as either malignant tumors or mature teratomatous lesions,[96] making the distinction between primary and metastatic neoplasms difficult. It also is important to rule out the possibility of an anterior mediastinal teratoma with extension into the lung parenchyma, because in some rare cases, the teratomatous lesion may exhibit both intrapulmonary and mediastinal involvement.[97]

Intrapulmonary teratomas have been described in the literature only in case reports.[98–113] No series of cases has been reported to date; thus, the exact incidence as a primary lung tumor is difficult to assess. Intrapulmonary teratomas have been described in both children and adults, ranging in age from 3 or 4 months to 60 years and beyond. The clinical presentation also is varied and includes signs and symptoms that are common to other pulmonary neoplasms, such as cough, hemoptysis, chest pain, fever, dyspnea, pneumonia, weight loss, and vomiting. One of the most pathognomonic signs of intrapulmonary teratoma is trichoptysis (expectoration of hair); however, this sign is present in less than 20% of the cases. A small number of patients may be asymptomatic on presentation. Although intrapulmonary teratomas are more common in females, they have been described in almost as many male patients.

Macroscopic Features

Intrapulmonary teratomas may occur as intraparenchymal or endobronchial tumors.[114–116] In many cases, the diagnosis becomes evident when hair is found during a bronchoscopic examination. Most often, the diagnosis of teratoma is confirmed by gross examination of the tumor. Intrapulmonary teratomas are cystic (Fig. 9-40) with focal solid areas; in a minority of cases, the tumor may appear predominantly solid. The size of the tumor varies and can reach more than 10 cm in greatest dimension. The cut surface may disclose the presence of hair, cartilage, teeth, and sebaceous material.

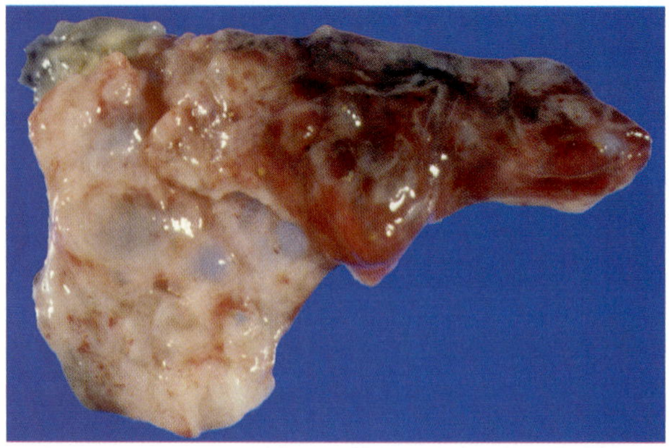

Figure 9-40 Intrapulmonary teratoma, gross specimen, with a cystic appearance.

Histopathologic Features

Intrapulmonary teratomas share the same diagnostic criteria as for gonadal teratomas, the most important being the presence of tissue from the three germinal layers. Like their counterparts in the gonads, intrapulmonary teratomas may consist of a wide variety of tissues. A majority of the cases reported have been of the mature type, variously containing appendage tissue, squamous epithelium, mature glial tissue, cartilage, bone, pancreatic tissue, or enteric epithelium (Figs. 9-41 and 9-42). In several cases, thymic tissue has also been present.

Malignant teratomas of the lung have been described in the literature[117–121] (Fig. 9-43). In some of these cases, only an undifferentiated malignant component has been reported, whereas in others, the malignant component has come from another germ cell tumor, such as a yolk sac

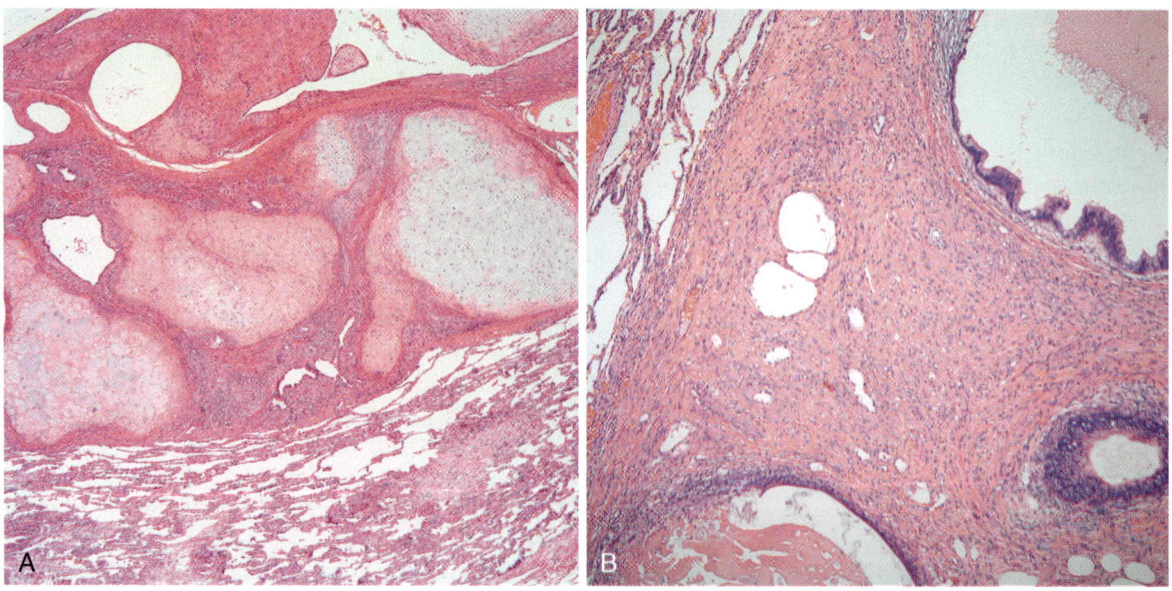

Figure 9-41 Intrapulmonary teratoma. **A**, Low-power view reveals a prominent cartilaginous component. **B**, This low-power view shows cystic changes, smooth muscle component, and a cyst lined by columnar epithelium.

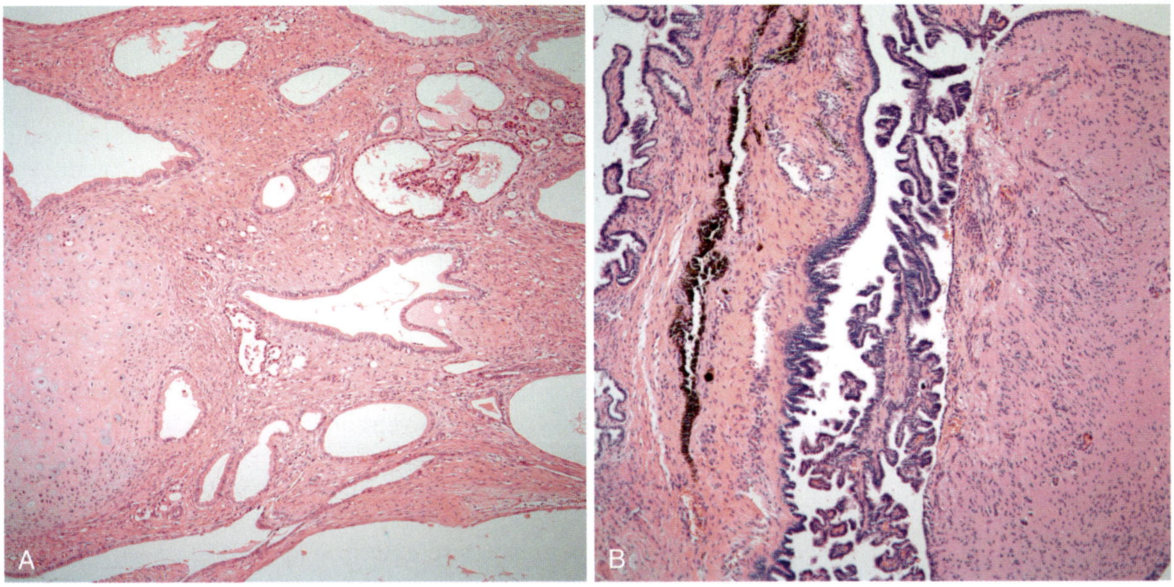

Figure 9-42 **A**, Intrapulmonary teratoma with mature elements composed of cartilage and benign glands. **B**, Mature elements composed of glial tissue and pigmented epithelium resembling ciliary body are better seen in this higher-power view.

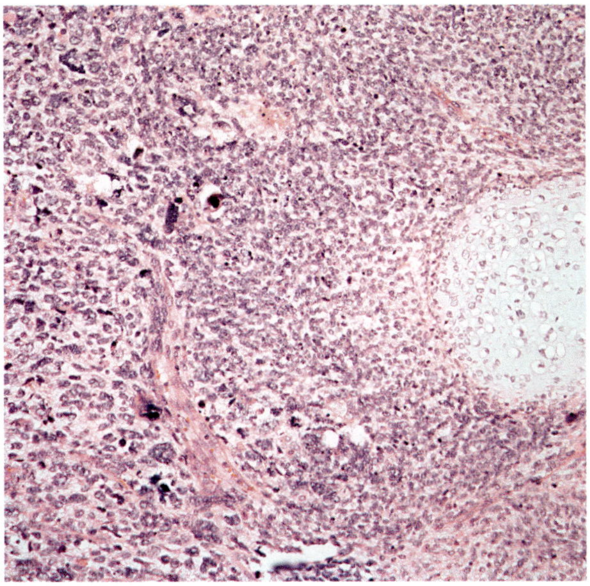

Figure 9-43 Intrapulmonary teratoma with a malignant sarcomatous component. Note adjacent mature cartilage.

tumor. A sarcomatous component in the form of malignant cartilage and an undifferentiated sarcomatous component have also been described. In a case described by Stair and associates[121] as teratocarcinoma, the tumor was composed of areas of adenocarcinoma with cartilage, as well as areas of spindle cell proliferation. These findings in an intrapulmonary neoplasm may indicate pulmonary carcinosarcoma or the so-called ex pleomorphic adenoma.

Differential Diagnosis

The diagnosis of teratoma is rather straightforward. With small biopsy specimens, however, numerous and diverse conditions may enter into the differential diagnosis, and a definitive diagnosis may be impossible to establish. Specific considerations in the differential diagnosis will be directly related to the sample of tissue obtained.

Immunohistochemical Features

The use of immunohistochemical stains in the diagnosis of teratomas will be limited to the identification of the specific tissues that make up the tumor. Neural markers such as S-100 protein, muscle markers such as desmin and actin, and vascular markers such as factor VIII, CD34, and CD31 may be of help in the identification of particular components. Otherwise, the diagnosis of intrapulmonary teratoma does not require immunohistochemical studies.

Treatment and Prognosis

Complete surgical resection by lobectomy or pneumonectomy is the treatment of choice and is curative for mature teratomas. Adjuvant therapy may be appropriate in selected patients. The behavior of teratoma with a malignant component may be aggressive, especially when a malignant mesenchymal component is present. Despite well-designed therapy, recurrences, metastatic disease, and fatal outcome all have been documented with malignant teratoma.

THYMOMA

Thymomas are more commonly found in the anterior mediastinum. The occurrence of thymomas outside of the mediastinal structures is well documented, however, and they have manifested as primary tumors in the neck and trachea and within the thyroid gland.[122–124] In the thoracic area, thymomas have been described as primary tumors in the pleura[125] and in the lung.[126–140] Before a definitive diagnosis of primary ectopic thymoma can be established, the presence of thymoma in the mediastinal compartment must be ruled out. Thymomas may become infiltrative tumors, spreading outside the mediastinal compartment into the pleura or lung, or outside of the thoracic cavity. Although capsular integrity is the most important assessment parameter used in guiding the management of mediastinal thymomas, it is irrelevant with tumors occurring in an intrapulmonary location. Histologic subtype also becomes irrelevant with intrapulmonary thymomas. Distinguishing thymoma from thymic carcinoma is important, however, because thymic carcinoma is a separate clinicopathologic entity that exhibits more aggressive behavior.

Different theories have been presented to account for the occurrence of intrapulmonary thymomas, but none of them provides a completely adequate explanation. Disturbance in the embryologic development of the thymus may be a factor, but this theory is more likely to explain the presence of ectopic thymic tissue in the neck, rather than in the lung. Thus, the occurrence of thymomas in an intrapulmonary location remains speculative.

Clinical Features

Intrapulmonary thymomas have been described in various age groups, comprising patients from teenagers to persons older than 70 years. A slight predilection for in females has been noted, but these tumors have been described in men and women in almost equal proportions. Patients may be completely asymptomatic or may present with a wide variety of clinical signs and symptoms including chest pain, fatigue, hemoptysis, dyspnea, dysphagia, dysarthria, nephrotic syndrome, cough, fever, and chills. Other reported manifestations include hyperhomocysteinemia and, more rarely, myasthenia gravis.

Macroscopic Features

Intrapulmonary thymomas occur in two different forms: hilar tumors and intrapulmonary peripheral tumors. Tumor size may range from 1 cm to more than 10 cm in greatest dimension. The tumors are seen to be well circumscribed and white to tan in color, with or without focal areas of hemorrhage or necrosis, and are of firm consistency. In unusual cases, additional tumor lesions may be visible in the pulmonary parenchyma.

Histopathologic Features

The histopathologic features of intrapulmonary thymomas are the same as those described for mediastinal thymomas. The tumor may show a biphasic cellular proliferation composed of lymphocytes and epithelial cells in differing proportions (Fig. 9-44). In some cases, either of these components may be predominant. The tumor may show the characteristic fibrous bands separating the cellular proliferation into differently sized islands of tumor cells. The epithelial cellular proliferation is composed of medium-sized cells with round to oval nuclei and small or inconspicuous nucleoli. Minimal mitotic activity may be seen in the epithelial component, and mitotic figures are visible in the lymphocytic component. The cellular proliferation of spindle cell thymoma is composed of fusiform cells with indistinct cell borders, elongated nuclei, and inconspicuous nucleoli (Fig. 9-45). The cells may be arranged in a subtle storiform pattern, with numerous, readily identifiable ectatic vessels. Mitotic figures and nuclear atypia are absent, and there are scattered lymphocytes.

Immunohistochemical Features

Although the diagnosis of thymoma is rather straightforward, immunohistochemical studies may be of help. Thymomas show positive staining for keratin, and when a lymphocytic component is present, the lymphocytes also may show positive staining for leukocyte common antigen (LCA) and T and B cell markers such as L-26 and terminal deoxynucleotidyl transferase (TdT). Although thymomas are epithelial tumors, staining for EMA may be only weakly positive and, in many cases, it is negative. Other markers for which thymomas may show positive staining include keratin 5/6, calretinin, CD5, and CD117.

Differential Diagnosis

Because of the prominent lymphocytic component and proliferation of T cells, lymphoblastic lymphoma is an important consideration in the differential diagnosis. The positive staining of markers for T cells (TdT) also may obscure the diagnosis of thymoma. In this setting, the use of epithelial markers, namely keratin, may be of great help in properly classifying the tumor as a thymoma. When epithelial cells predominate, the main consideration in the differential diagnosis is non–small cell carcinoma. The absence of marked nuclear atypia and mitotic activity, coupled with the presence of lobulation and perivascular spaces interspersed with the cellular proliferation, is a more common feature with thymomas. When a spindle cell growth pattern is apparent, the main differential diagnostic consideration will be a primary spindle cell sarcoma, which may display a hemangiopericytic

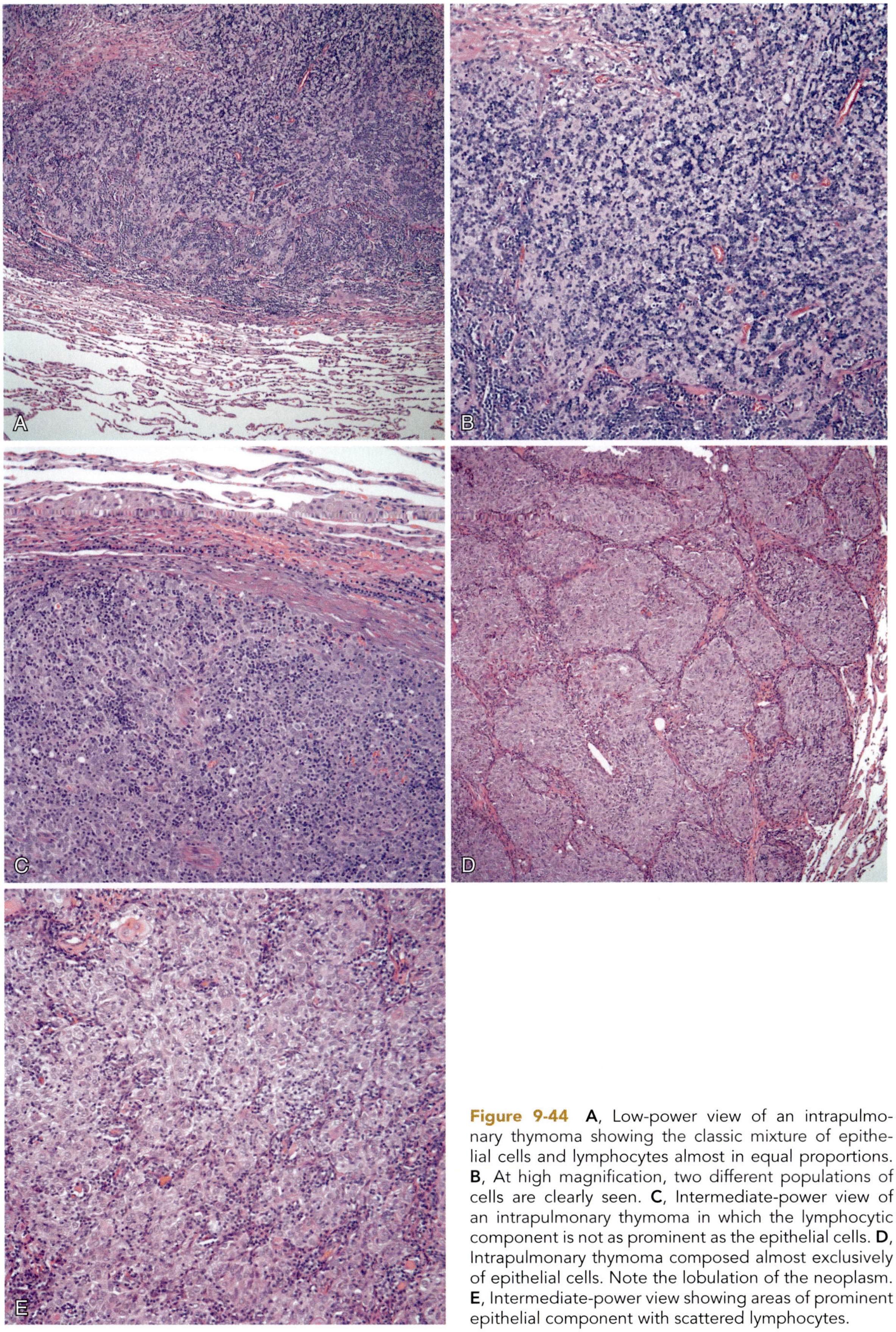

Figure 9-44 **A**, Low-power view of an intrapulmonary thymoma showing the classic mixture of epithelial cells and lymphocytes almost in equal proportions. **B**, At high magnification, two different populations of cells are clearly seen. **C**, Intermediate-power view of an intrapulmonary thymoma in which the lymphocytic component is not as prominent as the epithelial cells. **D**, Intrapulmonary thymoma composed almost exclusively of epithelial cells. Note the lobulation of the neoplasm. **E**, Intermediate-power view showing areas of prominent epithelial component with scattered lymphocytes.

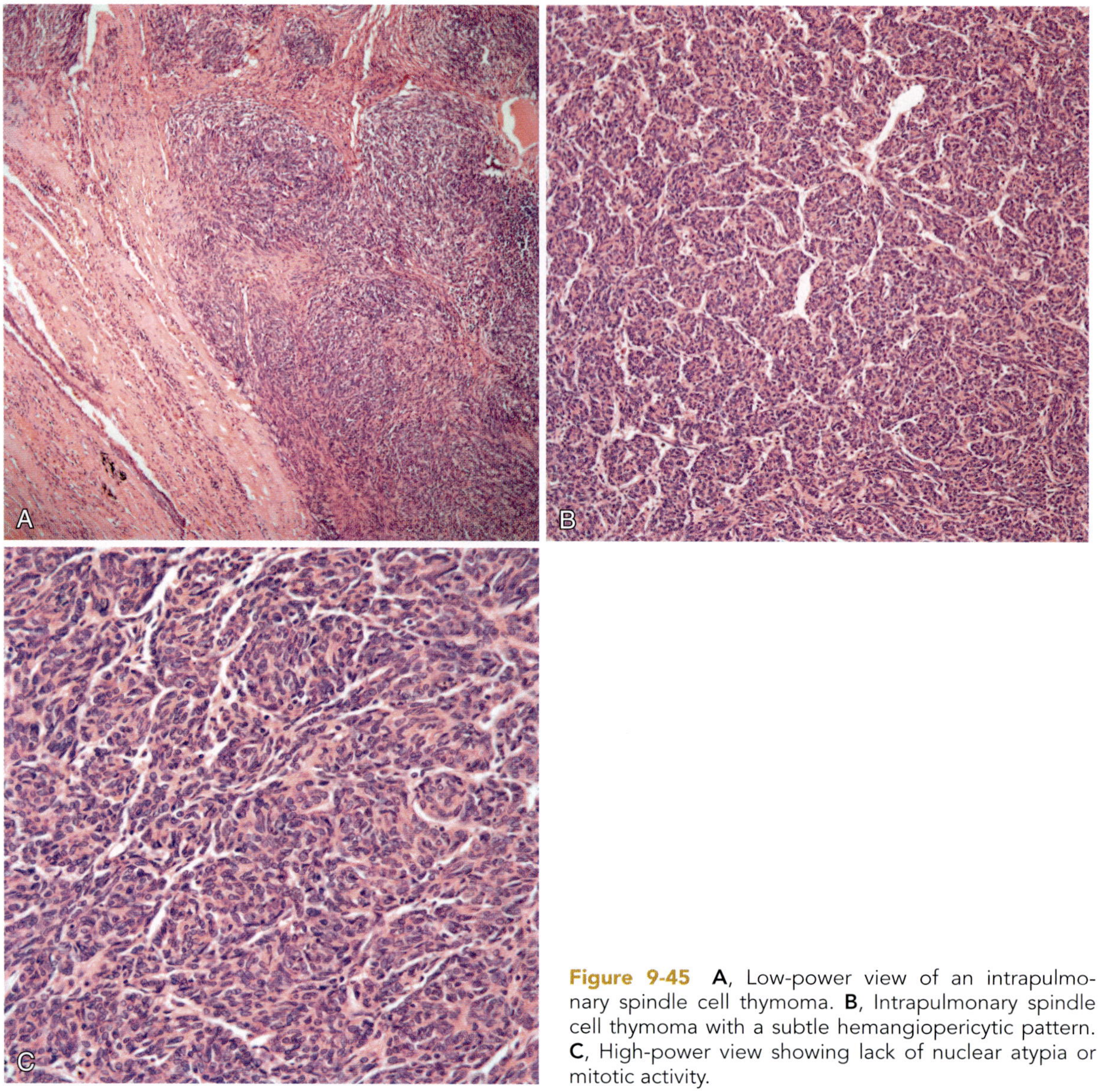

Figure 9-45 **A**, Low-power view of an intrapulmonary spindle cell thymoma. **B**, Intrapulmonary spindle cell thymoma with a subtle hemangiopericytic pattern. **C**, High-power view showing lack of nuclear atypia or mitotic activity.

pattern. Once again, the absence of marked nuclear atypia and mitotic activity, in addition to the positive staining of tumor cells for keratin, should indicate the correct diagnosis.

Treatment and Prognosis

The treatment of choice for intrapulmonary thymomas is complete surgical resection. In most of the cases reported, the behavior of the tumor has been indolent. In the largest series published to date,[140] comprising seven patients, follow-up periods ranged from 10 months to 8 years. Only one patient experienced a recurrence. In this particular case, the patient did not undergo complete surgical resection and was treated with radiation therapy. In the patients who died, however, the causes were unrelated to the intrapulmonary thymoma. Accordingly, the study authors concluded that intrapulmonary thymomas are slow-growing neoplasms with a favorable prognosis, so long as the tumor is amenable to complete surgical resection. For patients with nonresectable or invasive tumors, adjuvant treatment should be considered.

In a recent review of the literature, Myers and associates[139] concluded that complete resection appears to be sufficient treatment for intrapulmonary thymoma. These investigators also found that the presence of paraneoplastic syndromes decreases the likelihood of survival, whereas histologic type and tumor size do not appear to affect survival.

REFERENCES

1. Gerughty JM, Thomas RW. Glomus tumor of the palate: case report and review of the literature. *Br J Oral Maxillofac Surg.* 1992;30:398–400.
2. Hayes MM, van der Westhuizen N, Holden GP. Aggressive glomus tumor of the nasal region: report of a case with multiple local recurrences. *Arch Pathol Lab Med.* 1993;117:649–652.
3. Almagro UA, Schulte WJ, Norback DH. Glomus tumor of the stomach: histologic and ultrastructural features. *Am J Clin Pathol.* 1981;75:415–419.
4. Haque A, Modlin IM, West AB. Multiple glomus tumors of the stomach with intravascular spread. *Am J Surg Pathol.* 1992; 16:291–299.
5. Gould EW, Manivel JC, Albores-Saavedra J, Monteforte H. Locally infiltrative glomus tumors and glomangiosarcomas: a clinical, ultrastructural, and immunohistochemical study. *Cancer.* 1990;65:310–318.
6. Folpe AL, Fanburg-Smith JC, Miettienen M, Weiss SW. Atypical and malignant glomus tumors: analysis of 52 cases with proposal for the classification of glomus tumors. *Am J Surg Pathol.* 2001;25:1–12.
7. Watanabe M, Takagi K, Ono K, et al. Successful resection of a glomus tumor arising from the lower trachea: report of a case. *Jpn J Surg.* 1998;28:332–334.
8. Koskiken SK, Niemi PT, Ekfors TO, Sipilä J, Valavaara R, Dean PB. Glomus tumor of the trachea. *Eur Radiol.* 1998;8:364–366.
9. Altinok T, Cakir E, Gulhan E, Tastepe I. Tracheal glomus tumor. *J Thorac Cardiovasc Surg.* 2006;132:201–202.
10. Yu DK, Cho KH, Kim YJ, Heo DS. Tracheal glomangiosarcoma with multiple skin metastases. *J Dermatol.* 2004;31:776–778.
11. Tang CK, Toker C, Foris N, Trump BF. Glomangioma of the lung. *Am J Surg Pathol.* 1978;2:103–109.
12. Mackay B, Legha SS, Pickler GM. Coin lesion of the lung in a 19-year-old male. *Ultrastruct Pathol.* 1981;2:289–294.
13. Alt B, Huffer WE, Belchis DA. A vascular lesion with smooth muscle differentiation presenting as a coin lesion in the lung: glomus tumor versus hemangiopericytoma. *Am J Clin Pathol.* 1983;80:765–771.
14. Koss MN, Hochholzer L, Moran CA. Primary pulmonary glomus tumor: a clinicopathologic and immunohistochemical study of two cases. *Mod Pathol.* 1998;11:253–258.
15. Gaertner EM, Steinberg DM, Huber M, et al. Pulmonary and mediastinal glomus tumors—report of five cases including a pulmonary glomangiosarcoma: a clinicopathologic study with literature review. *Am J Surg Pathol.* 2000;24:1105–1114.
16. Kapur U, Helenowski M, Zayaad A, Ghai R, Vigeneswaran W, Rajan P. Pulmonary glomus tumor. *Ann Diagn Pathol.* 2007;11:457–459.
17. Lange TH, Magee MJ, Boley TM, Bell SW, Hazelrigg SR. Tracheobronchial glomus tumor. *Ann Thorac Surg.* 2000;70:292–295.
18. Oizumi S, Kon Y, Ishida T, et al. A rare case of bronchial glomus tumor. *Respiration.* 2001;68:95–98.
19. Hatori M, Aiba S, Kato M, et al. Expression of CD34 in glomus tumors. *Tohoku J Exp Med.* 1997;182:241–247.
20. Gromet MA, Ominsky SH, Epstein WL, Blois MS. The thorax as the initial site for systemic relapse in malignant melanoma. *Cancer.* 1979;44:776–784.
21. Paganopoulos E, Murray D. Metastatic malignant melanoma of unknown primary origin: a study of 30 cases. *J Surg Oncol.* 1983;23:8–10.
22. Carlucci GA, Schleussner RC. Primary melanoma of the lung. *J Thorac Surg.* 1942;11:643–649.
23. Kunkel OF, Torrey E. Report of a case of primary melanotic sarcoma of lung presenting difficulties in differentiating from tuberculosis. *N Y J Med.* 1916;16:198–201.
24. Todd FW. Two cases of melanotic tumors in the lung. *JAMA.* 1888;11:53–54.
25. Rosenberg LM, Polanco G, Blank S. Multiple tracheobronchial melanomas with ten-year survival. *JAMA.* 1965;192:133–135.
26. Reid JD, Mehta VT. Melanoma of the lower respiratory tract. *Cancer.* 1966;19:627–631.
27. Taboada CF, McMurray JD, Jordan RA, Seybold WD. Primary melanoma of the lung. *Chest.* 1972;62:629–631.
28. Allen SM, Drash EC. Primary melanoma of the lung. *Cancer.* 1968;21:154–159.
29. Mori K, Cho H, Som M. Primary "flat" melanoma of the trachea. *J Pathol.* 1977;121:101–105.
30. Robertson AJ, Sinclair DJM, Sutton PP, Guthrie W. Primary melanocarcinoma of the lower respiratory tract. *Thorax.* 1980; 35:158–159.
31. Gephardt GN. Malignant melanoma of the bronchus. *Hum Pathol.* 1981;12:671–673.
32. Cagle P, Mace ML, Judge DM, Teague RB, Wilson RK, Greenberg SD. Pulmonary melanoma: primary vs metastatic. *Chest.* 1984; 85:125–126.
33. Angel R, Prados M. Primary bronchial melanoma. *J La State Med Soc.* 1984;136:13–15.
34. Carstens PH, Kuhns JG, Ghazi C. Primary malignant melanoma of the lung and adrenal. *Hum Pathol.* 1984;15:910–914.
35. Demeter SL, Fuenning C, Miller JB. Primary malignant melanoma of the lower respiratory tract: endoscopic identification. *Cleve Clin J Med.* 1987;54:305–308.
36. Santos F, Entrenas LM, Sebastian F, et al. Primary bronchopulmonary malignant melanoma. Case report. *Scand J Thorac Cardiovasc Surg.* 1987;21:187–189.
37. Alhanem AA, Mehan J, Hassan AA. Primary malignant melanoma of the lung. *J Surg Oncol.* 1987;34:109–112.
38. Bertola G, Pasquotti B, Morassut S, Massarut S, Sigon R, Rossi C. Primary lung melanoma. *Ital J Surg Sci.* 1989;19:187–189.
39. Bagwell SP, Flynn SD, Cox PM, Davison JA. Primary malignant melanoma of the lung. *Am Rev Respir Dis.* 1989;139: 1543–1547.
40. Jennings TA, Axiotis CA, Kress Y, Carter D. Primary malignant melanoma of the lower respiratory tract: report of a case and literature review. *Am J Clin Pathol.* 1990;94:649–655.
41. Pasquini E, Rastelli E, Muretto P, et al. Primary bronchial malignant melanoma: a case report. *Pathologica.* 1994;86:546–548.
42. Farrell DJ, Kashyap AP, Ashcroft T, Morritt GN. Primary malignant melanoma of the bronchus. *Thorax.* 1996;51:223–224.
43. Ost D, Joseph C, Sogoloff H, Menezes G. Primary pulmonary melanoma: case report and literature review. *Mayo Clin Proc.* 1999;74:62–66.
44. Dountsis A, Zisis C, Karagianni E, Dahabreh J. Primary malignant melanoma of the lung: a case report. *World J Surg Oncol.* 2003;1:26–29.
45. Lie CH, Chao TY, Chung YH, Lin MC. Primary pulmonary malignant melanoma presenting with haemoptysis. *Melanoma Res.* 2005;15:219–221.
46. Kundranda MN, Clark CT, Chaudhry AA, Chan V, Daw HA. Primary malignant melanoma of the lung: a case report and review of the literature. *Clin Lung Cancer.* 2006;7:279–281.
47. Reddy VS, Mykytenko J, Giltman LI, Mansour KA. Primary malignant melanoma of the lung: review of the literature and report of a case. *Am Surg.* 2007;73:287–289.
48. Ozdemir N, Cangir AK, Kutlay H, Yavuzer S. Primary malignant melanoma of the lung in oculocutaneous albino patient. *Eur J Cardiothoracic Surg.* 2001;20:864–867.
49. Jensen OW, Egedorf J. Primary malignant melanoma of the lung. *Scand J Respir Dis.* 1967;48:127–135.
50. Wilson RW, Moran CA. Primary melanoma of the lung: a clinicopathologic and immunohistochemical study of eight cases. *Am J Surg Pathol.* 1997;21:1196–1202.
51. Littman CD. Metastatic melanoma mimicking primary bronchial melanoma. *Histopathology.* 1991;18:561–563.

52. De Wilt JHW, Farmer SE, Scolyer RA, McCaughan BC, Thompson JF. Isolated melanoma in the lung where there is no known primary site: metastatic disease or primary lung tumour? *Melanoma Res*. 2005;15:531–537.
53. Wick MR, Swanson PE, Rocamora A. Recognition of malignant melanoma by monoclonal antibody HMB-45. An immunohistochemical study of 200 paraffin-embedded cutaneous tumors. *J Cutan Pathol*. 1988;15:201–207.
54. Shuangshoti A, Panyathanya R. Ectopic meningiomas. *Arch Otolaryngol*. 1973;98:102–105.
55. Miller DC, Ojemann RG, Proppe KH, McGinnis BD, Grillo HC. Benign metastasizing meningioma. Case report. *J Neurosurg*. 1985;62:763–766.
56. Kodama K, Doi O, Higashiyama M, Horai T, Tateishi R, Nakagawa H. Primary and metastatic meningioma. *Cancer*. 1991;67:1412–1417.
57. Hoye SJ, Hoar CS, Murray JE. Extracranial meningioma presenting as a tumor of the neck. *Am J Surg*. 1960;100:486–489.
58. Kemnitz P, Spormann H, Heinrich P. Meningioma of lung: first report with light and electron microscopic findings. *Ultrastruct Pathol*. 1982;3:359–365.
59. Chumas JC, Lorelle CA. Pulmonary meningioma: a light and electron microscopic study. *Am J Surg Pathol*. 1982;6:795–801.
60. Strimlan CV, Golembiewski RS, Celko DA, Fino GJ. Primary pulmonary meningioma. *Surg Neurol*. 1988;29:410–413.
61. Robinson PG. Pulmonary meningioma: report of a case with electron microscopic and immunohistochemical findings. *Am J Clin Pathol*. 1992;97:814–817.
62. Piquet J, Valo I, Jousset Y, Enon B. Primary pulmonary meningioma first suspected of being a lung metastasis. *Ann Thorac Surg*. 2005;79:1407–1409.
63. Cesario A, Galetta D, Margaritora S, Granone P. Unsuspected primary pulmonary meningioma. *Eur J Cardiothorac Surg*. 2002;21:553–555.
64. Kaleem Z, Fitzpatrick MM, Ritter J. Primary pulmonary meningioma: report of a case and review of the literature. *Arch Pathol Lab Med*. 1997;121:631–636.
65. Maiorana A, Ficarra G, Fano RA, Spagna G. Primary solitary meningioma of the lung. *Pathologica*. 1996;88:457–462.
66. Falleni M, Roz E, Dessy E, et al. Primary intrathoracic meningioma: histological, immunohistochemical and ultrastructural study of two cases. *Virchows Arch*. 2001;439:196–200.
67. Incarbone M, Ceresoli GL, Tommaso L, et al. Primary pulmonary meningioma: report of a case and review of the literature. *Lung Cancer*. 2008;62:401–407.
68. Drlicek M, Grisold W, Lorber J, Hackl H, Wuketich S, Jellinger K. Pulmonary meningioma: immunohistochemical and ultratructural features. *Am J Surg Pathol*. 1991;15:455–459.
69. Flynn SD, Yousem SA. Pulmonary meningiomas: report of two cases. *Hum Pathol*. 1991;22:469–474.
70. Moran CA, Hochholzer L, Rush W, Koss MN. Primary intrapulmonary meningiomas: a clinicopathologic and immunohistochemical study of ten cases. *Cancer*. 1996;78:2328–2333.
71. Spinelli M, Claren R, Colombi R, Sironi M. Primary pulmonary meningioma may arise from meningothelial-like nodules. *Adv Clin Pathol*. 2000;4:35–39.
72. Gomez-Aracil V, Mayayo E, Alvira R, Arraiza A, Ramón y Cajal S. Fine needle aspiration cytology of primary pulmonary meningioma associated with minute meningothelial nodules. Report of a case with histologic, immunohistochemical, and ultrastructural studies. *Acta Cytol*. 2002;46:899–903.
73. Prayson RA, Farver CF. Primary pulmonary malignant meningioma. *Am J Surg Pathol*. 1999;23:722–726.
74. Van der Meij JJ, Boomars KA, van den Bosch JM, van Boven WJ, de Bruin PC, Seldenrijk CA. Primary pulmonary malignant meningioma. *Ann Thorac Surg*. 2005;80:1523–1525.
75. Rowsell C, Sirbovan J, Rosemblum MK, Perez-Ordonez B. Primary chordoid meningioma of lung. *Virchows Arch*. 2005;446:333–337.
76. Heppleston AG. A carotid-body-like tumour in the lung. *J Pathol Bacteriol*. 1958;75:461–464.
77. Prior JT. Minute peripheral pulmonary tumors: observations on their histogenesis. *Am J Pathol*. 1953;29:703–719.
78. Fawcett FJ, Husband EM. Chemodectoma of lung. *J Clin Pathol*. 1967;20:260–262.
79. Korn D, Bensch K, Liebow AA, Castleman B. Multiple minute tumors resembling chemodectomas. *Am J Pathol*. 1960;37:641–672.
80. Goodman ML, Laforet EG. Solitary primary chemodectomas of the lung. *Chest*. 1972;61:48–50.
81. Lee YT, Hori JM. Chemodectoma of the lung. *J Surg Oncol*. 1972;4:33–36.
82. Laustela E, Mattila S, Fransilla K. Chemodectoma of the lung. *Scand J Thorac Cardiovasc Surg*. 1969;3:59–62.
83. Prior JT, Jones DB. Minute peripheral pulmonary tumors. *J Thorac Surg*. 1952;23:224–236.
84. Spain DM. Intrapulmonary chemodectomas in subjects with organizing pulmonary thromboemboli. *Am Rev Respir Dis*. 1967;96:1158–1169.
85. Ichinose H, Hewitt RL, Drapanas T. Minute pulmonary chemodectoma. *Cancer*. 1971;28:692–700.
86. Saldana MJ, Salem LE, Travezan R. High altitude hypoxia and chemodectomas. *Hum Pathol*. 1973;4:251–263.
87. Zak FG, Chabes A. Pulmonary chemodectomatosis. *JAMA*. 1963;183:887–889.
88. Kuhn C, Askin FB. The fine structure of so-called minute pulmonary chemodectomas. *Hum Pathol*. 1975;6:681–691.
89. Churg AM, Warnock ML. So-called minute pulmonary chemodectoma: a tumor not related to paraganglioma. *Cancer*. 1976;37:1759–1769.
90. Gaffey MJ, Mills SE, Askin FB. Minute pulmonary meningothelial-like nodules: a clinicopathologic study of so-called minute pulmonary chemodectoma. *Am J Surg Pathol*. 1988;12:167–175.
91. Suster S, Moran CA. Diffuse pulmonary meningotheliomatosis. *Am J Surg Pathol*. 2007;31:624–631.
92. Ionescu DN, Sasatomi E, Aldeeb D, et al. Pulmonary meningothelial-like nodules: a genotypic comparison with meningiomas. *Am J Surg Pathol*. 2004;28:207–214.
93. Kuroki M, Nakata H, Masuda T, et al. Minute pulmonary meningothelial-like nodules: high-resolution computed tomography and pathologic correlations. *J Thorac Imaging*. 2002;17:227–229.
94. Sellami D, Gotway MB, Hanks DK, et al. Minute pulmonary meningothelial-like nodules: thin section CT appearance. *J Comp Assist Tomogr*. 2001;25:311–313.
95. Niho S, Yokose T, Nishiwaki Y, Mukai K. Immunohistochemical and clonal analysis of minute pulmonary meningothelial-like nodules. *Hum Pathol*. 1999;30:425–429.
96. Moran CA, Travis WD, Carter D, Koss MN. Metastatic mature teratoma in lung following testicular embryonal carcinoma and teratocarcinoma. *Arch Pathol Lab Med*. 1993;117:641–644.
97. Smith CJ. A teratoma of the lung containing teeth. *Am R Coll Surg Engl*. 1967;41:413–415.
98. Trivedi SA, Mehta KN, Nanavaty JM. Teratoma of the lung: report of a case. *Br J Dis Chest*. 1966;60:156–159.
99. Day DW, Taylor SA. An intrapulmonary teratoma associated with thymic tissue. *Thorax*. 1975;30:582–587.
100. Holt S, Deverall PB, Boddy JE. A teratoma of the lung containing thymic tissue. *J Pathol*. 1978;126:85–89.
101. Saruk M, Stern H, Tronic BS, Neumann RD, LiVolsi VA. Intrapulmonary benign cystic teratoma. *Conn Med*. 1980;44:687–690.
102. Prauer HW, Mack D, Babic R. Intrapulmonary teratoma 10 years after removal of a mediastinal teratoma in a young man. *Thorax*. 1983;38:632–634.

103. Berghout A, Mallens WM, te Velde J, Haak HL. Teratoma of the lung in a hemophilic patient. *Acta Haematol.* 1983;70:330–334.
104. Iwasaki T, Iuchi K, Matsumura A, Sueki H, Yamamoto S, Mori T. Intrapulmonary mature teratoma. *Jpn J Thorac Cardiovasc Surg.* 2000;48:468–472.
105. Groeger AM, Baldi A, Caputi M, et al. Intrapulmonary teratoma associated with thymic tissue. *Anticancer Res.* 2000;20:3919–3922.
106. Asano S, Hoshikawa Y, Yamane Y, Ikeda M, Wakasa H. An intrapulmonary teratoma associated with bronchiectasia containing various kinds of primordium: a case report and review of the literature. *Virchows Arch.* 2000;436:384–388.
107. Eren MN, Balci AE, Eren S. Benign intrapulmonary teratoma: report of a case. *J Thorac Cardiovasc Surg.* 2003;126:855–857.
108. Zenker D, Aleksic I. Intrapulmonary cystic benign teratoma: a case report and review of the literature. *Ann Thorac Cardiovasc Surg.* 2004;10:290–292.
109. Khan JA, Aslam F, Fatimi SH, Ahmed R. Cough, fever, and a cavitary lung lesion—an intrapulmonary teratoma. *J Postgrad Med.* 2005;51:330–331.
110. Alper F, Kaynar H, Kantarci M, et al. Trichoptysis caused by intrapulmonary teratoma: computed tomography and magnetic resonance imaging findings. *Australas Radiol.* 2005;49:53–56.
111. Faria RA, Bizon JA, Saad Jr RS, Dorgan Neto V, Botter M, Saieg MA. Intrapulmonary teratoma. *J Bras Pneumol.* 2007;33:612–615.
112. Agarwal R, Srinivas R, Saxena AK. Trichoptysis due to an intrapulmonary teratoma. *Respir Care.* 2007;52:1779–1781.
113. Rana SS, Swami N, Mehta S, Singh J, Biswal S. Intrapulmonary teratoma: an exceptional disease. *Ann Thorac Surg.* 2007;83:1194–1196.
114. Bateson EM, Hayes JA, Woo-Ming M. Endobronchial teratoma associated with bronchiectasis and bronchiolectasis. *Thorax.* 1968;23:69–75.
115. Jamieson MPG, McGowan AR. Endobronchial teratoma. *Thorax.* 1982;37:157–159.
116. Cai C, Zeng Y, Chen H, Gu Y, Zeng Q, Zhong N. Fibrobronchoscopic evidence of endobronchial hairs in intrapulmonary teratoma with hemoptysis but without trichoptysis. *Am J Med Sci.* 2008;336:441–444.
117. Pound AW, Willis RA. A malignant teratoma of the lung in an infant. *J Pathol.* 1969;98:111–114.
118. Kakkar N, Vasishta RK, Banerjee AK, Garewal G, Deodhar SD, Bambery P. Primary pulmonary malignant teratoma with yolk sac element associated with hematologic neoplasia. *Respiration.* 1996;63:52–54.
119. Gautam HP. Intrapulmonary malignant teratoma. *Am Rev Respir Dis.* 1969;100:863–865.
120. Maasilta PK, Ulla-Stina E, Salminen E, Taskinen EI. Malignant teratoma of the lung. *Acta Oncol.* 1999;38:1113–1115.
121. Stair JM, Stevenson R, Schaefer RF, et al. Primary teratocarcinoma of the lung. *J Surg Oncol.* 1986;33:262–267.
122. Asa SL, Dardick I, Van Nostrand AW, Bailey DJ, Gullane PJ. Primary thyroid thymoma: a distinct clinicopathologic entity. *Hum Pathol.* 1988;19:1463–1466.
123. Martin JME, Rundhawa G, Temple WJ. Cervical thymoma. *Arch Pathol Lab Med.* 1986;110:354–357.
124. Wadon A. Thymoma intratracheale. *Am J Pathol.* 1934; 60:308–312.
125. Moran CA, Travis WD, Rosado-de-Christenson M, Koss MN, Rosai J. Thymomas presenting as pleural tumors. Report of eight cases. *Am J Surg Pathol.* 1992;16:138–144.
126. McBurney RP, Clagett OT, McDonald JR. Primary intrapulmonary neoplasm (thymoma?) associated with myasthenia gravis: report of case. *Proc Staff Meet Mayo Clin.* 1951;26:345–353.
127. Thorburn JD, Stephens HB, Grimes OF. Benign thymoma in the hilus of the lung. *J Thorac Surg.* 1952;24:540–543.
128. Crane AR, Carrigan PT. Primary subpleural intrapulmonary thymoma. *J Thorac Surg.* 1953;25:600–605.
129. Kalish PE. Primary intrapulmonary thymoma. *N Y State J Med.* 1963;63:1705–1708.
130. Yeoh CB, Ford JM, Lattes R, Wylie RH. Intrapulmonary thymoma. *J Thorac Cardiovasc Surg.* 1966;51:131–136.
131. Kung IT, Loke SL, So SY, Lam WK, Mok CK, Khin MA. Intrapulmonary thymoma: report of two cases. *Thorax.* 1985;40:471–474.
132. Green WR, Pressoir R, Gumbs RV, Warner O, Naab T, Qayumi M. Intrapulmonary thymoma. *Arch Pathol Lab Med* 1987;111:1074–1076.
133. Fukayama M, Maeda Y, Funata N, et al. Pulmonary and pleural thymoma. Diagnostic application of lymphocyte markers to the thymoma of unusual site. *Am J Clin Pathol.* 1988;89:617–621.
134. James CL, Iyer PV, Leong ASY. Intrapulmonary thymoma. *Histopathology.* 1992;21:175–177.
135. Stefani A, Boulenger E, Mehaut S, Ciupea A, Alifano M. Primary intrapulmonary thymoma associated with congenital hyperhomocysteinemia. *J Thorac Cardiovasc Surg.* 2007;134:799–801.
136. Ishibashi H, Takahashi S, Tomoko H, Shibuya J, Suzuki S, Handa M. Primary intrapulmonary thymoma successfully resected with vascular reconstruction. *Ann Thorac Surg.* 2003;76:1735–1737.
137. Srivastava A, Padilla O, Alroy J, et al. Primary intrapulmonary spindle cell thymoma with marked granulomatous reaction: report of a case with review of literature. *Int J Surg Pathol.* 2003;11:353–356.
138. Veynovich B, Masetti P, Kaplan PD, Jasnosz KM, Yousem SA, Landreneau RJ. Primary pulmonary thymoma. *Ann Thorac Surg.* 1997;64:1471–1473.
139. Myers PO, Kritikos N, Bongiovanni M, et al. Primary intrapulmonary thymoma: a systematic review. *Eur J Surg Oncol.* 2007;33:1137–1141.
140. Moran CA, Suster S, Fishback NF, Koss MN. Primary intrapulmonary thymoma: a clinicopathologic and immunohistochemical study of eight cases. *Am J Surg Pathol.* 1995;19:304–312.

10

Lymphoproliferative Tumors of the Lung

Malignant primary lymphoproliferative tumors of the lung are rare and represent a small percentage of all primary malignant neoplasms of the lower respiratory tract. Much of the current knowledge regarding these tumors has been generated relatively recently—over the past 25 years or so—as a consequence of the widespread use of immunohistochemical studies and increased awareness of the occurrence of these neoplasms. By contrast, in the early 1980s, fewer than 200 cases had been reported, and in the previous 10 to 12 years, just over 100 cases were published.[1,2]

Subsequent to new developments and classification schemes, characterizations of such tumors as "pulmonary pseudolymphoma," "bronchus-associated lymphoid tissue (BALT)-type lymphoma," and "BALToma" have fallen out of favor as diagnostic entities. Bienenstock and coworkers[3,4] introduced the latter two terms in 1973, describing the morphologic and functional characteristics of bronchial lymphoid tissue. The designation *lymphoid interstitial pneumonitis* (LIP) is now confined to inflammatory lesions of the lung. Previously, it was thought that either pseudolymphoma or LIP represented a premalignant condition, because both have been reported to develop changes consistent with malignant transformation[5]; a more stratified histologic approach, however, has been advocated by some investigators.[6] Currently, the preferred designation is *marginal zone B cell lymphoma of the mucosa-associated lymphoid tissue (MALT) type*.

The criteria for diagnosing primary pulmonary lymphoma have also changed over the years. Initially, it was defined as a unilateral process, with or without hilar involvement, and with no mediastinal disease.[7] This definition, however, was recognized to eliminate cases with bilateral involvement.[2] Some investigators have found that the assessment between primary and secondary tumors is difficult to make on histologic grounds, because both processes may share similar histopathologic features. Therefore, "primary malignant lymphoma of the lung" represents an elusive diagnosis for the pathologist, who may not have access to the entire clinical history, which would tell whether the patient has enlarged lymph nodes elsewhere or tumor nodules in an extrathoracic location. Consequently, in this setting, assessment requires careful clinical and radiologic correlation.

For the practical assessment of lymphomas in the lung, the recognized clinical entities can be separated into two main families:

- Non-Hodgkin's lymphomas
  - Marginal zone B cell lymphoma, MALT type
  - Diffuse large cell B cell lymphoma
  - Anaplastic large cell lymphoma
  - Lyphomatoid granulomatosis
- Hodgkin's lymphoma

MARGINAL ZONE B CELL LYMPHOMA, MUCOSA-ASSOCIATED LYMPHOID TISSUE TYPE

Marginal zone B cell lymphoma of the MALT type may be the most common type of pulmonary lymphoma, accounting for more than 60% of all pulmonary lymphomas. Because the current terminology used to identify this tumor is new, frequency must be extrapolated from data available in previously published series.

In 1983, Koss and colleagues[8] presented a study of 161 patients with what the investigators called primary non-Hodgkin's lymphoma of the lung or, in a minority of the cases, pseudolymphoma of the lung. Although the tumors were classified according to the current schema of the time, it is likely that more than 70% of the non-Hodgkin's lymphoma cases may have represented MALT-type lymphomas, and probably less than 10% represented diffuse large cell lymphoma. As noted, also included in this study were so-called pseudolymphomas, accounting for 14% of the cases. Most of the patients in this study were in the sixth or seventh decade of life and were asymptomatic, with a solitary nodule or infiltrate in the lung found incidentally on a chest radiograph. Clinical signs and symptoms, when present, included cough, dyspnea, hemoptysis, and upper respiratory infection. More constitutional manifestations such as weight loss were documented in a minority of patients. Some patients had a history of Sjögren's syndrome or systemic lupus erythematosus. On radiologic examination, a pulmonary nodule of variable size (ranging from 2 to 8 cm) was the most common finding. Hilar adenopathy was present in a minority of cases.

In 1984, Herbert and associates[9] described nine cases of primary malignant lymphoma of the lung and suggested that these lymphomas arise from bronchus-associated lymphoid tissue, which would explain the histopathologic features as well as the clinical course (the tumor is confined to the lung for long periods of time). The patients in this study were between the ages of 30 and 68 years and presented with ill-defined consolidated areas in the lung that ranged from 2 to 8 cm in greatest dimension. Clonality was demonstrated by immunohistochemical analysis in four cases, suggesting that if these lymphomas of the lung were to disseminate, they might spread widely to other mucosal sites. Development of gastric lymphomas of the MALT type was documented in two of the cases.

L'Hoste and coworkers[10] reported a series of 36 primary lymphomas of the lung in which patient age ranged from 12 to 75 years; however, only one patient was younger than 30 years. These patients presented with unilateral or bilateral disease. At least 21 of the lymphomas were low-grade tumors and probably were of the MALT type. These workers were not able to discriminate on histopathologic grounds between tumors that recurred and eventually disseminated and those that followed a more indolent course.

Addis and colleagues[11] documented 15 primary pulmonary lymphomas, some of which had features that previously had been associated with the so-called pulmonary pseudolymphoma. These investigators suggested that pulmonary lymphomas arise from the centrocyte-like cells normally present in the bronchus-associated lymphoid tissue and warned that some of the cases previously identified as pseudolymphomas or LIP may in fact represent examples of pulmonary lymphoma. Similar findings also have been documented by different investigators.[12–15] An unusual case of MALT-type lymphoma has been reported in an HIV-positive 7-year-old child.[16] Tamura and associates[17] studied 12 cases of pulmonary B cell lymphoma for the presence of Epstein-Barr virus (EBV) infection and found that none of the cases showed signaling for the receptor EBER-1 using the antisense probe, suggesting that primary pulmonary MALT-type lymphoma is not associated with an EBV infection. In other unusual presentations, simultaneous involvement of the conjunctiva has been reported,[18] and the disorder also may manifest as chronic pneumonia.[19]

More recently, two studies have focused on the association of MALT-type pulmonary lymphoma with Sjögren's syndrome and other autoimmune disorders.[20,21] Sophisticated radiologic techniques have demonstrated that MALT-type lymphomas may manifest as a single nodule or in a consolidated pattern with multiple nodular areas of consolidation, bronchiectasis, or bronchiolitis, whereas on positron emission tomography (PET) scans, the lesions show heterogeneous (more common) or homogeneous fluorodeoxyglucose (FDG) uptake.[22,23] More recent series have confirmed previous clinical and histopathologic features of these tumors.[24–26]

Macroscopic Features

The tumors may be unilateral or bilateral and may present either as a distinct solitary pulmonary mass, localized pulmonary infiltrate, or diffuse pulmonary infiltrate. When these lesions manifest as a solitary mass, tumor size may range from 1 cm to more than 5 cm in greatest dimension.[8,9] In some series, tumors larger than 10 cm have been recorded.[10] They are whitish, without areas of necrosis or hemorrhage, and in some cases central scarring has been identified.

Histopathologic Features

The low-power view displays an atypical homogeneous lymphoid proliferation with cellular elements arranged in different growth patterns. A well-demarcated tumor nodule or mass that replaces and obliterates the normal lung parenchyma may be visible (Fig. 10-1), or the neoplastic cellular proliferation appears as multiple small, ill-defined nodules scattered in the lung parenchyma. Less commonly, the tumor may manifest as an ill-defined infiltrate tracking vascular structures. The tumor may be observed invading the pleura, or involving the bronchial cartilage (Fig. 10-2). The presence of tumor in the visceral pleura has been recognized as an unequivocal feature of malignancy in a lymphoid proliferation. Higher magnification shows lymphoid infiltrate invading epithelial structures such as the bronchial epithelium, and forming the so-called lymphoepithelial lesion characteristically seen in MALT-type lymphomas (Fig. 10-3). The neoplastic cellular proliferation is composed of small lymphocytes with mild nuclear irregularities admixed with scattered immunoblasts. The lymphoid proliferation may display a clear

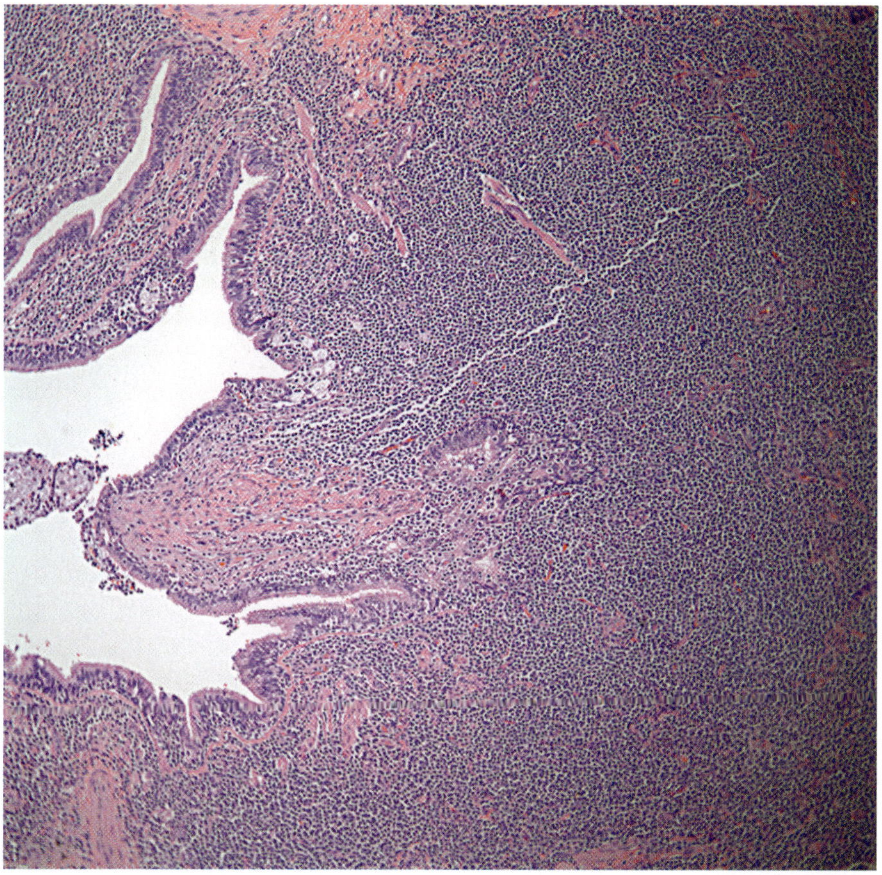

Figure 10-1 Mucosa-associated lymphoid tissue type lymphoma destroying lung parenchyma and growing along the main airway.

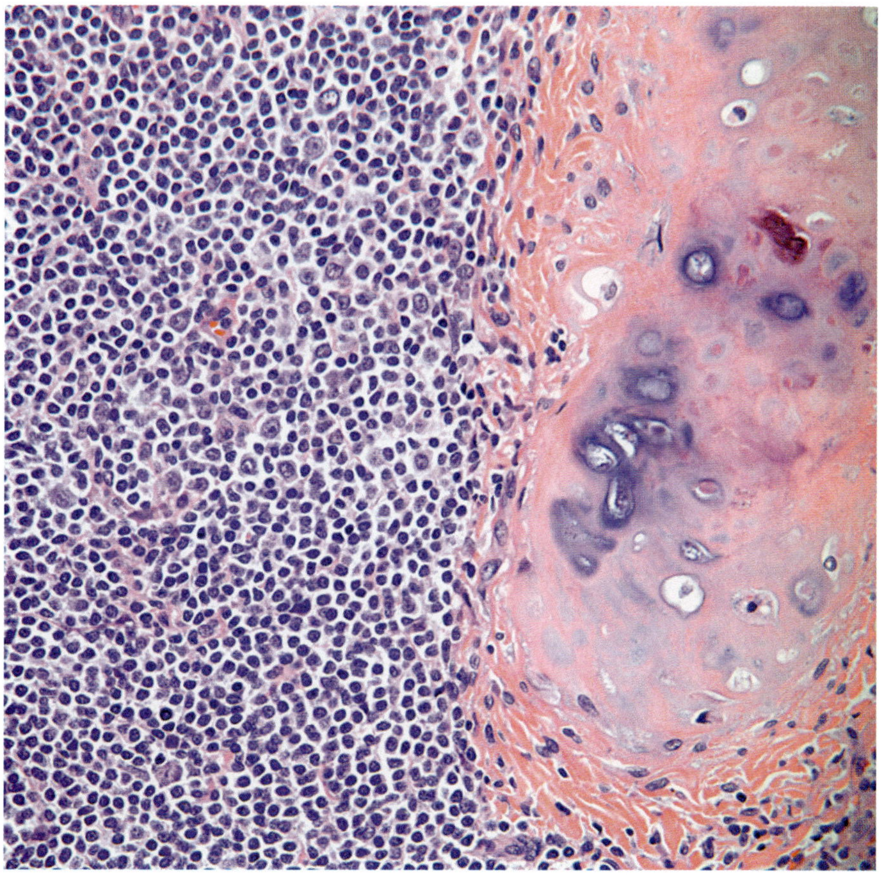

Figure 10-2 Mucosa-associated lymphoid tissue type lymphoma invading bronchial cartilage.

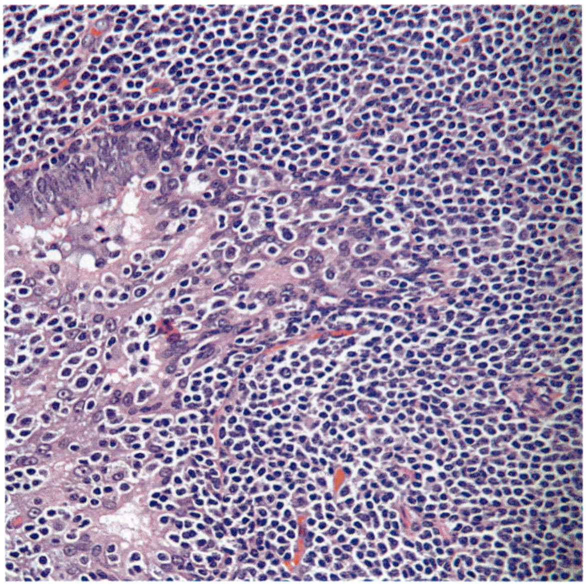

Figure 10-3 Mucosa-associated lymphoid tissue type lymphoma with a classic lymphoepithelial lesion.

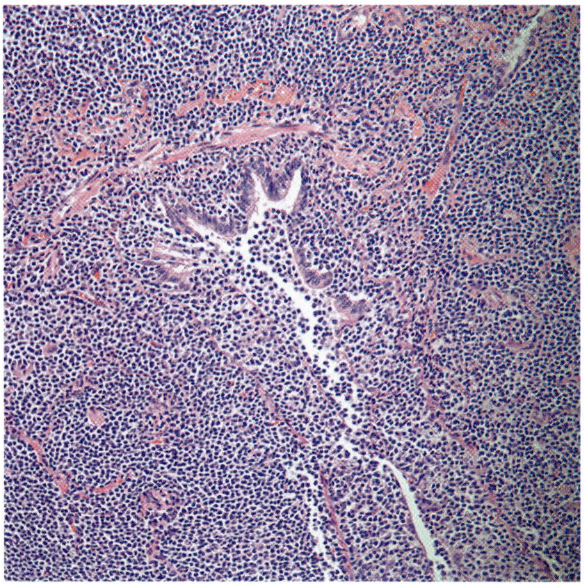

Figure 10-4 Mucosa-associated lymphoid tissue type lymphoma partially destroying and obliterating an airway.

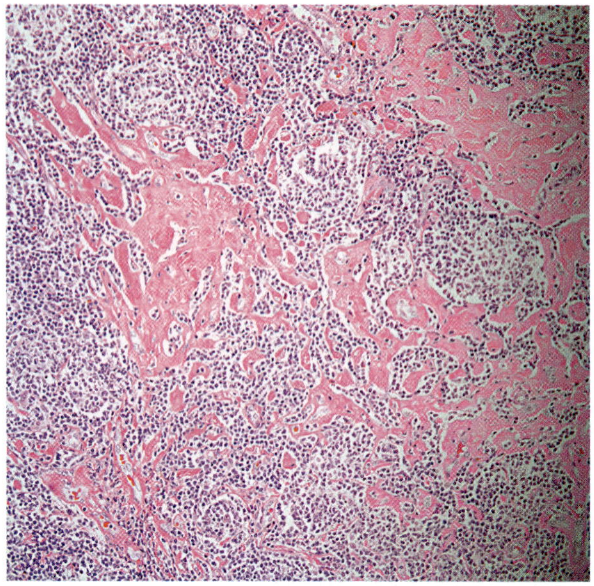

Figure 10-5 Mucosa-associated lymphoid tissue type lymphoma with amyloid-like stroma.

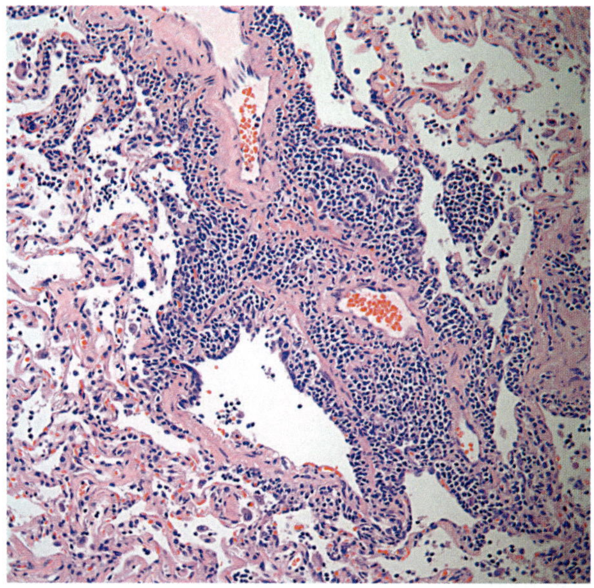

Figure 10-6 Mucosa-associated lymphoid tissue type lymphoma. Tracking of neoplastic cells into vascular structures can be seen.

halo surrounding the nucleus of the lymphoid cells, in a manner reminiscent of parafollicular B cells; while in other areas the lymphoid proliferation may appear plasmacytoid (Figs. 10-4 to 10-8). The presence of Dutcher bodies appears to correlate more often with malignant processes, rather than reactive ones.

Other features that may be present in differing proportions in MALT-type lymphomas are sarcoid-like granulomas, multinucleated giant cells, and cholesterol cleft granulomas. These unusual features may be seen in up to 50% of MALT-type lymphomas. Germinal centers also may be seen in these cases (Fig. 10-9); this feature was once considered a characteristic of the so-called pseudolymphoma. Lymph node involvement, another feature once considered an important indication of malignancy in lymphoid proliferations, may be present in less than one third of MALT-type lymphomas.

Malignant cells admixed with reactive follicles and polytypic plasma cells also may be observed.[12]

Immunohistochemistry

Because lymphoid proliferations may appear in the lung owing to a variety of conditions, immunohistochemical studies are vital to an accurate diagnosis. Flow cytometry

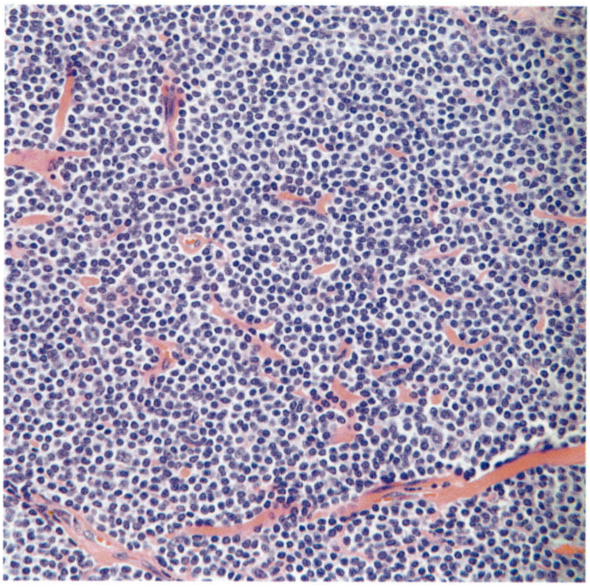

Figure 10-7 High-power view of a mucosa-associated lymphoid tissue type lymphoma showing a monotonous cellular proliferation.

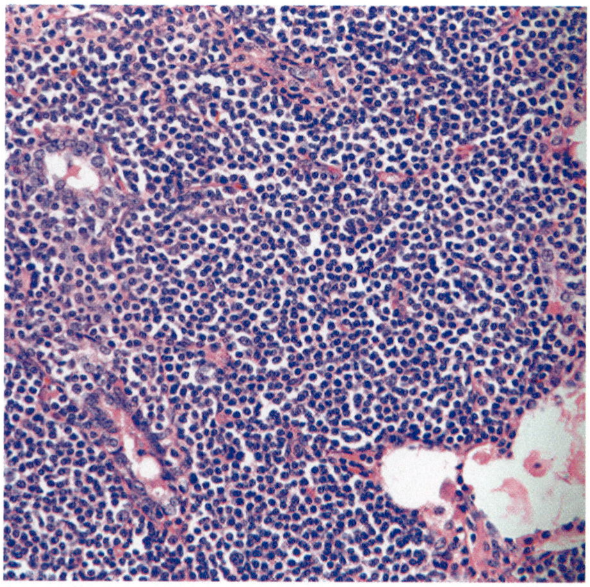

Figure 10-8 Mucosa-associated lymphoid tissue type lymphoma with plasmacytoid features.

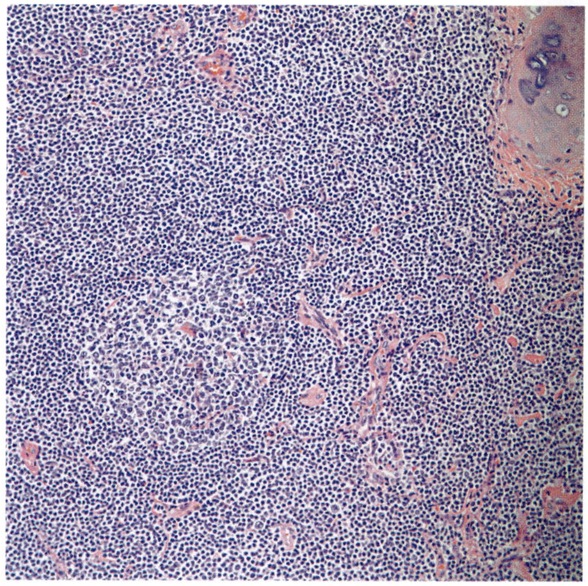

Figure 10-9 Residual germinal center present in a mucosa-associated lymphoid tissue type lymphoma.

and gene rearrangements may provide more insight into the true nature of the infiltrate in many difficult cases. Researchers have highlighted several different immunohistochemical features for these tumors, and as new antibodies are developed and their specificity and sensitivity are improved, the accepted immunohistochemical features continue to change. In a study of 45 cases of pulmonary lymphoma, Nicholson and coworkers[13] noted that all of the tumors studied by immunohistochemistry showed positive staining for CD20 (a B cell marker) with a variable number of reactive CD3 (a T cell marker)-positive cells. The investigators also found that CD21 can be used to document the presence of germinal centers, even when this morphologic feature was not apparent. In a study of 26 lymphoid lesions, Bégueret and colleagues[26] found that these tumors will express CD20 and CD43. MALT-type lymphomas usually express heavy chain for IgM or IgA and, less frequently, for IgG. Immunohistochemical studies also should be performed to document monoclonality; the use of κ and λ light chains may aid in the diagnosis, and polymerase chain reaction (PCR) analysis or gene rearrangement studies also should be considered. In general, MALT-type lymphomas demonstrate negative staining for CD23, CD5, Bcl-1, and Bcl-2.

Translocations have been reported in MALT-type lymphomas. The most common is t(11;18)(q21;q21), which can occur in 50% of these cases. Other translocations, including t(14;18)(q32;q21) and t(I;14)(p22;q32), have been recorded. More recently, a case with Bcl-10 expression and novel translocation t(1;2)(p22;p12) immunoglobulin κ chain–Bcl-10 has been documented.[27]

Differential Diagnosis

The most important considerations in the differential diagnosis are nodular (Figs. 10-10 and 10-11) and diffuse hyperplasia of the bronchial lymphoid tissue (Figs. 10-12 to 10-14) and secondary involvement of the lung by malignant lymphoma. In the past, the presence of germinal centers was used as a factor distinguishing between reactive and neoplastic lymphoid proliferations. Neoplastic lymphoid proliferation also may show the presence of germinal centers, however; thus, it is not a completely reliable feature of reactive lesions. These conditions share some clinical and radiologic features as well. In a

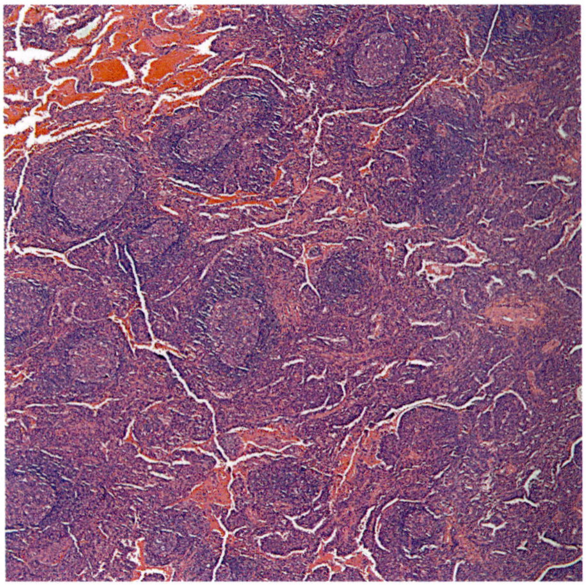

Figure 10-10 Nodular hyperplasia of the bronchial lymphoid tissue (pseudolymphoma). Numerous germinal centers are characteristic.

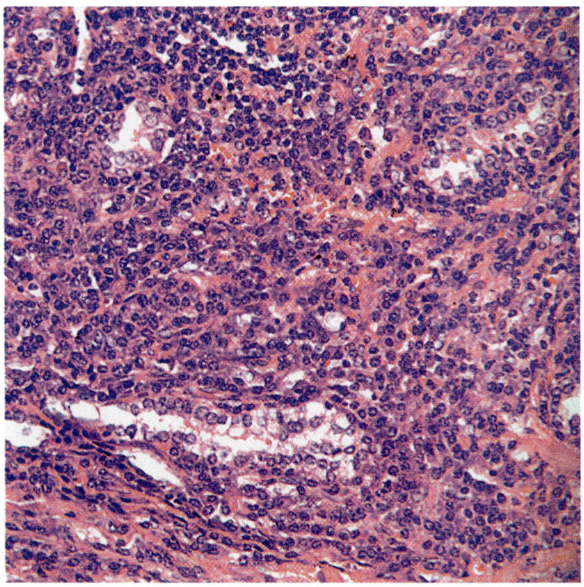

Figure 10-11 High-power view of nodular hyperplasia of the bronchus-associated lymphoid tissue type showing the presence of abundant plasma cells.

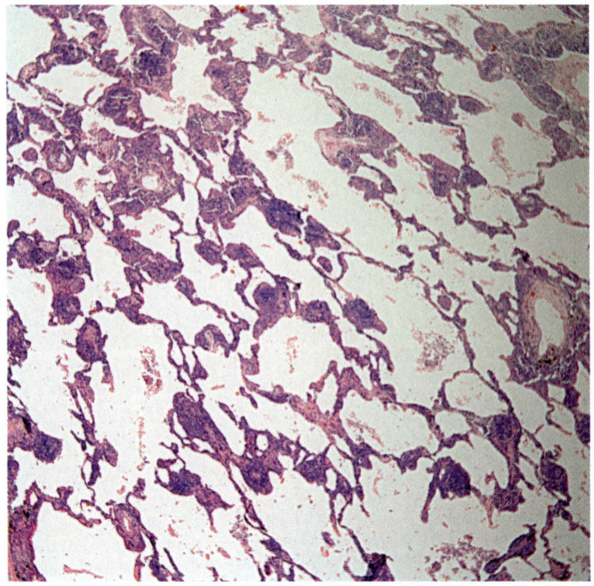

Figure 10-12 Low-power view of diffuse hyperplasia of the bronchus-associated lymphoid tissue type (lymphoid interstitial pneumonia) showing an extensive lymphoid component in the lung parenchyma.

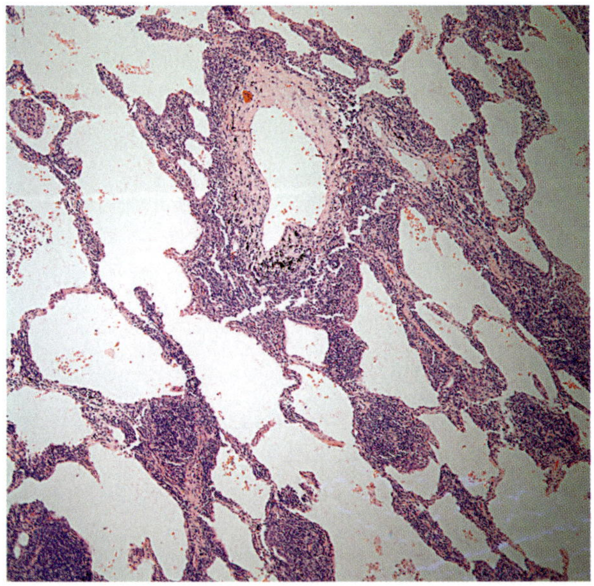

Figure 10-13 Intermediate-power view of diffuse hyperplasia of the bronchus-associated lymphoid tissue type showing perivascular lymphoid component.

study of 18 patients with LIP (diffuse hyperplasia of the bronchial lymphoid tissue), Koss and associates[28] found that the median age at diagnosis was 56 years, with clinical signs and symptoms of cough, dyspnea, or chest pain. Findings on the initial radiologic examination included patchy interstitial infiltrates or poorly defined pulmonary nodules. On histologic examination, the lesions displayed interstitial infiltrates composed of lymphocytes and plasma cells, with 47% of the cases showing germinal centers and 72% showing interstitial giant cells (see Figs. 10-10 to 10-12). In the cases studied by immunohistochemistry techniques, the investigators documented the presence of a polytypic infiltrate. In one case, the patient died of disseminated lymphoma, which raises the possibility that such lesions may develop into full-blown lymphomas. In this setting, mono- or polyclonality must be documented to properly classify the process as reactive or neoplastic.

Determining whether the tumor is a primary or a secondary lung neoplasm may be difficult on histopathologic

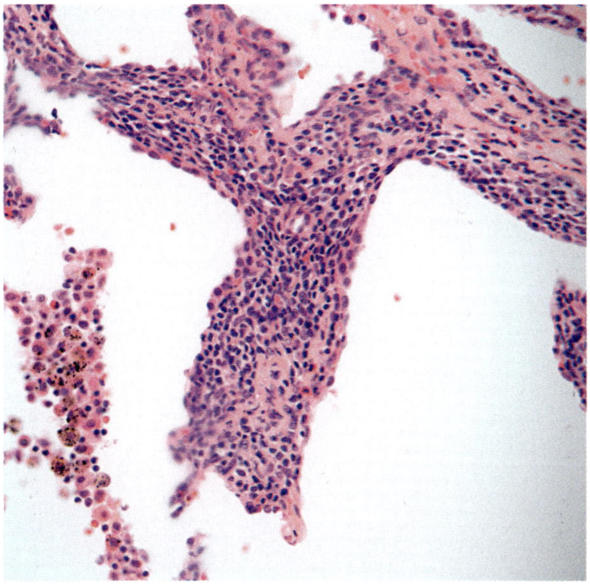

Figure 10-14 High-power view of diffuse hyperplasia of the bronchus-associated lymphoid tissue type showing a mixed cellularity composed of plasma cells and lymphocytes.

grounds alone. Costa and colleagues[29] published a study of 21,157 autopsies in which 414 of the cases represented systemic lymphoma, 85 showed lung involvement, and 43 represented B cell lymphomas. Five patterns of infiltration were documented: perivascular-peribronchial, nodular, alveolar, interstitial, and pleural. These patterns of involvement have been seen in primary pulmonary lymphomas, making the distinction very difficult on histologic grounds alone.

Prognosis and Treatment

The prognosis for patients with MALT-type pulmonary lymphoma is relatively good. Vallisa and associates[30] documented survival rates of 100% at 2 years and 93% at 5 years; they recommend that in cases of stable low-grade lymphoma, observation alone constitutes an appropriate management approach, whereas in cases that demonstrate progression of disease, the use of chemotherapy is indicated. Ferraro and coworkers[31] documented survival rates of 91%, 68%, and 53% for 1, 5, and 10 years, respectively. In this series, 19 of the patients (40%) underwent complete surgical resection.

Other researchers have questioned whether MALT-type lymphomas should be treated immediately. In a study by Koss and associates,[8] only 12 of 101 patients with lymphoma died in a period of 5 years, and only 18 died in a period of 15 years. In Herbert and coworkers' series,[9] only one of nine patients died within a follow-up period of 15 years. Survival rates of 88% at 5 years have been recorded by other investigators.[10] In a study of 11 patients, Troch and colleagues[32] suggested that MALT-type lymphoma of the lung is an indolent process with the potential for spontaneous regression. Accordingly, these workers suggested a watch-and-wait policy in stable cases. Other researchers have stated that when the tumor manifests as a single pulmonary mass, complete surgical resection may constitute optimal management.

DIFFUSE LARGE B CELL LYMPHOMA

In general, primary diffuse large B cell lymphomas of the lung are rare, accounting for no more than 10% to 15% of pulmonary lymphomas. It is likely that diffuse large B cell lymphomas represent less than 1% of all pulmonary neoplasms.

The clinical and radiologic features are similar to those of MALT-type pulmonary lymphoma. No gender predilection has been documented, and most patients are in their sixth decade of life. Patients may present with pulmonary symptomatology or with more systemic symptoms. A single mass or multiple unilateral or bilateral pulmonary nodules may be seen on radiographic studies, with or without lymph node involvement.

In 1982, Colby and Carrington[2] described 20 cases of pulmonary lymphoma, 10 of which represented primary tumors in the lung and 10 representing secondary pulmonary involvement. Although the description emphasized that primary and secondary pulmonary malignant lymphomas show similar histopathologic features, these cases probably were of the diffuse large B cell type. The investigators also stressed the presence of vascular lesions commonly associated with lymphomatoid granulomatosis. In Koss and coworkers' series of 161 cases,[8] it is possible that less than 10% of the cases described represented diffuse large B cell type lymphoma.

In a series of 45 cases of non-Hodgkin's lymphoma of the lung, Nicholson and associates[33] identified 6 cases associated with autoimmune disease. Three of these patients had cryptogenic fibrosing alveolitis treated with long-term immunosuppressive therapy. Five of the six cases corresponded to diffuse large B cell lymphoma and one to a low-grade lymphoma. The investigators suggested an association between autoimmune disease and lymphomas. Other workers also have reported the association of diffuse large B cell lymphoma and cryptogenic fibrosing alveolitis.[34] In Ferraro and coworkers'[31] account of 48 patients with primary non-Hodgkin's lymphoma of the lung, 13 cases may have been of the diffuse large B cell type, although the emphasis in this series was on the low-grade MALT-type lymphoma.

Macroscopic Features

Diffuse large B cell lymphomas may manifest as a solitary pulmonary mass or as unilateral or bilateral pulmonary nodules. Tumor size may range from 1 cm to more than 5 cm in greatest dimension, and necrosis may be present on the cut surface of the tumor, although it is not a consistent feature. The tumors are well circumscribed and light tan in color, with a soft consistency.

Histopathologic Features

The low-power view will show a homogeneous neoplastic cellular proliferation destroying and replacing normal pulmonary parenchyma (Fig. 10-15). The tumor may appear as a well-defined mass or may exhibit diffuse infiltration into the pulmonary interstitium with extension along vascular structures (Figs. 10-16 and 10-17).

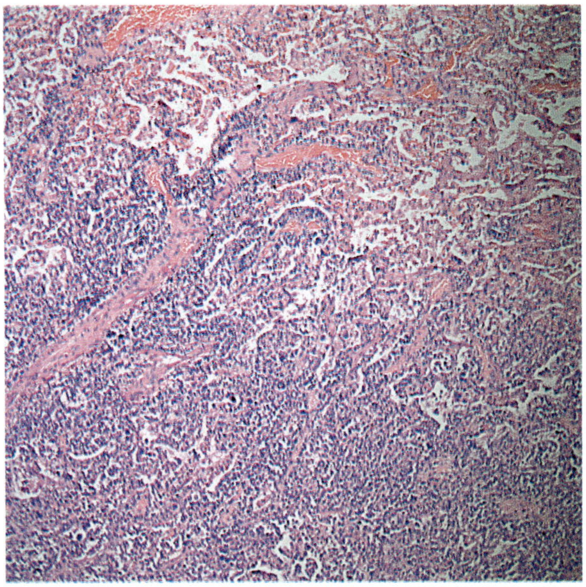

Figure 10-15 Diffuse large cell lymphoma. The neoplastic process is destroying lung parenchyma.

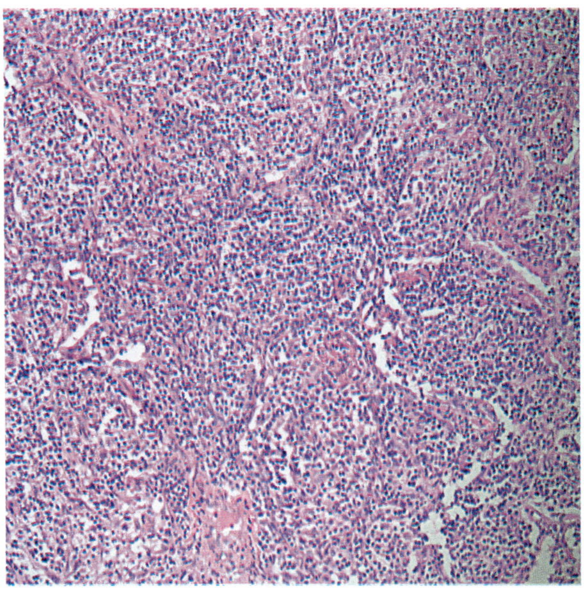

Figure 10-16 Diffuse large cell lymphoma of the lung with a subtle nested pattern.

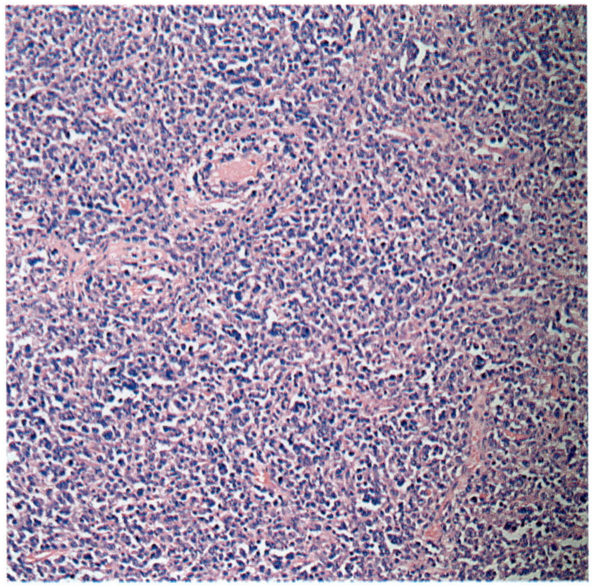

Figure 10-17 Diffuse large cell lymphoma. Sheets of neoplastic cells can be seen.

At higher magnification, a neoplastic cellular proliferation composed of larger cells with round to oval nuclei and prominent nucleoli can be seen (Fig. 10-18). Mitotic figures are commonly encountered, and areas of necrosis also may be present, ranging in extent from focal to more extensive. Invasion of normal pulmonary structures such as the bronchial wall and pleura is common. Some investigators have made special mention of the areas of low-grade MALT-type lymphoma undergoing transition to a high-grade process; thus, some of these tumors will be

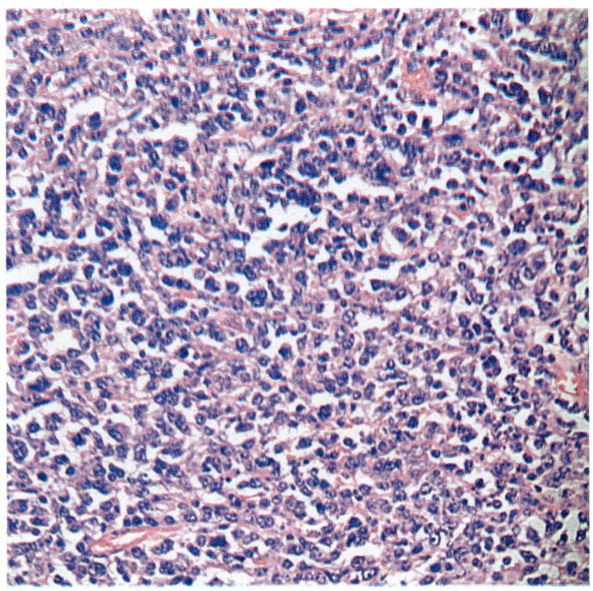

Figure 10-18 High-power view of the neoplastic cells in diffuse large cell lymphoma showing prominent nuclear atypia, nucleoli, and mitotic activity.

designated high-grade MALT-type lymphomas, although this term may not be appropriate.

Immunohistochemical Features

Because the neoplastic cellular proliferation may show cellular pleomorphism, it is important to rule out an epithelial tumor. Therefore, the use of epithelial markers, including keratins and epithelial membrane antigen (EMA), should be considered. A panel of immunohistochemical studies using B cell and T cell markers also should aid in the proper classification of these tumors. Neoplastic cells will show positive staining for B cell markers, CD20 (L-26) in particular, and negative staining for T cell markers. In some cases, some T-reactive cells may show positive staining using T cell markers. Other immunohistochemical studies to determine clonality or the use of molecular techniques should help in the final diagnosis.

Differential Diagnosis

Epithelial neoplasm, especially carcinoma, is an important consideration in the differential diagnosis. Some undifferentiated or pleomorphic carcinomas may mimic a lymphoid neoplasm. Therefore, use of a broader panel of immunohistochemical studies, including those utilizing keratins and EMA, should help in obtaining an accurate diagnosis. Other types of lymphomas also should be considered; however, use of additional immunohistochemical markers for B and T cells and other molecular techniques, including gene rearrangement studies, may permit more specific classification of these tumors.

Prognosis and Treatment

As indicated by data from some of the cases published in the literature, diffuse large B cell lymphomas may not share the favorable prognosis for MALT-type lymphomas. In the study reported by Colby and Carrington,[2] the outcome was poor, with one half of the patients dead by 24 months. In Nicholson and coworkers' study of six patients with this neoplasm,[33] three patients were evaluated at autopsy. Two of the three remaining patients died at 2 weeks and 6 months later, respectively, and only one patient survived 4 years. These patients also had an associated autoimmune condition that may have had an effect on overall survival. However, in the 13 cases described by Ferraro and colleagues[31] as non–MALT-type lymphoma, the survival rates at 1, 5, and 10 years were 85%, 65%, and 53%, respectively. Some researchers[30] have suggested that rituximab may improve the response to the CHOP regimen (cyclophosphamide, hydroxydaunomycin, vincristine [Oncovin], and prednisone) commonly used in the treatment of diffuse large B cell lymphomas.

ANAPLASTIC LARGE CELL LYMPHOMA

Anaplastic large cell lymphoma (ALCL) is far more common in lymph nodes, but it has been rarely reported in the lung as a primary neoplasm.[35,36] The tumor affects both male and female patients and may occur in any age group. Presenting clinical signs and symptoms may include cough, chest pain, dyspnea, or fever. A pulmonary mass with or without lymphadenopathy may be encountered on the chest radiograph. Because of the nonspecific clinical and radiologic findings, the only way to arrive at a specific diagnosis is by tissue analysis.

Histopathologic Features

The spectrum of morphologic features that may be seen in ALCL mimic those in other, more common epithelial tumors in the lung. The low-power view may show a neoplastic cellular proliferation with the tumor cells arranged in sheets or, in some unusual cases, a spindle cellular proliferation with a subtle storiform pattern (Figs. 10-19 to 10-21). Higher magnification reveals a neoplastic cellular proliferation composed of medium-sized to large cells with ample cytoplasm, round to oval nuclei, and prominent nucleoli. Multinucleated cells mimicking Reed-Sternberg cells, or multinucleated giant cells resembling Touton-type giant cells, are commonly seen (Figs. 10-22 and 10-23). The tumor may show pleomorphic features with marked nuclear atypia and mitotic activity, accompanied by areas of necrosis that may be focal or more extensive.

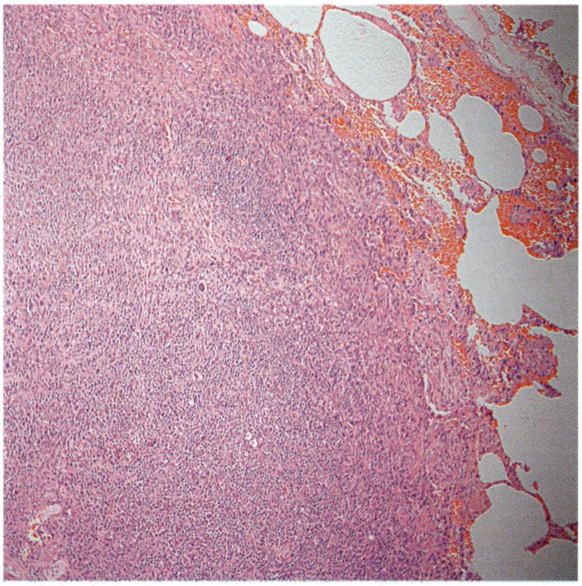

Figure 10-19 Anaplastic large cell lymphoma primary in the lung manifesting as a pulmonary mass.

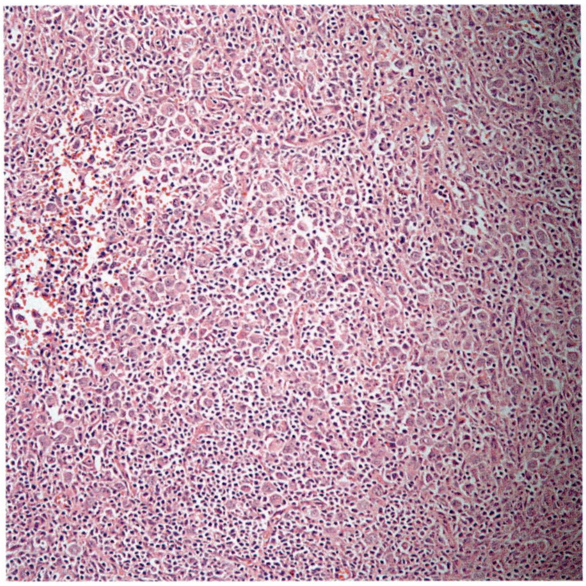

Figure 10-20 Sheets of pleomorphic cells in anaplastic large cell lymphoma.

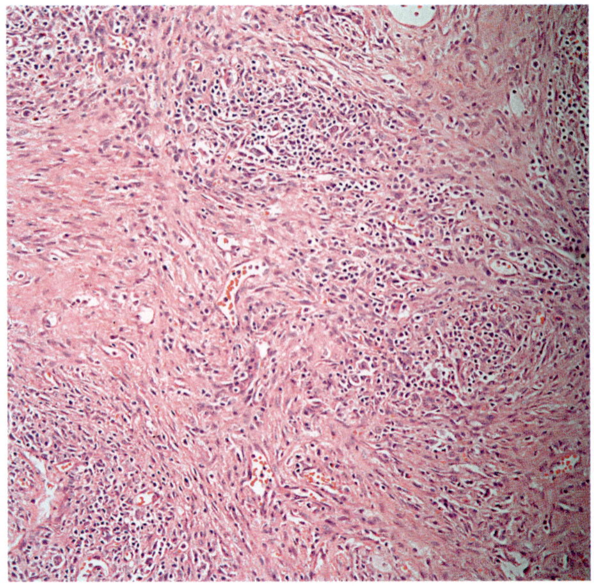

Figure 10-21 Subtle storiform pattern in anaplastic large cell lymphoma.

Immunohistochemical Features

ALCL typically will show positive staining for CD30 (Fig. 10-24), CD3, and ALK. In addition, the tumor may show positive staining for EMA but negative staining for CD15 (LeuM1). Because of the affinity of this tumor for positive staining for EMA, it is important to perform a wider panel of imunohistochemical studies, including other epithelial markers and lymphoid markers.

Prognosis and Treatment

Because of the presentation of this tumor as a pulmonary mass, some of these cases will require surgical resection

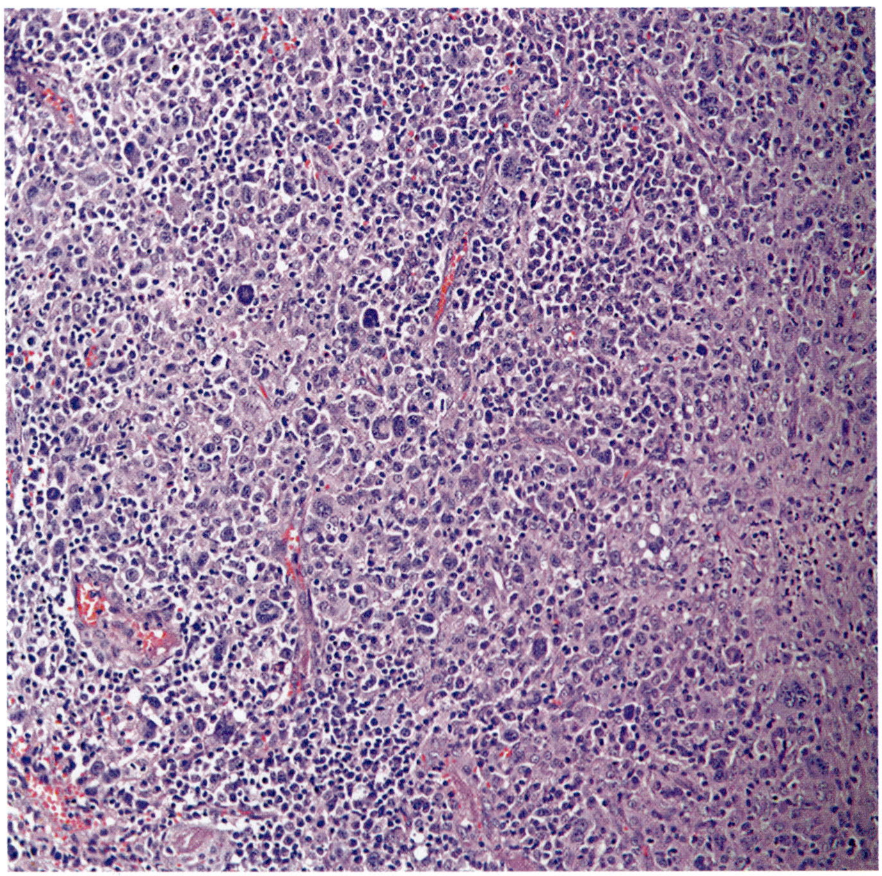

Figure 10-22 Anaplastic large cell lymphoma with prominent cellular pleomorphism.

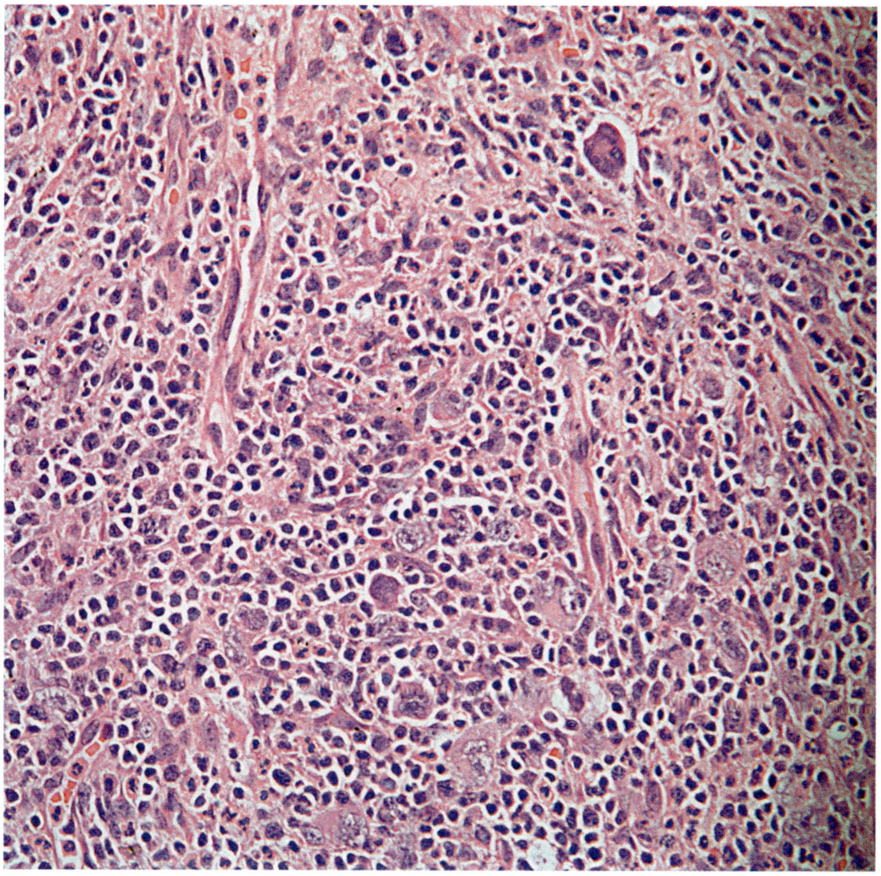

Figure 10-23 Anaplastic large cell lymphoma with multinucleated giant cells and Touton-type giant cells.

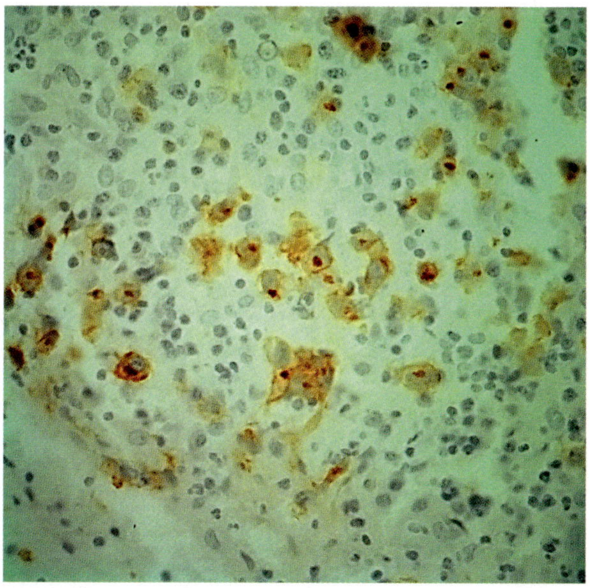

Figure 10-24 CD30 immunostaining is positive in anaplastic large cell lymphoma.

of the tumor, which is accomplished by lobectomy or other surgical procedure. These patients may be treated with chemotherapy, using protocols similar to those used with diffuse large B cell lymphomas. The number of cases published is relatively small, however, so it is difficult to draw meaningful conclusions regarding the pattern of clinical behavior of primary ALCL of the lung.

LYMPHOMATOID GRANULOMATOSIS

Lymphomatoid granulomatosis (LYG) is an angiocentric and angiodestructive lymphoid process of uncommon occurrence. The diagnosis of this neoplastic condition has been plagued by numerous controversies since its original description by Liebow and colleagues[37] in 1972, under the term *lymphomatoid granulomatosis*. These workers studied 40 patients with a tumoral condition that shared features of two different processes: lymphoma and Wegener's granulomatosis. LYG very rarely displays multinucleated giant cells on histopathologic examination, however. The histopathologic hallmark of this lesion, angiocentricity, also has been noted in other lymphomas of the lung.[2] In 1979, Katzenstein and associates[38] further analyzed 152 cases of LYG, including 36 of the 40 cases initially described in 1972 and 12 other cases that had already been reported in the literature. This study, which constitutes the largest series of patients with LYG to date, highlights several important characteristics of this process: Patient age spans a broad spectrum ranging from 7 to 85 years; 12 patients were younger than 20 years and 8 were older than 70 years. Although the tumors were more common in men than in women, the predominance was not marked (1.7:1). Clinical signs and symptoms in these patients ranged from pulmonary to more systemic manifestations, including cough, chest pain, shortness of breath, fever, weight loss, and malaise. Four patients were completely asymptomatic. A reticulonodular infiltrate was present on the initial chest radiograph in all patients, although unilateral involvement was seen in only 29 patients; bilateral lung disease was the most common finding. Extrapulmonary manifestations also were recorded: 39% of the patients had skin rash or nodules, 30% had neurologic involvement, and 30% had organomegaly (splenomegaly or hepatomegaly). Autopsy findings were available in 72 cases, disclosing renal involvement in one third of the cases. In four patients, results of a Monospot or heterophile antibody test were positive, although none of the patients exhibited the full-blown clinical picture of infectious mononucleosis, a condition that also has been linked to EBV infection. The investigators also noted that the giant cells that are commonly seen in Wegener's granulomatosis are absent in LYG.

With the use of modern immunohistochemistry, new discoveries were made, and in 1982, Nichols and associates[39] reported a single case in which they suggested the possibility that LYG is a T cell lymphoproliferative disorder. Similar findings were documented by other researchers.[40,41] Also in 1982, in a case report presented by Veltri and colleagues,[42] LYG manifested initially as a reactivated EBV infection. The investigators suggested a possible role for EBV in the pathogenesis of this condition.

Other groups of investigators, in describing a spectrum of differentiation for these lesions, had introduced the term *benign lymphocytic angiitis and granulomatosis*,[43–45] which was later modified to *angiocentric immunoproliferative lesion* (AIL), with a corresponding grading system.[46,47] This grading system depends on the presence of cytologic atypia and necrosis, with grade I representing a benign condition likely to respond to conservative treatment or chemotherapy and grades II and III more suggestive of malignancy.[47] In a study of 28 patients, Pisani and DeRemee[48] suggested that LYG may represent a histopathologic change that occurs transiently in several disease processes. In a subsequent editorial, LYG was presented in unequivocal terms as a specific clinicopathologic process, rather than a "transient" histopathologic finding.[49] More recently, Haque and associates[50] studied 11 patients with LYG who also were affected by the acquired immunodeficiency syndrome (AIDS). These investigators identified the presence of *EBV1*-encoded RNA and CD20-positive cells by double labeling and concluded that AIDS-associated LYG is a B cell neoplasm, and that it has a strong association with EBV infection.

In the World Health Organization's (WHO) latest edition of *Tumours of the Lung, Pleura, Thymus, and Heart*, LYG is defined as a lymphoproliferative disorder, composed of a polymorphous infiltrate of atypical-appearing EBV-infected B cells, and numerically more abundant admixed reactive T cells.[51] In addition, a histologic grading system based on the number of EBV-infected cells is provided. Grade 1 lesions contain fewer than 5 cells per high-power field and no necrosis; grade 2 lesions contain 5 to 20 EBV-infected cells per high-power field, with foci of necrosis; and grade 3 lesions show sheets of EBV-infected cells per high-power field, necrosis, and cellular monomorphism. Grade 3 lesions are considered to represent a subtype of diffuse large B cell lymphoma.

Histopathologic Features

Macroscopically, the lung parenchyma shows numerous intraparenchymal tumor nodules that may range in size from 1 cm to more than 5 cm in diameter. The nodules appear to be well circumscribed and are white to tan in color, with a firm consistency, with or without necrotic areas seen on the cut surface.

On histologic examination, the low-power view may demonstrate pulmonary nodules in a subpleural location (Fig. 10-25), an intraparenchymal nodule, or an ill-defined pulmonary interstitial infiltrate. On the high-power view, a polymorphous cellular infiltrate composed of large atypical lymphoid cells is seen admixed with small lymphocytes, plasma cells, and histiocytes. The larger cells have round to oval nuclei with prominent nucleoli. Binucleated cells also are commonly seen, and in some areas of the tumor they may resemble Reed-Sternberg cells. The most important feature of LYG is the presence of an angioinvasive and angiodestructive lesion that shows a malignant vasculitis with transmural infiltration of tumor cells in the walls of medium-sized and large vessels. Often, the transmural infiltration can be so marked that the tumor cells may obliterate the vascular lumen. Areas of necrosis also are an important feature for the diagnosis of LYG (Figs. 10-26 to 10-30).

Immunohistochemical Features

It is now accepted that LYG is a B cell clonal population expressing EBV (Fig. 10-31). In addition, the tumor shows numerous T polyclonal cells. In a study by Medeiros and coworkers,[52] eight cases were evaluated by molecular analysis to assess clonality, using restriction fragment analysis, the Southern blot technique, and probes to assess the configuration of the T cell receptor β, γ, and δ chain genes and the immunoglobulin heavy and κ light chain genes. These workers concluded that gene rearrangements are rare and identifed only one case (a grade III angiocentric immunoproliferative lesion) with rearrangement of the T cell receptor δ chain genes. In the remaining cases, no evidence of clonality was demonstrated. On the basis of these findings, the investigators concluded that angiocentric immunoproliferative lesions recapitulate other, similar lesions that occur in immunosuppressed patients.

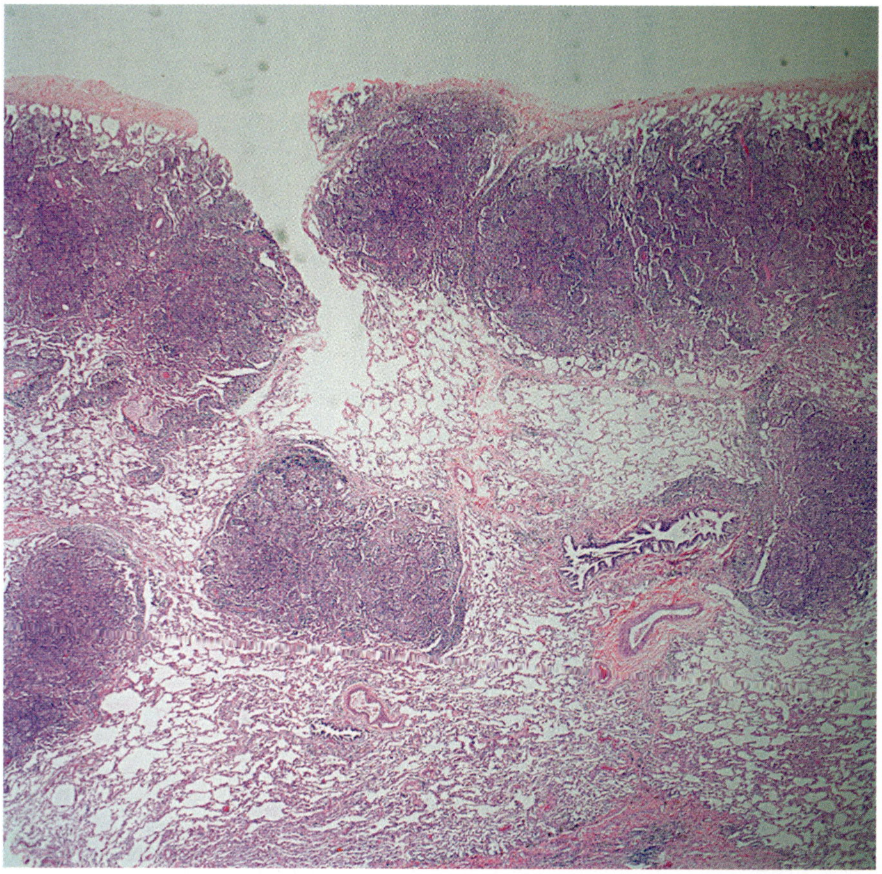

Figure 10-25 Lymphomatoid granulomatosis with several subpleural tumor nodules.

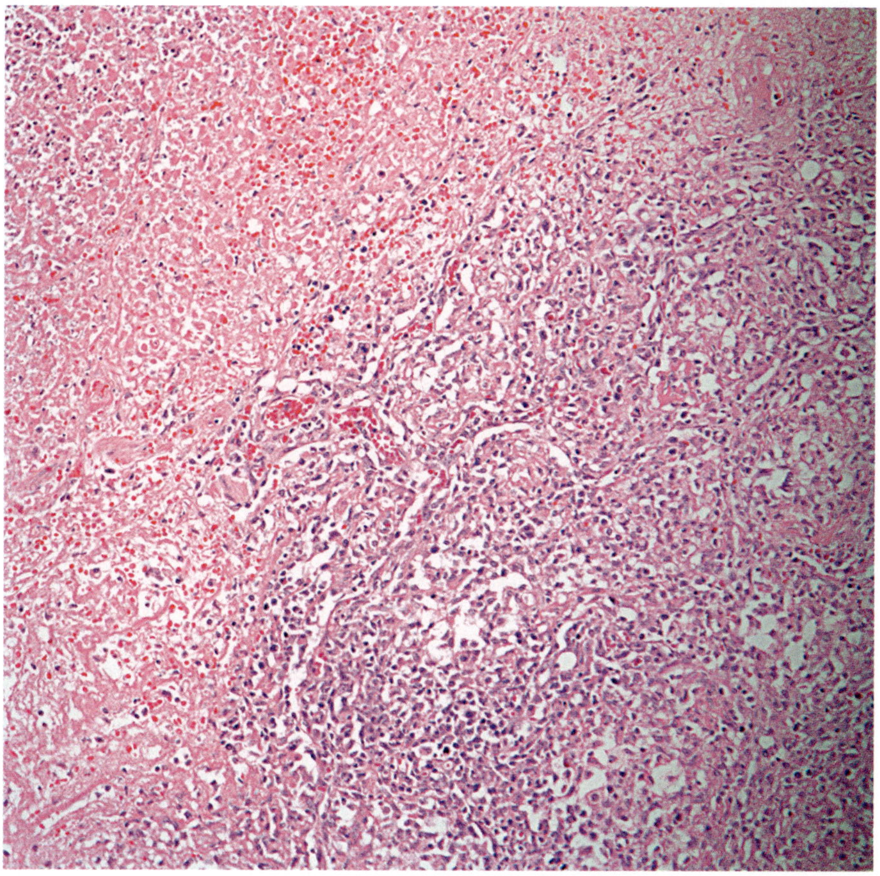

Figure 10-26 Lymphomatoid granulomatosis showing extensive necrosis.

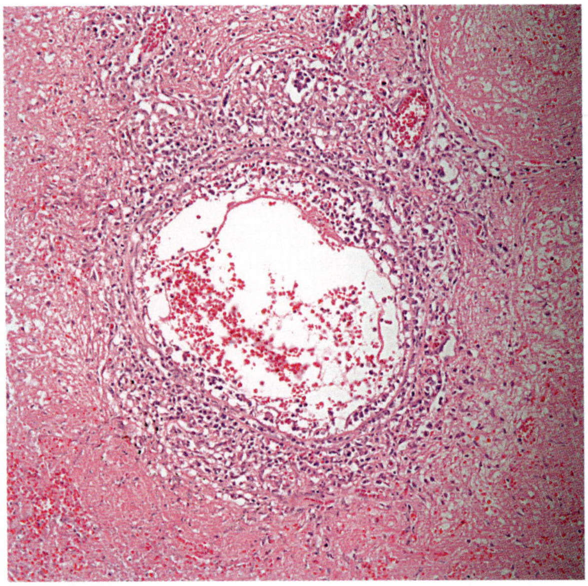

Figure 10-27 Lymphomatoid granulomatosis. Vascular structure in the middle of extensive necrosis shows neoplastic involvement.

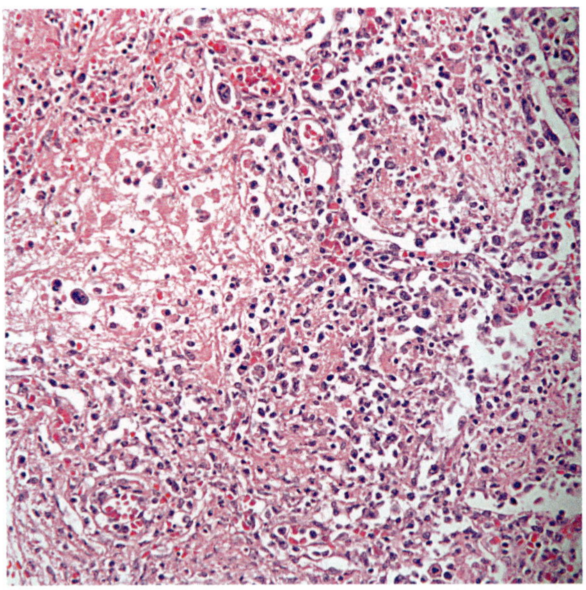

Figure 10-28 Lymphomatoid granulomatosis showing an atypical lymphoid proliferation with fibrinoid necrosis.

Differential Diagnosis

The most important considerations in the differential diagnosis are other types of lymphomas and an inflammatory benign infiltrate. When another lymphoproliferative tumor is suspected, a wider immunohistochemical panel of studies will aid in determining the correct interpretation. The presence of atypical cells, necrosis, and prominent angiocentric and angiodestructive changes should alert the pathologist to the possibility of a neoplastic process, rather than an inflammatory reaction. The possibility of a peripheral T cell lymphoma with involvement of the lung parenchyma also should be considered. Up to 20% of patients with peripheral T cell lymphomas may have pulmonary involvement at presentation, and in another 20%, pulmonary involvement will develop during the clinical course.[53] Therefore, good clinical and radiologic correlation is advised in this setting.

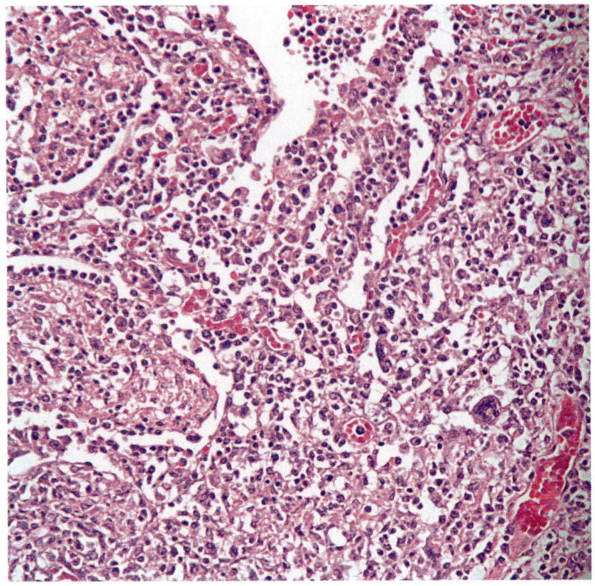

Figure 10-29 Lymphomatoid granulomatosis showing more viable areas of an atypical lymphoid proliferation. Note the presence of larger atypical cells.

Treatment and Prognosis

In the larger series of cases reported by Katzenstein and associates,[38] approximately two thirds of the patients died, with a median survival of 14 months. This study identified several favorable and unfavorable features for prognosis. Favorable clinical features included lack of symptoms and unilateral pulmonary involvement with histologic absence of atypical lymphoreticular cells. Unfavorable features included younger age at diagnosis (before the age of 25 years), neurologic manifestation, hepatomegaly, and the presence of atypical lymphoreticular cells. The investigators did not identify any particular mode of treatment, although the use of corticosteroids was suggested to be helpful. In a study of 42 patients, Koss and colleagues[51] documented that 38% of the patients died of their disease, most within 12 months of initial diagnosis. These workers did not find that increased atypical multinucleated cells in the initial biopsy were statistically significant predictors of survival.

Regarding therapy, Fauci and associates[54] described their 10-year experience with management of LYG in 15 patients, 13 of whom were treated with cyclophosphamide and prednisone. Of these 13 patients, 7 had complete remission lasting for approximately 5 years, whereas other

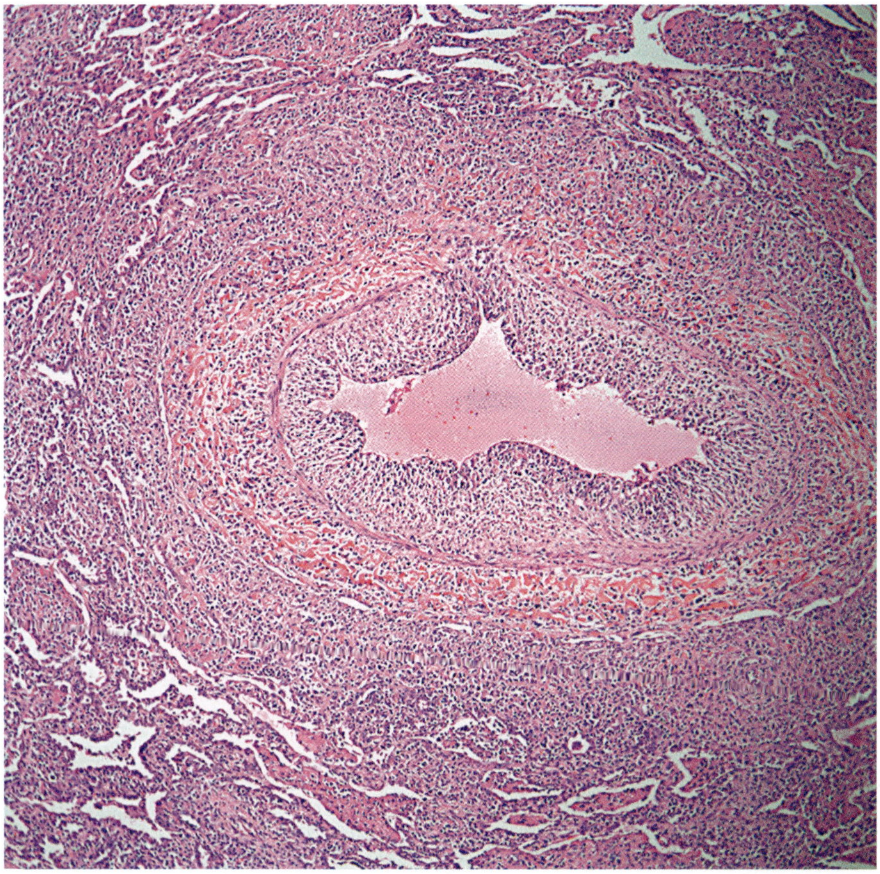

Figure 10-30 Extensive transmural involvement of a large vessel by lymphomatoid granulomatosis.

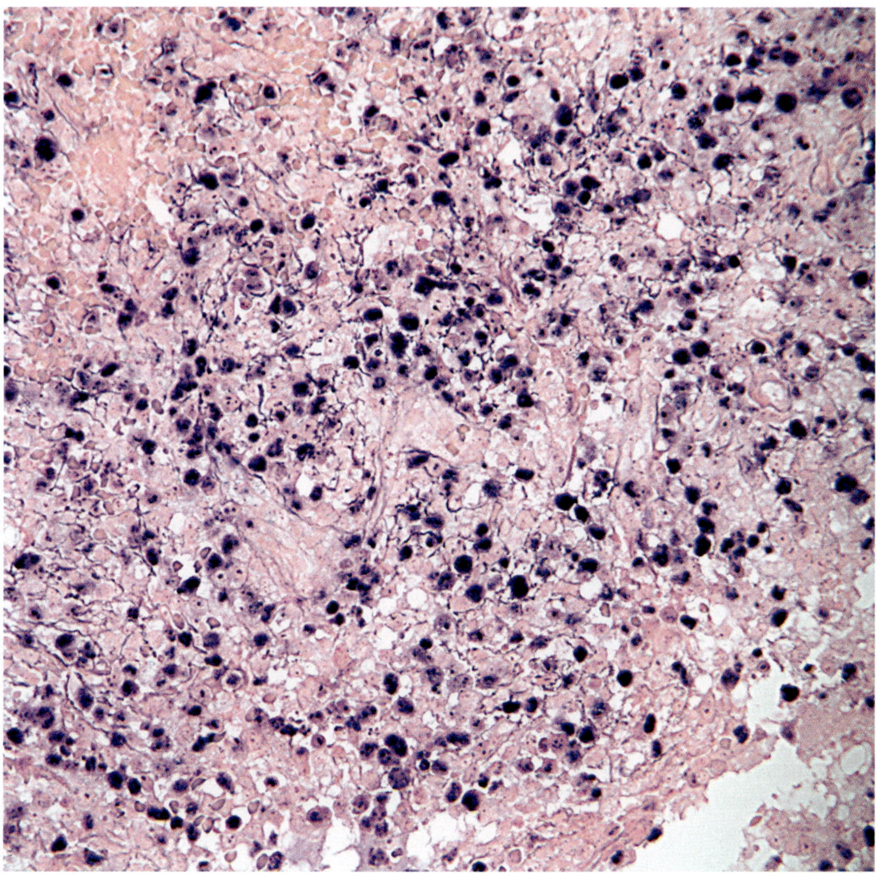

Figure 10-31 Immunohistochemical staining for Epstein-Barr virus is positive in numerous cells in lymphomatoid granulomatosis.

patients went on to develop lymphoma. These investigators suggested that early recognition and treatment might prevent the development of a "lymphoid neoplasm."

PRIMARY PULMONARY HODGKIN'S LYMPHOMA

The reported cases of primary pulmonary Hodgkin's lymphoma date back more than 70 years. It is possible that the pathologic process in these early reported cases may not necessarily have been a primary lung neoplasm, however, but may have been an extension of mediastinal or other extrathoracic tumors into the lung. In 1961, Kern and colleagues[55] documented four cases of primary pulmonary Hodgkin's lymphoma in the lung and carefully analyzed the current literature up to that year. These workers accepted only 14 previous cases as possible primary lung tumors, including only those for which the following data were available: histopathologic diagnosis, photomicrographs or microscopic description, and predominant disease in the lung with or without simultaneous involvement of hilar or mediastinal lymph nodes. Of their 4 reported cases and the 14 cases gathered from the literature, 8 were in men and 10 were in women between the ages of 18 and 75 years, with a median age of 40 years. Five patients were asymptomatic, and the tumor was discovered on a routine chest radiograph, whereas the remaining patients had clinical signs and symptoms including cough, chest pain, fever, and pruritus, among others. On radiologic evaluation, 15 patients were found to have a single pulmonary mass. In some of these patients, involvement of major bronchi was identified, suggesting more extensive disease. The resected specimens ranged in size from 3-cm tumor nodules to tumor masses occupying an entire lobe. In this review by Kern's group,[55] no lymph node involvement was identified, and the tumor was limited to the lung.

More than 20 years later, Yousem and associates[56] reported their experience with 15 cases thought to represent primary pulmonary Hodgkin's lymphoma. The study criteria for inclusion of cases were (1) histopathologic features of Hodgkin's lymphoma; (2) restriction of the process to the lung without hilar lymph node involvement; and (3) adequate clinical or pathologic exclusion of tumor at distant sites. Patient age ranged from 19 to 82 years, and women outnumbered men in a proportion of 2:1. The most common clinical signs and symptoms included cough, fever, and weight loss; two patients were asymptomatic. Of the 15 patients, 7 had unilateral involvement and the remaining 8 had bilateral involvement.

Radin[57] evaluated 155 cases of Hodgkin's lymphoma over an 8-year period in an attempt to estimate the incidence of Hodgkin's lymphoma in the lung. This investigator found that 88 patients (56%) had intrathoracic involvement at presentation; in 18 patients (11%) pulmonary parenchymal disease was evident, but the lymphoma was limited to the lung in only one patient. These previous studies highlight the unusual occurrence of Hodgkin's lymphoma as a primary lung neoplasm and speak in favor of complete clinical and radiologic evaluation in cases in which primary Hodgkin's lymphoma in the lung is suspected, to rule out a possible extrapulmonary tumor.

Histopathologic Features

On macroscopic examination, unilateral lung involvement may manifest as a single pulmonary mass; multiple pulmonary nodules are typical of bilateral disease (Fig. 10-32). The tumors may range in size from 2 cm to more than 5 cm and may involve extensive areas of a pulmonary lobe. The tumor nodule or mass may be soft in consistency, well circumscribed, and light tan or white; in some cases, areas of necrosis also have been documented.

On histologic examination, the growth patterns of Hodgkin's lymphoma of the lung are the same as those that have been recorded for extra-pulmonary Hodgkin's lymphoma—namely, nodular sclerosis, mixed cellularity, and lymphocyte predominance. Yousem and associates[56] documented several different growth patterns of Hodgkin's lymphoma in the lung, including nodular; diffuse, involving lymphatic routes; pneumonic; endobronchial; and subpleural. The histopathologic hallmark of Hodgkin's lymphoma, however, is the presence of Reed-Sternberg cells (Figs. 10-33 to 10-38). Immunohistochemical studies may prove helpful in the diagnosis of this lymphoma, and the use of CD15 (LeuM1) and CD30 will show positive staining in the Reed-Sternberg cells.

Differential Diagnosis

Anaplastic large cell lymphoma in the lung, occurring either as a primary neoplasm or as an extension from an extrathoracic tumor, is an important consideration in the differential diagnosis. The use of immunohistochemical stains for CD15, CD30, ALK, and EMA will be of help. Generally, ALCL shows negative staining

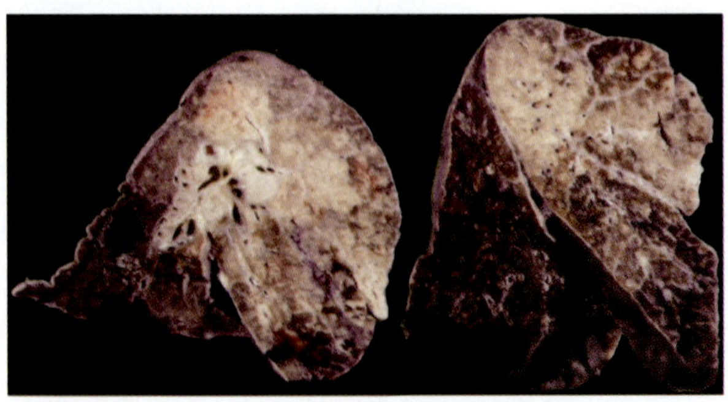

Figure 10-32 Lung showing numerous nodules of Hodgkin's lymphoma.

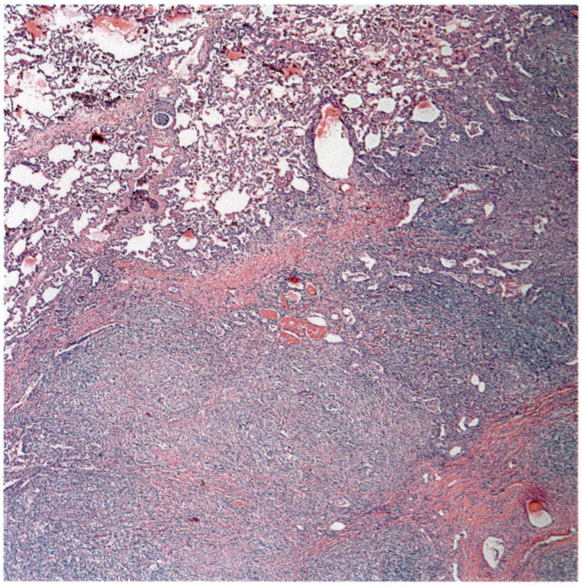

Figure 10-33 Hodgkin's lymphoma replacing normal lung parenchyma.

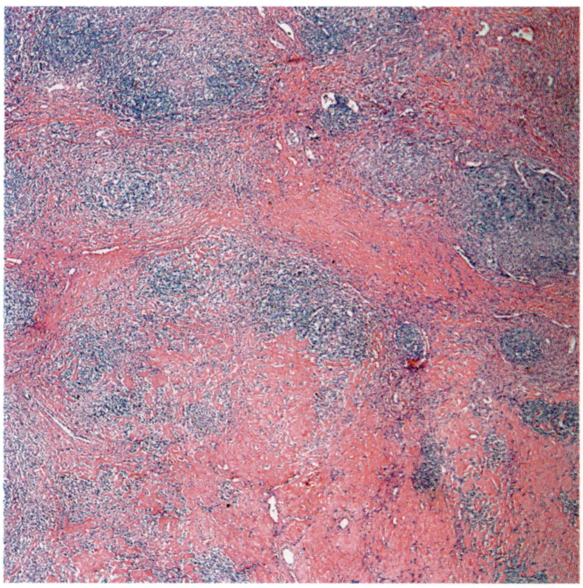

Figure 10-34 Hodgkin's lymphoma of the lung with extensive areas of collagen deposition, in keeping with the nodular sclerosing form of the disease.

for CD15, whereas the tumor may show positive staining for ALK, CD30, and EMA. Of course, other types of non-Hodgkin's lymphoma also should be considered, with proper histologic and immunohistochemical investigations. Use of a wider panel of immunostains including B cell and T cell markers should be of help.

Treatment and Prognosis

In the past, many patients diagnosed with primary Hodgkin's lymphoma of the lung were treated with surgery, which in some cases included radical procedures

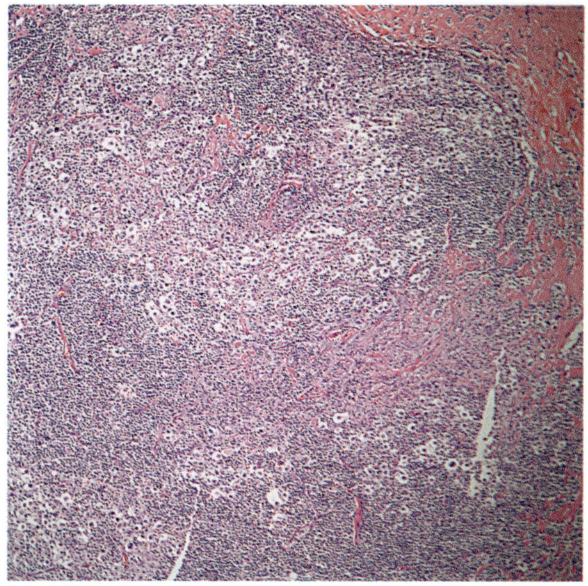

Figure 10-35 Hodgkin's lymphoma involving the lung. An atypical lymphoid proliferation can be seen.

such as pneumonectomy. In current practice, with more modern radiographic and histopathologic tools, it is possible in a majority of cases to arrive at a diagnosis with more limited procedures. Thus, many patients can be treated with chemotherapy instead of surgical resection. In some cases with extensive lung involvement, however, surgery may still be necessary. In cases reported by Yousem and associates,[56] the follow-up period in these patients has been variable. Some patients have remained alive without disease for up to 80 months, some patients have experienced recurrences, and some patients have died of their disease in follow-up periods ranging from 3 to 49 months.

MISCELLANEOUS TUMORS

Primary lung neoplasms that do not belong in the category of MALT-type lymphoma or LYG are exceedingly rare. Nevertheless, two such neoplasms have been described: plasmacytoma and mast cell tumor. Because these tumors may be associated with conditions such as multiple myeloma or mast cell disease, it is imperative to detect systemic involvement.

Plasmacytoma

The occurrence of primary plasmacytomas in the lung is extremely rare, and a few cases have been reported in the literature. It has been estimated that extramedullary plasmacytomas may occur in the lung in no more than 5% or 6% of all cases. A majority of the cases have been presented as single case reports.[58–67] These reports have documented an association with myeloma in only some of the cases; thus, it

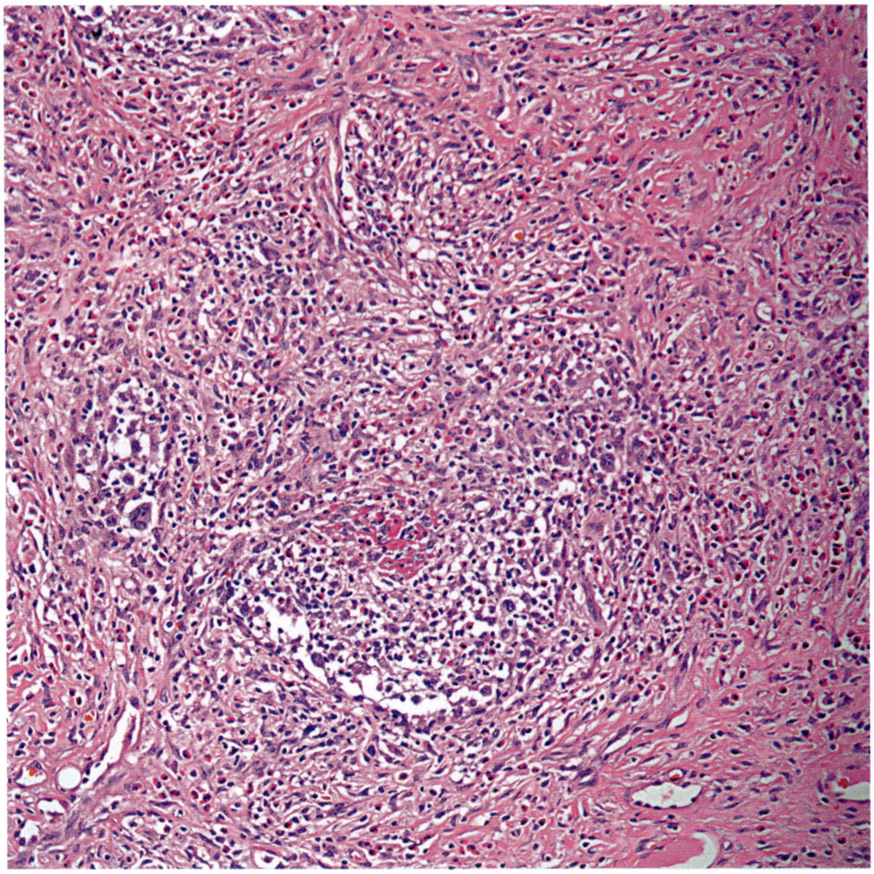

Figure 10-36 Hodgkin's lymphoma involving the lung. A tumor nodule composed of atypical cells can be seen associated with a large number of eosinophils.

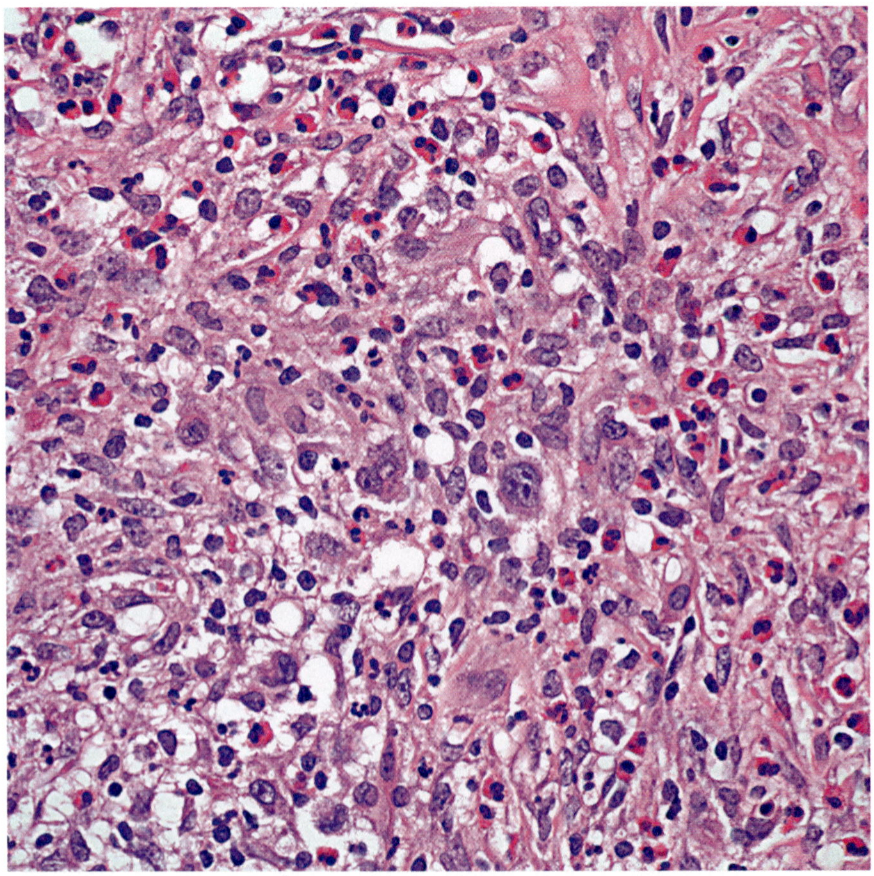

Figure 10-37 Hodgkin's lymphoma involving the lung. The Reed-Sternberg cells are associated with eosinophils.

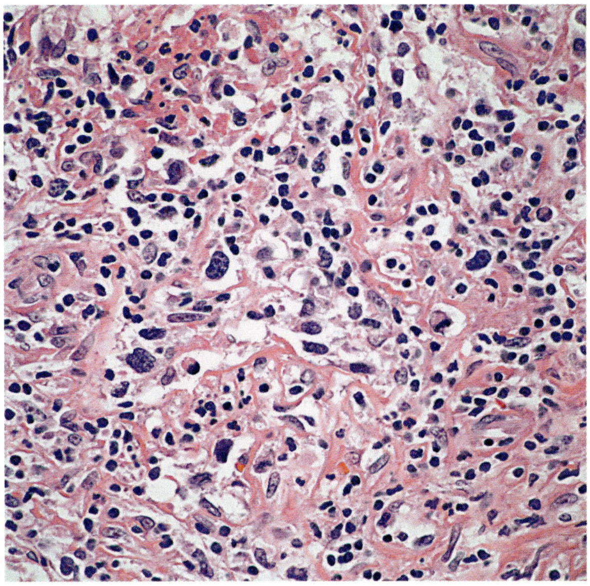

Figure 10-38 Hodgkin's lymphoma involving the lung. Reed-Sternberg cells can be seen without the presence of eosinophils.

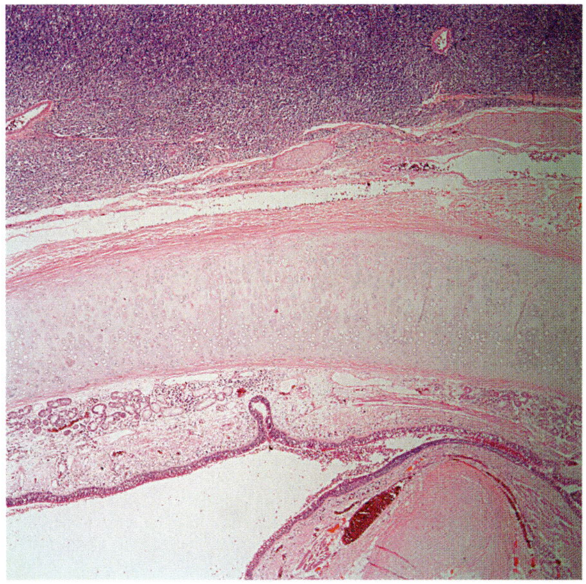

Figure 10-39 Primary plasmacytoma of the lung manifesting as a central tumor.

is imperative to properly rule out this possibility in cases in which the patient presents with a pulmonary tumor. All of the cases described in the single reports have been in adult patients older than 50 years of age.

Koss and associates[62] reported a study of five patients with pulmonary plasmacytoma (four men and one woman between the ages of 50 and 79 years). Two of the patients presented with pulmonary signs and symptoms, including cough, dyspnea, and hemoptysis. One patient had a monoclonal gammopathy, IgG-κ chain, but the bone marrow biopsy did not show myeloma; one patient was asymptomatic. In two additional patients, findings on bone marrow examination and serum protein electrophoresis were normal.

Pathological Features

The anatomic location of these tumors may be in the hilum or within the lung parenchyma. Tumor size ranges from 2 to 8 cm in greatest dimension. They appear to be yellowish or gray in color and well circumscribed, with a firm consistency.

On histologic examination, the tumors are characterized by a homogeneous cellular proliferation destroying lung parenchyma (Fig. 10-39). In focal areas, the tumor appears to show a subtle nested pattern (Fig. 10-40), whereas in other areas, a vascular-like growth pattern is apparent (Fig. 10-41). Higher magnification shows a fairly homogeneous cellular proliferation composed of medium-sized cells with light eosinophilic cytoplasm and eccentrically placed nuclei (Figs. 10-42 to 10-44). Nuclear atypia ranging from mild to moderate in degree can be seen in these cases. Areas of necrosis, amyloid deposition, and mitotic activity also may be features. Peribronchial lymph nodes may or may not be involved. Immunohistochemically, the plasma cell proliferation shows monoclonality using stains for κ and λ light chains, and the plasma cells also may show focal positive staining for EMA.

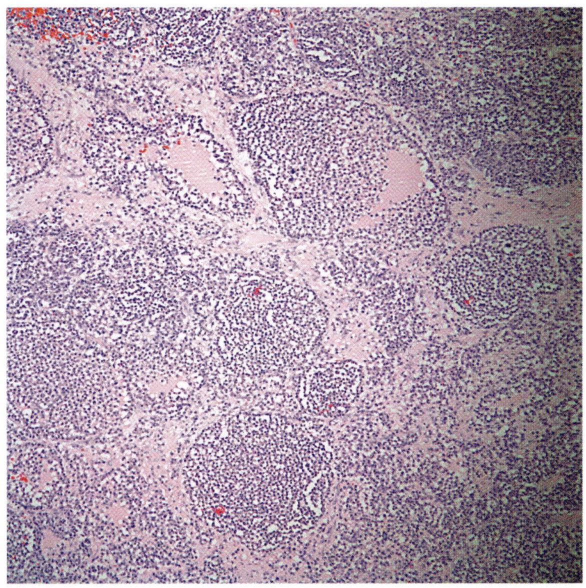

Figure 10-40 Plasmacytoma with a subtle nested pattern of growth.

Treatment and Prognosis

In the series of cases presented by Koss and associates,[62] the patients underwent surgical resection of the tumor,

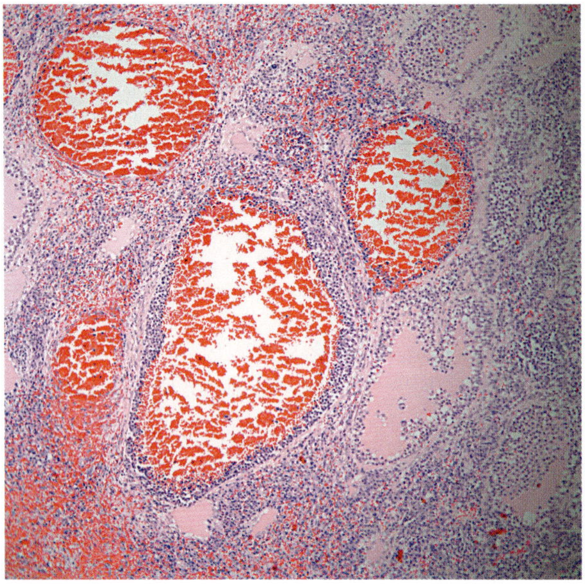

Figure 10-41 Plasmacytoma with a vascular-like pattern of growth.

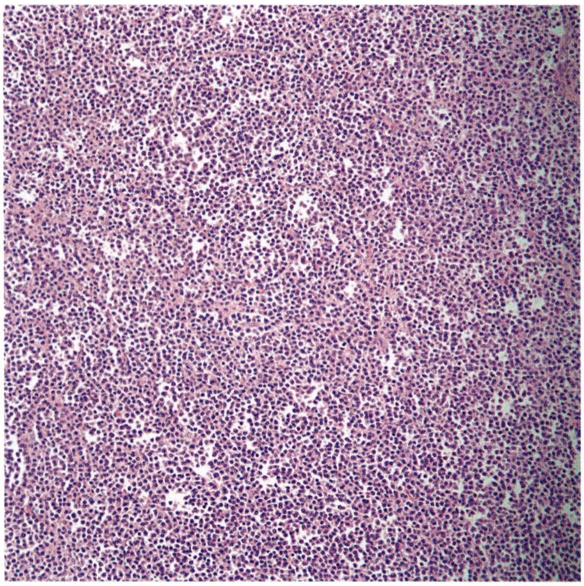

Figure 10-42 Plasmacytoma with sheets of a homogeneous cellular proliferation.

with procedures ranging from segmentectomy to lobectomy to pneumonectomy. The median follow-up period was 36 months; two patients who survived longer than 20 years died of unrelated conditions, whereas two other patients died 28 months after surgery. The investigators also compared their cases with those previously reported in the literature and estimated overall 2- and 5-year survival rates for patients with pulmonary plasmacytoma to be 66% and 40%, respectively. Thus, as noted by Koss and associates, patients with pulmonary plasmacytoma have the potential for long-term survival.

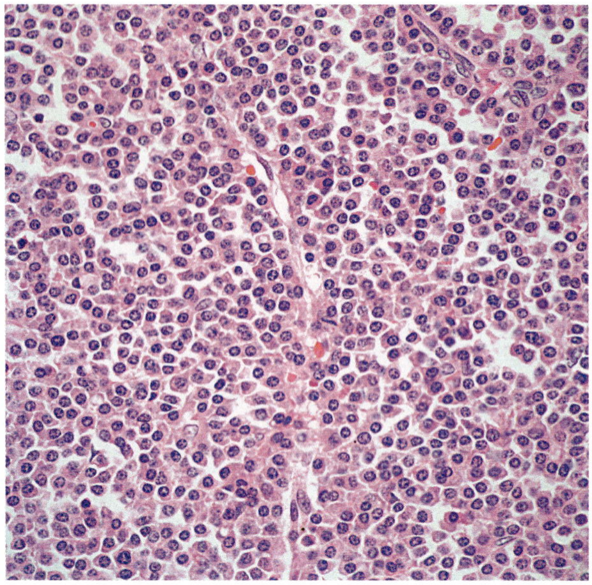

Figure 10-43 High-power view of a plasmacytoma of the lung showing a homogeneous cellular proliferation with mild nuclear atypia.

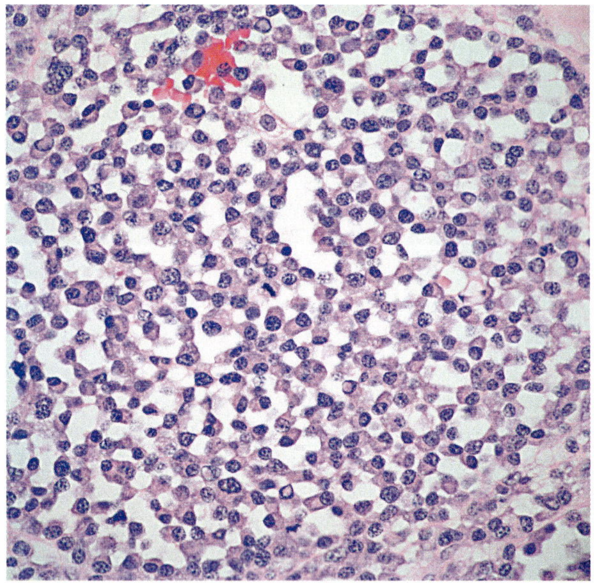

Figure 10-44 High-power view of a primary plasmacytoma of the lung showing moderate cellular atypia and scattered mitotic figures.

Mast Cell Tumor

Only a few cases of mast cell tumor have been reported in the literature.[68,69] Charrette and associates[68] described a 68-year-old man who presented with a 2-cm lung mass but was otherwise asymptomatic, and in whom findings on physical examination were within normal limits. A similar case, in a 53-year-old man, was presented by Kudo and coworkers.[69] Surgical resection of the mass was performed in both patients.

Histologically, the tumors were characterized by a diffuse proliferation of mononuclear cells with basophilic cytoplasm and abundant granules, and small hyperchromatic nuclei. Nuclear atypia, mitotic activity, and necrosis are usually not seen in these tumors. Immunohistochemical studies have been reported to show negative staining for keratin, lysozyme, and surfactant protein. Before a definitive diagnosis of mast cell tumor can be established, it is important to rule out other possibilities, such as plasmacytoma or another lymphoproliferative disorder. Thus, the use of a wider panel of immunohistochemical stains is important.

Owing to the unusual occurrence of this tumor in the lung, its pattern of clinical behavior is difficult to assess.

REFERENCES

1. Rabiah FA. Primary lymphocytic lymphoma (lymphosarcoma) of the lung. *Am Surg.* 1968;34:275.
2. Colby TV, Carrington CB. Pulmonary lymphomas simulating lymphomatoid granulomatosis. *Am J Surg Pathol.* 1982;6:19–32.
3. Bienenstock J, Johnston N, Perey DY. Bronchial lymphoid tissue. I. Morphologic characteristics. *Lab Invest.* 1973;28:688.
4. Bienenstock J, Johnston N, Perey DY. Bronchial lymphoid tissue. II. Functional characteristics. *Lab Invest.* 1973;28:695.
5. Saltzstein SL. Pulmonary malignant lymphoma and pseudolymphoma: classification, therapy and prognosis. *Cancer.* 1963;16:928.
6. Kradin RL, Mark EJ. Benign lymphoid disorders of the lung, with a theory regarding their development. *Hum Pathol.* 1983;14:857–867.
7. Papaioannou AN, Watson WL. Primary lymphoma of the lung: an appraisal of its natural history and a comparison with other localized lymphomas. *J Thorac Cardiovasc Surg.* 1965;49:373–386.
8. Koss MN, Hochholzer L, Nichols PW, Wehunt WD, Lazarus AA. Primary non-Hodgkin's lymphoma and pseudolymphoma of lung: a study of 161 patients. *Hum Pathol.* 1983;14:1024–1038.
9. Herbert A, Wright DH, Isaacson PG, Smith JL. Primary malignant lymphoma of the lung: histopathologic and immunohistochemical evaluation of nine cases. *Hum Pathol.* 1984;15:415–422.
10. L'Hoste RJ, Filipa DA, Lieberman PH, Bretsky S. Primary pulmonary lymphoma: a clinicopathologic study of 36 cases. *Cancer.* 1984;54:1397–1406.
11. Addis BJ, Hyjek E, Isaacson PG. Primary pulmonary lymphoma: a re-appraisal of its histogenesis and its relationship to pseudolymphoma and lymphoid interstitial pneumonia. *Histopathology.* 1988;13:1–17.
12. Elenitoba K, Medeiros LJ, Khorsand J, King TC. Lymphoma of the mucosa-associated lymphoid tissue of the lung. *Am J Clin Pathol.* 1995;103:341–345.
13. Nicholson AG, Wotherspoon AC, Diss TC, et al. Pulmonary B-cell non-Hodgkin's lymphomas. The value of immunohistochemistry and gene analysis in diagnosis. *Histopathology.* 1995;26:395–403.
14. Tamura A, Komatsu H, Yanai N, et al. Primary pulmonary lymphoma: relationship between clinical features and pathologic findings in 24 cases. The Japan National Chest Hospital Study Group for Lung Cancer. *Jpn J Clin Oncol.* 1995;25:140–152.
15. Li G, Hansmann ML, Zwingers T, Lennert K. Primary lymphomas of the lung: morphological, immunohistochemical and clinical features. *Histopathology.* 1990;16:519–531.
16. Teruya-Feldstein J, Temeck BK, Sloas MM, et al. Pulmonary malignant lymphoma of mucosa-associated lymphoid tissue (MALT) arising in a pediatric HIV-positive patient. *Am J Surg Pathol.* 1995;19:357–363.
17. Tamura A, Kitagawa M, Komatsu H, et al. Does an Epstein-Barr viral infection influence the pathogenesis of a primary pulmonary B-cell lymphoma? *Lung.* 1995;173:385–387.
18. Motoishi M, Enokibori T, Katsuki Y, Tsuchiya M, Hatakenaka R. Mucosa-associated lymphoid tissue lymphoma involving lung and conjunctiva. *J Thorac Cardiovasc Surg.* 2008;56:246–248.
19. Chow WH, Ducheine Y, Hilfer J, Brandstetter RD. Primary malignant non-Hodgkin's lymphoma of the lung arising in mucosa-associated lymphoid tissue. *Chest.* 1996;110:838–840.
20. Váróczy L, Gergely L, Illés A. Diagnostics and treatment of pulmonary BALT lymphoma: a report of four cases. *Ann Hematol.* 2003;82:363–366.
21. Papiris SA, Kalomenidis I, Malagari K, et al. Extranodal marginal zone B-cell lymphoma of the lung in Sjögren's syndrome patients: reappraisal of clinical, radiological and pathology findings. *Respir Med.* 2007;101:84–92.
22. Wislez M, Cadranel J, Antoine M, et al. Lymphoma of pulmonary mucosa-associated lymphoid tissue: CT scan findings and pathological correlations. *Eur Respir J.* 1999;14:423–429.
23. Bae YA, Lee KS, Han J, et al. Marginal zone B-cell lymphoma of bronchus-associated lymphoid tissue: imaging findings in 21 patients. *Chest.* 2008;133:433–440.
24. Ahmed S, Kussick SJ, Siddiqui A, et al. Bronchial-associated lymphoid tissue lymphoma: a clinical study of a rare disease. *Eur J Cancer.* 2004;40:1320–1326.
25. Zinzani PL, Tani M, Gabriele A, et al. Extranodal marginal zone B-cell lymphoma of MALT type of the lung: single-center experience with 12 patients. *Leuk Lymphoma.* 2003;44:821–824.
26. Béguerel H, Vergier B, Parrens M, et al. Primary lung small B-cell lymphoma versus lymphoid hyperplasia: evaluation of diagnostic criteria in 26 cases. *Am J Surg Pathol.* 2002;26:76–81.
27. Chuang SS, Liu H, Ye H, et al. Pulmonary mucosa–associated lymphoid tissue lymphoma with strong nuclear 10 (BCL10) expression and novel translocation t(1;2)(p22;p12)/immunoglobulin kappa chain-BCL10. *J Clin Pathol.* 2007;60:727–728.
28. Koss MN, Hochholzer L, Langloss JM, Wehunt WD, Lazarus AA. Lymphoid interstitial pneumonia: clinicopathological and immunohistochemical findings in 18 cases. *Pathology.* 1987;19:178–185.
29. Costa MB, Siqueira SA, Saldiva PH, Rabe KF, Mauad T. Histologic patterns of lung infiltration of B-cell, T-cell, and Hodgkin's lymhoma. *Am J Clin Pathol.* 2004;121:718–726.
30. Vallisa D, Trabacchi E, Cavanna L. Primary lung lymphoma. *Curr Drug Targets Inflamm Allergy.* 2004;3:469–471.
31. Ferraro P, Trastek VF, Adlakha H, Deschamps C, Allen MS, Pairolero PC. Primary non-Hodgkin's lymphoma of the lung. *Ann Thorac Surg.* 2000;69:993–997.
32. Troch M, Streubel B, Petkov V, Turetschek K, Chott A, Raderer M. Does MALT lymphoma of the lung require immediate treatment? An analysis of 11 untreated cases with long-term follow up. *Anticancer Res.* 2007;27:3633–3638.
33. Nicholson AG, Wotherspoon AC, Jones AL, Sheppard MN, Isaacson PG, Corrin B. Pulmonary B-cell non-Hodgkin's lymphoma associated with autoimmune disorders: a clinicopathological review of six cases. *Eur Respir J.* 1996;9:2022–2025.
34. Orchard TR, Eraut CD, Davison AG. Non-Hodgkin's lymphoma arising in cryptogenic fibrosing alveolitis. *Thorax.* 1998;53:228–229.
35. Rush WL, Andriko JA, Taubenberger JK, et al. Primary anaplastic large cell lymphoma of the lung: a clinicopathologic study of five patients. *Mod Pathol.* 2002;13:1285–1292.
36. Yang HB, Li J, Shen T. Primary anaplastic large cell lymphoma of the lung: report of two cases and literature review. *Acta Haematol.* 2007;118:188–191.
37. Liebow AA, Carrington CR, Friedman PJ. Lymphomatoid granulomatosis. *Hum Pathol.* 1972;3:457–558.
38. Katzenstein AL, Carrington CB, Liebow AA. Lymphomatoid granulomatosis: a clinicopathologic study of 152 cases. *Cancer.* 1979;43:360–373.
39. Nichols PW, Koss MN, Levine AM, Lukes RJ. Lymphomatoid granulomatosis: a T-cell disorder? *Am J Med.* 1982;72:467–471.

40. Gaulard P, Henni T, Marolleau JP, et al. Lethal midline granuloma (polymorphic reticulosis) and lymphomatoid granulomatosis. Evidence for a monoclonal T-cell lymphoproliferative disorder. *Cancer*. 1988;62:705–710.
41. Whitaker S, Foroni L, Luzzatto L, et al. Lymphomatoid granulomatosis—evidence of a clonal T-cell origin and an association with lethal midline granuloma. *Q J Med.* 1988;68:645–655.
42. Veltri RW, Raich PC, McClung JE, Shah SH, Sprinkle PM. Lymphomatoid granulomatosis and Epstein-Barr virus. *Cancer*. 1982;50:1513–1517.
43. Saldana MJ, Patchefsky AS, Israel AI, Atkinson GW. Pulmonary angiitis and granulomatosis. The relationship between histological features, organ involvement, and response to treatment. *Hum Pathol.* 1977;8:392–409.
44. Weiss MA, Rolfes DB, Alvira MA, Cohen LJ. Benign lymphocytic angiitis and granulomatosis: a case report with evidence of an autoimmune etiology. *Am J Clin Pathol.* 1984;81:110–116.
45. Gracey DR, DeRemee RA, Colby TV, Unni KK, Weiland LH. Benign lymphocytic angiitis and granulomatosis: experience with three cases. *Mayo Clin Proc.* 1988;63:323–331.
46. Jaffe ES. Pathologic and clinical spectrum of post-thymic T-cell malignancies. *Cancer*. 1984;2:413.
47. Lipford EH, Margolick JB, Longo DL, Fauci AS, Jaffe ES. Angiocentric immunoproliferative lesions: a clinicopathologic spectrum of post-thymic T-cell proliferations. *Blood.* 1988;72:1674–1681.
48. Pisani R, DeRemee R. Clinical implications of the histopathologic diagnosis of pulmonary lymphomatoid granulomatosis. *Mayo Clin Proc.* 1990;65:151–163.
49. Myers JL. Lymphomatoid granulomatosis: past, present, …future? *Mayo Clin Proc.* 1990;65:274–278.
50. Haque AK, Myers JL, Hudnall SD, et al. Pulmonary lymphomatoid granulomatosis in acquired immunodeficiency syndrome: lesions with Epstein-Barr virus infection. *Mod Pathol.* 1998;11:347–356.
51. Koss MN, Harris NL. Lymphomatoid granulomatosis. In: Travis WD, Brambilla E, Müller-Hermelink HK, Harris CC, eds. *Tumours of the Lung, Pleura, Thymus, and Heart. World Health Organization Classification of Tumours*. Lyon, France: IARC Press; 2004:92–94.
52. Medeiros LJ, Peiper SC, Elwood L, Yano T, Raffeld M, Jaffe ES. Angiocentric immunoproliferative lesions: a molecular analysis of eight cases. *Hum Pathol.* 1991;22:1150–1157.
53. Harrison NK, Twelves C, Addis BJ, Taylor AJ, Souhami RL, Isaacson PG. Peripheral T-cell lymphoma presenting with angioedema and diffuse pulmonary infiltrates. *Am Rev Respir Dis.* 1988;138:976–980.
54. Fauci AS, Haynes BF, Costa J, Katz P, Wolff SM. Lymphomatoid granulomatosis: prospective clinical and therapeutic experience over 10 years. *N Engl J Med.* 1982;306:68–74.
55. Kern WH, Crepeau AG, Jones JC. Primary Hodgkin's disease of the lung: report of 4 cases and review of the literature. *Cancer*. 1961;14:1151–1165.
56. Yousem SA, Weiss LM, Colby TV. Primary pulmonary Hodgkin's disease: a clinicopathologic study of 15 cases. *Cancer*. 1986;57:1217–1224.
57. Radin AI. Primary pulmonary Hodgkin's disease. *Cancer*. 1990;65:550–563.
58. Kazzas B, Dewar A, Corrin B. An unusual pulmonary plasmacytoma. *Histopathology*. 1992;21:285–287.
59. Piard F, Yaziji N, Jarry O, et al. Solitary plasmacytoma of the lung with light chain extracellular deposits: a case report and review of the literature. *Histopathology*. 1998;32:356–361.
60. Chen KY, Wu HD, Chang YL, Shih JY, Yang PC. Primary pulmonary plasmacytoma with lobar consolidation: an unusual presentation. *J Formos Med Assoc.* 1998;97:507–510.
61. Koss MN, Hocholzer L, Moran CA, Frizzera G. Pulmonary plasmacytomas: a clinicopathologic and immunohistochemical study of five cases. *Ann Diagn Pathol.* 1998;2:1–11.
62. Wise JN, Schaefer RF, Read RC. Primary pulmonary plasmacytoma. *Chest.* 2001;120:1405–1407.
63. Lattin BH, Blanke CD, Deloughery TG. Pulmonary and intracerebral plasmacytoma in a patient without multiple myeloma: a case report. *Am J Hematol.* 2003;73:131–134.
64. Niitsu N, Kohri M, Hayama M, et al. Primary pulmonary plasmacytoma involving bilateral lungs and marked hypergammaglobulinemia: differentiation from extranodal marginal zone B-cell lymphoma of mucosa-associated lymphoid tissue. *Leukemia Res.* 2005;29:1361–1364.
65. Marisavljevic D, Markovic O, Martinovic VC, Ponomarev D. Plasmacytoma of the lung: an indolent disease resistant to conventional myeloma treatment. *Med Oncol.* 2005;2:207–210.
66. Chang CC, Chang YL, Lee LN, Lee YC. Primary pulmonary plasmacytoma with immunoglobulin G/lambda light chain monoclonal gammopathy. *J Thorac Cardiovasc Surg.* 2006; 132:984–985.
67. Thoennissen NH, Schliemann C, Hungermann D, et al. Solitary plasmacytoma of the lung with coexisting sarcoid-like lesions. *Ann Hematol.* 2008;87:417–420.
68. Charrette EE, Mariano AV, Laforet EG. Solitary mast cell tumor of lung. *Arch Intern Med.* 1966;118:358–362.
69. Kudo H, Morinaga S, Shimosato Y, et al. Solitary mast cell tumor of the lung. *Cancer*. 1988;61:2089–2094.

11

Lung Tumors of Uncertain Histogenesis

CLEAR CELL "SUGAR" TUMOR OF THE LUNG
GRANULAR CELL TUMOR
INFLAMMATORY PSEUDOTUMOR
SCLEROSING HEMANGIOMA (PNEUMOCYTOMA)

This chapter describes a group of lung tumors characterized by uncertain histogenesis and very rare occurrence. Despite current advances in immunohistochemistry and molecular biology, definitive conclusions regarding the cellular origins of these neoplasms are still lacking. Although researchers have made progress in correcting erroneous concepts about the histogenesis of some of these tumors, very little information is available on others. The following tumors are discussed:

- Clear cell "sugar" tumor
- Granular cell tumor
- Inflammatory pseudotumor (IPT)
- Sclerosing hemangioma (pneumocytoma)

The most important clinical and immunohistochemical features for these entities are summarized in Tables 11-1 and 11-2, respectively.

CLEAR CELL "SUGAR" TUMOR OF THE LUNG

Benign clear cell tumors of the lung are unusual neoplasms that have been reported sporadically in the literature. Since its original description, this neoplasm has been described mainly in individual case reports or in small series that emphasize the elucidation of its histogenesis. Although several theories have been advanced, the true histogenesis of this neoplasm is not universally agreed upon.

Historical Aspects

The original description of the clear cell "sugar" tumor of the lung appeared in 1963, when Liebow and Castleman presented this new entity in an abstract.[1] In 1971, the same investigators[2] presented one of the largest series to date, consisting of 12 cases, and outlined most of the currently available information on these tumors. These workers noted that the colloquial name of "sugar tumor" derived from a chemical analysis in one case that demonstrated the presence of glycogen hexose—hence the term *sugar*. The clinical, macroscopic, and microscopic features presented in these 12 cases have been largely echoed in more recent descriptions of this particular tumor. Although Liebow and Castleman did not offer an explanation for its occurrence, they did acknowledge the possibility of a myoid origin by demonstrating histologic features that were similar to those of clear cell leiomyomas of the stomach and uterus.

A wide array of explanations for the origin of these tumors have been proposed. Becker and Soifer[3] described the tumor's ultrastructural features in a case in which glycogen was detected, comparing its distribution with that of glycogen in the livers of patients with Pompe's disease, and noting dense core neurosecretory granules in 2% to 5% of the cells. They suggested that these tumors derived from Kulschitzky cells. Andrion and colleagues[4] presented a case in which the tumor cells did not react with neuroendocrine markers and suggested a possible origin from epithelial nonciliated bronchiolar (Clara) cells or epithelial serous cells. In a series of nine cases, Gaffey and associates[5] documented melanogenesis by showing positive staining in tumor cells for HMB-45 and HMB-50, and demonstrating premelanosomes by electron microscopy. Lantuejoul and coworkers[6] reported two cases in which the tumor cells showed positive staining not only for HMB-45 but also for CD34, which they interpreted as pericytic differentiation.

More recently, a group of tumors sharing some of the histologic and immunohistochemical features of clear cell sugar tumors have been introduced into the literature under the designation *PEComas*.[7] Clear cell tumors with histopathologic features similar to those of tumors found in the lung also have been described in extrathoracic locations.[8–15] It has been stated that clear cell tumors, angiomyolipoma, and lymphangioleiomyomatosis may belong to the family of lesions known as PEComas.

TABLE 11-1 CLINICAL FEATURES

Tumor	Symptoms	Location: Central	Location: Peripheral	Clinical Behavior
Clear cell "sugar" tumor	Asymptomatic	Rare	Common	Complete resection curative
Granular cell tumor	Asymptomatic Airway obstruction	Common	Rare	Complete resection curative
Inflammatory pseudotumor	Airway obstruction	Common	Common	Recurrence if not completely resected
Sclerosing hemangioma	Asymptomatic	Rare	Common	Complete resection curative Metastasis to lymph nodes in rare cases

TABLE 11-2 IMMUNOHISTOCHEMICAL FEATURES

Antibody	Clear Cell "Sugar" Tumor	Granular Cell Tumor	Inflammatory Pseudotumor	Sclerosing Hemangioma
Cytokeratin	−	−	−, +	−, +
Keratin 7	−	−	−	+, −
S-100 protein	+	+	−	−
TTF-1	−	−	−	+
HMB-45	+	−	−	−
Surfactant protein	−	−	−	+
CD34	+	−	−	−
EMA	−	−	−	+
Vimentin	−	−, +	+	+
CD1a	+, −	−	−	−
HMB-50	+	−	−	−
Factor XIIIa	+	−	−	−
NSE	+, −	−, +	−	−
Leu7	−	+, −	−	−
ALK-1	−	−	+	−

ALK-1, anaplastic lymphoma kinase antibody-1; EMA, epithelial membrane antigen; NSE, neuron-specific enolase; TTF-1, thyroid transcription factor-1.

Clinical Features

The clear cell sugar tumor does not appear to have any gender or age predilection. Although a majority of cases have been described in adults, the tumor also has been reported in children.[16] A majority of patients are asymptomatic, and the tumor is discovered during a routine chest radiographic examination. Clinical and laboratory signs and symptoms, if present, may include fever, anemia, elevated erythrocyte sedimentation rate, presence of C-reactive protein, elevated platelet count, pneumonia, and chest or back pain.[2,17] Rarely, the tumor may be associated with unusual manifestations such as hemoptysis[18] or other pathologic conditions such as lymphangioleiomyomatosis and tuberous sclerosis.[19] The anatomic location of the tumor generally is in the periphery of the lung.

Macroscopic Features

In the vast majority of cases, tumor size ranges from 1 to 7 cm in greatest dimension, but larger sizes up to 12 cm also have been reported.[20] The tumors usually are well circumscribed but not encapsulated and of solid consistency, with variable color ranging from pink to red, gray, or brown (Fig. 11-1). Rarely, tumors have been described as cystic.[20] The cut surface may be slightly granular or glistening and smooth in appearance.

Histopathologic Features

The low-power view shows a cellular proliferation replacing normal lung parenchyma, which appears to be composed of cells with predominantly clear cytoplasm (Figs. 11-2 and 11-3). The cells may be arranged in cords or sheets, with minimal intervening connective tissue and prominent ectatic blood vessels with thin walls (Figs. 11-4 and 11-5). Higher magnification reveals oval to polygonal cells with distinct cell borders, clear cytoplasm, small nuclei, and inconspicuous nucleoli (Figs. 11-6 to 11-8). In other areas, histologic features may consist of a mixture of clear cells and spindle cells characterized by an elongated nucleus, inconspicuous nucleoli, and rather light eosinophilic cytoplasm (Fig. 11-9). The spindle cell component may be prominent in some areas of the tumor. One important characteristic of this tumor

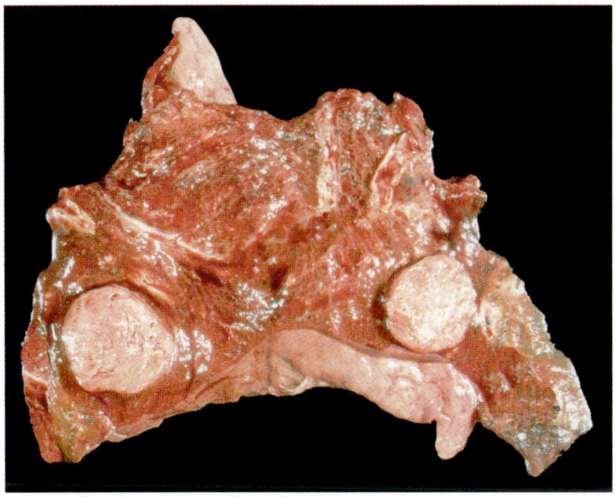

Figure 11-1 Intrapulmonary clear cell "sugar" tumor, gross specimen. The well-circumscribed, white to tan tumor shows no evidence of necrosis.

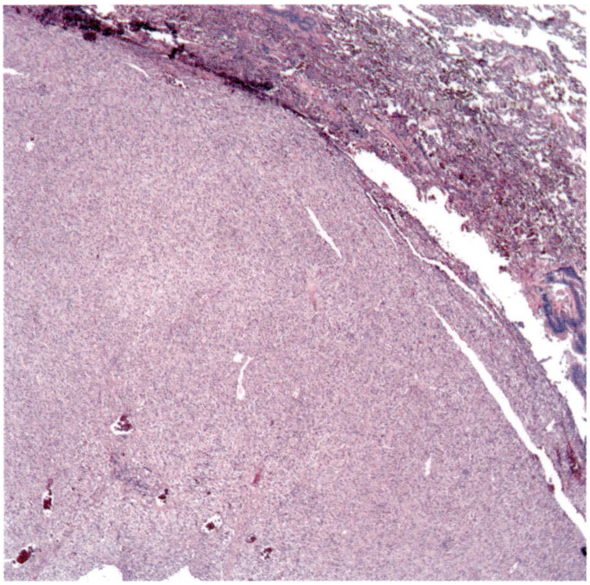

Figure 11-2 Low-power view of a sugar tumor of the lung. Note the clear demarcation of the tumor margins.

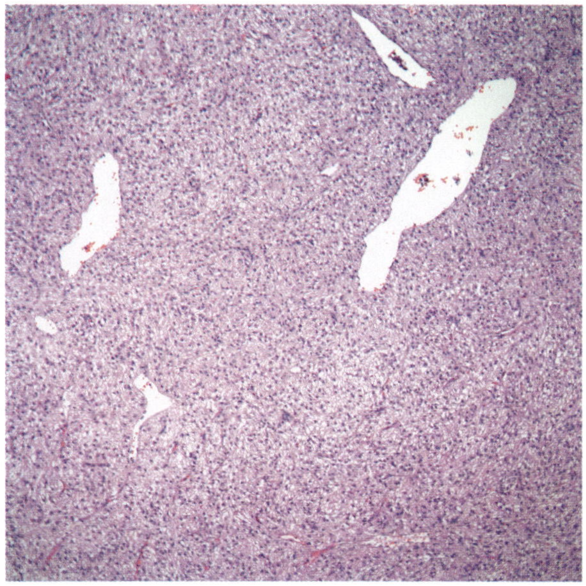

Figure 11-3 Intermediate-power view of a sugar tumor, showing the classic clear cell proliferation accompanied by numerous ectatic vessels.

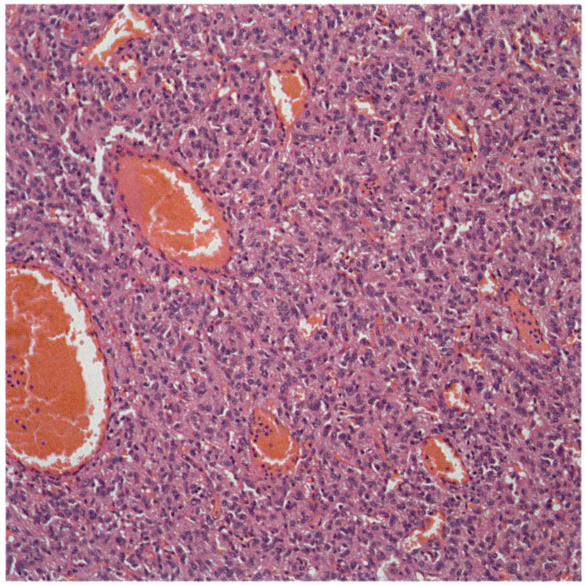

Figure 11-4 Sugar tumor in which the cells have a light eosinophilic cytoplasm. Note the presence of ectatic vessels filled with red cells.

is the presence of "spider cells," larger cells with granules in a linear arrangement that radiate from the nucleus (see Fig. 11-9B). In some areas, ectatic vessels with pools of red cells may be present (Fig. 11-10A), whereas in others, the presence of ectatic vessels and spindle cells imparts a hemangiopericytic pattern (Fig. 11-10B). In unusual cases, Touton-type giant cells or otherwise multinucleated giant cells may be present (Fig. 11-11). Neuroid cells also may be prominent (Fig. 11-12), and focal areas may show a neurotization-like process (Fig. 11-13). The clear cell component may show an inflammatory infiltrate (Fig. 11-14). The tumor does not characteristically show increased mitotic activity; and although rare mitotic figures may be seen, in most cases mitotic activity, cellular pleomorphism, and necrosis and hemorrhage are lacking. Although most of these features are more readily seen in resected specimens, the diagnosis of sugar tumor of the lung also can be accomplished by cytologic analysis and examination of core biopsy material.[21]

Histochemical-Immunohistochemical and Ultrastructural Features

The use of periodic acid–Schiff reagent (PAS) is helpful in identifying glycogen in the clear cells, whereas stains for mucin are negative. The tumor characteristically shows negative staining for epithelial markers such as keratin

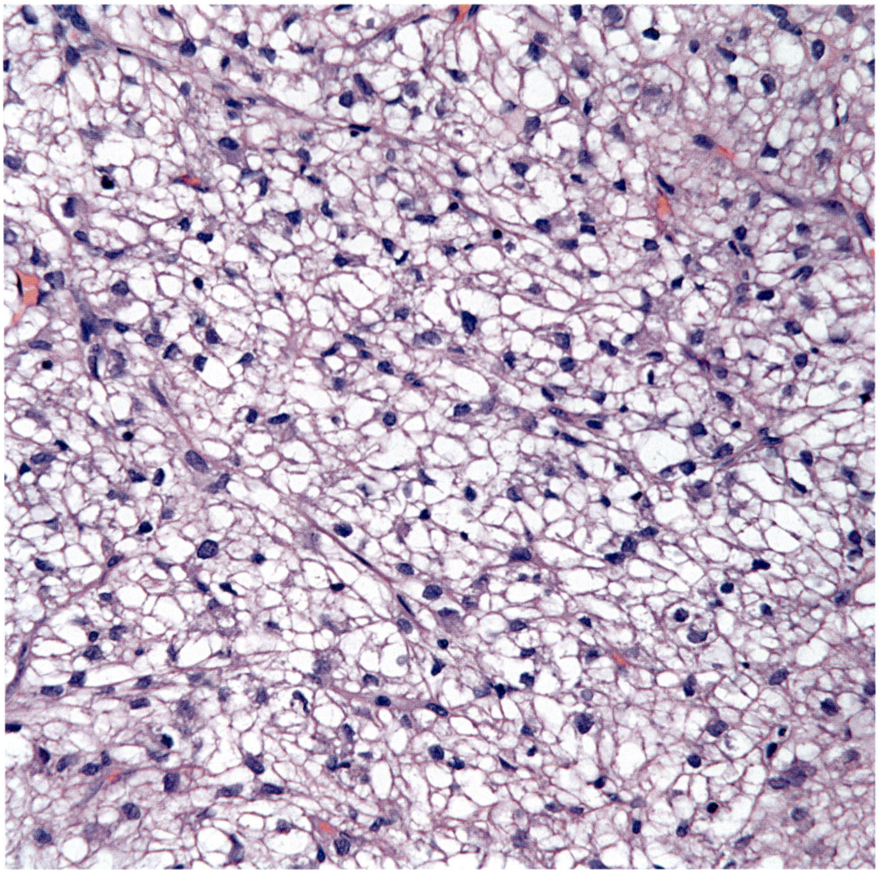

Figure 11-5 High-power view of a sugar tumor with the characteristic clear cells, small nuclei, and lack of cellular pleomorphism.

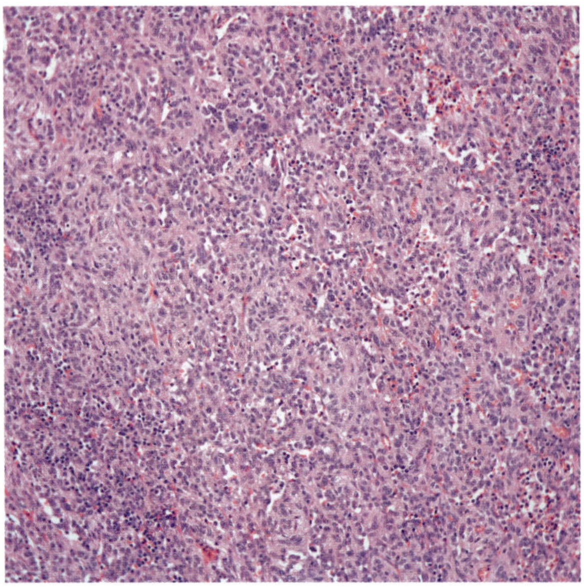

Figure 11-6 Sugar tumor with solid areas with inconspicuous vessels.

and epithelial membrane antigen (EMA), as well as neuroendocrine markers including chromogranin. Tumor cells have shown positive staining for S-100 protein, synaptophysin, CD34, CD1a, HMB-45, HMB-50, NKIC3, HAM-56, cathepsin B, factor XIIIa, and neuron-specific enolase.[5,6,22–24] At the ultrastructural level, various findings have been reported, including neurosecretory granules, pericytic differentiation, and premelanosomes.[5,6]

Differential Diagnosis

The most important considerations in the differential diagnosis are primary lung carcinoma and metastatic carcinomas (such as carcinomas of the kidney and thyroid), both with clear cell features. In this setting, the use of immunohistochemical stains, especially keratin, may lead to a correct interpretation. Clinical history of a kidney tumor is strongly suggestive of metastatic disease.

Treatment and Clinical Behavior

The treatment of choice for these tumors is complete surgical resection, accomplished with a wedge resection or lobectomy. In some unusual circumstances involving large tumors, pneumonectomy has been performed.[20] The clinical course typically is uneventful, with an excellent outcome; in one reported case, however, metastatic disease developed and the patient died 10 years after initial diagnosis.[24] The tumor was described as a "sugar tumor" of the lung with necrosis and an unusual histologic feature of columnar cells with clear cytoplasm, raising the possibility that it may have represented a different neoplasm.[25–27]

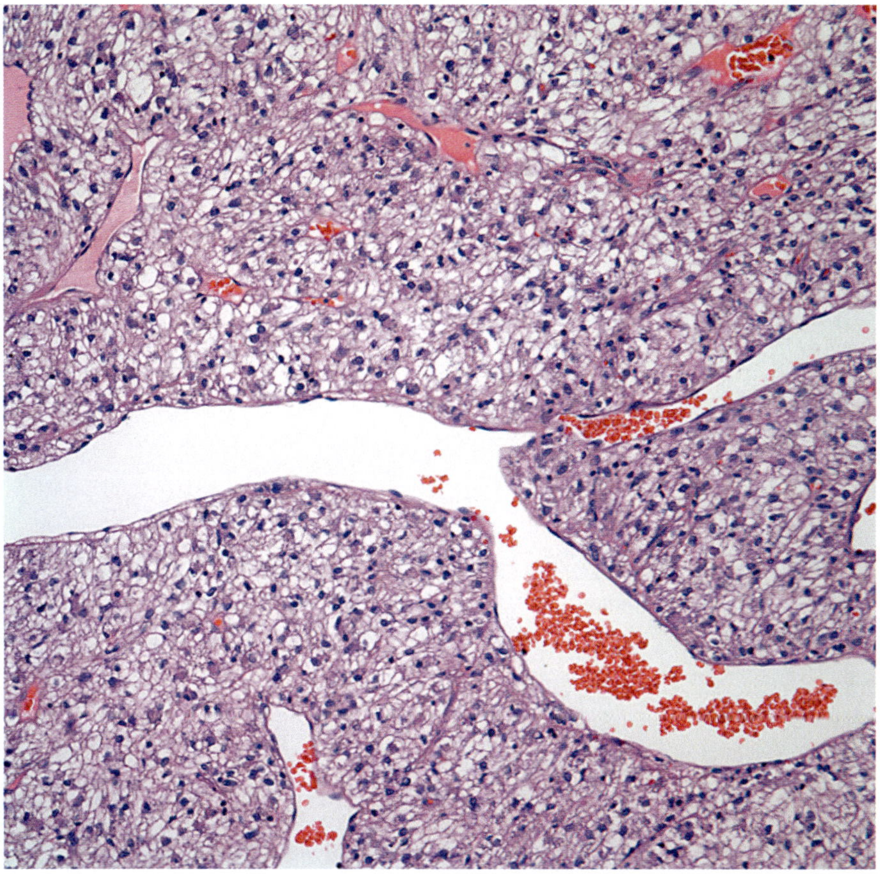

Figure 11-7 Clear cells in a sugar tumor approaching the walls of ectatic vessels.

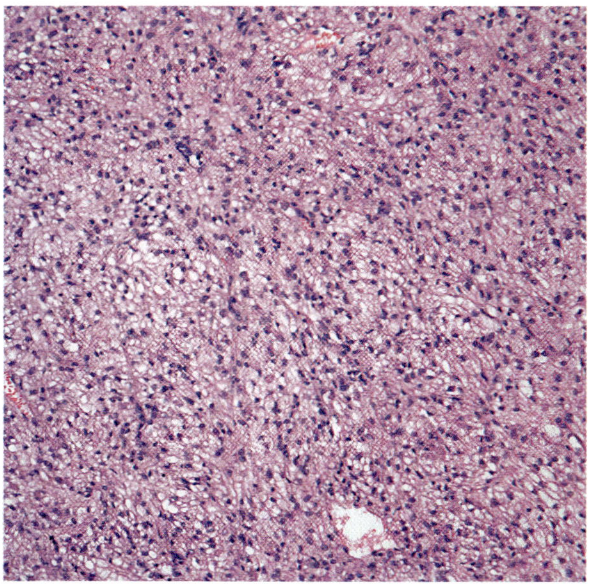

Figure 11-8 Sugar tumor with the classic clear cells and features mimicking those of a neural tumor.

GRANULAR CELL TUMOR

Granular cell tumors are neoplasms of rare occurrence and ubiquitous distribution that appear to be more common in the head and neck area (accounting for approximately 50% of all tumors of this type). These neoplasms have been described in multiple anatomic locations, however, including soft tissues, the breast, and the gastrointestinal, biliary, genitourinary, and lower respiratory tracts. The vast majority of these tumors are benign; however, a malignant counterpart has been described.[28–33] Despite the well-known occurrence of these tumors, their histogenesis remains unsettled.

Historical Aspects

Abrikossoff is credited with the initial description of this tumor in 1926. He initially argued that it represented degenerative skeletal muscle and later modified his opinion, suggesting an origin from myoblasts and referring to the tumor as "myoblastoma."[34,35] With the development of techniques such as ultrastructural and immunohistochemical studies, different theories have been proposed to explain the histogenesis of these tumors, including origins from histiocytes, fibroblasts, and Schwann cells.[36–38] Although some researchers have argued in favor of the Schwann cell as the cell of origin, granular cell tumors and schwannomas do not necessarily share similar ultrastructural, immunohistochemical, and karyotypic features. Currently, the granular cell tumor is regarded as a "specific" clinicopathologic entity without a known histogenetic mechanism.

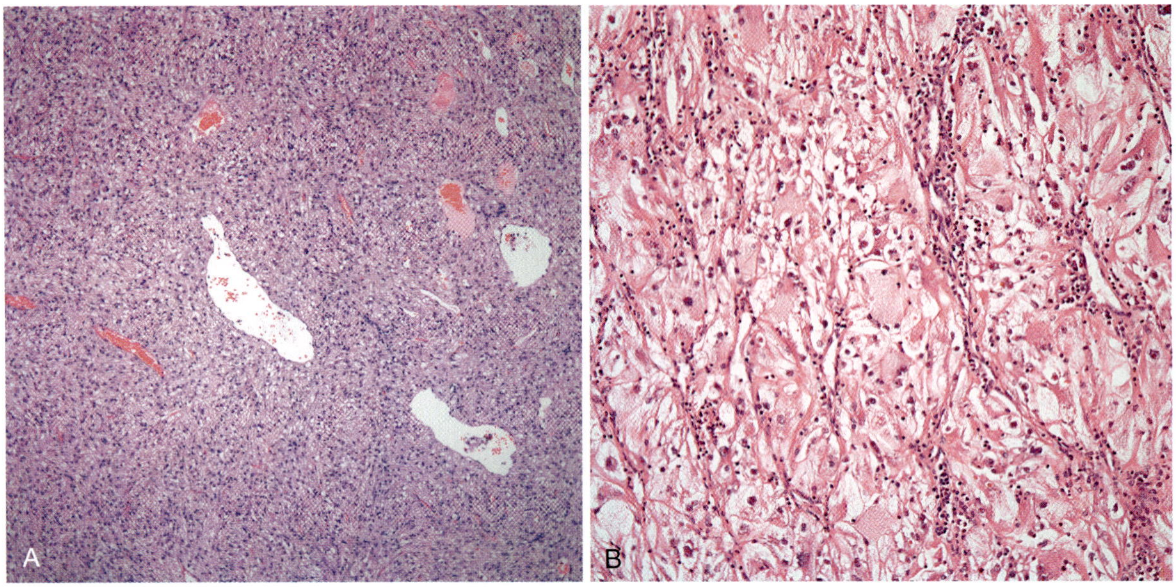

Figure 11-9 **A**, Sugar tumor showing a prominent spindle cell proliferation with ectatic vessels, mimicking a hemangiopericytic pattern. **B**, Sugar tumor composed of large cells with ample light eosinophilic cytoplasm and so-called spider cells.

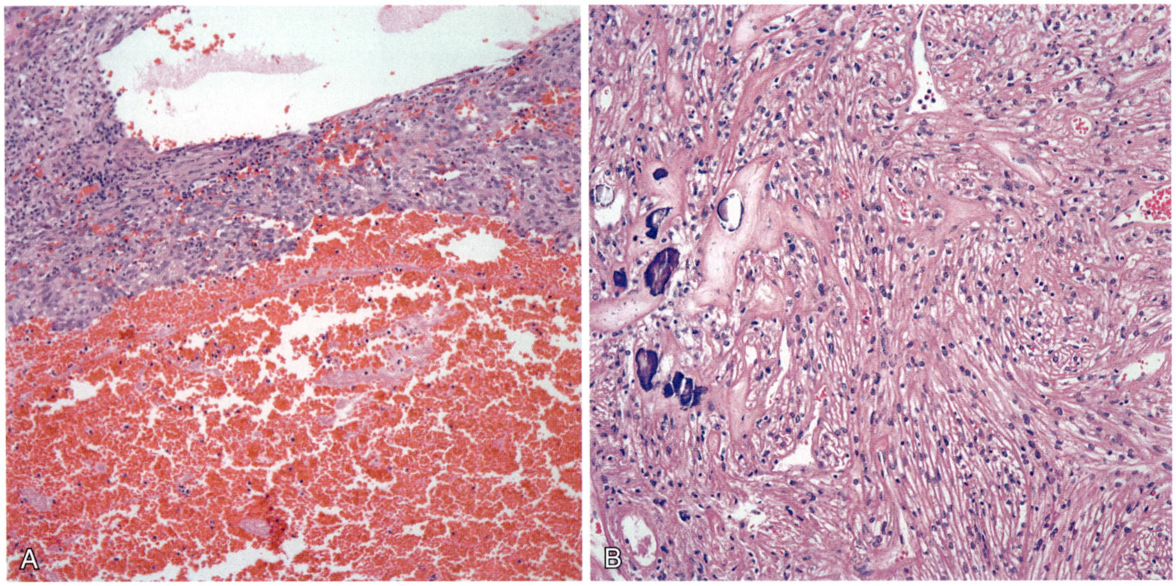

Figure 11-10 **A**, Sugar tumor with prominent dilated vessels filled with blood, giving the appearance of a vascular neoplasm. **B**, Sugar tumor with prominent spindle cell component and adjacent calcifications (dark areas).

Kramer published the initial description of the granular cell tumor in the bronchus.[39] By the late 1960s, the occurrence of this tumor in the lower respiratory tract was noted mostly in case reports, as a mere curiosity.[40–45]

Clinical Aspects

Like granular cell tumors appearing outside of the thoracic cavity, the bronchial tumor has been described mainly in adult patients, with a median age of 47 years, who may present with a history of cough, hemoptysis, wheezing, obstructive pneumonia, or weight loss. In unusual cases, the patient is completely asymptomatic and the tumor is discovered during a routine radiographic examination.[46–50] Bronchial granular cell tumors also have been described in children, who exhibit symptoms similar to those in adults.[51,52] Although in a majority of patients a single bronchial tumor is present, the presence of multiple, multifocal tumors within the bronchial tree has been reported.[45,53–55] In their study of 20 patients with granular cell tumor of the lung, Deavers and coworkers[46] documented that multifocal tumors were present in approximately 25% of the cases. In contrast with these findings, a study of 31 tumors of the lower respiratory tract reported

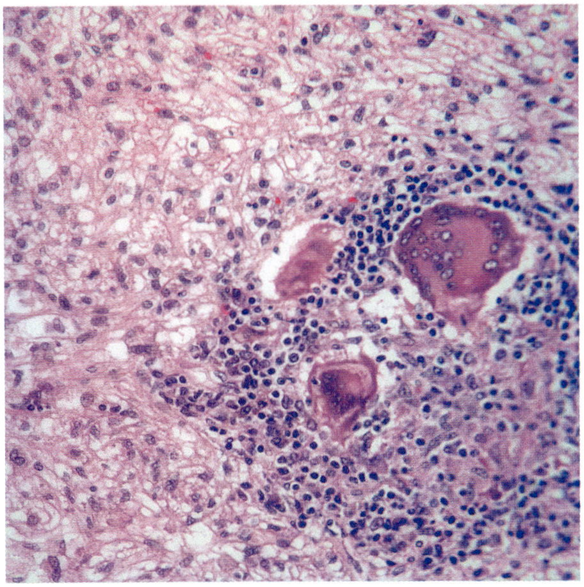

Figure 11-11 Sugar tumor with areas of giant cell granulomatous reaction.

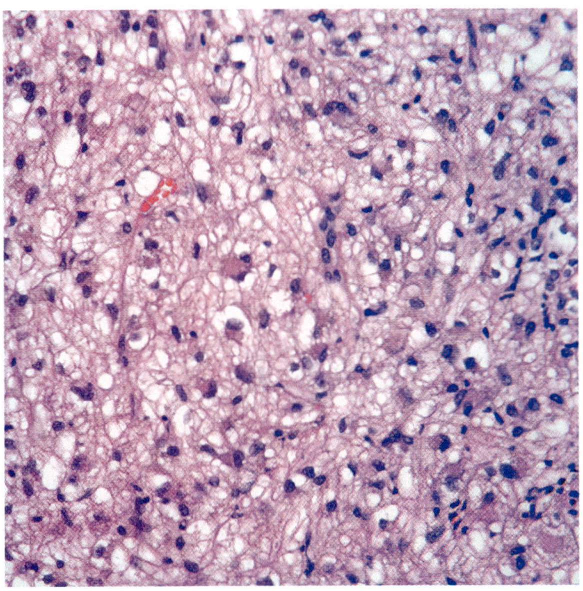

Figure 11-12 Sugar tumor with numerous "neuroid-like" cells.

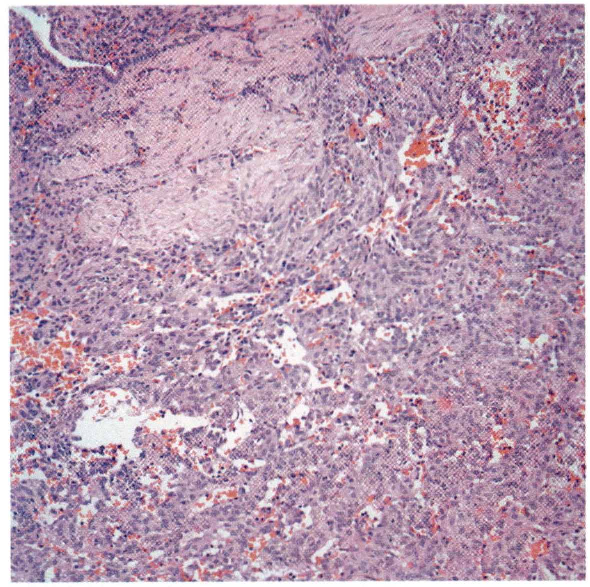

Figure 11-13 Sugar tumor with focal areas of a neurotization-like process.

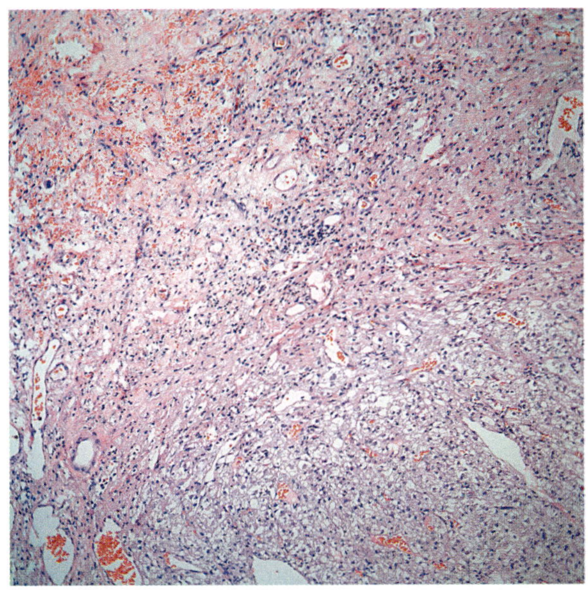

Figure 11-14 Sugar tumor with areas of inflammatory reaction.

by van der Maten and associates[47] found that 19 of the tumors originated from the bronchus; in approximately 61% of the patients, the tumor was found incidentally during the workup for lung carcinoma. This association has been reported in cases in which granular cell tumor coexists with bronchogenic carcinoma.[56]

Macroscopic Features

The tumors generally are centrally located and involve the airway. Size is variable and ranges from less than 1 cm up to 5 cm in greatest dimension. The tumor has a firm consistency and ranges in color from tan to whitish to yellowish (Fig. 11-15). It may take on the appearance of a polypoid tumor obstructing the airway or of a coin lesion.[46,50] In a case described by Schulster and colleagues,[50] the tumor had a coin lesion appearance and was found to involve the wall of a segmental bronchus. In general, the cut surface does not show evidence of necrosis or hemorrhage, so documentation of these features, when present, is important, because they indicate more aggressive behavior.

Histopathologic Features

The low-power view shows a tumor cell proliferation growing underneath the bronchial epithelium in sheets, replacing or growing around the normal bronchial

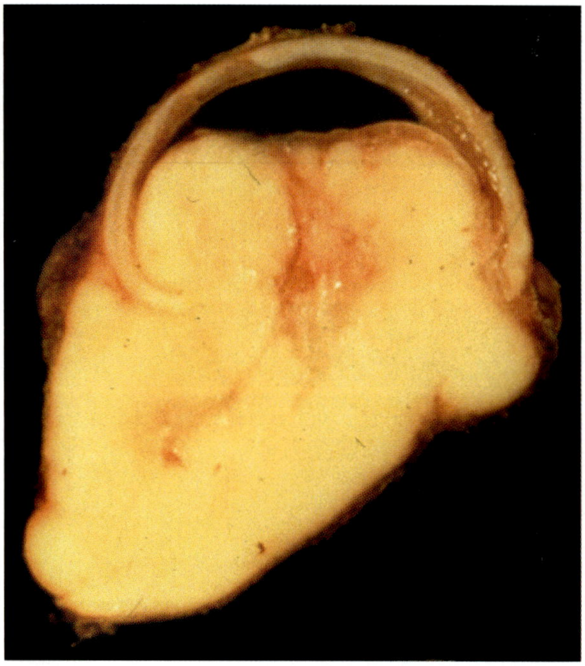

Figure 11-15 Gross specimen of a granular cell tumor growing in a polypoid fashion and obstructing the airway.

structures (Fig. 11-16). In some cases, the epithelium may display squamous metaplasia or ulceration (Fig. 11-17). At higher magnification, the tumor is seen to be composed of medium-sized, round to polygonal cells with ample light eosinophilic and granular cytoplasm. The nuclei may be centrally or peripherally located, with inconspicuous nucleoli (Fig. 11-18). High-power examination should provide definitive evidence of the granular nature of the cytoplasm. The tumors are not encapsulated and often show infiltrative borders (Fig. 11-19). Perineural invasion is common (Fig. 11-20). Some tumors may have a prominent spindle cell component (Fig. 11-21) with cytologic features similar to those of the round or polygonal cell component; however, when the spindle cell component is prominent, areas with a desmoplastic-like reaction may be visible. In some unusual cases, the tumor extends into lymph nodes (Fig. 11-22), may show cystic changes (Fig. 11-23), or displays metaplastic bone formation (Fig. 11-24). When the tumor is not endobronchially located, it may appear well circumscribed, replacing the lung parenchyma.

Mitotic activity, necrosis, and hemorrhage are absent in benign tumors. Although the great majority of granular cell tumors of the lung are benign, malignant tumors have been reported.[57] The histologic features of malignant tumors are similar, with the addition of nuclear pleomorphism, mitotic activity (Fig. 11-25), and necrosis.[58–61] When a single biopsy specimen is available for review, the presence of these features should alert the pathologist to the possibility of a malignant granular cell tumor.

Histochemical, Immunohistochemical, and Ultrastructural Features

The granules present in the cytoplasm of granular cell tumors react positively with PAS. On immunohistochemical studies, the most consistent marker is S-100 protein.[62–64] Researchers also have reported positive staining for neuron-specific enolase, vimentin, actin, myelin basic protein, Leu7, cathepsin B, and antichymotrypsin.[47–49] Granular cell tumors demonstrate negative staining for keratin, EMA, glial fibrillary acidic protein (GFAP), chromogranin, lysozyme, neurofilament protein, HMB-45, desmin, myoglobin, and carcinoembryonic antigen (CEA). One case of a granular cell tumor arising in soft tissue with DNA ploidy has been reported.[59]

Differential Diagnosis

Although the histologic features of granular cell tumors allow for a light microscopic diagnosis, in some cases the tumor can be confused with other entities, such as melanoma or sarcoma. Both granular cell tumors and melanoma may show positive staining for S-100 protein, but granular cell tumors will not display positive staining for HMB-45 or Melan-A. Some mesenchymal neoplasms also may show positive staining for S-100 protein; however, in doubtful cases, the use of a wider panel of immunohistochemical studies may provide better evidence for a specific diagnosis. In addition, the use of PAS histochemical stains may prove to be useful. Malignant granular cell tumors of extrathoracic origin may metastasize to the lungs, so reliable clinical information is required for accurate designation as primary or metastatic.

Treatment and Prognosis

The treatment of choice for granular cell tumors of the lung is complete surgical resection. Bronchoscopic extirpation, laser therapy, sleeve resection, lobectomy, or transbronchoscopic surgical resection all have been used.[46,65] The choice of a particular procedure will depend on the location, size, and other features of the tumor. Reported instances of recurrence may be related to incomplete resection of the tumor. If the tumor is completely resected and the histologic picture is benign, the treatment is curative. When the tumor is malignant, an aggressive clinical course, with development of metastatic disease, is likely.

INFLAMMATORY PSEUDOTUMOR

Inflammatory pseudotumor of the lung is a controversial term for a pulmonary growth that destroys normal lung parenchyma and is believed in many cases to follow an inflammatory process. This neoplasm has the potential to

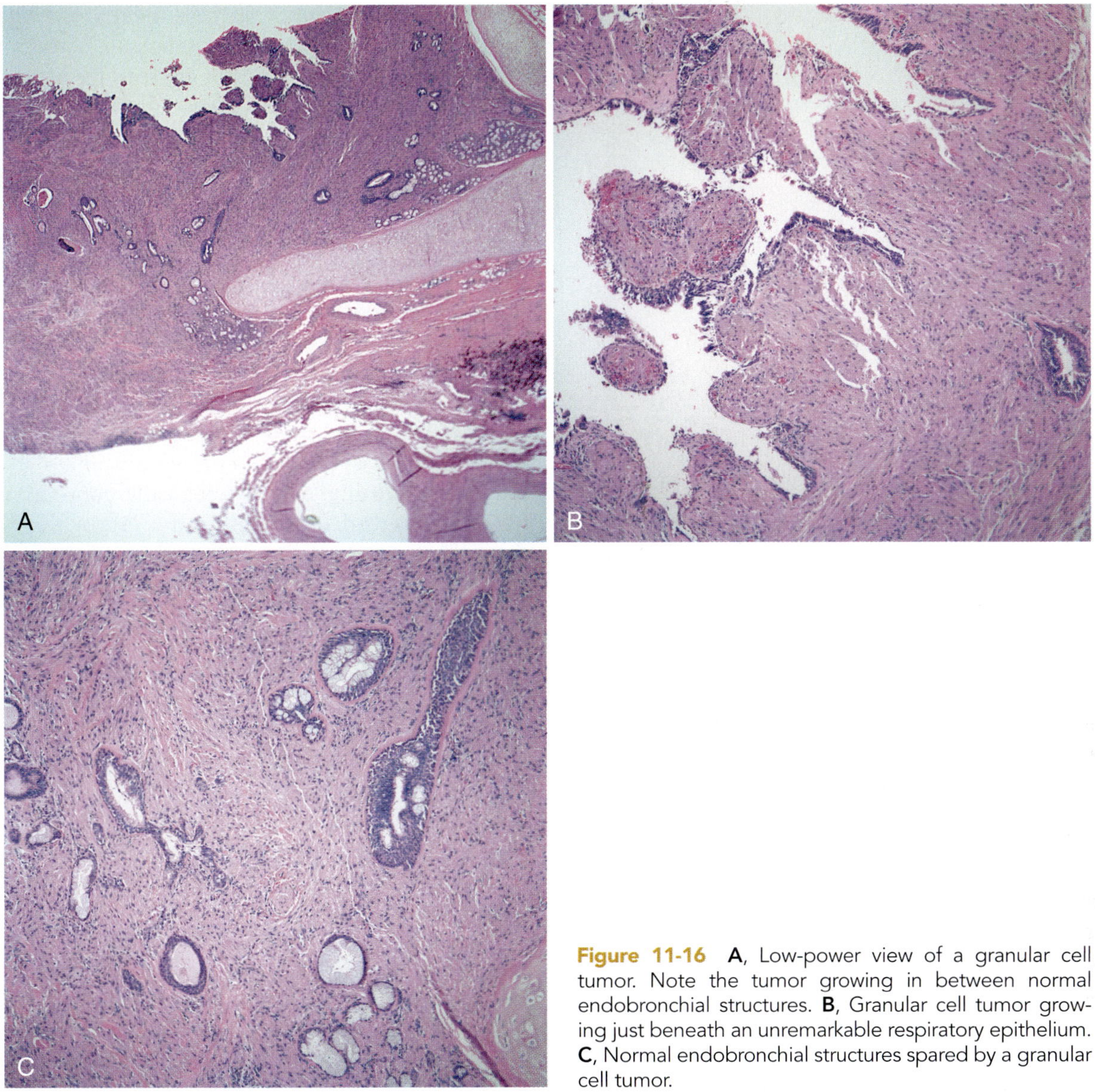

Figure 11-16 **A**, Low-power view of a granular cell tumor. Note the tumor growing in between normal endobronchial structures. **B**, Granular cell tumor growing just beneath an unremarkable respiratory epithelium. **C**, Normal endobronchial structures spared by a granular cell tumor.

recur and invade adjacent structures, such as the pleura, mediastinum, and diaphragm, and it may not necessarily display an inflammatory component (i.e., a pneumonic process). The term *inflammatory myofibroblastic tumor* has been used as an alternative designation for these lesions but does not completely explain their true nature in that some tumors are composed almost exclusively of plasma cells. Accordingly, the more accurate term *inflammatory pseudotumor* is retained here.

Historical Aspect

In the view of many investigators, IPT may represent an inflammatory response to a previous insult. In some cases, the clinical history includes an upper respiratory infection or a resolving pneumonic process. This possibility is potentially supported by the finding that in some cases, IPT has expressed human herpesvirus-8 genes.[66,67] Some workers, however, have argued that IPT may be a true tumor and have demonstrated cytogenetic evidence supporting a clonal origin.[68] In addition, the fact that many of these lesions recur[69] also indicates that it may be a true tumor, rather than a postinflammatory response. This neoplasm may originate from pulmonary myofibroblasts, however, and the presence of myofibroblasts in conditions such as diffuse alveolar damage may indicate that IPT does in fact follow an inflammatory response.[70] Regardless of the histologic type encountered, no known etiology for these lesions has been recognized.

Clinical Features

IPT has been estimated to represent less than 1% of all pulmonary tumors. The true incidence is uncertain, however, because a wide variety of lesions have been included

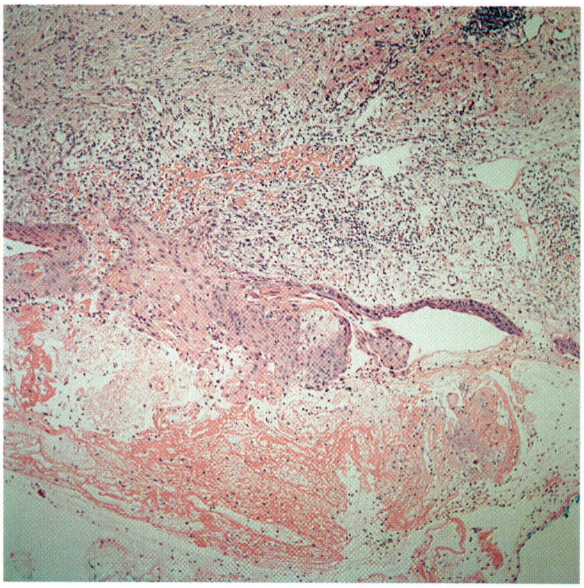

Figure 11-17 Granular cell tumor with ulceration of the respiratory epithelium showing squamous metaplasia.

under this designation.[69,71–101] Other conditions that have been mistakenly identified as IPT include organizing pneumonia, sclerosing hemangioma, and pseudolymphoma, among others. In most cases IPT manifests as a solitary "coin lesion" in a relatively young patient, usually before the age of 40 years. IPT is not restricted to younger patients, however, and also has been described in patients older than 40 years.

Although a history of cough, chest pain, and fever is common, IPT also has been described in patients who have been completely asymptomatic, in whom the lung abnormality has been discovered during a routine radiographic study. Patients also may present in a more acute state with massive hemoptysis.[89] Agrons and colleagues[88] analyzed data for 61 patients ranging in age from 17 to 61 years, with a slight male predominance (male-to-female ratio of 36:25). In 52 patients, the tumor manifested as a peripheral solitary nodule or mass, and in 11 of these, extrapulmonary involvement was evident in the hilum, mediastinum, and airway. Thus, these workers concluded that IPT typically is a solitary pulmonary lesion that can involve extrapulmonary structures. Ishida and associates[80] documented pleural involvement in three of seven patients with IPT. Kim and coworkers[97] described the radiographic features of IPT in ten patients, in three of whom the lesion was endobronchial in location.

Classification

Although most pathologists would not categorize organizing pneumonia as IPT, Matsubara and colleagues[101] described 32 cases of IPT of the lung in which they alluded to the possible progression of organizing pneumonia to fibrous histiocytoma or to plasma cell granuloma. They stated that most or all of the cases of IPT are believed to originate as organizing pneumonia and noted a considerable overlap of histopathologic features among organizing pneumonia, fibrous histiocytoma, and plasma cell granuloma. In this report, 44% of the cases corresponded to organizing pneumonia.

One of the problems in classifying organizing pneumonia as IPT is that in bronchiolitis obliterans, findings may include radiologic evidence of an intrapulmonary nodule with airspace consolidation,[102] similar to that in some of the cases referred to as IPT. If cases of bronchiolitis obliterans are included in this category of lesions, then any "benign" mass lesion in the lung that is unclassified will automatically be labeled as an IPT. Because of these problems, some investigators have determined this entity as a whole to be etiologically enigmatic, nosologically confusing, and histologically unpredictable and have recommended restricting the use of this designation to pulmonary lesions.[103] Bahadori and Liebow[72] preferred the term *plasma cell granuloma* for this entity; use of this nomenclature, however, denies the existence of lesions that are composed almost entirely of a fibrohistiocytic proliferation. In a description of an endobronchial case of IPT, Buell and associates[73] documented the presence of plasma cells and spindle cells, which on electron microscopy resembled those of fibrocytic derivation. Spencer[76] documented 27 cases of IPT, finding that all of the lesions incorporated features of both plasma cell granuloma and histiocytoma; he proposed the pulmonary plasma cell–histiocytoma complex. Two cases in these series were categorized as tumors that had undergone malignant transformation. Pettinato and colleagues,[81] however, described 20 cases of "inflammatory myofibroblastic tumor (plasma cell granuloma)" in which the lesions were seen to be composed of variable proportions of plasma cells, histiocytes, and spindle cells. Of interest, the investigators documented that in 5% of the cases, more than one lesion was present in the lung. Also, in 5% of the cases, the inflammatory process had involved the mediastinum and thoracic wall.

Other workers have focused their attention on lesions with fibrohistiocytic histology. Gal and coworkers[87] analyzed the prognostic factors for fibrohistiocytic lesions of the lung, classifying them as IPT, fibrohistiocytic type; borderline fibrohistiocytic lesions; or malignant fibrous histiocytoma. In this study, 15 lesions were identified as IPT and 3 as borderline lesions. Only 2 of the patients with IPT experienced recurrence. In a study of 23 patients with IPT, Cerfolio and associates[93] concluded that regardless of the histologic findings, the most important prognostic factor is whether the tumors are circumscribed or locally invasive.

Based on the many descriptions of IPT in the lung, two distinct histopathologic subtypes generally are accepted: fibrohistiocytic type and plasma cell type. It is important for prognostic purposes to determine whether these

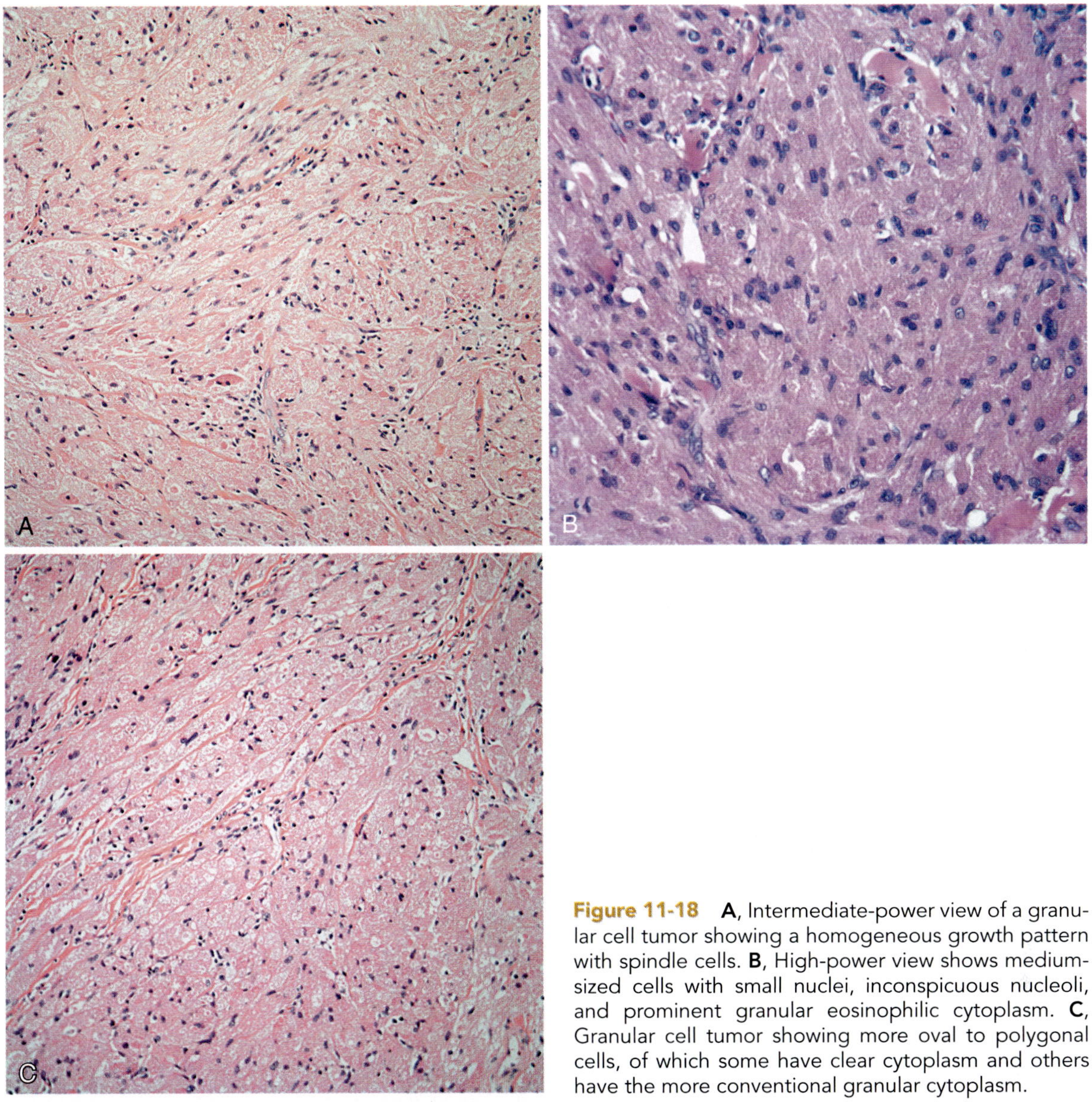

Figure 11-18 **A**, Intermediate-power view of a granular cell tumor showing a homogeneous growth pattern with spindle cells. **B**, High-power view shows medium-sized cells with small nuclei, inconspicuous nucleoli, and prominent granular eosinophilic cytoplasm. **C**, Granular cell tumor showing more oval to polygonal cells, of which some have clear cytoplasm and others have the more conventional granular cytoplasm.

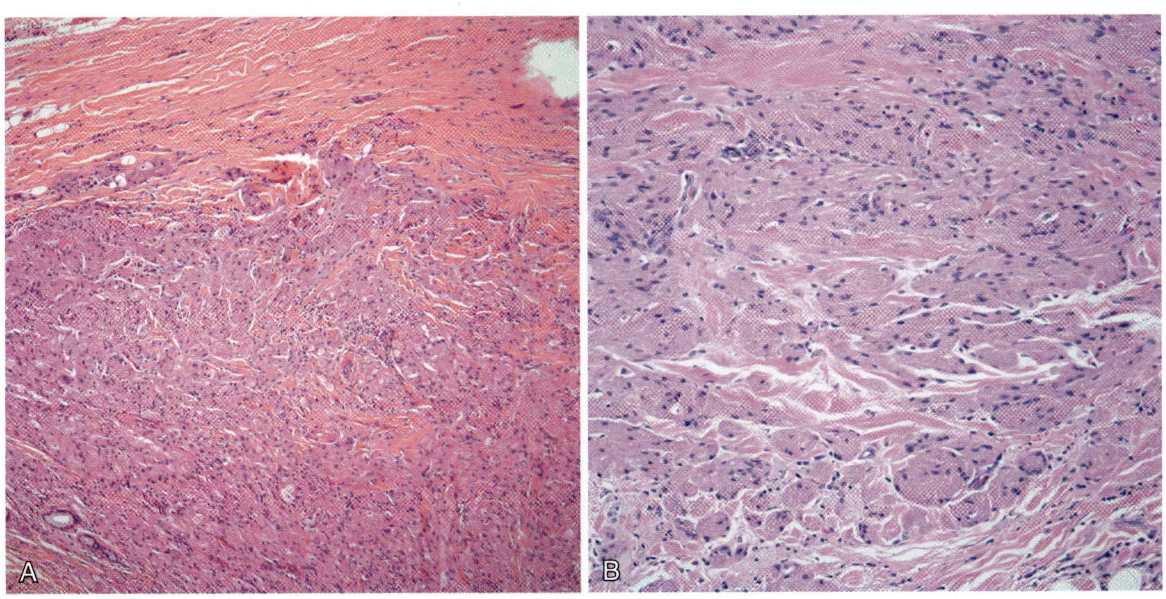

Figure 11-19 **A**, Granular cell tumor with infiltrative borders. **B**, At higher magnification, tumor cells dissecting fibroconnective tissue can be seen, although the tumor initially appeared to be well circumscribed.

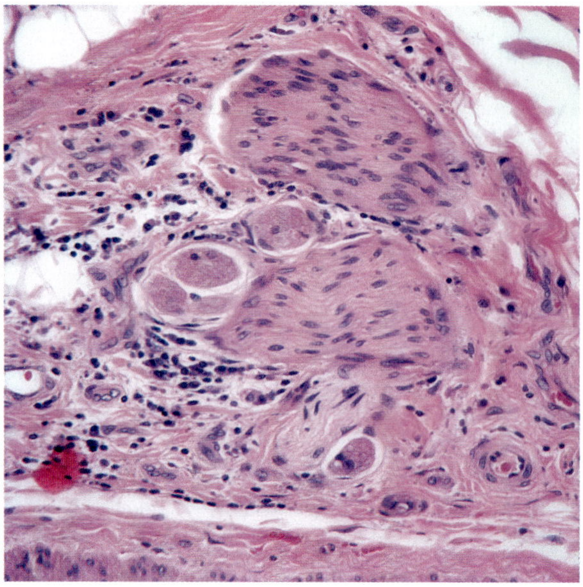

Figure 11-20 Granular cell tumor showing perineural invasion.

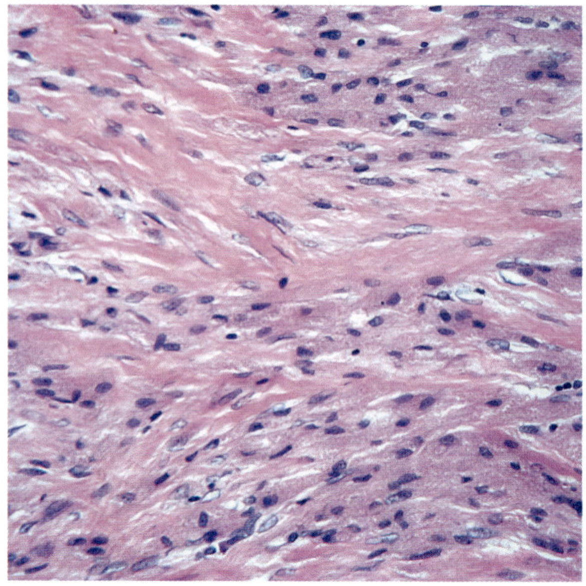

Figure 11-21 Granular cell tumor with prominent spindle cell arrangement.

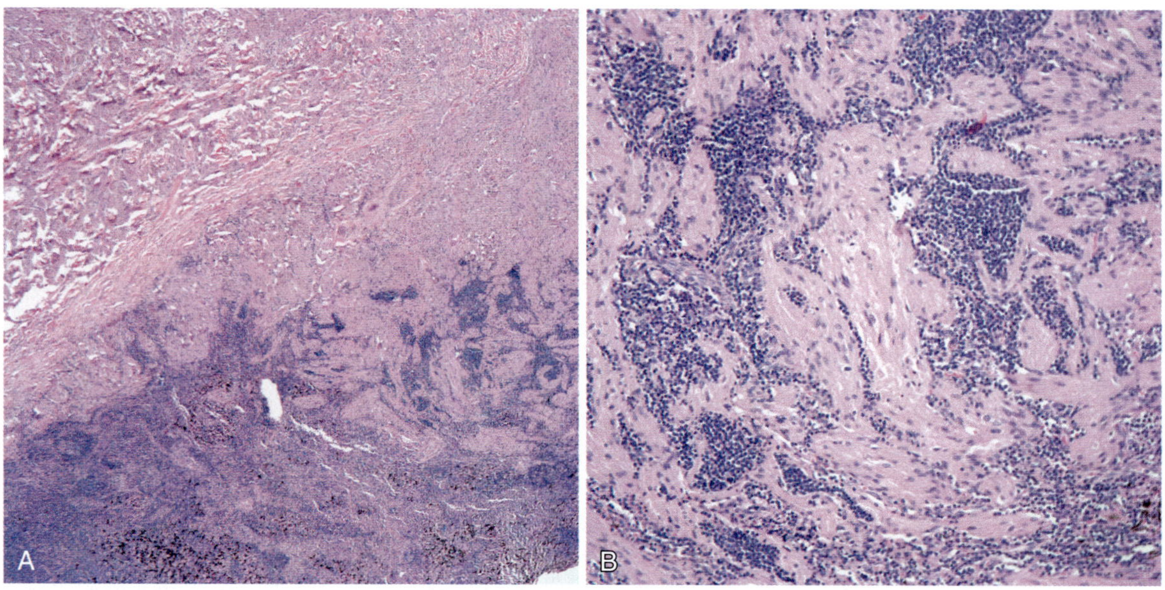

Figure 11-22 Granular cell tumor. **A**, Tumor invading peribronchial lymph node. **B**, At higher magnification, infiltration of the tumor into nodal tissue can be seen.

tumors are invasive. Painstaking analysis of the radiologic features and careful sectioning of the tumor are important aspects of the evaluation and final classification of these lesions.

Macroscopic Features

As with other intrapulmonary neoplasms, the lesion may be either centrally or peripherally located (Fig. 11-26), which in turn may determine symptomatology. With peripheral lesions, tumor size may range from 1 cm to more than 10 cm in diameter. The lesions are well circumscribed but not encapsulated. Cut surface is rather homogeneous in appearance and may have a yellowish color. Endobronchial tumors may show similar features; however, they may not be as large as those occurring in the periphery of the lung parenchyma. Centrally located tumors may show some ulceration of the overlying epithelial surface and appear to have infiltrative borders. Rare cases of cystic lesions also have been described.[82]

Histopathologic Features

Although the two major histologic growth patterns—the fibrohistocytic type and the plasma cell type—may be visible in a particular IPT, in many instances, focal

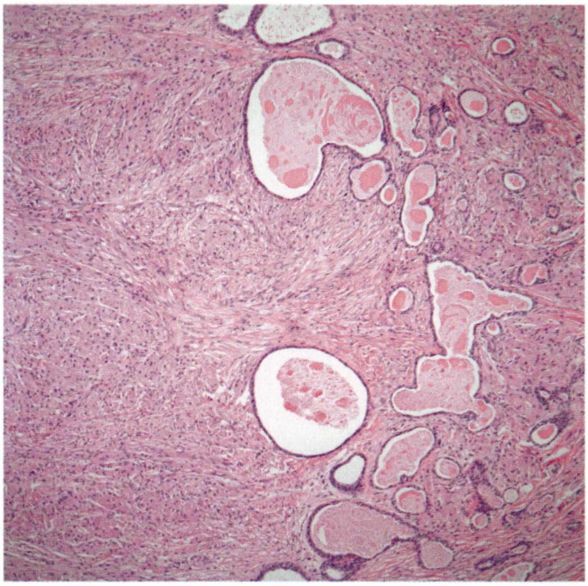

Figure 11-23 Cystically dilated glands present in a granular cell tumor.

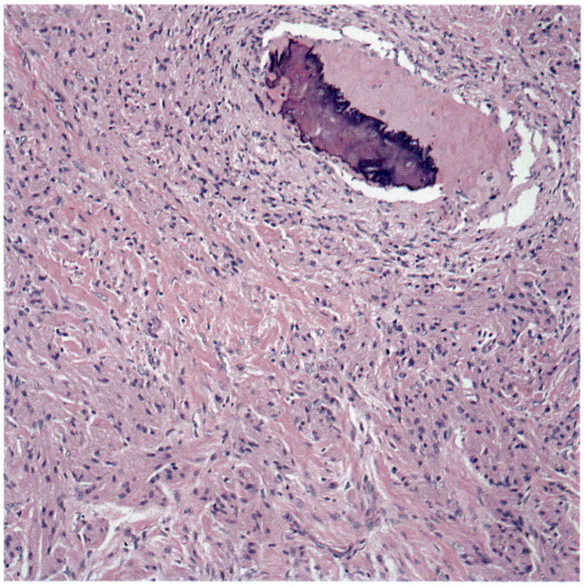

Figure 11-24 Granular cell tumor with metaplastic bone formation.

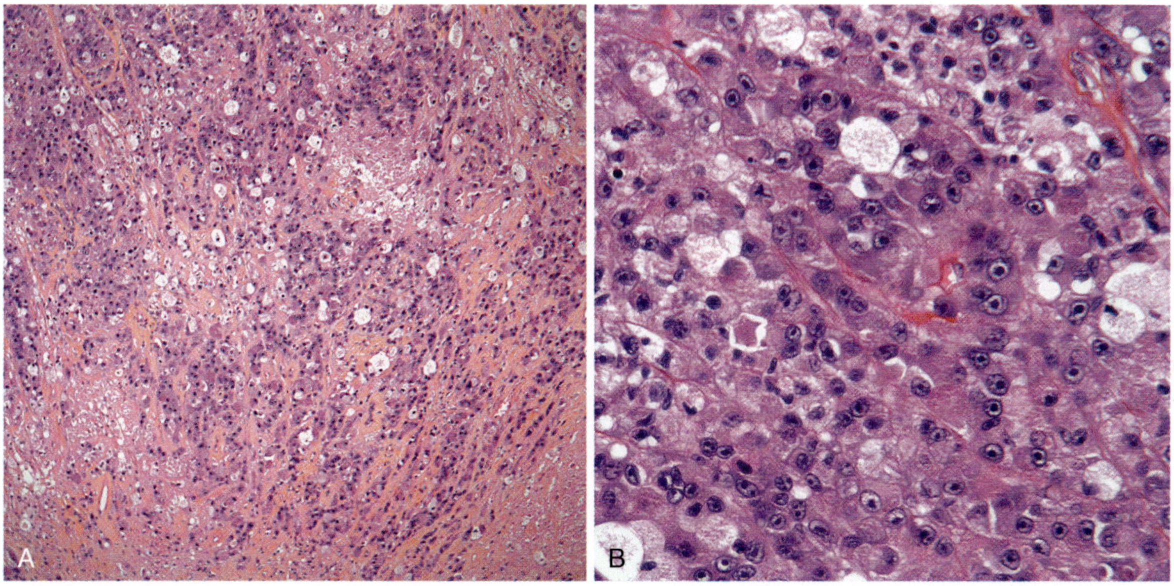

Figure 11-25 Malignant granular cell tumor. **A**, The tumor is composed of cells that are similar to those of the benign counterpart, but with cellular pleomorphism. **B**, At higher magnification, granular cells with round to oval nuclei and prominent nucleoli are evident. Mitotic figures also are present.

or even more extensive areas of one particular histologic pattern may be seen. In lesions of the fibrohistocytic type, low-power magnification shows a well-organized spindle cell proliferation with a subtle or well-formed storiform pattern (Figs. 11-27 to 11-29). At higher magnification, the spindle cell proliferation may show sprinkled inflammatory cells, particularly lymphocytes and plasma cells (Fig. 11-30). The spindle cells have a fusiform appearance with moderate amounts of eosinophilic cytoplasm, elongated nuclei, and inconspicuous nucleoli (Fig. 11-31). At the periphery of the lesion, it is possible to identify conglomerates of foamy "xanthoma" cells admixed with the spindle cells (Fig. 11-32). Touton-type giant cells may be present, admixed with the histiocytic proliferation (Fig. 11-33). Cholesterol cleft granulomas also may be observed in this tumor (Fig. 11-34). Nuclear atypia is absent or mild, and mitotic activity also is lacking; mitotic figures, if present, are few and far apart.

In some of these lesions, no inflammatory component may be present, giving the impression of a true malignant neoplasm. In unusual cases in which the neoplasm is

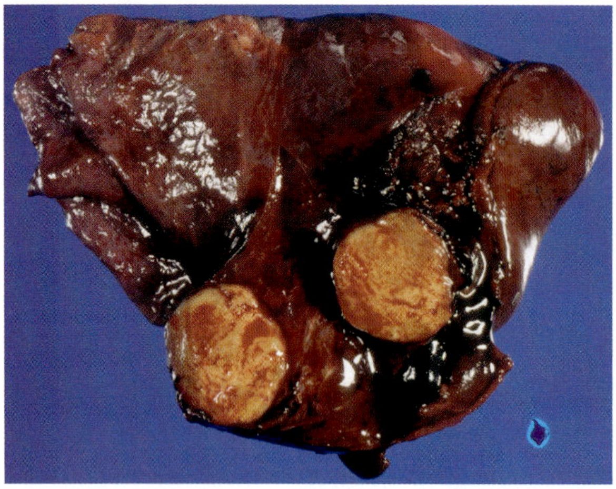

Figure 11-26 Gross specimen of an intrapulmonary peripheral inflammatory pseudotumor. The tumor is well circumscribed, with a deep yellow hue.

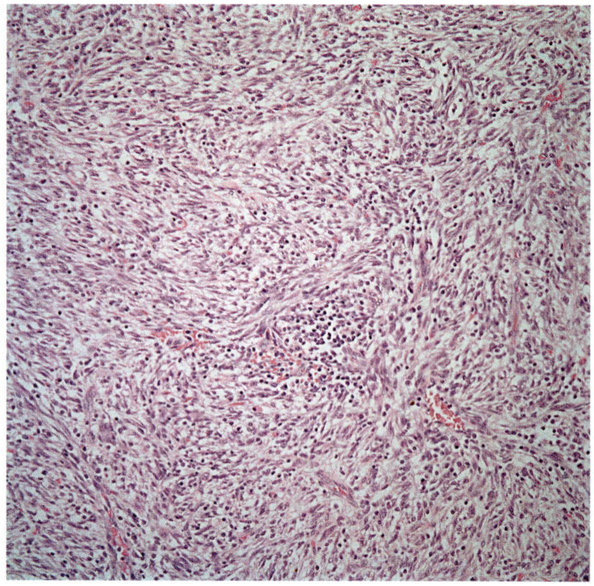

Figure 11-28 Inflammatory pseudotumor showing a prominent spindle cell proliferation sprinkled with inflammatory cells.

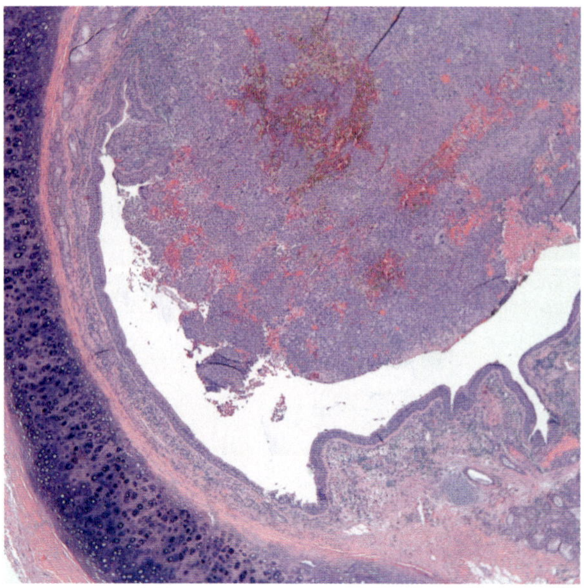

Figure 11-27 Low-power view of an inflammatory pseudotumor obstructing the airway.

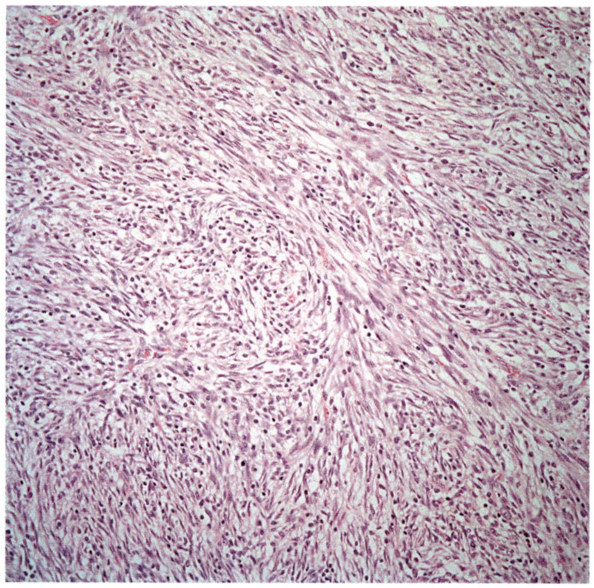

Figure 11-29 Fibrohistiocytic inflammatory pseudotumor with a subtle storiform pattern.

in an endobronchial location, a superimposed inflammatory reaction may be present, and it occasionally may be possible to identify an infectious origin. The plasma cell variant may show a predominance of plasma cells (Fig. 11-35). Areas of remaining alveolar parenchyma may be present (Fig. 11-36), as well as areas in which spindle fibroblastic cells are admixed with inflammatory cells (mainly plasma cells) (Fig. 11-37). In some instances, areas of calcification and ossification may be present, whereas in others, extensive areas of hyalinized stroma may be a major component of the lesion (Fig. 11-38). In this subtype of IPT, mitotic activity is absent. Focal necrosis occasionally may be present.

Immunohistochemical Features

The histopathologic features observed may determine the immunohistochemical studies requested. In general, however, the plasma cell population will exhibit a polyclonal cellular proliferation when stained for κ and λ light chains. The spindle cell proliferation may show positive staining for smooth muscle actin and vimentin. More

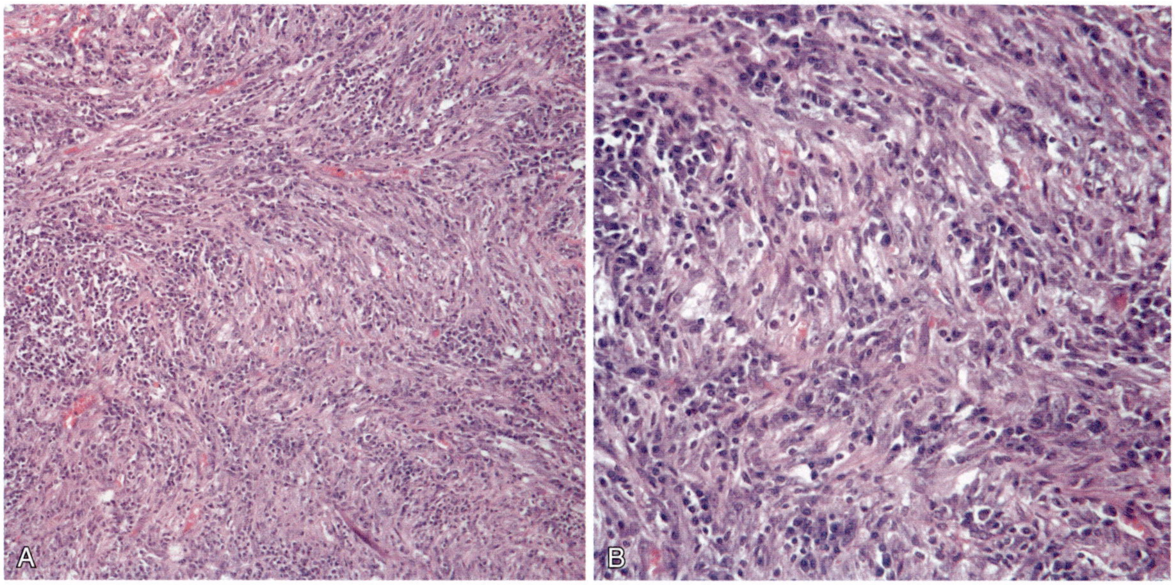

Figure 11-30 **A**, Inflammatory pseudotumor with prominent spindle cell proliferation and a more obvious inflammatory component. **B**, Higher-power view shows both the spindle and the inflammatory components.

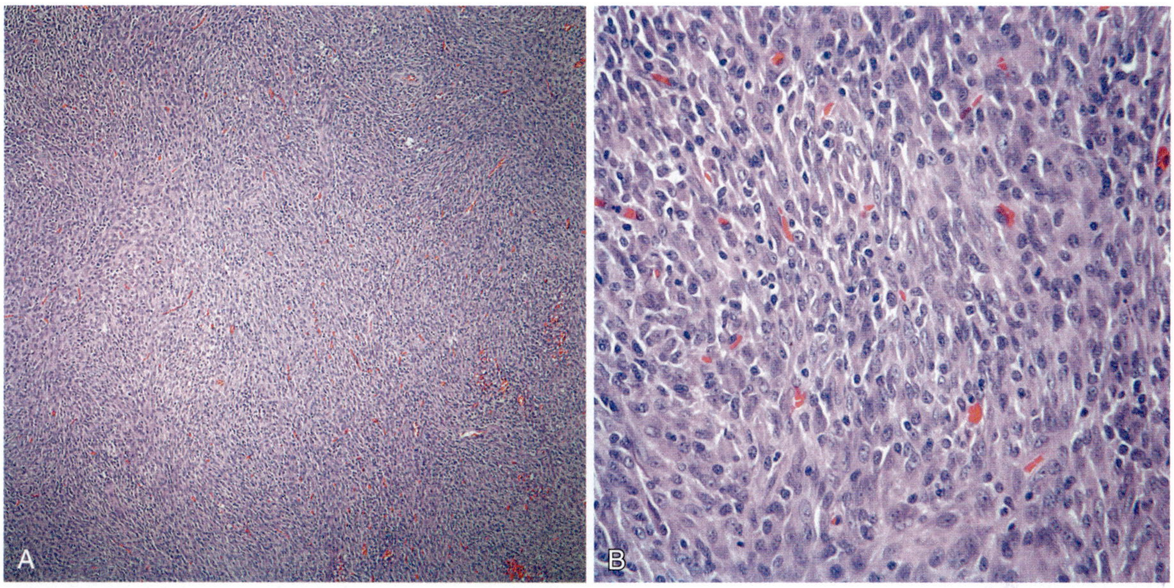

Figure 11-31 **A**, Fibrohistiocytic-type inflammatory pseudotumor showing a spindle cellular proliferation with only scattered inflammatory cells. **B**, Higher-power view shows additional features of a fibrohistiocytic proliferation; however, no mitotic activity or marked cellular pleomorphism is present.

recently, the anaplastic lymphoma kinase antibody-1 (ALK-1) has been reported to produce a positive stain in IPT.[104–106] In a study by Coffin and associates,[104] ALK positivity was observed in only 36% of cases and p80 positivity in 34% of the same cases, whereas fluorescence in situ hybridization (FISH) showed ALK rearrangement in 9 of 22 cases examined (47%). The investigators concluded that abnormalities of ALK and p80 are more common in abdominal and intrapulmonary IPTs in the first decade of life, and that these abnormalities are associated with a higher frequency of recurrence. Other workers, however, have encountered negative results with these studies, limiting the true value of immunohistochemical techniques in the diagnosis of these lesions.[98]

Differential Diagnosis

The specific clinical entities considered in the differential diagnosis for IPT may depend on the histopathologic pattern observed. In cases in which inflammatory cells are predominant, the possibility of an infectious condition with superimposed organizing pneumonia needs to be

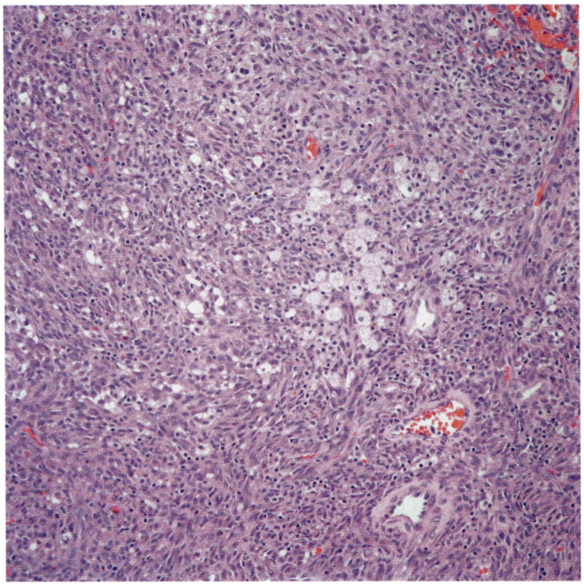

Figure 11-32 Inflammatory pseudotumor showing a spindle cell proliferation with collections of foamy macrophages.

considered. The use of histochemical studies for organisms or tissue cultures may lead to the correct interpretation. Owing to the marked presence of plasma cells, pulmonary plasmacytoma also needs to be considered. In this setting the use of immunohistochemical stains for κ and λ light chains may be useful. When the IPT is composed predominantly of spindle cells, malignant fibrous histiocytoma and sarcomatoid carcinoma must be ruled out.[87,107] In tumors with marked cellular atypia visible by light microscopy, observation of increased mitotic activity with atypical mitosis generally will lead to the correct interpretation. Immunohistochemical studies are of limited value in this setting.

Treatment and Prognosis

The treatment of these lesions is largely surgical; however, the diagnosis is made by histopathologic means. Biopsy and cytologic analysis will be of limited value in the diagnosis of this neoplasm. Therefore, the identification of a coin lesion may require a more radical surgical approach. In a study of 955 resected coin lesions in patients ranging in age from 16 to 81 years, Toomes and associates[75] reported that 74% of the patients were asymptomatic and 49% had malignant neoplasms. Patients were treated with different surgical procedures ranging from pneumonectomy to tumor enucleation. Among the 51% diagnosed as benign neoplasms, tuberculosis and "benign tumors" had the highest incidence. Unfortunately, a breakdown of the diagnoses by age group was not available. It is expected, however, that malignant neoplasms are more likely to occur in the older population.

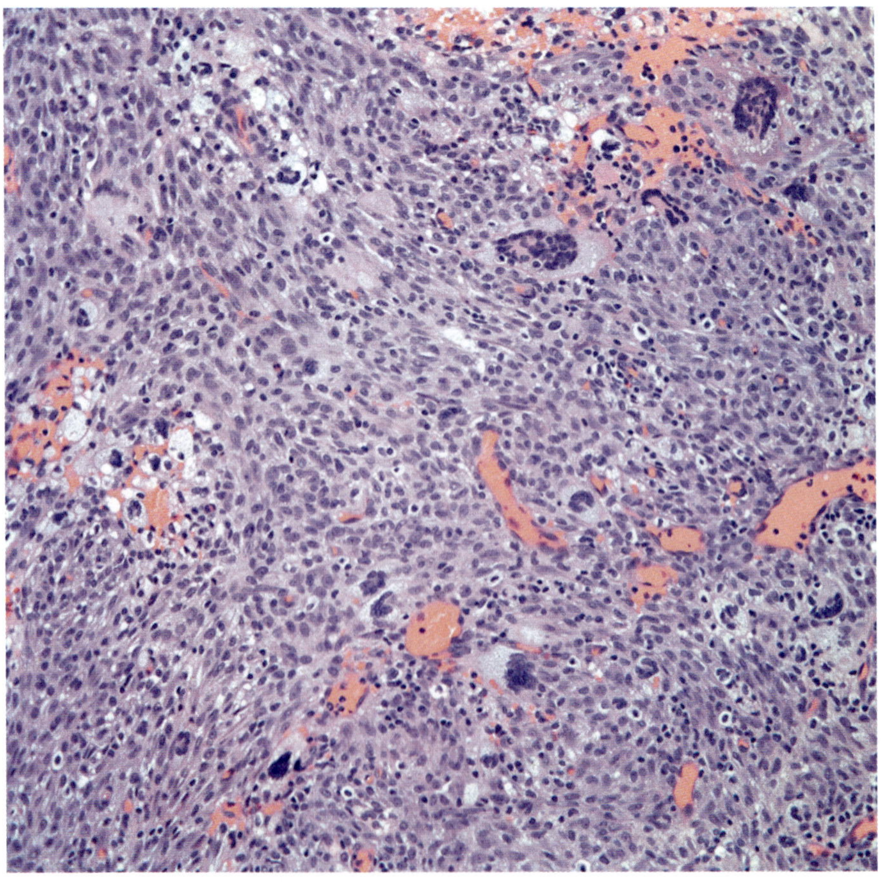

Figure 11-33 Inflammatory pseudotumor with scattered giant cells.

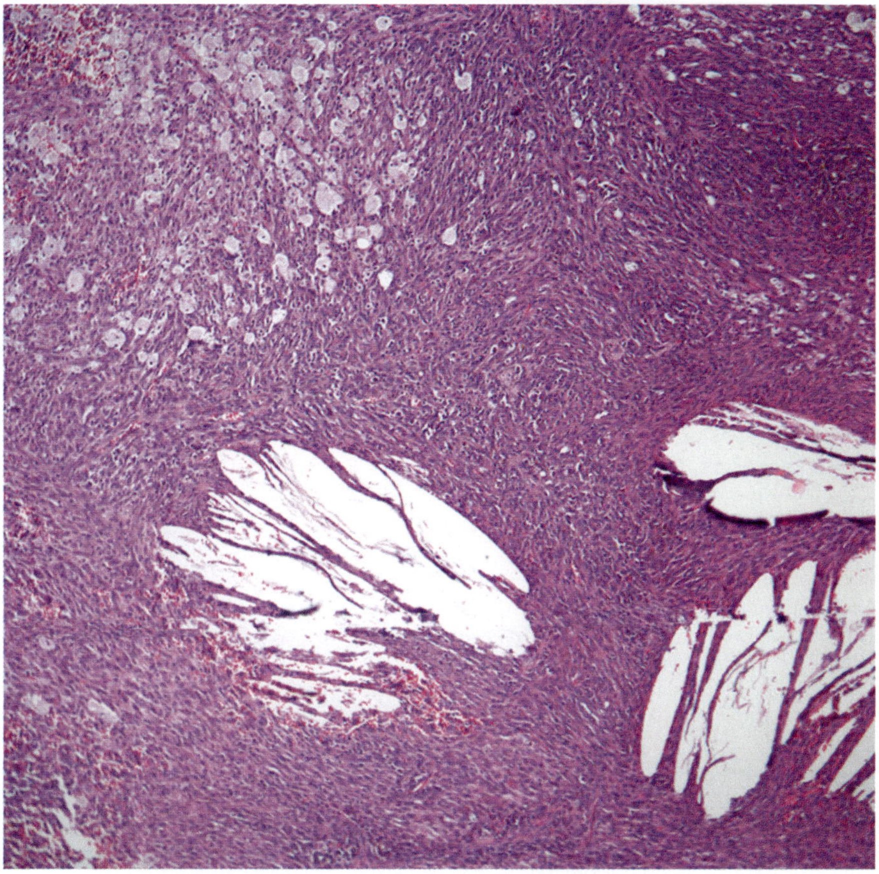

Figure 11-34 Inflammatory pseudotumor with prominent spindle cell component and cholesterol cleft granulomas.

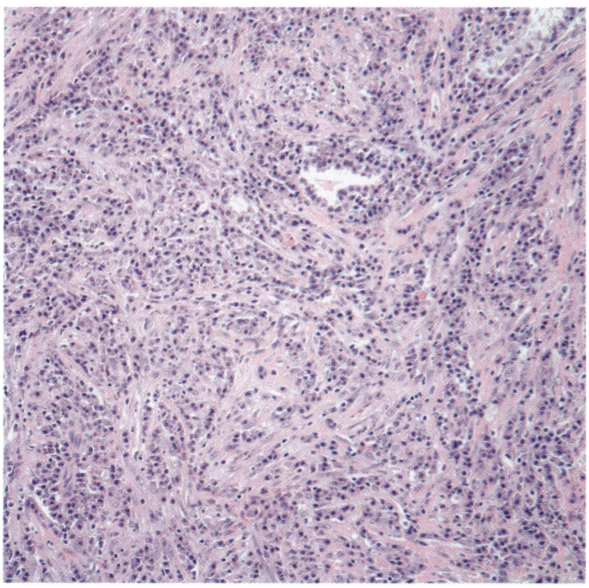

Figure 11-35 Inflammatory pseudotumor composed predominantly of plasma cells, with very limited spindle cell component.

In a recent study from the Mayo Clinic, Cerfolio and colleagues[93] evaluated 23 cases of IPT treated surgically and noted an overall survival rate at 5 years of 91%. Fatal outcome was unrelated to the IPT. Surgical treatment varied, ranging in extent from wedge resection to pneumonectomy. In three patients with incomplete surgical resection, the tumor recurred. In four patients who were initially treated with irradiation or chemotherapy, the lesion did not regress and had to be removed surgically. Other investigators also have argued that surgical approach with close follow-up is the treatment of choice.[90,94,96]

SCLEROSING HEMANGIOMA (PNEUMOCYTOMA)

Based on the available information, it is clear that the term *sclerosing hemangioma* is a misnomer, and that this benign tumor is not a true vascular neoplasm. Several theories have attempted to explain the origin of the cells involved in this tumor, including histiocytic, endothelial, epithelial, and mesothelial origins.[108–121] Although the epithelial origin is favored by many investigators, some unsettled issues remain regarding the two components that are present in these tumors. Although sclerosing hemangioma is essentially an intrapulmonary tumor, a tumor with the same characteristics has been described more recently in the anterior mediastinum.[122]

Historical Aspects

The original description of sclerosing hemangioma of the lung is credited to Liebow and Hubbell. In 1956, they described a series of seven cases of an intrapulmonary

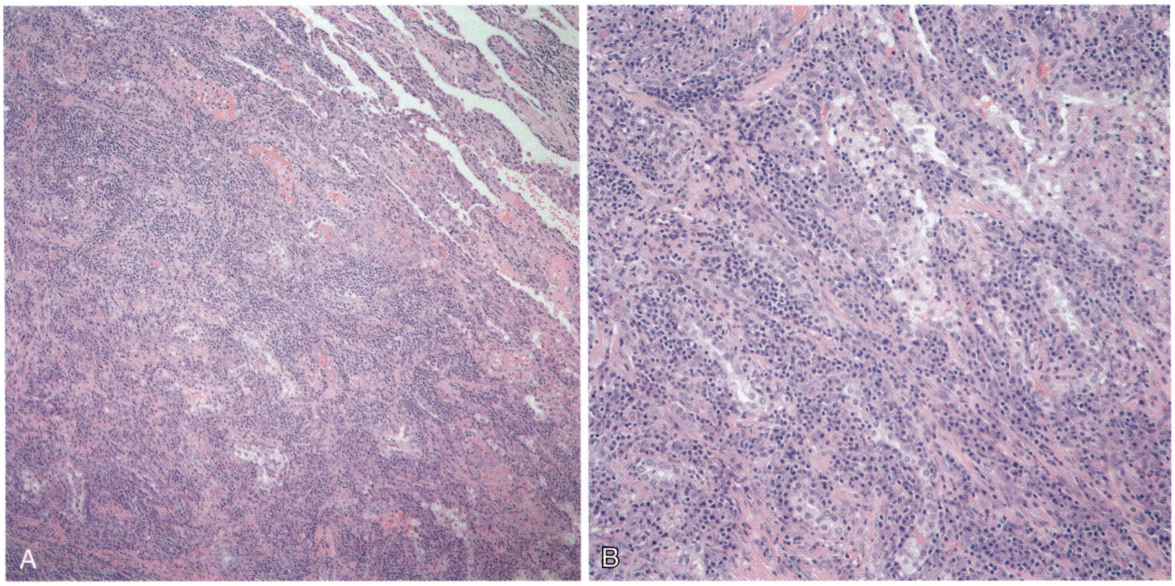

Figure 11-36 **A**, Well-circumscribed peripheral inflammatory pseudotumor. Note that residual alveolar structures also are present within the tumor. **B**, Higher-power view of the plasma cell proliferation and residual alveolar structures.

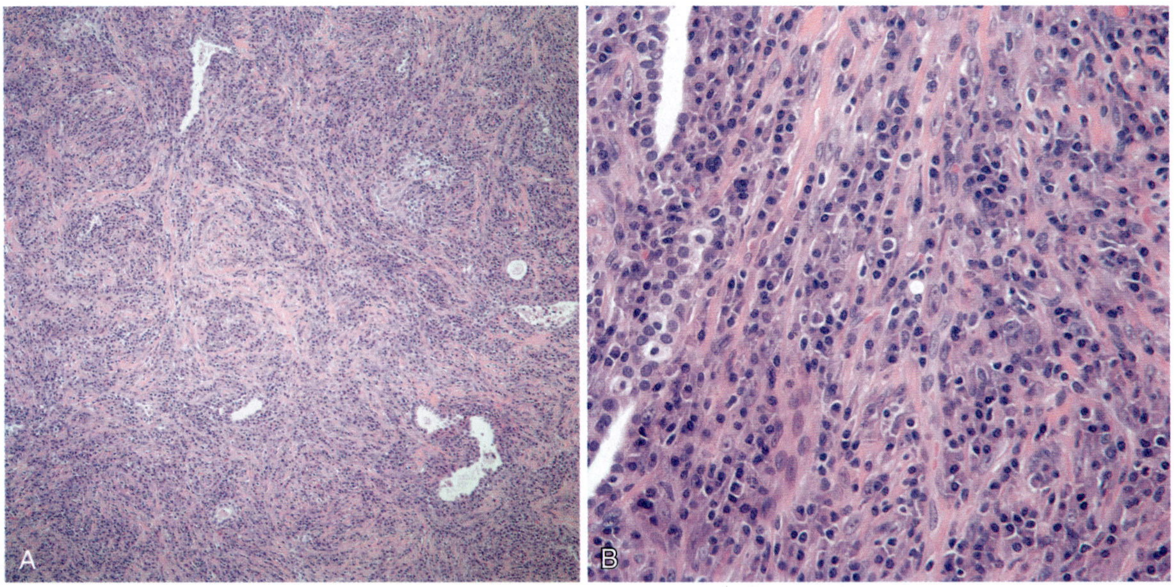

Figure 11-37 **A**, Inflammatory pseudotumor showing both spindle cell and plasma cell components. **B**, Higher-power view clearly showing both components.

neoplasm with features similar to those of some tumors occurring in the skin, designating it "sclerosing hemangioma."[108] Even though these tumors are now believed not to be of vascular origin, these investigators identified many anatomic, demographic, and clinical features that are highly relevant in the current assessment of these tumors.[108] These investigators determined that sclerosing hemangioma is more common in young adult females, that some patients are symptomatic, and that it is a slow-growing tumor with an affinity for the lower lobes. Their report also provided a basic histopathologic description of these tumors, including (1) proliferation of vessels with tendency to sclerosis; (2) papillary infoldings; (3) hemorrhage; and (4) presence of a large number of histiocytes. On this basis, these workers decided that the tumors had not only a vascular origin but also a possible histiocytic or xanthomatous component.

In 1972, after the use of electron microscopy had become widespread, Hill and Eggleston[111] described a similar tumor occurring in a 19-year-old female patient and suggested an epithelial origin from primitive respiratory epithelium. In 1973, Kennedy and colleagues docu-

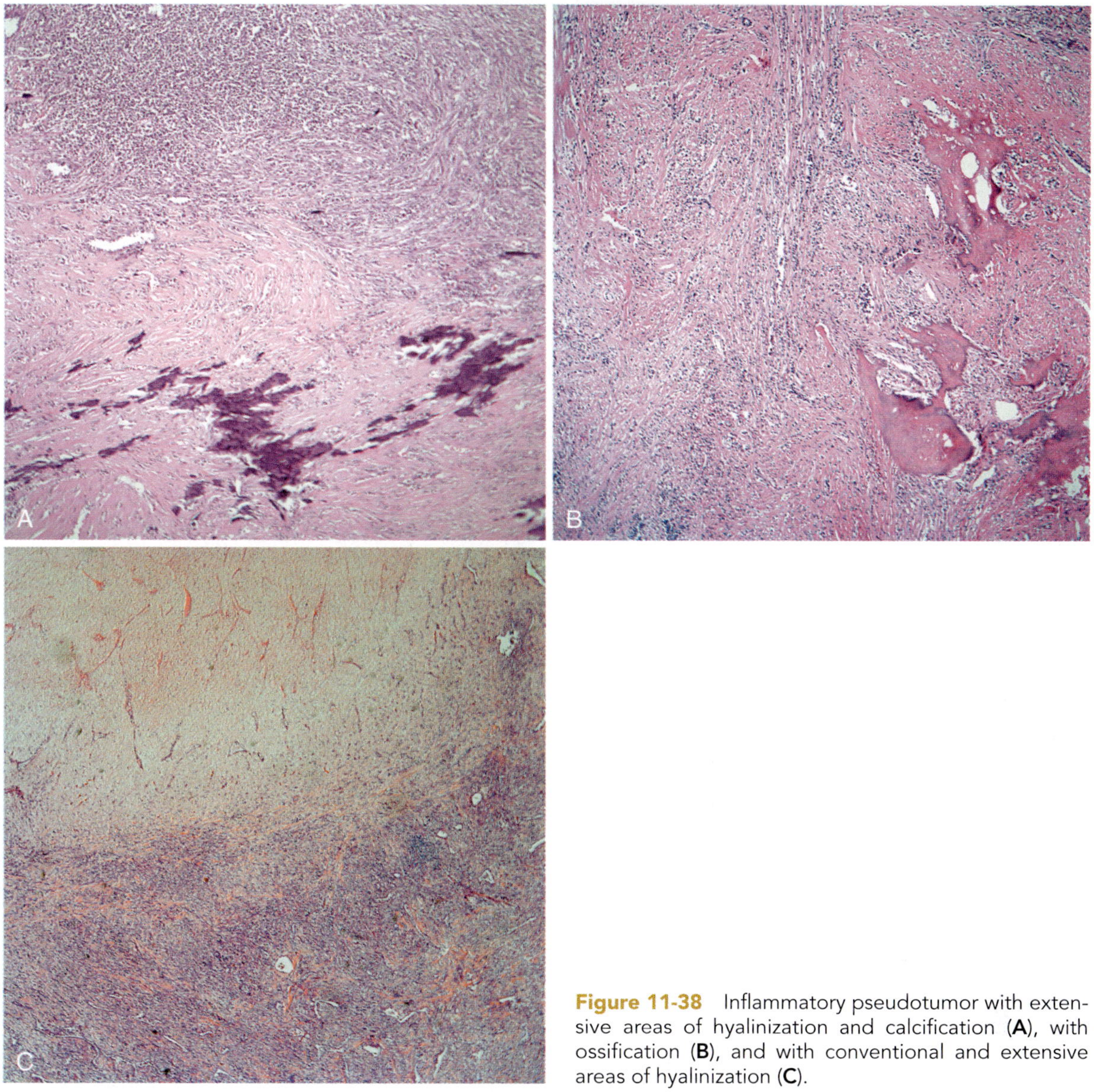

Figure 11-38 Inflammatory pseudotumor with extensive areas of hyalinization and calcification (**A**), with ossification (**B**), and with conventional and extensive areas of hyalinization (**C**).

mented two additional cases in which the histopathologic description included presence of granular pneumocytes, thus evincing the proposed term *papillary pneumocytoma* for this clinical entity. Alvares and Escalona[115] arrived at a similar conclusion, suggesting that sclerosing hemangioma represents a proliferation of distal respiratory epithelium with characteristics of immature type II pneumocytes. In their study of 13 cases of sclerosing hemangioma, Nagata and associates[114] demonstrated the presence of surfactant apoprotein in the cytoplasm of stromal and papillary cells, thereby providing more support for an epithelial origin with differentiation toward type II pneumocytes. Nagata's group[120] analyzed an additional 16 cases and concluded that in view of the different staining pattern, the stromal cells may represent heterogeneous epithelial cells. Satoh and coworkers[121] acheived similar results after studying three cases, demonstrating differentiation toward type II pneumocytes. Kay and associates[110] reported a case with a suggested endothelial origin. In 1983, Katzenstein and colleagues[119] presented data on nine cases of sclerosing hemangiomas studied by immunohistochemical and electron microscopic techniques and suggested a mesothelial origin. Various investigators have raised the possibility of mesenchymal origin.[123,124] Some workers consider sclerosing hemangioma to be a type of hamartoma, whereas others argue that it may be related to the so-called alveolar adenoma.[125,126]

Clinical Features

Sclerosing hemangioma appears to occur with highest frequency among young adult women in the fourth or fifth decade of life. Approximately 80% of the reported cases are in women. Although the tumor may be more common in Asian women, no large series of cases has confirmed that assessment. In a majority of patients, the tumor is found incidentally during a routine radiographic examination as a coin lesion. In a few patients, presenting signs and symptoms of chest pain, cough, and hemoptysis have been described.[125,127–130] In some unusual cases, sclerosing hemangiomas have been described in association with other conditions, such as familial adenomatosis polyposis.[131] Although sclerosing hemangiomas more commonly affect young adult patients, these tumor also have been described in children.[132]

Macroscopic Features

In a majority of cases, the tumor is a single mass in a subpleural location in the periphery of the lung. The tumor is well circumscribed and tan in color, with a homogeneous-appearing surface; in some cases, focal areas of hemorrhage can be identified (Fig. 11-39). Tumor size ranges from less than 1 cm to 8 cm in greatest dimension. Although sclerosing hemangiomas may occur in any lung or lung segment, they appear to have a predilection for the lower lobes. In some unusual cases, the tumor can manifest as multifocal within the same lung or, more rarely, as bilateral multiple pulmonary nodules.[133–135] In other rare occurrences, sclerosing hemangioma may manifest as a cystic intrapulmonary tumor[136] or in an endobronchial location.[137]

Histopathologic Features

The histopathologic features of these tumors can vary widely. Four major histopathologic patterns have been described for sclerosing hemangiomas[127]: solid, hemorrhagic, papillary, and sclerosing. A majority of tumors will display an admixture of two or more of these patterns in differing proportions. In the *solid* pattern, the tumor is characterized by sheets of a monotonous-appearing cellular proliferation composed of oval to polygonal cells with open nuclei and distinct nucleoli, surrounded by a rim of amphophilic to lightly eosinophilic cytoplasm (Fig. 11-40). Focal collections of macrophages can be identified between these sheets of tumor cells (Fig. 11-41). The *hemorrhagic* growth pattern is characterized by dilated vascular spaces filled with blood (Fig. 11-42). The *papillary* pattern demonstrates papillary structures lined by small cuboidal cells with dark nuclei, reminiscent of alveolar lining cells. The stroma is populated by a monotonous cellular proliferation composed of large, round to polygonal cells similar to those present in the solid growth pattern (Fig. 11-43). In the *sclerosing* pattern, the tumor shows focal or extensive areas of hyalinization, mainly around vessels (Fig. 11-44). In some areas, tumor cells may have a signet ring cell–like or clear cell appearance; collections of foamy macrophages often can be identified (Fig. 11-45). Sclerosing hemangiomas also may display mast cells, cholesterol cleft granulomas (Fig. 11-46), calcifications (Fig. 11-47), adipose tissue (Fig. 11-48), necrosis, and a prominent giant cell component[130,138] (Fig. 11-49).

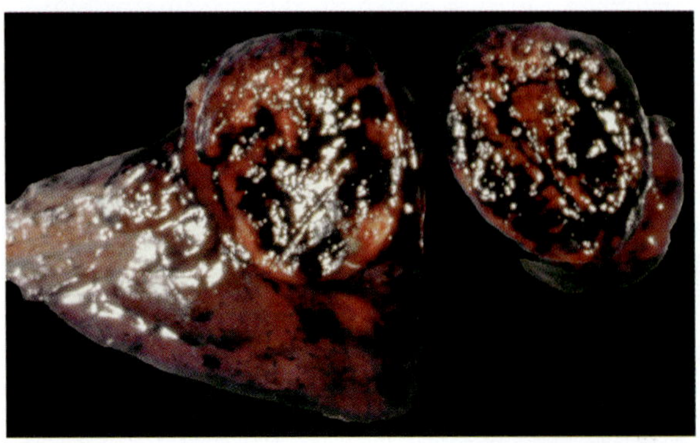

Figure 11-39 Gross specimen of a sclerosing hemangioma. Note the presence of hemorrhagic areas.

Immunohistochemical and Molecular Biology Features

Despite the rarity of sclerosing hemangioma, numerous studies have been conducted to investigate its histogenesis. The increasing knowledge and availability of antibodies as applied to tumor pathology have contributed to the available information. For instance, the initial notion that sclerosing hemangiomas were of endothelial origin (vascular tumors) has been ruled out because they have not shown positive staining for vascular markers such as CD31, CD34, *Ulex europaeus agglutinin*, and factor VIII. With use of newer antibodies that appear to be more specific for certain cells, positive staining in some of the components of sclerosing hemangiomas has been described. Several studies have reported conflicting results, however.[129,139–149] In some early reports using immunohistochemical techniques, positive staining for EMA, vimentin, CD68, cytokeratins (CAM5.2 and MNF116), S-100 protein, α-smooth muscle actin, secretory component, CEA, surfactant apoprotein, and Clara cell antigen was noted,[129,140,141] whereas other studies have documented neuroendocrine differentiation.[139] Previous findings have been augmented by descriptions of newly discovered antibodies, with positive staining reported for thyroid transcription factor-1 (TTF-1), cytokeratin 7, CAM5.2, surfactant apoproteins A and B, Clara cell antigen, estrogen and progesterone receptors, pro–surfactant protein C, and hepatocyte nuclear factor-3 (HNF-3) α and β.[130,144–148] Because of the dual cellular population present in sclerosing hemangiomas, however, these antibodies may label only one of the components. In general, EMA and TTF-1 appear to show positive staining in surface and stromal cells, whereas stromal cells usually are

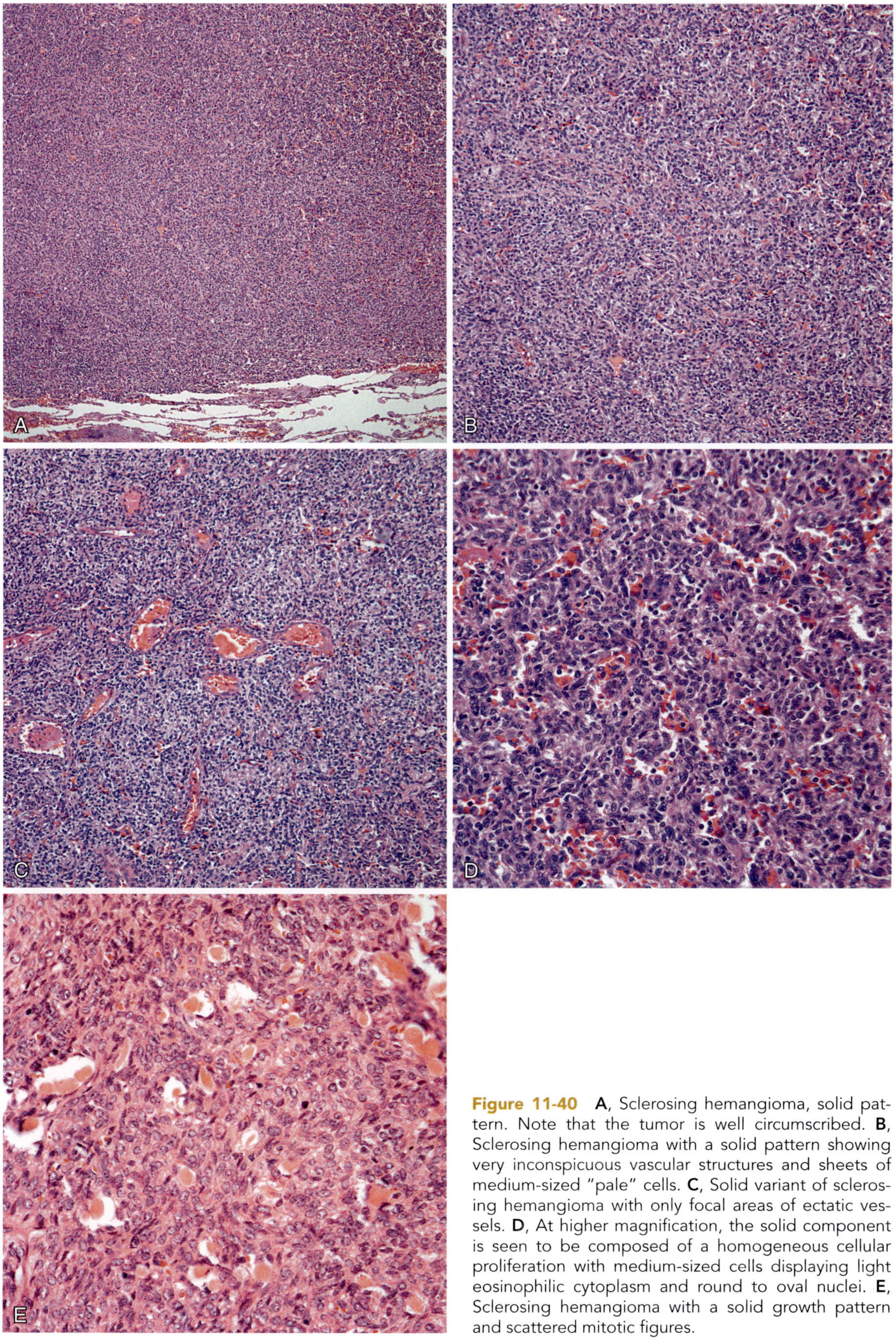

Figure 11-40 **A**, Sclerosing hemangioma, solid pattern. Note that the tumor is well circumscribed. **B**, Sclerosing hemangioma with a solid pattern showing very inconspicuous vascular structures and sheets of medium-sized "pale" cells. **C**, Solid variant of sclerosing hemangioma with only focal areas of ectatic vessels. **D**, At higher magnification, the solid component is seen to be composed of a homogeneous cellular proliferation with medium-sized cells displaying light eosinophilic cytoplasm and round to oval nuclei. **E**, Sclerosing hemangioma with a solid growth pattern and scattered mitotic figures.

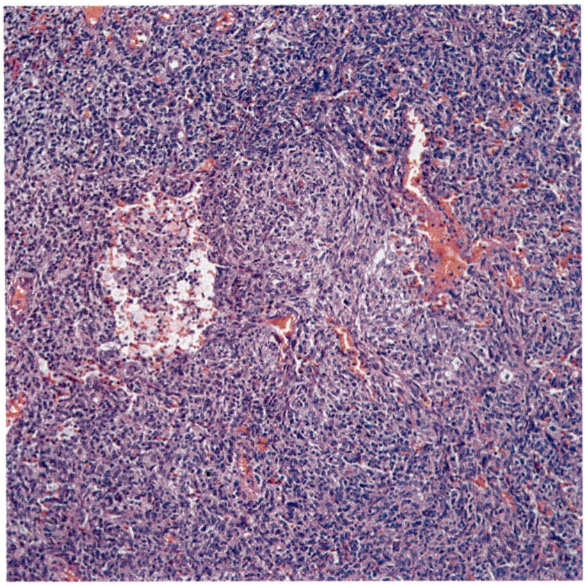

Figure 11-41 Sclerosing hemangioma with collections of foamy macrophages at the periphery of the tumor.

negative or weakly and focally positive for pan-keratin. Stromal tumor cells appear to react positively with cytokeratin 7 and CAM-5.2 low-molecular-weight keratin. Positive staining for surfactant proteins A and B and Clara cell antigen may be seen only in the surface epithelium and not in the stromal cells. These stromal cells also can demonstrate positive staining for vimentin and TTF-1.[130,149] Some studies have reported positive cell membrane and cytoplasmic staining for MIB-1, whereas others have documented no significant staining with p53.[150,151]

In addition to the multiple immunohistochemical studies available, some molecular biology studies have been performed, with interesting findings. Niho and coworkers[152] extracted DNA for clonal analysis based on an X-chromosome–linked polymorphic marker, human androgen receptor (HUMARA), and found monoclonality in both cellular components, suggesting that sclerosing hemangioma represents neoplasia and that both cells (cuboidal and stromal) are derived from the same origin. Using proteomic analysis, Jin and associates[153] documented that apolipoprotein A-1, antizyme inhibitor, the 27-kDa heat shock protein, and antioxidant proteins such as peroxiredoxin II (Prx II) and glutathione *S*-transferase (GST) are present in the down-regulated proteins in this tumor. More recently, Sartori and colleagues[154] documented that epithelial growth factor receptor (EGFR), human epidermal growth factor receptor 2 (HER2), and K-Ras sequencing did not reveal molecular alterations, whereas allelic losses at p16 and Rb loci with identical microsatellite allelic loss patterns were present in both cellular components.

Differential Diagnosis

With small biopsy specimens, making a definitive diagnosis of sclerosing hemangioma may prove to be challenging, because this neoplasm can be confused with any other epithelial malignancy. In addition, positive staining for epithelial markers, mainly keratin-7 and EMA, may lead to an incorrect interpretation. If the tumor has a prominent spindle cell component or demonstrates the presence of vascular structures, it may be confused with a low-grade sarcoma. A lymph node positive for tumor cells found during a staging procedure may indicate carcinoma with metastasis. The diagnosis becomes more obvious with complete surgical resection, which provides adequate tissue for identification of the different growth patterns.

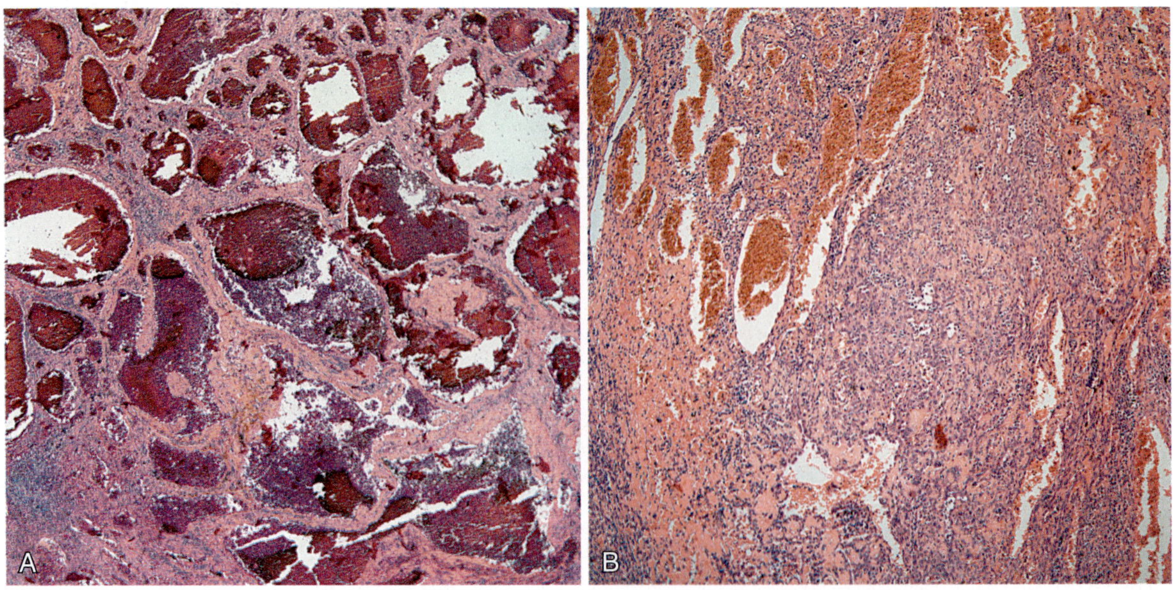

Figure 11-42 **A**, Low-power view of sclerosing hemangioma with prominent pools of red cells. **B**, Ectatic vessels filled with blood. The solid stromal proliferation characteristic of sclerosing hemangioma is visible.

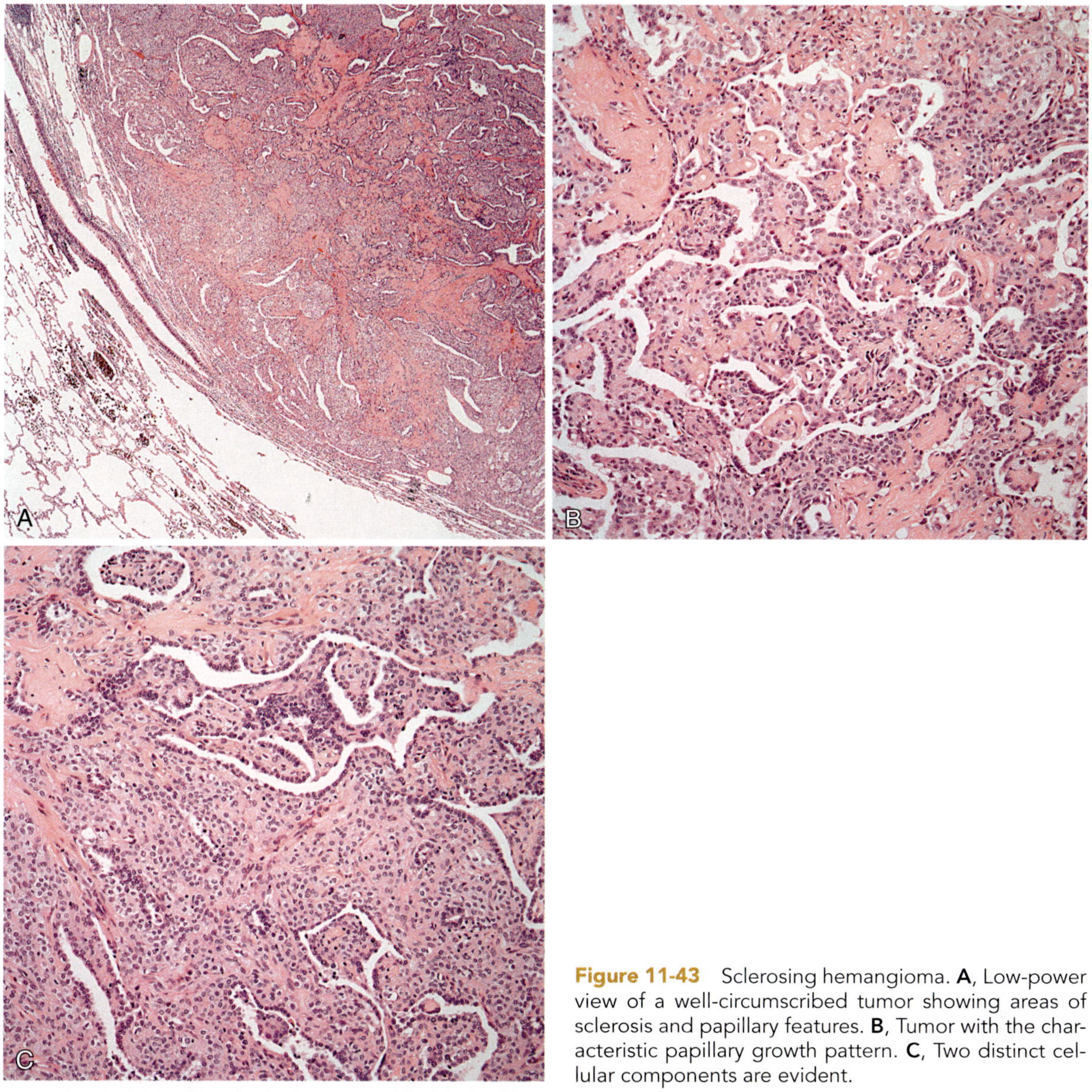

Figure 11-43 Sclerosing hemangioma. **A**, Low-power view of a well-circumscribed tumor showing areas of sclerosis and papillary features. **B**, Tumor with the characteristic papillary growth pattern. **C**, Two distinct cellular components are evident.

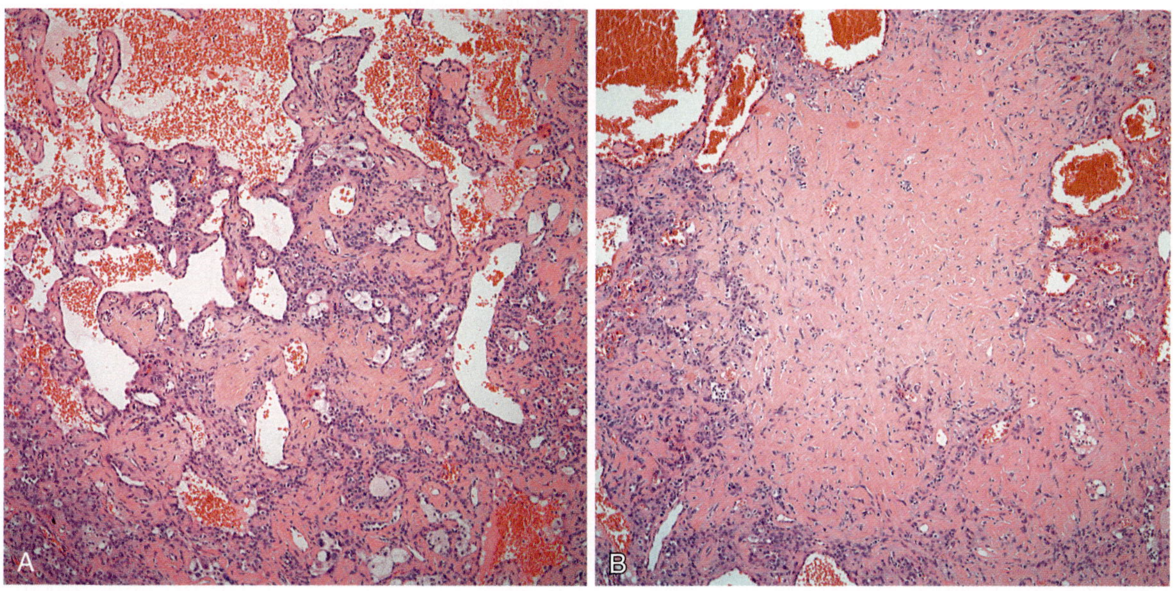

Figure 11-44 Sclerosing hemangioma. **A**, More discrete sclerotic areas are seen in between tumor cells. **B**, More extensive areas of sclerosis.

Continued

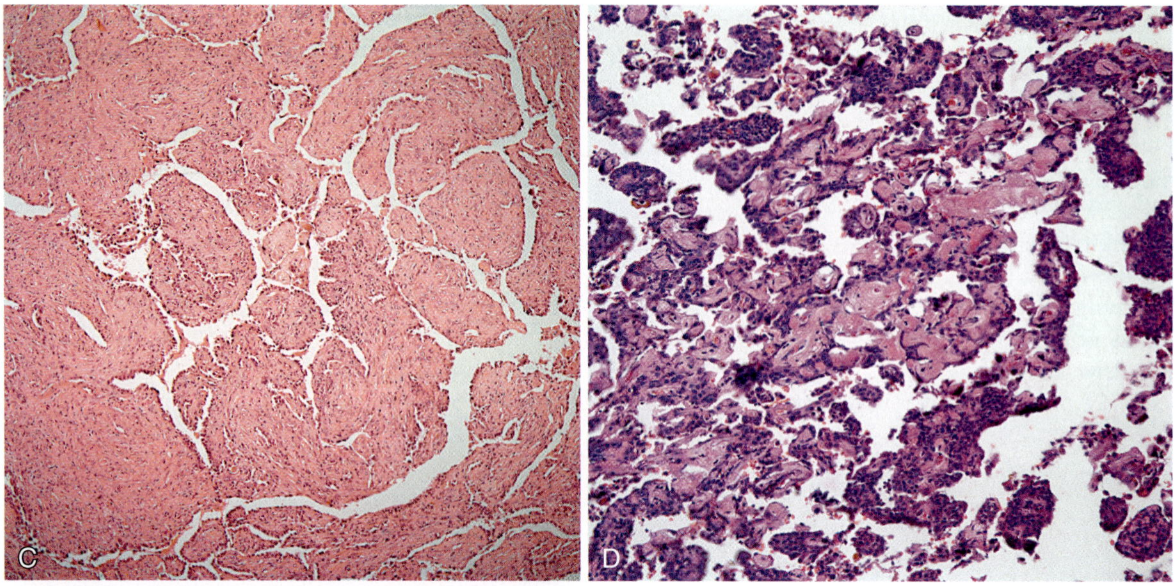

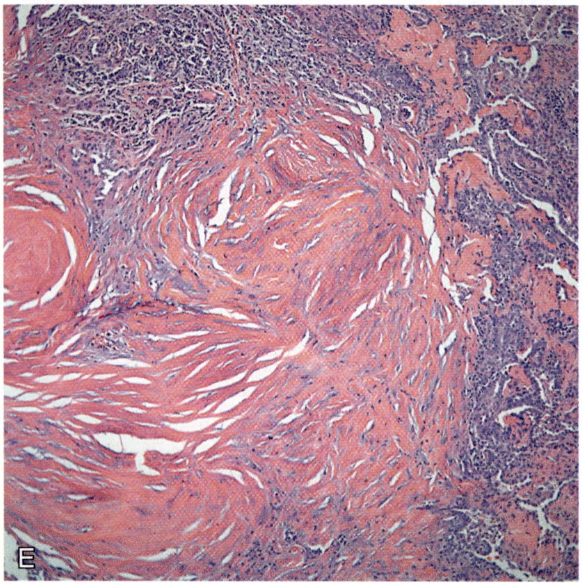

Figure 11-44—cont'd **C**, Extensive hyalinization is present, but papillary areas are still visible. **D**, Papillary areas with sclerosis mimicking angiosarcoma. **E**, In some cases, only focal solid areas and extensive hyalinization may be visible.

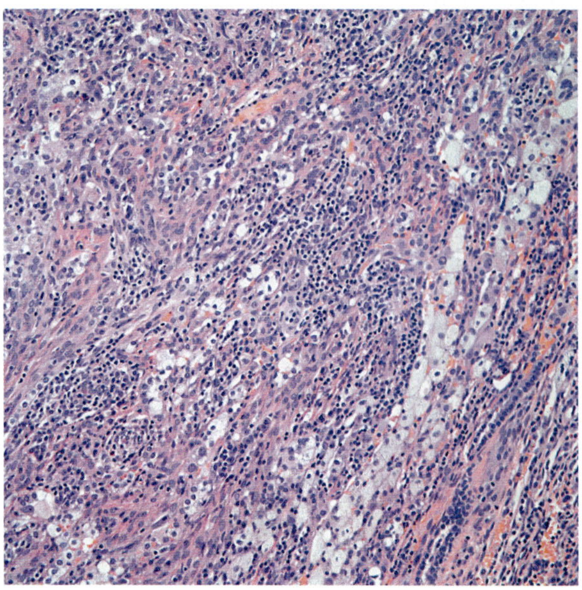

Figure 11-45 Sclerosing hemangioma with prominent collections of foamy macrophages.

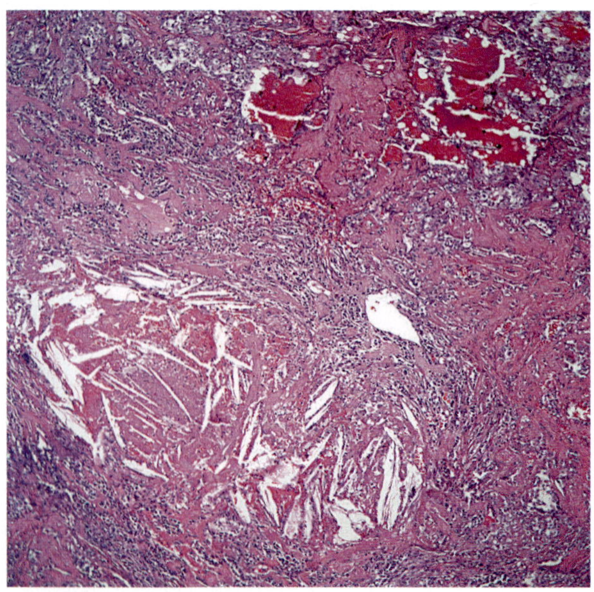

Figure 11-46 Sclerosing hemangioma with areas of cholesterol cleft granulomas.

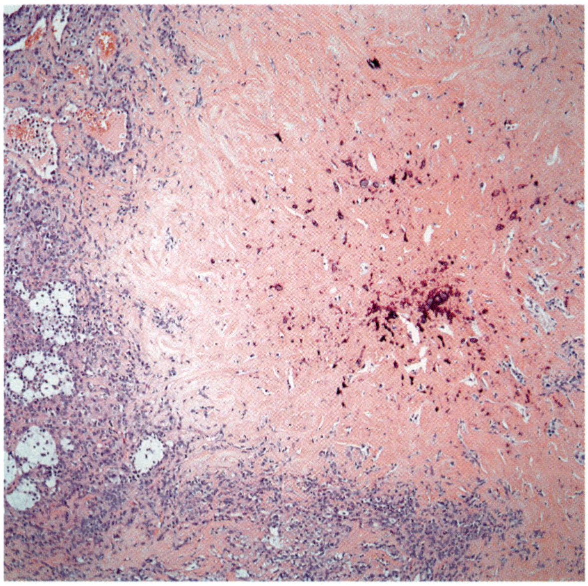

Figure 11-47 Sclerosing hemangioma with areas of calcifications.

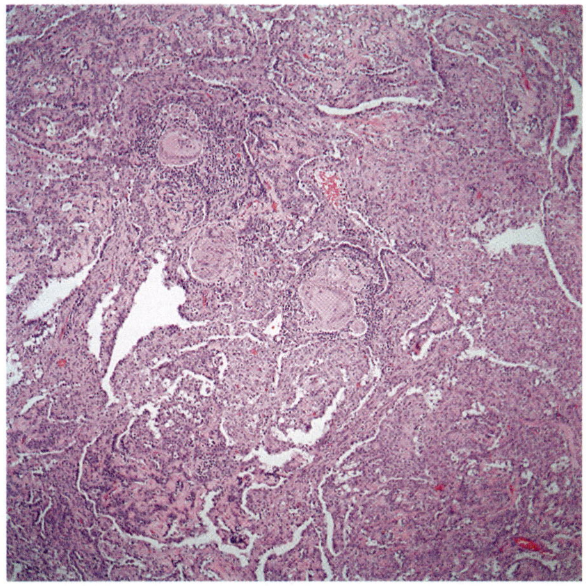

Figure 11-49 Sclerosing hemangioma with prominent granulomatous reaction.

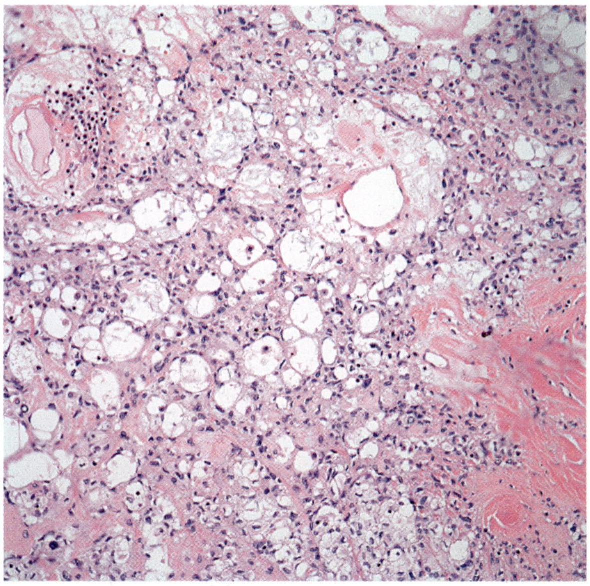

Figure 11-48 Sclerosing hemangioma with adipose tissue, which in some cases may mimic signet ring cells.

Treatment and Prognosis

The treatment of choice for sclerosing hemangioma is complete surgical resection by wedge resection or lobectomy, depending on the clinical and radiologic features of the tumor. Although sclerosing hemangiomas are thought to be benign, in some unusual cases the tumor follows a more aggressive course, and numerous instances of pleural and lymph node metastatic involvement have been described (Fig. 11-50), as well as tumor recurrence.[155–158] Therefore, close follow-up is recommended for these patients.

REFERENCES

1. Liebow AA, Castleman B. Benign "clear cell tumors" of the lung [abstract]. *Am J Pathol*. 1963;43:13a–14a.
2. Liebow AA, Castleman B. Benign clear cell ("sugar") tumors of the lung. *Yale J Biol Med*. 1971;43:213–222.
3. Becker NH, Soifer I. Benign clear cell tumor ("sugar tumor") of the lung. *Cancer*. 1971;27:712–719.
4. Andrion A, Mazzucco G, Gugliotta P, Monga G. Benign clear cell ("sugar") tumor of the lung: a light microscopic, histochemical, and ultrastructural study with a review of the literature. *Cancer*. 1985;56:2657–2663.
5. Gaffey MJ, Mills SE, Zarbo RJ, Weiss LM, Gown AM. Clear cell tumor of the lung. Immunohistochemical and ultrastructural evidence of melanogenesis. *Am J Surg Pathol*. 1991;15:644–653.
6. Lantuejoul S, Isaac S, Pinel N, Negoescu A, Guibert B, Brambilla E. Clear cell tumor of the lung: an immunohistochemical and ultrastructural study supporting a pericytic differentiation. *Mod Pathol*. 1997;10:1001–1008.
7. Bonetti F, Pea M, Martignoni G, Zamboni G. PEC and sugar. *Am J Surg Pathol*. 1992;16:307–308.
8. Govender D, Sabaratnam RM, Essa A. Clear cell "sugar" tumor of the breast. *Am J Surg Pathol*. 2002;26:670–675.
9. Tanaka Y, Ijiri R, Kato K, et al. HMB-45/Melan-A and smooth muscle actin–positive clear-cell epithelioid tumor arising in the ligament teres hepatis: additional example of clear cell "sugar" tumors. *Am J Surg Pathol*. 2000;24:1295–1299.
10. Tazelaar HD, Batts K, Srigley JR. Primary extrapulmonary sugar tumor (PEST): a report of four cases. *Mod Pathol*. 2001;14:615–622.
11. Kung M, Landa JF, Lubin J. Benign clear cell tumor ("sugar tumor") of the trachea. *Cancer*. 1984;54:517–519.
12. Sawyer JR, Nicholas RW, Parham DM. A novel t(X;2)(q13;q35) in clear cell sugar tumor of bone. *Cancer Genet Cytogenet*. 2004;154:77–80.
13. Adachi Y, Horie Y, Kitamura Y, et al. CD1a expression in PEComas. *Pathol Int*. 2008;58:169–173.
14. Hornick JL, Fletcher CDM. Sclerosing PEComa: clinicopathologic analysis of a distinctive variant with a predilection for the retroperitoneum. *Am J Surg Pathol*. 2008;32:493–501.

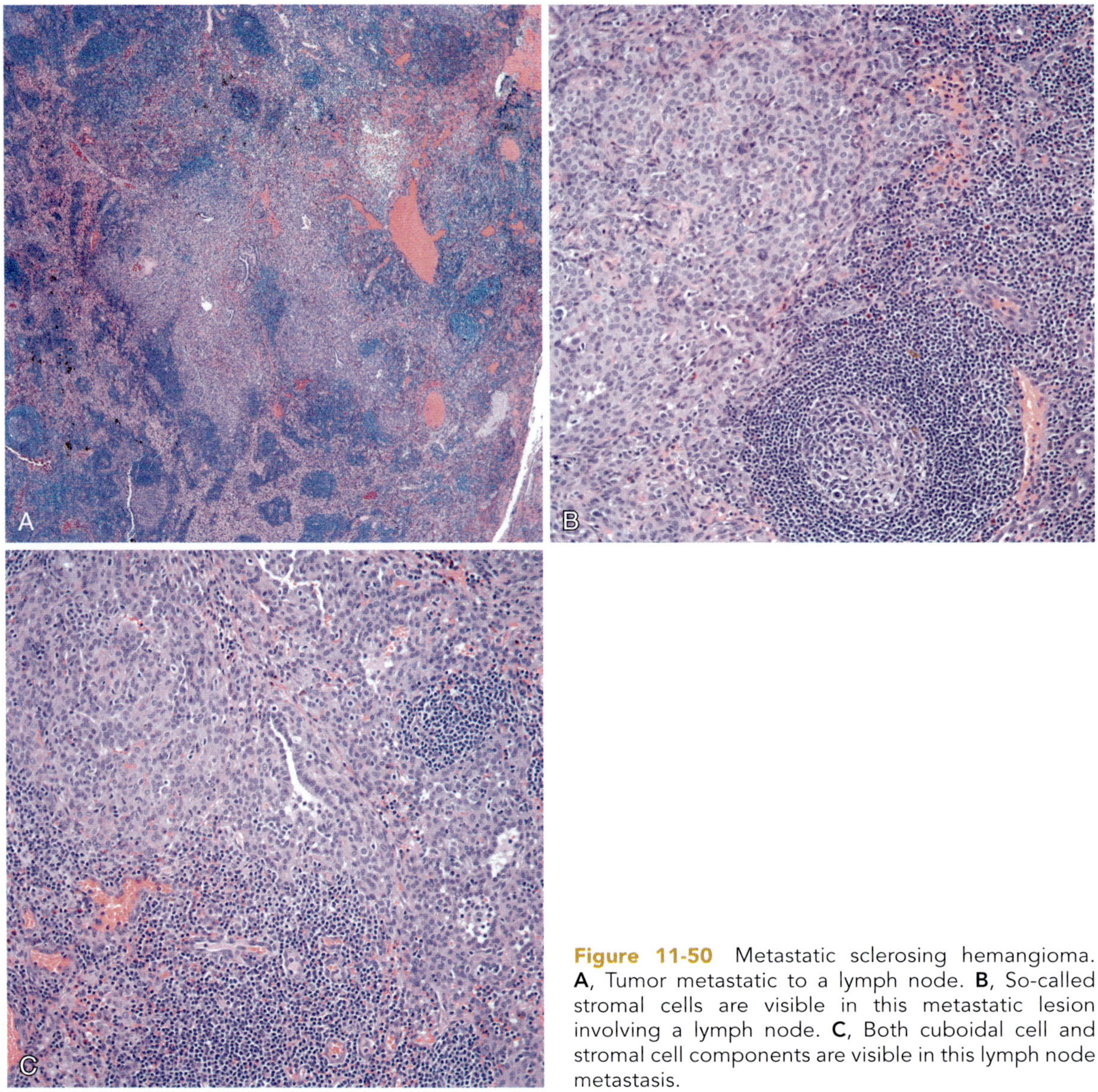

Figure 11-50 Metastatic sclerosing hemangioma. **A**, Tumor metastatic to a lymph node. **B**, So-called stromal cells are visible in this metastatic lesion involving a lymph node. **C**, Both cuboidal cell and stromal cell components are visible in this lymph node metastasis.

15. Fetsch P, Fetsch JF, Marincola FM, Travis W, Batts KP, Abati A. Comparison of melanoma antigen recognized by T cells (MART-1) to HMB-45: additional evidence to support a common lineage for angiomyolipoma, lymphangiomyomatosis, and clear cell sugar tumor. *Mod Pathol.* 1998;11:699–703.
16. Fukuda T, Machinami R, Joshita T, Nagashima K. Benign clear cell tumor of the lung in an 8 year old girl. *Arch Pathol Lab Med.* 1986;110:664–666.
17. Gora-Gebka M, Liberek A, Bako W, Szumera M, Korzon M, Jaskiewicz K. The "sugar" clear cell tumor of the lung—clinical presentation and diagnostic difficulties of an unusual lung tumor in youth. *J Pediatr Surg.* 2006;41:e27–e29.
18. Santana ANC, Nunes FS, Ho N, Takagaki TY. A rare cause of hemoptysis: benign sugar (clear) cell tumor of the lung. *Eur J Cardiothoracic Surg.* 2004;25:652–654.
19. Flieder DB, Travis WD. Clear cell "sugar" tumor of the lung: association with lymphangioleiomyomatosis and multifocal micronodular pneumocyte hyperplasia in a patient with tuberous sclerosis. *Am J Surg Pathol.* 1997;21:1242–1247.
20. Kavunkal A, Pandiyan MS, Philip MA, et al. Large clear cell tumor of the lung mimicking malignant behavior. *Ann Thorac Surg.* 2007;83:310–312.
21. Edelweiss M, Gupta N, Rosetkova E. Preoperative diagnosis of clear cell "sugar" tumor of the lung by computed tomography–guided fine needle biopsy and core needle biopsy. *Ann Diagn Pathol.* 2007;11:421–426.
22. Adachi Y, Kitamura Y, Nakamura H, et al. Benign clear (sugar) cell tumor of the lung with CD1a expression. *Pathol Int.* 2006;56:453–456.
23. Shiran MS, Arunachalam N, Sabariah AR, Pathmanathan R. Clear cell "sugar" tumor of the lung: a case report. *Malays J Pathol.* 2006;28:113–116.
24. Gal AA, Koss MN, Hochholzer L, Chejfec G. An immunohistochemical study of benign clear cell ("sugar") tumor of the lung. *Arch Pathol Lab Med.* 1991;115:1034–1038.
25. Sale GF, Kulander BG. Benign clear cell tumor of lung with necrosis. *Cancer.* 1976;37:2355–2358.
26. Sale GE, Kulander BG. "Benign" clear cell tumor (sugar tumor) of the lung with hepatic metastases ten years after resection of pulmonary primary [letter]. *Arch Pathol Lab Med.* 1988;112:1177–1178.

27. Dail D. Benign clear cell ("sugar") tumor of the lung [letter]. *Arch Pathol Lab Med*. 1988;113:573–574.
28. Lack EE, Worsham GF, Callihan MD, et al. Granular cell tumor: a clinicopathologic study of 110 patients. *J Surg Oncol*. 1980;13:301–316.
29. Chaudhry AP, Jacobs MS, SunderRaj M, Yamane GM, Jain R, Scharlock SE. A clinicopathologic study of 50 adult oral granular cell tumors. *J Oral Med*. 1984;39:97–103.
30. Allaire GS, Laflamme P, Bourgouin P. Granular cell tumors of the orbit. *Can J Ophthalmol*. 1995;30:151–155.
31. Vance SF, Hudson RP. Granular cell myoblastoma: clinicopathologic study of forty-two patients. *Am J Clin Pathol*. 1969;52:208–211.
32. Ordonez NG, Mackay B. Granular cell tumor: a review of the pathology and histogenesis. *Ultrastruct Pathol*. 1999;23:207–222.
33. Ordonez NG. Granular cell tumor: a review and update. *Adv Anat Pathol*. 1999;6:186–203.
34. Abrikossoff A. Uber Myome, ausgehen von der quergestreiften willkurlichen Muskulatur. *Virchows Arch Pathol Anat Physiol*. 1926;260:215–233.
35. Abrikossoff A. Weitere Untersuchungen uber Myoblastenmyome. *Virchows Arch Pathol Anat*. 1931;280:723–740.
36. Azzopardi JG. Histogenesis of granular cell "myoblastoma." *J Pathol Bacteriol*. 1956;71:85–94.
37. Pearse AG. The histogenesis of granular cell myoblastoma (granular cell perineural fibroblastoma). *J Pathol Bacteriol*. 1950;62:351–362.
38. Fisher ER, Wechsler H. Granular cell myoblastoma: misnomer, electron microscopic and histochemical evidence concerning its Schwann cell derivation and nature (granular cell schwannoma). *Cancer*. 1962;15:936–954.
39. Kramer R. Myoblastoma of the bronchus. *Ann Otol*. 1939;48:1083–1085.
40. Frenckner P. The occurrence of so-called myoblastoma in the mouth and upper air passages. *Acta Otolaryngol*. 1938;26:689–693.
41. Greenberg SD, Beall AC, Gonzales-Angulo A. Granular cell myoblastoma producing bronchial obstruction. *Dis Chest*. 1963;44:320–323.
42. Hebert WM, Seale RH, Samson PC. Primary granular cell myoblatoma of the bronchus: report of a case with resection. *J Thorac Surg*. 1957;34:409–411.
43. Jones ER, MacArthur AM. Benign granular cell myoblatoma of the bronchus. *Br J Surg*. 1959;46:420–422.
44. Kraus AR, Melnick PJ, Weinberg JA. Myoblastoma of the bronchus. *J Thorac Surg*. 1948;17:382–384.
45. Benson WR. Granular cell tumors (myoblastomas) of the tracheobronchial tree. *J Thorac Cardiovasc Surg*. 1966;52:17–29.
46. Deavers M, Guinee D, Koss MN, Travis WD. Granular cell tumors of the lung: clinicopathologic study of 20 cases. *Am J Surg Pathol*. 1995;19:627–635.
47. van der Maten J, Blaauwgeers JL, Sutedja TG, Kwa HB, Postmus PE, Wagenaar SS. Granular cell tumors of the tracheobronchial tree. *J Thorac Cardiovasc Surg*. 2003;126:740–743.
48. De Clercq D, van der Straeten M, Roels H. Granular cell myoblastoma of the bronchus. *Eur J Respir Dis*. 1983;64:72–76.
49. Alvarez-Fernandez E, Carretero-Albinama L. Bronchial granular cell tumor. *Arch Pathol Lab Med*. 1987;111:1065–1069.
50. Schulster P, Khan FA, Azueta V. Asymptomatic pulmonary granular cell tumor presenting as a coin lesion. *Chest*. 1975;68:256–258.
51. Vaos G, Zavras N, Priftis K, Pierrakos P. Bronchial granular cell tumor in a child: impact of diagnostic delay on the type of surgical resection. *J Pediatr Pathol*. 2006;41:1326–1328.
52. Oparah SS, Subramanian VA. Granular cell myoblastoma of the bronchus: report of 2 cases and review of the literature. *Ann Thorac Surg*. 1976;22:199–202.
53. Redje B, Rohatgi PK, Herman MA. Multicentric endobronchial granular cell myoblastoma. *Chest*. 1990;98:945–948.
54. Garancis JC, Komorowski RA, Kuzma JF. Granular cell myoblastoma. *Cancer*. 1970;25:542–550.
55. Young CD, Gay RM. Multiple endobronchial granular cell myoblastomas discovered at bronchoscopy. *Hum Pathol*. 1984;15: 193–194.
56. Cutlan RT, Eltorky M. Pulmonary granular cell tumor coexisting with bronchogenic carcinoma. *Ann Diagn Pathol*. 2001;5:74–79.
57. Jiang M, Anderson T, Nwogu C, Tan D. Pulmonary malignant granular cell tumor. *World J Surg Oncol*. 2003;1:22.
58. Callejo SA, Kronish JW, Decker SJ, Cohen GR, Rosa Jr RH. Malignant granular cell tumor metastatic to the orbit. *Ophthalmology*. 2000;107:550–554.
59. Parayno PP, August CZ. Malignant granular tumor: report of a case with DNA ploidy analysis. *Arch Pathol Lab Med*. 1996;120:296–300.
60. Khanzur T, Balducci L, Tavassoli M. Granular cell tumor: clinical spectrum of benign and malignant entity. *Cancer*. 1987;60:220–222.
61. Fanbur-Smith JC, Meis-Kindblom JM, Fante R, Kindblom LG. Malignant granular cell tumor of soft tissue: diagnostic criteria and clinicopathological correlation. *Am J Surg Pathol*. 1998;22:779–794.
62. Nakazato Y, Ishizeki J, Takahashi K, Yamaguchi H. Immunohistochemical localization of S-100 protein in granular cell myoblastoma. *Cancer*. 1982;49:1624–1628.
63. Miettinen M, Lehtonen E, Lehtola H, Ekblom P, Lehto VP, Virtanen I. Histogenesis of granular cell tumour—an immunohistochemical and ultrastructural study. *J Pathol*. 1984;142:221–229.
64. Mazur M, Shultz J, Myers JL. Granular cell tumor: immunohistochemical analysis of 21 benign tumors and one malignant tumor. *Arch Pathol Lab Med*. 1990;114:692–696.
65. Daniel TM, Smith RH, Faunce HF, Sylvest VM. Transbronchoscopic versus surgical resection of tracheobronchial granular cell myoblastoma. *J Thorac Cardiovasc Surg*. 1980;80:898–903.
66. Gomez-Roman JJ, Sanchez-Velasco P, Ocejo-Vinyals G, Hernandez-Nieto E, Leyva-Cobian F, Val-Bernal JF. Human herpesvirus-8 genes are expressed in pulmonary inflammatory myofibroblastic tumor (inflammatory pseudotumor). *Am J Surg Pathol*. 2001;25(5):624–629.
67. Farris AB, Kradin RL. Follicular localization of dendritic cells in a xanthomatous inflammatory tumor of lung associated with human herpes virus-8 infection. *Virchows Arch*. 2006;449:726–729.
68. Su LD, Atayde-Perez A, Sheldon S, Fletcher JA, Weiss SW. Inflammatory myofibroblastic tumor: cytogenetic evidence supporting clonal origin. *Mod Pathol*. 1998;11(4):364–368.
69. Janik JS, Janik JP, Lovell MA, Hendrickson RJ, Bensard DD, Greffe BS. Recurrent inflammatory pseudotumors in children. *J Pediatr Surg*. 2003;38(10):1491–1495.
70. Pache JC, Christakos PG, Gannon DE, Mitchell JJ, Low RB, Leslie KO. Myofibroblasts in diffuse alveolar damage of the lung. *Mod Pathol*. 1998;11(11):1064–1070.
71. Roscher AA, Endlich HH. Inflammatory pseudotumor of the lung. *Int Surg*. 1970;53(4):261–278.
72. Bahadori M, Liebow AA. Plasma cell granuloma. *Cancer*. 1973;31(1):191–208.
73. Buell R, Wang NS, Seemayer TA, Ahmed MN. Endobronchial plasma cell granuloma (xanthomatous pseudotumor). *Hum Pathol*. 1976;7(4):411–426.
74. Yu H, Dawel Z, Zhengyan W. Inflammatory pseudotumor of the lung: an analysis of 41 cases. *Chinese Med J*. 1979;92(8):548–554.
75. Toomes H, Delphendahl A, Manke HG, Vogt-Moykopf I. The coin lesion of the lung: a review of 955 resected coin lesions. *Cancer*. 1983;51(3):534–537.
76. Spencer H. The pulmonary plasma cell/histiocytoma complex. *Histopathology*. 1984;8:903–916.

77. Chen HP, Lee SS, Berardi RS. Inflammatory pseudotumor of the lung: ultrastructural and light microscopic study of a myxomatous variant. *Cancer*. 1984;54:861–865.
78. Maples MD, Adkins RB, Graham BS, Dao AH, Scott Hw. Pseudotumor of the lung. *Am Surg*. 1985;51(2):84–88.
79. Scott L, Blair G, Taylor G, Dimmick J, Fraser G. Inflammatory pseudotumors in children. *J Pediatr Surg*. 1988;23(8):755–758.
80. Ishida T, Oka T, Nishino T, Tateishi M, Mitsudomi T, Sugimachi K. Inflammatory pseudotumor of the lung in adults: radiographic and clinicopathological analysis. *Ann Thorac Surg*. 1989;48:90–95.
81. Pettinato G, Manivel JC, Rosa ND, Dehner LP. Inflammatory myofibroblastic tumor (plasma cell granuloma): clinicopathologic study of 20 cases with immunohistochemical and ultrastructural observations. *Am J Clin Pathol*. 1990;94:538–546.
82. Vujanic GM, Dojcinov D. Inflammatory pseudotumor of the lung in children. *Pediatr Hematol Oncol*. 1991;8:121–129.
83. Daudi FA, Lees GM, Higa TE. Inflmmatory pseudotumours of the lung: two cases and review. *Chinese J Surg*. 1991;34(5):461–464.
84. Nonomura A, Mizukami Y, Matsubara F, et al. Seven patients with plasma cell granuloma (inflammatory pseudotumor) of the lung, including two with intrabronchial growth: an immunohistochemical and electron microscopic study. *Intern Med*. 1992;31:756–765.
85. Souid AK, Ziemba MC, Dubansky AS, et al. Inflammatory myofibroblastic tumor in children. *Cancer*. 1993;72(6):2042–2048.
86. McGinnis M, Jacobs G, el-Naggar A, Redline RW. Congenital peribronchial myofibroblastic tumor (so-called "congenital leiomyosarcoma"). A distinct neonatal lung lesion associated with nonimmune hydrops fetalis. *Mod Pathol*. 1993;6(4):487–492.
87. Gal AA, Koss MN, McCarthy WF, Hochholzer L. Prognostic factors in pulmonary fibrohistiocytic lesions. *Cancer*. 1994;73:1817–1824.
88. Agrons GA, Rosado-de-Christenson ML, Kirejczyk WM, Conran RM, Stocker JT. Pulmonary inflammatory pseudotumor: radiologic features. *Radiology*. 1998;206:511–518.
89. Alexiou C, Obuszko Z, Beggs D, Morgan WE. Inflammatory pseudotumors of the lung. *Ann Thorac Surg*. 1998;66:948–950.
90. Messineo A, Mognato G, D'Amore ESG, Antoniello L, Guglielmi M, Checchetto G. Inflammatory pseudotumor of the lung in children: conservative or aggressive approach? *Med Pediatr Oncol*. 1998;31:100–104.
91. Zennaro H, Laurent F, Vergier B, et al. Inflammatory myofibroblastic tumor of the lung (inflammatory pseudotumor): uncommon cause of solitary pulmonary nodule. *Eur Radiol*. 1999;9:1205–1207.
92. Jubrail D, Charalambos Z, Niki A, Konstantinos K. Inflammatory pseudotumor: a controversial entity. *Eur J Cardiothorac Surg*. 1999;16:670–673.
93. Cerfolio RJ, Allen MS, Nascimento AG, et al. Inflammatory pseudotumors of the lung. *Ann Thorac Surg*. 1999;67:933–936.
94. Topçu S, Taştepe I, Alper A, et al. Inflammatory pseudotumors of the lung: a clinical study of eleven patients. *J Thorac Cardiovasc Surg*. 2000;119(1):180–182.
95. Karnak I, Senocak ME, Ciftci AO, et al. Inflammatory myofibroblastic tumor in children: diagnosis and treatment. *J Pediatr Surg*. 2001;36(6):908–912.
96. Kim JH, Cho JH, Park MS, et al. Pulmonary inflammatory pseudotumor—a report of 28 cases. *Korean J Intern Med*. 2002;17(4):252–258.
97. Kim TS, Ham J, Kim GY, Lee KS, Kim H, Kim J. Pulmonary inflammatory pseudotumor (inflammatory myofibroblastic tumor): CT features with pathologic correlation. *J Comput Assist Tomogr*. 2005;29(5):633–639.
98. Kobashi Y, Fukuda M, Nakata M, Irei T, Oka M. Inflammatory pseudotumor of the lung: clinicopathological analysis in seven adult patients. *Int J Clin Oncol*. 2006;11:461–466.
99. Kovach SJ, Fischer AC, Katzman PJ, et al. Inflammatory myofibroblastic tumors. *J Surg Oncol*. 2006;94(5):385–391.
100. Travis WD, Koss MN, Colby TV. Miscellaneous diseases of uncertain etiology. In: Travis WD, Koss MN, Colby TV, et al., eds. *Non Neoplastic Disorders of the Lower Respiratory Tract*. Washington, DC: American Registry of Pathology and Armed Forces Institute of Pathology; 2002.
101. Matsubara O, Tan-Liu NS, Kenney RM, Mark EJ. Inflammatory pseudotumor of the lung: progression from organizing pneumonia to fibrous histiocytoma or to plasma cell granuloma in 32 cases. *Hum Pathol*. 1988;19:807–814.
102. King TE. Bronchiolitis obliterans. *Lung*. 1989;167:69–93.
103. Batsakis JG, Luna MA, el-Naggar AK, Goepfert H. "Inflammatory pseudotumor": What is it? How does it behave? *Ann Otol Rhinol Laryngol*. 1995;104:329–331.
104. Coffin CM, Patel A, Perkins S, Elenitoba-Johnson KS, Perlman E, Griffin CA. ALK1 and p80 expression and chromosomal rearrangements involving 2p23 in inflammatory myofibroblastic tumor. *Mod Pathol*. 2001;14(6):569–576.
105. Debelenko LV, Arthur DC, Pack SD, Helman LJ, Schrump DS, Tsokos M. Identification of CARS-ALK fusion in primary and metastatic lesions of an inflammatory myofibroblastic tumor. *Lab Invest*. 2003;83(9):1255–1265.
106. Kinoshita Y, Tajiri T, Ieiri S, et al. A case of an inflammatory myofibroblastic tumor in the lung which expressed *TPM3-ALK* gene fusion. *Pediatr Surg Int*. 2007;23:595–599.
107. Wick MR, Ritter J, Nappi O. Inflammatory sarcomatoid carcinoma of the lung: report of three cases and clinicopathologic comparison with inflammatory pseudotumors in adult patients. *Hum Pathol*. 1995;26:1014–1021.
108. Liebow AA, Hubbell DS. Sclerosing hemangioma (histiocytoma, xanthoma) of the lung. *Cancer*. 1956;9:53–75.
109. Haas JE, Yunis EJ, Totten RS. Ultrastructure of sclerosing hemangioma of the lung. *Cancer*. 1972;30:512–518.
110. Kay S, Still WJS, Borochovitz D. Sclerosing hemangioma of the lung: an endothelial or epithelial neoplasm? *Hum Pathol*. 1977;8:468–474.
111. Hill GS, Eggleston JC. Electron microscopic study of the so-called "pulmonary sclerosing hemangioma." Report of a case suggesting epithelial origin. *Cancer*. 1972;30:1092–1106.
112. Palacios JJ, Escribano PM, Toledo J, Garzon A, Larrú E, Palomera J. Sclerosing hemangioma of the lung: an ultrastructural study. *Cancer*. 1979;44:949–955.
113. Kennedy A. "Sclerosing haemangioma" of the lung: an alternative view of its development. *J Clin Pathol*. 1973;26:792–799.
114. Nagata N, Dairaku M, Ishida T, Sueishi K, Tanaka K. Sclerosing hemangioma of the lung: immunohistochemical characterization of its origin as related to surfactant apoprotein. *Cancer*. 1985;55:116–123.
115. Alvarez-Fernandez E, Escalona-Zapata J. Sclerosing hemangioma of the lung. A histochemical, electron-microscopic, tissue culture, and time-lapse cinematographic study. *Histopathology*. 1981;5:579–588.
116. Mikuz G, Szinicz G, Fischer H. Sclerosing hemangioma of the lung. Case report and electron microscopic investigation. *Virchows Arch A Pathol Anat Histol*. 1979;385:93–101.
117. Eggleston JC. The intravascular bronchioloalveolar tumor and the sclerosing hemangioma of the lung: misnomers of pulmonary neoplasia. *Semin Diagn Pathol*. 1985;2:270–280.
118. Shimosato Y. Lung tumors of uncertain histogenesis. *Semin Diagn Pathol*. 1995;12:181–192.
119. Katzenstein AL, Weise DL, Fulling K, Battifora H. So-called sclerosing hemangioma of the lung: evidence for mesothelial origin. *Am J Surg Pathol*. 1983;7:3–14.
120. Nagata N, Dairaku M, Sueishi K, Tanaka K. Sclerosing hemangioma of the lung: an epithelial tumor composed of immunohistochemically heterogeneous cells. *Am J Clin Pathol*. 1987;88:552–559.
121. Satoh Y, Tsuchiya E, Weng SY, et al. Pulmonary sclerosing hemangioma of the lung. A type II pneumocytoma by immunohistochemical and immunoelectron microscopic studies. *Cancer*. 1989;64:1310–1317.

122. Sakamoto K, Okita M, Kumagiri H, Kawamura S, Takeuchi K, Mikami R. Sclerosing hemangioma isolated to the mediastinum. *Ann Thorac Surg*. 2003;75:1021–1023.
123. Huszar M, Suster S, Herczeg E, Geiger B. Sclerosing hemangioma of the lung: immunohistochemical demonstration of mesenchymal origin using antibodies to tissue specific intermediate filaments. *Cancer*. 1986;58:2422–2427.
124. Ling W, Ma L. Is sclerosing hemangioma of lung an alveolar mixed tumor? *Pathology*. 1983;15:205–211.
125. Spencer H, Nambu S. Sclerosing hemangioma of the lung. *Histopathology*. 1986;10:477–487.
126. Semeraro D, Gibbs AR. Pulmonary adenoma: a variant of sclerosing haemangioma of lung. *J Clin Pathol*. 1989;42:1222–1223.
127. Katzenstein AL, Gmelich JT, Carrington CB. Sclerosing hemangioma of the lung: a clinicopathological study of 51 cases. *Am J Surg Pathol*. 1980;4:343–356.
128. Chan KW, Gibbs AR, Lo WS, Newman GR. Benign sclerosing pneumocytoma of lung (sclerosing hemangioma). *Thorax*. 1982;37:404–412.
129. Leong ASY, Chan KW, Seneviratne HSK. A morphological and immunohistochemical study of 25 cases of so-called sclerosing hemangioma of the lung. *Histopathology*. 1995;27:121–128.
130. Devouassoux-Shisheboran M, Hayashi T, Linnoila RI, Koss MN, Travis WDA. clinicopathologic study of 100 cases of pulmonary sclerosing hemangioma with immunohistochemical studies: TTF-1 is expressed in both round and surface cells, suggesting an origin from primitive respiratory epithelium. *Am J Surg Pathol*. 2000;24:906–916.
131. Hosaka N, Sasaki T, Adachi K, et al. Pulmonary sclerosing hemangioma associated with familial adenomatous polyposis. *Hum Pathol*. 2004;35:764–768.
132. Batinica S, Gunek G, Raos M, Jelasić D, Bogović M. Sclerosing hemangioma of the lung in a 4-year-old child. *Eur J Pediatr Surg*. 2002;12:192–194.
133. Hishida T, Yoshida J, Nishimura M, Ishii G, Nishiwaki Y, Nagai K. Multiple sclerosing hemangioma with a 10-year history. *Jpn J Clin Oncol*. 2005;35:37–39.
134. Noguchi M, Kodama T, Morinaga S, Shimosato Y, Saito T, Tsuboi E. Multiple sclerosing hemangiomas of the lung. *Am J Surg Pathol*. 1986;10:429–435.
135. Hanaoka J, Ohuchi M, Inoue S, Sawai S, Tezuka N, Fujino S. Bilateral multiple pulmonary slcerosing hemangioma. *Jpn J Thorac Cardiovasc Surg*. 2005;53:157–161.
136. Khoury JD, Shephard MN, Moran CA. Cystic sclerosing hemangioma of the lung. *Histopathology*. 2003;43:239–243.
137. Devouassoux-Shisheboran M, de la Fouchardière A, Thivolet-Béjui F, Sourisseau-Millan ML, Guerin JC, Travis WD. Endobronchial variant of sclerosing hemangioma of the lung: histologic and cytological features of endobronchial material. *Mod Pathol*. 2004;17:252–257.
138. Moran CA, Zeren H, Koss MN. Sclerosing hemangioma of lung: granulomatous variant. *Arch Pathol Lab Med*. 1994; 118:1028–1030.
139. Xu HM, Li WH, Hou N, et al. Neuroendocrine differentiation in 32 cases of so-called sclerosing hemangioma of the lung: identified by immunohistochemical and ultrastructural study. *Am J Surg Pathol*. 1997;21:1013–1022.
140. Haimoto H, Tsutsumi Y, Nagura H, Nakashima N, Watanabe K. Immunohistochemical study of so-called sclerosing haemangioma of the lung. *Virchows Arch A Pathol Anat Histopathol*. 1985;407:419–430.
141. Yousem SA, Wick MR, Singh G, et al. So-called sclerosing hemangioma of lung. An immunohistochemical study supporting a respiratory epithelial origin. *Am J Surg Pathol*. 1988;12:582–590.
142. Fukayama M, Koike M. So-called sclerosing hemangioma of the lung: an immunohistochemical, histochemical and ultrastructural study. *Acta Pathol Jpn*. 1988;38:627–642.
143. Alvarez-Fernandez E, Carretero-Albinana L, Menarguez-Palanca J. Sclerosing hemangioma of the lung: an immunohistochemical study of intermediate filaments and endothelial markers. *Arch Pathol Lab Med*. 1989;13:121–124.
144. Rodriguez-Soto J, Colby TV, Rouse RV. A critical examination of the immunophenotype of pulmonary sclerosing hemangioma. *Am J Surg Pathol*. 2000;24:442–450.
145. Chan ACL, Chan JKC. Pulmonary sclerosing hemangioma consistently expresses thyroid transcription factor (TTF-1). A new clue to its histogenesis. *Am J Surg Pathol*. 2000;24:1531–1536.
146. Illei PB, Rosai J, Klimstra DS. Expression of thyroid transcription factor-1 and other markers in sclerosing hemangioma of the lung. *Arch Pathol Lab Med*. 2001;125:1335–1339.
147. Nicholson AG, Magkou C, Snead D, et al. Unusual sclerosing haemangiomas and sclerosing haemangioma-like lesions, and the value of TTF-1 in making the diagnosis. *Histopathology*. 2002;41:404–413.
148. Yamazaki K. Type II pneumocyte differentiation in pulmonary sclerosing hemangioma: ultrastructural differentiation and immunohistochemical distribution of lineage-specific transcription factors (TTF-1, HNF3 alpha, and HNF-3 beta) and the surfactant proteins. *Virchows Arch*. 2004;445:45–53.
149. Wang E, Lin D, Wang Y, Yuan X. Immunohistochemical and ultrastructural markers suggest different origins for cuboidal and polygonal cells in pulmonary sclerosing hemangioma. *Hum Pathol*. 2004;35:503–508.
150. Hattori H. Sclerosing hemangioma of the lung is positive for MIB-1 in cell membrane and cytoplasmic staining pattern. *Histopathology*. 2002;40:291–293.
151. Iyoda A, Hiroshima K, Shiba M, et al. Clinicopathological analysis of pulmonary sclerosing hemangioma. *Ann Thorac Surg*. 2004;78:1928–1931.
152. Niho S, Suzuki K, Yokose T, Kodama T, Nishiwaki Y, Esumi H. Monoclonality of both pale cells and cuboidal cell of sclerosing hemangioma of the lung. *Am J Pathol*. 1998;152:1065–1069.
153. Jin LJ, Shin BK, Jung WY, et al. Proteomic analysis of pulmonary sclerosing hemangioma. *Proteomics*. 2006;6:4877–4883.
154. Sartori G, Bettelli S, Schirosi L, et al. Microsatellite and EGFR, HER2, and K-RAS analyses in sclerosing hemangioma of the lung. *Am J Surg Pathol*. 2007;31:1512–1520.
155. Chan NG, Melega DE, Inculet R, Shepherd JG. Pulmonary sclerosing hemangioma with lymph node metastases. *Can Respir J*. 2003;10:391–392.
156. Komatsu T, Fukuse T, Wada H, Sakurai T. Pulmonary sclerosing hemangioma with pulmonary metastasis. *Thorac Cardiovasc Surg*. 2006;54:348–355.
157. Kim KH, Sul HJ, Kang DY. Sclerosing hemangioma with lymph node metastasis. *Yonsei Med J*. 2003;44:150–154.
158. Wei S, Tian J, Song X, Chen Y. Recurrence of pulmonary sclerosing hemangioma. *Thorac Cardiovasc Surg*. 2008;56:117–122.

12

Benign Tumors and Tumor-like Lesions of the Lung

A wide range of conditions may manifest as tumors or tumor-like lesions in the lung parenchyma. Although space limitations prevent the inclusion of every single clinical entity that may manifest as a pulmonary growth, this chapter covers some of the most common lesions that may require the expertise of the pathologist for accurate diagnosis. As a simple classification scheme, they have been separated into histiocytic and nonhistiocytic lesions.

NONHISTIOCYTIC LESIONS

Nonhistiocytic lesions comprise a wide range of rare conditions that may pose some difficulty in diagnosis, especially when only a small biopsy specimen is available for histologic analysis. Although these conditions are unusual, it is important to be able to properly diagnose and classify them. The following conditions are addressed in this section:

- Alveolar adenoma
- Mucous gland adenoma
- Amyloid tumor
- Alveolar proteinosis
- Placental transmogrification
- Pulmonary alveolar microlithiasis
- Pulmonary metastatic calcification
- Lymphangioleiomyomatosis
- Dirofilariasis

Alveolar Adenoma

Alveolar adenoma is a benign tumor of unusual occurrence in the lung parenchyma. Although the tumor may have been reported earlier under a different designation,[1] Yousem and Hochholzer coined the term *alveolar adenoma* in their report of six cases, which included four women and two men between the ages of 45 and 74 years. All of the patients were asymptomatic or displayed clinical signs and symptoms unrelated to the pulmonary tumor. All of the lesions were solitary pulmonary nodules, and all of the patients underwent surgical resection of the tumor.

Histopathologic Features

On gross inspection, these tumors generally are seen to be solitary coin lesions within the lung parenchyma. Size ranges from 1 to 3 cm in greatest dimension; they may be cystic and hemorrhagic.

On histologic examination, at low magnification the tumors appear to be well circumscribed, with prominent large cystic spaces that contain a clear acellular fluid (Fig. 12-1). At the periphery of the lesion, the tumor appears to be more cellular and glandular, with a microcystic-like pattern (Fig. 12-2). Higher magnification reveals a discrete inflammatory infiltrate composed of lymphocytes and plasma cells in the septa separating cystic glandular areas. These cystic spaces are lined by medium-sized cuboidal cells with a hobnail appearance resembling that

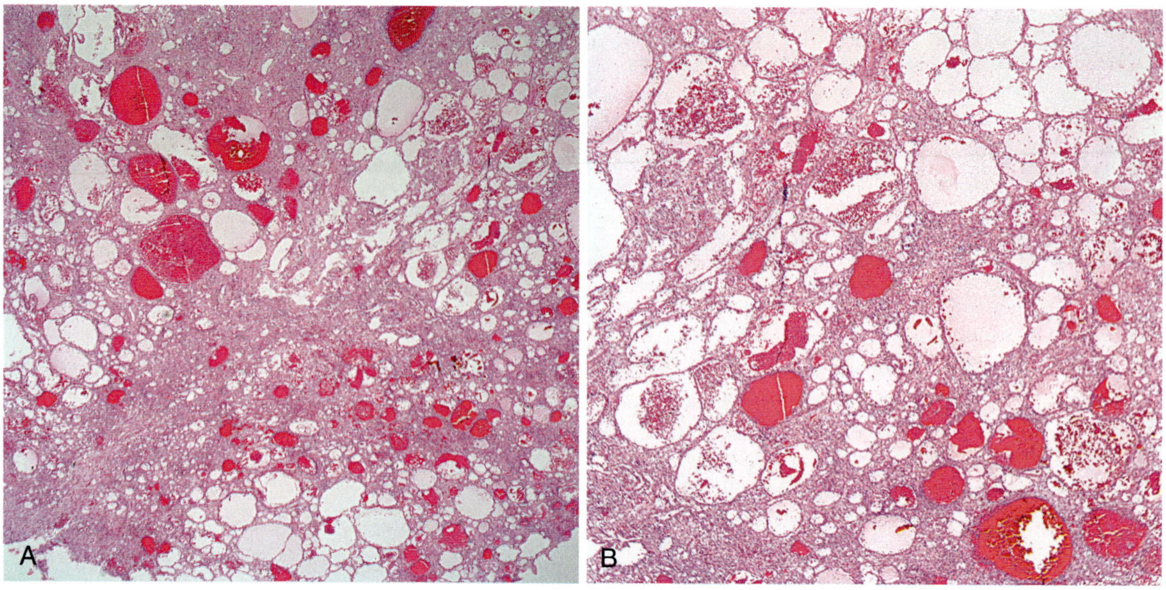

Figure 12-1 Alveolar adenoma. **A**, Low-power view showing classic solid and cystic areas. **B**, Cystic areas containing clear acellular fluid and fresh blood.

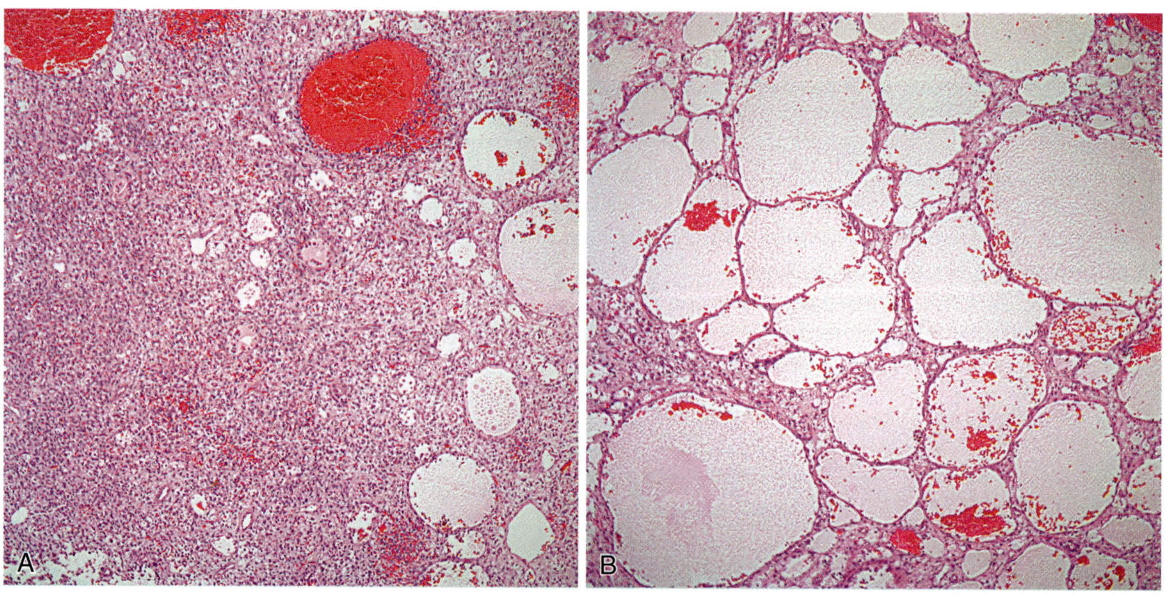

Figure 12-2 **A**, Alveolar adenoma with prominent solid areas. **B**, Alveolar adenoma with prominent cystic areas.

of pneumocytes, whereas in the peripheral areas with a more glandular appearance, the cells lining the alveolar spaces constitute a pneumocyte type II proliferation (Fig. 12-3). Mitotic activity is rare or nonexistent in these lesions, and necrosis is not a feature (Fig. 12-4). Periodic acid–Schiff (PAS) histochemical stain shows a positive reaction in the fluid contained in the cystic spaces.

Immunohistochemical studies have been performed in these lesions, and as might be expected, use of epithelial markers such as keratin and EMA gives a positive reaction. Surfactant apoprotein staining also has been found to be positive.[2,3] The tumor demonstrates negative staining for vascular markers including CD31, CD34, and factor VIII.

Differential Diagnosis

Inadequate biopsy specimens constitute the biggest obstacle to a correct diagnosis. Because of the glandular proliferation with prominent type II pneumocytes, the most important consideration in the differential diagnosis is adenocarcinoma with a bronchioloalveolar pattern. Both adenocarcinoma and bronchioloalveolar carcinoma may show positive staining for conventional markers including thyroid transcription factor 1 (TTF-1), surfactant, and epithelial markers. Thus, an unequivocal diagnosis of alveolar adenoma cannot be achieved with use of a small biopsy specimen but will require analysis of material obtained at complete resection of the tumor.

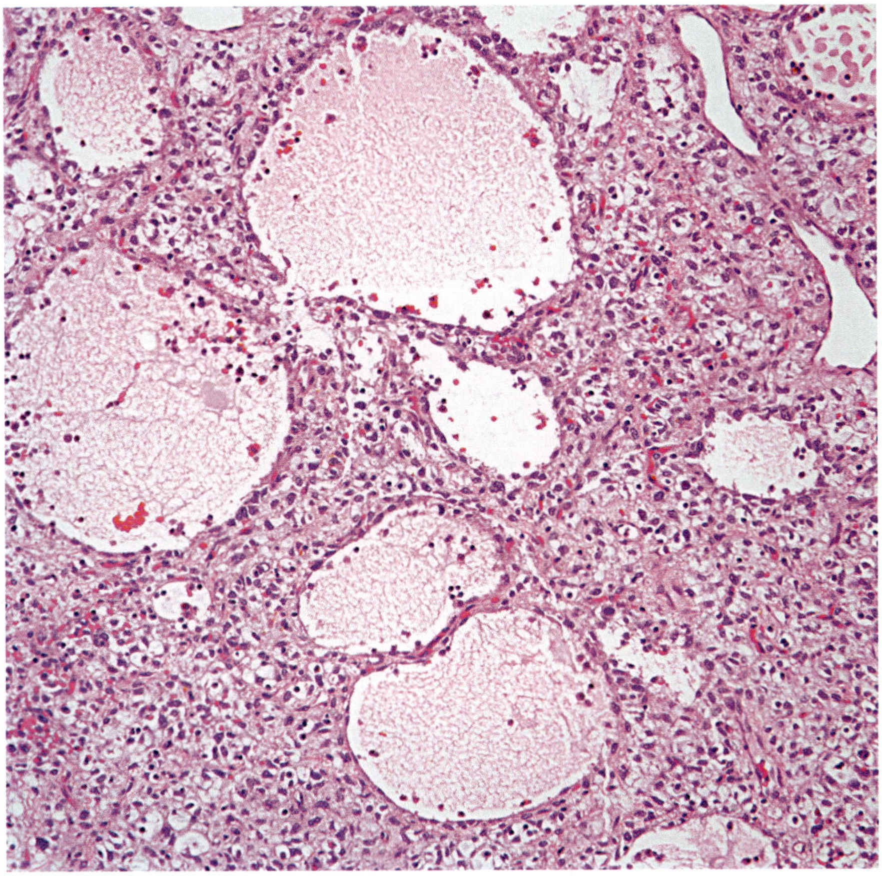

Figure 12-3 Alveolar adenoma with alternating cystic and solid areas.

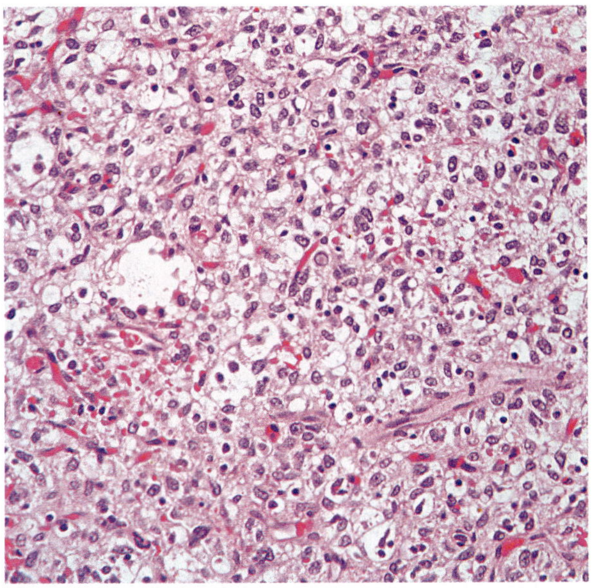

Figure 12-4 Solid areas of alveolar adenoma showing homogeneous cellular proliferation lacking mitotic activity and cellular atypia.

Because of the large cystic spaces present in these lesions, one other possibility to be considered is lymphangioma. In this instance, however, the epithelial lining of type II pneumocytes and the negative staining for vascular markers would indicate the correct interpretation.

Treatment and Prognosis

Surgical resection is the treatment of choice for alveolar adenomas and is curative. Procedures used have ranged in extent from wedge resection to lobectomy, although a more conservative approach may be warranted in some cases. Nevertheless, when it is difficult to assess the true nature of this tumor from limited biopsy material, resection is indicated. The available follow-up data have indicated that this is an indolent benign process.

Mucous Gland Adenoma

Mucous gland adenomas are benign tumors that have been recognized for some time[4–12] but formerly were classified with other so-called adenomas, not of this type, that corresponded to different types of tumors. Thus, it is difficult to determine the exact incidence of mucous gland adenomas. The tumor has been suggested to originate from the submucosal seromucous glands and ducts of the proximal airways and may represent an overdilatation of the normal structures. England and Hochholzer in 1995[13] presented 10 cases, summarizing the previous names for this tumor and identifying only 41 previous cases.

Clinical Features

The tumor appears to affect men and women equally, without any gender predilection, and has been documented to occur in adults between the ages of 25 and 67. The patients may be asymptomatic or may present with clinical signs and symptoms of bronchial obstruction such as cough, dyspnea, chest pain, or hemoptysis, reflecting the central location of the tumor.

Macroscopic Features

Mucous gland adenomas may manifest as polypoid, exophytic endobronchial tumors obstructing the pulmonary lumen. Size ranges from less than 1 cm to more than 5 cm in greatest dimension. These lesions are well circumscribed with a soft consistency and a mucoid appearance, with cystic changes. Areas of hemorrhage and necrosis are not common in these tumors.

Histopathologic Features

The hallmark histopathologic feature of mucous gland adenoma is the limitation of tumor growth between the bronchial epithelium and the bronchial cartilaginous plate (Fig. 12-5). The tumor is circumscribed within that particular space, without invasion into adjacent lung parenchyma or beyond the bronchial cartilage (Fig. 12-6). The low-power view shows an exuberant dilatation of the normal submucosal seromucinous glands of the lung, with areas of inflammatory reaction, and mucoid material filling the dilated glandular structures (Figs. 12-7 to 12-9). The tumor also may show a prominent papillary growth pattern. A higher-power view reveals a gamut of histopathologic change ranging from a glandular component with predominantly mucous epithelium, with little intervening stromal tissue, to compact glandular proliferation of seromucinous glands (Figs. 12-10 to 12-13). In other areas, the tumor may display cystically dilated glands of different sizes lined by squamous epithelium and separated by fibrocollagenous stroma (Fig. 12-14). In most cases, it is possible to identify an admixture of patterns that range from cystic to solid. Areas of cholesterol cleft granulomas, an inflammatory process composed predominantly of plasma cells, and areas of squamous metaplasia are commonly seen (Fig. 12-15). The glandular proliferation does not involve the adjacent lung parenchyma.

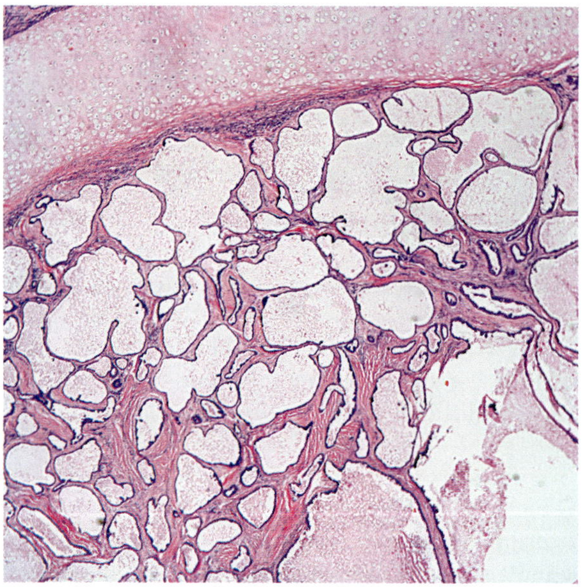

Figure 12-5 Mucous gland adenoma with exuberant dilatation of the submucosal glands.

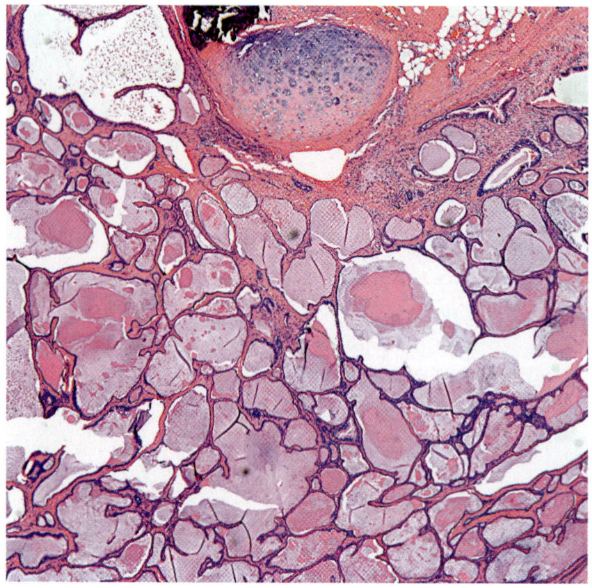

Figure 12-6 Mucous gland adenoma in which the proliferation of glands is limited to the bronchial cartilaginous plate.

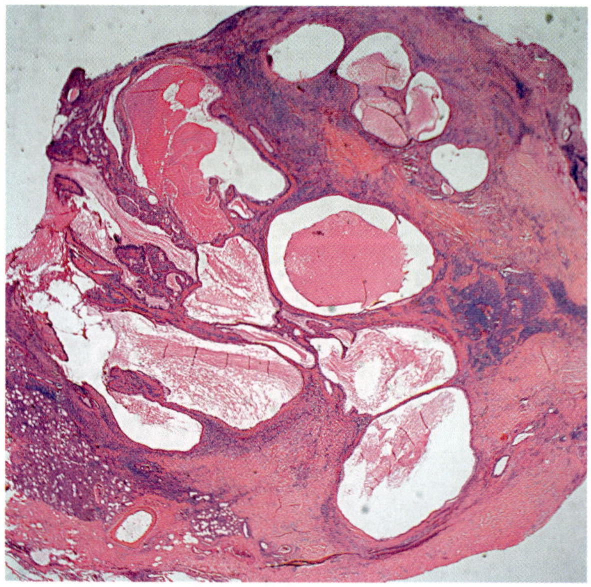

Figure 12-7 Low-power view of mucous gland adenoma with cystically dilated submucosal glands.

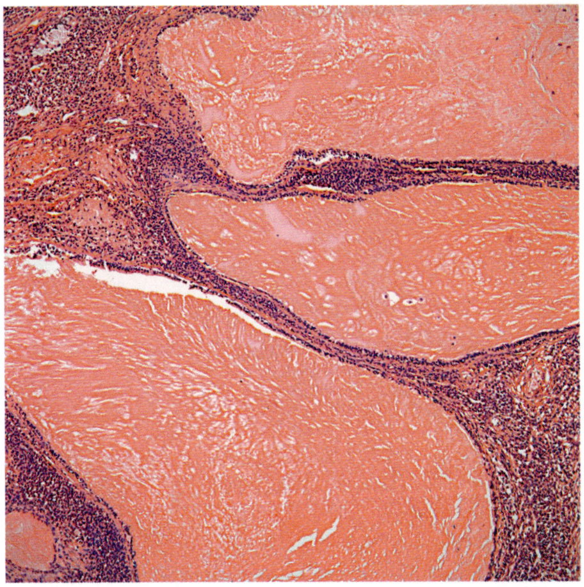

Figure 12-8 Mucous gland adenoma with dilated glands and inflammatory reaction.

Although the diagnosis of mucous gland adenoma is essentially a morphologic diagnosis, immunohistochemical studies have been performed in some reported cases. As might be expected, the tumor shows positive staining for epithelial markers including keratins, epithelial membrane antigen (EMA), and carcinoembryonic antigen (CEA). Proliferative markers such as Ki-67 will label only scattered cells.

Differential Diagnosis

The most important considerations in the differential diagnosis are low-grade mucoepidermoid carcinoma and adenocarcinoma. In small biopsy specimens, an unequivocal diagnosis may prove difficult to obtain; however, the presence of an exuberant dilatation of normal endobronchial glands should alert the pathologist to the possibility of a mucous gland adenoma. If the biopsy tissue is from an area of glandular proliferation, the diagnosis may be very difficult, if not impossible. In a resected specimen, the presence of a process limited to the space between surface respiratory epithelium and the bronchial cartilage indicates an adenoma, rather than a mucoepidermoid carcinoma. Abnormal dilatation of glands with acellular mucoid material within the glandular lumen also should point to the correct interpretation; in adenocarcinoma, an atypical glandular proliferation not limited to the bronchial cartilage, and showing nuclear pleomorphism or mitotic activity, or both, may be observed.

Treatment and Prognosis

The treatment of choice is complete surgical resection, and the prognosis is excellent. The choice of surgical procedure will depend on the anatomic distribution of

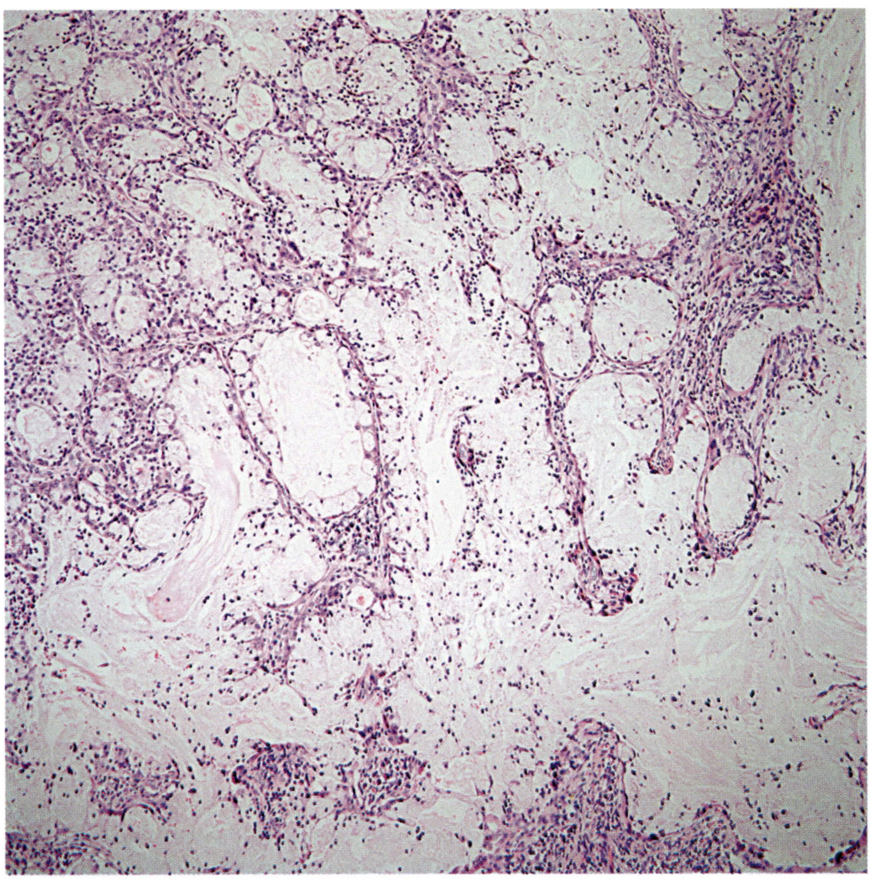

Figure 12-9 Mucous gland adenoma with prominent mucus-secreting glands.

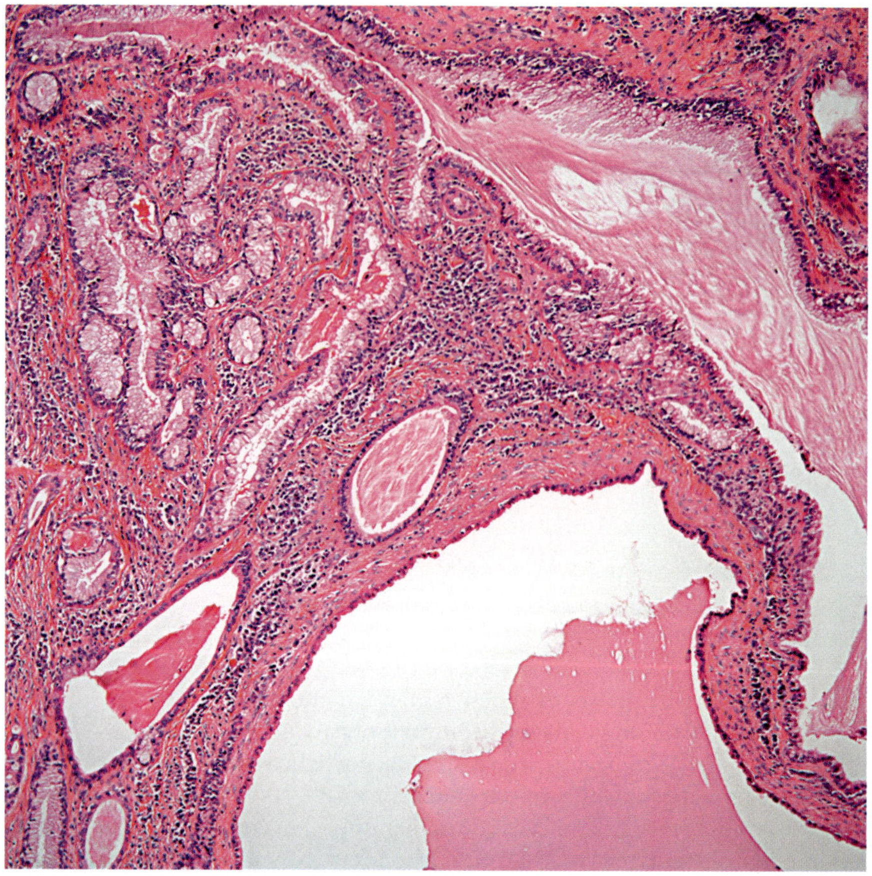

Figure 12-10 Mucous gland adenoma with dilated glands of different sizes.

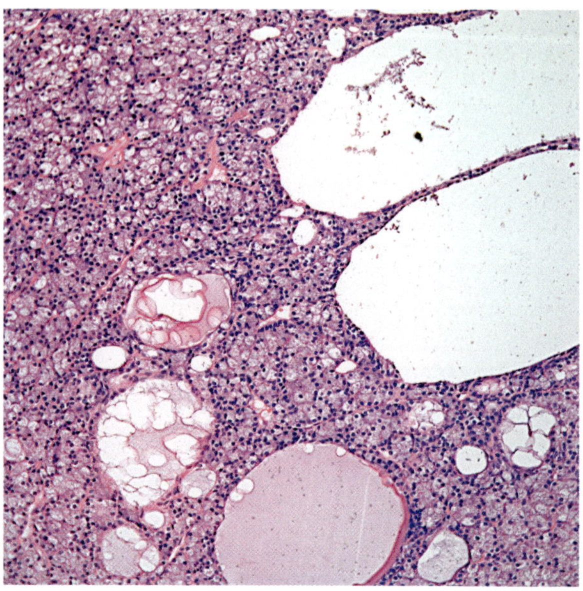

Figure 12-11 Mucous gland adenoma with dilated glands and prominent solid areas of serous glands.

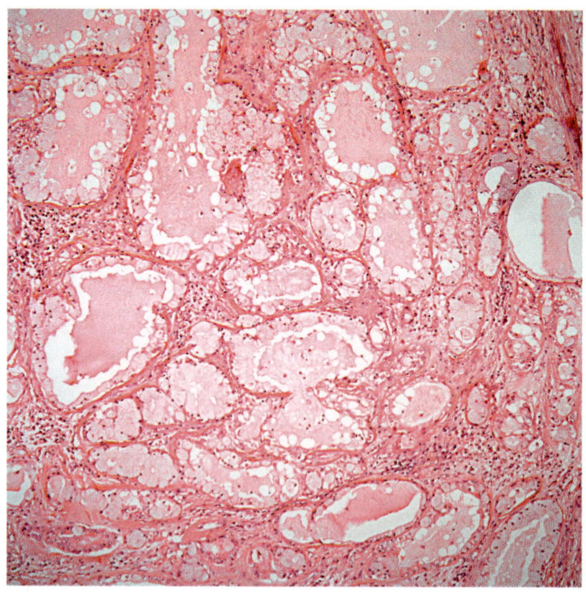

Figure 12-12 Mucous gland adenoma with hyperplasia of mucous glands.

the tumor, the surgeon's level of confidence in the initial biopsy results, and radiologic findings. Therefore, even though the tumor is completely benign, the surgical approach may entail a more radical procedure such as lobectomy.

Amyloid Tumor (Amyloidoma)

Amyloid deposition within the lung parenchyma is a well-known phenomenon, recognized for many decades. The deposition may be secondary to systemic amyloidosis or

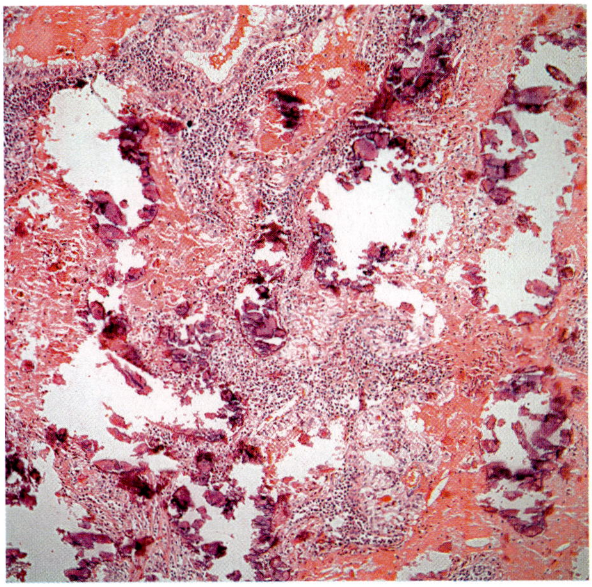

Figure 12-13 Mucous gland adenoma. Prominent mucous glands exhibit extensive calcification.

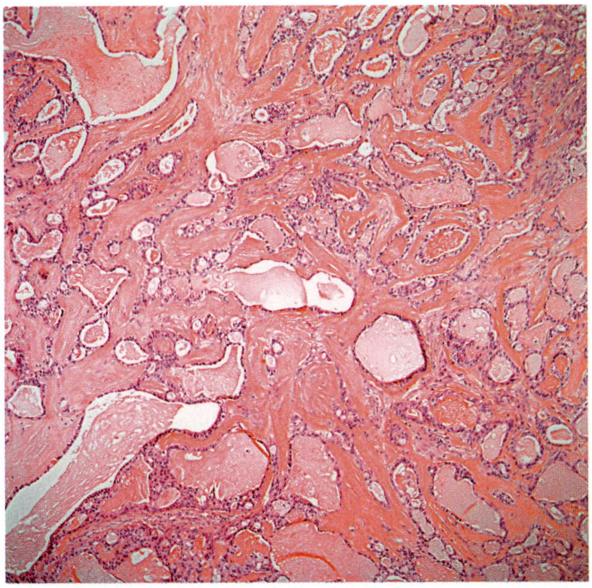

Figure 12-14 Mucous gland adenoma with proliferation of glandular structures separated by fibrocollagenous stroma and focal squamous metaplasia.

to various other conditions. Several studies analyzing the presence of amyloid in the respiratory tract, including the tracheobronchial area and lung parenchyma, have been reported.[14-16] Celli and associates[15] described 22 autopsy cases of patients with systemic amyloidosis; 12 of the patients had primary systemic amyloidosis, 3 patients had amyloidosis secondary to myeloma or Waldenström's macroglobulinemia, and 7 patients had secondary amyloidosis. Cordier and colleagues[16] reported their findings in 21 patients with systemic amyloidosis involving the lower respiratory tract. In this series, the lung and tracheobronchial tree manifested different patterns of involvement, including diffuse, nodular, interstitial, and plaque-like. The

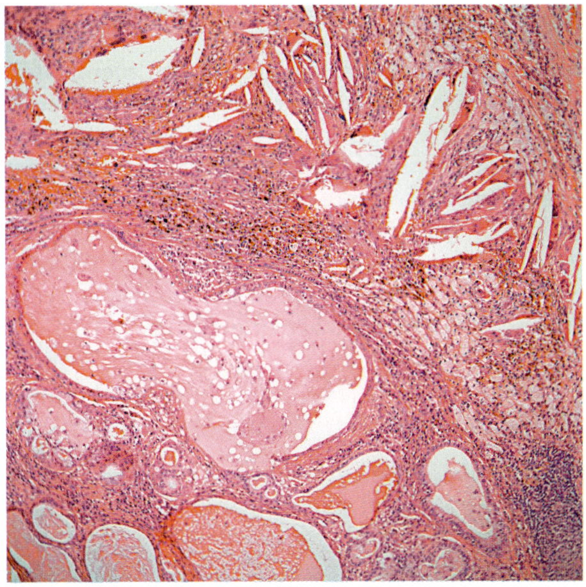

Figure 12-15 Mucous gland adenoma with prominent foamy histiocytic reaction and cholesterol cleft granulomas.

investigators emphasized that the lung may show amyloid deposition in conditions such as myeloma, Waldenström's macroglobulinemia, familial neuropathy, and Niemann-Pick or Gaucher's disease; senile cardiac forms of this condition also have been documented. Although these conditions are important, the focus of the following discussion is solely on the presence of amyloid in the respiratory tract without evidence of systemic disease, because in some cases the pulmonary nodules may raise the clinical possibility of a pulmonary malignancy.

Nodular deposits of amyloid in the lung parenchyma, also known as amyloidomas, are well known to occur, and their presence has been reported in the literature. Possible etiologic factors such as light chain immunoglobulin or the presence of abundant plasma cells often seen adjacent to amyloid tumors have been suggested as the cause of amyloid deposition. The potassium permanganate oxidation technique, which appears to separate amyloid type AA from other forms of amyloid, has provided results that may support the immunoglobulin-derived amyloid by excluding the protein A-amyloid. The etiology is still unknown, however. In some cases, the amyloid tumor has been associated with other conditions such as Sjögren's syndrome[17,18] and pulmonary lymphoma, mucosa-associated lymphoid tissue (MALT) type,[19] whereas other cases have been characterized by extensive lung involvement[20] or presence of a solitary nodule.[21] In 1986, Hui and coworkers[22] presented 48 cases of amyloidosis restricted to the lower respiratory tract. These workers encountered 14 cases involving the tracheobronchial tree, 24 cases with solitary or multiple pulmonary nodules, and 6 cases with diffuse interstitial parenchymal pattern. Patients with tracheobronchial involvement are most likely to present with symptoms such as dyspnea, whereas those with nodular parenchymal involvement usually are asymptomatic.

Macroscopic Findings

Pulmonary amyloid may be present in different forms. The tracheobronchial involvement may be diffuse or localized, whereas parenchymal amyloidosis may manifest as single or multiple nodules (Fig. 12-16), ranging in size from 1 cm to more than 10 cm in diameter. These tumors may be unilateral or bilateral and have been described as of soft consistency, well circumscribed, and grayish in color. Those in the tracheobronchial tree have been described as plaque-like or polypoid.

Histopathologic Features

The low-power view of lung involved in nodular amyloidosis (amyloidoma) shows a well-circumscribed but unencapsulated amorphous eosinophilic tumor nodule replacing lung parenchyma (Fig. 12-17). Higher magnification reveals this nodule to be composed of an acellular amorphous material; however, in the periphery of the nodule, an inflammatory infiltrate rich in plasma cells and numerous multinucleated giant cells can be seen (Figs. 12-18 to 12-22). In some cases, the process is diffuse, with some preservation of the normal architecture. The amyloid is deposited in an interstitial pattern (Fig. 12-23), with widening of the interstitium, and involving the pulmonary vasculature. In this pattern, the inflammatory infiltrate is not as prominent as in the nodular pattern, and multinucleated giant cells may be only scattered or absent.

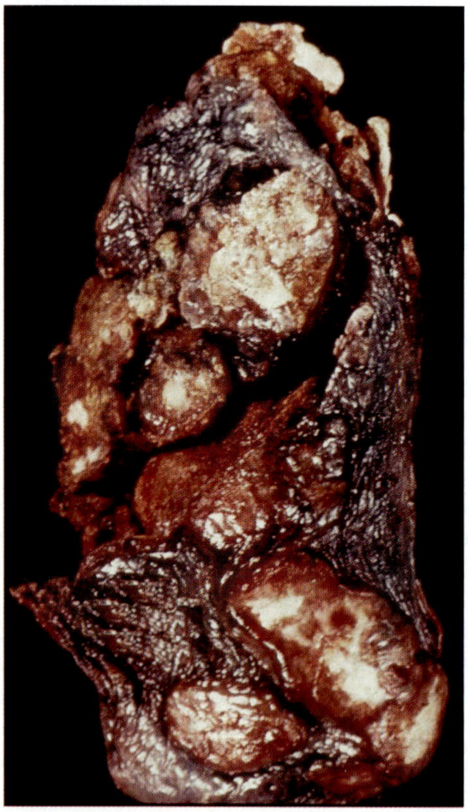

Figure 12-16 Amyloid tumor, gross specimen. Several nodules are present in the lung parenchyma.

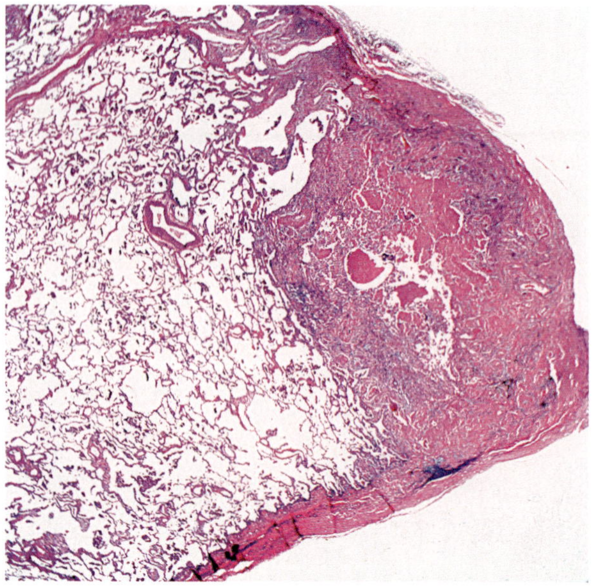

Figure 12-17 Low-power view of an amyloid tumor of the lung in a subpleural location.

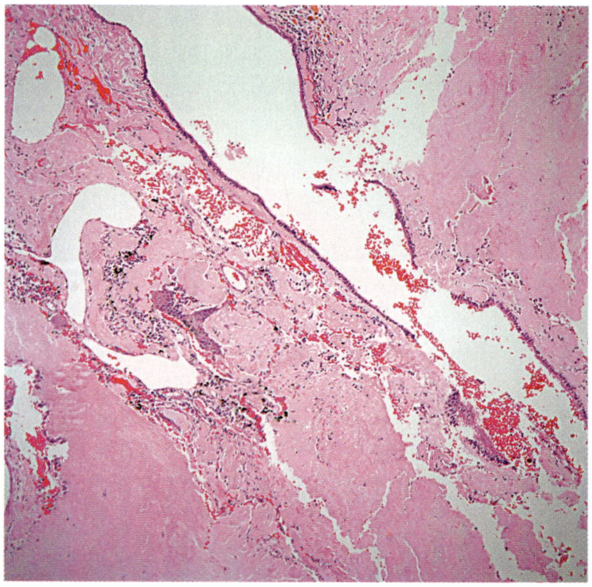

Figure 12-18 Pulmonary amyloid tumor. Entrapment of respiratory epithelium can be seen.

Special Studies

Even though the morphologic presence of amyloid is rather characteristic, histochemical staining studies using Congo red may be of help in small biopsy specimens, or in cases with subtle changes suggesting presence of amyloid in the lung parenchyma. Congo red displays a birefringent apple-green color under polarized light microscopy. Amyloid may show a λ light chain immunohistochemical

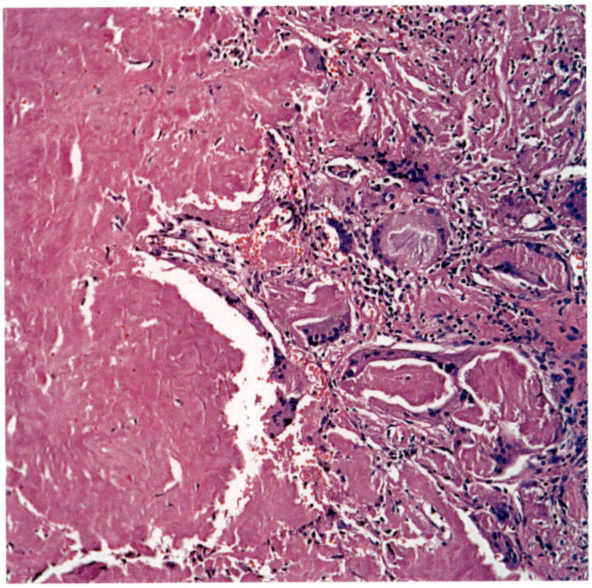

Figure 12-19 Amyloid tumor with multinucleated giant cells of the Touton type.

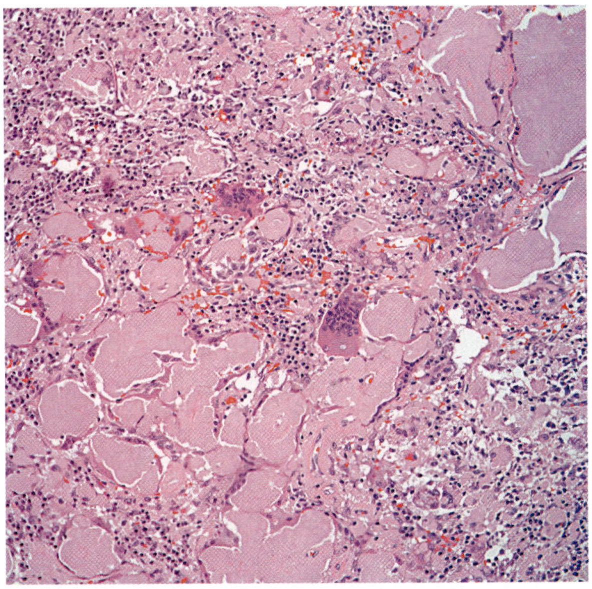

Figure 12-20 Amyloid tumor with prominent inflammatory reaction and osteoclast-like giant cells.

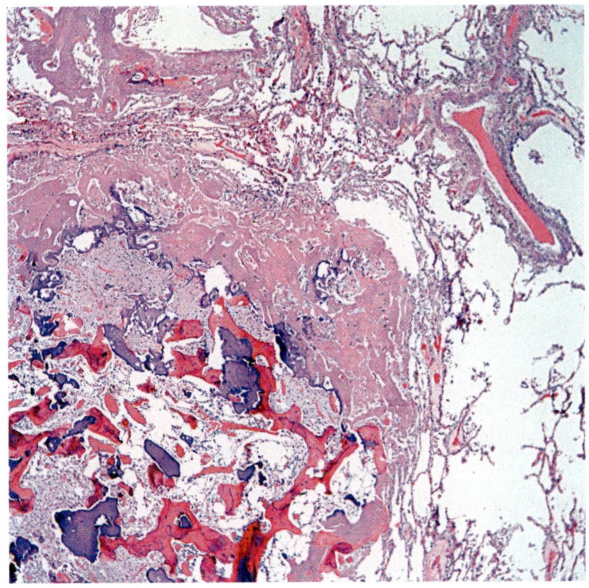

Figure 12-21 Amyloid tumor with extensive bone formation.

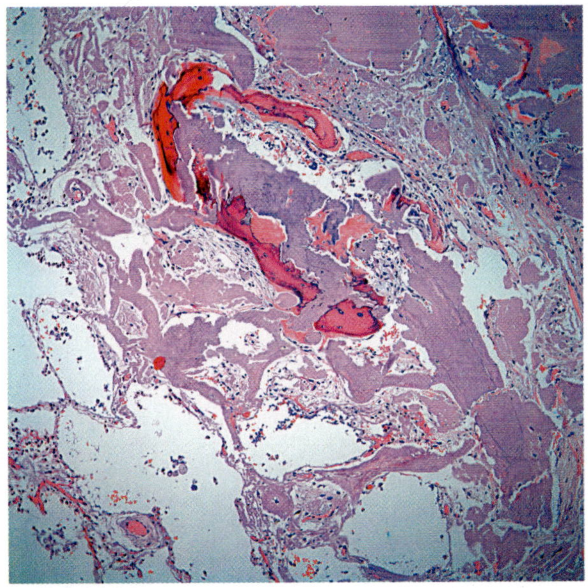

Figure 12-22 Amyloid tumor with focal ossification.

reaction and serum amyloid P. Immunohistochemical studies in the plasma cells present in amyloid tumors have shown a polytypical cellular proliferation. Recently, Rodriguez and colleagues[23] performed spectrometric studies in proteinaceous deposits in neural tissue and concluded that liquid chromatography-electrospray tandem mass spectrometry is a novel application for characterization of proteinaceous deposits, including amyloid.

Differential Diagnosis

One important non-neoplastic condition that may be confused with amyloid tumor is the so-called hyalinizing granuloma of lung. In this condition, extensive areas of hyalinization with inflammatory reaction may closely mimic amyloid. Hyalinizing granuloma of the lung is a rare condition, probably related to sclerosing mediastinitis, retroperitoneal fibrosis, sclerosing cholangitis, and other similar lesions. It usually occurs in adults and may manifest as a pulmonary mass, potentially giving rise to signs and symptoms of pulmonary obstruction. On histologic examination, this lesion is seen to be a well-demarcated tumor mass with extensive fibrosis and thick collagen bundles admixed with an inflammatory reaction (Figs. 12-24 to 12-26). Histochemical staining with Congo red is negative in these cases. Another diagnostic possibility is intrapulmonary solitary fibrous tumor, especially with lesions showing extensive areas of collagenization. Once again,

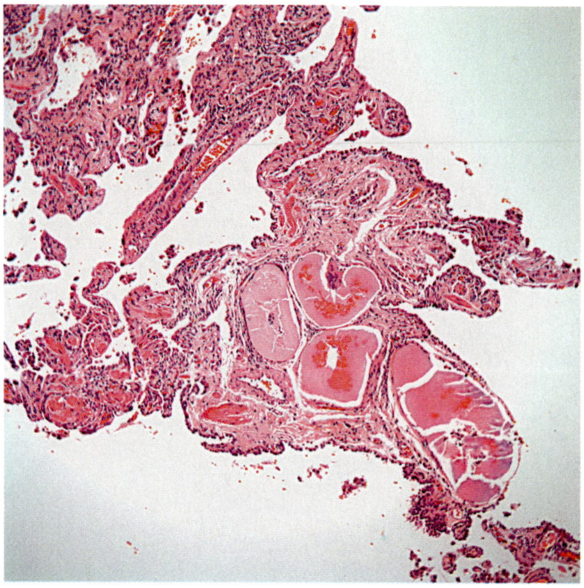

Figure 12-23 Amyloid tumor with interstitial deposition.

Congo red or immunohistochemical studies for CD34 and Bcl-2 should lead to the correct interpretation.

Treatment and Prognosis

The treatment of choice for amyloidosis manifesting as a pulmonary mass is surgical resection. The prognosis appears to be good for patients with this form of the disease, in contrast to patients with diffuse pulmonary involvement, in whom surgical resection may not be possible. The pattern of diffuse involvement appears to be associated with progression to respiratory insufficiency eventuating in death.

Alveolar Proteinosis

Rosen and coworkers[24] are credited for describing this condition in 27 patients, in whom the alveoli were filled by a PAS-positive proteinaceous material rich in lipid. The investigators speculated that the alveolar proteinaceous material was produced by the lining cells, which slough into the lumen, ultimately becoming necrotic and yielding granules and variably laminated bodies to the alveolar content. In addition, the investigators noted the resemblance of this condition to the changes seen with *Pneumocystis jiroveci (carinii)* infection in the lung.

Alveolar proteinosis also has been associated with immunosuppression. Bedrossian and colleagues[25] reported eight cases of alveolar proteinosis associated with hematologic malignancies and acknowledged that all of the cases reported in the literature were associated with either infectious processes or with hematologic malignancies. Three radiologic patterns of involvement with alveolar proteinosis have been documented: reticulonodular, small acinar nodules mimicking miliary disease, and coalescence of various-sized acinar nodules leading to focal consolidation.[26]

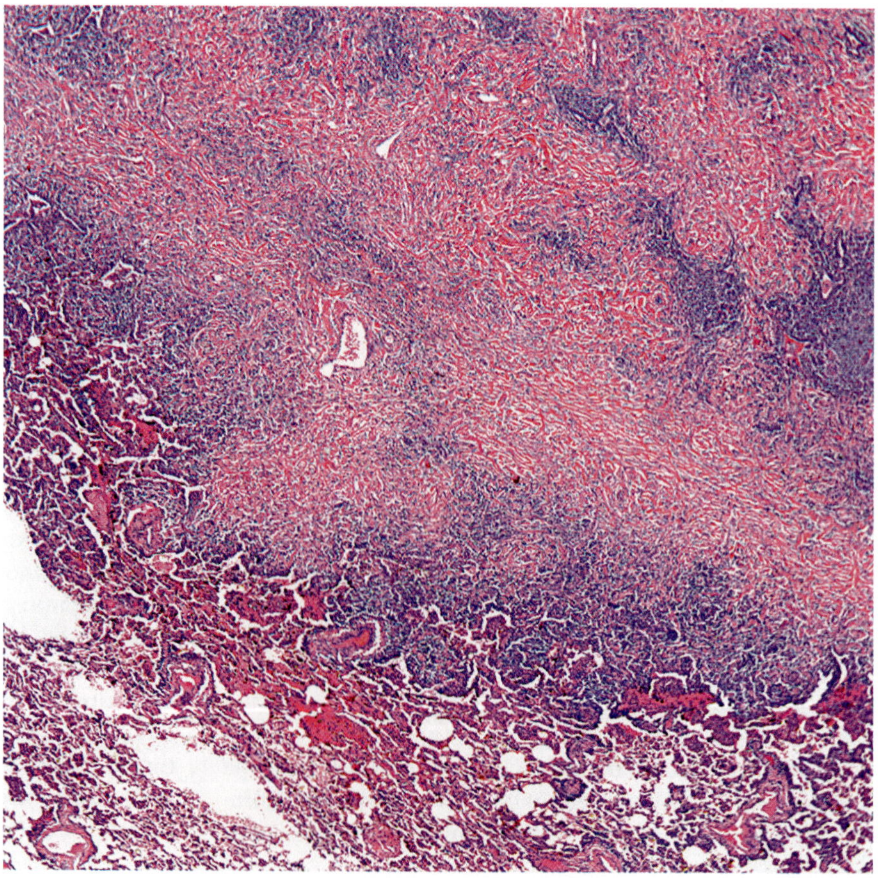

Figure 12-24 Low-power view of a hyalinizing granuloma showing extensive areas of sclerosis and inflammatory reaction.

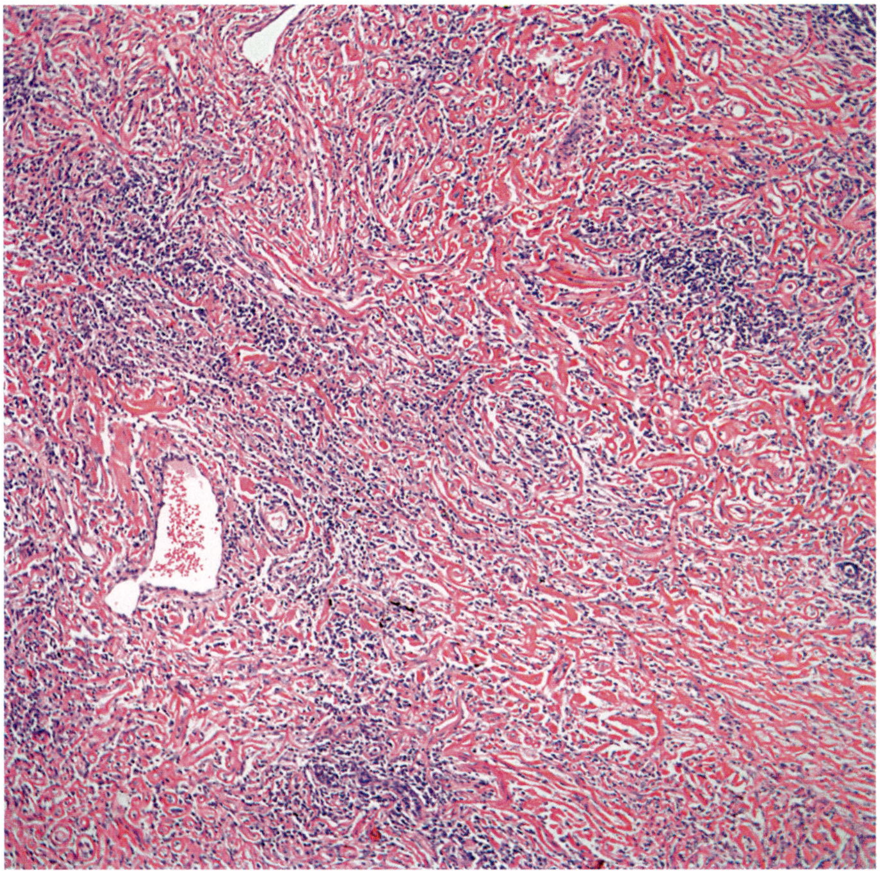

Figure 12-25 Intermediate-power view of a hyalinizing granuloma showing extensive deposition of collagen admixed with ectatic vessels.

A majority of patients will present with clinical signs and symptoms of cough, dyspnea, chest pain, or fever.[27]

Histopathologic Features

The histopathologic hallmark of alveolar proteinosis is filling of the alveoli by a proteinaceous acellular material, which characteristically demonstrates reactivity with periodic acid–Schiff (PAS) histochemical stain. The pulmonary architecture is preserved, with only minimal changes in the interstitium (Figs. 12-27 to 12-29). By electron microscopy, annular inclusions, lamellar osmiophilic inclusions, dense granules, and myeloid bodies have been identified.

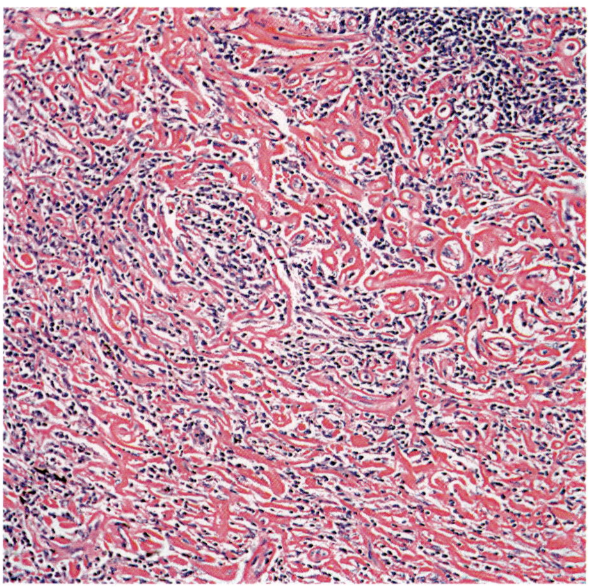

Figure 12-26 High-power view of a hyalinizing granuloma showing collagen admixed with inflammatory cells.

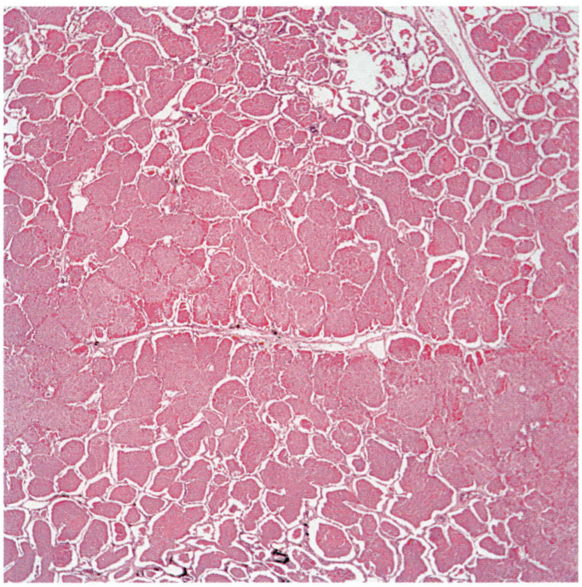

Figure 12-27 Low-power view of lung involved in alveolar proteinosis showing extensive filling of alveolar spaces by an acellular material.

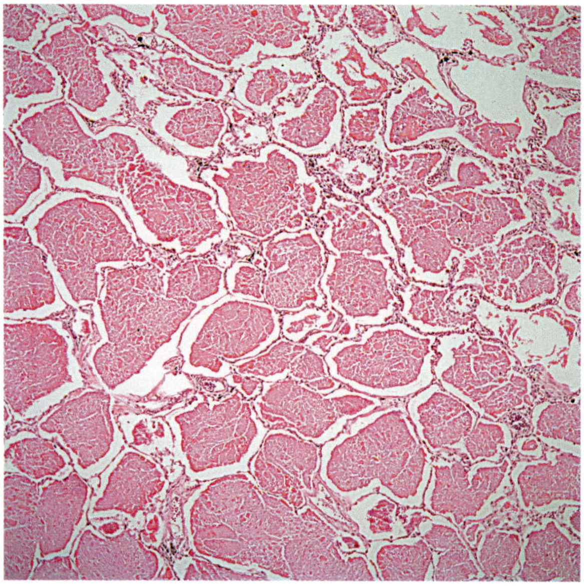

Figure 12-28 Alveolar proteinosis. Alveolar spaces are filled by a proteinaceous material, with preservation of the alveolar architecture.

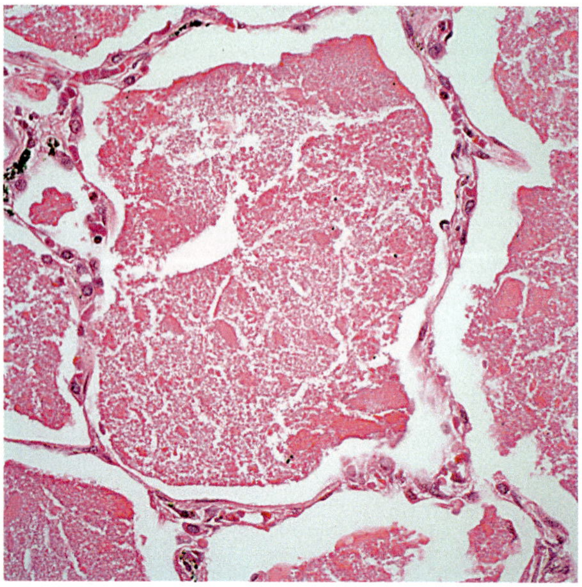

Figure 12-29 Alveolar proteinosis. High-power view shows the proteinaceous intra-alveolar material. Note the granularity of the material.

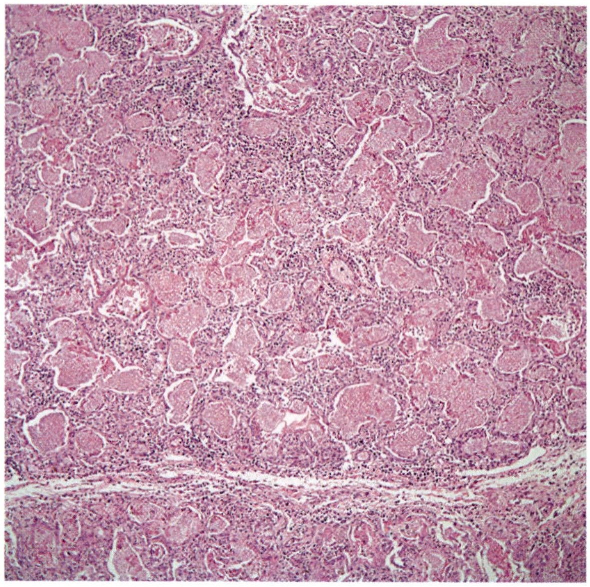

Figure 12-30 *Pneumocystis* pneumonia. Alveoli are filled by an acellular exudate.

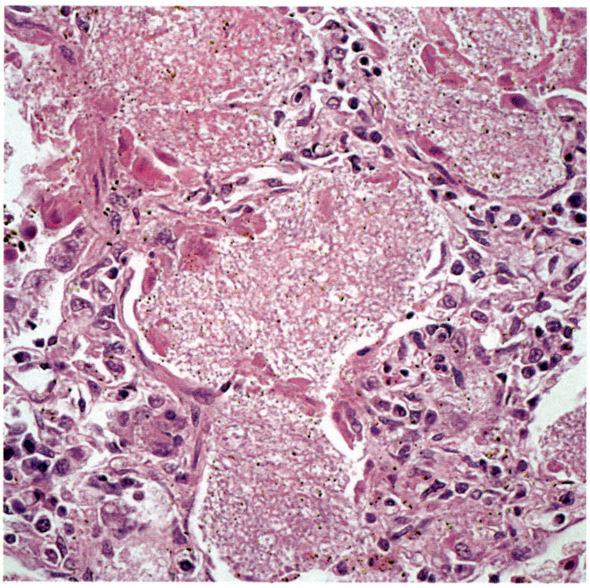

Figure 12-31 Higher-power view showing the intra-alveolar exudate in *Pneumocystis* pneumonia. Note the associated inflammatory changes.

Differential Diagnosis

The most important consideration in the differential diagnosis is *Pneumocystis carinii* pneumonia (PCP; *P. jiroveci*) (Figs. 12-30 to 12-32). Given that both of these processes may take place in immunocompromised persons, staining with PAS or Gomori-methenamine silver (GMS) may help to confirm the diagnosis. Lung involved in alveolar proteinosis will show positive staining with PAS and negative staining with GMS, which is contrary to what would occur in *Pneumocystis* pneumonia. Another condition that may be considered is pulmonary edema; however, the use of PAS histochemical stain will lead to the correct interpretation.

Treatment and Prognosis

Pulmonary lavage has been used with some success. Kariman and associates[28] studied 28 patients with alveolar proteinosis and divided them into two groups in accordance with their clinical course. Approximately 24% of the patients exhibited spontaneous remission with no treatment, whereas the remaining 76% underwent pulmonary lavage. In this latter group of patients, 21% did not respond to treatment.

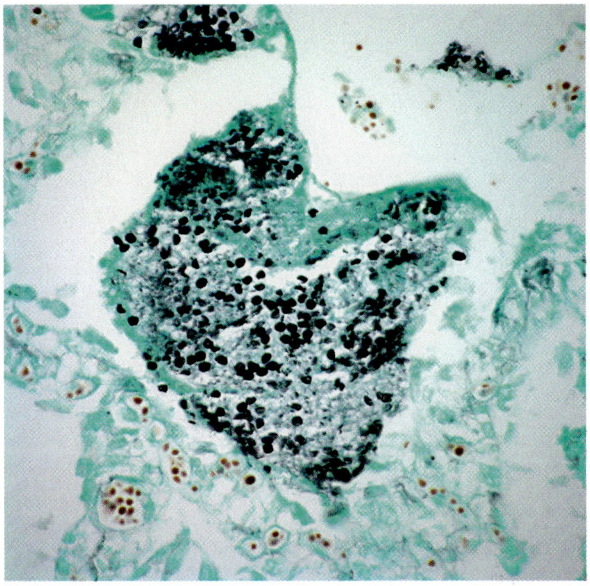

Figure 12-32 Staining with Gomori-methenamine silver shows the *Pneumocystis jiroveci (carinii)* organisms.

Placental Transmogrification of the Lung

The term *transmogrify* means "to change into a different form or shape, especially one that is fantastic or bizarre." This definition clearly indicates the grotesque nature of the process that takes place within the lung parenchyma during placental transmogrification of the lung. Since the original description by McChesney,[29] presented in abstract form, only a few additional cases have appeared in the literature, using different names or designating variants of the condition.[30–32] Careful analysis of these descriptions reveals that all of them represent the same condition, with a spectrum of histopathologic features. Mark and associates[31] described this condition under the designation placentoid bullous lesion of the lung in four adult patients with "unilateral multicystic lung disease." Two of the patients had a history of repeated childhood pneumonias. Almost simultaneously, Flider and colleagues[30] reported the cases of three patients, ranging in ages from 24 to 33 years, with cystic lesions of the lung. These workers' interpretation of this process was as a variant of giant bullous emphysema. In a more recent case report,[32] this condition was interpreted as pulmonary lipomatosis, a variant of placental transmogrification, in an adult patient with history of bronchopneumonia and a cystic intrapulmonary lesion.

On the basis of those reports, it is evident that this process should be classified as a single lesion with variable histopathologic features. The best terminology for these extremely rare lesions is *placental transmogrification of the lung*. Despite the broad spectrum of histopathologic features that may be seen in these lesions, it is apparent that, in previous reports, different designations refer to the same entity.

Clinical Features

The process appears to affect adult patients, especially young adults, with a history of pneumonic process. History of tobacco use also has been recorded in some cases. In all cases, the chest radiograph displayed a unilateral intrapulmonary cystic lesion, which may appear as a bulla or an enlarging cystic lesion.

Macroscopic Features

Invariably, the gross descriptions of the resected lesions are similar, including degenerated intrapulmonary lesions with cystic degeneration, papillary-like areas, or grape-like structures resembling molar placental tissue. The normal lung parenchyma appears collapsed, with total destruction of the normal macroscopic features of lung tissue (Fig. 12-33).

Histopathologic Features

The spectrum of histopathologic features encountered in placental transmogrification of the lung includes variable features. The lung parenchyma is replaced by a proliferation of papillary-like structures lined by cuboidal epithelial cells (Figs. 12-34 and 12-35). The core of these papillary structures may contain variable amounts of inflammatory cells—namely, lymphocytes. They may appear edematous, and in some cells, degeneration of these papillary structures may take place, giving the impression of degenerated placental villi (Figs. 12-36 to 12-40). In other areas, the papillary structures may contain smooth muscle or may be replaced by mature adipose tissue or a mixture of both. In focal areas, airway structures are preserved and may constitute the only visible normal anatomic architecture.

Treatment and Prognosis

The treatment for these unusual lesions is surgical resection, which has been performed in all cases described; the final diagnosis also is made at the time of surgery. Diagnosis on limited biopsy material or cytology may be difficult, and in such cases, findings are of limited value. No recurrences have been reported in any of the reported cases. Thus, complete surgical resection appears to be curative.

Pulmonary Alveolar Microlithiasis

The etiology of pulmonary alveolar microlithiasis, an unusual condition in the lung, is unknown, and although the composition of the microliths points to an abnormal chemical process, none of the patients described has had a primary metabolic abnormality. The process does not seem to have a predilection for either gender and may follow a protracted clinical course. Owing to the rarity of this condition, most of the information in the literature is presented in case reports, with only a couple of short series.[33,34]

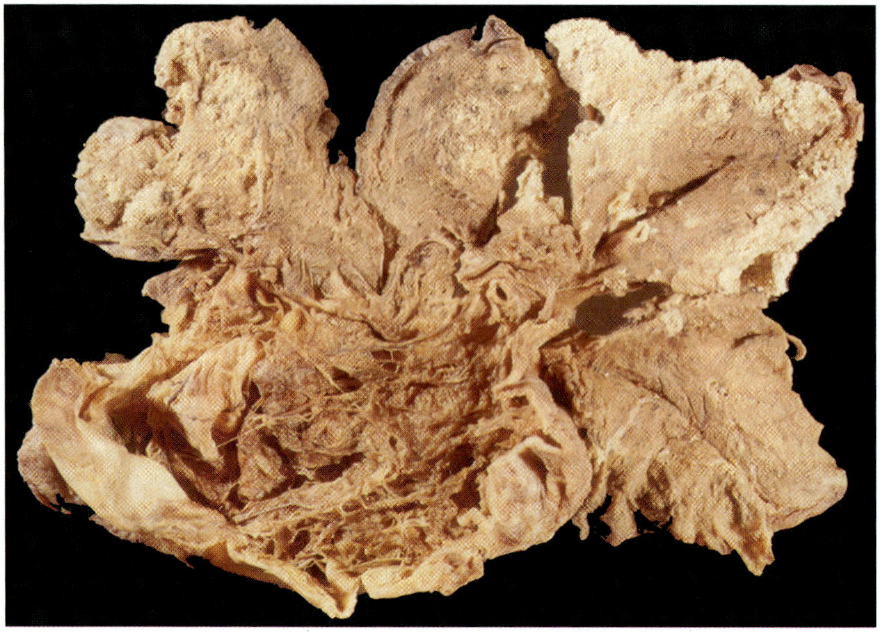

Figure 12-33 Gross specimen of lung that has undergone placental transmogrification, with total destruction of the lung parenchyma.

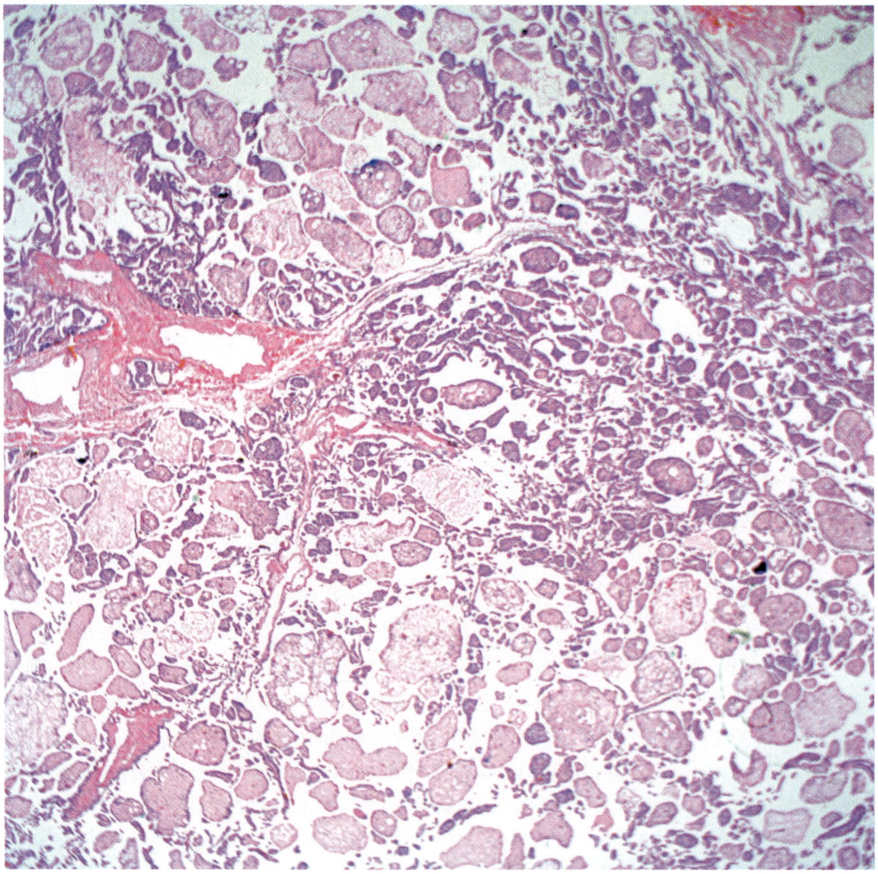

Figure 12-34 Placental transmogrification. Low-power view shows destruction of normal parenchymal architecture with replacement by placentoid-like structures.

Clinical Features

As indicated by findings in the larger series, pulmonary alveolar microlithiasis displays no gender predilection and can affect anyone at any age, having been documented in small children and older adults. A familial pattern has been observed in approximately one half of the cases described.[34] Patients may present with shortness of breath or complaints of gradual decrease in respiratory performance.[33] On radiographic evaluation, a diffuse bilateral pulmonary infiltrate that resembles a "sand

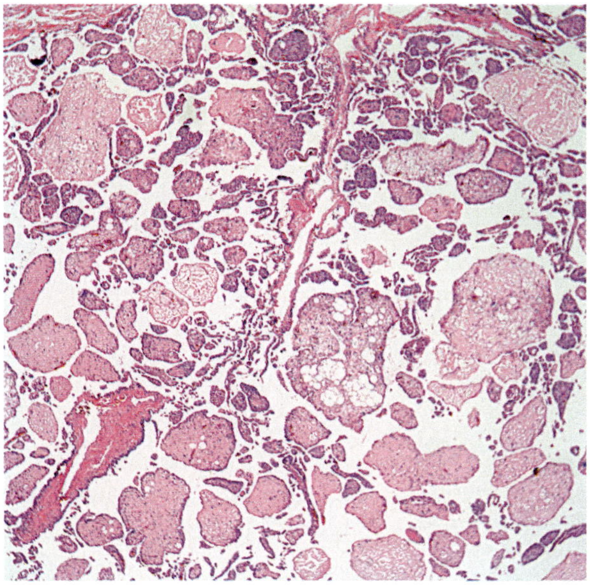

Figure 12-35 Placental transmogrification. The characteristic papillary-like structures replacing lung parenchyma are evident.

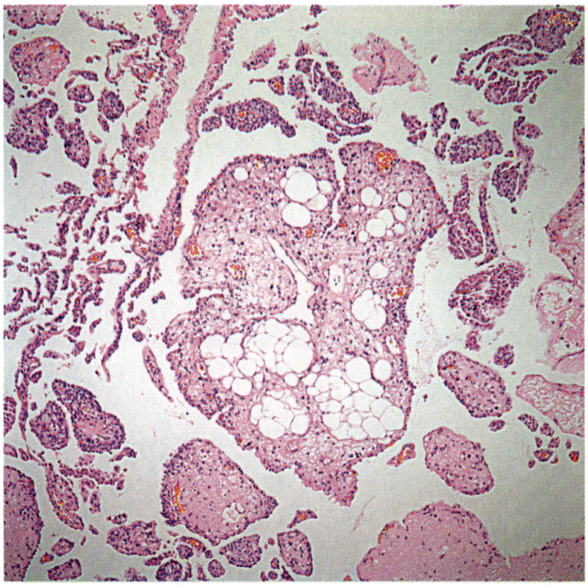

Figure 12-36 Placental transmogrification. High-power view of a characteristic papillary-like structure composed of adipose and myxoid tissue.

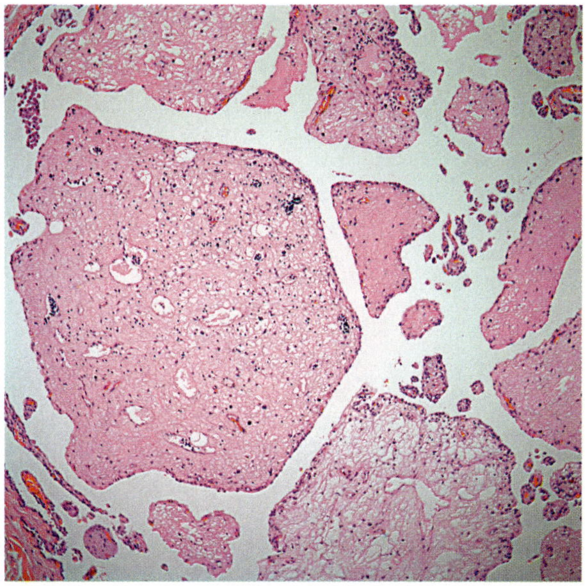

Figure 12-37 Placental transmogrification with papillary-like structure composed of only myxoid tissue.

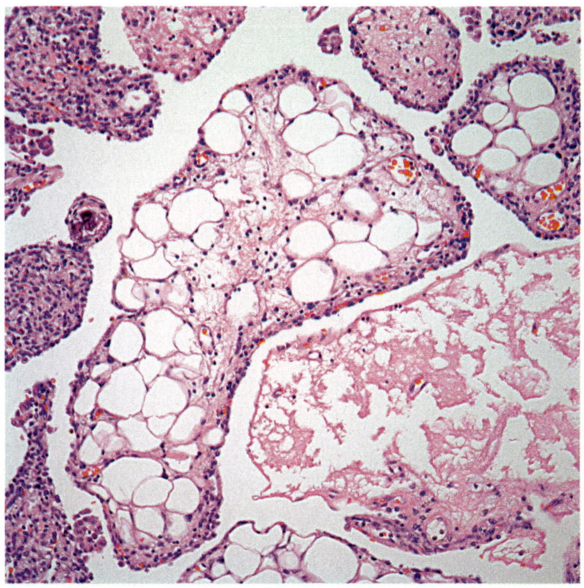

Figure 12-38 Placental transmogrification. The papillary-like structure is composed almost exclusively of mature adipose tissue with a rim of epithelial cells.

storm" typically is seen on the chest film[33] (Fig. 12-41). No metabolic abnormality related to disturbances of phosphorus or calcium has been associated with this condition; however, chemical analysis of the microliths shows that they are composed of calcium and phosphorus salts.[33] Macroscopically, the lung may show features mimicking pulmonary fibrosis (Fig. 12-42).

Histopathologic Features

Alveolar microlithiasis typically is characterized by numerous spherical bodies filling the alveolar spaces (Figs. 12-43 and 12-44). Each of these calcospherites measures approximately 250 to 750 μm in diameter. Morphologically, they appear to be laminated bodies with an onion layer–like appearance (Figs. 12-45 and 12-46). In some cases, focal ossification may be present (Fig. 12-47).

Differential Diagnosis

Although the histopathologic features of pulmonary alveolar microlithiasis are fairly straightforward, there are a few lesions that may enter into the differential diagnosis. Pulmonary "blue bodies" may have a similar shape and composition; however, they do not fill the alveolar spaces and are few in number. In addition, blue bodies are

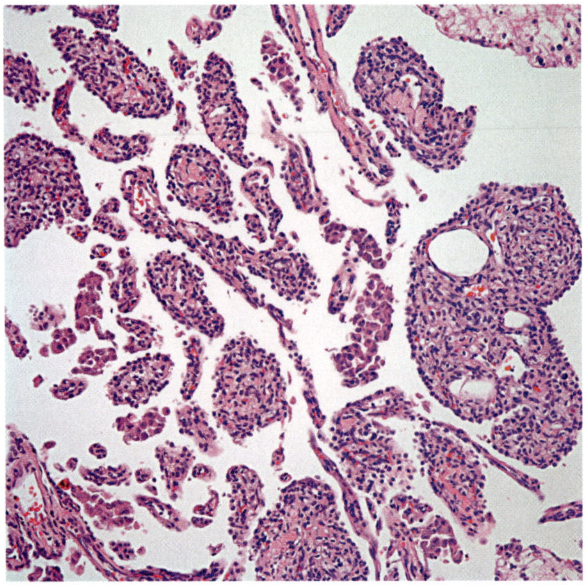

Figure 12-39 Placental transmogrification with papillary-like structures composed of collapsed pneumocytes.

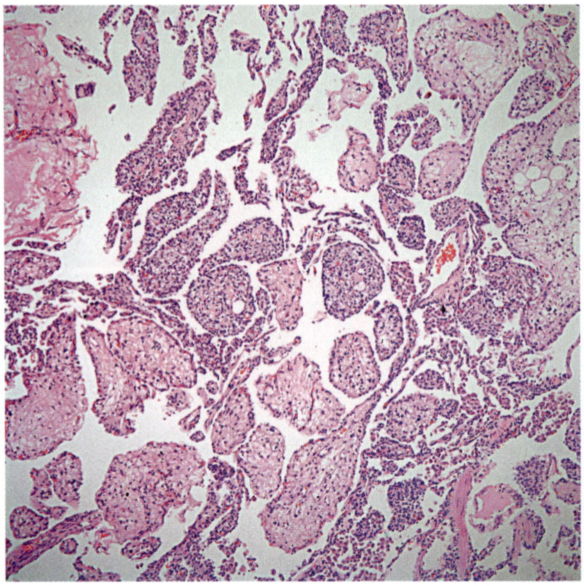

Figure 12-40 Placental transmogrification with admixture of papillary-like structures composed of adipose, myxoid, and collapsed pneumocytes.

commonly associated with inflammatory lesions, pneumoconiosis, or interstitial pneumonitis.[35] Diffuse pulmonary ossification and heterotopic ossification also may enter into the differential diagnosis.[36,37] Both of these conditions cause lamellar bone formation, and the distribution is interstitial. In addition, light microscopy shows round calcospherites, in sharp contrast with the irregular bone formation present in pulmonary ossification. If multiple corpora amylacea are present, their round shape may erroneously suggest the presence of microliths. Diffuse corpora amylacea filling alveolar spaces would be a highly unusual finding, however. Pulmonary metastatic calcification also may be considered; this entity is discussed further on.

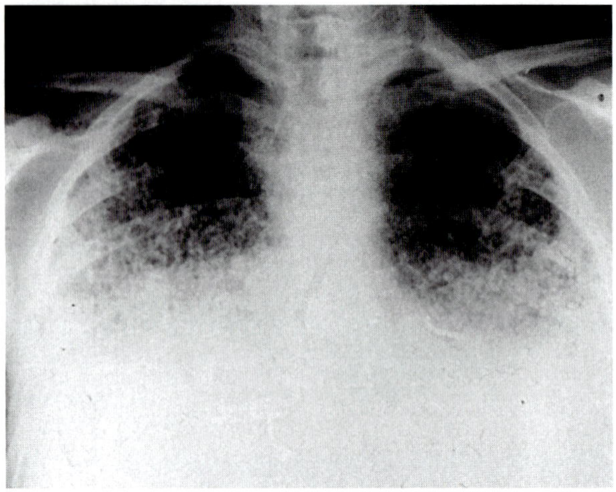

Figure 12-41 Chest radiograph of a patient with alveolar microlithiasis showing the classic "sandstorm" feature.

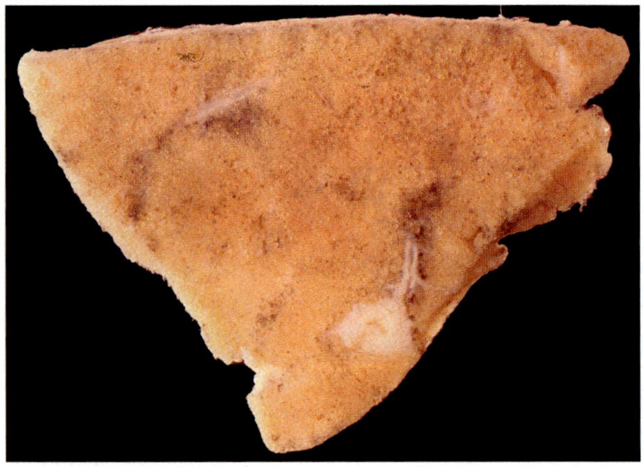

Figure 12-42 Section of a lung affected by alveolar microlithiasis, with numerous small cyst-like structures.

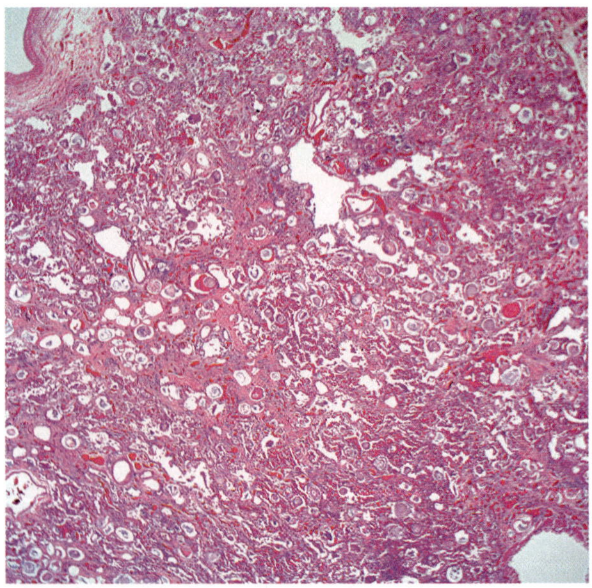

Figure 12-43 Alveolar microlithiasis. In this low-power view, note the presence of calcifications filling alveolar spaces.

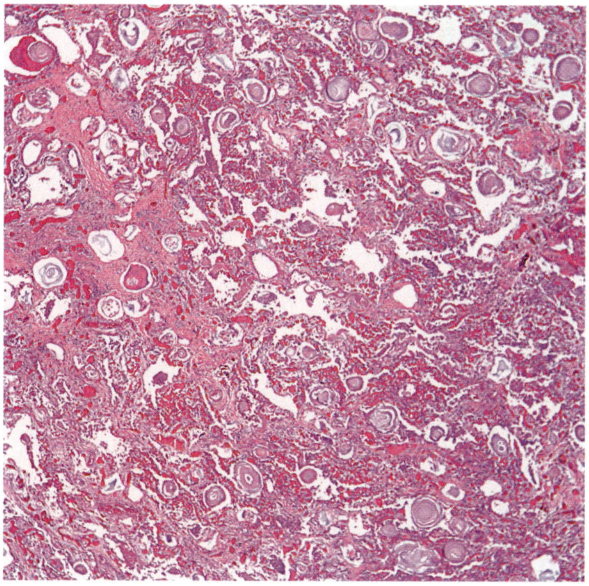

Figure 12-44 Alveolar microlithiasis. Higher-power view shows the microliths filling alveolar spaces.

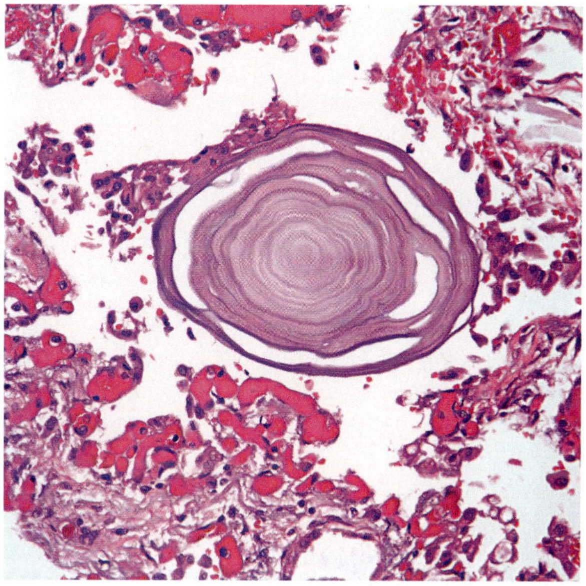

Figure 12-46 Alveolar microlithiasis. High-power view of a microlith reveals an onion slice–like appearance.

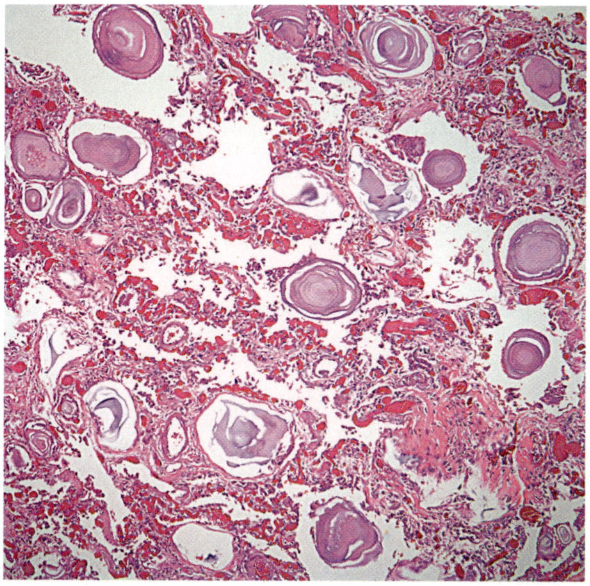

Figure 12-45 Alveolar microlithiasis. Numerous microliths filling the alveolar spaces are visible. Note also the destruction of normal lung parenchyma.

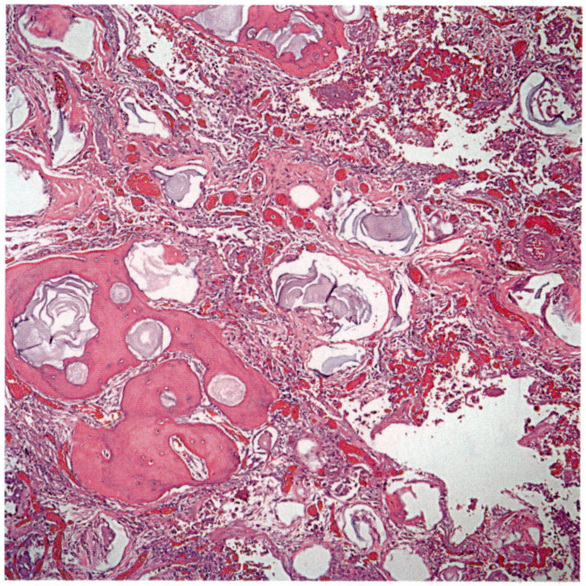

Figure 12-47 Alveolar microlithiasis with focal areas of ossification.

Treatment and Prognosis

No specific treatment for pulmonary alveolar microlithiasis is available. The condition may follow a protracted course, but eventually most patients succumb to respiratory failure. Some patients may live with this condition for long periods, from 5 to 40 years.[33]

Pulmonary Metastatic Calcification

Pulmonary metastatic calcification is an unusual phenomenon that may pose a diagnostic problem because the clinical presentation may mimic that of a neoplastic process. Metastatic calcification may be seen in patients with various disorders and conditions including patients who have undergone treatment for malignancies such as parathyroid carcinoma, those with lymphoproliferative disorders, transplant recipients, and patients with abnormal renal function.[38–46] Metastatic calcification may occur in any age group and in both male and female patients. Conventional chest radiographs may not be as accurate as CT scans (Fig. 12-48). On radiologic examination, the process is seen to be bilateral, dense, and asymmetrical.[47,48] Some researchers have suggested that dual-energy digital radiography is a more sensitive modality than conventional chest radiography for the diagnosis of metastatic calcification.[61]

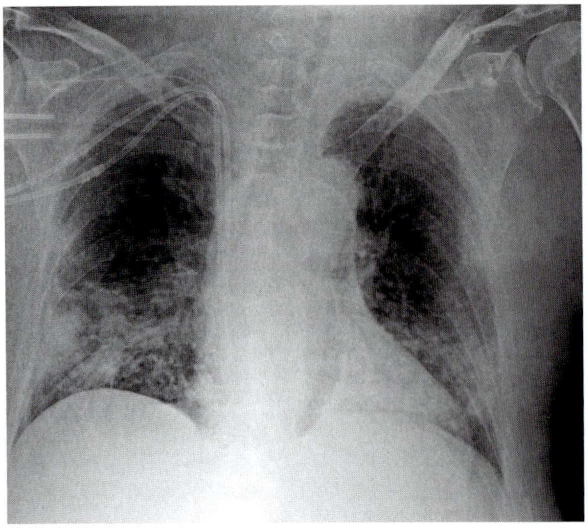

Figure 12-48 Lung with metastatic calcification. Chest radiograph shows diffuse bilateral pulmonary infiltrates.

The exact mechanism for metastatic calcification is not known; however, it may be influenced by serum calcium and phosphate concentrations, alkaline phosphatase activity, and local physicochemical conditions such as pH.[49] In contrast to the process of dystrophic calcification, metastatic calcification does not require a previous tissue injury.[46]

Histopathologic Features

On gross examination, the lung may appear congested, with a gritty-looking cut surface (Fig. 12-49). Unlike alveolar microlithiasis, in which the calcospherites fill the alveolar spaces, metastatic calcification follows a more haphazard pattern, in which the calcified material is deposited in the interstitum, bronchial wall, and airways. In many cases, the pattern of calcification follows the outlines of the alveoli (Figs. 12-50 to 12-52).

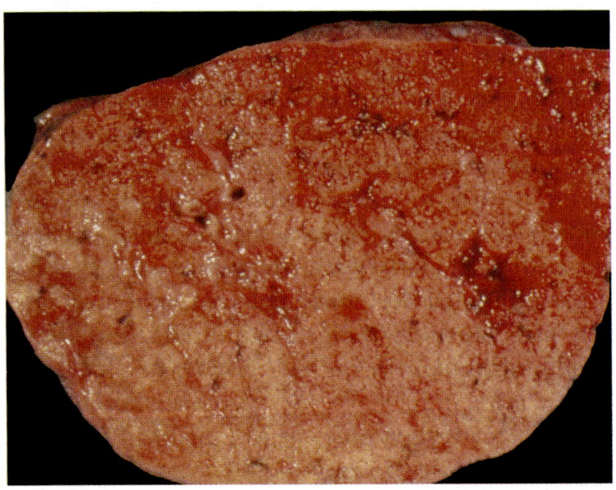

Figure 12-49 Lung with metastatic calcification, gross specimen. Note the gritty appearance with congestion.

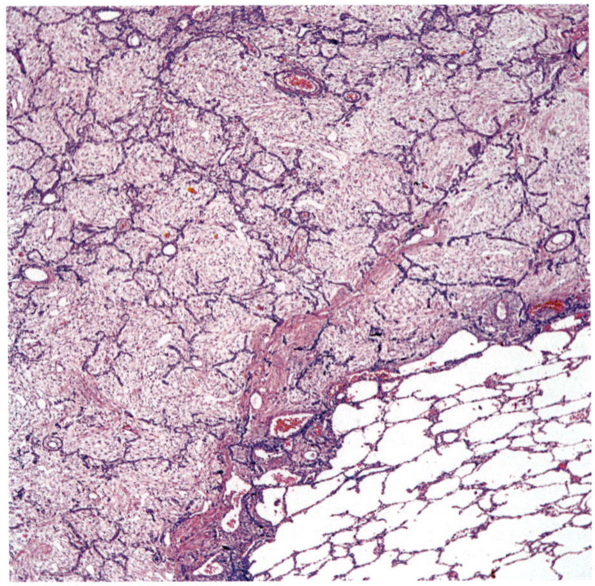

Figure 12-50 Lung with metastatic calcification. This low-power view shows a dendritic process with areas mimicking organized alveolar damage.

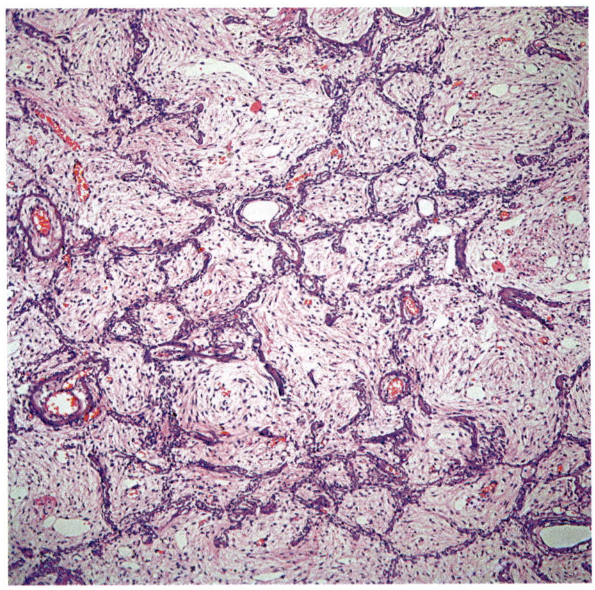

Figure 12-51 Lung with metastatic calcification. Calcification can be seen around the walls of the alveoli.

Treatment and Prognosis

The treatment and prognosis of metastatic calcification will be determined by the underlying condition. In some patients, the pathologic process may end in respiratory failure and death.

Lymphangioleiomyomatosis

Lymphangioleiomyomatosis (LAM) is an unusual disorder of unknown etiology that predominantly affects premenopausal women but also has been described, albeit rarely,

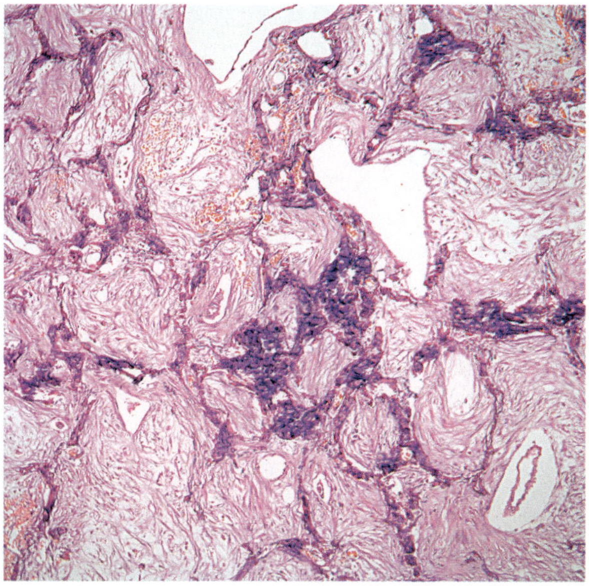

Figure 12-52 Lung with metastatic calcification. The areas of calcification are prominent in this image.

in children, men, and postmenopausal women.[50–54] This disorder may occur without evidence of another disease process or in association with tuberous sclerosis complex (TSC). LAM has been estimated to occur at a rate of 1 to 2 cases per 1 million women; however, it may be underreported. Although the pathogenesis of the disorder has not yet been elucidated, LAM and TSC may share a genetic relationship. The *TSC2* tumor suppressor gene at chromosomal locus 16p13 has been implicated in the pathogenesis of LAM. This particular abnormality also has been identified in approximately one half of renal angiomyolipomas in patients with LAM or tuberous sclerosis. Although these are two distinct disorders, the pulmonary changes in TSC, which may occur in less than 5% of these patients, are difficult to distinguish from those in LAM, not only histologically but also clinically and radiologically. TSC affects both genders, however. Some researchers also have argued that tuberous sclerosis has a relatively increased frequency in families, whereas LAM does not.[55,56] In addition, tuberous sclerosis has an autosomal dominant transmission, with neurologic and cutaneous manifestations.[57] Other investigators have suggested, however, that pulmonary LAM and Bourneville's tuberous sclerosis may represent two forms of the same process.[58]

Clinical Features

Presenting clinical signs and symptoms of LAM may include recurrent pneumothorax, chylous effusion, dyspnea, cough, and hemoptysis. Characteristic radiologic findings consist of multiple bilateral nodular and cystic changes in the lung parenchyma seen on CT scans.[59] Cases of unilateral pulmonary involvement have been described, however.[60] The mean age at onset of symptoms was estimated in one study to be 32 years.[61] Open lung biopsy used to be the procedure of choice to establish the diagnosis, but more recently, transbronchial biopsies have yielded some satisfactory results.[62–64]

Histopathologic Features

Grossly, the lungs of patients with LAM are characterized by multiple cysts with a honeycomb appearance (Fig. 12-53). The cysts are of different sizes with variable wall thickness. On microscopic examination, the low-power view shows numerous cysts, which may appear as emphysematous changes and may be filled with pools of blood or with pigmented macrophages (Figs. 12-54 and 12-55). At higher magnification, it is possible to identify a cellular

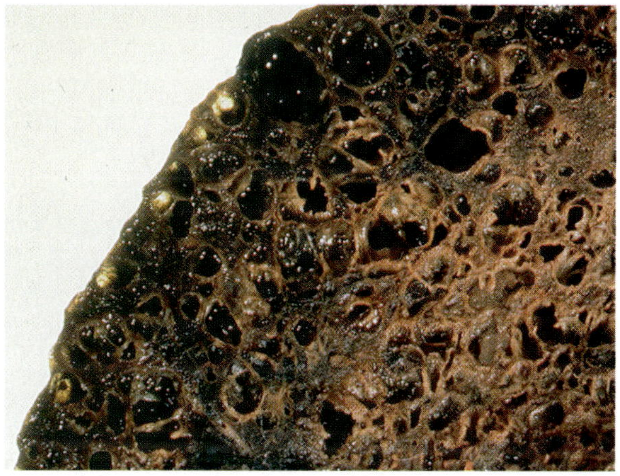

Figure 12-53 Gross specimen of a portion of a lung exhibiting multiple pulmonary cysts of different sizes. This variability is typical of lymphangioleiomyomatosis.

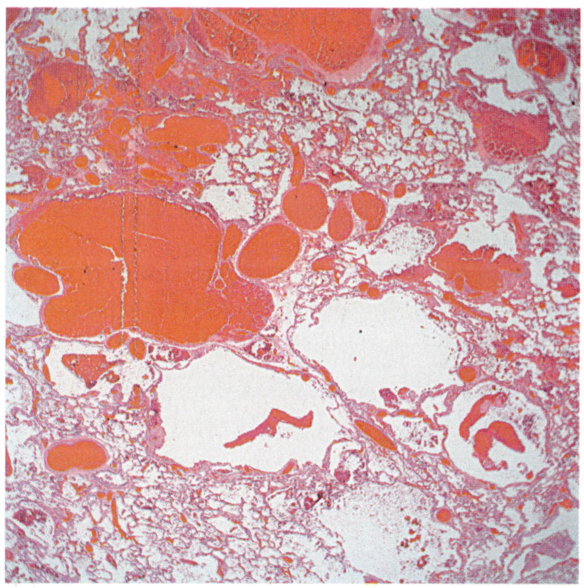

Figure 12-54 Lymphangioleiomyomatosis. On this low-power view, note the presence of numerous cysts, some of them filled with hemorrhage.

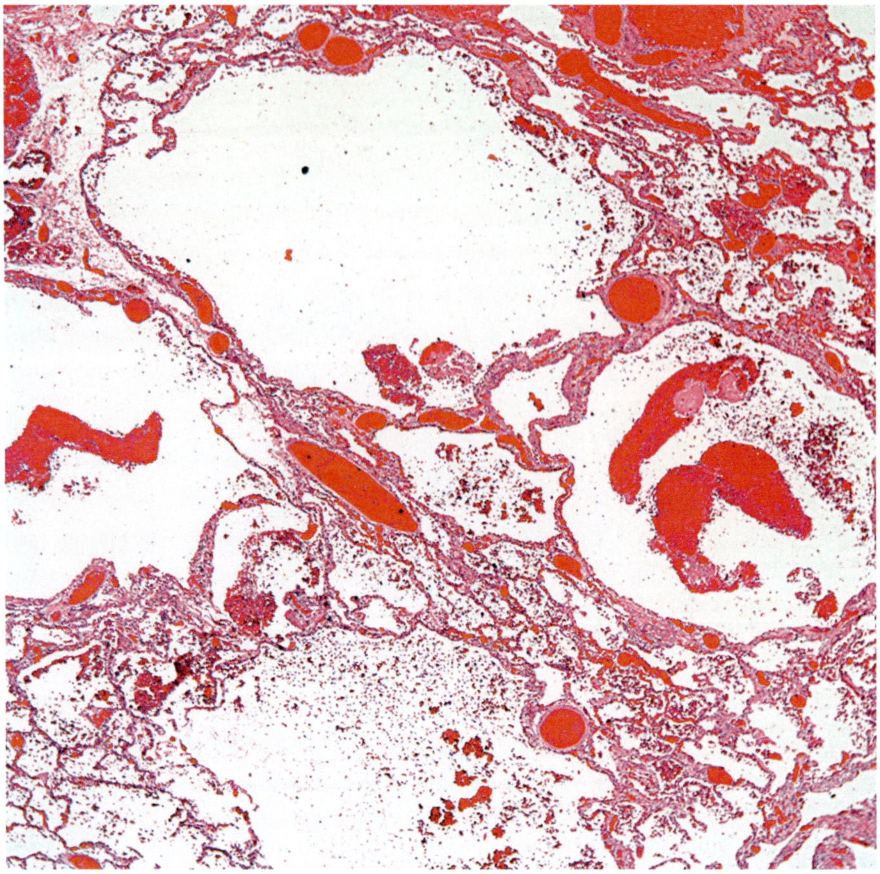

Figure 12-55 Lymphangioleiomyomatosis. Cystic structures can be seen admixed with normal lung parenchyma.

proliferation composed of spindle cells with elongated nuclei, inconspicuous nucleoli, and scanty cytoplasm and areas of more ovoid cells with clear cytoplasm (Figs. 12-56 and 12-57). This cellular proliferation appears to partially line some of the cystic structures and also may be visible in the interstitium of the lung parenchyma. It does not show evidence of nuclear atypia or mitotic activity. In adjacent areas, the lung parenchyma also may show hyperplasia with type II pneumocytes, which may be arranged in a micronodular pattern.[65,66] Some workers have divided LAM into two separate histologic groups, one predominantly cystic and the other predominantly muscular, and have argued that this classification has prognostic importance.[67]

On immunohistochemical studies, lung involved by LAM shows positive staining for muscle markers including smooth muscle actin and desmin. Positive staining also has been reported with estrogen and progesterone receptors, HMB-45,[68] insulin-like growth factor (IGF), and matrix metalloproteinases (MMPs).

Treatment and Prognosis

No specific treatment for LAM is available. Hormonal manipulation with antiestrogen therapy or with progesterone treatment, oophorectomy, and lung transplantation has been used with various degrees of success.[69–71] Some investigators have correlated histopathologic findings with prognosis, noting a poor prognosis for patients with lesions exhibiting predominantly cystic changes.[67] Other workers have combined and scored these two features and have estimated that the survival rate, from biopsy to lung transplantation or death, is approximately 85% at 5 years and 71% at 10 years.[72] The cause of death generally is respiratory insufficiency.

Pulmonary Dirofilariasis

Pulmonary dirofilariasis is an infectious process produced by a helminth common in dogs, *Dirofilaria immitis*, for which humans are an accidental host. Pulmonary dirofilariasis usually manifests as one or more coin nodules affecting both children and adults. Because of the clinical and radiologic presentation, it often is mistaken for a neoplastic process, and diagnosis is accomplished by tissue examination. Since the initial descriptions by Dashiell[73] and Goodman,[74] numerous instances of this entity have been presented, mostly as case reports or short series.[75–79] As happens in dogs, the worms may lodge in the heart; however, they may die before reaching maturity and pass into the pulmonary arteries. This infectious process is rather rare and may account for only a very small percentage of cases presenting as a granulomatous reaction in the lung.

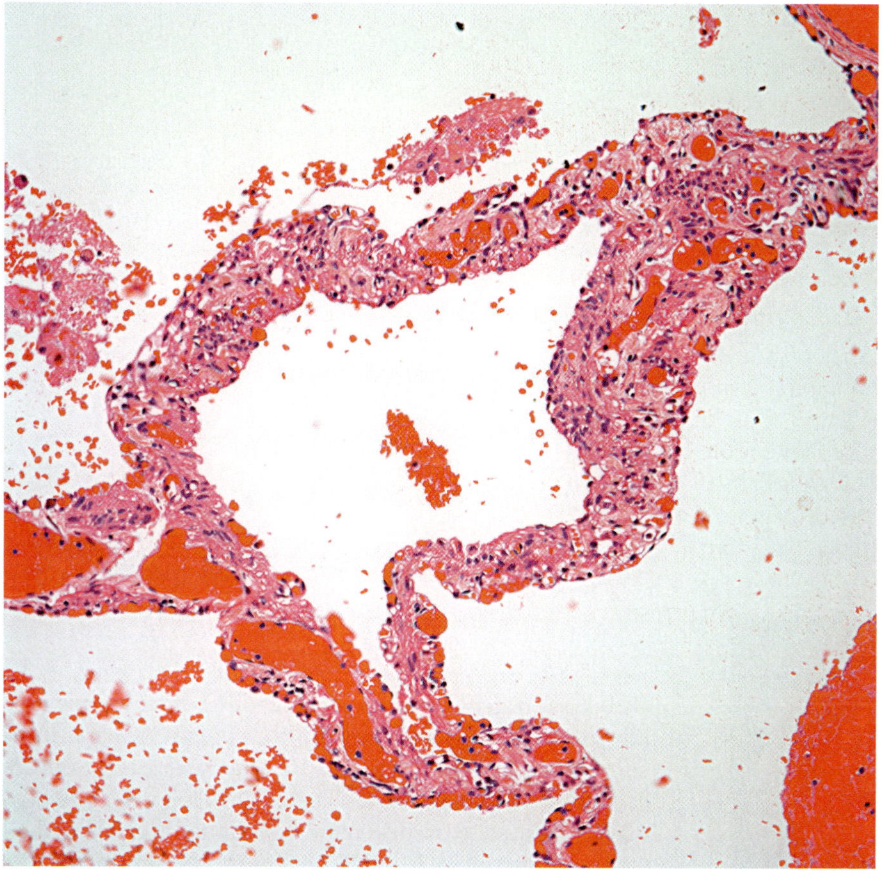

Figure 12-56 Lymphangioleiomyomatosis. Note the cystic structure lined by smooth muscle.

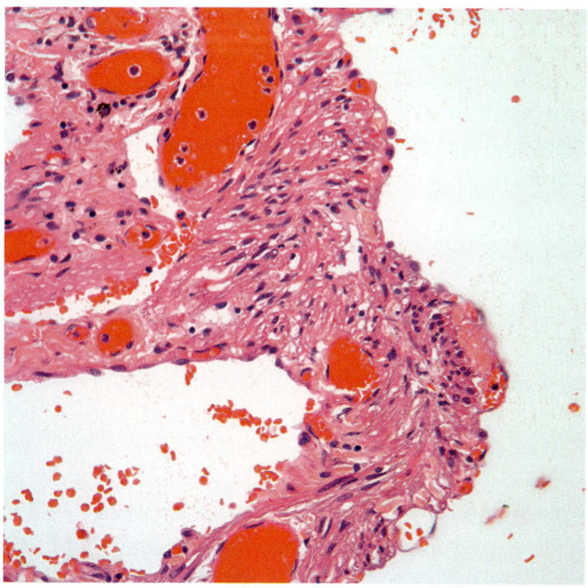

Figure 12-57 Higher-power view of smooth muscle in lymphangioleiomyomatosis showing focal clear cell changes.

Ulbright and Katzenstein[80] reported a study of 86 cases of solitary pulmonary granuloma in the lung and identified fungal or acid-fast organisms in 60 cases. In 25 cases an infectious etiology could not be determined, and in only one case could fragments of a helminth be identified. The investigators noted that microbiologic cultures were less productive than direct tissue examination. Therefore, it seems clear that in daily practice, pulmonary dirofilariasis is an unusual occurrence. The largest series of cases was reported by Flieder and associates,[81] who summarized the entire spectrum of histopathologic changes that this infectious process may elicit in the lung parenchyma by studying 41 lesions in 39 patients.

Clinical Features

Pulmonary dirofilariasis may be seen in patients ranging in age from 8 to 80 years, with a median of 58 years. The infection appears to be more common in men than in women, and it is not necessarily associated with immunosuppression, although in some patients a history of a previous malignancy may be elicited. At least one half of the patients are asymptomatic, and the pulmonary nodule is discovered on a routine chest radiograph. Among those patients who present with signs and symptoms, cough, dyspnea, chest pain, fever, and wheezing are common; hemoptysis is rare. Eosinophilia may be present in up to 15% of these patients. On the chest radiograph, dirofilariasis manifests more commonly as a solitary pulmonary nodule; in some cases, however, multiple nodules may be seen. The right lung appears to be more commonly affected than the left, and although these nodules may be seen more frequently in the periphery of the lung, central lesions also may occur.

Macroscopic Features

The pulmonary nodules may range in size from 0.5 to 4 cm in diameter. They are well circumscribed, of soft consistency, granular in appearance, and gray (Fig. 12-58). They are more commonly seen in a subpleural location, and the cut surface is necrotic but does not show any identifiable worms. The adjacent lung parenchyma exhibits a normal appearance.

Histopathologic Features

The low-power view of these nodules is that of a well-defined but unencapsulated necrotic granuloma with destruction of normal lung parenchyma (Fig. 12-59). At higher magnification, a thrombosed artery containing fragments of nonviable worm, surrounded by an inflamed fibrous capsule, may be observed. In some cases, the worm is present within necrotic lung parenchyma, and not within the vascular spaces (Fig. 12-60A). The worms usually are immature and thus do not contain ova and measure approximately 125 to 250 µm long, whereas the cuticle ranges in thickness from 5 to 25 µm (Figs. 12-60B and 12-61). These parasites may be highlighted using histochemical stains such as PAS or Movat. In a study by Flieder and associates,[81] the granulomatous reaction was found to contain a round, geographic necrosis, or wedge-shaped lesion in approximately one third of the cases; caseous necrosis was present in 41% and Charcot-Leyden crystals were present in 27%. In most cases, the nodules have a rim composed of dense hyalinized tissue with an inflammatory reaction composed of lymphocytes, plasma cells, and histi-

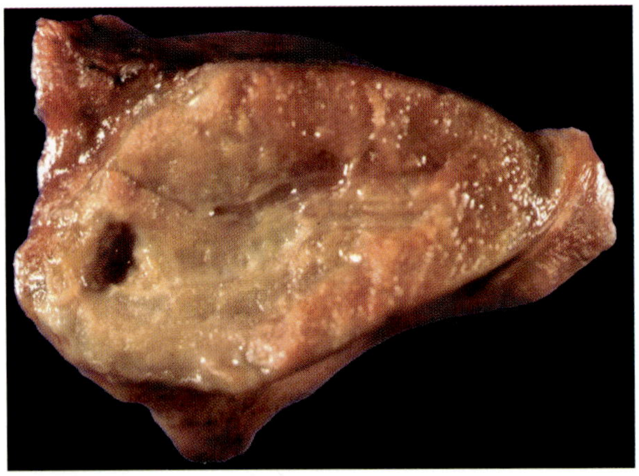

Figure 12-58 Gross specimen of lung involved by dirofilariasis. An intrapulmonary mass is evident.

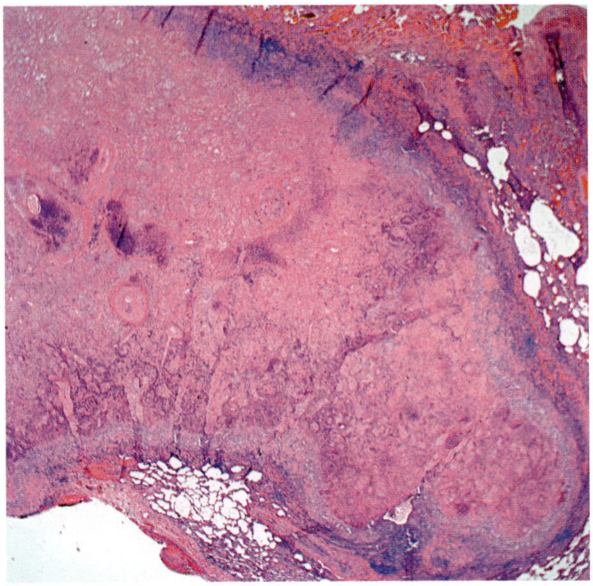

Figure 12-59 Necrotic pulmonary nodule typical of dirofilariasis.

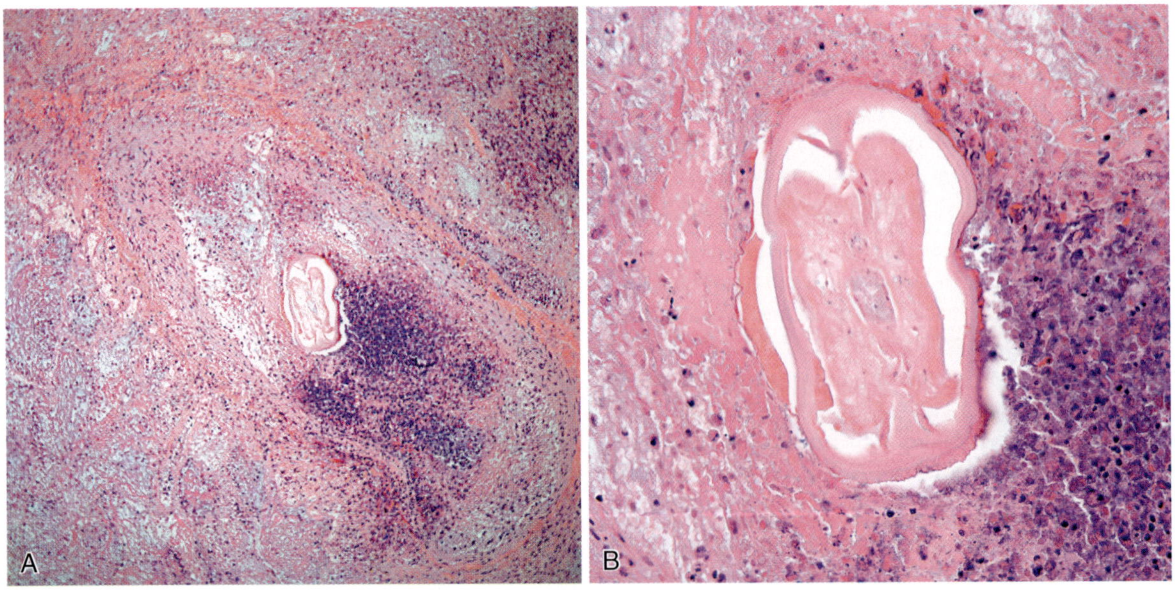

Figure 12-60 Pulmonary dirofilariasis. **A**, Low-power view of the parasite embedded in necrotic material. **B**, Higher-power view of the parasite (*Dirofilaria immitis*).

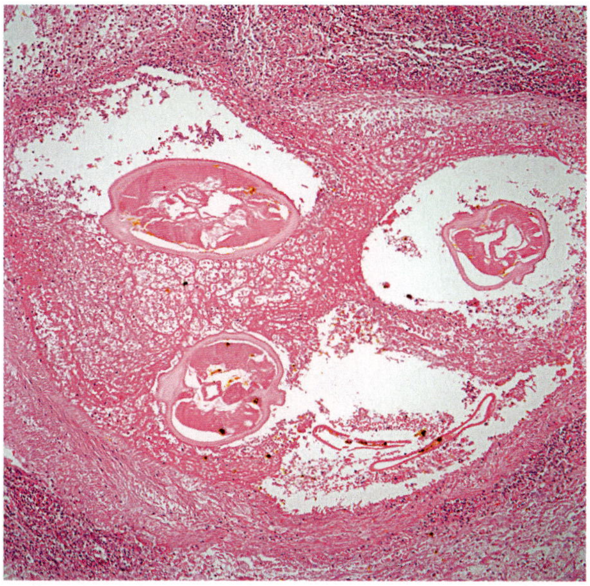

Figure 12-61 In some cases of pulmonary dirofilariasis, it is possible to identify several organisms.

ocytes. Langerhans giant cells, neutrophils, and non-necrotizing granulomatous reaction also may be present. On the other hand, adjacent lung parenchyma may show features of desquamative interstitial pneumonitis (DIP)–like areas, follicular bronchiolitis, or organizing pneumonia. Focal areas showing vasculitis and capilaritis also may be seen in some cases. Other features that may be observed in association with pulmonary dirofilariasis include microcalcifications, cholesterol cleft granulomas, amyloid-like stromal areas, and fibrinous pleuritis. The most important diagnostic criterion is identification of the worm.

Differential Diagnosis

Examination of serial sections may be required to identify the worm, because it may not be present in initial superficial sections. In cases in which material for evaluation is limited, the differential diagnosis will include any other infectious process due to fungal or acid-fast bacilli, Wegener's granulomatosis, Churg-Strauss syndrome, and possibly pulmonary lymphoma. Depending on the setting, special stains or tissue culture will rule out these possibilities. If the material available for evaluation was taken from areas adjacent to the granulomatous reaction, other entities such as bronchiolitis obliterans with organizing pneumonia (BOOP), extrinsic allergic alveolitis, or desquamative interstitial pneumonitis may be considered in the differential diagnosis.

Treatment and Prognosis

Surgical excision of the nodules is curative; in cases with multiple nodules, however, all nodules should be sampled, because dirofilariasis may be associated with other, less benign processes, including primary carcinomas of the lung.

HISTIOCYTIC LESIONS

The broad spectrum of histiocytic disorders that may manifest as pulmonary tumors or tumor-like lesions encompasses lesions of infectious, metabolic, environmental, and unknown etiology, among others. This section focuses on lesions that may manifest as either a pulmonary mass or lung nodules. Even with this subgrouping, however, coverage of the extensive range of pathologic conditions would be impossible here. It is well known that systemic disorders, including storage diseases such as Fabry's disease,[82] infantile G_{M1}-gangliosidosis,[83] Gaucher's disease,[84,85] and Niemann-Pick disease,[86,87] may involve the lung. In these conditions, however, a previous diagnosis typically has been established, and the lung is involved secondarily. Other systemic conditions, such as Whipple's disease, also may involve the lung[88,89]; these conditions are therefore not covered here because the pulmonary involvement is secondary to systemic disease. A select group of lesions, which may share similar histopathologic and immunohistochemical features, will be presented, including the following:

- Langerhans cell histiocytosis
- Erdheim-Chester disease
- Rosai-Dorfman disease
- Juvenile xanthogranuloma
- Crystal-storing histiocytosis
- Xanthoma
- Malakoplakia

Pulmonary Langerhans Cell Histiocytosis

Pulmonary Langerhans cell histiocytosis (PLCH) has also been referred to as primary pulmonary histiocytosis X, eosinophilic granuloma of the lung, and Langerhans cell granulomatosis. This type of histiocytosis may involve the lung either as a solitary lung process or secondarily as part of a systemic process. It is well known that Langerhans cell histiocytosis may manifest in adults as either single organ involvement or as multisystem disease. The focus here is on single organ involvement in the pulmonary region.

Although numerous reviews and case series have been reported,[90–108] the rate of occurrence of PLCH is difficult to determine, and hard data on its prevalence are lacking. In a study of 502 patients who underwent lung biopsy, 17 (3.4%) were diagnosed with this disease.[109] Approximately 25% of the cases are initially identified during routine chest radiographs, which may disclose pulmonary abnormalities. Although the exact pathogenesis of PLCH is unknown, Soler and colleagues[90] suggested an uncontrolled immune reaction.

Clonality has been determined in some cases of this disease.[100–103] Using a human androgen receptor assay (HUMARA), Willman and coworkers[103] identified clonality in 9 of 10 cases of Langerhans cell histiocytosis (none of which were in the lung). Yu and colleagues[101] also documented clonality. Yousem and associates[100] also used HUMARA to study 24 nodules in 13 patients, finding that 29% showed clonality and 71% were nonclonal. These workers concluded that PLCH appears to be primarily a reactive process.

Clinical Features

PLCH occurs most often in adult patients in their third or fourth decade of life; however, it also has been reported in children.[106] The process is more common in whites than in African Americans. Several different studies have variously determined equal rates of occurrence in men and women, higher incidence in men, and higher incidence in women. One consistent association has been with cigarette smoking, which is documented in approximately 80% of patients. Presenting signs and symptoms may include cough, chest pain, dyspnea, hemoptysis, or pneumothorax. Approximately 20% of the patients may be completely asymptomatic, however, and the process may be first detected on a routine chest radiograph. The characteristic radiographic feature is a reticulonodular bilateral infiltrate, although in some cases the radiologic findings may be nonspecific. The diagnosis typically is made by means of open lung biopsy; in some studies, however, transbronchial biopsy has been used.

PLCH also has been associated with neoplastic conditions including non-Hodgkin's lymphoma, Hodgkin's lymphoma, and carcinoma.[95–97] Close clinical, radiologic, and histopathologic correlation will be necessary to establish the nature of these associations.

Macroscopic Features

Specimens obtained by open lung biopsy or wedge resection will show multiple parenchymal nodules of different sizes, ranging from less than 1 cm to more than 3 cm in diameter (Fig. 12-62). These nodules are whitish, of firm consistency, and well circumscribed but not encapsulated. Areas of necrosis or hemorrhage are not common but may be present.

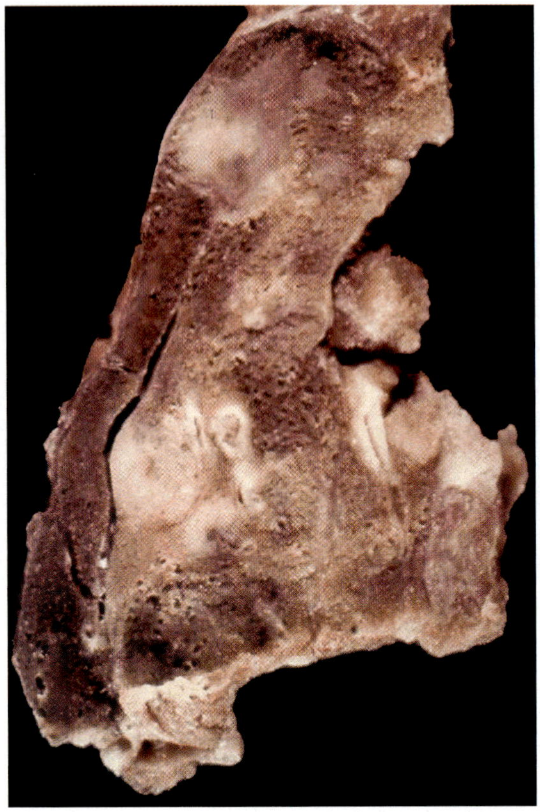

Figure 12-62 Lung involved in Langerhans cell histiocytosis, gross specimen. Several nodules of different sizes are present in the lung parenchyma.

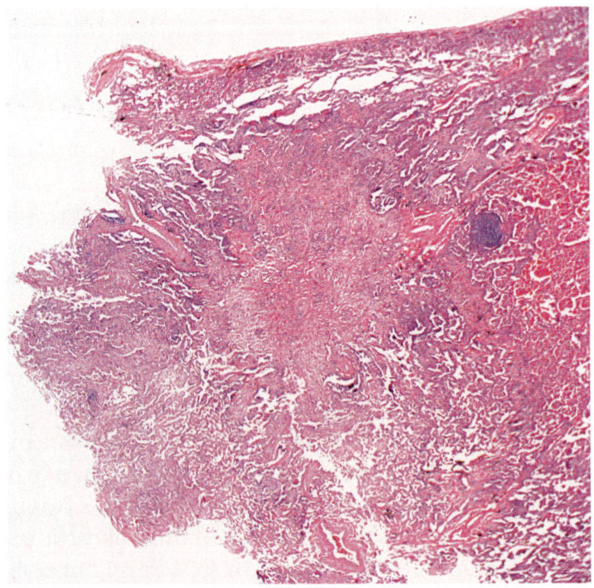

Figure 12-63 Low-power view of lung involved in Langerhans cell histiocytosis. Note the intraparenchymal nodule.

Histopathologic Features

The low-power view shows parenchymal nodules of differing sizes obliterating normal lung parenchyma. These nodules often have a stellate shape, with the so-called Medusa's head profile; however, some may have a round contour (Figs. 12-63 and 12-64). Necrosis or cavitations may be seen in approximately 20% to 25% of the cases. At high magnification, a proliferation of histiocytes can be seen admixed with inflammatory cells, which in a majority of cases will show numerous eosinophils (Figs. 12-65 and 12-66). In some nodules, fibrotic changes will be seen, rather than a marked inflammatory infiltrate with only scattered eosinophils. The presence of eosinophils is helpful in making the diagnosis but is not required. The histiocytes

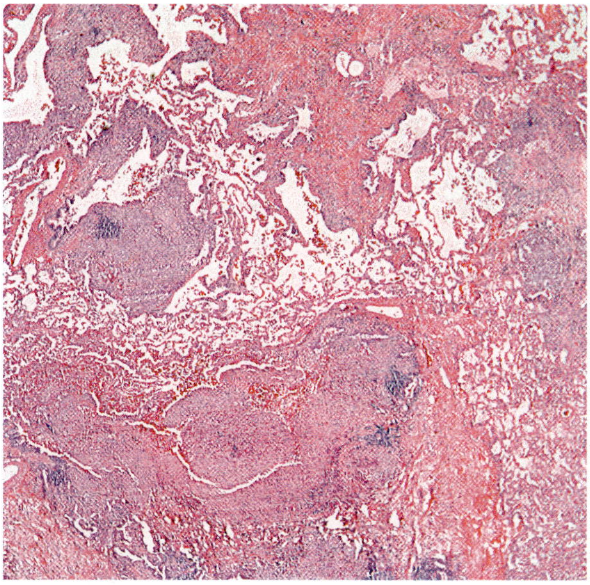

Figure 12-64 Pulmonary Langerhans cell histiocytosis. Low-power view of involved lung shows intraparenchymal nodules in different stages of disease, with more prominent fibrosis in some and increased cellularity in others.

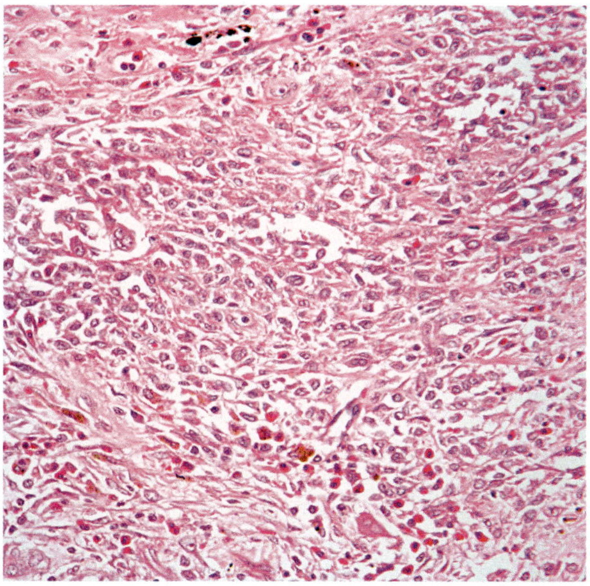

Figure 12-65 Pulmonary Langerhans cell histiocytosis. The histiocytic cellular proliferation is admixed with eosinophils.

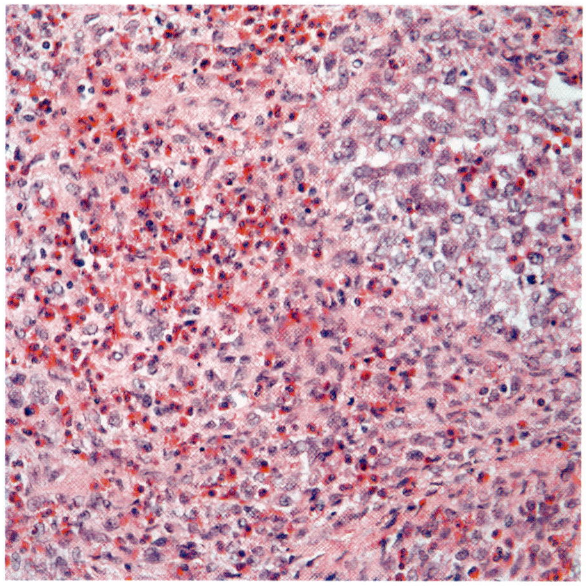

Figure 12-66 Pulmonary Langerhans cell histiocytosis with a more prominent eosinophilic infiltrate.

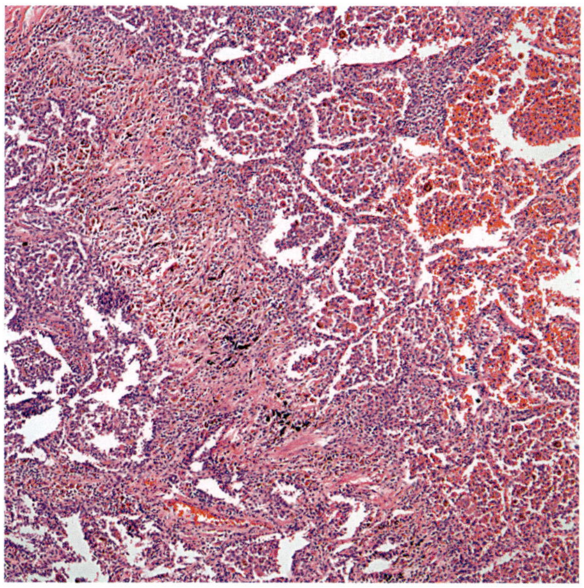

Figure 12-67 Adjacent lung parenchyma in pulmonary Langerhans cell histiocytosis with desquamative interstitial pneumonitis–like changes.

characteristically show indented or grooved nuclei. The histiocytic proliferation may in some instances extend into the alveolar wall without forming a nodule and also may involve blood vessels and the airway. Some changes may be observed in the noninvolved lung parenchyma, including a DIP-like reaction (Fig. 12-67), indicated by the accumulation of pigment-laden macrophages within alveolar spaces with mild interstitial fibrosis.

On immunohistochemical studies, involved lung shows positive staining for S-100 protein, CD1a, human leukocyte antigen (HLA)-DR, langerin (CD207), and E-cadherin. Ultrastructural imaging of the Langerhans cells will show the typical Birbeck granules—the racket- or rod-shaped organelles characteristic of this disease.

Differential Diagnosis

Although PLCH is rather a straightforward diagnosis, in some cases the characteristic features are not readily visible, and other conditions may be considered, including Erdheim-Chester disease, malignant lymphoma, and eosinophilic pneumonia.[107] With any of these conditions, the use of immunohistochemical studies and correlation with the radiographic findings may help in arriving at the correct diagnosis.

Treatment and Prognosis

Several approaches to the treatment of PLCH, including cessation of smoking, steroids, chemotherapy, and lung transplantation, have been tried. Transplantation usually is reserved for patients with severely compromised lung function. Recurrences of PLCH have been documented in the transplanted lung.

The treatment approach will depend largely on the clinical situation and respiratory function of the individual patient. Smoking cessation is very important in the management of these patients. Although many studies have suggested a good prognosis, some patients go on to develop respiratory insufficiency resulting in death. Vassallo and associates[105] reviewed the cases of 102 adults with PLCH over follow-up periods ranging from 0 to 23 years (median, 4 years). The investigators noted 33 deaths, 15 of which were attributed to respiratory failure, with an overall median survival of 12.5 years. They also identified six patients with malignant lymphoproliferative disorders and five patients with lung carcinoma. These workers concluded that the survival of adults with PLCH is shorter than that of persons in the general population.

Erdheim-Chester Disease

Erdheim-Chester disease is a rare type of histiocytosis, with only a few series of cases reported in the literature.[110–115] William Chester and Jacob Erdheim described this condition in 1930 as a form of lipoid granulomatosis different from other lipidosis entities.[110] The authors described two autopsy cases in which the histiocytic process was present in bone and viscera. In 1973, Jaffe[111] reported an additional case and coined the term *Erdheim-Chester disease*.

Clinical Features

The clinical presentation in Erdheim-Chester disease varies considerably, depending on the organs involved. Although the emphasis here is on pulmonary symptoms, an important point is that the lung is not necessarily the only site involved, and a search for evidence of disease in other sites is strongly recommended. Erdheim-Chester disease usually is a multisystem process that may involve several anatomic regions. One of the most common presentations is skeletal abnormalities, including expansile lesions of the ribs, symmetrical patchy sclerosis, thickening of the metaphyses of long tubular bones, and patchy sclerosis of the calcaneus. Other extraskeletal manifestations may include dyspnea, radiologic evidence of pulmonary infiltrates and pleural effusion, pulmonary fibrosis, congenital megacalices, hydronephrosis, hydroureter, chronic lipogranulomatous pyelonephritis, retroperitoneal xanthogranulomas, ophthalmic abnormalities, and hyperlipidemia. In patients with pulmonary manifestations, the best way to arrive at a precise diagnosis is to perform an open lung biopsy.

Histopathologic Features

The histopathologic features of Erdheim-Chester disease are rather characteristic. The low-power view displays a histiocytic process involving pleura and pulmonary septum (Fig. 12-68). In some cases the involvement is more extensive, with pleural, septal, and parenchymal changes (Fig. 12-69). The histiocytic proliferation is composed of small to medium-sized histiocytes with foamy or finely granular cytoplasm (Figs. 12-70 to 12-72), and the

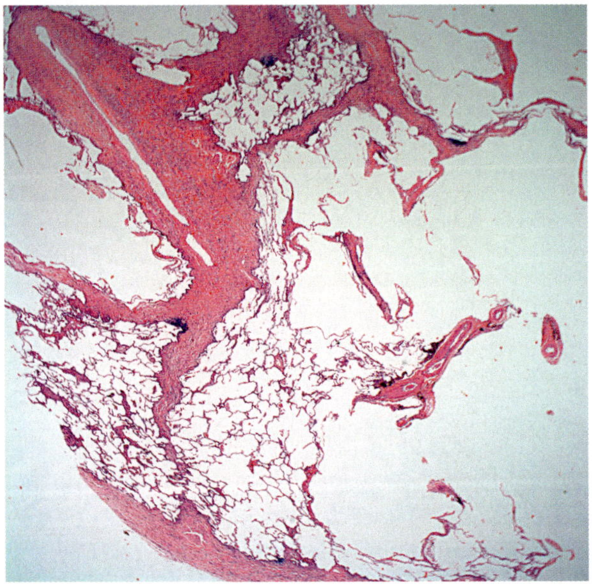

Figure 12-68 Erdheim-Chester disease. In this low-power view, note the involvement of pleura and pulmonary septum with adjacent emphysematous changes in lung parenchyma.

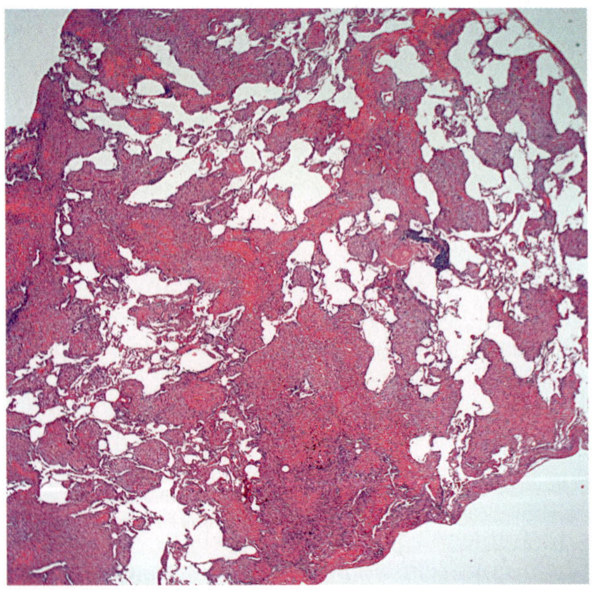

Figure 12-69 Erdheim-Chester disease involving pleura, septum, and lung parenchyma.

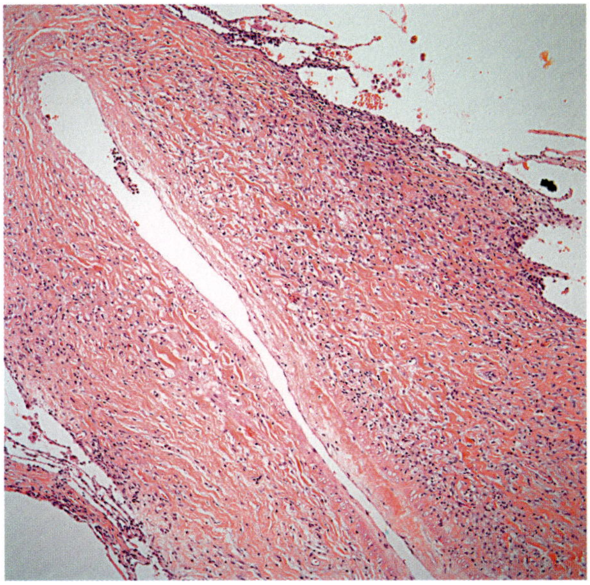

Figure 12-70 Involvement of pulmonary septum in Erdheim-Chester disease.

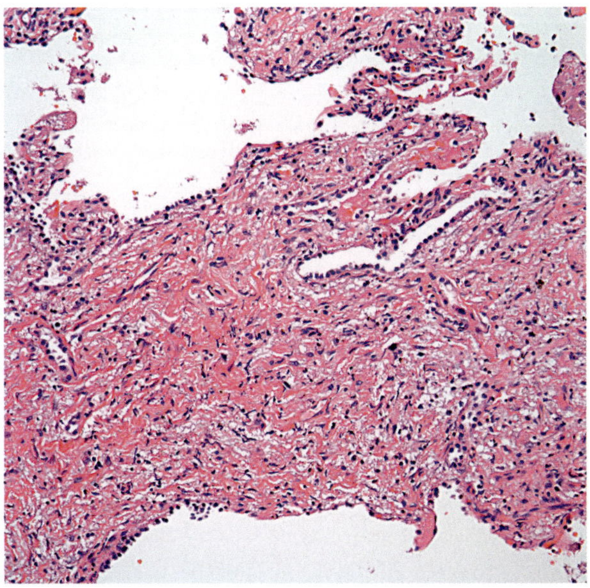

Figure 12-71 Entrapped alveolar elements in Erdheim-Chester disease.

nuclei do not show the grooving characteristic of PLCH. Granulomatous changes are not a feature of Erdheim-Chester disease. The histiocytic infiltrate usually involves the pleura and pulmonary septum; the lung parenchyma, by contrast, manifests changes more in keeping with interstitial lung disease or emphysematous changes. The histiocytic proliferation may also show a discrete inflammatory infiltrate composed of lymphocytes and plasma cells but rarely shows a marked inflammatory component, and eosinophils are not increased in number, when present.

On immunohistochemical studies, the histiocytic proliferation shows positive staining for CD68 (Kp-1) and factor XIIIa, whereas staining for CD1a is negative.

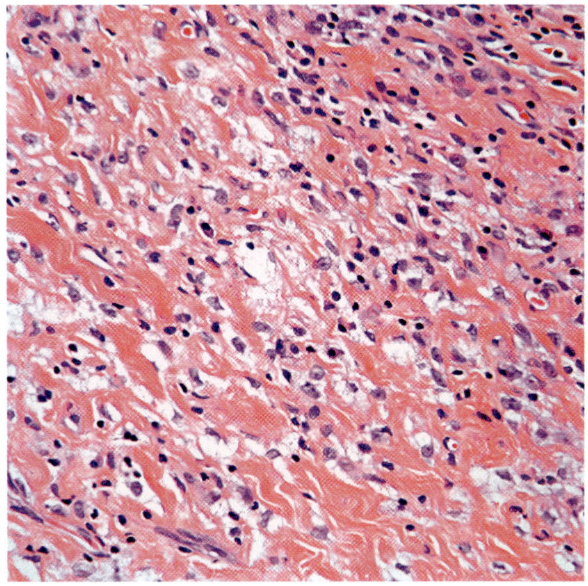

Figure 12-72 High-power view of the histiocytic proliferation in Erdheim-Chester disease.

S-100 protein may show variable staining—both negative and positive staining have been documented.

Treatment and Prognosis

No specific treatment for this condition is available, and different approaches have been attempted, including corticosteroids, interferon α-2a, surgical debulking, and chemotherapy. The prognosis for patients with Erdheim-Chester disease with pulmonary involvement is rather poor, because progression to respiratory failure eventuating in death is the usual course.

Rosai-Dorfman Disease

Rosai-Dorfman disease, also known as sinus histiocytosis with massive lymphadenopathy (SHML), is a process of ubiquitous distribution—it has been described essentially everywhere in the body.[116-122] Although the etiology of this condition is still unknown, different theories have been proposed to explain its occurrence, including an immunologic response and an infectious origin. Paulli and coworkers[121] evaluated two cases using HUMARA and found that the histiocytic proliferation was polyclonal. The process, as originally described, is more often encountered in young adults, and the most common anatomic site is the lymph nodes. Rosai-Dorfman disease may involve an extranodal site in approximately 20% of the cases; however, the lung and pleura are among the most unusual sites of occurrence. In some of the cases of disease involving lung parenchyma, the lung disease occurred in addition to disease at other sites, namely, lymph nodes. Thus, it is exceedingly rare for this condition to occur solely and primarily in the lung parenchyma or pleura. When this condition affects the lung parenchyma, the patient may

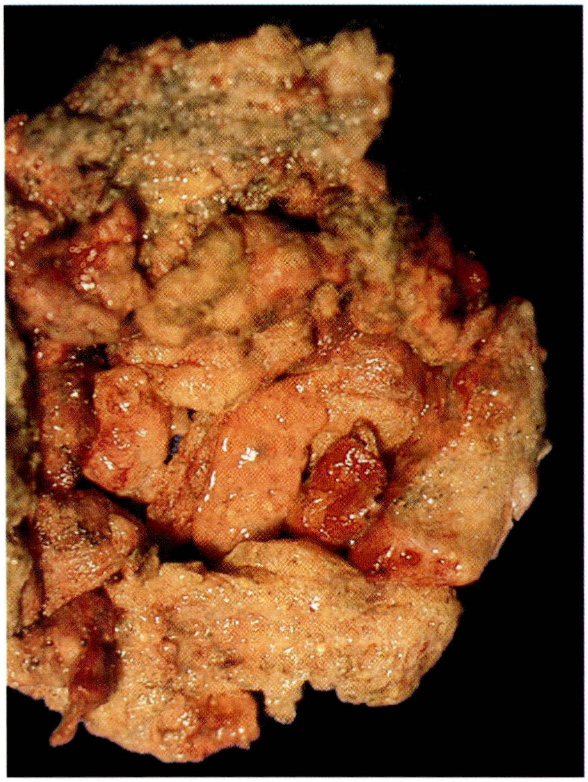

Figure 12-73 Gross specimen of lung in Rosai-Dorfman disease, manifesting as a pulmonary mass with yellowish color and soft consistency.

present with an intrapulmonary mass (Fig. 12-73), which may be indistinguishable clinically or radiologically from other neoplastic processes. Therefore, tissue diagnosis is the best approach.

Histopathologic Features

The microscopic features of Rosai-Dorfman disease in the lung are similar to those described in the lymph nodes. The main histologic hallmark of the process is the proliferation of large histiocytes, which may have one or more nuclei and contain ample pale cytoplasm (Figs. 12-74 to 12-77). Some of these lymphocytes may show the presence of lymphophagocytosis or emperipolesis; however, this finding may not be readily apparent. The histiocytic proliferation is usually seen on the background of a prominent inflammatory response, consisting predominantly of plasma cell and lymphocytes. In general, the two most important cellular components in Rosai-Dorfman disease are large histiocytes and plasma cells. The pulmonary parenchyma is clearly replaced by the process, and the adjacent uninvolved lung parenchyma may show features of interstitial lung disease.

Immunohistochemical studies may be of help in the diagnosis of this condition, because the histiocytes show positive staining for S-100 protein, CD68, CD15, CD163, and α_1-antichymotrypsin and are negative for CD1a and factor XIIIa.

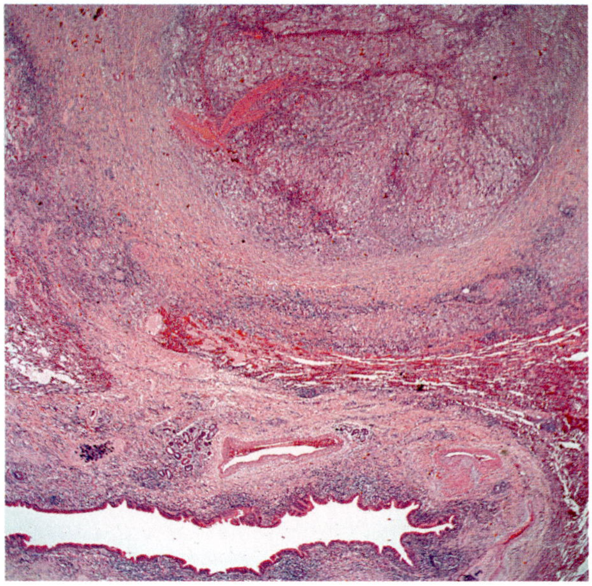

Figure 12-74 Low-power view of lung involved in Rosai-Dorfman disease showing a pulmonary mass destroying normal lung architecture.

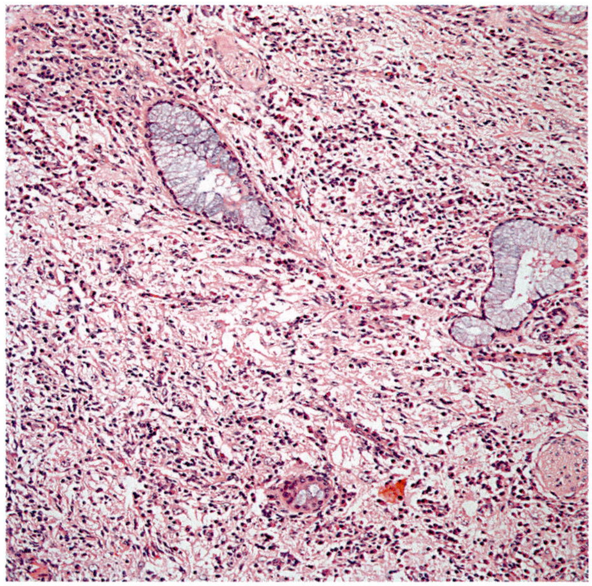

Figure 12-75 Rosai-Dorfman disease in the lung. Note adjacent mucous bronchial glands.

Treatment and Prognosis

No specific treatment for Rosai-Dorfman disease is available, and the prognosis may be related to the extent of involvement at the time of diagnosis. In more limited cases, surgical resection of the tumor mass may be accomplished, followed by observation, whereas in cases with more systemic involvement, surgical resection followed by adjuvant treatment can be attempted. Chemotherapy has not been shown to be of meaningful benefit, however.

In a follow-up study of 238 patients with Rosai-Dorfman disease, Foucar and colleagues[116] found that 21 had died—4 as a result of the disease, 13 with the disease

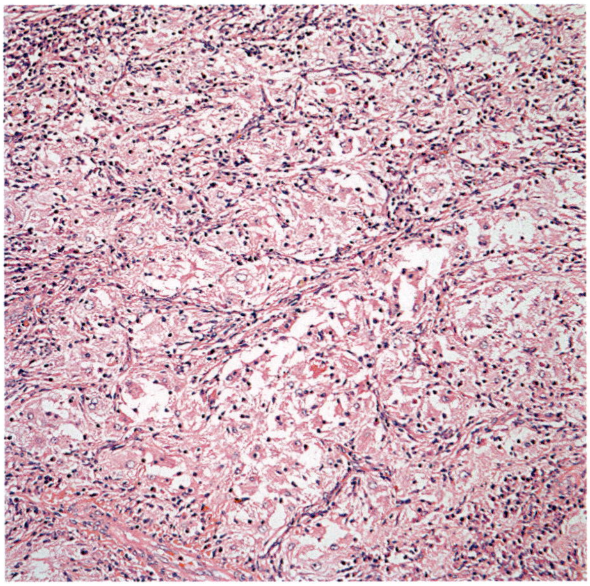

Figure 12-76 Rosai-Dorfman disease in the lung. Histiocytic proliferation is admixed with inflammatory cells.

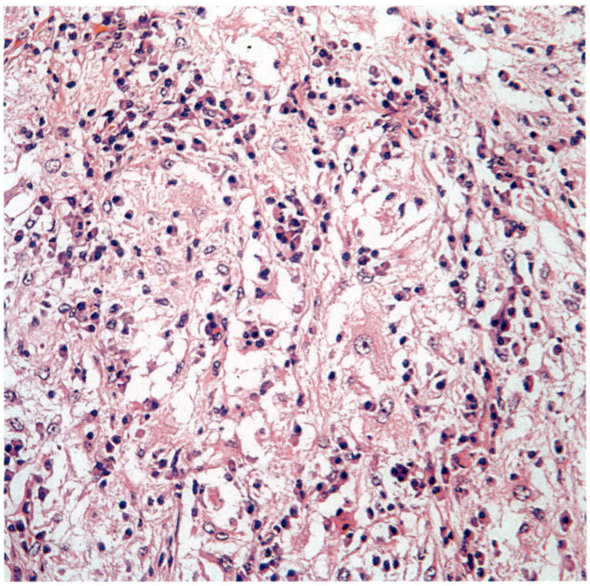

Figure 12-77 Rosai-Dorfman disease in the lung. High-power view reveals large histiocytes with prominent nucleoli admixed with plasma cells.

in whom death presumably was due to other causes, and 4 with no evidence of disease. At 1 year, 49 patients were alive without disease, whereas 36 had persistent disease. Whether lung involvement affects the survival rate among patients with this disease is difficult to determine, owing to its rare occurrence in the lung.

Pulmonary Juvenile Xanthogranuloma

Pulmonary juvenile xanthogranuloma (PJXG) is grouped among the non–Langerhans cell histiocytoses. This is an unusual condition of rare occurrence in the lung parenchyma, and only a few cases have been reported in the literature.[123-129] Unlike in Langerhans cell histiocytosis, in PJXG the putative cell of origin is unknown. The dermal dendrocyte has been proposed as a possibility; however, this theory would not explain lesions that occur primarily in deep-seated tissues or in viscera. Therefore, some authors have speculated that a plasmacytoid monocyte may be the cell of origin.[125]

PJXG is more common in children and young adults and affects the lung only rarely. When the lung is involved, the lesion may be bilateral or unilateral and multiple or single. A single lesion rarely is the presenting manifestation, although this has been reported sporadically. Patients often exhibit dermal involvement or experience symptoms of involvement of other organs and viscera.

Histopathologic Features

On gross inspection, this lesion may manifest as a solitary lung nodule or mass of variable size, which ranges from less than 1 cm to more than 3 cm in greatest dimension. The lesions are soft and yellowish and well-demarcated but not encapsulated.

On histologic examination, the low-power view is that of a well-circumscribed but unencapsulated mass (Figs. 12-78 and 12-79) destroying lung parenchyma. Higher magnification reveals a proliferation of histiocytes, which may range from small to medium in size, with or without prominent nuclei (Fig. 12-80). The histiocytic proliferation may be accompanied by an inflammatory infiltrate composed of lymphocytes and plasma

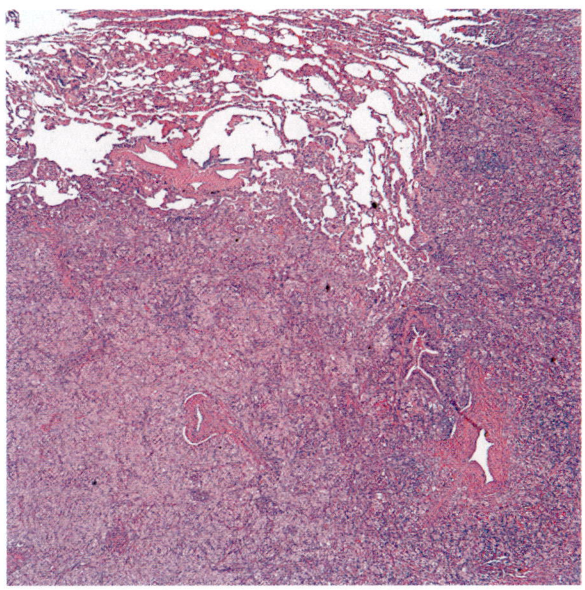

Figure 12-78 Pulmonary juvenile xanthogranuloma. Low-power view shows destruction of lung parenchyma.

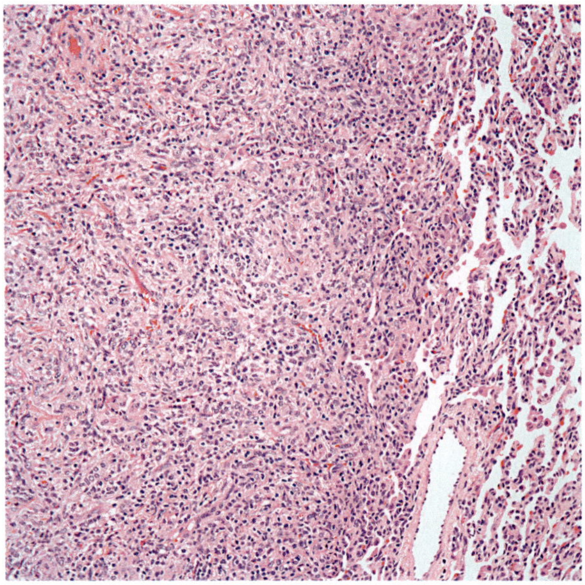

Figure 12-79 Pulmonary juvenile xanthogranuloma. The tumor is well circumscribed but not encapsulated.

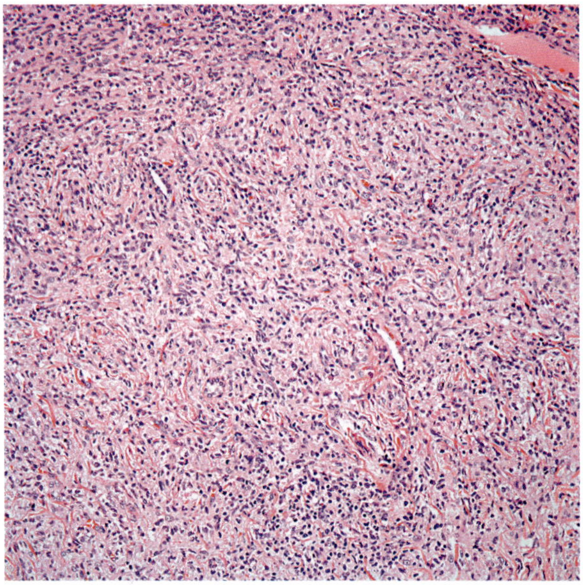

Figure 12-80 Pulmonary juvenile xanthogranuloma with a prominent histiocytic proliferation admixed with inflammatory cells.

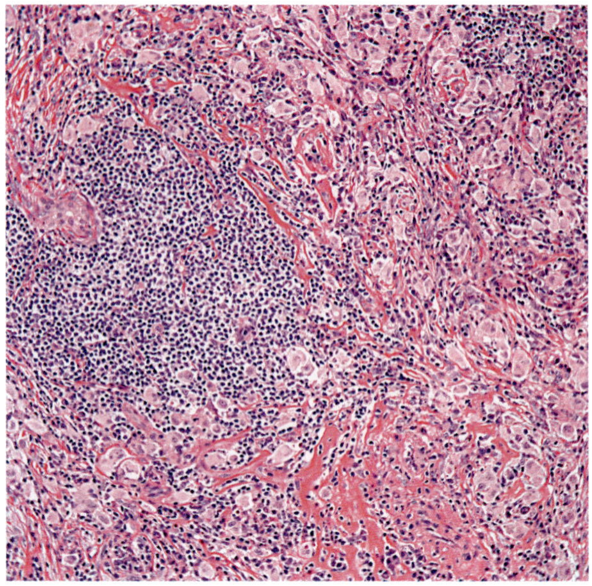

Figure 12-81 Pulmonary juvenile xanthogranuloma with a prominent histiocytic proliferation associated with a cluster of lymphocytes.

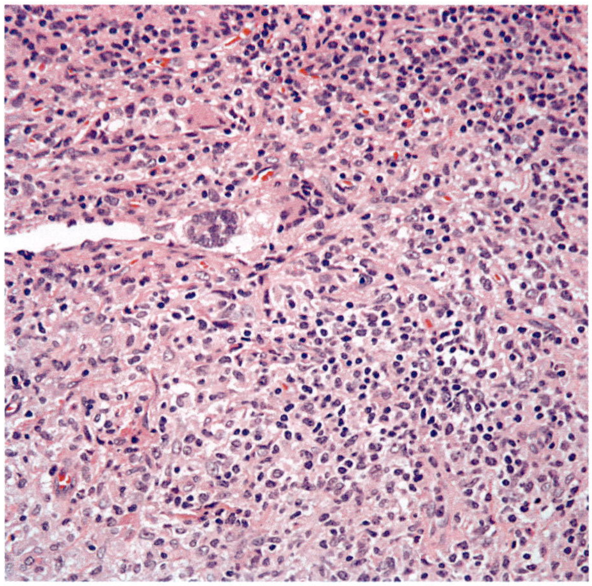

Figure 12-82 Scattered giant cells may be seen in pulmonary juvenile xanthogranuloma.

cells. Nodular collections of lymphocytes may be seen in some areas (Fig. 12-81). Also in focal areas, scattered multinucleated giant cells may be seen admixed with the histiocytic proliferation (Fig. 12-82). These giant cells are difficult to find, and in many cases they are absent. Nuclear atypia, mitotic activity, and necrosis or hemorrhage are not common in this process.

Immunohistochemical studies in patients with dermal juvenile xanthogranuloma have shown positive staining of histiocytes for CD68, factor XIIIa, HLA-DR, leukocyte common antigen (LCA), CD4, and S-100 protein. Staining for CD1a, CD3, CD21, CD34, and CD35 is negative. In addition, ultrastructural imaging studies are negative for the presence of Birbeck granules.

Treatment and Prognosis

Because of the rarity of this lesion in the lung parenchyma, unequivocal determination of whether it has an impact on patient survival is not possible. Most likely, it is the extent of the disease at the time of diagnosis that determines clinical outcome. Surgical resection of the pulmonary lesions appears to be a logical approach, when this procedure can be accomplished.

Crystal-Storing Histiocytoma or Histiocytosis

Crystal-storing histiocytoma is an unusual process that can manifest with or without an association with lymphoproliferative disorders. The most common lymphoproliferative process involved is multiple myeloma. *Crystal-storing histiocytoma* has been suggested as a term to describe this process when it occurs without any association with a lymphoproliferative disorder. This process is believed to be reactive in nature, in contrast with that associated with a lymphoproliferative disorder. If the process is associated with a lymphoproliferative disorder, the more generic name *crystal-storing histiocytosis* should be used. This type of process has been identified in several organ systems, including the gastrointestinal, genitourinary, hematopoietic, and respiratory systems. Three different storage components have been identified in this process: (1) crystallized immunoglobulins, (2) phagocytosed clofazimine in patients receiving treatment for leprosy, and (3) Charcot-Leyden crystals. Regardless of the material accumulated, the basic histopathologic process is similar and includes a histiocytic proliferation.[130–146]

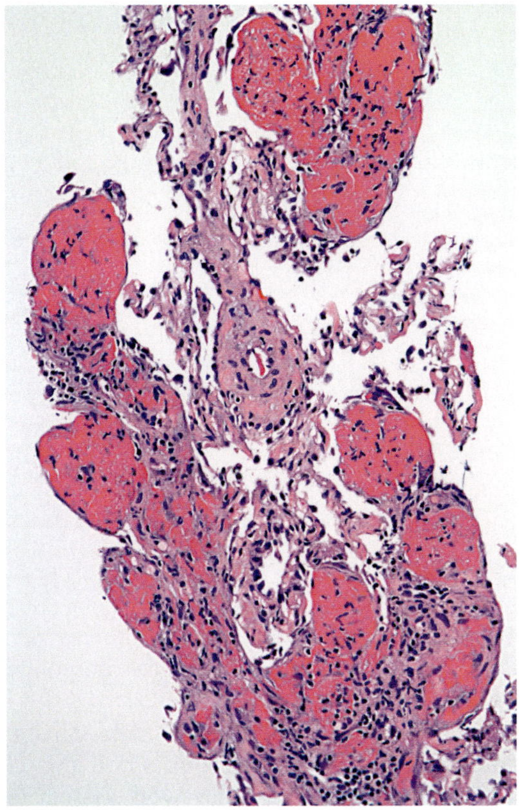

Figure 12-83 Crystal-storing histiocytoma. Lung parenchyma harbors deposits of intra-alveolar histiocytes.

Pathologic Features

At low magnification, the lung parenchyma in crystal-storing histiocytosis appears to keep its basic architecture; however, the alveoli are seen to be filled with an eosinophilic material that in some areas spills into the interstitium, giving the appearance of a fibrinous-type exudate (Figs. 12-83 and 12-84). At higher magnification, the material filling the alveoli is characterized by a histiocytic proliferation composed of larger histiocytes with ample cytoplasm and small round nuclei. The cytoplasm of the histiocytes is filled with crystalloid material, representing crystallized immunoglobulin. Crystal-storing histiocytoma manifests as a pulmonary mass or nodule replacing lung parenchyma (Figs. 12-85 to 12-87). The histiocytic proliferation may have the appearance of "muscle" proliferation, as seen in some rhabdomyomas. In some cases the histiocytes appear to contain a rather granular, noncrystallized immunoglobulin.

Immunohistochemical studies may help to identify histiocytic proliferation, because the cells show positive staining for CD68 and also may show a monoclonal arrangement of immunoglobulin using κ or λ stains. The histiocytes demonstrate negative staining for CD1a and factor XIIIa. Electron microscopy will ultimately determine the type of crystal material present in the cytoplasm.

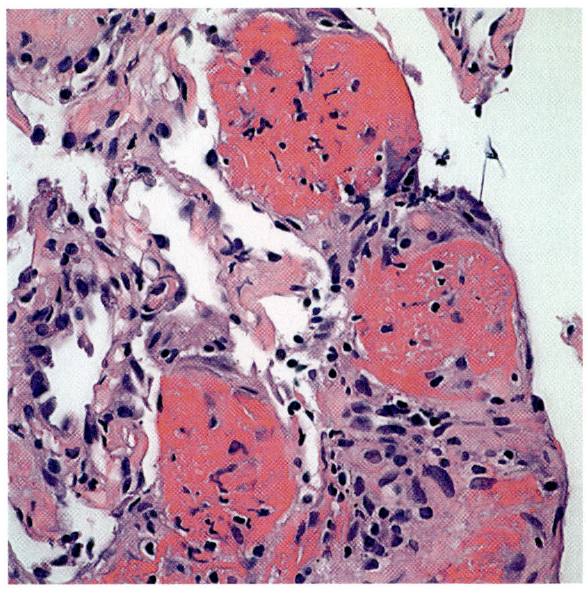

Figure 12-84 Crystal-storing histiocytoma. High-power view reveals intra-alveolar histiocytes containing crystalloid material.

Treatment and Prognosis

Surgical resection for the tumor-like lesion present in the lung parenchyma appears to be the treatment of choice; however, recurrences have been documented. Nevertheless, the prognosis will be determined by the underlying condition. It is imperative that in cases limited to the pulmonary parenchyma, without an obvious lymphoproliferative process, a complete clinical evaluation should be undertaken to rule out an occult neoplasm.

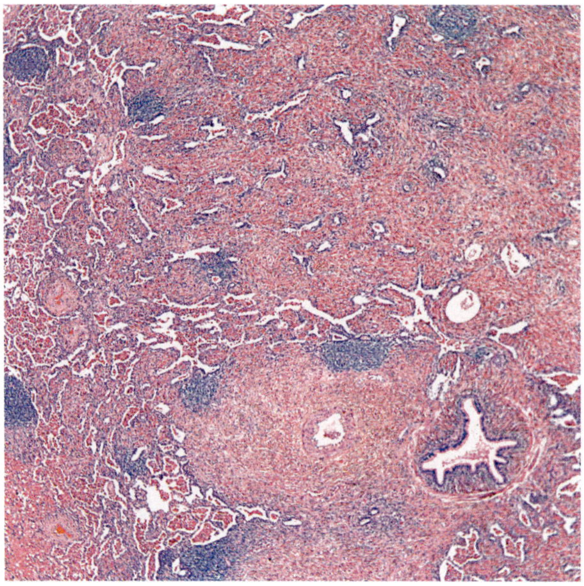

Figure 12-85 Crystal-storing histiocytoma involving and replacing lung parenchyma.

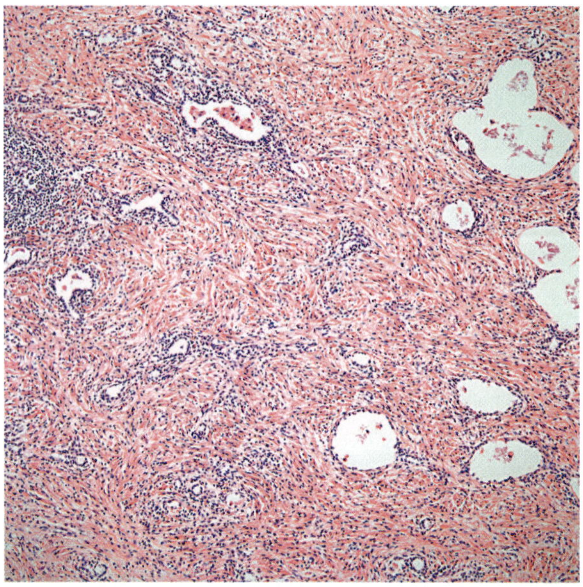

Figure 12-86 Crystal-storing histiocytoma. The histiocytic proliferation mimics muscle proliferation.

Pulmonary Xanthoma

Pulmonary xanthoma is an unusual benign tumor of the lung that appears only once in the literature. Andrianopoulos and colleagues[147] described the only case reported to date. The patient was a 32-year-old asymptomatic man without any pertinent clinical history. During a routine chest radiograph, a solitary pulmonary mass of 4 cm in greatest dimension was detected. On immunohistochemical studies, the tumor demonstrated negative reactivity for EMA, keratin, S-100 protein, chromogranin, PAS and

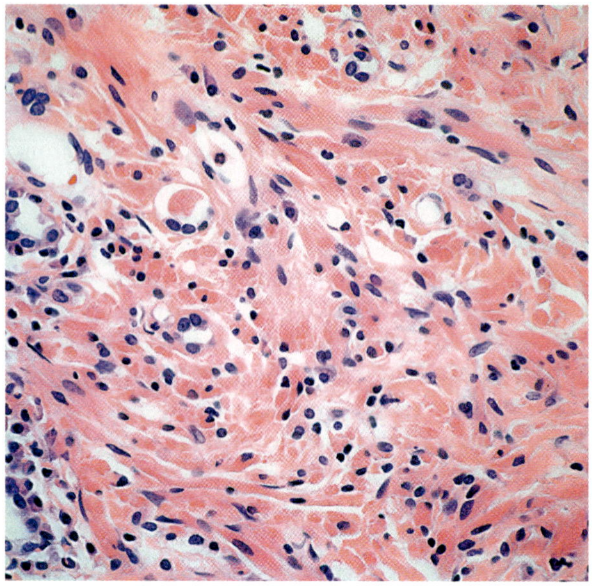

Figure 12-87 Crystal-storing histiocytoma. High-power view of the histiocytic proliferation shows intracytoplasmic crystalloid material.

D-PAS (i.e., with diastase pretreatment), mucicarmine, and oil red O. Electron microscopic findings were nonspecific, and the DNA histogram revealed a diploid cell population. Although this is the only case described in the literature, it is possible that similar cases have not been reported. The authors of this text subsequently identified a case in their files that was histologically and immunohistochemically similar to that in the published report (unpublished data).

Histopathologic Features

The low-power view of this lesion shows a well-circumscribed but unencapsulated subpleural process that replaces normal lung parenchyma. The homogeneous cellular proliferation is composed of medium-sized cells with ample clear or pale cytoplasm and nuclei displaced toward the periphery of the cells (Figs. 12-88 and 12-89). Higher magnification reveals that the cellular proliferation is composed of these xanthoma cells without any evidence of mitotic activity, nuclear atypia, necrosis, or hemorrhage (Fig. 12-90). Admixed with this xanthomatous component are sprinkled inflammatory cells—namely, lymphocytes and scattered plasma cells.

On immunohistochemical studies, the process demonstrates negative staining for epithelial, neuroendocrine, and neural markers; however, it is possible that staining for CD68 may be positive.

The treatment of choice for this process is surgical resection, which may be accomplished by wedge resection or segmentectomy. Complete surgical resection appears to be curative.

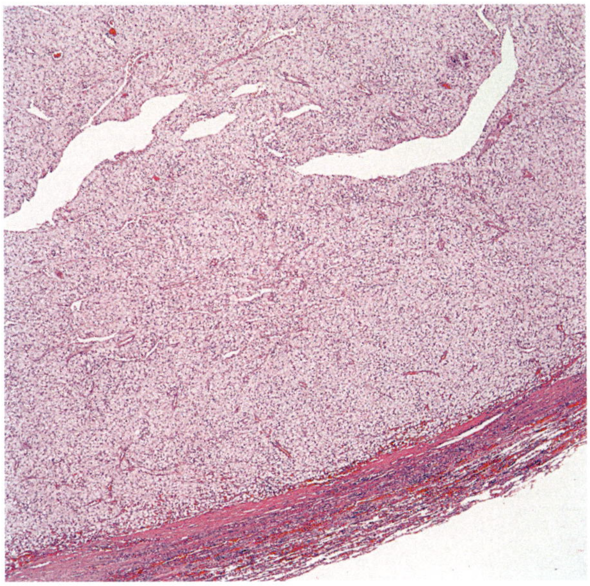

Figure 12-88 Low-power view of a pulmonary xanthoma. Note the well-circumscribed tumor.

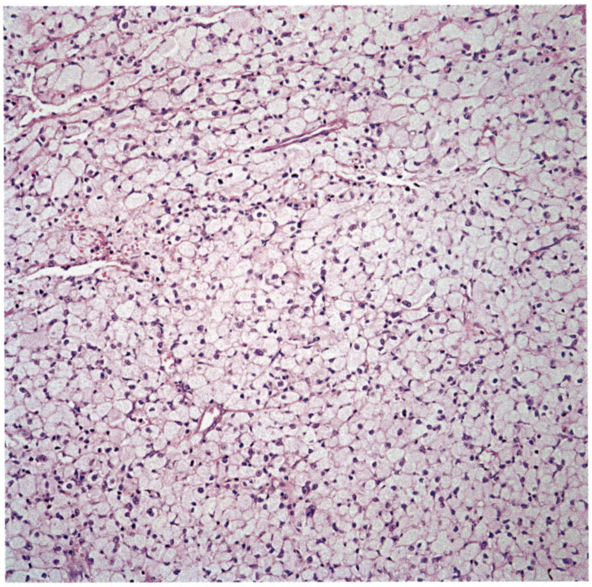

Figure 12-89 Pulmonary xanthoma with a homogeneous cellular proliferation.

Pulmonary Malakoplakia

Pulmonary malakoplakia is not a bona fide histiocytic process but rather an infectious process that may elicit a histiocytic response. Therefore, it is discussed here among other lesions of a histiocytic nature.

Malakoplakia is a process of ubiquitous distribution that has been described in many organ systems, including the genitourinary, central nervous, and gastrointestinal systems. Although some authors have suggested that the process is secondary to infection with *E. coli*, in the lung, it commonly has been associated with AIDS or other immunosuppressive states and has been linked to infections

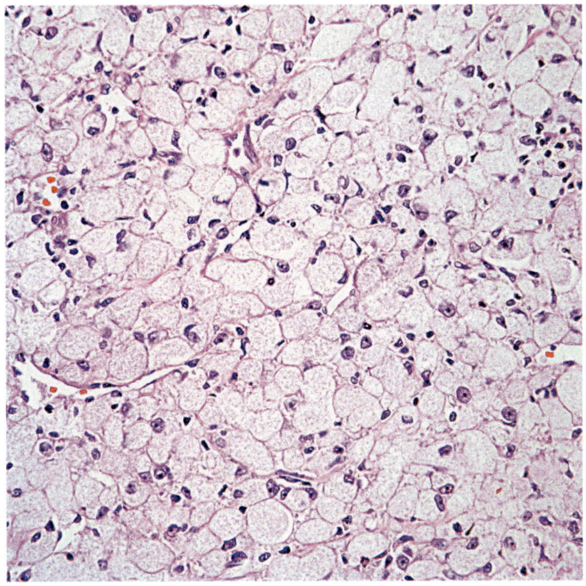

Figure 12-90 High-power view of a pulmonary xanthoma showing larger cells with pale cytoplasm and lack of cytologic atypia.

by agents such as *Rhodococcus equi* and *Pasteurella*.[148–152] Clinical and radiologic features of pulmonary malakoplakia are rather nonspecific. Tissue examination is required for final diagnosis.

Pathologic Features

Malakoplakia in the lung can manifest as an endobronchial nodule or as an intraparenchymal pulmonary mass with destruction of the lung parenchyma and necrosis (Fig. 12-91), indistinguishable from that seen with another pulmonary neoplasm.

The lung parenchyma may harbor one or more pulmonary nodules of differing sizes. The pathognomonic feature of malakoplakia is a histiocytic proliferation admixed with plasma cells and scattered Michaelis-Gutmann bodies (Figs. 12-92 to 12-94). In some instances, however, malakoplakia in the lung may be seen as a proliferation of spindle cells in a fibroblastic background admixed

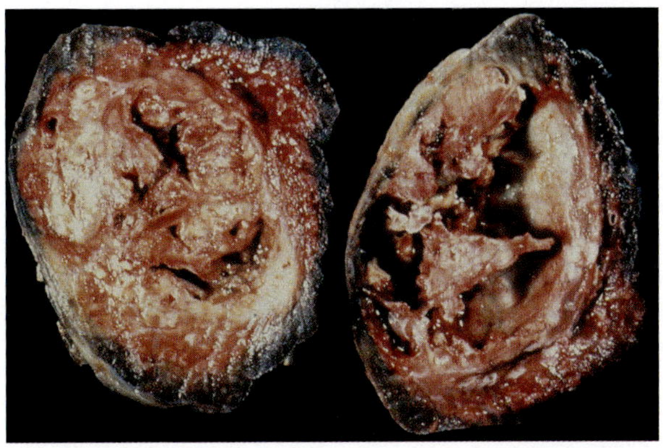

Figure 12-91 Resected lung specimen. The pulmonary mass was secondary to malakoplakia.

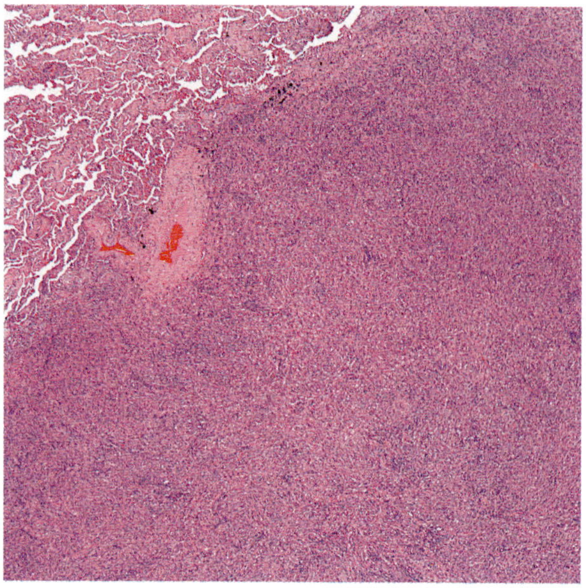

Figure 12-92 Malakoplakia manifesting as a pulmonary mass. Note the well-circumscribed tumor nodule.

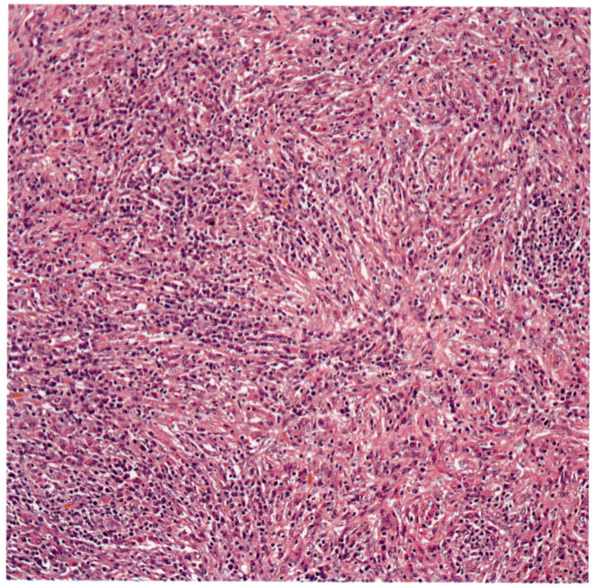

Figure 12-93 Malakoplakia with prominent histiocytic and plasma cell proliferation mimicking features of organizing pneumonia.

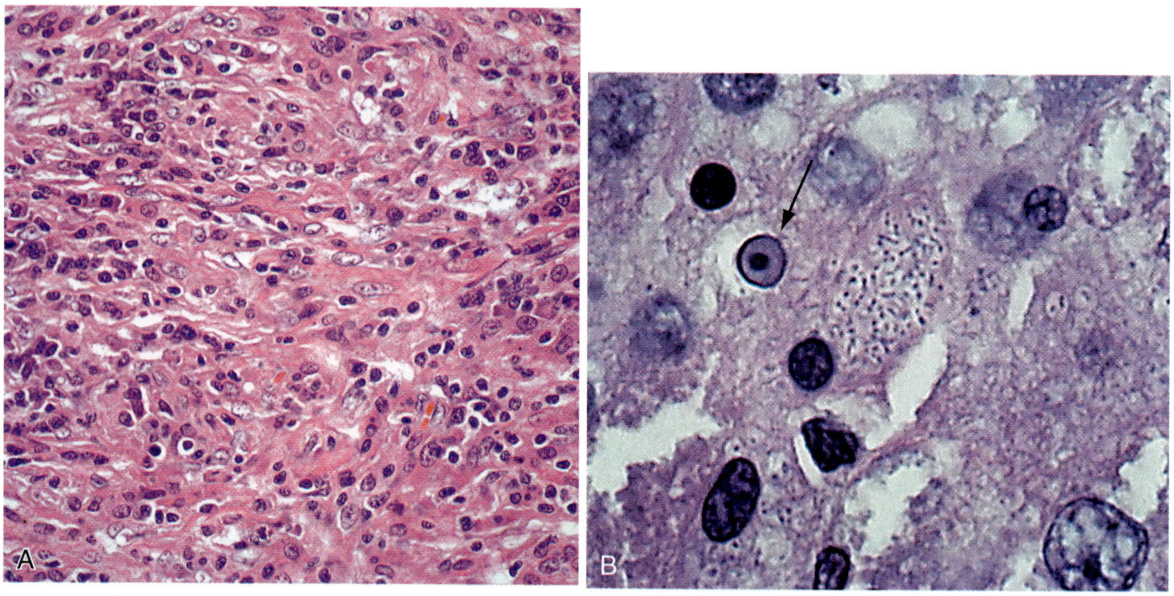

Figure 12-94 Malakoplakia. **A**, At higher magnification, the histocytic and plasma cell infiltrate is seen to be admixed with numerous Michaelis-Gutmann bodies. **B**, High-power view of a Michaelis-Gutmann body *(arrow)*.

with lymphocytes, plasma cells, and numerous Michaelis-Gutmann bodies. This pattern may be easily confused with the low-power appearance of BOOP or with inflammatory pseudotumor of the lung. The use of special histochemical stains for iron or von Kossa stain can be helpful in identification of the Michaelis-Gutmann bodies. Ultrastructural studies of Michaelis-Gutmann bodies may show a fingerprint-like pattern in some cases of malakoplakia.

Treatment and Prognosis

If the lesion is a pulmonary nodule, complete surgical resection is curative. Any specific infection associated with this process will require appropriate treatment. Although this process is benign, the underlying condition is the one that will determine the outcome in patients with pulmonary malakoplakia.

REFERENCES

1. Wada A, Tateishi R, Terazawa T, et al. Lymphangioma of the lung. *Arch Pathol Lab Med.* 1974;98:211.
2. Yousem SA, Hochholzer L. Alveolar adenoma. *Hum Pathol.* 1986;17:1066–1071.
3. Burke LM, Rush WI, Khoor A, et al. Alveolar adenoma: a histochemical, immunohistochemical, and ultrastructural analysis of 17 cases. *Hum Pathol.* 1999;30:158–167.

4. Weinberger MA, Katz S, Davis EW. Peripheral bronchial adenoma of mucous gland type: clinical and pathologic aspects. *J Thorac Surg.* 1955;29:626–635.
5. Ramsey JH, Reimann DL. Bronchial adenomas arising in mucous glands: illustrative case. *Am J Pathol.* 1953;29:339–345.
6. Pritchett PS, Key BM. Mucous gland adenoma of the bronchus: ultrastructural and histochemical studies. *Ala J Med Sci.* 1978;15:44–48.
7. Allen MS, Marsh WL, Geissinger WT. Mucous gland adenoma of the bronchus. *J Thorac Cardiovasc Surg.* 1974;67:966–968.
8. Edwards CW, Matthews HR. Mucous gland adenoma of the bronchus. *Thorax.* 1981;36:147–148.
9. Emory WB, Mitchell WT, Hatch HB. Mucous gland adenoma of the bronchus. *Am Rev Respir Dis.* 1973;108:1407–1410.
10. Gilman RA, Klassen KP, Scarpelli DG. Mucus gland adenoma of bronchus. *Am J Clin Pathol.* 1956;26:131–154.
11. Heard BE, Corrin B, Dewar A. Pathology of seven mucous cell adenomas of the bronchial glands with particular reference to ultrastructure. *Histopathology.* 1985;9:687–701.
12. Kroe DJ, Pitcock JA. Benign mucous gland adenoma of the bronchus. *Arch Pathol.* 1967;84:539–542.
13. England DM, Hochholzer L. Truly benign "bronchial adenoma:" report of 10 cases of mucous gland adenoma with immunohistochemical and ultrastructural findings. *Am J Surg Pathol.* 1995;19:887–899.
14. Attwood HD, Price CG, Riddell RJ. Primary diffuse tracheobronchial amyloidosis. *Thorax.* 1972;27:620–624.
15. Celli BR, Rubinow A, Cohen AS, Brody JS. Patterns of pulmonary involvment in systemic amyloidosis. *Chest.* 1978;74:543–547.
16. Cordier JF, Loire R, Brune J. Amyloidosis of the lower respiratory tract: clinical and pathologic features in a series of 221 patients. *Chest.* 1986;90:827–831.
17. Bonner H, Ennis RS, Geelhoed GW, Tarpley TM. Lymphoid infiltration and amyloidosis of lung in Sjögren's syndrome. *Arch Pathol.* 1973;95:42–44.
18. Kobayashi H, Matsuoka R, Kitamura S, Tsunoda N, Saito K. Sjögren's syndrome with multiple bullae and pulmonary nodular amyloidosis. *Chest.* 1988;94:438–440.
19. Lantuejoul S, Moulai N, Quetant S, et al. Unusual cystic presentation of pulmonary nodular amyloidosis associated with MALT-type lymphoma. *Eur Respir J.* 2007;30:589–592.
20. Laden SA, Cohen ML, Harley RA. Nodular pulmonary amyloidosis with extrapulmonary involvement. *Hum Pathol.* 1984;15:594–597.
21. Chaudhuri MR, Parker DJ. A solitary amyloid nodule in the lung. *Thorax.* 1970;25:382–386.
22. Hui AN, Koss MN, Hochholzer L, Wehunt WD. Amyloidosis presenting in the lower respiratory tract. *Arch Pathol Lab Med.* 1986;110:212–218.
23. Rodriguez FJ, Gamez JD, Vrana JA, et al. Immunoglobulin derived depositions in the nervous system: novel mass spectrometry application for protein characterization in formalin-fixed tissues. *Lab Invest.* 2008;88:1024–1037.
24. Rosen SH, Castleman B, Liebow AA. Pulmonary alveolar proteinosis. *N Engl J Med.* 1958;258:1123–1142.
25. Bedrossian CWM, Luna M, Conklin RH, Miller WC. Alveolar proteinosis as a consequence of immunosuppression. *Hum Pathol.* 1980;11:527–535.
26. McCook TA, Kirks DR, Merten DF, Osborne DR, Spock A, Pratt PC. Pulmonary alveolar proteinosis in children. *AJR Am J Roentgenol.* 1981;137:1023–1027.
27. Prakash UB, Barham SS, Carpenter HA, Dines DE, Marsh HM. Pulmonary alveolar phospholipoproteinosis: experience with 34 cases and a review. *Mayo Clin Proc.* 1987;62:499–518.
28. Kariman K, Kylstra JA, Spock A. Pulmonary alveolar proteinosis: prospective clinical experience with 23 patients for 15 years. *Lung.* 1984;162:223–231.
29. McChesney T. Placental transmogrification of the lung: a unique case with remarkable histopathologic features. *Lab Invest.* 1979;40:245–246.
30. Fidler ME, Koomen M, Sebek B, Greco MA, Rizk CC, Askin FB. Placental transmogrification of the lung, A histologic variant of giant bullous emphysema. *Am J Surg Pathol.* 1995;19:563–570.
31. Mark EJ, Muller KM, McChesney T, Dong-Hwan S, Honig C, Mark MA. Placentoid bullous lesion of the lung. *Hum Pathol.* 1995;26:74–79.
32. Hochholzer L, Moran CA, Koss MN. Pulmonary lipomatosis: a variant of placental transmogrification. *Mod Pathol.* 1997;10:846–849.
33. Moran CA, Hochholzer L, Hasleton PS, Johnson FB, Koss MN. Pulmonary aleolar microlithiasis: a clinicopathological and chemical analysis of seven cases. *Arch Pathol Lab Med.* 1997;121:607–611.
34. Prakash UB, Barham SS, Rosenow 3rd EC, Brown ML, Payne WS. Pulmonary alveolar microlithiasis. A review including ultrastructural and pulmonary function studies. *Mayo Clin Proc.* 1983;58:290–300.
35. Koss MN, Johnson FB, Hochholzer L. Pulmonary blue bodies. *Hum Pathol.* 1981;12:258–266.
36. Kanne JP, Godwin D, Takasugi JE, Schmidt RA, Stern EJ. Diffuse pulmonary ossification. *J Thorac Imaging.* 2004;19:98–102.
37. Bossche LV, Vanderstraeten G. Heterotopic ossification: a review. *J Rehabil Med.* 2005;37:129–136.
38. Nakamura M, Ohishi A, Watanabe R, et al. Adult T-cell leukemia with hypercalcemia-induced metastatic calcification in the lungs due to production of parathyroid hormone–related protein. *Intern Med.* 2001;40:409–413.
39. Liou JH, Cho LC, Hsu YH. Paraneoplastic hypercalcemia with metastatic calcification. *Kaohsiung J Med Sci.* 2006;22:85–88.
40. Valdivielso P, Lopez-Sanchez J, Garrido A, Sanchez-Carrillo JJ. Metastatic calcifications and severe hypercalcemia in a patient with parathyroid carcinoma. *J Endocrinol Invest.* 2006;29:641–644.
41. Alfrey AC. The role of abnormal phosphorus metabolism in the progression of chronic kidney disease and metastatic calcification. *Kidney Int.* 2004;66(Suppl):s13–s17.
42. Lingam RK, The J, Sharma A, Friedman E. Metastatic pulmonary calcification in renal failure: a new HRCT pattern. *Br J Radiol.* 2002;75:74–77.
43. Cherng SC, Cheng CY, Chen CY, Hsu HH, Chu P. Metastatic pulmonary calcification in renal failure mimicking pulmonary embolism on lung scan. *Clin Nucl Med.* 2005;30:322–323.
44. Kobayashi T, Satoh K, Nakano S, Toyama Y, Ohakawa M. A case of metastatic pulmonary calcification after transient acute renal failure. *Radiat Med.* 2005;23:435–438.
45. Ullmer E, Borer H, Sandoz P, Mayr M, Dalquen P, Soler M. Diffuse pulmonary nodular infiltrates in a renal transplant recipient. *Chest.* 2001;120:1394–1398.
46. Eggert C, Albright RC. Metastatic pulmonary calcification in a dialysis patient. *Hemodial Int.* 2006;10:551–555.
47. Guermazi A, Esperou H, Selimi F, Gluckman E. Imaging of diffuse metastatic and dystrophic pulmonary calcification in children after haematopoietic stem cell transplantation. *Br J Radiol.* 2005;78:708–713.
48. Marchiori E, Muller NL, Soares A, Escuissato DL, Gasparetto EL, Cerqueira EM. Unusual manifetations of metastatic pulmonary calcification. *J Thorac Imaging.* 2005;20:66–70.
49. Chan ED, Morales DV, Welsh CH, McDermott MT, Schwarz MI. Calcium deposition with or without bone formation in the lung. *Am J Respir Crit Care Med.* 2002;165:1654–1669.
50. Kelly J, Moss J. Lymphangioleiomyomatosis. *Am J Med Sci.* 2001;321:17–25.
51. Ferrans VJ, Yu ZX, Nelson WK, et al. Lymphangioleiomyomatosis (LAM): a review of clinical and morphological features. *J Nippon Med Sch.* 2000;67:311–329.
52. Hohman DW, Noghrehkar D, Ratnayake S. Lymphangioleiomyomatosis: a review. *Eur J Intern Med.* 2008;19:319–324.

53. Kalassian KG, Doyle R, Kao P, Ruoss S, Raffin TA. Lymphangioleiomyomatosis: new insights. *Am J Respir Crit Care Med.* 1997;155:1183–1186.
54. Schiavina M, Di Scioscio V, Contini P, et al. Pulmonary lymphangioleiomyomatosis in a karyotypically normal man without tuberous sclerosis complex. *Am J Respir Crit Care Med.* 2007;176:96–98.
55. Basset F, Soler P, Marsac J, Corrin B. Pulmonary lymphangiomyomatosis: three new cases studied with electron microscopy. *Cancer.* 1976;38:2357–2366.
56. Stovin PG, Lum LC, Flower CD, Darke CS, Beeley M. The lungs in lymphangioleiomyomatosis and in tuberous sclerosis. *Thorax.* 1975;30:497–509.
57. Urban T, Lazor R, Lacronique J, et al. Pulmonary lymphangioleiomyomatosis. A study of 69 patients. Groupe d'Etudes et de Recherche sur les Maladies "Orphelines" Pulmonaires (GERM"O"P). *Medicine (Baltimore).* 1999;78:321–337.
58. Capron F, Ameille J, Leclerc P, et al. Pulmonary lymphangioleiomyomatosis and Bourneville's tuberous sclerosis with pulmonary involvement: the same disease? *Cancer.* 1983;52:851–855.
59. McCormack F, Brody A, Meyer C, et al. Pulmonary cysts consistent with lymphangioleiomyomatosis are common in women with tuberous sclerosis. *Chest.* 2002;121(3 Suppl):61S.
60. Wenaden AE, Copley SJ. Unilateral lymphangioleiomyomatosis. *J Thorac Imaging.* 2005;20:226–228.
61. Oh YM, Mo EK, Jang SH, et al. Pulmonary lymphangioleiomyomatosis in Korea. *Thorax.* 1999;54:618–621.
62. Delgrange E, Delgrange B, Wallon J, Rosoux P. Diagnostic approach to pulmonary lymphangioleiomyomatosis. *J Intern Med.* 1994;236:461–464.
63. Bonetti F, Chiodera PL, Pea M, et al. Transbronchial biopsy in lymphangiomyomatosis of the lung. HMB45 for diagnosis. *Am J Surg Pathol.* 1993;17:1092–1102.
64. Guinee DG, Feuerstein I, Koss MN, Travis WD. Pulmonary lymphangioleiomyomatosis. Diagnosis based on results of transbronchial biopsy and immunohistochemical studies and correlation with high-resolution computed tomography findings. *Arch Pathol Lab Med.* 1994;118:846–849.
65. Matsui K, Riemenschneider W, Hilbert SL, et al. Hyperplasia of type II pneumocytes in pulmonary lymphangioleiomyomatosis. *Arch Pathol Lab Med.* 2000;124:1642–1648.
66. Maruyama H, Seyama K, Sobajima J, et al. Multifocal micronodular pneumocyte hyperplasia and lymphangioleiomyomatosis in tuberous sclerosis with *TSC2* gene. *Mod Pathol.* 2001;14:609–614.
67. Kitaichi M, Nishimura K, Itoh H, Izumi T. Pulmonary lymphangioleiomyomatosis: a report of 46 patients including a clinicopathologic study of prognostic factors. *Am J Respir Crit Care Med.* 1995;151:527–533.
68. Tanaka H, Imada A, Morikawa T, et al. Diagnosis of pulmonary lymphangioleiomyomatosis by HMB45 in surgically treated spontaneous pneumothorax. *Eur Repir J.* 1995;8:1879–1882.
69. Bittmann I, Dose TB, Müller C, Dienemann H, Vogelmeier C, Löhrs U. Lymphangioleiomyomatosis: recurrence after single lung transplantation. *Hum Pathol.* 1997;28:1420–1423.
70. Dishner W, Cordasco EM, Blackburn J, Demeter S, Levin H, Carey WD. Pulmonary lymphangiomyomatosis. *Chest.* 1984;85:796–799.
71. El-Allaf D, Borlee G, Hadjoudj H, Henrard L, Marcelle R, van Cauwenberge H. Pulmonary lymphangiomyomatosis. *Eur J Respir Dis.* 1984;65:147–152.
72. Beasly MB, Matsui K, Yu ZX, et al. Histologic predictors of survival in 101 cases of pulmonary lymphangioleiomyomatosis (LAM): prognostic significance of histology score [abstract]. *Am J Respir Crit Care Med.* 2000;161:A15.
73. Dashiell GF. A case of dirofilariasis involving the lung. *Am J Trop Med Hyg.* 1961;10:37–38.
74. Goodman ML, Gore I. Pulmonary infarct secondary to *Dirofilaria* larva. *Arch Intern Med.* 1964;113:702–705.
75. Asimacopoulos PJ, Katras A, Christie B. Pulmonary dirofilariasis. The largest single-hospital experience. *Chest.* 1992;102:851–855.
76. Milanez de Campos JR, Barbas CS, Filomeno LT, et al. Human pulmonary dirofilariasis: analysis of 24 cases from São Paulo, Brazil. *Chest.* 1997;112:729–733.
77. Ro JY, Tsakalakis PJ, White VA, et al. Pulmnary dirofilariasis: the great imitator of primary or metastatic lung tumor. A clinicopathologic analysis of seven cases and a review of the literature. *Hum Pathol.* 1989;20:69–76.
78. Kahn FW, Wester SM, Agger WA. Pulmonary dirofilariasis and transitional cell carcinoma: benign lung nodules mimicking metastatic malignant neoplasms. *Arch Intern Med.* 1983;143:1259–1260.
79. Neafie RC, Piggott J. Human pulmonary dirofilariasis. *Arch Pathol.* 1971;92:342–349.
80. Ulbright TM, Katzenstein ALA. Solitary necrotizing granulomas of the lung. Differentiating features and etiology. *Am J Surg Pathol.* 1980;4:13–28.
81. Flieder DB, Moran CA. Pulmonary dirofilariasis: a clinicopathologic study of 41 lesions in 39 patients. *Hum Pathol.* 1999;30:251–256.
82. Brown LK, Miller A, Bhuptani A, et al. Pulmonary involvement in Fabry disease. *Am J Respir Crit Care Med.* 1997;155:1004–1010.
83. Matsumoto T, Matsumori H, Taki T, Takagi T, Fukuda Y. Infantile GM1-gangliosidosis with marked manifestation of lungs. *Acta Pathol Jpn.* 1979;29:269–276.
84. Amir G, Ron N. Pulmonary pathology in Gaucher's disease. *Hum Pathol.* 1999;30:666–670.
85. Miller A, Brown LK, Pastores GM, Desnick RJ. Pulmonary involvement in type 1 Gaucher disease: functional and exercise findings in patients with and without clinical interstitial lung disease. *Clin Genet.* 2003;63:368–376.
86. Minai OA, Sullivan EJ, Stoller JK. Pulmonary involvement in Niemann-Pick disease: case report and literature review. *Respir Med.* 2000;94:1241–1251.
87. Nicholson AG, Florio R, Hansell DM, et al. Pulmonary involvement by Niemann-Pick disease. A report of six cases. *Histopathology.* 2006;48:596–603.
88. Muir-Padilla J, Myers JB. Whipple disease: a case report and review of the literature. *Arch Pathol Lab Med.* 2005;129:933–936.
89. Kelly CA, Egan M, Rawinson J. Whipple's disease presenting with lung involvement. *Thorax.* 1996;51:343–344.
90. Soler P, Kambouchner M, Valeyre D, Hance AJ. Pulmonary Langerhans' cell granulomatosis. *Annu Rev Med.* 1992;43:105–115.
91. Marcy TW, Reynolds HY. Pulmonary histiocytosis X. *Lung.* 1985;163:129–150.
92. Vassallo R, Ryu JH, Colby TV, Hartman T, Limper AH. Pulmonary Langerhans' cell histiocytosis. *N Engl J Med.* 2000;342:1969–1978.
93. Colby TV, Lombard C. Histiocytosis X in the lung. *Hum Pathol.* 1983;14:847–856.
94. Allen TC. Pulmonary Langerhans cell histiocytosis and other pulmonary histiocytic diseases. *Arch Pathol Lab Med.* 2008;132:1171–1181.
95. Lombard CM, Medeiros J, Colby TV. Pulmonary histocytosis X and carcinoma. *Arch Pathol Lab Med.* 1987;111:339–341.
96. Neumann MP, Frizzera G. The coexistence of Langerhans' cell granulomatosis and malignant lymphoma may take different forms: report of seven cases with a review of the literature. *Hum Pathol.* 1986;17:1060–1065.
97. Sajjad SM, Luna MA. Primary pulmonary histiocytosis X in two patients with Hodgkin's disease. *Thorax.* 1982;37:110–113.
98. O'Donnell AE, Tsou E, Awh C, Fallat ME, Patterson K. Endobronchial eosinophilic granuloma: a rare cause of total lung atelectasis. *Am Rev Respir Dis.* 1987;136:1478–1480.
99. Meier B, Rhyner K, Medici TC, Kistler G. Eosinophilic granuloma of the skeleton with involvement of the lung: a report of three cases. *Eur J Respir Dis.* 1983;64:551–556.

100. Yousem SA, Colby TV, Chen YY, Chen WG, Weiss LM. Pulmonary Langerhans' cell histiocytosis: molecular analysis of clonality. *Am J Surg Pathol.* 2001;25:630–636.
101. Yu RC, Chu C, Buluwela L, Chu AC. Clonal proliferation of Langerhans cells in Langerhans cell histiocytosis. *Lancet.* 1994;343:767–768.
102. Willman CL. Detection of clonal histiocytosis in Langerhans cell histiocytosis: biology and clinical significance. *Br J Cancer.* 1994;70:S29–S33.
103. Willman CL, Busque L, Griffith BB, et al. Langerhans' cell histiocytosis (histiocytosis X)—a clonal proliferative disease. *N Engl J Med.* 1994;331:154–160.
104. Travis WD, Borok Z, Roum JH, et al. Pulmonary Langerhans cell granulomatosis (histiocytosis X): a clinicopathologic study of 48 cases. *Am J Surg Pathol.* 1993;17:971–986.
105. Vassallo R, Ryu JH, Schroeder DR, Decker PA, Limper AH. Clinical outcomes of pulmonary Langerhans'-cell histocytosis in adults. *N Engl J Med.* 2002;346:484–490.
106. McDowell HP, Macfarlane PI, Martin J. Isolated pulmonary histiocytosis. *Arch Dis Child.* 1988;63:423–426.
107. Pomeranz SJ, Proto AV. Histiocytosis X: unusual confusing features of eosinophilic granuloma. *Chest.* 1986;89:88–92.
108. Friedman PJ, Liebow AA, Sokoloff J. Eosinophilic granuloma of lung: clinical aspects of primary pulonary histiocytosis in the adult. *Medicine (Baltimore).* 1981;60:385–396.
109. Gaenler EA, Carrington CB. Open biopsy for chronic diffuse infiltrative lung disease: clinical, roentgenographic, and physiologic correlations in 502 patients. *Ann Thorac Surg.* 1980;30:411–426.
110. Chester WD. Uber Lipoidgranulomatose. *Virchows Arch Pathol Anat.* 1930;279:561–602.
111. Jaffe HL. Lipid (cholesterol) granulomatosis. In: Jaffe HL, ed. *Metabolic, Degenerative, and Inflammatory Disease of Bone.* Philadelphia: Lea & Febiger; 1972:535–541.
112. Veyssier-Belot C, Cacoub P, Caparros-Lefebvre D, et al. Erdheim-Chester disease. Clinical and radiological characteristics of 59 cases. *Medicine (Baltimore).* 1996;75:157–169.
113. Shamburek RD, Brewer B, Gochuico BR. Erdheim-Chester disease: a rare multisystem histiocytic disorder associated with interstitial lung disease. *Am J Med Sci.* 2001;321:66–75.
114. Egan AJ, Boardman LA, Tazelaar HD, et al. Erdheim-Chester disease: clinical, radiological, and histopathological findings in five patients with interstitial lung disease. *Am J Surg Pathol.* 1999;23:17–26.
115. Rush WL, Andriko JA, Galateau-Salle F, et al. Pulmonary pathology of Erdheim-Chester disease. *Mod Pathol.* 2000;13:747–754.
116. Foucar E, Rosai J, Dorfman R. Sinus histocytosis with massive lymphadenopathy (Rosai-Dorfman disease): review of the entity. *Semin Diagn Pathol.* 1990;7:19–73.
117. Wright DH, Richards DB. Sinus histiocytosis with massive lymphadenopathy (Rosai-Dorfman disease): report of a case with widespread nodal and extranodal dissemination. *Histopathology.* 1981;5:697–709.
118. Huang Q, Change KL, Weiss LM. Extranodal Rosai-Dorfman disease involving the bone marrow: a case report. *Am J Surg Pathol.* 2006;30:1189–1192.
119. Ben Ghorbel I, Naffati H, Khanfir M, et al. Disseminated form of Rosai-Dorfman disease: a case report. *Rev Med Interne.* 2005;26:415–419.
120. Ohori P, Yu J, Landreneau RJ, Thaete FL, Kane K. Rosai-Dorfman disease of the pleura: a rare extranodal presentation. *Hum Pathol.* 2003;34:1210–1211.
121. Paulli M, Bergamaschi G, Tonon L, et al. Evidence of polyclonal nature of the cell infiltrate in sinus histiocytosis with massive lymphadenopathy (Rosai-Dorfman disease). *Br J Haematol.* 1995;91:415–418.
122. Bonetti F, Chilosi M, Menestrina F, et al. Immunohistological analysis of Rosai-Dorfman histiocytosis. A disease of S-100+CD1a–histiocytes. *Virchows Arch A Pathol Anat Histopathol.* 1987;411:129–135.
123. Bakir B, Unuvar E, Terzibasioglu E, Guven K. Atypical lung involvement in a patient with systemic juvenile xanthogranuloma. *Pediatr Radiol.* 2007;37:325–327.
124. Matcham NJ, Andronikou S, Sibson K, Ramani P, Grier D. Systemic juvenile xanthogranulomatosis imitating a malignant abdominal wall tumor with lung metastases. *J Pediatr Hematol Oncol.* 2007;29:72–73.
125. Kraus MD, Haley JC, Ruiz R, Essary L, Moran CA, Fletcher CD. Juvenile xanthogranuloma: an immunophenotypic study with a reappraisal of histogenesis. *Am J Dermatopathol.* 2001;23:104–111.
126. Guthrie JA, Arthur RJ. Juvenile xanthogranuloma with pulmonary, subcutaneous, and hepatic involvement. *Clin Radiol.* 1994;49:498–500.
127. Lottsfeldt FI, Good RA. Juvenile xanthogranuloma with pulmonary lesions. A case report. *Pediatrics.* 1964;33:233–238.
128. Kourilsky S, Piéron R, Renault P, Parrot R, Demay C. Isolated round intrapulmonary mass in a young person: xanthogranuloma. *J Fr Med Chir Thorac.* 1965;19:307–319.
129. Diard F, Cadier L, Billaud C, Trojani M. Neonatal juvenile xanthogranulomatosis with pulmonary, extrapleural and hepatic involvement. One case report. *Ann Radiol (Paris).* 1982;25:113–118.
130. Ionescu DN, Pierson DM, Qing G, Li M, Colby TV, Leslie KO. Pulmonary crystal-storing histiocytoma. *Arch Pathol Lab Med.* 2005;129:1159–1163.
131. Jones D, Renshaw AA. Recurrent crystal-storing histiocytosis of the lung in a patient without a clonal lymphoproliferative disorder. *Arch Pathol Lab Med.* 1996;120:978–980.
132. Pais AV, Pereira S, Garg I, Stephen J, Antony M, Inchara YK. Intra-abdominal, crystal-storing histiocytosis due to clofazimine in a patient with lepromatous leprosy and concurrent carcinoma of the colon. *Lepr Rev.* 2004;75:171–176.
133. Lewis JT, Candelora JN, Hogan RB, Briggs FR, Abraham SC. Crystal-storing histiocytosis due to massive accumulation of Charcot-Leyden crystals: a unique association producing colonic polyposis in a 78-year-old woman with eosinophilic colitis. *Am J Surg Pathol.* 2007;31:481–485.
134. Pitman SD, Wang J, Serros E, Zuppan C. A 70-year-old woman with acute renal failure. *Arch Pathol Lab Med.* 2006;130:1077–1078.
135. Joo M, Kwak JE, Chang SH, et al. Localized gastric crystal-storing histiocytosis. *Histopathology.* 2007;51:116–119.
136. Keane C, Gill D. Multi-organ involvement with crystal-storing histiocytosis. *Br J Haematol.* 2008;141:750.
137. Prassad ML, Charney DA, Sarlin J, Keller SM. Pulmonary immunocytoma with massive crystal storing histiocytosis: a case report with review of literature. *Am J Surg Pathol.* 1998;22:1148–1153.
138. Kusakabe T, Watanabe K, Mori T, Iida T, Suzuki T. Crystal-storing histiocytosis associated with MALT lymphoma of the adnexa: a case report with review of literature. *Virchows Arch.* 2007;450:103–108.
139. Pock L, Stuchlik D, Hercogova J. Crystal storing histiocytosis of the skin associated with multiple myeloma. *Int J Dermatol.* 2006;45:1408–1411.
140. Chantranuwat C. Noncrystallized form of immunoglobulin-storing histiocytosis as a cause of chronic lung infiltration in multiple myeloma. *Ann Diagn Pathol.* 2007;11:220–222.
141. Fairweather PM, Williamson R, Tsikleas G. Pulmonary extranodal marginal zone lymphoma with massive crystal storing histiocytosis. *Am J Surg Pathol.* 2006;30:262–267.
142. Papla B, Spolnik P, Rzenno E, et al. Generalized crystal-storing histiocytosis as a presentation of multiple myeloma: a case with a possible pro-aggregation defect in the immunoglobulin heavy chain. *Virchows Arch.* 2004;445:83–89.
143. Sun Y, Tawfiqul B, Valderrama E, Kline G, Kahn LB. Pulmonary crystal-storing histiocytosis and extranodal marginal zone B-cell lymphoma associated with a fibroleiomyomatous hamartoma. *Ann Diagn Pathol.* 2003;7:47–53.

144. Zioni F, Giovanardi P, Bozzoli M, Artusi T, Bonacorsi G, Sighinolfi P. Massive bone marrow crystal-storing histiocytosis in a patient with IgA-lambda multiple myeloma and extensive extramedulary disease: a case report. *Tumori.* 2004;90:348–351.
145. Galed-Placed I. Immunoglobulin crystal-storing histiocytosis in a pleural effusion from a woman with IgA κ multiple myeloma. *Acta Cytol.* 2006;50:539–541.
146. Stokes MB, Aronoff B, Siegel D, D'Agati VD. Dysproteinemia-related nephropathy associated with crystal-storing histiocytosis. *Kidney Int.* 2006;70:597–602.
147. Andrianopoulos E, Lautides G, Kormas P, Mugolias J, Mavrogeorgis A. Pulmonary xanthoma. A case report with immunohistologic study and DNA-image analysis. *Eur J Cardiothorac Surg.* 1995;9:534–536.
148. Guerrero MF, Ramos JM, Renedo G, Gadea I, Alix A. Pulmonary malacoplakia associated with *Rhodococcus equi* infection in patients with AIDS: case reports and review. *Clin Infect Dis.* 1999;28:1334–1336.
149. Hodder RV, St George-Hyslop P, Chalvardjian A, Bear RA, Thomas P. Pulmonary malakoplakia. *Thorax.* 1984;39:70–71.
150. Bastas A, Markou N, Botsi C, et al. Malakoplakia of the lung caused by *Pasteurella multocida* in a patient with AIDS. *Scand J Infect Dis.* 2002;34:53–538.
151. Shin MS, Allen Jr JA, Ho KJ. Pulmonary malacoplakia associated with *Rhodococcus equi* infection in a patient with AIDS. *Chest.* 1999;115:889–892.
152. Colby TV, Hunt S, Pelzmann K, Carrington DB. Malakoplakia of the lung: a report of two cases. *Respiration.* 1980;39:295–299.

13

Tumors of the Pleura

The pleura can be seeded by a wide spectrum of primary and metastatic tumoral conditions. Primary neoplasms affecting the pleura include epithelial, mesenchymal, and lymphoid neoplasms; of these categories, epithelial malignancies are the most common. The focus of this chapter is on primary lesions of the pleura.

EPITHELIAL TUMORS

Primary epithelial or epithelioid tumors of the pleura comprise various clinical entities, of which mesotheliomas are the most common, although a number of other conditions should be considered in the assessment of pleural biopsy material or resected specimens. These tumors, which may range in degree of malignant potential from benign to low-grade to high-grade malignant neoplasms, include the following:

- Malignant mesothelioma
- Pseudomesotheliomatous adenocarcinoma
- Thymoma
- Adenomatoid tumor
- Mucoepidermoid carcinoma
- Endometriosis

MALIGNANT MESOTHELIOMA

The most common primary malignant tumor of the pleura is malignant mesothelioma, a condition that nevertheless can be difficult to diagnose. Owing to the legal implications of asbestos exposure and its link with pathogenesis of these lesions and because of their variable histopathologic appearance, they have been the subject of extensive studies. Malignant mesotheliomas are relatively unusual tumors, and the annual incidence in the United States has been estimated to be approximately 3 to 7 cases per 1 million persons, but this rate may be rising.[1,2] Although mesotheliomas have been associated with exposure to asbestos fibers, approximately 50% of persons affected by mesotheliomas do not report asbestos exposure, indicating that the etiology may be multifactorial.[1–5]

A careful analysis of radiologic findings along with histopathologic evaluation of appropriate material should provide clinicians and pathologists with the necessary information to make a specific diagnosis. In many instances the clinical and radiologic aspects are clear-cut but the available material for histopathologic examination is not adequate. In such circumstances, any attempt to make a definitive diagnosis should be deferred until additional material is obtained if clinically indicated. Surgical treatment for mesothelioma can be extreme; thus, an unequivocal diagnosis is imperative. Furthermore, other pleural conditions of an inflammatory nature may mimic malignant mesothelioma. Therefore, the clinical and radiologic information should be used not to make a diagnosis per se but rather to guide decisions about a diagnostic approach using immunohistochemical or electron microscopic techniques. Ultimately, the diagnosis of mesothelioma is a histopathologic one.

Historical Aspects

Wagner may have been the first to describe this tumor in the pleura, in 1870[6]; in subsequent years, however, great controversy emerged regarding the characterization of tumors with diffuse pleural involvement. Many of these tumors were assigned different designations, including endothelial carcinoma, sarcoma, lymphangitis proliferans, sarcocarcinoma, and endothelioma.[7,8] It was not until 1920 that Dubray and Rosson proposed the designation *mesothelioma*,[9] a term in common use today. Although early reports had questioned the existence of primary pleural tumors, in time, well-documented cases were reported.[8,10] In 1931, Klemperer and Rabin[8] classified pleural tumors by their macroscopic appearance into localized and diffuse conditions. This distinction gave rise to the current terms *diffuse pleural mesothelioma* and *solitary fibrous tumor of the pleura*.

In 1960, Wagner and associates[11] described 33 patients with mesothelioma and suggested the association with asbestos fibers. According to these investigators, all of the patients except one had a history of probable exposure to asbestos. Hirsch and colleagues[12] described 28 cases, in which asbestos exposure was established in 17 cases. Some investigators presented larger series of cases with more emphasis on the association of mesothelioma and asbestos exposure,[4,5] whereas others explored the histopathologic variability of mesotheliomas.[13] In the past, the diagnosis was established using conventional histologic examination and histochemical stains, such as periodic acid–Schiff reagent (PAS) with and without diastase and mucicarmine, but today the emphasis has shifted to newer modalities such as electron microscopic and immunohistochemical techniques. Nevertheless, the numerous clinicopathologic correlations have contributed greatly to the current understanding of mesotheliomas.[14–22]

Clinical Features

Clinical and radiologic findings are of great importance in establishing the diagnosis. Thus, every effort should be made to correlate histologic features with clinical and radiological information. In general, mesotheliomas are more common in adults older than 50 years of age, but these tumors also may occur in children.[23,24] History of long-standing exposure to asbestos, whether confirmed or not, should prompt a careful analysis of the biopsy tissue. Mesotheliomas can occur without a history of asbestos exposure, as evidenced by cases described in children and housewives. Other possible etiopathologic factors in the development of mesothelioma include radiation exposure, chronic inflammation, viral infections, and diethylstilbestrol.[25]

If mesothelioma is suspected, a thorough search for evidence of the following diagnostic criteria is warranted:

- Diffuse involvement of the pleura
- Intraparenchymal tumor nodules or masses (peripheral)
- Diffuse thickening of the pleura
- Encasement of the lung
- Unilateral or bilateral pleural involvement
- Pleura-based tumor mass

Patients with mesothelioma may present with nonspecific signs and symptoms such as chest pain, dyspnea, cough, weight loss, and pleural effusions.

Macroscopic Findings

Mesotheliomas are tumors with a characteristic gross appearance, rarely posing a diagnostic problem on gross examination. The tumor will display diffuse pleural involvement with thickening of the pleural lining encasing the entire lung (Fig. 13-1). In some cases, tumor growth follows the intrapulmonary septum, and in rare instances the tumor may involve the lung parenchyma,

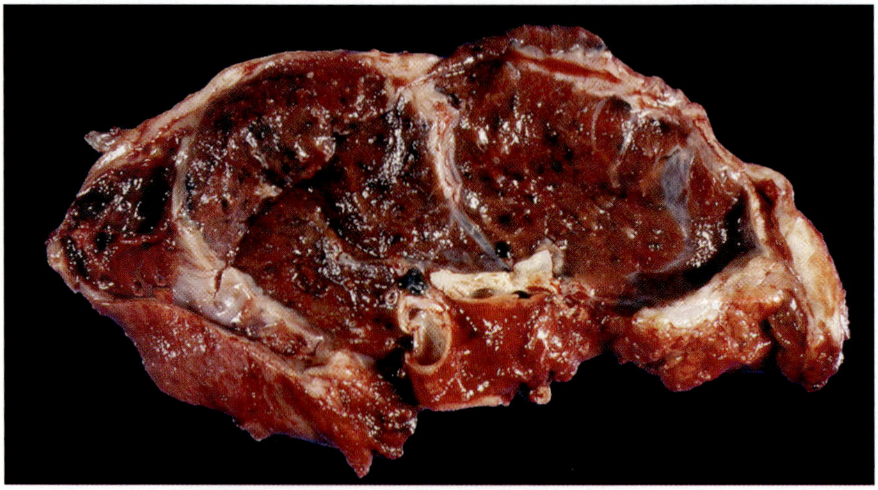

Figure 13-1 Extrapulmonary pneumonectomy specimen exhibiting diffuse thickening of the pleura.

forming small nodules on the surface. The presence of a well-defined tumor mass in the periphery of the lung, even if diffuse pleural involvement also is evident, should alert the pathologist to the possibility of an adenocarcinoma with diffuse involvement of the pleura.

Histopathologic Features

Mesotheliomas may show a variety of histopathologic growth patterns, but the three most common are epithelioid, sarcomatoid, and biphasic (a combination of the epithelioid and sarcomatoid types).

Epithelioid Mesothelioma

Epithelioid mesothelioma probably is the most common of the three variants, accounting for approximately 70% of all mesotheliomas. Several distinct histopathologic growth patterns of epithelioid malignant mesothelioma have been described, and occasionally, distinguishing among them may pose a diagnostic challenge.[26–29] These subvariants include the following:

Tubulopapillary. This is the most common growth pattern in epithelioid mesotheliomas. The tumor may show the characteristic papillary growth pattern consisting of medium-sized round to oval cells, with moderate amounts of eosinophilic cytoplasm, round nuclei, and conspicuous nucleoli. In other areas, this cellular proliferation may show elongated tubular structures that appear to anastomose with one another. The tumor is fairly uniform in appearance, with very mild nuclear atypia and minimal mitotic activity. Areas of necrosis and hemorrhage are not commonly seen (Figs. 13-2 to 13-13).

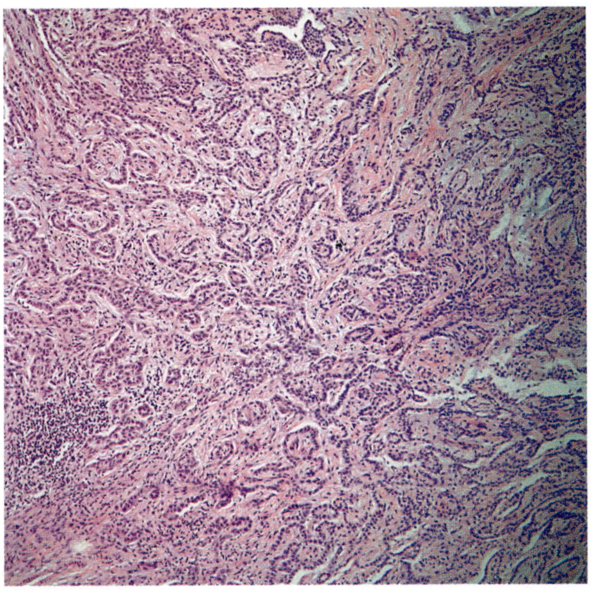

Figure 13-2 Malignant mesothelioma with a tubulopapillary growth pattern.

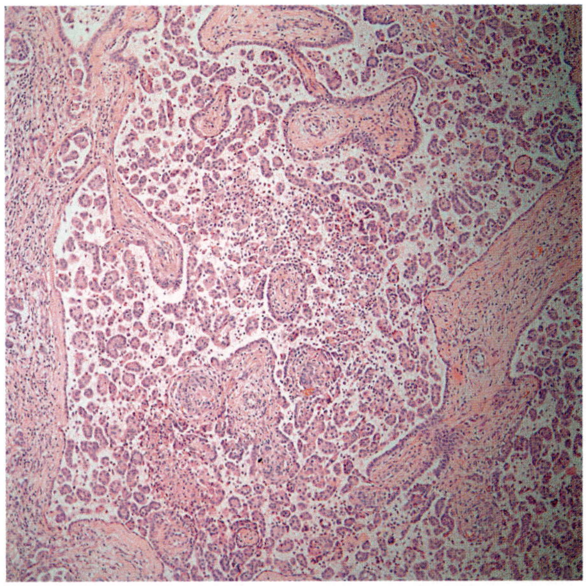

Figure 13-3 Mesothelioma with a prominent papillary growth pattern.

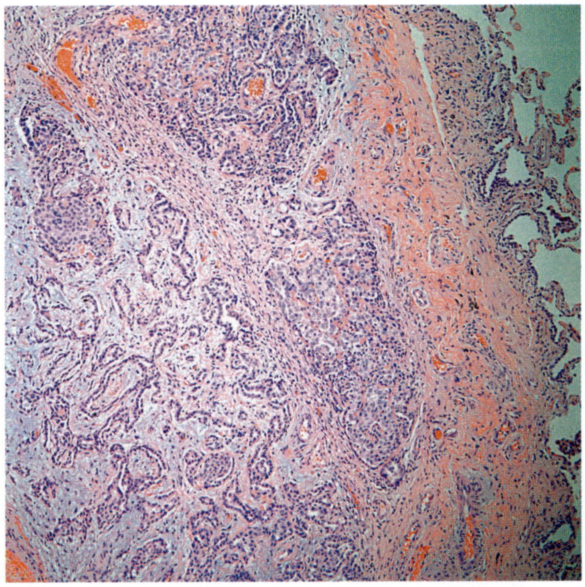

Figure 13-4 Mesothelioma with thickening of the pleura and a desmoplastic reaction.

Clear cell. This growth pattern is characterized by a cellular proliferation composed of medium-sized, round to oval cells with round nuclei and conspicuous nucleoli, and clear cytoplasm. A diffuse cellular proliferation dissecting fibroconnective tissue is visible. Mitotic activity, although present, is not prominent, and focal areas of necrosis may be seen. This growth pattern mimics clear cell carcinoma of renal origin (Figs. 13-14 to 13-17).

Glandular. This growth pattern is characterized by the presence of well-formed glands similar to those seen in adenocarcinoma. The glandular proliferation appears to dissect fibroconnective tissue, and in some cases, a desmoplastic reaction with inflammatory infiltrate may be present. This growth pattern closely resembles that in adenocarcinoma (Figs. 13-18 and 13-19).

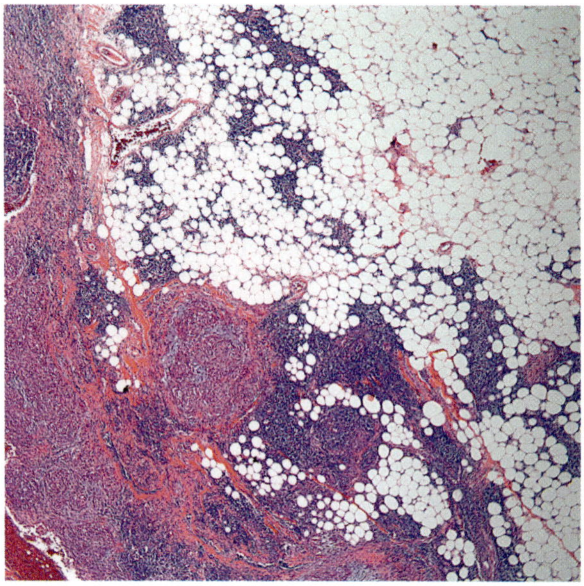

Figure 13-5 Mesothelioma with infiltration into adjacent adipose tissue. Note the presence of a lymphoid reaction.

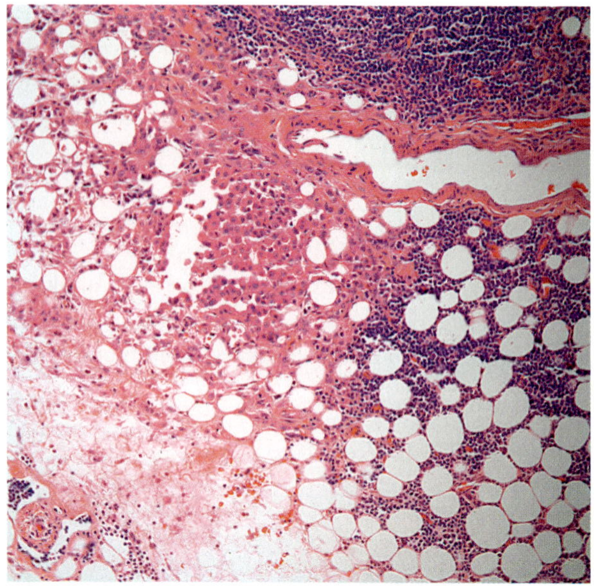

Figure 13-6 Higher-power view of the adipose infiltration by mesothelioma.

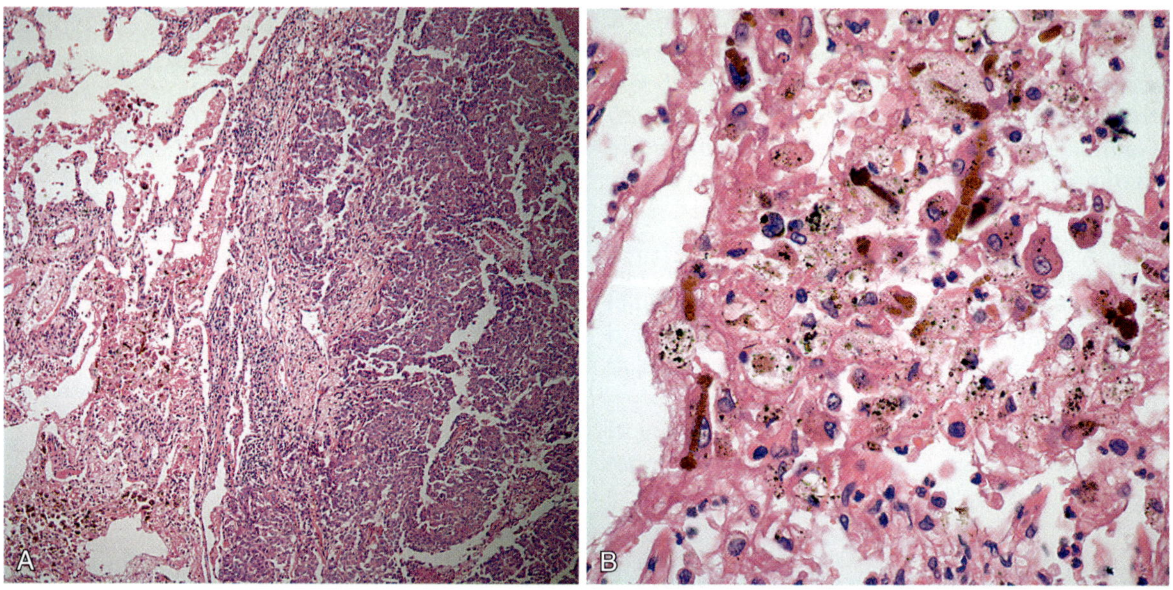

Figure 13-7 **A**, Mesothelioma with infiltration into the lung parenchyma. Note adjacent ferruginous bodies. **B**, High-power view of ferruginous bodies in the lung parenchyma.

Myxoid/mucoid. This growth pattern consists of a neoplastic cellular proliferation embedded in a myxoid or mucoid matrix, which may show glandular differentiation or the conventional tubulopapillary growth pattern. In some cases, the tumor may display abundant mucoid matrix; this appearance may be confused with that of a mucinous adenocarcinoma. With this pattern, mucicarmine staining does not show intracellular mucin production (Figs. 13-20 to 13-22).

Adenomatoid. This growth pattern closely resembles that of the conventional adenomatoid tumor and is characterized by cords of medium-sized cells with clear cytoplasm and displacement of the nuclei toward the periphery of the cells. Nuclear atypia, mitotic activity, necrosis, and hemorrhage are not common (Figs. 13-23 to 13-25).

Deciduoid. This growth pattern is characterized by a cellular proliferation composed of medium-sized cells with eosinophilic cytoplasm, displaying a "deciduoid" appearance similar to that seen in endometrial cyclic changes (Figs. 13-26 and 13-27).

Cartilaginous and osseous metaplasia. This unusual variant of mesothelioma may pose a diagnostic challenge. The tumor shows areas of formation of "osteoid" or immature cartilage that may be confused with a primary orthopedic tumor. Along with the osseous or

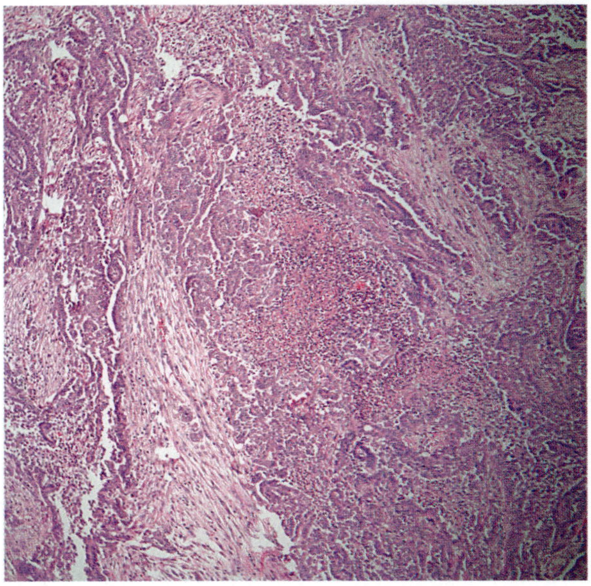

Figure 13-8 Mesothelioma with a tubulopapillary growth pattern and focal areas of necrosis.

cartilaginous changes, a cellular proliferation composed of medium-sized cells with round to oval nuclei and conspicuous nucleoli is characteristic. In some areas the cellular proliferation may exhibit spindle cell features or a mixture of spindle and epithelioid cells (Figs. 13-28 and 13-29).

Among these histopathologic growth patterns, the easiest to recognize, tubulopapillary, is the most common. Nevertheless, at least a theoretical familiarity with the other growth patterns is essential to permit a proper differential diagnosis. Regardless of the histopathologic growth pattern, whether the tumor shows clear cell change, myxoid areas, glandular differentiation, or an adenomatoid pattern, an important radiologic feature that cannot be overlooked is diffuse involvement of the pleura by tumor. This finding should always prompt consideration of the possibility of mesothelioma. In the great majority of cases, only a small biopsy specimen is available for diagnostic analysis.

Recently, Arrossi and coworkers[30] evaluated 56 cases of extrapleural pneumonectomy to correlate the original subtype of mesothelioma in the biopsy specimen with that determined using the resected specimen. These workers found that in many cases, mesotheliomas must be reclassified after more complete sectioning is accomplished.

Histochemical Features

Before the advent of immunohistochemistry, histochemical studies played an important role in the diagnosis of mesothelioma. Currently, they can offer an easy solution in more routine cases. PAS, with and without diastase digestion and mucicarmine, and hyaluronic acid, with and without diastase digestion, have been used in the past

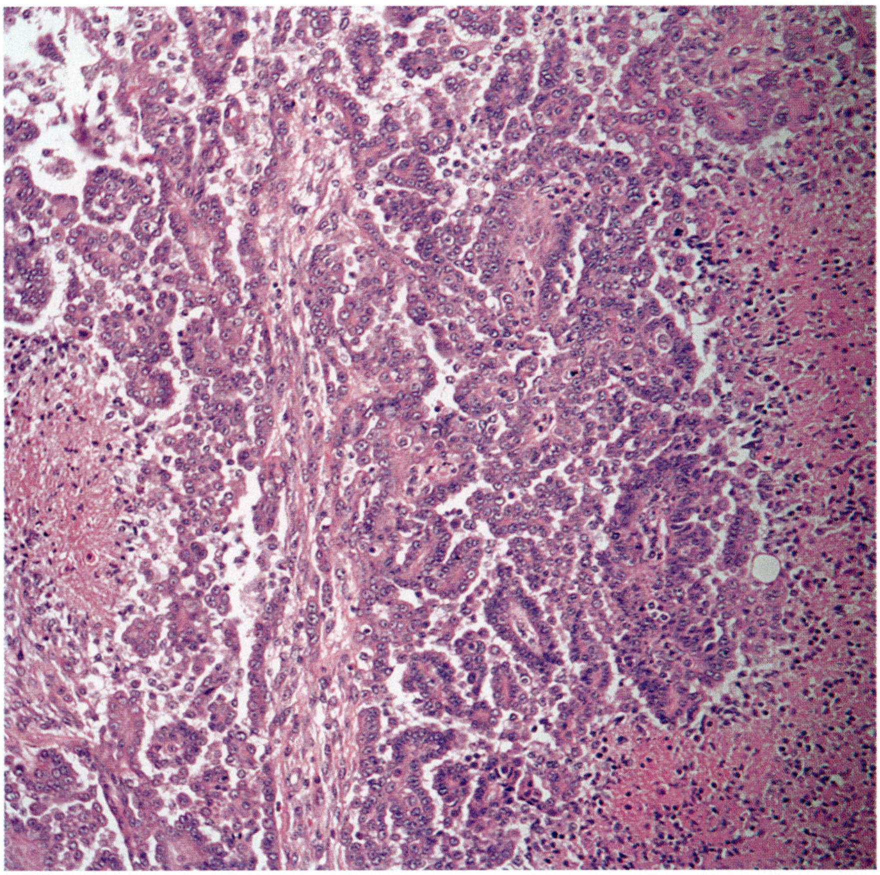

Figure 13-9 Higher-power view of a mesothelioma with a papillary growth pattern, with adjacent areas of necrosis.

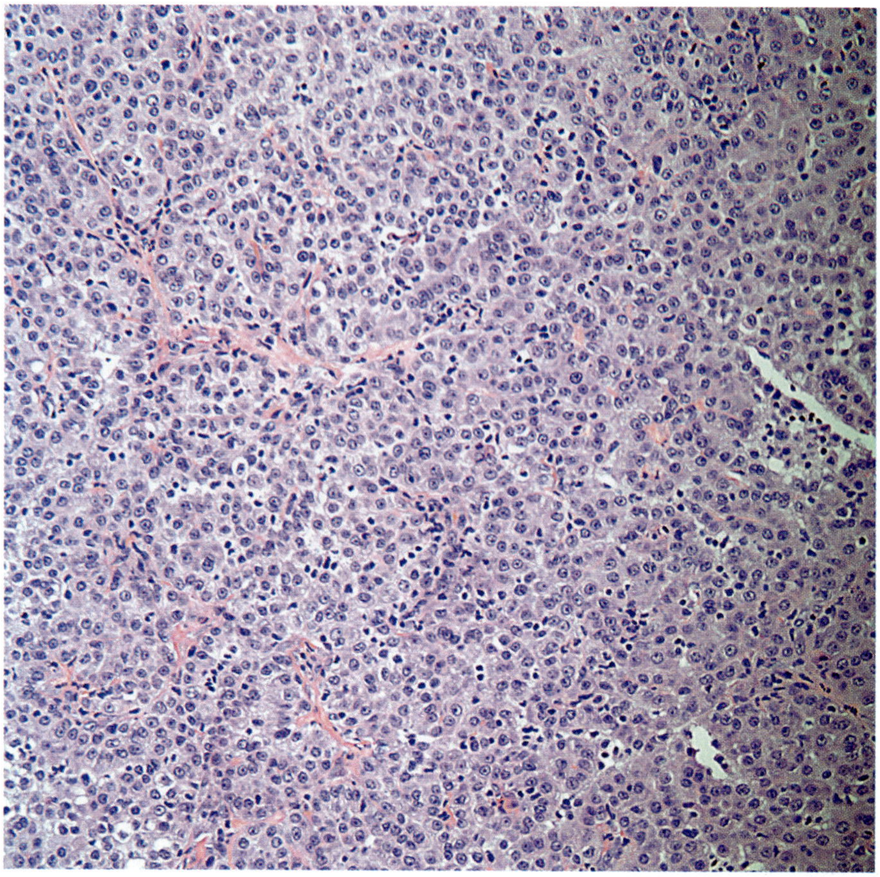

Figure 13-10 Solid component of an epithelioid mesothelioma composed of sheets of a homogeneous neoplastic cellular proliferation.

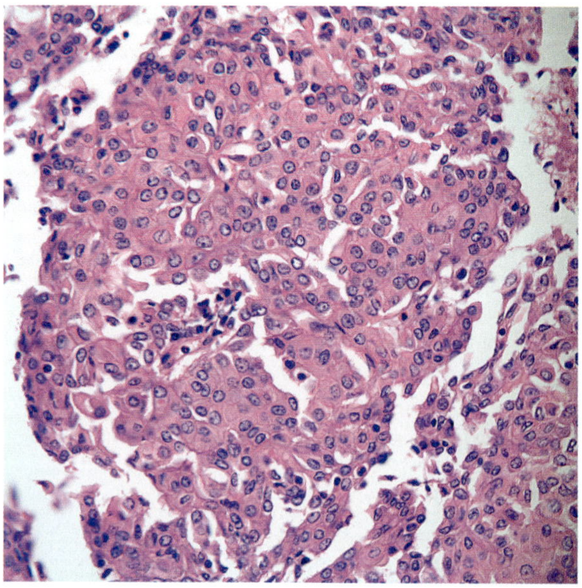

Figure 13-11 Higher-power view of an epithelioid mesothelioma showing a homogeneous cellular proliferation without marked nuclear atypia or mitotic activity.

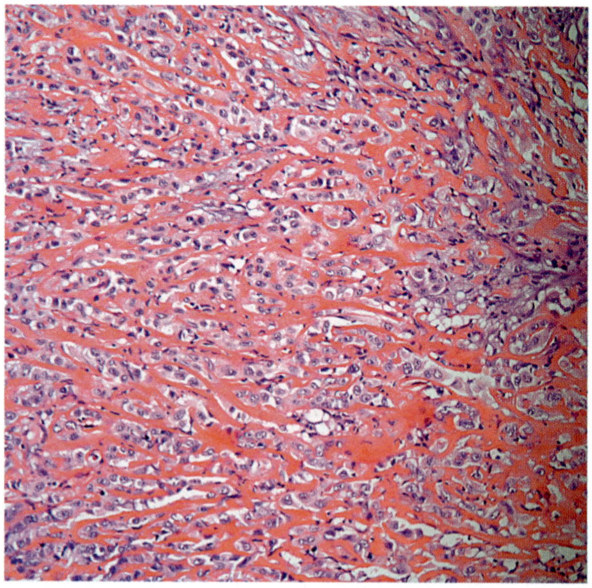

Figure 13-12 Epithelioid mesothelioma with prominent collagen bundles.

with some success. Although both histochemical techniques are very useful, only one is necessary to provide sufficient data for evaluating a particular lesion. As noted, presence of intracellular mucin is strongly indicative of adenocarcinoma, but this finding also has been reported in some mesotheliomas (in up to 5% of the cases). Some mesotheliomas will exhibit abundant extracellular but not intracellular mucin. Thus, in current practice, histochemical techniques often are bypassed in favor of immunohistochemical studies.

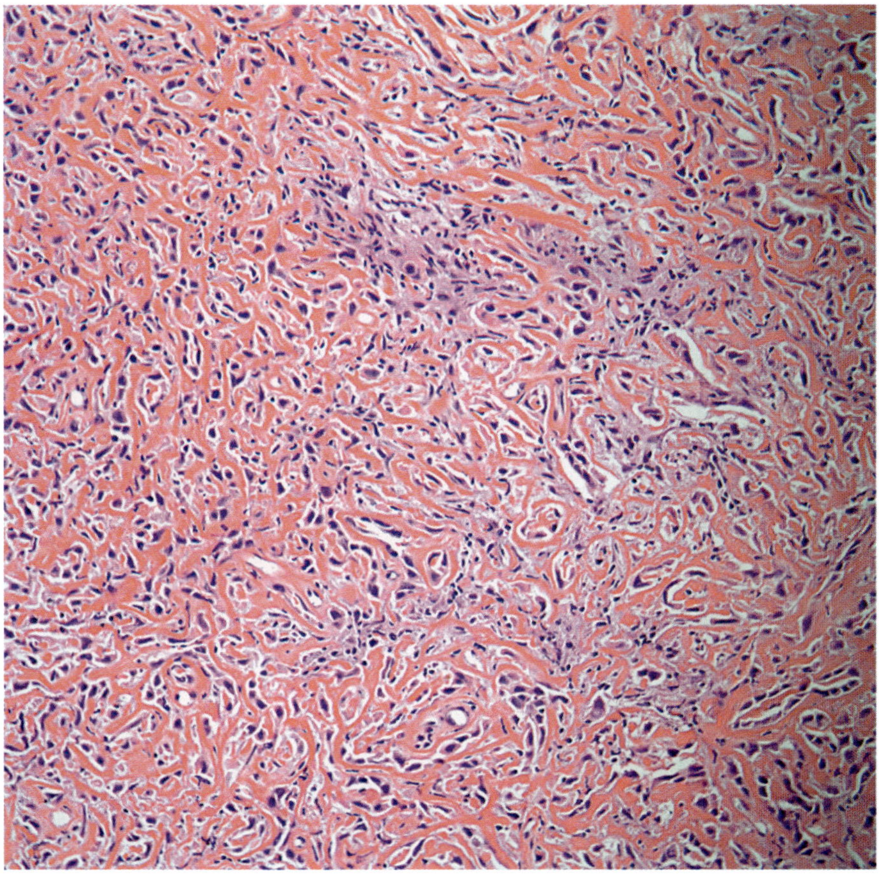

Figure 13-13 Epithelioid mesothelioma with extensive collagen deposition with neoplastic cells dissecting collagen.

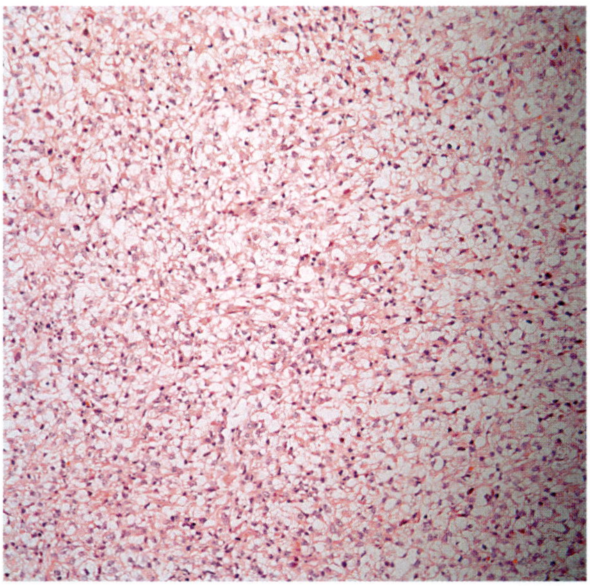

Figure 13-14 Low-power view of a mesothelioma with prominent clear cell features.

Immunohistochemical Features

A great deal of information regarding immunohistochemical studies in the evaluation of mesotheliomas is available. Recent attempts to define the application and limitation of these studies have been reviewed to discover important practical information in the evaluation of mesotheliomas.[31–33] Numerous studies attempting to positively identify mesotheliomas have been published, some of which have provided useful information, whereas others have merely attempted to identify adenocarcinoma in order to rule out mesothelioma. Thus, the diagnosis of mesothelioma has in the past been considered one of exclusion. Although many different kinds of immunohistochemical markers are available that may help in the diagnosis of mesothelioma, only a few are used in practice (Table 13-1). These can be classified as positive or negative markers for mesothelioma. The *positive markers* for mesothelioma include keratin 5/6, calretinin, the Wilms tumor susceptibility gene product (WT-1), HBME-1, thrombomodulin, and mesothelin.

Keratin 5/6 labels epithelioid mesotheliomas in approximately 90% of cases (Fig. 13-30). It is considered a valuable marker for mesothelioma[34–37]; however, staining for this antibody also may be positive in carcinomas of extrathoracic origin[34,38] and in squamous cell carcinoma of the lung. Therefore, this antibody's value depends largely on the context in which it is used. Calretinin is part of a large family of cytoplasmic calcium-binding proteins and labels approximately 85% of epithelioid mesotheliomas (Fig. 13-31). Of the three antibodies in this family, only calretinin labels mesothelioma and non-neoplastic mesothelium.[39–41] WT-1 is the product of the Wilms tumor gene, a tumor suppressor gene located at 11p13 in

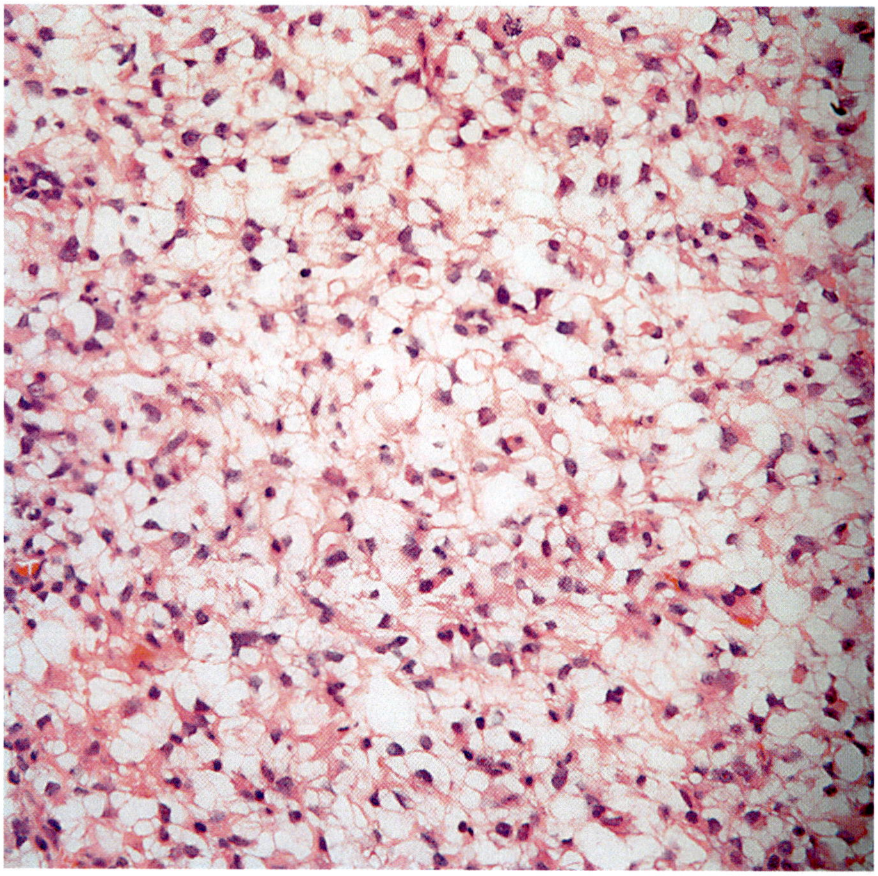

Figure 13-15 Higher-power view of clear cell mesothelioma showing absence of cellular atypia or mitotic activity.

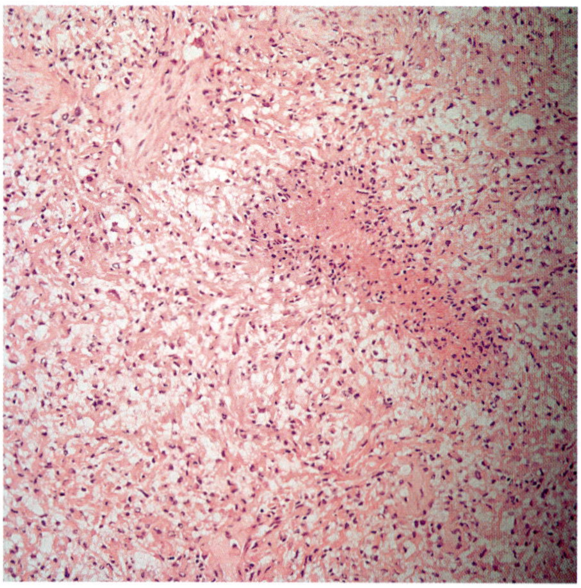

Figure 13-16 Clear cell mesothelioma with focal areas of necrosis.

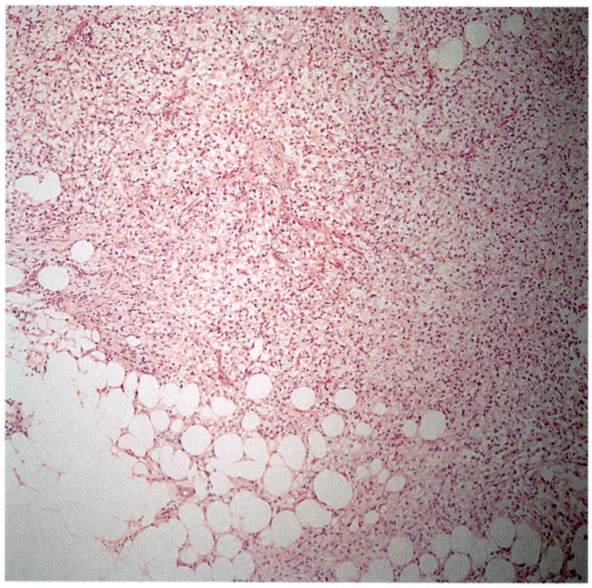

Figure 13-17 Clear cell mesothelioma. Tumor can be seen infiltrating adipose tissue.

mesangial cells of the kidney. WT-1 shows a strong positive reaction in mesotheliomas; however, it also may react positively in tumor cells of other neoplasms, including ovarian and peritoneal serous carcinomas, malignant melanoma, and renal cell carcinoma.[42–48] HBME-1 was generated from a human cell line derived from a patient with malignant mesothelioma. This antibody decorates the membrane of mesothelial cells, as opposed to cytoplasmic staining in adenocarcinomas.[49] HBME-1 may not be a highly reliable marker of mesothelioma, however, because a notable percentage of adenocarcinomas and serous tumors of the ovary also may show positive staining.[49,50]

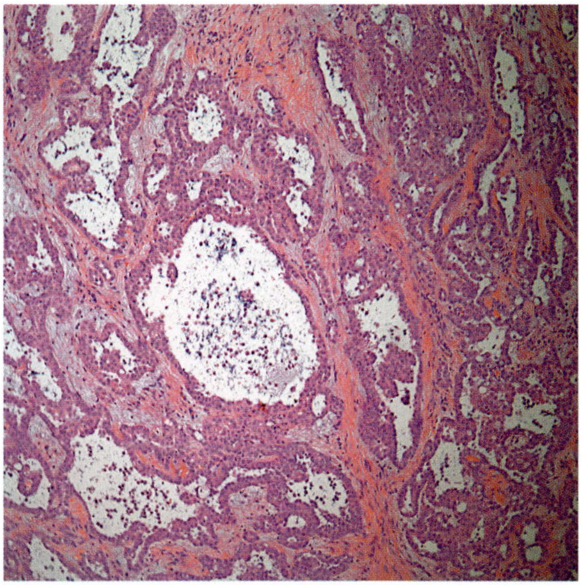

Figure 13-18 Malignant mesothelioma with a prominent glandular pattern.

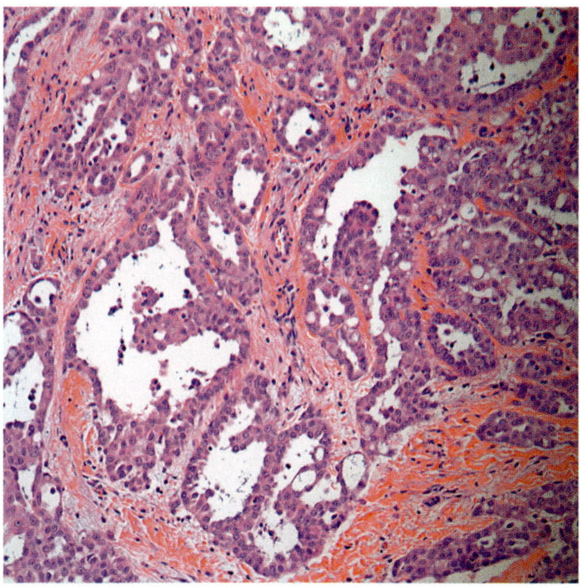

Figure 13-19 Glandular pattern of mesothelioma. Nuclear pleomorphism and mitotic activity are absent.

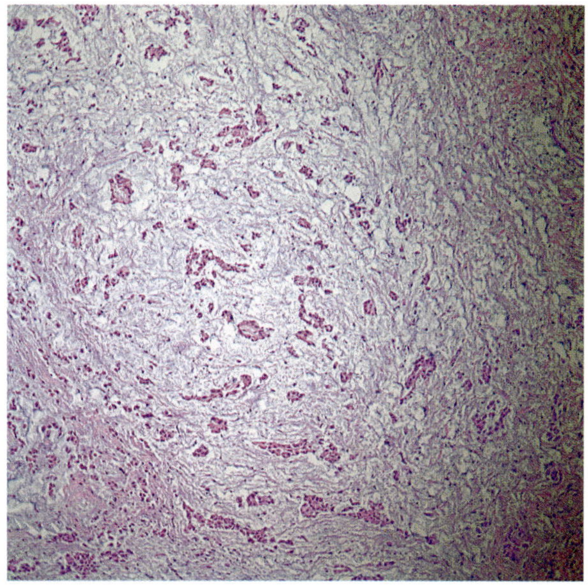

Figure 13-20 Mesothelioma with abundant mucoid substance and scattered clusters of cells.

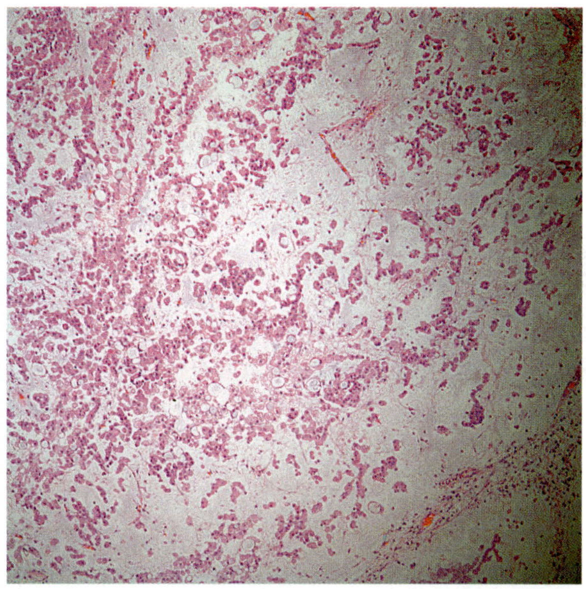

Figure 13-21 Mesothelioma with a more obvious neoplastic cellular proliferation embedded in a mucoid substance.

Thrombomodulin (CD141) is a glycoprotein expressed in endothelial cells and in a variety of other cell types, including mesothelial cells. Several studies have been presented in the literature with claims of 60% to 100% staining in malignant mesotheliomas. This marker also may give positive staining in approximately 75% of adenocarcinomas; therefore, its usefulness is limited.[51–53] Mesothelin is a surface protein that is expressed in the membrane of neoplastic cells in mesotheliomas and in non-neoplastic mesothelial cells. However, mesothelin also may give positive staining in serous carcinomas of the ovary, pancreatic adenocarcinomas, cholangiocarcinoma, colonic adenocarcinoma, and pulmonary adenocarcinoma.[54–57]

A plethora of markers have been used in the diagnosis of mesothelioma, but mainly to rule it out. When the differential diagnosis is between mesothelioma and adenocarcinoma, the most commonly used *negative markers* are carcinoembryonic antigen (CEA), MOC31, thyroid transcription factor-1 (TTF-1), Leu-M1 (CD15), and B72.3. Other markers that have been used include Ber-Ep4 and BG-8. The ideal is a positive marker that excludes the possibility of mesothelioma.

CEA is considered one of the most reliable markers for distinguishing adenocarcinoma from mesothelioma, because the vast majority of mesotheliomas demonstrate

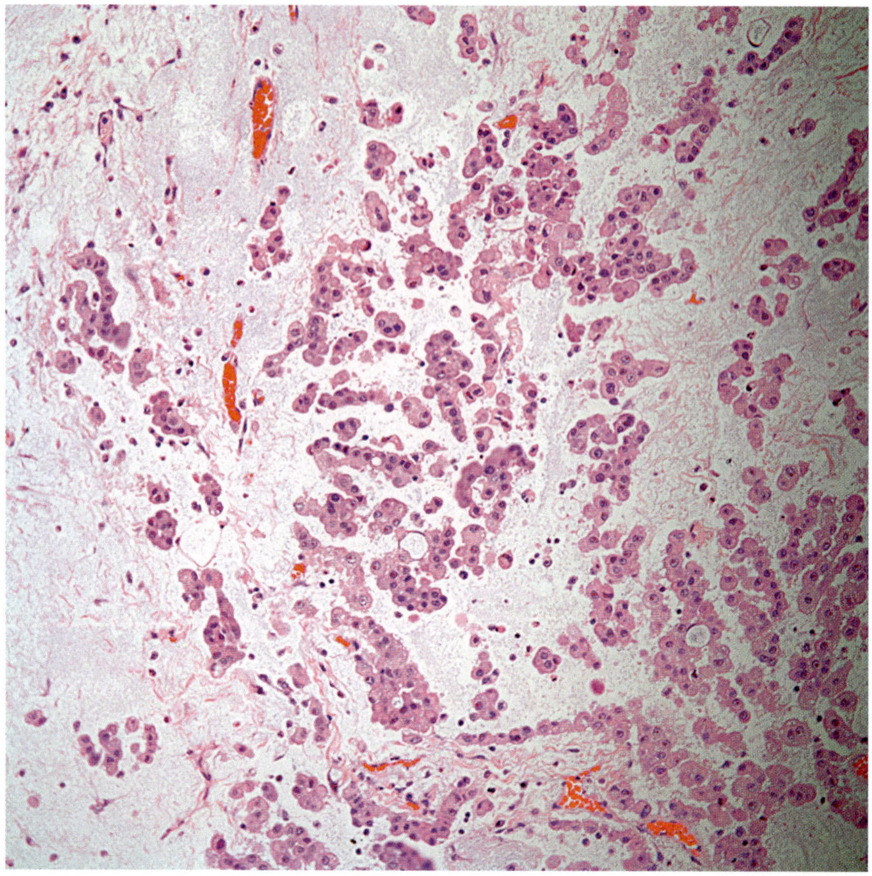

Figure 13-22 Mucoid mesothelioma in which the neoplastic cells appear somewhat oncocytic.

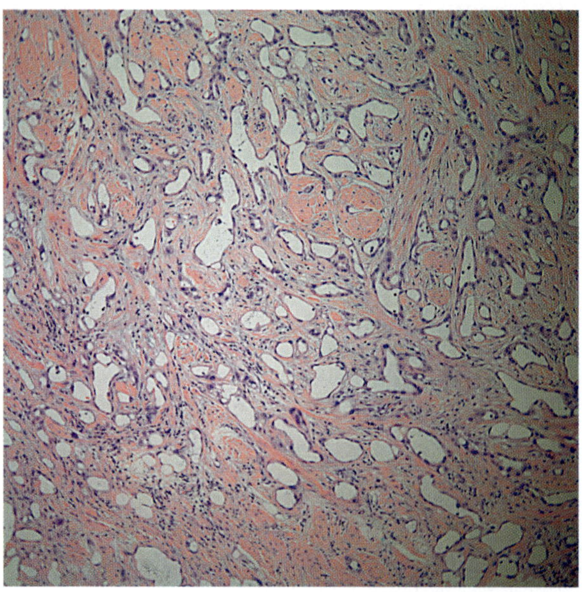

Figure 13-23 Mesothelioma with an adenomatoid-like pattern of growth.

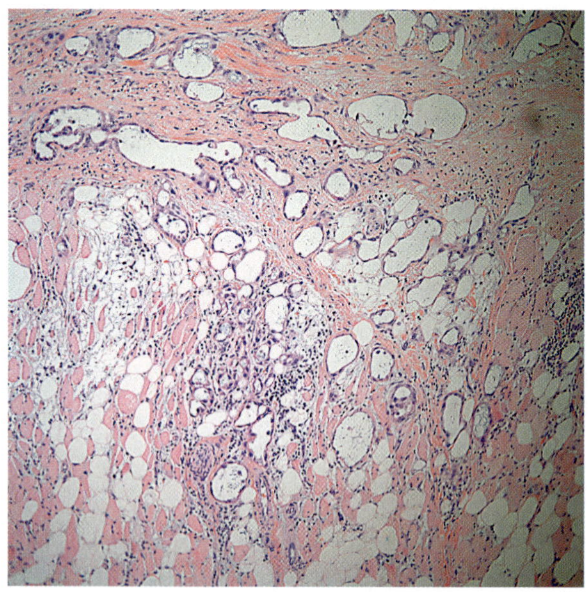

Figure 13-24 Mesothelioma infiltrating into muscle.

negative reactivity for this antibody. Some studies have suggested that the 5% positivity observed in some mesotheliomas may be due to the use of a heteroantiserum unabsorbed by CEA, which may label unrelated epitopes. In this setting, the use of monoclonal antibodies to specific CEA epitopes is more reliable.[58–65] MOC31 has been reported in several studies as an important marker for distinguishing mesothelioma from adenocarcinoma, because it purportedly gives positive staining in adenocarcinoma cells.[66–68] In some cases of mesothelioma, however, MOC31 may give focal and spotty positive staining. TTF-1 is expressed in normal lung and in

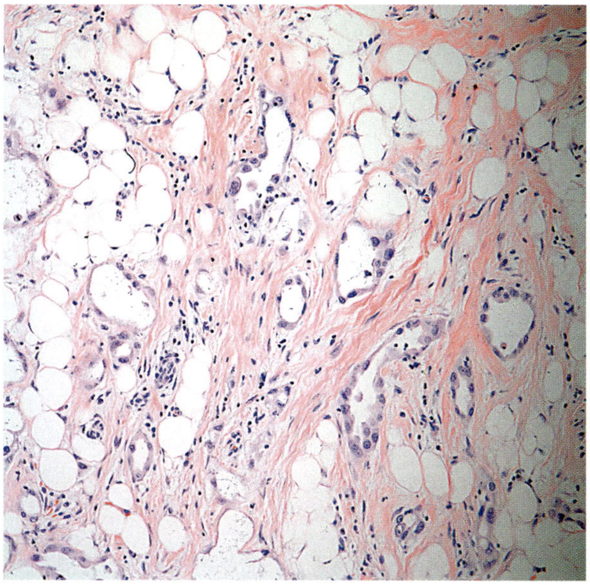

Figure 13-25 Mesothelioma with adenomatoid-like pattern. Tumor can be seen infiltrating adipose tissue.

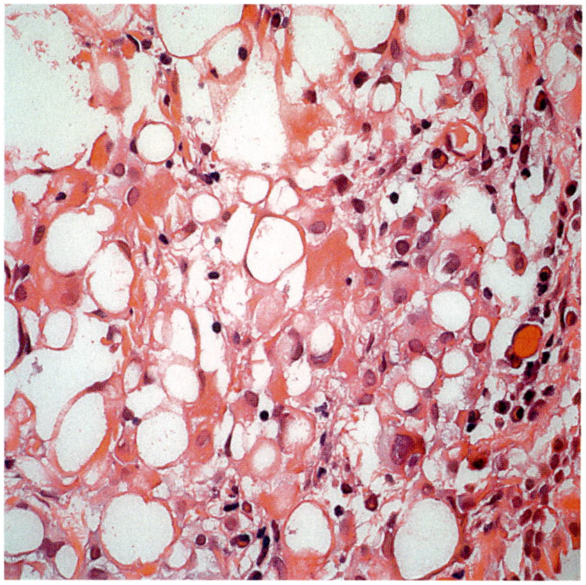

Figure 13-27 Higher-power view of a deciduoid mesothelioma.

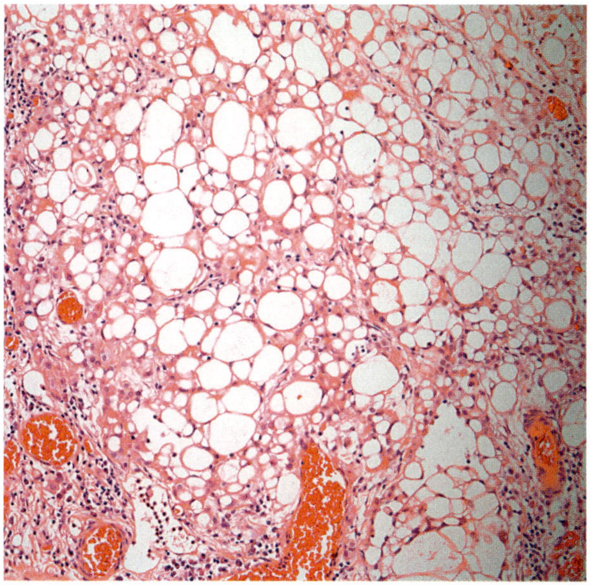

Figure 13-26 Mesothelioma with prominent deciduoid-like changes.

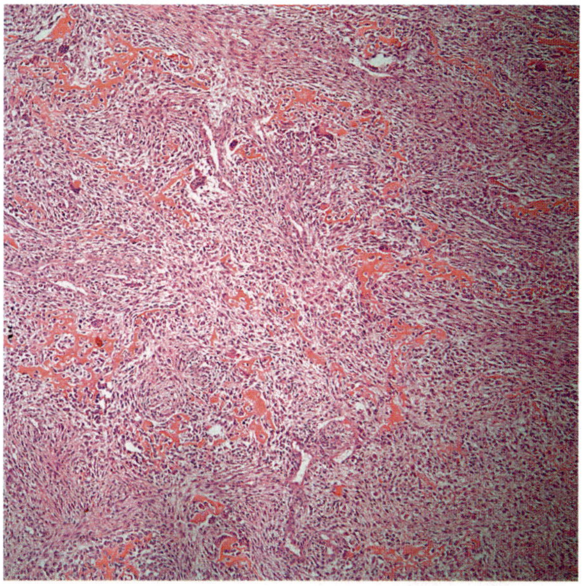

Figure 13-28 Low-power view of mesothelioma with osseous metaplasia mimicking osteosarcoma.

thyroid epithelial cells. TTF-1 shows high specificity for lung adenocarcinoma, and so far, staining for TTF-1 has been reported to be negative in mesotheliomas. Thus, it is one of the most important markers to separate pulmonary adenocarcinoma from mesothelioma.[69–71] Leu-M1 (CD15) has a high level of specificity for adenocarcinoma; however, some mesotheliomas, namely peritoneal mesotheliomas, also may demonstrate positive staining in tumor cells.[72,73] B72.3 is a generic epithelial determinant (tumor-associated glycoprotein-72) that is a high-molecular-weight cell membrane glycoprotein. Although it is a good marker for adenocarcinoma, some mesotheliomas also may demonstrate focal positive staining.[64,74]

As mentioned earlier, many more antibodies have been presented in the literature as very specific for the distinction between adenocarcinoma and mesothelioma; over time, however, these antibodies have proved unreliable. One such antibody, Ber-Ep4, originally was presented as specific for adenocarcinoma but also has been shown to react with mesotheliomas in more than 20% of the cases.[73] BG-8 is another antibody that may react strongly in cases of adenocarcinoma; however, some mesotheliomas also may show positive staining.[75]

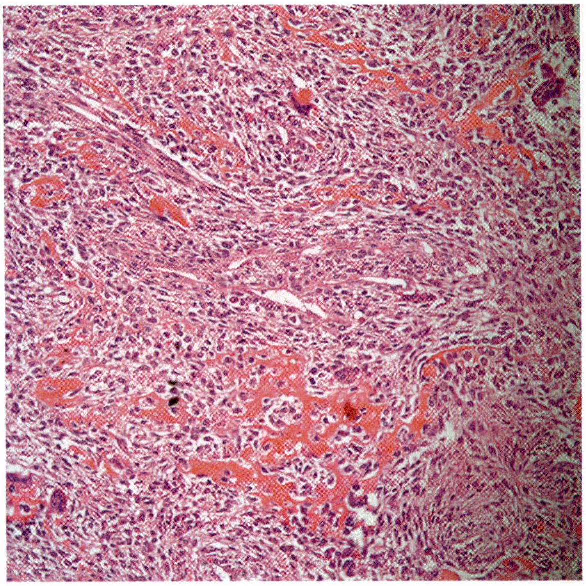

Figure 13-29 Mesothelioma. Higher-power view clearly shows the osseous metaplasia and epithelioid areas.

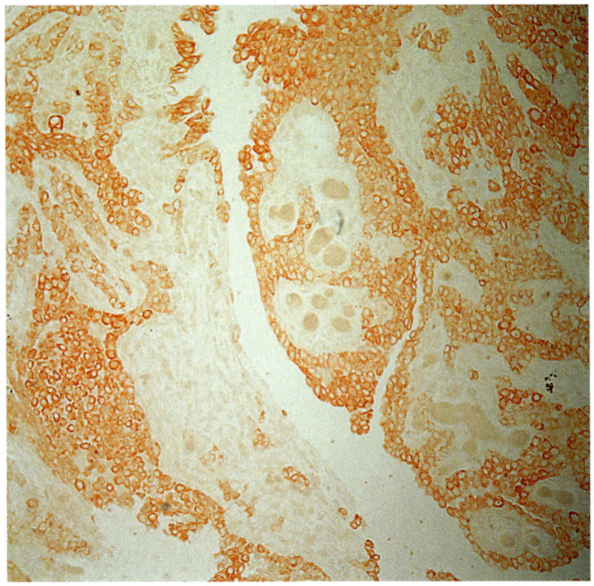

Figure 13-30 Immunohistochemical staining for keratin 5/6 gives a positive reaction in tumor cells.

TABLE 13-1 COMMONLY USED IMMUNOHISTOCHEMICAL STAINS FOR DISTINGUISHING BETWEEN MESOTHELIOMA AND ADENOCARCINOMA

Antibody	Adenocarcinoma	Mesothelioma
CEA	+	–
Leu-M1	+	–
B72.3	+	–
TTF-1	+	–
Calretinin	–/+*	+
Keratin 5/6	0	+
Broad-spectrum keratin	+	+
EMA	+	+
Ber-Ep4	+	–/+

*Some adenocarcinomas may show positive staining for calretinin.
CEA, carcinoembryonic antigen; EMA, epithelial membrane antigen; TTF-1, thyroid transcription factor-1.

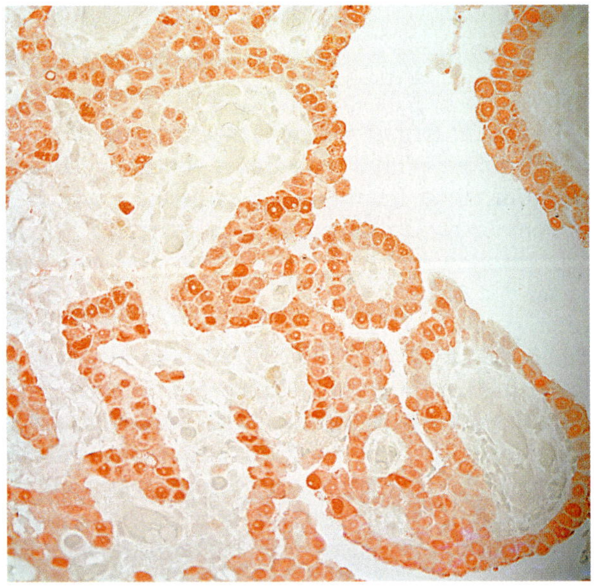

Figure 13-31 Immunohistochemical staining for calretinin gives a nuclear positive reaction in tumor cells.

Electron Microscopy

Ultrastructural studies are very important in the diagnosis of mesothelioma; however, in many cases the utility of such studies is hampered by lack of material when it is needed the most. Often, sufficient material does not become available until a more extensive procedure has been performed, but in a majority of the cases, the initial biopsy specimen is the only material available for diagnosis. Electron microscopic features are helpful for evaluation of better-differentiated tumors; but when the tumor is poorly differentiated, the ultrastructural findings are rarely helpful. In most cases when immunohistochemical analysis has failed to provide a clear interpretation, findings on electron microscopy also will be questionable. Nevertheless, the latter study can be very helpful, and every effort should be made to obtain a sample for this examination. The finding of long, slender microvilli is a histopathologic hallmark of mesothelioma.

Differential Diagnosis

In the setting of an atypical epithelial cellular proliferation, the most important condition to rule out is either pulmonary adenocarcinoma extending into the pleura, metastatic epithelial tumor of other origin, or most important, mesothelial hyperplasia (Table 13-2). If the cellular proliferation has been deemed to be malignant, then immunohistochemical studies, especially carcinomatous epitopes, will be the next step. A similar approach is appropriate with a metastatic epithelial neoplasm from

TABLE 13-2 CONTRASTING FEATURES OF MESOTHELIOMA AND MESOTHELIAL HYPERPLASIA

Feature	Mesothelioma	Hyperplasia
Penetration into adipose tissue or muscle	+	0
Stromal invasion	+	0
Inflammation	Often 0	+
Cellular atypia	+	+
Mitoses	+	+
Cellular proliferation in surface	Often 0	+
Granulation tissue	Often 0	+
Fibrin	Often 0	+

another source to the pleura; however, the interpretation can be more difficult in cases of mesothelial hyperplasia. In this setting, no available immunohistochemical stain can separate a neoplastic cellular proliferation from a hyperplastic one. Thus, even though the necessary steps have been followed, it is imperative not only to correlate the histopathologic findings with the clinical and radiologic features but also to provide an accurate interpretation of the results of the immunohistochemical studies. Even electron microscopic studies would fail to separate such cellular proliferations. In essence, the diagnosis is a morphologic one that requires careful attention to specific histopathologic features, such as invasion into adipose tissue or skeletal muscle, that are associated with malignant mesothelioma (see Tables 13-1 and 13-2).

Sarcomatoid Mesothelioma

The sarcomatoid variant of mesothelioma is less common than the epithelial variant and probably accounts for less than 15% of mesotheliomas in its pure form. As its name implies, the characteristic tumor growth pattern is one of spindle cells with elongated nuclei and inconspicuous nucleoli, mimicking sarcoma of soft tissues. In a study of spindle cell tumors of the pleura, Carter and Otis[76] proposed three types, ranging from low grade (possibly benign) to high grade: fibroma (keratin-negative tumor), sarcomatoid mesothelioma (keratin-positive tumor), and sarcoma, or malignant spindle cell tumor (keratin-negative). Because in some cases the histopathologic features may overlap, immunohistochemical studies play an important role in diagnosis.

Malignant spindle cell tumors (keratin-positive) of the pleura can be further subdivided into three distinct categories based on their growth pattern:

Spindle cell type (fibrosarcoma-like or malignant fibrous histiocytoma–like). The histopathologic diagnosis of either one of these variants is rather straightforward. In the fibrosarcoma-like pattern, the tumor is composed of a spindle cellular proliferation that may show the so-called herringbone pattern with interdissecting fascicles of spindle cells with indistinguishable cell membranes, moderate amounts of light eosinophilic cytoplasm, elongated nuclei, and inconspicuous nucleoli. Nuclear atypia is present, and mitotic activity is readily visible. In the malignant fibrous histiocytoma–like pattern, the tumor displays features of a high-grade sarcoma with a fascicular growth pattern characterized by the presence of spindle or oval cells, or both, with elongated or round nucleus and conspicuous nucleoli. In addition, the tumor also may exhibit multinucleated malignant giant cells intermixed with the spindle cell proliferation. Nuclear atypia is prominent, and mitotic activity is readily visible (Figs. 13-32 to 13-40).

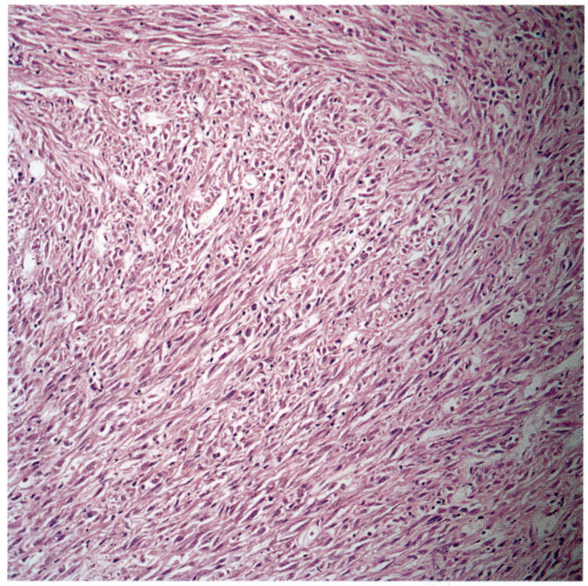

Figure 13-32 Low-power view of a sarcomatoid mesothelioma, fibrosarcoma-like.

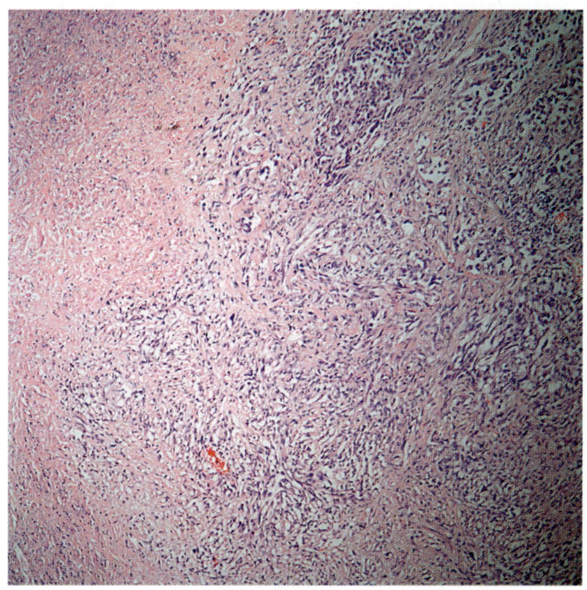

Figure 13-33 Sarcomatoid mesothelioma with areas of necrosis.

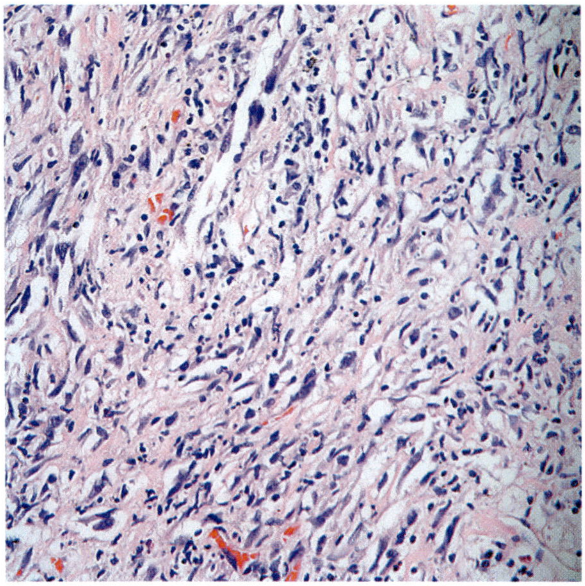

Figure 13-34 Sarcomatoid mesothelioma composed of spindle cells with prominent atypical features.

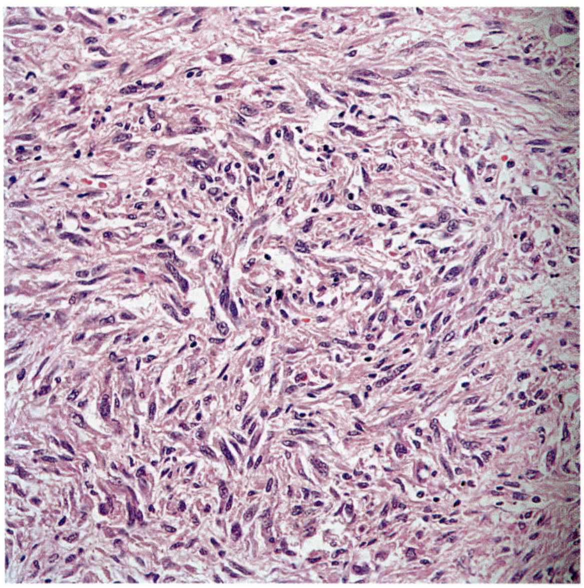

Figure 13-35 Higher-power view of sarcomatoid mesothelioma showing nuclear atypia and mitotic activity.

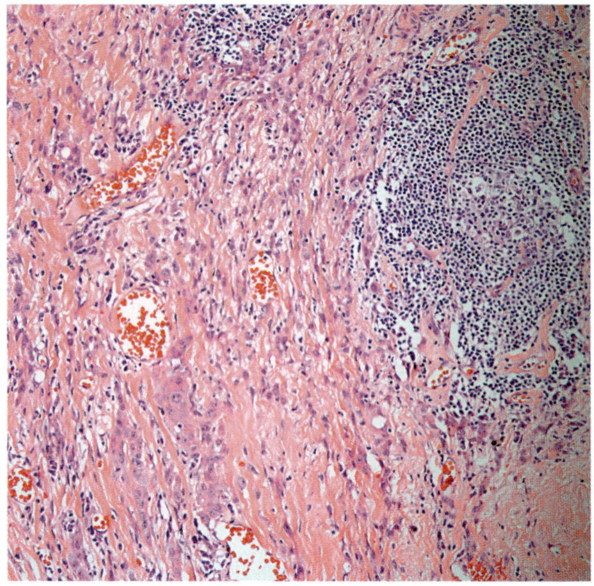

Figure 13-36 Sarcomatoid mesothelioma with adjacent inflammatory reaction.

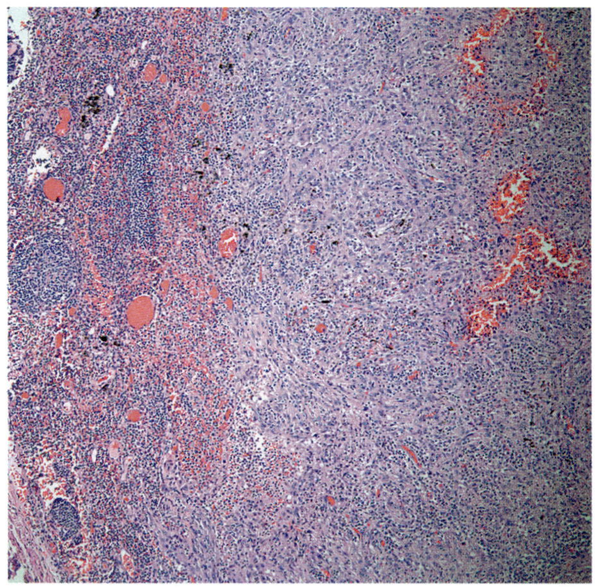

Figure 13-37 Lymph node with metastatic sarcomatoid mesothelioma.

Desmoplastic mesothelioma. This variant is the one that poses a challenge in diagnosis, mainly when only a small biopsy specimen is available for interpretation. The initial description by Kannerstein and Churg[77] in 1980 has been followed by a few more series. Cantin and associates[78] reported 27 cases in which the clinical course was often rapid, and the mean survival for cases of pure sarcomatoid tumor was approximately 6.18 months. In their experience, desmoplastic mesothelioma also showed a greater tendency toward metastatic disease at 60%, compared with 40% of the nondesmoplastic variant. Mangano and coworkers[79] reported a series of 31 cases in which the emphasis was on separating desmoplastic mesotheliomas from fibrous pleurisy. These workers noted the presence of p53 in these two conditions and concluded that reactivity for this marker can be positive in both, and that although p53 is more commonly seen in desmoplastic mesothelioma, the difference was not statistically significant. Histologically, these tumors may show extensive areas of collagenization with a very discrete spindle cell proliferation that may be missed in a cursory review of the histologic sections. The following are the most important histopathologic features[79,80]

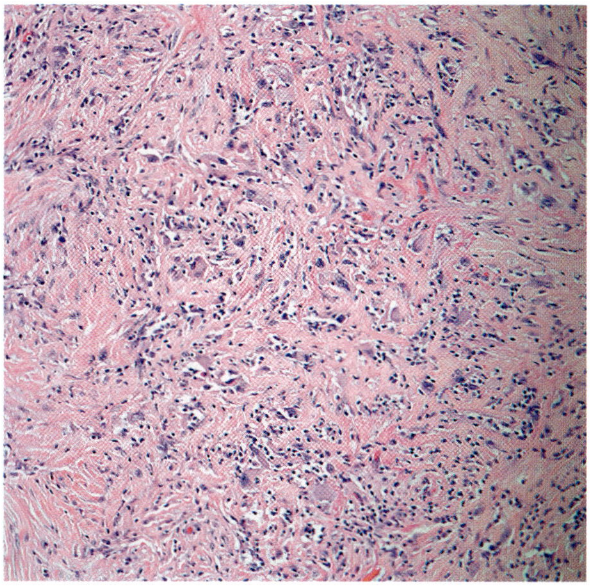

Figure 13-38 Low-power view of a malignant fibrous histiocytoma–like sarcomatoid mesothelioma.

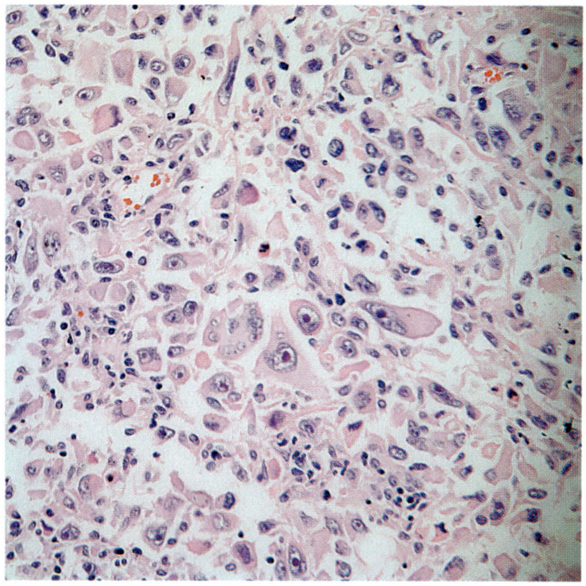

Figure 13-40 High-power view of malignant fibrous histiocytoma–like mesothelioma. Note the the presence of pleomorphic cells.

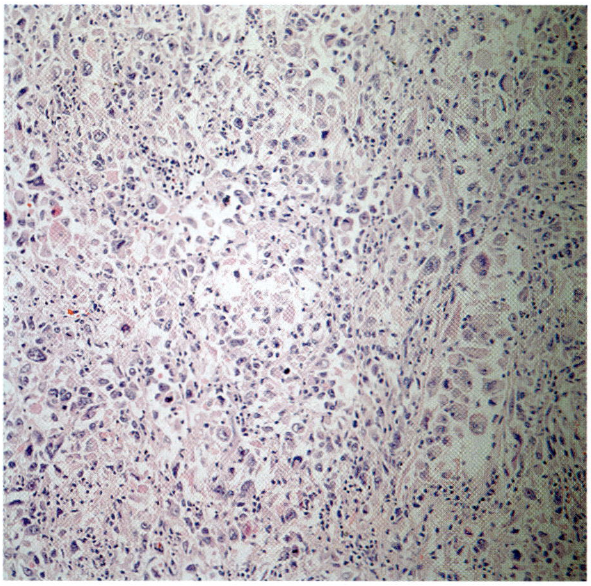

Figure 13-39 Malignant fibrous histiocytoma–like sarcomatoid mesothelioma with prominent cellular pleomorphism.

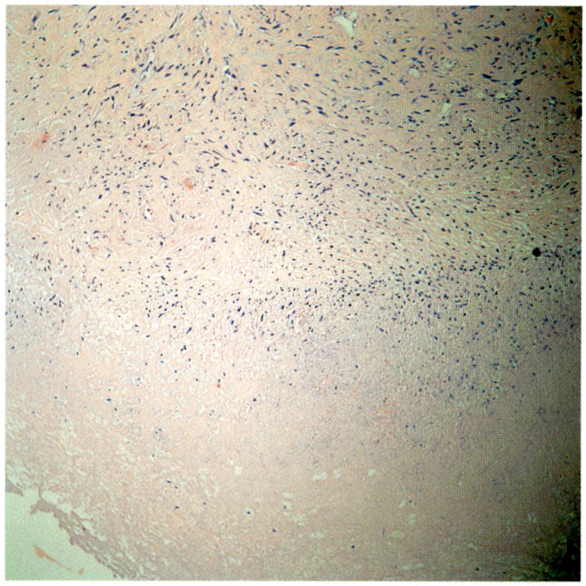

Figure 13-41 Desmoplastic mesothelioma with adjacent necrosis.

that have been associated with the diagnosis of desmoplastic mesothelioma:

- Invasion of chest wall or lung
- Foci of bland necrosis
- Frank sarcomatoid foci
- Distant metastasis

These criteria apply mainly to resected specimens (Figs. 13-41 to 13-44), pleural peeling, or a very generous pleural biopsy specimen. In a small sample, establishing this diagnosis may prove to be very difficult, if not impossible. Colby[80] has warned about the care that must be exercised in making such a diagnosis and has stated that because no proven therapy for desmoplastic mesothelioma is recognized, underdiagnosis is preferable to overdiagnosis. This is especially true nowadays, because the current trend is to perform extrapleural pneumonectomies for the treatment of mesothelioma.

Lymphohistiocytoid. This type of mesothelioma is included in the subcategory of sarcomatoid mesotheliomas,[81] although in some cases the epithelioid component may be formed by oval cells instead of by spindle cells. This subtype is unusual and is characterized by a prominent lymphoid component admixed with a cellular proliferation composed of epithelial cells with a "histiocytoid appearance" (Figs. 13-45 to 13-47).

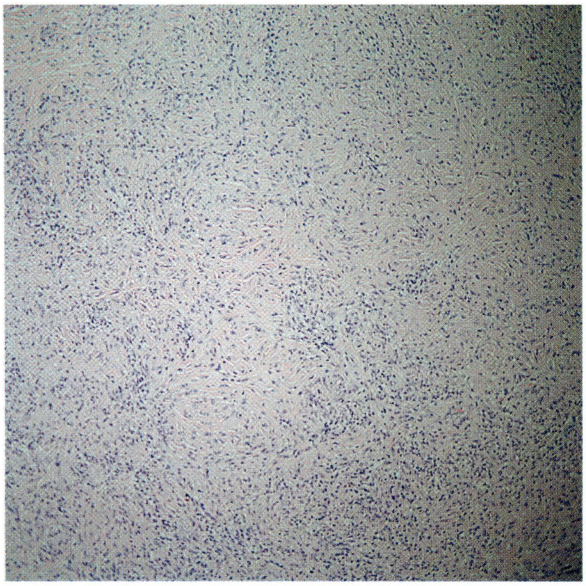

Figure 13-42 Desmoplastic mesothelioma with spindle cells mixed with a collagenous stroma.

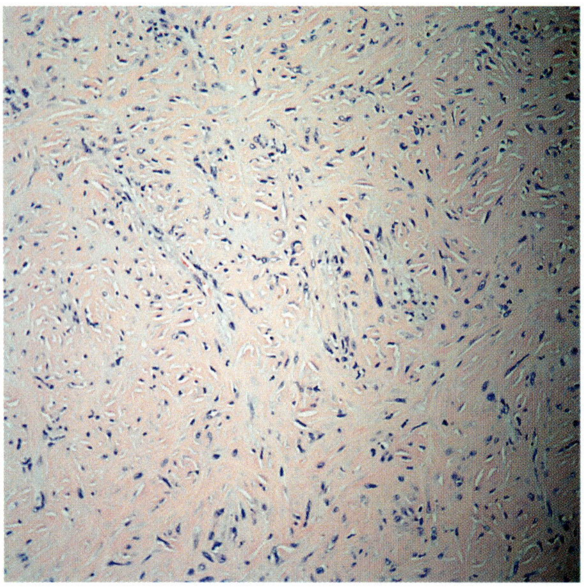

Figure 13-43 Desmoplastic mesothelioma with spindle cell component and collagenous stroma.

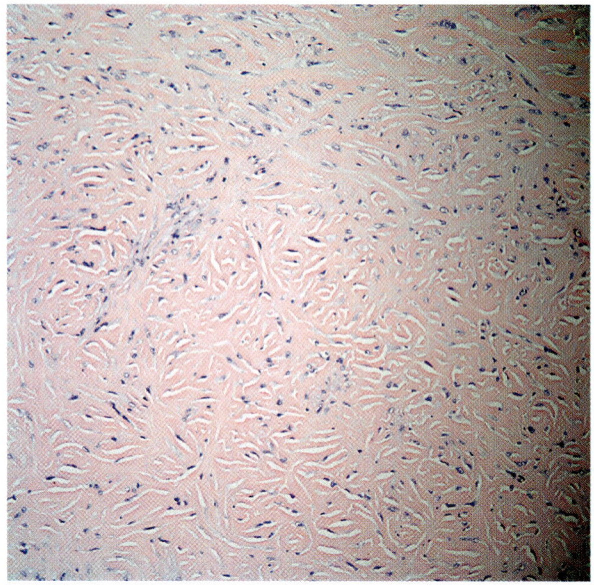

Figure 13-44 Desmoplastic mesothelioma. Note the scattered spindle cells present.

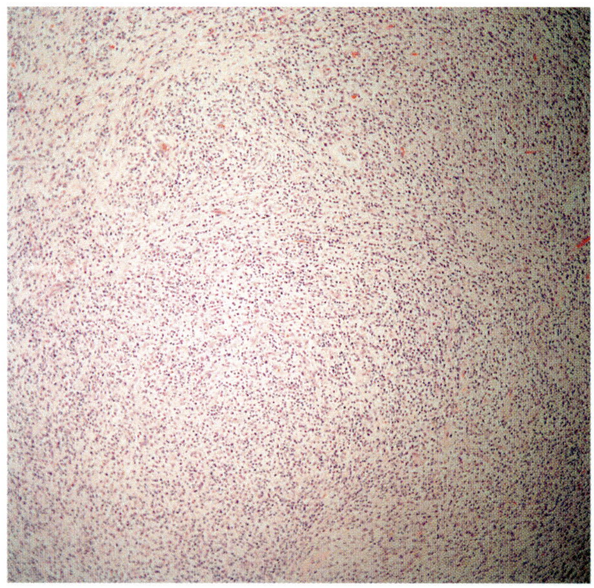

Figure 13-45 Lymphohistiocytoid mesothelioma with a prominent lymphohistiocytic component.

Histochemical Studies

Histochemical studies, such as those using PAS with and without diastase, mucicarmine, or hyaluronic acid with and without diastase digestion, have no role in the diagnosis of these tumors.

Immunohistochemical Studies

In the setting of a spindle cell mesothelioma, the role of immunohistochemical studies is relatively limited whether the tumor is desmoplastic or not, because most of the antibodies used in diagnosis of conventional epithelioid mesotheliomas have no practical use in identification of sarcomatoid mesotheliomas. Broad-spectrum keratin is by far the most important (Fig. 13-48). All other carcinomatous epitopes are known not to react with sarcomatoid tumors. The use of calretinin and keratin 5/6 is rather limited because positivity may vary, and negative results do not mean that the tumor in question is not a mesothelioma. Fibrous pleurisy cannot be distinguished from desmoplastic mesothelioma by means of immunohistochemical techniques, because both lesions may react with keratin antibodies. Use of immunohistochemical studies is relevant to rule out other spindle cell tumors of different lineage, including leiomyosarcomas, malignant fibrous histiocytoma, and other mesenchymal tumors.

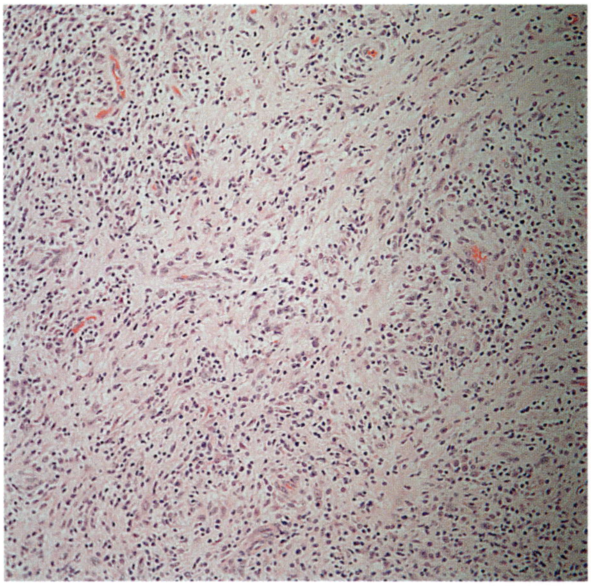

Figure 13-46 Lymphohistiocytoid mesothelioma exhibiting an admixture of epithelial cells and lymphohistiocytic cells.

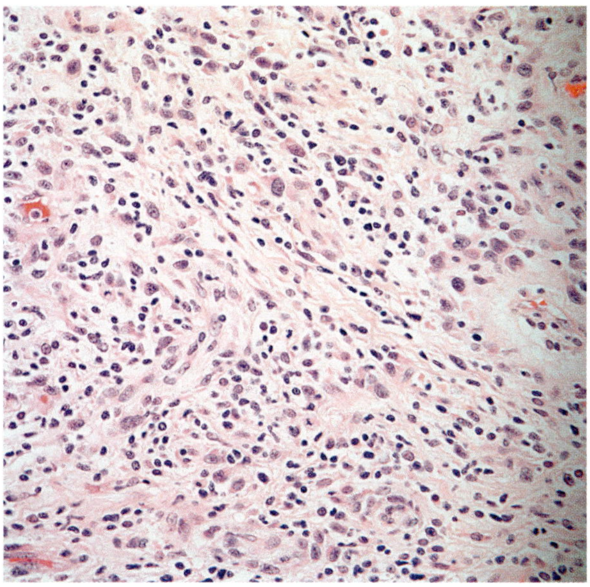

Figure 13-47 Lymphohistiocytoid mesothelioma. Marked cellular atypia and mitotic activity are lacking.

Differential Diagnosis

When the neoplastic nature of the tumor is not in question, the most important distinction is that with another spindle cell neoplasm of mesenchymal origin. In this setting, immunohistochemical studies or electron microscopy will lead to the appropriate interpretation. In cases of sarcomatoid carcinoma involving the pleura in a diffuse manner, the radiographic finding of an intrapulmonary tumor mass will lead to the appropriate interpretation. This distinction may prove to be very difficult on histopathologic grounds, however. By far the most challenging entities to rule out in the differential diagnosis are fibrinous pleuritis and fibrous pleurisy of a reactive or inflammatory nature. With these processes, the diagnosis is based on morphologic grounds, because immunohistochemistry cannot solve the problem (Table 13-3).

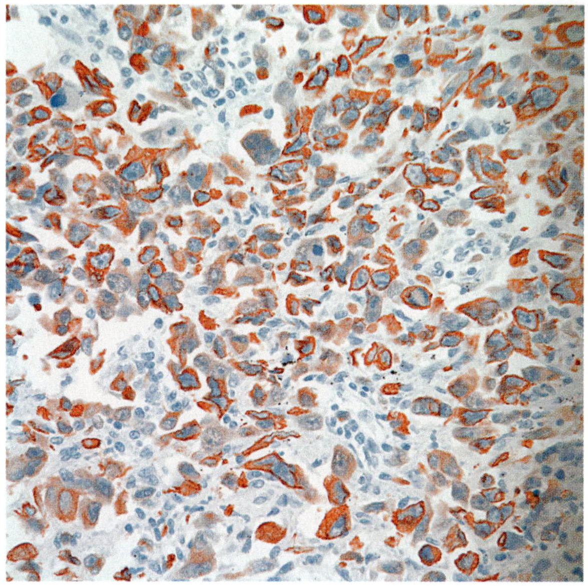

Figure 13-48 Immunohistochemical staining for broad-spectrum keratin gives a positive reaction in tumor cells of a malignant fibrous histiocytoma–like mesothelioma.

Biphasic Mesotheliomas

As their name implies, biphasic mesotheliomas are composed of a mixture of epithelial and sarcomatoid areas (Figs. 13-49 to 13-52). As a rule, presence of unequivocal sarcomatoid areas or epithelial areas, or both, is necessary to identify these tumors as biphasic; however, the material available may vary in composition, with biopsy and resected specimens differing in cellularity. In a more recent study on the usefulness of biopsy versus resection, a considerable number of cases

TABLE 13-3 COMMON HISTOPATHOLOGIC AND IMMUNOHISTOCHEMICAL FEATURES OF SARCOMATOID MESOTHELIOMA AND FIBROUS PLEURISY

Feature	Mesothelioma	Fibrous Pleurisy
Histologic Examination		
Zonation	0	+
Cellular atypia	+	+
Granulation tissue	Often 0	+
Fibrin	Often 0	+
Inflammatory reaction	Often 0	+
Mitotic activity	+	+
Immunohistochemical Staining		
Broad-spectrum keratin	+	+
Keratin 5/6	+/−	−/+
Calretinin	−/+	−/+
Smooth muscle actin	+	+

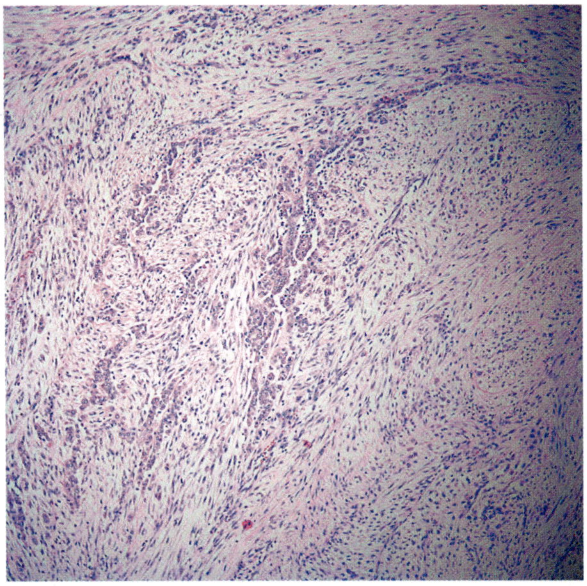

Figure 13-49 Biphasic mesothelioma showing sarcomatoid and epithelioid areas.

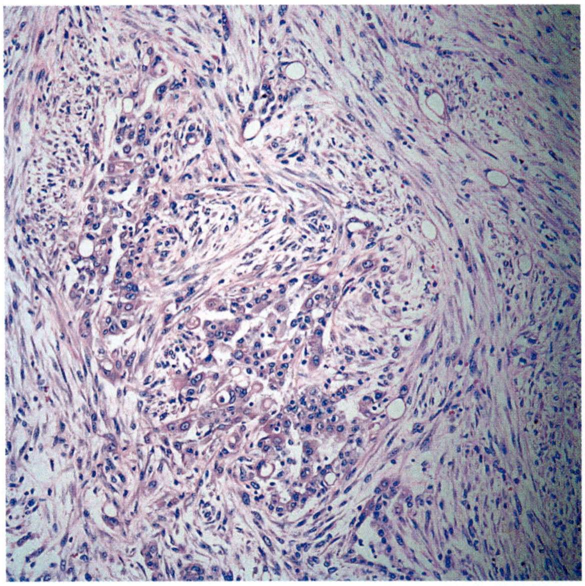

Figure 13-50 Biphasic mesothelioma with epithelioid and sarcomatoid components present in almost equal proportions.

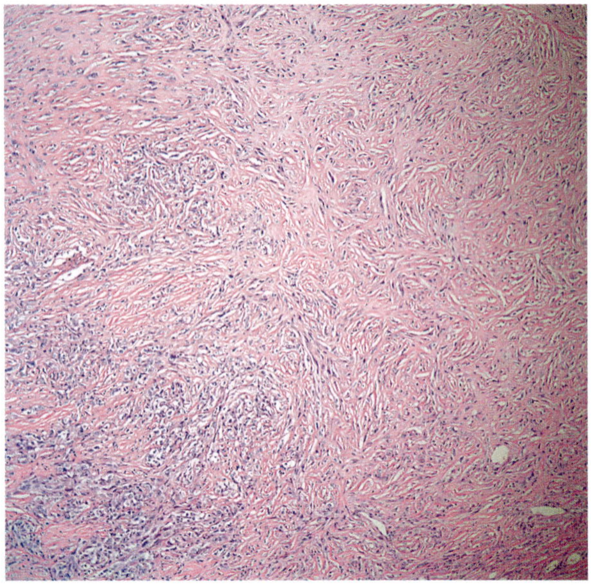

Figure 13-51 Biphasic mesothelioma with epithelioid and desmoplastic areas.

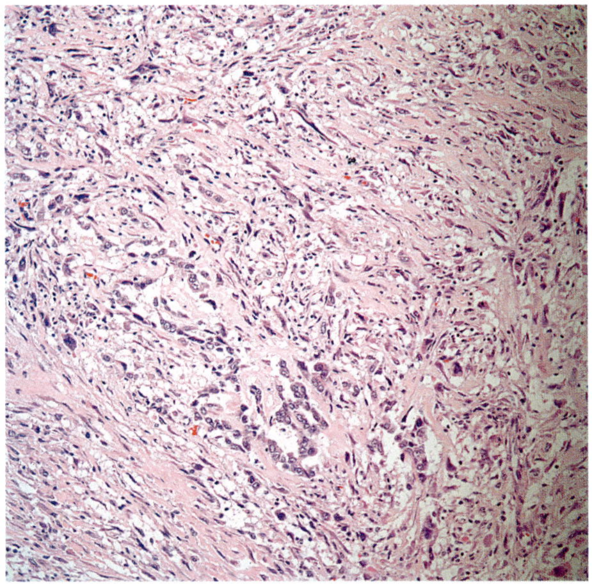

Figure 13-52 Biphasic mesothelioma with a prominent sarcomatoid component.

were found in which the biphasic nature of the specimen was not easily determined in the original biopsy material.[30] One important consideration in the differential diagnosis for biphasic mesothelioma is primary synovial sarcoma of the pleura; the latter tumor, however, is a pleura-based mass without diffuse involvement of the pleura. Once again, close clinical and radiologic correlation is strongly recommended.

Treatment and Prognosis

One of the most common modalities of treatment is extrapulmonary pneumonectomy. Rice[82] recently reviewed this subject, noting that despite improvements in the operative mortality rate, surgery alone is associated with high rates of local failure; thus, the use of neoadjuvant modalities including radiation therapy and chemotherapy may be indicated. Nevertheless, in a majority of cases the prognosis is still poor, with survival for no longer than 12 to 18 months after initial diagnosis. In view of the widespread acceptance of these modalities in the treatment of mesothelioma, now more than ever, the diagnosis requires careful attention not only to the histologic features of the tumor but also to its clinical and radiologic aspects.

Practical Approach

Because the diagnosis of mesothelioma is multifactorial, a conceptual and more practical approach has been formulated that can be applied in a majority of the cases, especially when the diagnosis is in some doubt. This approach consists of the following:

- Detailed clinical history
- Detailed radiologic information
- Adequate biopsy material (preferably containing adipose tissue or skeletal muscle in order to evaluate invasion)
- Immunohistochemical studies
- Electron microscopy

Clinical Setting

- If the tumor is epithelioid, a battery of immunohistochemical studies should be performed, including staining for keratin 5/6, calretinin, CEA, Leu-M1, B72.3, MOC31, and TTF-1.
- If the tumor is sarcomatoid, immunohistochemical studies can be limited to use of broad-spectrum keratin. Keratin 5/6 and calretinin can be added; however, it is well known that reactivity for those antibodies may be negative in sarcomatoid mesotheliomas. Immunohistochemical studies to rule out other mesenchymal neoplasms may be included, depending on the degree of suspicion.
- When the differential diagnosis is between mesothelioma and mesothelial hyperplasia, the diagnosis is made on histopathologic grounds by determining presence and extent of invasion, and the use of immunohistochemical studies is not reliable.
- When the differential diagnosis is between sarcomatoid mesothelioma and fibrous pleurisy, the use of immunohistochemical stains is not reliable, and the diagnosis is based on histopathologic grounds by demonstrating invasion.

PSEUDOMESOTHELIOMATOUS ADENOCARCINOMA

The presence of adenocarcinomas growing along the pleural surface is fairly uncommon and constitutes the basis for extensive use of ancillary tools in the diagnosis of mesothelioma. In 1976, Harwood and colleagues[83] described six cases of pulmonary carcinoma that were characterized by diffuse pleural thickening, in a manner similar to that described in malignant mesothelioma. Owing to the gross and microscopic characteristics of the tumor, these investigators classified this type of lung carcinoma as a specific variant that they termed *pseudomesotheliomatous carcinoma*. Over the past 25 years or so, several series of cases have been described, highlighting not only the similarities of this tumor to malignant mesothelioma but also providing the necessary tools to distinguish between these two conditions, in view of considerations regarding treatment and legal implications of the diagnosis.[84–90]

Clinical Features

No specific features are recognized to differentiate pseudomesotheliomatous adenocarcinoma of the pleura from malignant mesothelioma. A majority of patients are men older than 50 years of age with a history of tobacco use. Some of these tumors have been reported in patients exposed to asbestos, iron, and stone dust. The most common clinical signs and symptoms include weight loss, dyspnea, cough, chest pain, and pleural effusion. On radiographic examination, the pleura may appear thickened, whereas at thoracotomy, the findings may include extensive thickening of the pleura or multiple pleural nodules studding the pleural surface.

Macroscopic Features

The gross features associated with pseudomesotheliomatous adenocarcinoma may mimic those seen in pleural mesotheliomas, especially the extensive pleural thickening that may encase the entire lung and extend into the pulmonary septum (Fig. 13-53). In some cases a small peripheral intrapulmonary nodule may be seen, but this feature may not be easily identified. The tumor also may extend to involve diaphragm or pericardium.

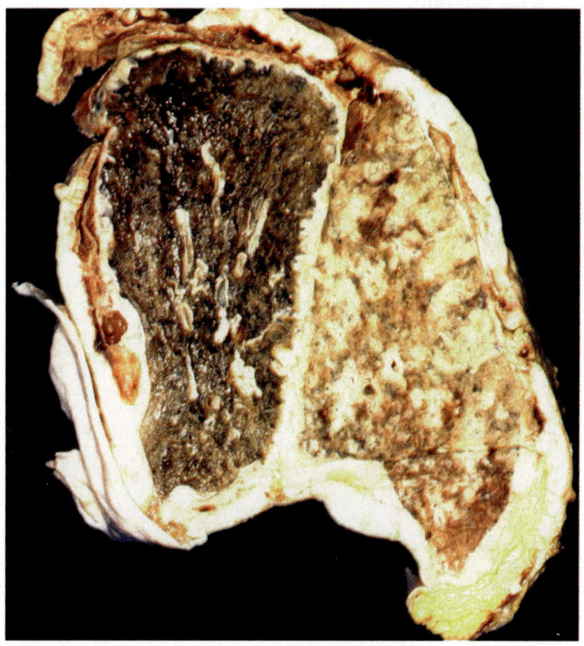

Figure 13-53 Pseudomesotheliomatous adenocarcinoma mimicking mesothelioma. Note the encasement of the lung parenchyma.

Histopathologic Features

The tumor more closely mimics the epithelioid variant of malignant mesothelioma. Pseudomesotheliomatous adenocarcinoma characteristically shows areas of glandular, tubular, or papillary features embedded in a collagenous stroma. The neoplastic proliferation may appear embedded, in more haphazard fashion, in a background of collagenous stroma, which in some cases exhibits a desmoplastic reaction mimicking a biphasic mesothelioma. This desmoplastic reaction also may display an inflammatory reaction (Figs. 13-54 to 13-57).

Histochemical and Immunohistochemical Features

Histochemical staining with PAS with and without diastase digestion, as well as mucicarmine, may be of help, because the presence of intracellular mucin indicates the correct interpretation. This finding may not be present in all cases; therefore, the use of immunohistochemical stains may be necessary. In this setting, the carcinomatous epitopes CEA (Fig. 13-58), B72.3, MOC31, and TTF-1 may be of help. Although a wider variety of antibodies

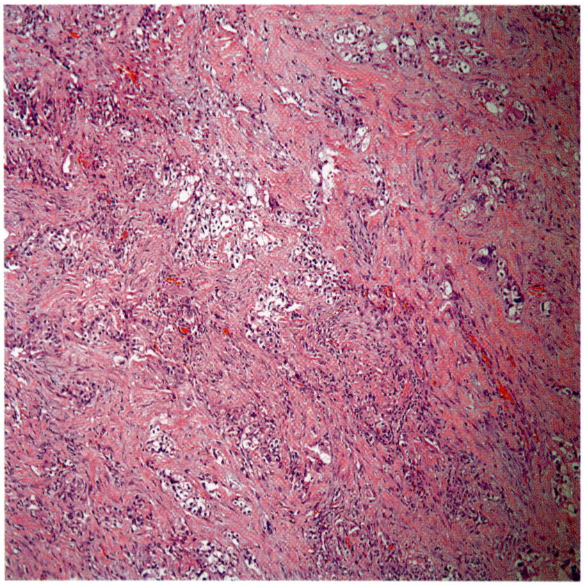

Figure 13-54 Pseudomesotheliomatous adenocarcinoma with extensive collagen deposition infiltrated by clusters of malignant cells.

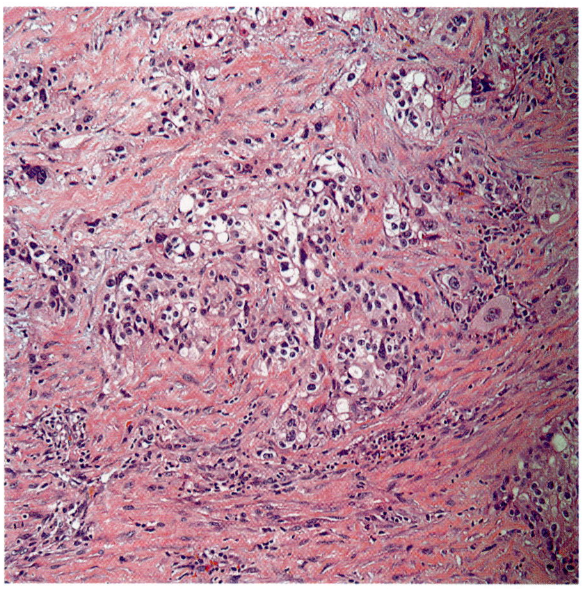

Figure 13-55 Pseudomesotheliomatous adenocarcinoma. A malignant epithelial cell proliferation can be seen within fibroconnective tissue.

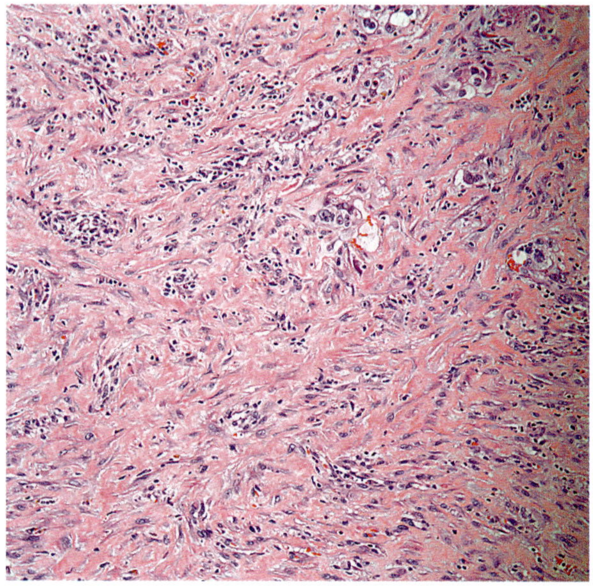

Figure 13-56 Pseudomesotheliomatous adenocarcinoma. Only clusters of malignant cells are present, embedded in fibroconnective tissue with an inflammatory reaction.

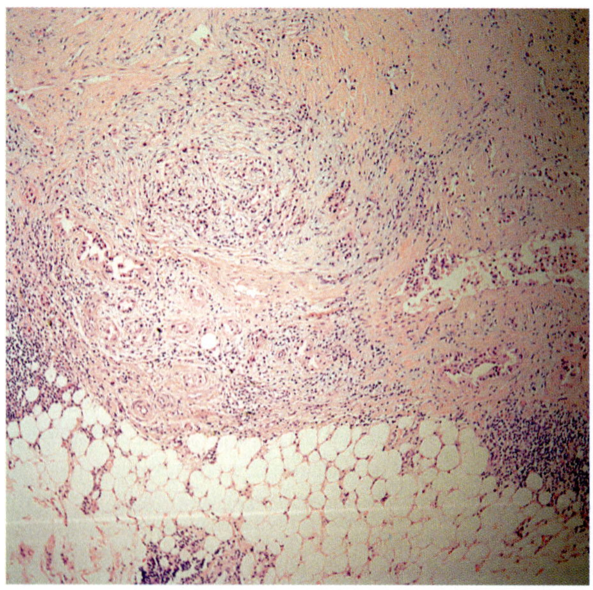

Figure 13-57 Pseudomesotheliomatous adenocarcinoma. Tumor can be seen infiltrating adjacent pleural adipose tissue.

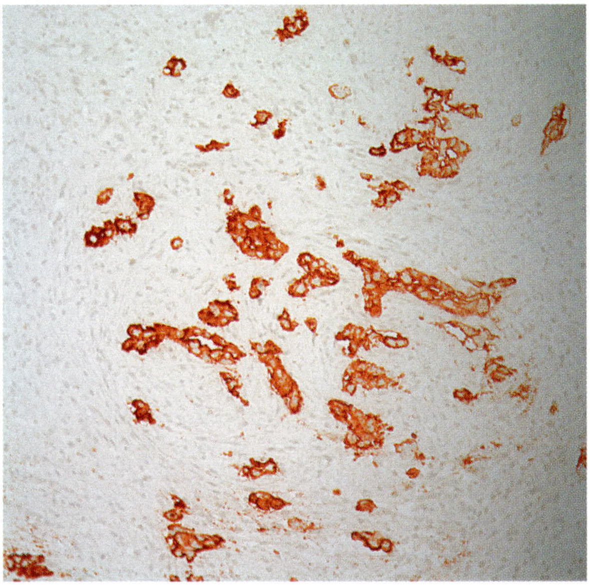

Figure 13-58 Immunohistochemical stain for carcinoembryonic antigen gives a positive reaction in tumor cells of this pseudomesotheliomatous adenocarcinoma.

can be used, these are the ones essential to the practical evaluation of mesothelioma versus adenocarcinoma. If pulmonary adenocarcinoma metastatic to the pleura is not suspected, the use of a wider group of antibodies will be required.

Treatment and Prognosis

Patients with pseudomesotheliomatous adenocarcinomas of the pleura are not candidates for extrapulmonary pneumonectomy. Therefore, it is important to establish the correct interpretation, and to separate pseudomesotheliomatous adenocarcinoma from mesotheliomas. Pseudomesotheliomatous adenocarcinomas are advanced-stage neoplasms (stage IIIb disease). The most common treatment is chemotherapy, and the prognosis is rather poor, with reported survival in larger series of less than 18 months.

THYMOMAS

Thymomas are epithelial tumors more commonly seen in the anterior mediastinum; however, they may occur ectopically in different sites including the head and neck, trachea, thyroid, and lung. In unusual circumstances, the tumor may diffusely involve the pleural surface in a manner similar to that seen with mesotheliomas.[91–95] Anterior mediastinal thymomas may invade the pleura, however; thus, it is important to rule out this possibility before rendering the diagnosis of primary ectopic pleural thymoma. Thymomas growing on the pleural surface in a manner mimicking that of mesotheliomas have been reported sporadically.[96,97] In the recent past, more attention has been given to this unusual presentation of thymomas.[98–105]

Clinical Features

The tumor appears to affect adults, with a mean patient age of 54 years, without predilection for either gender. Patients may present with clinical signs and symptoms of cough, chest pain, fever, or shortness of breath or, more unusually, with myasthenia gravis, or may be completely asymptomatic. On radiographic examination, the tumor may appear as a pleura-based mass or as diffuse pleural thickening similar to that seen in malignant mesothelioma.

Macroscopic Features

The gross appearance of pleural thymomas will depend on the anatomic distribution of the tumor. Tumors that manifest as pleura-based lesions may appear attached to the pleura in a broad-based fashion. The tumor is well circumscribed, of solid consistency, and light tan in color. The cut surface may show a slightly nodular or lobulated appearance. Areas of hemorrhage or necrosis are not common. When the tumor involves the pleura in a diffuse manner, thickening of the pleura by a whitish lesion that appears to spread along the pleural surface is visible.

Histopathologic Features

The histopathologic features of pleural thymomas recapitulate those seen in anterior mediastinal tumors. The tumor may exhibit an admixture of epithelial cells and lymphocytes, predominantly lymphocytic tumor, predominantly epithelial, or a spindle cell tumor (Figs. 13-59 and 13-60). The tumor also may demonstrate lobulation, in which the tumor lobules are separated by fibrous bands and perivascular spaces. In the spindle cell growth pattern, the tumor exhibits a spindle cellular proliferation in a manner reminiscent of hemangiopericytoma. Regardless of growth pattern, increased nuclear atypia and mitotic activity are not features of these tumors.

Immunohistochemical Features

Like thymomas in other locations, the tumor will display positive staining in the epithelial component with keratin antibodies, whereas the lymphocytic component demonstrates positive staining for lymphoid markers, including B cell and T cell markers. In addition, the tumor may occasionally display positive staining in the epithelial component for calretinin or keratin 5/6. Use of epithelial membrane antigen may give either only focal weak staining in thymomas or, in many cases, completely negative reaction in epithelial cells.

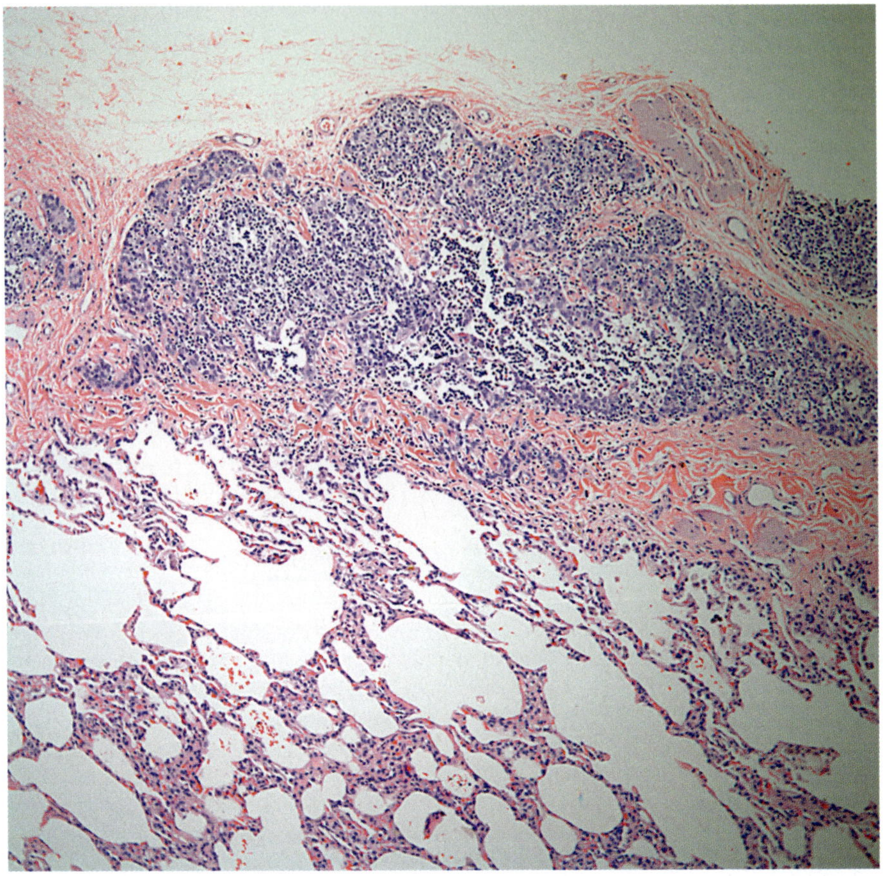

Figure 13-59 Low-power view of a pleural thymoma.

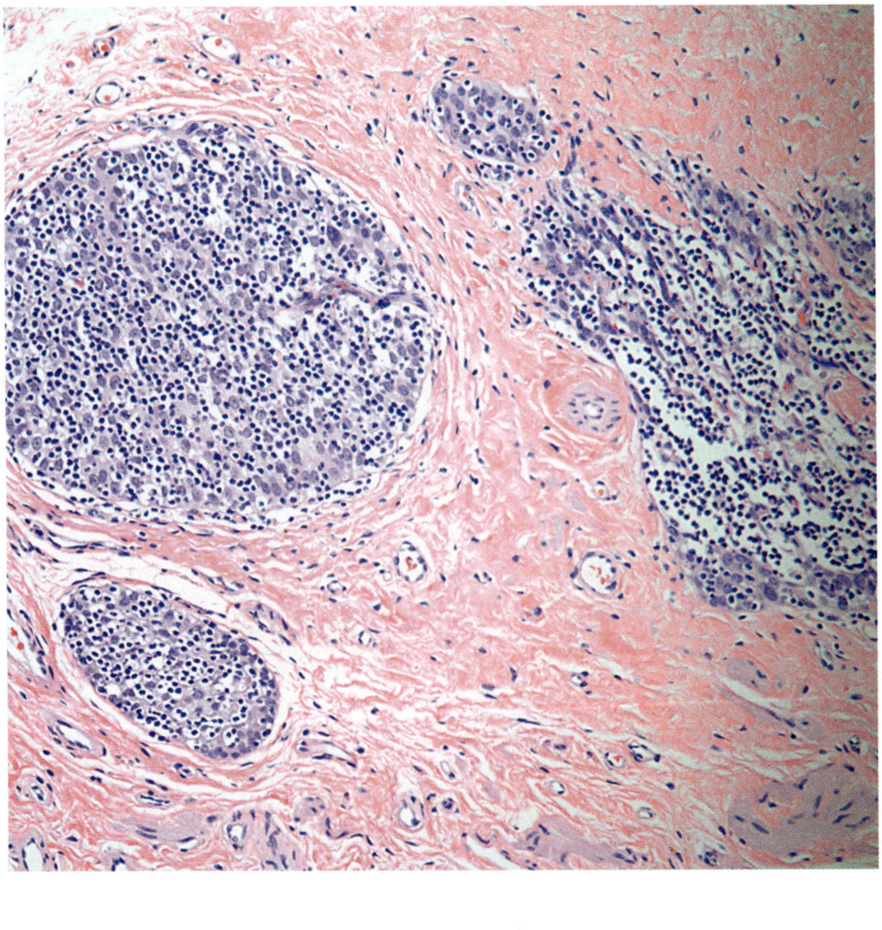

Figure 13-60 Pleural thymoma with classic features of a mixture of lymphocytes and epithelial cells.

Differential Diagnosis

The most important considerations in the differential diagnosis for primary pleural thymomas are mesothelioma and metastatic carcinoma to the pleura. In both cases recognition of a biphasic cellular proliferation composed of lymphocytes and epithelial cells may lead to the correct interpretation. One of the histopathologic variants of mesothelioma, the so-called lymphohistiocytoid mesothelioma, may pose a more difficult diagnostic problem. In this setting, calretinin and keratin 5/6 may cross-react with thymomas. On histopathologic examination, most lymphohistiocytoid mesotheliomas exhibit a spindle cell component embedded in a lymphoid stroma. This finding is unusual for a spindle cell thymoma, which characteristically demonstrates very little lymphoid component. In cases of carcinoma, the absence of marked nuclear atypia or mitotic activity, and of evidence for a pulmonary mass, may lead to the correct interpretation. Lymphomas involving the pleura also may enter into the differential diagnosis; however, the use of keratin antibodies will be of help in this setting. When flow cytometry is performed, it is likely that the results will point to an immature T cell proliferation, which should not be misinterpreted as a T cell neoplasm, because T cells also are components of thymomas.

Treatment and Prognosis

The treatment for pleural thymoma is surgical resection of the tumor. The extent of the surgical procedure will be determined by the extent of disease. When the tumor is a pleura-based mass, it is more amenable to complete resection by a conservative surgical procedure; however, in cases of diffuse pleural involvement, a more radical procedure such as pneumonectomy may be required. The prognosis also will depend on the extent of disease and the status of resectability of the tumor. When the tumor is a pleura-based mass that has been completely removed, the prognosis may be better; for patients with diffuse pleural involvement, in whom the tumor is not amenable to complete surgical resection, the prognosis may not be as good.

ADENOMATOID TUMOR

Adenomatoid tumors can be interpreted as benign mesothelial lesions, which more often occur in the genital tract. In the thoracic cavity, the tumor may appear in the mediastinal compartment or on the pleural surface.[106–108] Adenomatoid tumors occur rarely in the pleura.

Clinical Features

The few cases described to date have been identified in adults at follow-up evaluation for another condition. In the two cases described by Kaplan,[108] one patient had an adenocarcinoma of the lung, and the other had histoplasmosis. Their tumors were found incidentally during surgery and were described as pleural nodules ranging in size from 0.5 to 2.5 cm in greatest dimension.

Histopathologic Features

Like adenomatoid tumors in other sites, pleural tumors are characterized by cords or sheets of medium-sized cells with vacuolated cytoplasm and nuclei displaced to the periphery, almost mimicking a signet ring cell appearance (Figs. 13-61 and 13-62). In other areas, the tumor

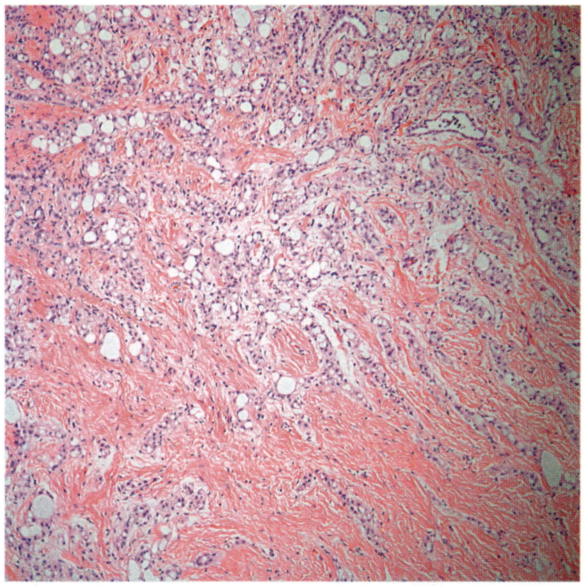

Figure 13-61 Adenomatoid tumor with cords of cells dissecting fibrocollagen.

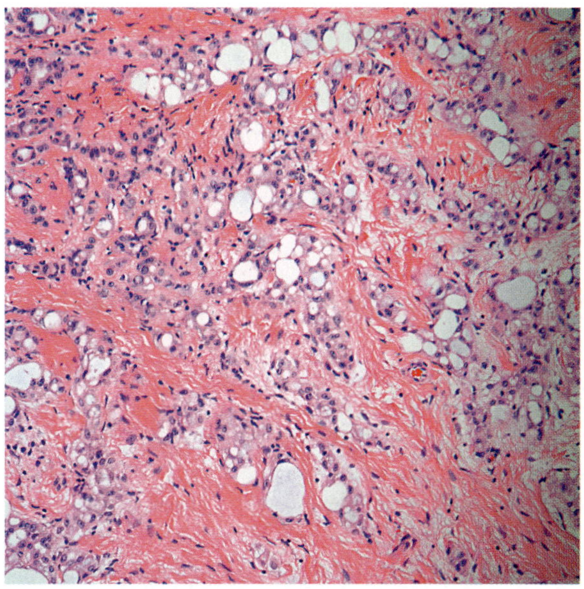

Figure 13-62 Adenomatoid tumor with the classic morphology, almost mimicking a signet ring cell carcinoma.

may exhibit sheets of medium-sized cells with light eosinophilic cytoplasm and round nuclei; in some cells, nucleoli may be seen. The cellular proliferation is embedded in a fibrous stroma, and the cords of cells may be separated by thin fibrocollagenous tissue. The tumor does not exhibit nuclear pleomorphism or increased mitotic activity. Areas of hemorrhage or necrosis are not commonly observed.

Immunohistochemical Features

Adenomatoid tumors and mesotheliomas may share a similar immunohistochemical profile. Adenomatoid tumors may show positive staining for keratin and calretinin, and in some cases for keratin 5/6 as well. The tumor demonstrates negative staining for CEA, CD15, B72.3, and MOC31.

Differential Diagnosis

Adenomatoid tumors should not pose a problem in diagnosis; however, malignant mesotheliomas may show adenomatoid-like areas. This possibility must be assessed by careful documentation of the extent of disease. In malignant mesothelioma, a characteristic finding is diffuse pleural involvement, which has not been the case in documented cases of adenomatoid tumors. Adenocarcinoma also is a possibility; in this setting, however, the use of carcinomatous epitopes such as CEA, CD15, B72.3, and MOC31 would point to the correct interpretation. When epithelioid hemangioendothelioma (EH) is suspected, use of vascular markers such as CD34, CD31, and factor VIII may lead to the correct diagnosis, because adenomatoid tumors demonstrate negative staining for vascular markers.

Treatment and Prognosis

The treatment of choice for these tumors is surgical resection. Because the condition is considered to be benign, complete surgical resection is curative. No cases of metastasis or recurrence have been described.

MUCOEPIDERMOID CARCINOMA

Salivary gland–type tumors have been well documented in the lung parenchyma; however, the presence of similar tumors on the pleural surface is unusual. Thus far, two cases of mucoepidermoid carcinoma manifesting as pleural tumors have been described.[109] Both of the patients were adults, with no previous history of a head and neck neoplasm. Both presented with symptoms of chest pain and shortness of breath. On radiologic examination, the two tumors were described as pleura-based.

Histopathologic Features

In the cases described, histopathologic features were similar to those of tumors arising in the salivary glands. An epithelial cellular proliferation is evident, composed of medium-sized cells with eosinophilic cytoplasm, round nuclei, and in some cases prominent nucleoli. The cellular proliferation has epidermoid features; however, keratinization is not present. Presence of mucus-secreting cells admixed with intermediate cells and epidermoid cells is the hallmark feature in these tumors. Areas of fibrinous pleuritis also may be seen in these cases. The tumor also may contain prominent sclerotic areas, composed of a prominent spindle fibroblastic cellular proliferation with islands of cells that display the classic features of intermediate or epidermoid cells admixed with mucus-secreting cells (mucocytes). This particular pattern is that of the so-called sclerosing mucoepidermoid carcinoma (Figs. 13-63 to 13-65).

Immunohistochemical Features

The diagnosis of mucoepidermoid carcinoma does not require immunohistochemical analysis; however, the tumor may demonstrate positive staining for keratin 5/6, p63, CEA, keratin, and epithelial membrane antigen. This immunophenotype may be seen with either primary or metastatic tumors of the pleura.

Treatment and Prognosis

The treatment of choice is complete surgical resection. Owing to the rarity of this tumor in the pleura, the true pattern of its biologic behavior is difficult to establish. In the cases described, however, both were of low-grade histology; thus, complete surgical resection may be the only treatment needed, and the clinical behavior may be that of an indolent neoplasm.

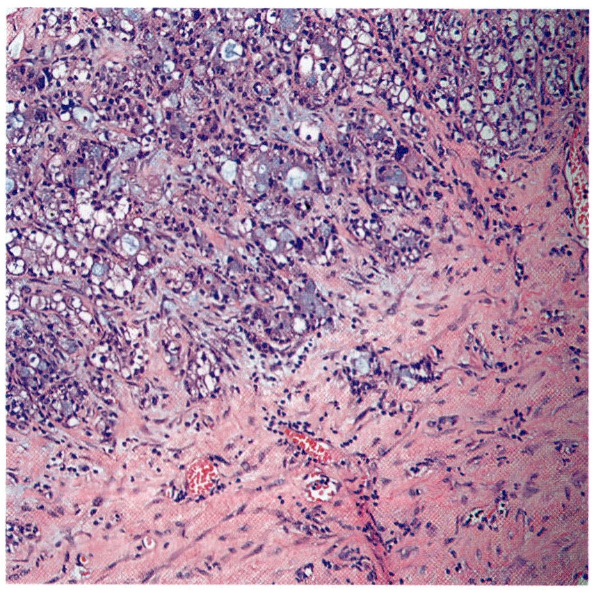

Figure 13-63 Pleural mucoepidermoid carcinoma. Epidermoid cells are seen admixed with mucus-secreting cells.

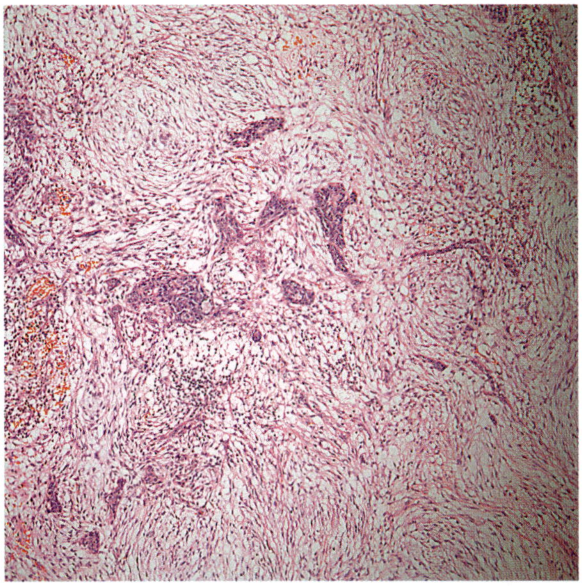

Figure 13-64 Sclerosing mucoepidermoid carcinoma with islands of epithelial cells embedded in a spindle cell fibroblastic stroma.

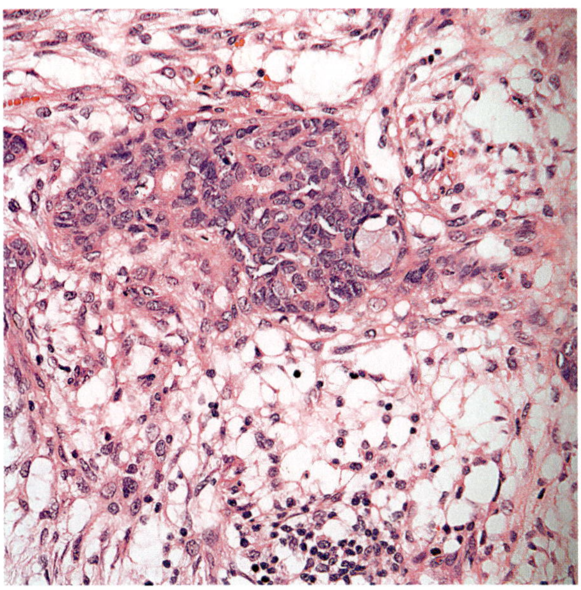

Figure 13-65 Higher-power view of a sclerosing mucoepidermoid carcinoma showing epithelial cells admixed with mucus-secreting cells embedded in a fibroblastic stroma.

PLEUROPULMONARY ENDOMETRIOSIS

The occurrence of ectopic endometrial tissue in the thoracic cavity, mainly along the pleural surface, has been recognized for some time. Although in many cases ectopic endometrial tissue may be an incidental finding, in others it may appear as a pleura-based tumor.[110–114] The endometriosis occasionally may involve only the pleura, or disease of the lung parenchyma may predominate.

Clinical Features

Endometriosis predominantly affects women of reproductive age; however, cases of pleuropulmonary endometriosis have been reported in older women. In the cases described by Flieder and associates,[110] the age range was 27 to 74 years. The most common clinical signs and symptoms include shortness of breath, cough, pleuritic chest pain, and hemoptysis. In some cases, the pleura may be the only affected site, without involvement of pelvic tissues.

Some affected women have no previous history of pregnancy or gynecologic surgery but have received hormonal therapy. On radiologic evaluation, findings in cases limited to the pleura may include evidence of pneumothorax, pulmonary infiltrates, or a distinct pleural nodule (Fig. 13-66). Lesions within the pulmonary parenchyma typically appear as intraparenchymal tumor nodules.

Macroscopic Features

On gross examination, macroscopic features in pulmonary endometriosis may range from strips of hemorrhagic tissue to well-formed small tumors ranging in size from smaller than 1 cm to 3 cm in greatest dimension (Fig. 13-67). Some cases have manifested with large pulmonary masses, however.[114] In general, the lesions may appear cystic and hemorrhagic and well circumscribed but not encapsulated.

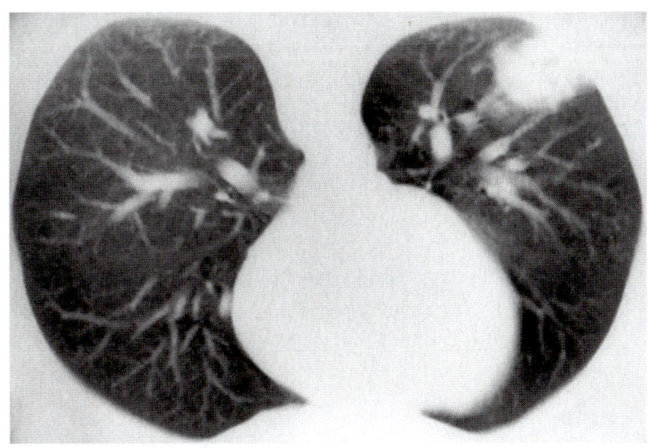

Figure 13-66 Computed tomography scan of the thorax showing a pleural lesion of endometriosis.

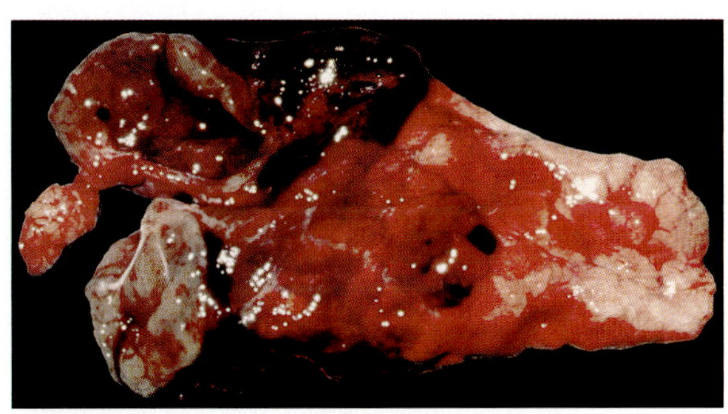

Figure 13-67 Pleural endometriosis in resected specimen. Note the cystic and hemorrhagic lesion.

Histopathologic Features

On histologic examination, pleuropulmonary endometriosis is characterized by proliferative endometrial, glands, in which the glands are lined by columnar, cuboidal, or pseudostratified epithelium with oval nuclei, inconspicuous nucleoli, and scant eosinophilic or clear cytoplasm. Periglandular myxoid changes may be seen in some areas, whereas mitotic activity is invariably present. The stromal tissue is characterized by areas of fibrocollagenous tissue with inflammatory cells, especially plasma cells, although lymphocytes, eosinophils, and macrophages may be seen. The pleural lesions may display a broad-based attachment to the visceral pleura without involvement of the underlying lung parenchyma. Stromal proliferation of vessels may or may not be seen in these cases (Figs. 13-68 to 13-71).

Immunohistochemical Features

Use of immunohistochemical stains may help in the diagnosis of endometriosis, especially in cases in which only a small biopsy specimen is available for evaluation. The glandular and stromal components may show positive staining for estrogen (Fig. 13-72A) and progesterone receptors, broad-spectrum keratin, keratin-7, and WT-1 (Fig. 13-72B). In some cases, the glands also may show positive staining for CEA and for Her-2neu; however, staining for other carcinomatous epitopes, such as CD-15 and B72.3, and neuroendocrine markers appears to be negative.

Differential Diagnosis

Clinical entities to be considered in the differential diagnosis may depend largely on the material available for evaluation, and on the location of the lesion. When the lesion is intrapulmonary and a small, limited biopsy specimen is available, the main consideration will be a malignant glandular proliferation of adenocarcinoma. In this setting, immunohistochemical markers may be of help. When the lesions are in the pleura, the differential diagnosis also will include adenocarcinoma or biphasic mesothelioma, especially when a marked stromal reaction is present. The finding of a small pleura-based nodule would be most unusual for mesothelioma, however. This is another setting in which use of immunohistochemical stains may be of help. Although most cases of endometriosis occur in adult females, one last possible condition to be considered would be pleuropulmonary blastoma. Some cases of endometriosis may manifest with prominent cystic changes and stromal growth, which can be confused with the histopathologic picture in pleuropulmonary

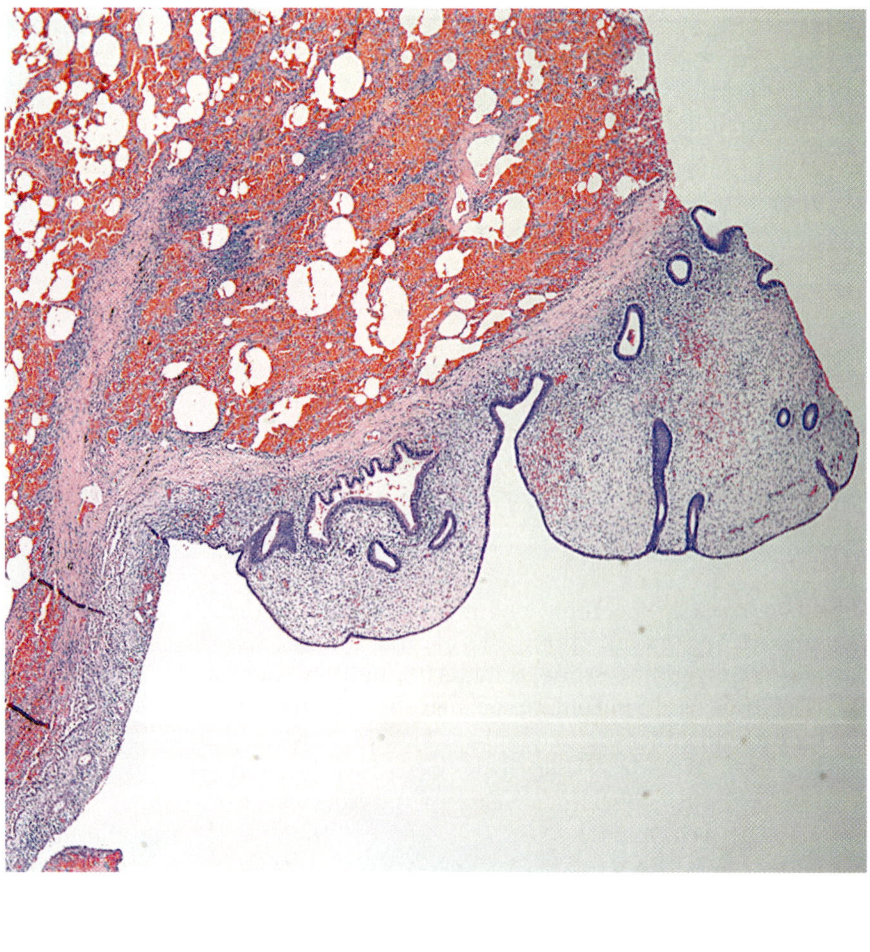

Figure 13-68 Low-power view of endometriosis involving the pleural surface.

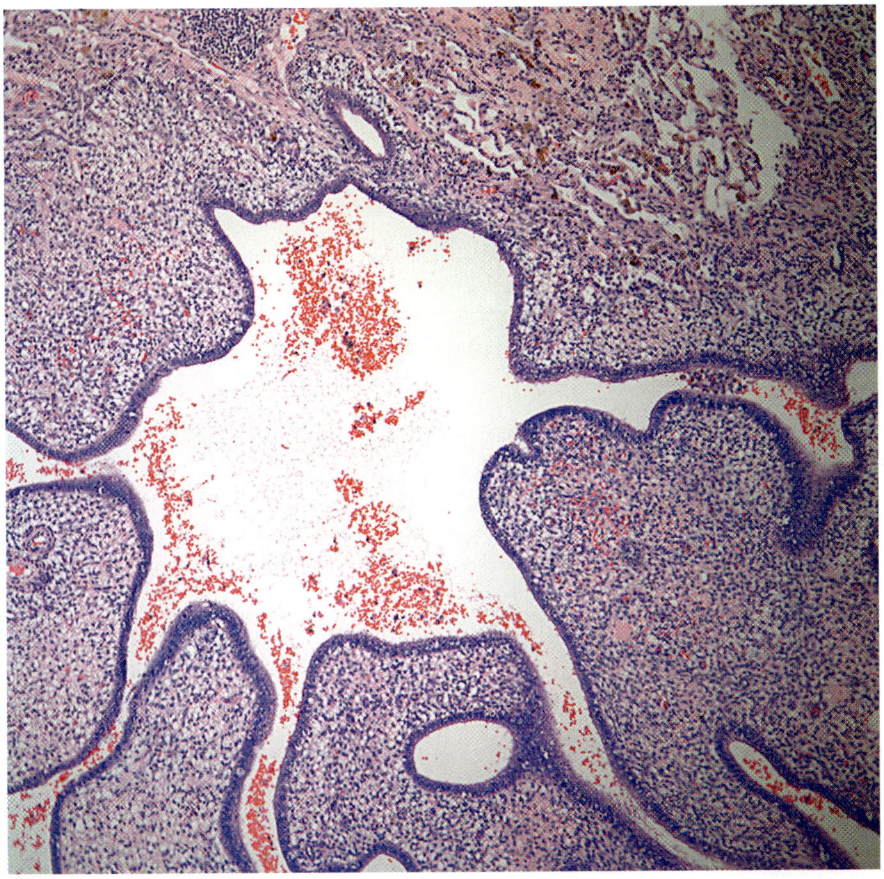

Figure 13-69 Pleural endometriosis showing distended glands.

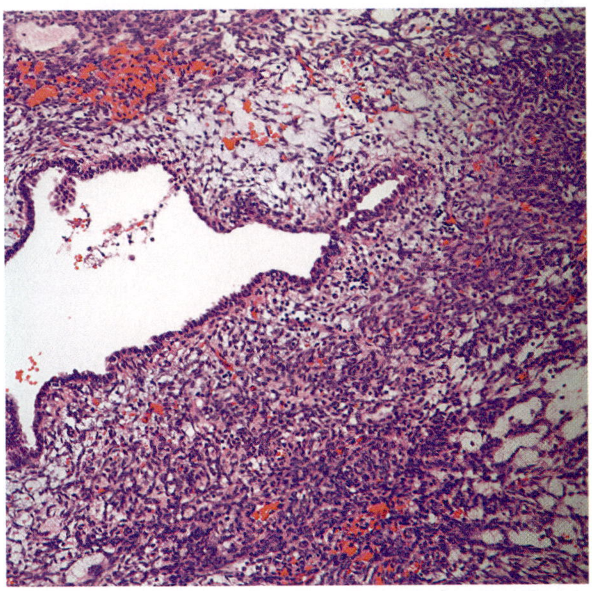

Figure 13-70 Pleural endometriosis showing distended gland with periglandular stromal and myxoid changes.

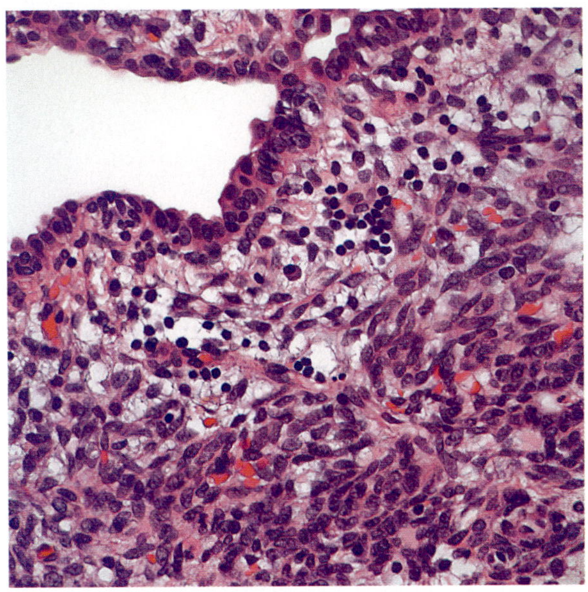

Figure 13-71 Pleural endometriosis. Plasma cells are scattered throughout areas of the stroma.

blastoma. The presence of glands more akin to the proliferative phase of endometrium and the presence of inflammatory cells, especially plasma cells in the stroma, should indicate endometriosis. In addition, the positive staining for estrogen and progesterone receptors, as well as for WT-1, would be most unusual for pleuropulmonary blastoma.

NEUROENDOCRINE TUMORS

Although the vast majority of neuroendocrine tumors occur in an intrapulmonary location, in certain unusual circumstances, so-called carcinoid tumorlets may appear as either a single pleural nodule or multiple pleural nodules (Figs. 13-73 and 13-74). When such tumorlets

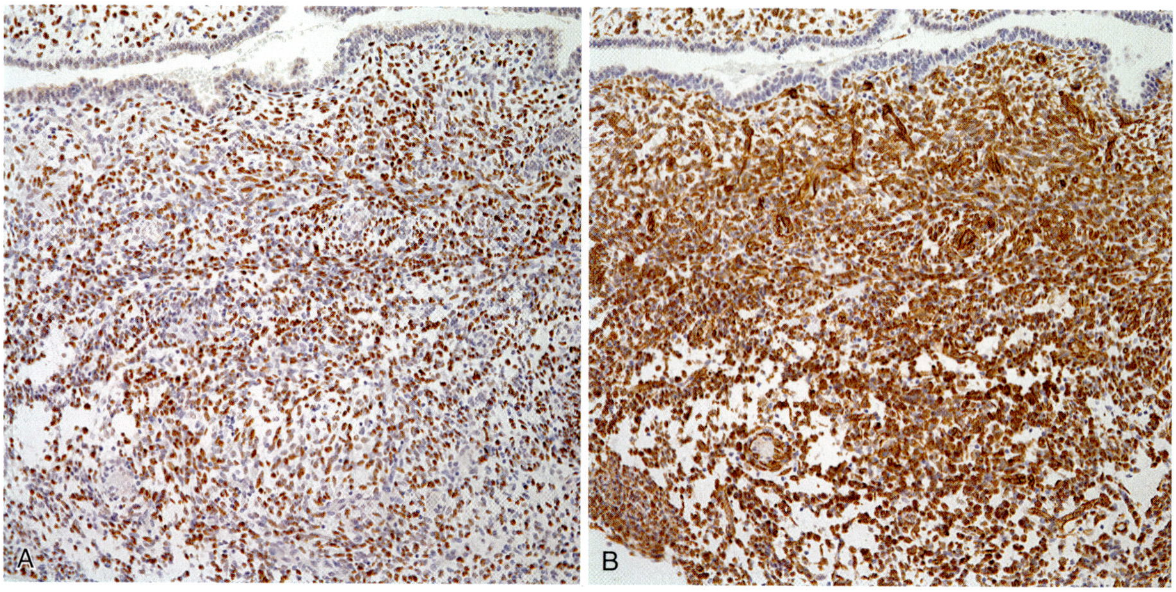

Figure 13-72 **A**, Immunostain for estrogen receptor gives a strong nuclear positive reaction. **B**, Immunohistochemical stain for WT1 gives a positive reaction.

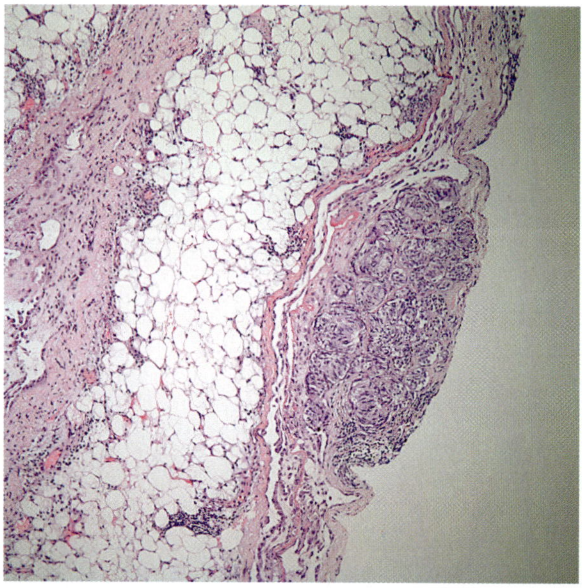

Figure 13-73 Pleura with a neuroendocrine carcinoid tumorlet.

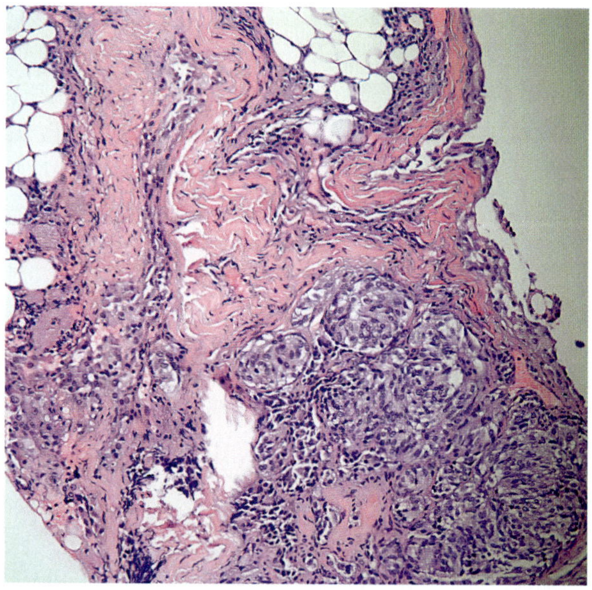

Figure 13-74 High-power view of a pleural carcinoid tumorlet.

are identified, it is important to assess whether an intrapulmonary mass with metastasis to the pleura is present. Otherwise, the diagnostic criteria for pleural carcinoid tumorlets are similar to those for tumors in an intrapulmonary location. The tumor lesions measure less than 0.5 cm in greatest dimension. If the identification is made radiologically, clinical differentiation between primary tumors of the pleura and metastatic disease to the pleura may be more challenging. Nevertheless, the size of the lesions and their immunohistochemical profile will lead to an accurate interpretation.

NON-EPITHELIAL TUMORS OF THE PLEURA

The occurrence of non-epithelial tumors of the pleura is well documented. This category of pleural neoplasms encompasses tumors of differing etiology and a wide spectrum of differentiation, including vascular, muscle, fibrous, neural, and neuroectodermal tumors, among others. Their diagnosis requires familiarity with the histopathologic features of the individual tumors, as well as an appropriate level of clinical suspicion, because most of these tumors are rarely seen as primary pleural neoplasms. Therefore, it is important to consider them in the differential diagnosis for tumors of the pleura, despite their rarity.

VASCULAR TUMORS

The two most important vascular tumors are angiosarcoma and EH. Although these tumors share a common immunophenotype, the histopathologic features may be different enough to permit proper classification. Because of the manner in which these tumors involve the pleura, some investigators have linked them to epithelial tumors of similar presentation identified as pseudomesotheliomatous adenocarcinoma, using terms such as *pseudomesotheliomatous angiosarcoma* or *hemangioendothelioma*. Such attempts at analogy illustrate the difficulty in use of clinical and radiologic criteria to distinguish these tumors from conventional mesotheliomas or adenocarcinomas involving the pleural surface.

Epithelioid Hemangioendothelioma

The classic presentation of EH is one of multiple bilateral pulmonary nodules; less commonly, however, involvement of the pleura may closely resemble that seen with mesothelioma. The tumor appears to affect men and women older than 45 years of age, who present with clinical signs and symptoms that may include chest pain, weight loss, cough, fever, or pleural effusion. Such constellations of clinical manifestations are rather nonspecific and may be seen with diverse lung or pleural tumors. Radiologic features that have been reported in cases of EH include unilateral pleural effusions and nodular pleural thickening, similar to that seen in cases of mesothelioma.[115] In some instances, even though the patient may present with a pleural effusion, the tumor may not necessarily be located in the pleura, but may be seen to involve adjacent structures such as the diaphragm.[116]

In addition, patients with pleural EH may have a history of asbestos exposure.[117] In most of these cases, microscopic study has not disclosed the presence of the ferruginous bodies that would be seen in cases of mesothelioma; therefore, the association of asbestos and EH of the pleura remains undetermined. This neoplasm also may manifest with unusual features such as bilateral pleural tumor with extension into the peritoneum,[118] or as a primary pleural tumor with metastasis to the skin.[119] In 1996, Lin and colleagues[120] reported 14 cases of what they termed malignant vascular tumors of the serous membranes mimicking mesothelioma, 8 of which occurred in the pleura. The mean patient age was 52 years, and all were male, except for two female patients with peritoneal tumors. In all patients with pleural tumors, radiologic examination revealed diffuse pleural thickening and pleural effusion, and in one of these patients a 1.5-cm solitary subpleural tumor also was identified, whereas another had a previous history of EH involving bone and at presentation was found to have pleural disease mimicking mesothelioma. At least two patients had a history of asbestos exposure, which could not be confirmed by histologic means.

Histopathologic Features

The histopathologic features of pleural EH are the same as those observed when the tumor occurs in the lung or outside of the thoracic cavity. Essentially, the tumor is composed of strands, cords, or solid areas of epithelioid cells composed of round to oval to spindle cells with a myxoid or hyalinized stromal component. The cells may show a nucleus toward the periphery, giving the appearance of signet ring–like cells. Mitotic index is not high and nuclear pleomorphism is mild. In some cases, areas forming intracellular lumens containing red cells may be seen. A case of pleural EH with prominent rhabdoid features has been described.[121] The cellular proliferation appears to be embedded in a collagenous background, and in some instances it may extend into adjacent adipose tissue, in a manner similar to that for epithelioid mesotheliomas (Figs. 13-75 to 13-78).

Immunohistochemical Features

The use of vascular markers such as CD34, CD31 (Fig. 13-79), and factor VIII is important and will help in demonstrating the vascular nature of this tumor; in some cases, however, the tumor cells also may demonstrate focally

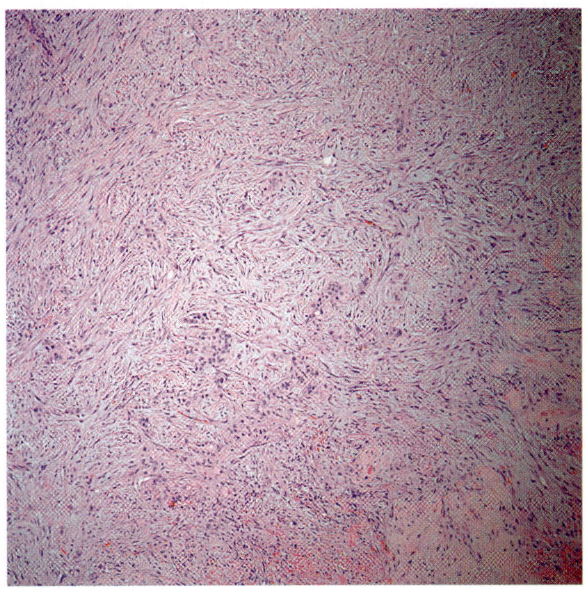

Figure 13-75 Low-power view of a pleural epithelioid hemangioendothelioma. Note the presence of abundant collagenous material.

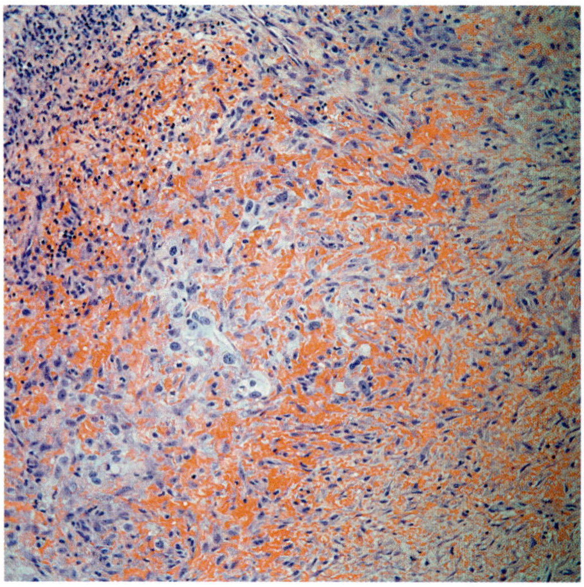

Figure 13-76 Pleural epithelioid hemangioendothelioma exhibiting spindle cells admixed with red cells.

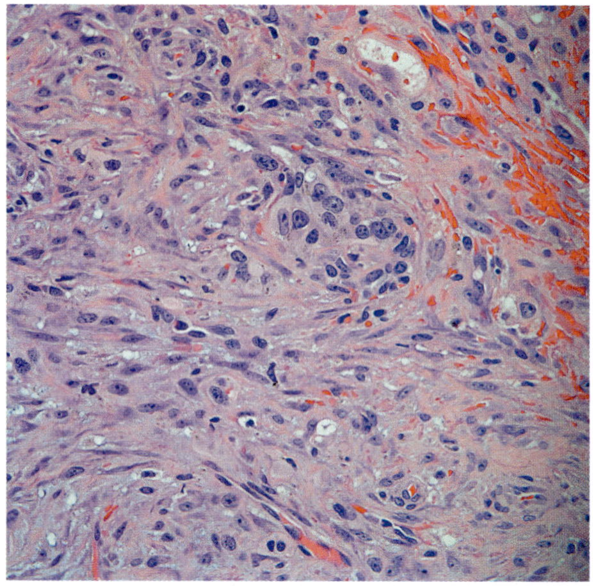

Figure 13-77 High-power view of the spindle cell component of a pleural epithelioid hemangioendothelioma showing absence of mitotic activity and marked nuclear atypia.

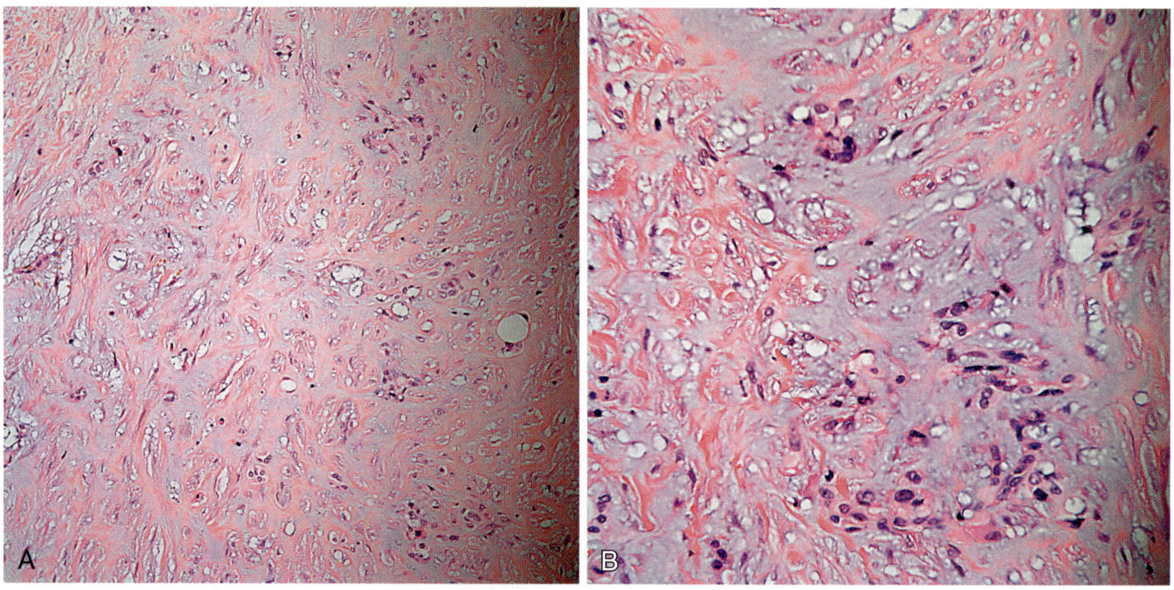

Figure 13-78 Epithelioid hemangioendothelioma. **A**, Tumor exhibiting the classic features of a chondroid-like background. **B**, High-power view of the epithelioid cells embedded in a chondroid-like stroma.

or weakly positive staining for epithelial markers such as keratin. Therefore, it is crucial that the staining for the vascular markers previously mentioned be included in the panel of immunohistochemical studies whenever this tumor is suspected. In addition, EH appears to show strong positive reaction for vimentin.

Differential Diagnosis

Because of the similarity of clinical and radiologic findings for EH and epithelial tumors, it is important to rule out the possibility of an epithelial tumor, especially mesothelioma or adenocarcinoma involving the pleural surface. In this setting, immunohistochemical studies including vascular and epithelial markers should lead to the correct interpretation. Histopathologic diagnosis may be more challenging with small biopsy specimens, in which the characteristic microscopic features of EH may not be apparent. In such instances, the use of immunohistochemical studies may be more helpful, mainly in cases in which reactivity for the conventional epithelial markers is negative and the histologic character of the tumor is not the conventional one of mesothelioma or adenocarcinoma. One other condition that may present a diagnostic chal-

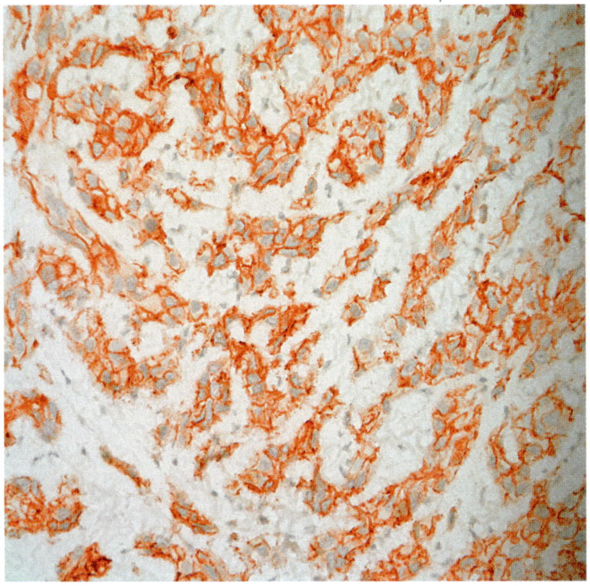

Figure 13-79 Immunohistochemical staining for CD31 gives a strong positive reaction in tumor cells of this epithelioid hemangioendothelioma.

lenge is adenomatoid tumor. Once again, adenomatoid tumor may demonstrate positive staining for markers such as calretinin and keratin and negative staining for vascular markers including CD31, CD34, and factor VIII.

Treatment and Prognosis

The treatment of choice for these tumors is surgical resection; however, the issue may be more complicated when the pathologic findings include extensive involvement of the pleura with encasement of the lung, which may necessitate use of extrapleural pneumonectomy or adjuvant treatment with chemotherapy. Such decisions are based on patient factors, such as age and comorbidity, and on the radiologic findings.

The prognosis will be defined by the extent of the tumor. A pleura-based nodule or mass that is amenable to complete surgical resection carries a better prognosis than cases with extensive involvement of the pleura. In the cases reported by Lin and coworkers,[120] a majority of the patients died of their disease.

Angiosarcoma

Angiosarcomas more commonly are seen as primary tumors of the soft tissues, which may include the chest wall. They also have been reported as primary pleural tumors that clinically and radiologically may mimic pleural mesothelioma. Therefore, a histopathologic assessment is necessary to arrive at this particular diagnosis.

In 1997, Falconieri and asociates[122] reported two autopsy cases of "diffuse pleuropulmonary angiosarcoma simulating mesothelioma." According to the clinical description, the tumors grew along the serosal surfaces, and were characterized by thick rinds of tissue encasing the lung. Thus, the investigators concluded that on rare occasions, angiosarcomas may involve the pleura in a manner similar to that described for mesotheliomas. Clinical signs and symptoms associated with pleural angiosarcoma may include hemothorax, chest pain, cough, hemoptysis, and shortness of breath.[123–128] Pleural angiosarcomas described in the Japanese literature have been linked with tuberculous pyothorax.[129,130] In a radiologic investigation, Frate and colleagues[131] reported computed tomography (CT) and positron emission tomography (PET) features of an angiosarcoma in which the chest films showed circumferential right-sided pleural thickening. A PET scan performed for staging purposes showed multiple lobulated focal areas of increased uptake, similar to those seen on the CT scan.

In a series of 5 cases of epithelioid angiosarcomas of the pleura, Zhang and coworkers[132] reported an age range of 22 to 79 years, with a male-to-female ratio of 9:1. In Western cases diagnosed as pleural angiosarcomas, no history of tuberculous pyothorax was present, in contrast with the Japanese cases, whereas a history of asbestos exposure was available for some of the Western patients. The investigators also raised some questions about cases in which the neoplasm had been identified as pleural EH, noting that some if not all of those cases may represent epithelioid angiosarcoma.

Histopathologic Features

The histopathologic features of pleural angiosarcomas are similar to those described for such tumors in the soft tissues. The tumor may be composed of sheets, strands, or cords of epithelioid cells embedded in a collagenous or hyalinized stroma. The neoplastic cellular proliferation is composed of round to oval cells with a moderate amount of light eosinophilic cytoplasm, round nuclei, and small nucleoli. The cells appear to be plump in comparison with those in a histiocytic or epithelioid cellular proliferation. Necrosis or areas of hemorrhage may be present. Mitotic figures may be readily seen, and nuclear atypia is common. The neoplastic cellular proliferation also may be seen infiltrating adjacent adipose tissue (Figs. 13-80 to 13-85).

Immunohistochemical Features

Angiosarcomas display similar immunophenotype to EH. Staining for vascular markers including CD31, CD34, and factor VIII usually is positive in tumor cells; however, staining for cytokeratin and CEA may be focal or weakly positive.[132] Therefore, the use of a complete panel including vascular and epithelial markers is indicated for tumor evaluation when pleural angiosarcoma is suspected.

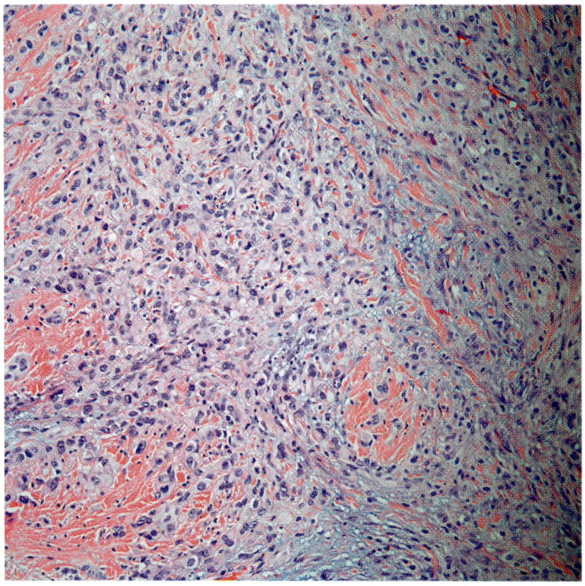

Figure 13-80 Pleural angiosarcoma with sheets of epithelioid cells.

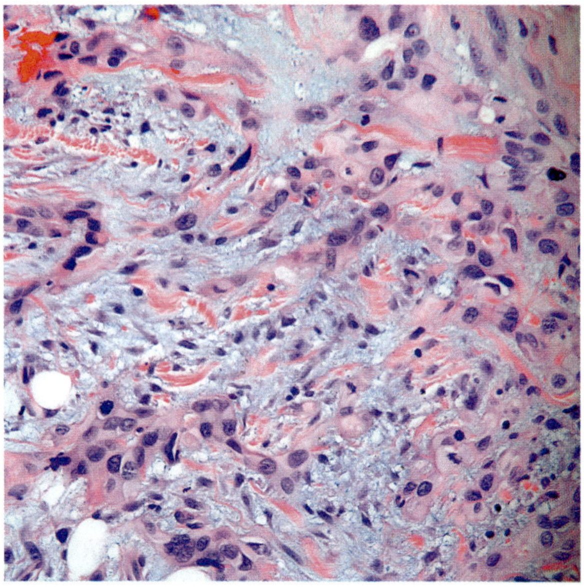

Figure 13-81 Pleural angiosarcoma with readily identifiable mitotic figures.

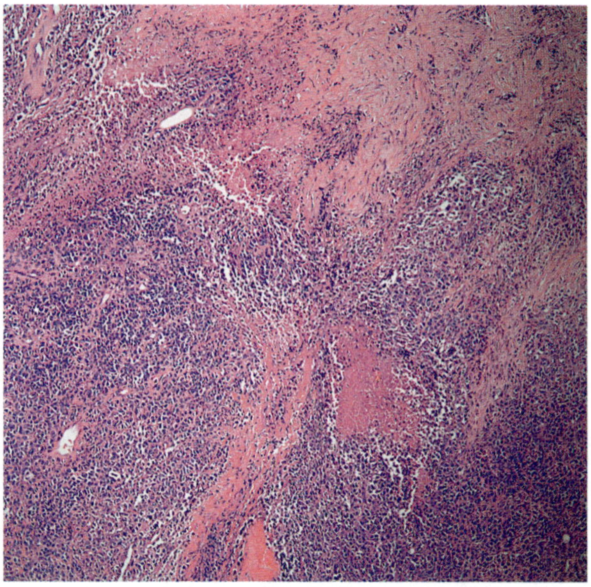

Figure 13-82 Pleural angiosarcoma with areas of necrosis.

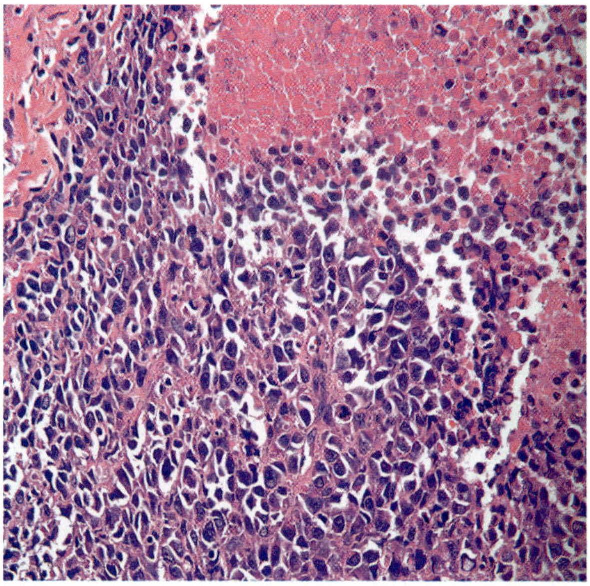

Figure 13-83 High-grade angiosarcoma of the pleura with prominent nuclear atypia and mitotic figures.

Treatment and Prognosis

Surgical resection of the tumor and chemotherapy have been attempted; however, the prognosis is still poor. Metastasis to distant organs, including brain, has been documented in some cases.

FIBROBLASTIC TUMORS

The following tumors are the three most important clinical entities in the family of fibroblastic neoplasms:

- Solitary fibrous tumor (SFT)
- Calcifying fibrous pseudotumor (CFPT)
- Desmoid tumor

Solitary Fibrous Tumor

SFT is a tumor of ubiquitous distribution, and it has been described in diverse anatomic areas including the thorax, head and neck, soft tissue, and viscera.[133–136] Several terms have been coined for this tumor, including *localized fibrous mesothelioma*, *submesothelial fibroma*, and *fibrous mesothelioma*. Recognition of this tumor as a separate clinicopathologic

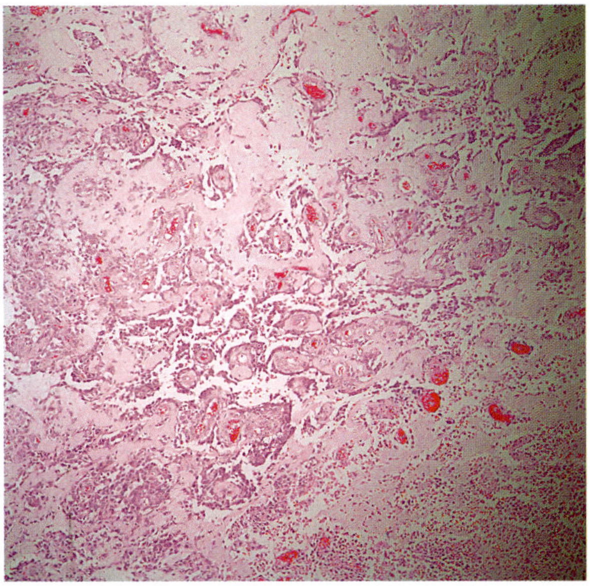

Figure 13-84 Pleural angiosarcoma with more conventional features.

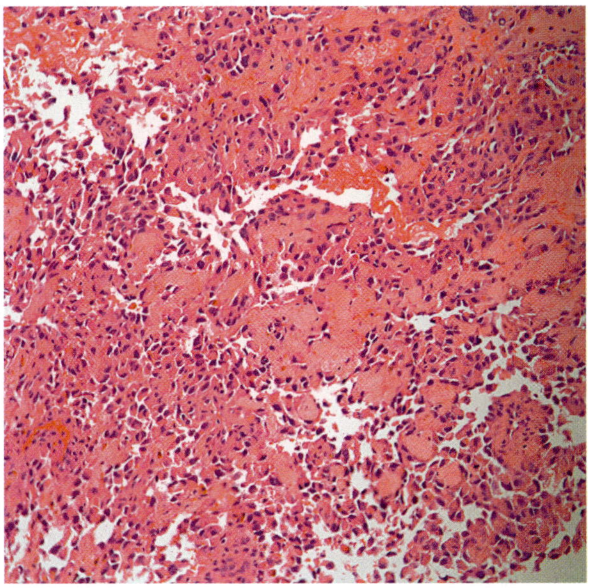

Figure 13-85 Vascular spaces can still be identified in this pleural angiosarcoma.

entity in the pleura is credited to Klemperer and Rabin,[8] who distinguished SFT from the conventional diffuse pleural tumors, and stated that its behavior also differed from tumors involving the pleura in a diffuse manner. Although some debate has emerged regarding the histogenesis of these tumors, ultrastructural studies have suggested a fibroblastic origin, rather than a mesothelial origin. Currently, the tumor is well recognized as a distinct clinicopathologic entity, but only a few large series documenting its clinical, histopathologic, immunohistochemical, and behavioral features have been published.[137–145]

Clinical Features

SFT does not have any predilection for either gender and has been described in patients of various ages ranging from younger than 10 years to older than 80 years; however, the tumor appears to be most common in the sixth decade of life. Presenting signs and symptoms may include cough, chest pain, pleural effusion, shortness of breath, hemoptysis, and general malaise. One important clinical finding in patients with SFT is hypoglycemia, which may be present in approximately 10% of cases. Approximately 25% of patients present with no symptoms, and the tumor is detected during a routine radiographic examination. On radiographic evaluation, SFT, as the "solitary" in its name implies, is seen to be a pleura-based tumor that appears to involve the visceral pleura more often and also may involve the parietal pleura.

Macroscopic Features

A majority of these neoplasms are described as sharply circumscribed or encapsulated polypoid tumors attached to the pleura by a short pedicle (Fig. 13-86). Tumor size may range from 1 cm to more than 25 cm in greatest dimension. The cut surface is tan-white and whorled in appearance, with a rubbery consistency, and exhibits areas of fibrosis. Other features may include necrosis, hemorrhage, and cystic changes, which have been associated with malignant tumors. Some tumors are attached to the pleura not by a pedicle but rather by a broad base (Fig. 13-87), whereas some other tumors are described as exhibiting inward growth with compression and displacement of the lung.

Histopathologic Features

SFT has a wide range of microscopic features, and in many cases more than one pattern may be observed. The two main growth patterns are solid spindle and diffuse sclerosing. Of these two patterns, the solid spindle is the most versatile, because the tumors may exhibit a wide range of

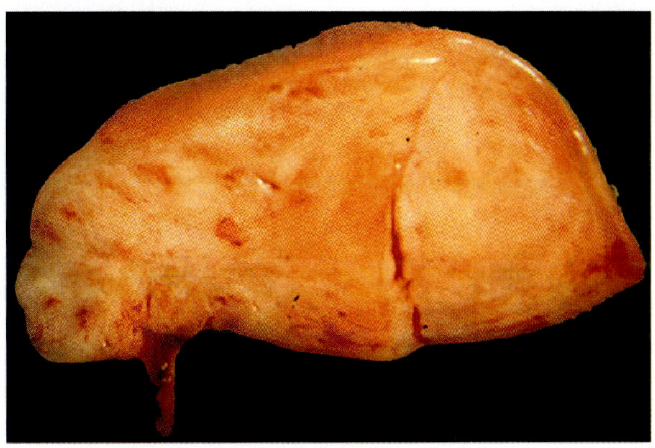

Figure 13-86 Solitary fibrous tumor of the pleura in resected specimen. Note the short pedicle.

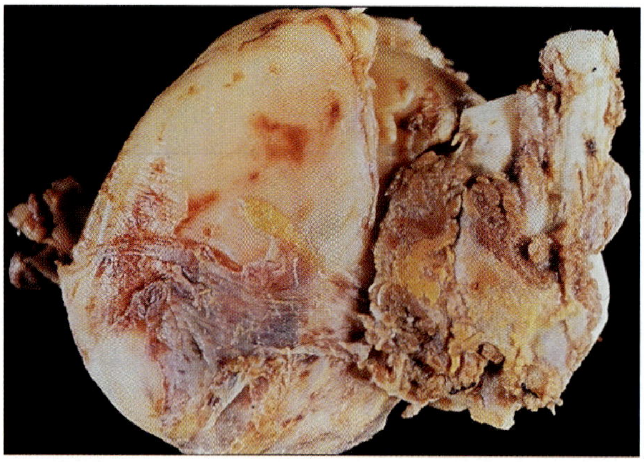

Figure 13-87 Solitary fibrous tumor of the pleura, gross specimen. Note the broad-based attachment with compression of lung parenchyma.

microscopic features that are commonly observed in other mesenchymal neoplasms, including short storiform (the so-called patternless pattern), angiofibroma-like, hemangiopericytoma-like, fibrosarcoma-like (herringbone pattern), monophasic synovial sarcoma–like, and neural-like (Figs. 13-88 to 13-94).[144] Other tumors are characterized by extensive collagenization, which often has a rope-like appearance. Based on these histopathologic growth patterns, the finding of a tumor showing hypo- and hypercellular areas, ectatic blood vessels, spindle cells mimicking any known spindle cell sarcoma, and areas of extensive collagenization would indicate SFT. These different histopathologic patterns are more readily apparent in material obtained at complete surgical resection than in small limited biopsy specimens. In some cases, the tumor may infiltrate into the peripheral lung parenchyma or mediastinal structures.

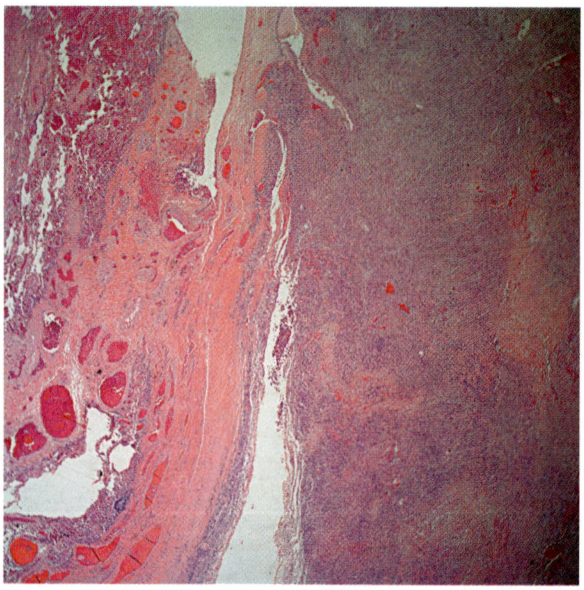

Figure 13-88 Low-power view of a solitary fibrous tumor of the pleura. Note the pleura-based location of the tumor.

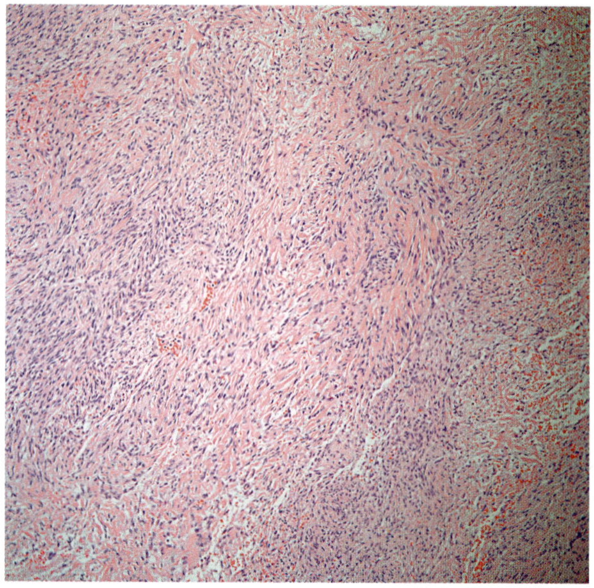

Figure 13-89 Solitary fibrous tumor of the pleura with the classic spindle cell component admixed with collagen fibers.

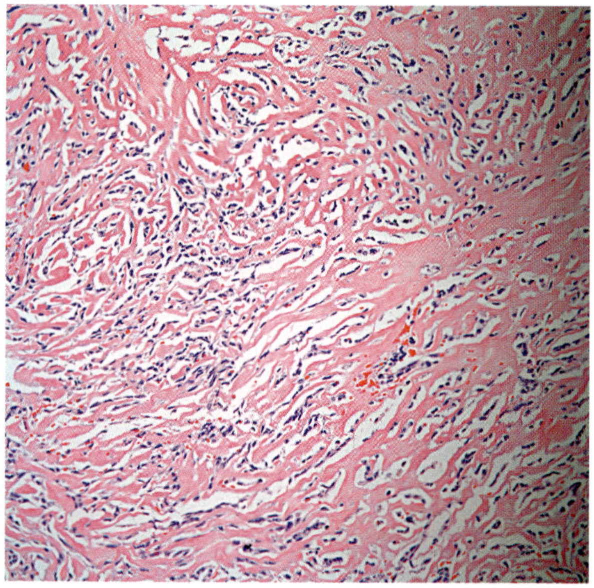

Figure 13-90 Solitary fibrous tumor of the pleura with extensive areas of rope-like collagen.

England and colleagues[140] divided SFTs into histologically benign and malignant tumors on the basis of the presence of mitotic activity (more than 4 mitotic figures per 10 high-power fields), high degree of cellularity, pleomorphism, hemorrhage, and necrosis. Of the 223 cases presented in this study, 141 were classified as benign and 82 were classified as malignant. Other criteria, such as size of the tumor and clinical findings, may not completely correlate with clinical behavior; however, a logical assumption is that the larger the tumor, the more likely it is to infiltrate adjacent structures and therefore be less amenable to complete surgical resection.

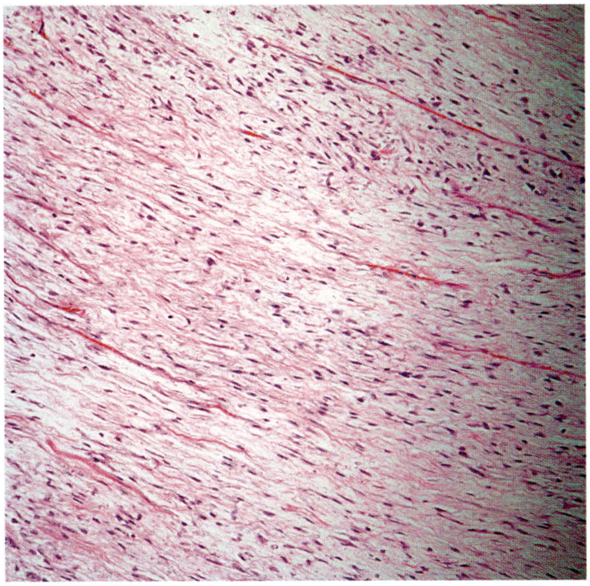

Figure 13-91 Solitary fibrous tumor with a neurofibroma-like pattern.

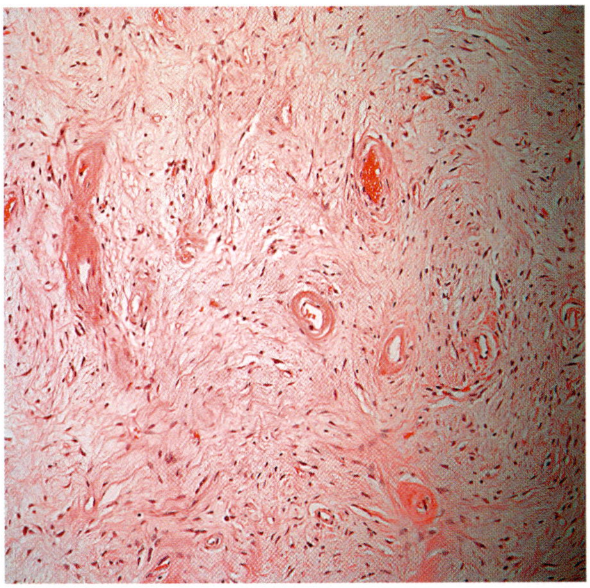

Figure 13-92 Solitary fibrous tumor of the pleura with an angiofibroma-like pattern.

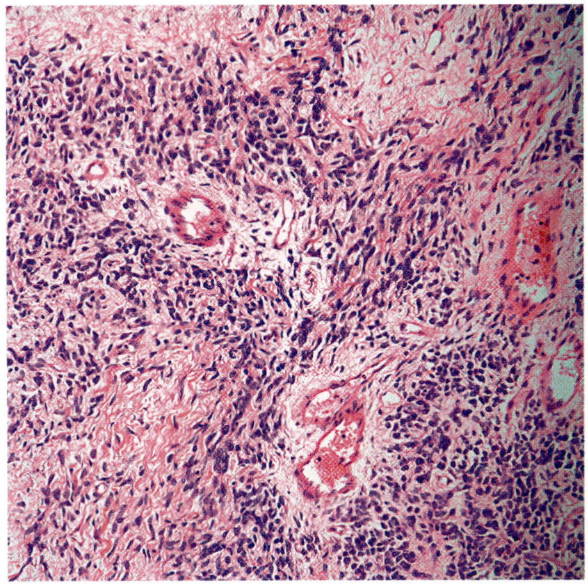

Figure 13-93 Solitary fibrous tumor of the pleura with neural-like features.

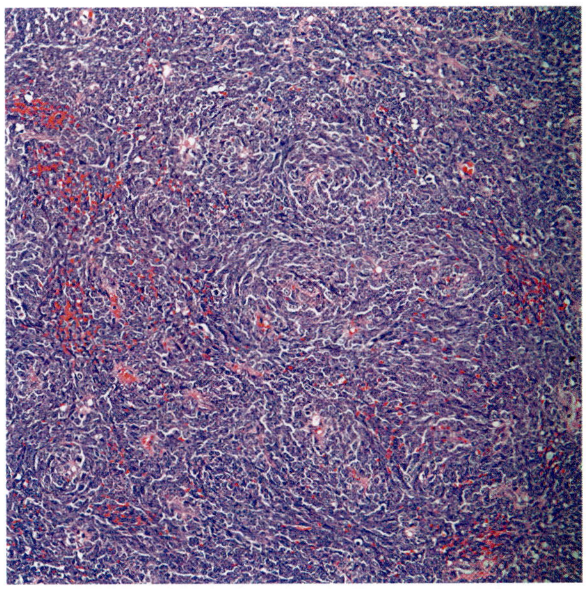

Figure 13-94 Solitary fibrous tumor of the pleura with a monophasic synovial sarcoma–like growth pattern.

Immunohistochemical Features

The most consistently positive immunohistochemical stains in SFT include those for vimentin, CD34, and Bcl-2; however, staining for smooth muscle actin and desmin may be weakly positive or affect only scattered cells. Immunohistochemical staining for keratin, EMA, S-100 protein, factor VIII, and CD31 generally is negative. When the tumor infiltrates the periphery of the lung, entrapment of lung parenchyma may occur that will show positive staining for keratin antibodies.

Differential Diagnosis

The histopathologic features of SFT may mimic those of several mesenchymal neoplasms, including synovial sarcoma, angiofibroma, and neural tumors. The presence of more than one growth pattern in the same tumor and the use of immunohistochemical markers, especially CD34 and Bcl-2, and negative staining for S-100 protein and epithelial or other vascular markers should aid in the diagnosis of SFT. With limited biopsy material, the nature of the lesion may not be readily recognized;

therefore, extensive sampling is recommended in evaluation of these tumors to permit appreciation of the different growth patterns.

Treatment and Prognosis

The treatment of choice for SFT is complete surgical resection. The tumor's behavior can be estimated according to its resectability, as well as the histologic evaluation. Tumors that are attached to the pleura by a pedicle, despite the worrisome histology, may not follow an aggressive course. In 45% of the cases designated as malignant tumors by England and associates,[140] the patients apparently were cured by complete surgical resection. These patients were described as having pedunculated, well-circumscribed tumors. Of those patients in whom the tumors were designated as malignant, 55% died after a clinical course marked by recurrence and metastasis. As noted by the investigators, these findings suggest that resectability is the single most important indicator of clinical behavior. Similarly, Briselli and colleagues[139] concluded that nuclear pleomorphism and high mitotic rate do not necessarily indicate poor prognosis if the tumor is circumscribed.

Desmoid Tumor

Desmoid tumors are neoplasms of ubiquitous distribution that are commonly seen in intra-abdominal locations or involving the musculature of the shoulder, chest wall, or back.[145,146] Tumors in the chest wall usually are in extrathoracic locations, and patients present with a palpable mass. Desmoid tumors of the chest wall with pleural involvement have been reported[147]; however, primary pleural desmoid tumors are rather rare and have been recorded in only a few series of cases.[148,149]

Clinical Features

The tumor appears to affect persons ranging in age from 16 to 66 years, without gender predilection. Patients may present with clinical signs and symptoms of chest pain, shortness of breath, and cough. In some cases, a history of trauma has been obtained. On radiologic examination, the tumors appear as pleura-based neoplasms that may involve either visceral or parietal pleura.

Macroscopic Features

The tumors are well circumscribed and not pedunculated and have a glistening surface and firm consistency. The tumors range in size from 5 cm to more than 15 cm in greatest dimension (Fig. 13-95). The cut surface is white-grayish and bosselated in appearance, and areas of necrosis and hemorrhage are not common.

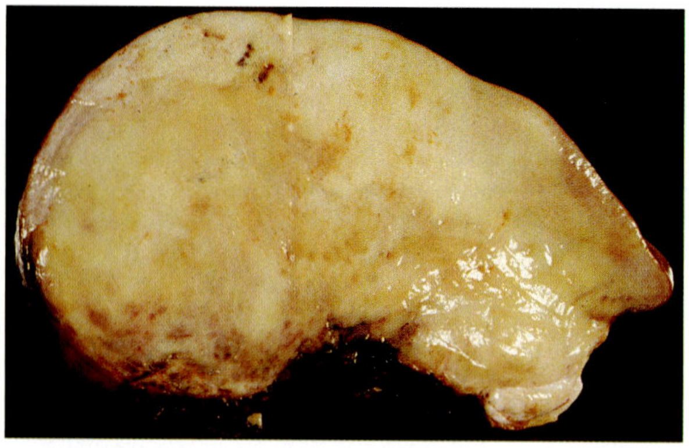

Figure 13-95 Desmoid tumor of the pleura, gross specimen. The tumor is well circumscribed, with a firm consistency.

Histopathologic Features

The morphologic features of desmoid tumors of the pleura are essentially the same as those described for desmoid tumors in other locations. The tumor characteristically shows intersecting fascicles of spindle cells with tapered, wavy to elongated nuclei and without nuclear atypia. The cells are seen in a background of a collagenous or finely fibrillary matrix (Fig. 13-96). Numerous blood vessels with either thin or thick walls are invariably present. These tumors appear to have infiltrative borders; however, they usually do not exhibit prominent nuclear atypia, mitotic activity, hemorrhage, or necrosis.

Immunohistochemical Features

Pleural tumors have been shown to demonstrate positive staining for vimentin and actin and also may show focal positive staining for desmin. Positive staining for B-catenin and cytoplasmic staining for cyclin D1 also have been reported. In general, desmoid tumors demonstrate negative staining for epithelial markers, CD34, and S-100 protein.

Differential Diagnosis

The most important consideration in the differential diagnosis is SFT. In this setting, the use of immunohistochemical studies may prove beneficial, because desmoid tumors generally demonstrate negative staining for CD34 and Bcl-2, whereas SFT usually demonstrates positive staining for these markers. Although SFT may show focal positive staining for actin, desmoid usually will show a strong positive reaction.

Treatment and Prognosis

The treatment of choice is complete surgical resection with negative margins. Therefore, complete surgical resection is the most important parameter in the evaluation of clinical behavior. Those patients with tumors that are not amenable to complete resection eventually will experience recurrence of their disease.

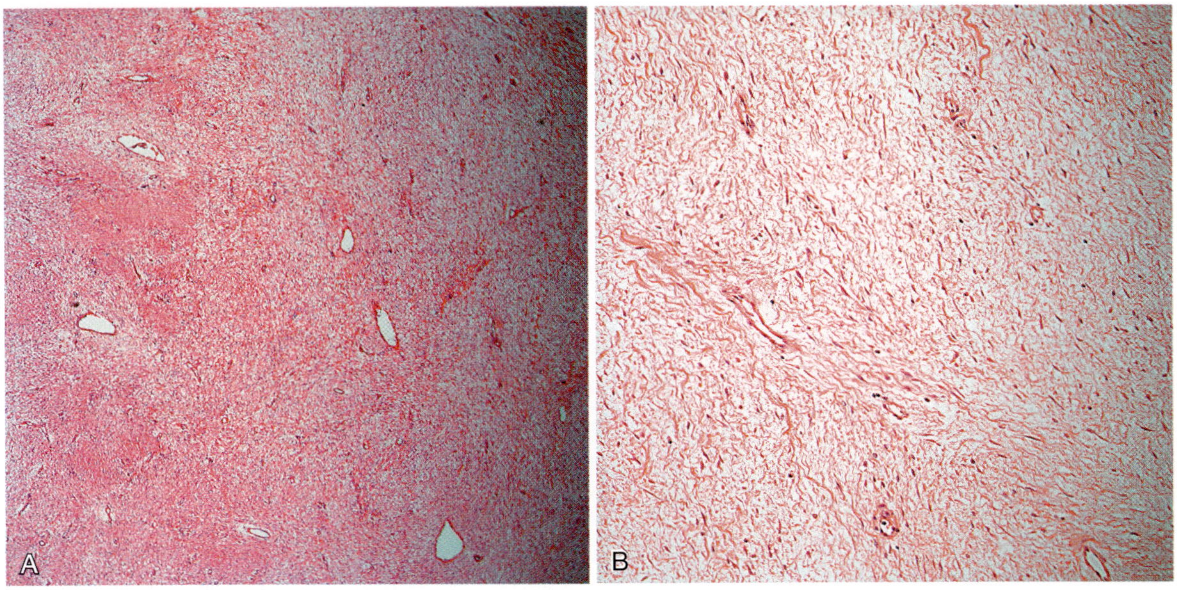

Figure 13-96 **A**, Low-power view of a desmoid tumor of the pleura showing "gapping" ectatic blood vessels and spindle cell proliferation. **B**, High-power view of the spindle fibroblastic proliferation with absence of nuclear atypia and mitotic activity.

Calcifying Fibrous Pseudotumor

CFPT initially was described by Fetsch and colleagues[150] as a tumor of soft tissues with distinct morphologic features, characterized by abundant hyalinized collagen with psammomatous or dystrophic calcifications and a lymphoplasmacytic infiltrate. According to these investigators, this condition probably is fibroinflammatory or reactive in nature. Some workers[151] have suggested that the tumor represents a late sclerosing stage of inflammatory myofibroblastic tumor in at least some cases. Others have failed to find convincing evidence to support an association with inflammatory myofibroblastic tumor and have confirmed the designation of calcifying fibrous tumor.[152]

Tumors originating in the thoracic cavity are extremely rare and have been reported to occur in the chest wall and the lung.[153–155] Pinkard and coworkers[156] are credited with the first description of these tumors in the pleura. These investigators reported three cases with characteristics similar to those described in the soft tissues, and this series was followed by several single reports.[157–163]

Clinical Features

The tumors appear not to have any gender predilection and have been described in patients from age 23 to 55 years. Clinical signs and symptoms have included chest pain, shortness of breath, and cough; some patients are asymptomatic. Chest radiographs show well-marginated, noncalcified pleural tumors, with calcifications evident on CT scans.[164]

Macroscopic Features

The tumors can be single or multiple lesions evident on the pleural surface. They are well circumscribed, of firm consistency, tan, and lobulated, and the cut surface may have a gritty appearance. Tumor size ranges from 1 cm to more than 10 cm in greatest dimension (Fig. 13-97).

Histopathologic Features

Pleural CFPT is similar to the corresponding condition described in soft tissues. The histopathologic hallmark of these tumors is extensive hyalinization with a discrete spindle cell proliferation, with numerous calcifications of different sizes, and a discrete lymphoplasmacytic infiltrate (Figs. 13-98 and 13-99). The tumor does not show necrosis, hemorrhage, cellular atypia, or mitotic activity.

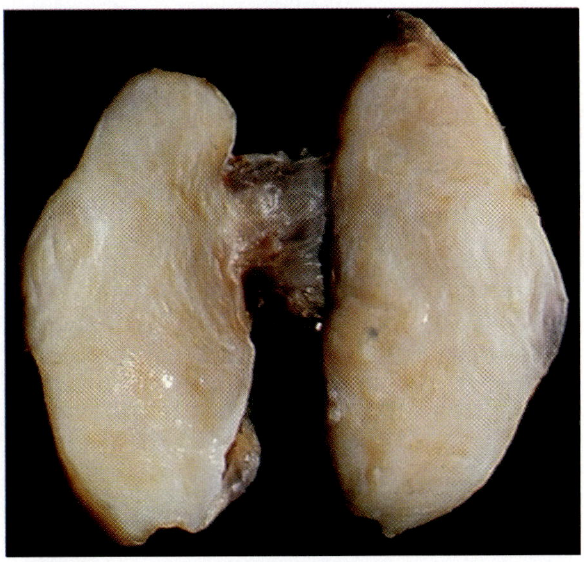

Figure 13-97 Calcifying fibrous pseudotumor of the pleura, gross specimen. The tumor is well circumscribed.

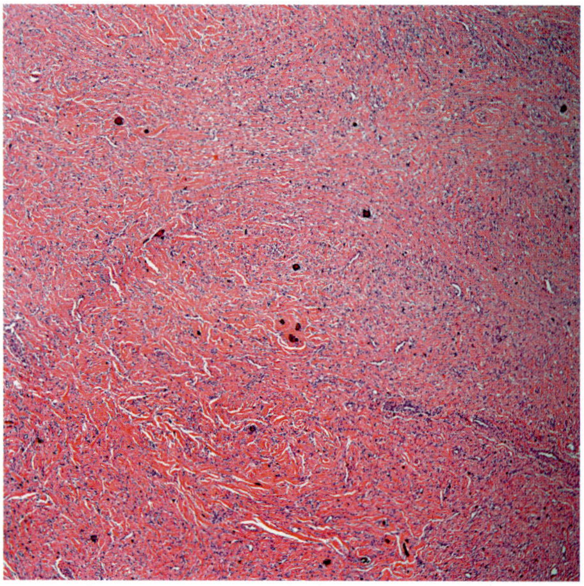

Figure 13-98 Low-power view of a calcifying fibrous pseudotumor showing extensive fibrocollagen and scattered calcifications.

Immunohistochemical Features

Because only a few cases of CFPT in a pleural location have been reported, information about immunohistochemical studies is limited. These tumors demonstrate positive staining for CD34, with negative staining for epithelial markers.

Differential Diagnosis

The most important consideration in the differential diagnosis is SFT. In this setting, the presence of psammomatous or dystrophic calcifications in a tumor with abundant collagen and lymphoplasmacytic infiltrate should lead to the correct interpretation. In contrast with SFT, which may show different patterns of growth in the same tumor, CFPT exhibits a fairly uniform growth pattern. Both of these tumors may show CD34-positive staining.[165] The immunohistochemical reaction for Bcl-2 currently is unknown.

Treatment and Prognosis

Complete surgical resection is the treatment of choice. When multiple pleural tumors are present, however, a more complex surgical approach may be necessary. Local recurrences have been described in a few patients who had soft tissue tumors; thus, similar behavior for tumors occurring on the pleura surface might be expected.

NEUROECTODERMAL TUMORS

Neuroectodermal tumors, the extraosseous round cell tumors that bear features similar to those of the skeletal neoplasms collectively designated Ewing's sarcoma, rarely occur in the thoracopulmonary region. Over the years, these tumors have been known by a variety of names, including extraskeletal Ewing's sarcoma, malignant small cell tumor of the thoracopulmonary region, Askin's tumor, paravertebral round cell tumor, and primitive neuroectodermal tumor (PNET). Currently, PNET is the designation used for almost all of these tumors.[166–175]

Historical Aspects

The existence of a group of soft tissue neoplasms characterized by round cells with scant cytoplasm, moderate amounts of chromatin in the nuclei, inconspicuous nucleoli,

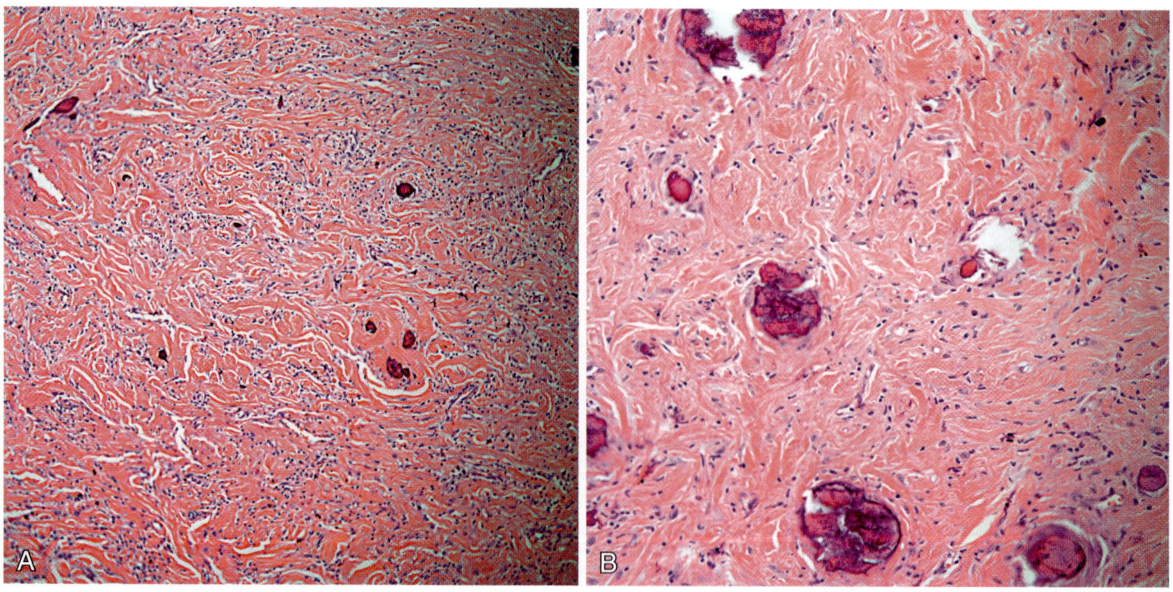

Figure 13-99 **A**, Calcifying fibrous pseudotumor showing abundant fibrocollagen, inflammatory cells, and calcifications. **B**, High-power view of the calcification in calcifying fibrous pseudotumor.

mitosis, rosettes, hemorrhage, and necrosis was first recognized by Angerval and Enzinger[166] in their description of 39 cases. Some of these tumors occurred in the thoracic area, and all of them displayed the distinctive feature of intracellular glycogen. At the time of their report, this feature was considered to be a characteristic of extraskeletal Ewing's sarcoma but not of other neoplasms, such as neuroblastoma and Askin's tumor. It is well known, however, that some neuroblastomas also may contain glycogen in their cytoplasm[176]; thus, the finding of glycogen alone does not indicate a particular neoplasm. Askin and colleagues[167] are credited for the description of these tumors in the thoracopulmonary region. The investigators described 20 cases designated under the name of malignant small cell tumor of the thoracopulmonary region. None of the cases described showed glycogen in the cytoplasm of the cells, but on histologic examination, the tumors were very similar to those previously described by Angerval and Enzinger as extraskeletal Ewing's sarcoma. The absence of glycogen was one of the parameters used to separate the two entities. Ultrastructural studies also have been controversial, with some indicating that the features of extraskeletal Ewing's sarcoma are distinctive enough to allow separation from other small cell tumors[177] and others implying that the spectrum of ultrastructural features of these tumors is broad, with some overlap.[178]

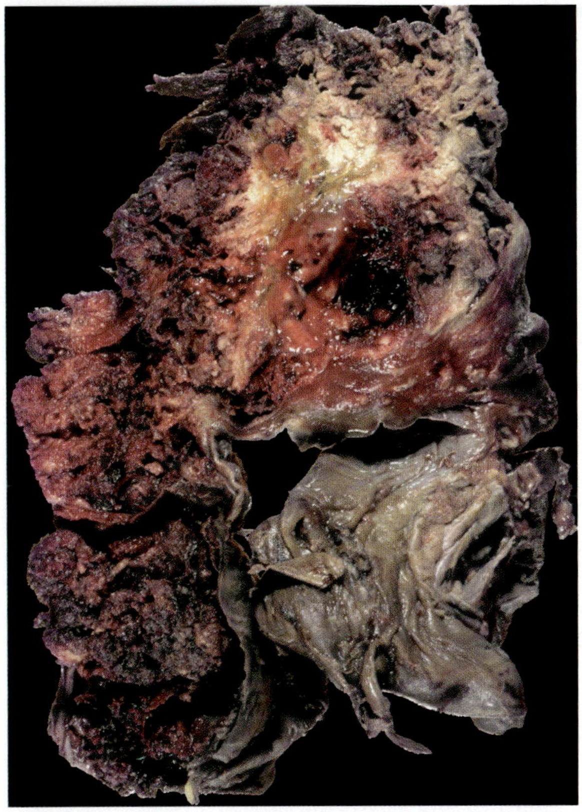

Figure 13-100 Primitive neuroectodermal tumor (Askin tumor), gross specimen. Note the areas of necrosis and hemorrhage.

Clinical Features

Clinically, the tumors appear to be more common in the younger population, and patients may present with diverse clinical signs and symptoms, including chest pain, shortness of breath, and pneumothorax. On radiologic examination, the tumor may be observed toward one side of the chest involving pleura or chest wall. Similar tumors also have been described as primary lung neoplasms, arising within the lung parenchyma.[179–182]

Macroscopic Features

These tumors may range in size from 2 cm to more than 10 cm in greatest dimension. They are tan-white with a firm consistency and have a homogeneous-appearing surface. Areas of hemorrhage or necrosis may be present. Areas of calcification also have been reported. The tumor may involve the pleura or invade lung or rib. These tumors occasionally may be located at the hilum of the lung or in the paraspinal region or chest wall (Fig. 13-100).

Histopathologic Features

Morphologically, these tumors are characterized by a neoplastic cellular proliferation, visible at low magnification, which can be separated into lobules by thin fibroconnective tissue in some areas, whereas in others it is distributed in sheets of neoplastic cells, cords, or nests. Cystic areas filled with red cells may also be seen. At higher magnification, the neoplastic cellular population is fairly homogeneous, composed of round cells with indistinct cell borders, scant cytoplasm, round to elongated nuclei, and inconspicuous small nucleoli. In some areas the tumor cells have a tendency to be distributed around vessels. Mitotic activity can be brisk, and necrosis and hemorrhage are invariably present. In better-differentiated tumors, the presence of rosettes helps in the diagnosis; however, rosettes are not always a feature. Necrosis and hemorrhage may be so prominent that the tumor cells are difficult to visualize. In other tumors, the so-called Azzopardi phenomenon may be seen (Figs. 13-101 to 13-106).

Histochemical and Immunohistochemical Features

Use of PAS histochemical stains may aid in the diagnosis; however, results of such histochemical studies may be negative, and positive staining may be seen in other types of neoplasms occurring in the same anatomic location.

Immunohistochemical techniques have shaped current views regarding these tumors, to some extent. Initially, the use of neuron-specific enolase (NSE) was considered specific for the neural derivation of these tumors; however, that notion faded rapidly after NSE was proved to stain several other tumors that were not necessarily of

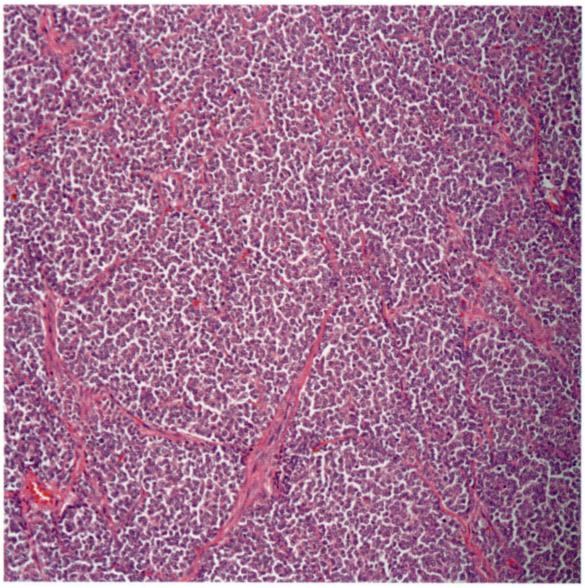

Figure 13-101 Primitive neuroectodermal tumor with a nested pattern of growth.

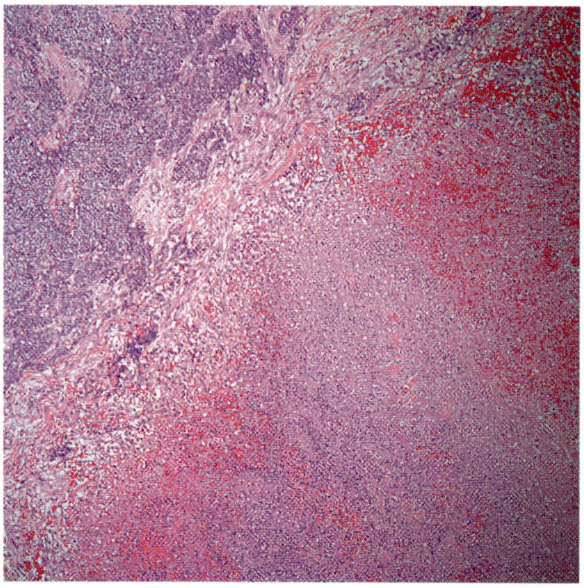

Figure 13-102 Primitive neuroectodermal tumor with extensive areas of hemorrhage.

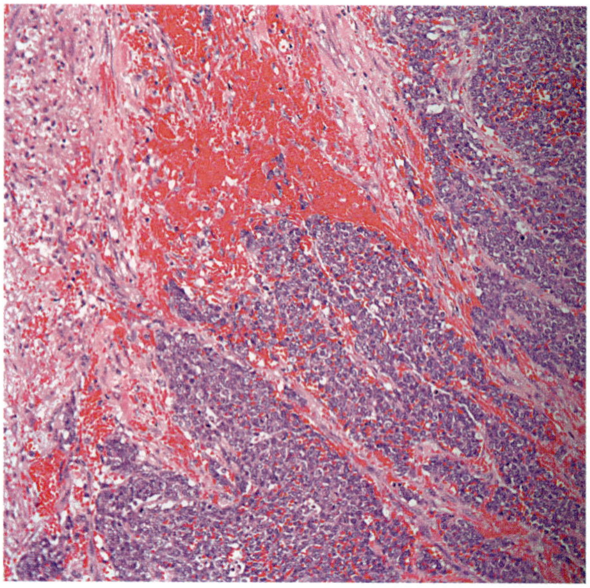

Figure 13-103 Primitive neuroectodermal tumor. Tumor cells are admixed with areas of hemorrhage.

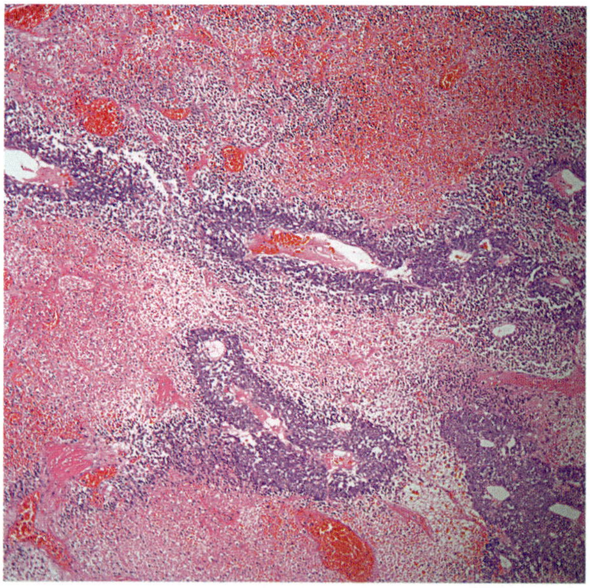

Figure 13-104 Primitive neuroectodermal tumor with a prominent perivascular tumor arrangement.

neural origin.[183,184] Another marker that has been used in the evaluation of these tumors is S-100 protein; however, the results obtained have been controversial.[169,185] More recently, the use of CD99 (HBA-71, or the MIC2 gene product [i.e., Ewing's marker]) has been viewed as an important immunohistochemical tool for diagnosis; however, staining for CD99 also may be positive in other tumors of epithelial and mesenchymal origin. Synaptophysin, which is more widely used as a neuroendocrine marker, can be of help in the proper clinical setting; it appears to stain these tumors more consistently.[186] WT-1 also has been used with some success for identification of small round cell tumors and has been claimed to reliably differentiate desmoplastic small round cell tumor from Ewing's sarcoma/PNET.[187] Staining for NB84 also appears to be positive in some cases of PNET but is more commonly positive in neuroblastomas.[188]

Molecular Biology Features

Recent advances in molecular techniques have established a closer relationship between Ewing's sarcoma and PNET. Today, little doubt exists that those tumors are closely related. Chromosomal translocations t(11;22)(q24;q12) and t(21;22)(q22;1q12) and the related oncoproteins have been found in cases of Ewing's sarcoma and PNET.[189–191]

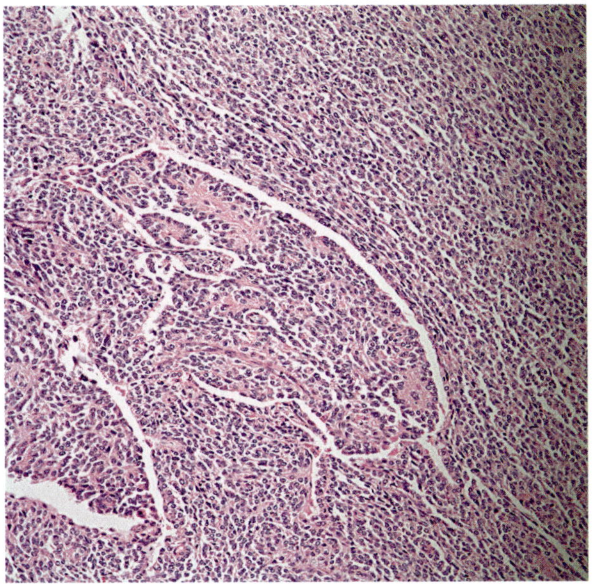

Figure 13-105 Primitive neuroectodermal tumor with areas of pseudorosettes.

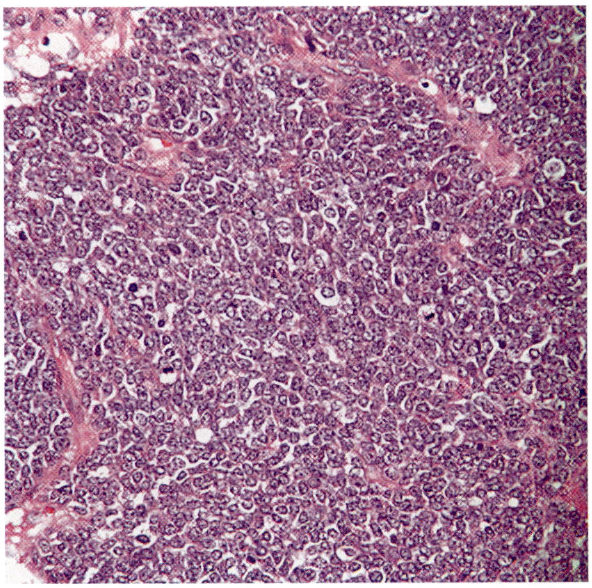

Figure 13-106 High-power view of a primitive neuroectodermal tumor showing nuclear atypia and mitotic activity.

Differential Diagnosis

The differential diagnosis for PNET in the thoracic cavity can be quite challenging because other sarcomas and neural tumors can occur in this location. By far the most difficult determinations involve differentiating those from rhabdomyosarcoma, neuroblastoma, lymphoma or leukemia, and more rarely, metastatic small cell carcinoma or metastatic sarcoma from an osseous primary. The last two conditions can be dealt with by a careful clinical history and radiologic evaluation; however, a careful histologic and immunohistochemical analysis is required to rule out the former.

In cases of rhabdomyosarcoma, the presence of rhabdomyoblast in better-differentiated tumors may lead to a correct interpretation. When the histologic picture is less characteristic, the use of a panel of immunohistochemical studies including muscle markers can resolve any diagnostic dilemma. Neuroblastoma can be more challenging to identify because these tumors also vary in their immunohistochemical profile. Positive staining for NSE and S-100 protein may be a feature of both tumors; however, synaptophysin and CD99 positivity coupled with characteristic histopathologic features of this tumor indicates a PNET (Table 13-4). In cases of lymphoma or leukemia, the histopathologic features and the presence of positive staining in tumor cells for LCA and B cell or T cell markers should lead to the correct interpretation.

Treatment and Prognosis

The treatment of choice for PNET is chemotherapy; however, the prognosis is relatively poor. In a study of 30 cases by Contesso and associates,[192] the overall survival rate was 38% at 2 years and 14% at 6 years.

MISCELLANEOUS TUMORS OF THE PLEURA

This section focuses on a group of miscellaneous lesions associated with neoplastic or pseudoneoplastic conditions that are more common in other anatomic areas such as skin and soft tissues, or with systemic conditions, but in

TABLE 13-4 IMMUNOHISTOCHEMICAL FEATURES OF SMALL CELL TUMORS

Tumor	Gly	Ker	Chr	NSE	S-100	Mb	LCA	Syn	Des	SMA	CD99
Rhabdomyosarcoma	+/−	−	−	−	−	+	−	−	+	+	+/−
Neuroblastoma	+/−	−	−	+	+/−	−	−	−	−	−	−
Small cell carcinoma	−	+	+/−	+	−	−	−	+/−	−	−	+/−
Lymphoma/leukemia	−	−	−	−	−	−	+	−	−	−	−
PNET	+/−	+/−	−	+	+/−	−	−	+	−	−	+

Chr, chromogranin; Des, desmin; Gly, glycogen; Ker, keratin; LCA, leukocyte common antigen; Mb, myoglobin; NSE, neuron-specific enolase; PNET, primitive neuroectodermal tumor; SMA, smooth muscle actin; Syn, synaptophysin.

unusual circumstances manifest as pleural lesions. The following tumors are described:

- Synovial sarcoma
- Smooth muscle tumors
- Melanoma
- Liposarcoma
- Amyloid tumors

BIPHASIC SYNOVIAL SARCOMA

Biphasic synovial sarcoma is more common in the soft tissues, but rarely may manifest as a primary pleural neoplasm. Gaertner and colleagues[193] reported five cases, three in female patients and two in males between the ages of 9 and 50 years. The patients presented with clinical signs and symptoms of dysphagia, chest pain, fever, or pneumothorax. In four patients the findings were those of a pleural mass; however, in one of the patients pleural thickening also was detected. The tumors ranged in size from 5 cm to more than 20 cm in greatest dimension. All of the patients were treated with surgery, and at least three also underwent chemoradiation therapy. According to this report, four of the patients died within a follow-up period of 12 to 30 months. Only one patient in this series was alive with disease 8 years after the initial diagnosis.

Histopathologic Features

The morphologic features of biphasic synovial sarcoma are the same as those described for the corresponding tumor of the soft tissues. The characteristic histopathologic features include a spindle cell proliferation of tightly arranged fascicles of neoplastic cells with fusiform nuclei and inconspicuous nucleoli. Mitotic figures are readily identifiable. This spindle cell proliferation may display a fibrosarcomatous or hemangiopericytic growth pattern and is intermixed with a glandular epithelial component composed of glandular structures lined by either low cuboidal epithelium or tall columnar epithelium, which may show intraluminal secretion and papillary arrangement (Figs. 13-107 to 13-109). Mitotic activity in this glandular component is not readily identifiable. In addition, the tumor may exhibit an inflammatory infiltrate composed of mast cells, lymphocytes or plasma cells, metaplastic bone formation, or calcifications.

Histochemical and Immunohistochemical Features

The use of PAS with and without diastase and mucicarmine may help demonstrate positive staining for mucin, mainly in the glandular component of the tumor. On immunohistochemical studies, staining for the epithelial markers keratin and EMA, as well as CEA in the glandular component, may be positive. Focal staining for keratin and EMA may be evident in the spindle cell component. Staining for S-100 protein and Bcl-2 also may be positive in the spindle cell component of the tumor.

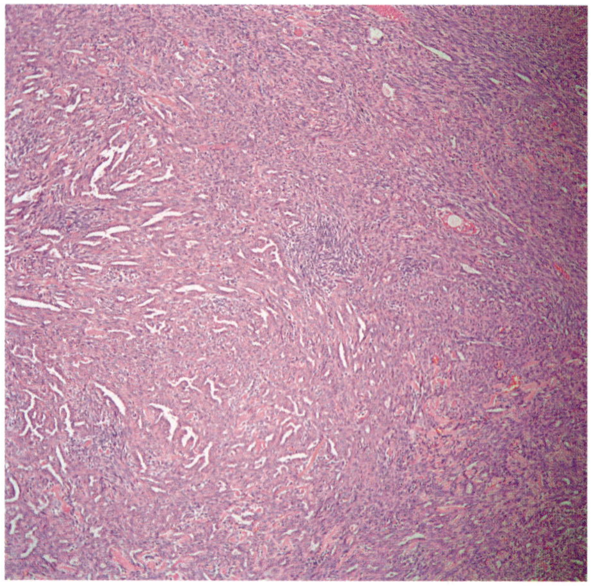

Figure 13-107 Low-power view of a pleural biphasic synovial sarcoma.

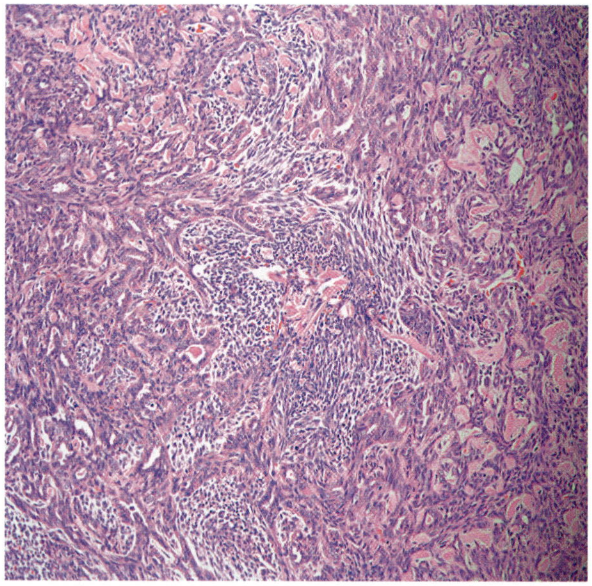

Figure 13-108 Pleural biphasic synovial sarcoma. A spindle cell proliferation is seen admixed with glandular structures.

Differential Diagnosis

Because of the biphasic nature of these tumors, the most important consideration in the differential diagnosis is biphasic malignant mesothelioma. Although rare, malignant mesotheliomas have been described in a few cases in which the tumor manifests as a pleural mass. Positive staining for CEA in the glandular component of the tumor will indicate the diagnosis of synovial sarcoma.

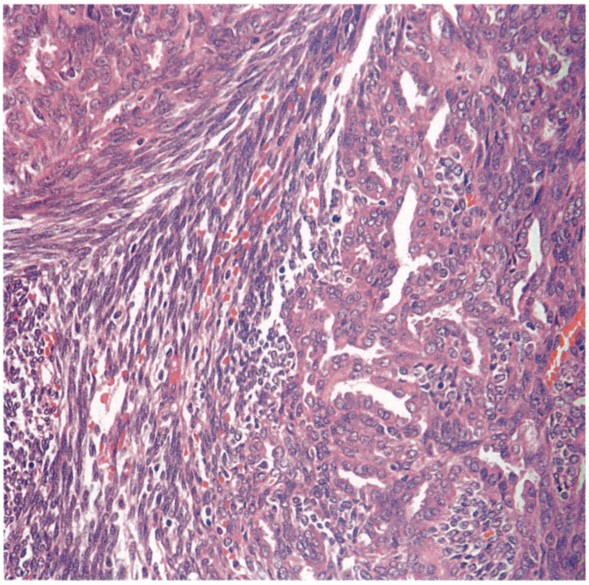

Figure 13-109 High-power view of a pleural biphasic synovial sarcoma showing glandular and spindle components. Mitotic figures are present.

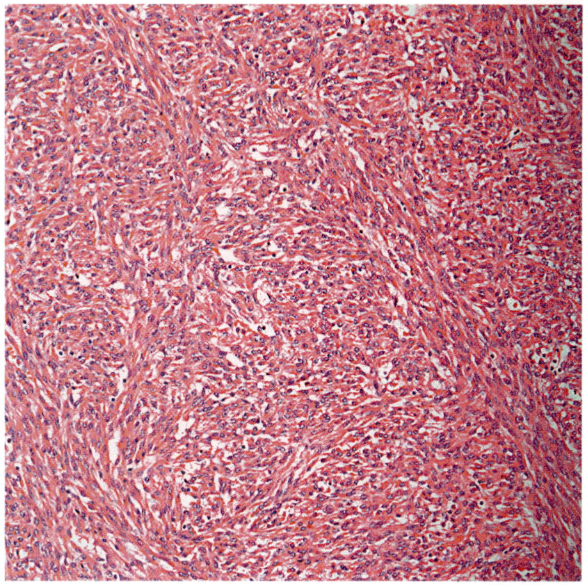

Figure 13-110 Pleural low-grade smooth muscle tumor.

The positive reaction of tumor cells for epithelial markers, especially keratin and EMA, is rather focal in synovial sarcomas, in contrast with the more global strongly positive reaction in mesotheliomas. The other important differential diagnostic possibility is metastatic synovial sarcoma of soft tissue origin. In this setting, a complete clinical history and radiologic evaluation should help in establishing a definitive diagnosis.

SMOOTH MUSCLE TUMORS

Smooth muscle tumors rarely manifest as primary pleural neoplasms. In a series of five cases,[194] consisting of three women and two men ranging in age from 21 to 69 years, presenting signs and symptoms included chest pain and empyema; one patient was asymptomatic. In four patients, the tumor manifested as a solitary pleura-based mass, whereas in another, the tumor appeared to encase the lung in a manner similar to that observed for malignant mesothelioma. Tumor size ranged from 10 to 18 cm in greatest dimension. All patients underwent surgical resection; however, in two patients the surgical removal of the tumor was incomplete. The follow-up period (2–12 months) was not long enough to provide meaningful information on the behavior of these tumors.

Histopathologic Features

The tumors described in the literature range from the smooth muscle tumor of uncertain malignant potential to leiomyosarcoma of low-, intermediate-, and high-grade histology (Figs. 13-110 and 13-111). Tumors of low-grade histology were characterized by interlacing fascicles of elongated cells intersecting at right angles. The spindle cellular proliferation displayed cigar-shaped nuclei and a moderate amount of eosinophilic cytoplasm. No areas of hemorrhage or necrosis were present, and nuclear atypia was mild, with only rare mitotic figures. In the tumors of intermediate- and high-grade histology, the basic arrangement of the neoplastic cellular proliferation was similar to that seen in low-grade tumors; however, areas of necrosis and hemorrhage were present. In addition, nuclear atypia and mitotic figures were readily identified and numerous.

Immunohistochemical Features

Use of immunohistochemical stains is helpful in the assessment of these tumors. Smooth muscle actin and desmin tend to give a positive reaction. In some smooth muscle tumors of the pleura, keratin antibodies also may give a positive reaction; thus, a wider panel of antibodies should be used when smooth muscle tumor is suspected.

Differential Diagnosis

The most important considerations in the differential diagnosis for primary smooth muscle tumors of the pleura are malignant mesothelioma and metastatic smooth muscle tumor. In the former, immunostaining for keratin and calretinin may lead to the correct diagnosis; however, some smooth muscle tumors of the pleura may react positively for keratin antibodies. Nevertheless, it would be unusual for a mesothelioma to show a strong positive reaction for smooth muscle actin or desmin. When metastatic smooth muscle tumor is suspected, a complete clinical history and radiologic evaluation play the most important role.

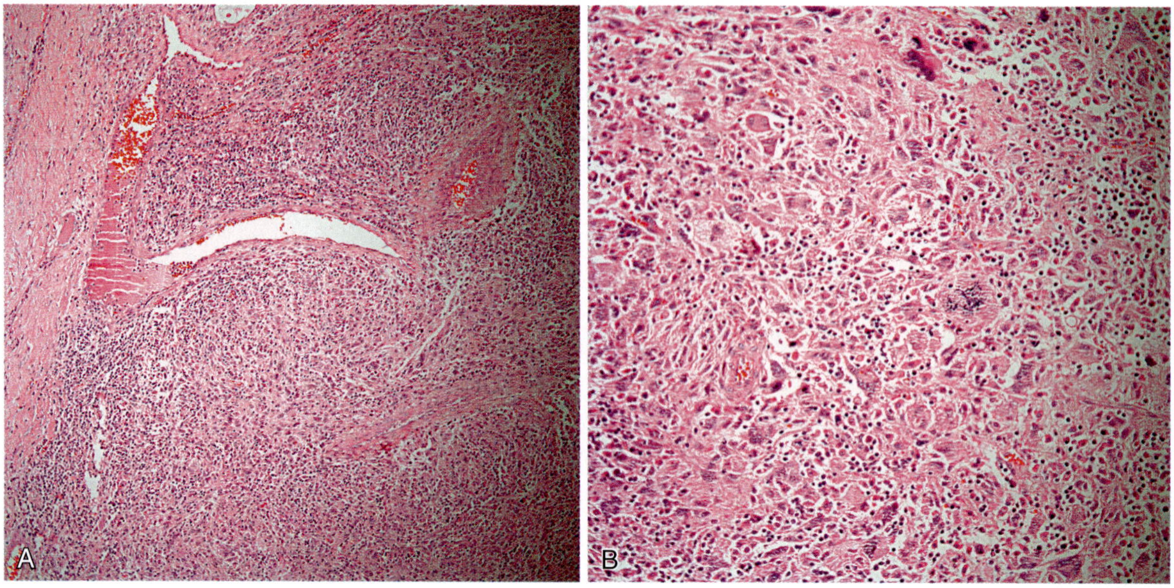

Figure 13-111 **A**, Low-power view of a high-grade pleural smooth muscle tumor. **B**, At higher magnification, prominent nuclear atypia and mitotic activity are evident.

MELANOMA

The presence of melanomas in the thoracic cavity, especially on the pleural surface, usually indicates metastatic disease. In some cases, the metastatic tumors may even encase the lung in a manner similar to that for pleural mesothelioma.

Primary melanoma of the pleura has only rarely been described in the literature. Smith and colleagues[195] reported a unique case of a 49-year-old man who presented with dyspnea and productive cough. The patient had a history of tobacco used but did not report hemoptysis. The patient denied any skin lesions. The chest films revealed opacification of the right lower lung field, and at fluoroscopy, an extrapleural mass effect was noted. The patient died 10 months after diagnosis; however, his death was unrelated to the tumor. At autopsy, no evidence of other organ involvement was observed.

On histologic examination, the tumor was characterized by melanin pigment and a neoplastic cellular proliferation composed of larger cells with vesicular nuclei and prominent nucleoli. Warthin-Starry histochemical stains demonstrated the presence of melanin. Although no immunohistochemical information was provided for this particular case, in current practice the use of immunohistochemical studies for S-100 protein, Melan A, and HMB-45 would lead to a correct interpretation.

Because most cases of melanoma in the thoracic cavity represent metastatic disease, proper evaluation for ocular melanoma or a regressed melanoma of the skin is imperative.

LIPOSARCOMA

These tumors are by far more common in the soft tissues and only rarely manifest as thoracic tumors. In the thorax, the mediastinal compartment is the most common site. However, cases of primary liposarcoma of the pleura also have been reported.[196–198] A majority of the reported cases have been in adults, with an age range of 19 to 61 years. Presenting clinical signs and symptoms have included shortness of breath, cough, and pleurisy. Tumor size has ranged from 3 cm to more than 10 cm in greatest dimension. All of the patients described underwent surgical resection of the tumor. The histologic picture varies, ranging from well-differentiated to myxoid to pleomorphic type, and the clinical course also has been variable, with some patients experiencing no recurrence and others experiencing metastasis, local recurrence, or death from their disease. The treatment of choice for these tumors, especially those of low malignant potential, is complete surgical resection ensuring tumor-free margins. In cases of high-grade histology, adjuvant therapies may be considered.

AMYLOID TUMORS

Amyloid tumors are more commonly seen in the thoracic cavity as intrapulmonary neoplasms. In unsual circumstances, however, amyloid may be seen coating the pleural surface, with thickening of the pleura resembling that in malignant mesothelioma[199] (Fig. 13-112). On histologic examination, the presence of eosinophilic amorphous material admixed with an inflammatory infiltrate, cholesterol cleft granulomas, and giant cells are common features (Fig. 13-113). Histochemical staining with Congo red should help in the diagnosis, because the stain shows apple-green birefringence under polarized light.

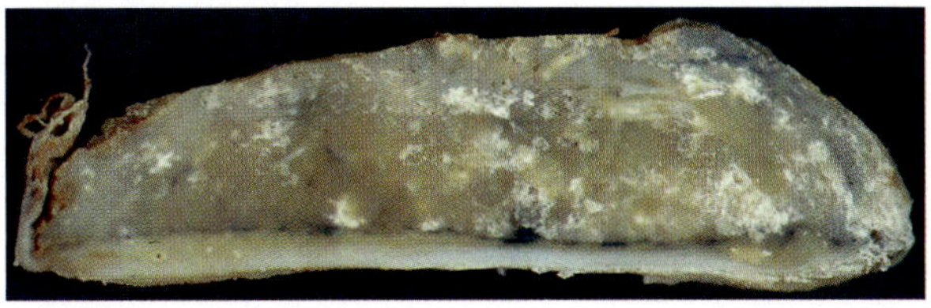

Figure 13-112 Diffuse pleural involvement by amyloid.

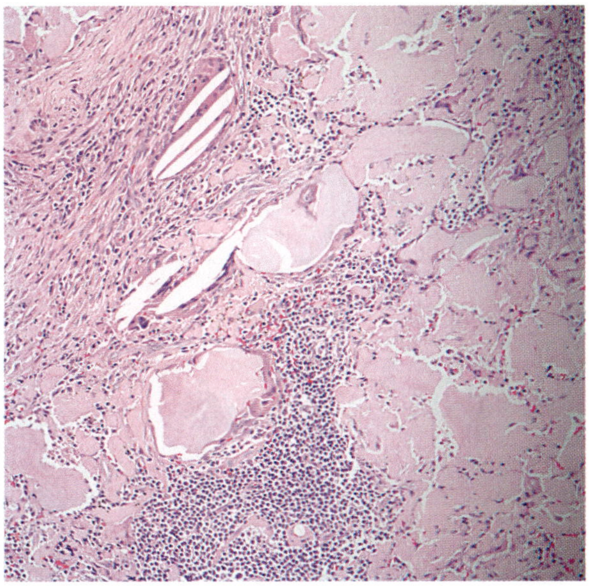

Figure 13-113 Pleural amyloid. Note the presence of amorphous material and cholesterol cleft granulomas with scattered giant cells.

REFERENCES

1. Hinds MW. Mesothelioma in the United States. Incidence in the 1970's. *J Occup Med*. 1978;20:469–471.
2. *SEER Cancer Statistics Review 1975–2003*. Bethesda, MD: National Cancer Institute; Available at http://seer.cancer.gov/csr/1975_2003/results_merged/sect_17mesothelioma.pdf.
3. Craighead JE. The epidemiology and pathogenesis of malignant mesothelioma. *Chest*. 1989;96:92–93.
4. Wright WE, Sherwin RP. Histological types of malignant mesothelioma and asbestos exposure. *Br J Ind Med*. 1984;41:514–517.
5. Borow M, Conston A, Livornese L, Schalet N. Mesothelioma following exposure to asbestos: a review of 72 cases. *Chest*. 1973;64:641–646.
6. Wagner E. Das tuberkelahuliche Lymphadenom. *Arch F Heilk*. 1870;11:497–525.
7. Robertson HE. Endothelioma of the pleura. *J Cancer Res*. 1923–1924;8:317.
8. Klemperer P, Rabin CB. Primary neoplasms of the pleura. *Arch Pathol*. 1931;11:385–412.
9. DuBray ES, Rosson FB. Primary mesothelioma of the pleura: a clinical and pathological contribution to the pleural malignancy, with report of a case. *Arch Intern Med*. 1920;26:715–737.
10. Godwin MC. Diffuse mesotheliomas: with comment on their relation to localized fibrous mesotheliomas. *Cancer*. 1957;10:298–319.
11. Wagner JC, Sleggs CA, Marchand P. Diffuse pleural mesothelioma and asbestos exposure in the North Western Cape Town province. *Br J Ind Med*. 1960;17:260–271.
12. Hirsch A, Brochard P, De Cremoux H, et al. Features of asbestos-exposed and unexposed mesothelioma. *Am J Ind Med*. 1982;3:413–422.
13. McCaughey WTE. Criteria for the diagnosis of diffuse mesothelial tumors. *Ann N Y Acad Sci*. 965;132:603–613.
14. Huncharek M, Kelsey K, Mark EJ, et al. Treatment and survival in diffuse malignant pleural mesothelioma: a study of 83 cases from Massachusetts General Hospital. *Anticancer Res*. 1996;16:1265–1268.
15. Aaisner J, Wiernik PH. Malignant mesothelioma: current status and future prospects. *Chest*. 1978;74:438–444.
16. Gardner MJ, Acheson ED, Winter PD. Mortality from mesothelioma of the pleura during 1968–78 in England and Wales. *Br J Cancer*. 1982;46:81–88.
17. Oels HC, Harrison EG, Carr DT, Bernatz PE. Diffuse malignant mesothelioma of the pleura: a review of 37 cases. *Chest*. 1971;60:564–570.
18. Chahinian AP, Pajak TF, Holland JF, Norton L, Ambinder RM, Mandel EM. Diffuse malignant mesothelioma. Prospective evaluation of 69 patients. *Ann Intern Med*. 1982;96:746–755.
19. Brenner J, Sordillo PP, Magill GB, Golbey RB. Malignant mesothelioma of the pleura: review of 123 patients. *Cancer*. 1982;49:2431–2435.
20. Law MR, Hodson ME, Heard BE. Malignant mesothelioma of the pleura: relation between histological type and clinical behavior. *Thorax*. 1982;37:810–815.
21. Qua JC, Rao UMN, Takita H. Malignant pleural mesothelioma: a clinicopathological study. *J Surg Oncol*. 1993;54:47–50.
22. Suzuki Y. Pathology of human malignant mesothelioma. *Semin Oncol*. 1980;8:268–282.
23. Grundy GW, Miller RW. Malignant mesothelioma in childhood: report of 13 cases. *Cancer*. 1972;30:1216–1218.
24. Moran CA, Suster S, Albores-Saavedra J. Peritoneal mesotheliomas in children: a clinicopathologic study of 8 cases. *Histopathology*. 2008;52:824–830.
25. Peterson JT, Greenberg DS, Buffler PA. Non-asbestos related malignant mesothelioma. A review. *Cancer*. 1984;54:951–960.
26. Ordoñez NG. Epithelial mesothelioma with deciduoid features: report of four cases. *Am J Surg Pathol*. 2000;24:816–823.
27. Ordoñez NG, Mackay B. Clear cell mesothelioma. *Ultrastruct Pathol*. 1996;20:331–336.
28. Henderson DW, Attwood HD, Constance TJ, Shilkin KB, Steele RH. Lymphohistiocytoid mesothelioma: a rare lymphomatoid variant of predominantly sarcomatoid mesothelioma. *Ultrastruct Pathol*. 1988;12:367–384.
29. Yousem SA, Hochholzer L. Malignant mesothelioma with osseous and cartilaginous differentiation. *Arch Pathol Lab Med*. 1987;111:62–66.
30. Arrossi AV, Lin E, Rice D, Moran CA. Histologic assessment and prognostic factors of malignant pleural mesothelioma treated with extrapleural pneumonectomy. *Am J Clin Pathol*. 2008;130:754–764.
31. Moran CA, Wick MR, Suster S. The role of immunohistochemistry in the diagnosis of malignant mesothelioma. *Semin Diagn Pathol*. 2000;17:178–183.
32. Suster S, Moran CA. Applications and limitations of immunohistochemistry in the diagnosis of malignant mesothelioma. *Adv Anat Pathol*. 2006;13:316–329.
33. Wick MR, Moran CA, Mills SE, Suster S. Immunohistochemical differential diagnosis of pleural effusions with emphasis on malignant mesothelioma. *Curr Opin Pulm Med*. 2001;7:187–192.

34. Ordonez NG. Value of cytokeratin 5/6 immunostain in distinguishing epithelial mesothelioma of the pleura from lung adenocarcinoma. *Am J Surg Pathol.* 1998;22:1215–1221.
35. Ordonez NG. In search of a positive immunohistochemical marker for mesothelioma: an update. *Adv Anat Pathol.* 1998;5:53–60.
36. Moll R, Dhouailly D, Sun TT. Expression of keratin 5 as a distinctive feature of epithelial and biphasic mesotheliomas: an immunohistochemical study using monoclonal antibody AE14. *Virchows Arch B Cell Pathol Incl Mol Pathol.* 1989;58:129–145.
37. Clover J, Oates J, Edwards C. Anti-cytokeratin 5/6: a potential marker for epithelioid mesothelioma. *Histopathology.* 1997;31:140–143.
38. Chu PG, Weiss LM. Expression of cytokeratin 5/6 in epithelial neoplasms: an immunohistochemical study of 509 cases. *Mod Pathol.* 2002;15:6–10.
39. Gotzos V, Vogt P, Celio MR. The calcium binding protein calretinin is a selective marker for malignant mesothelial proliferation using formalin-fixed paraffin sections. *J Pathol.* 1992;192:137–147.
40. Doglioni C, Dei Tos AP, Laurino L, et al. Calretinin: a novel immunocytochemical marker for mesothelioma. *Am J Surg Pathol.* 1996;20:1037–1046.
41. Dei Tos AP, Doglioni C. Calretinin: a novel tool for diagnostic immunohistochemistry. *Adv Anat Pathol.* 1998;5:61–66.
42. Oates J, Edwards C. HBME-1, MOC31, WT1 and calretinin: an assessment of recently described markers for mesothelioma and adenocarcinoma. *Histopathology.* 2000;36:341–347.
43. Foster MR, Johnson JE, Olson SJ, Allred DC. Immunohistochemical analysis of nuclear versus cytoplasmic staining of WT1 in malignant mesothelioma and primary pulmonary adenocarcinoma. *Arch Pathol Lab Med.* 2001;125:1316–1320.
44. Kumar-Singh S, Segers K, Rodeck U, et al. WT1 mutation in malignant mesothelioma and WT1 immunoreactivity in relation to p53 and growth factor receptor expression, cell-type transition, and prognosis. *J Pathol.* 1997;181:67–74.
45. Yaziji H, Battifora H, Barry TS, et al. Evaluation of 12 antibodies for distinguishing epithelioid mesothelioma from adenocarcinoma: identification of a three antibody immunohistochemical panel with maximal sensitivity and specificity. *Mod Pathol.* 2006;19:514–523.
46. Amin KM, Litzky LA, Smythe WR, et al. Wilm's tumor-1 susceptibility (WT1) gene products are selectively expressed in malignant mesothelioma. *Am J Pathol.* 1995;146:344–356.
47. Walker C, Rutten F, Yuan X, Pass H, Mew DM, Everitt J. Wilms' tumor suppressor gene expression in rat and human mesothelioma. *Cancer Res.* 1994;54:3101–3106.
48. Ordonez NG. The value of thyroid transcription factor-1, E-cadherin, BG8, WT1, and CD44S immunostaining in distinguishing epithelial pleural mesothelioma from pulmonary and nonpulmonary adenocarcinoma. *Am J Surg Pathol.* 2000;24:598–606.
49. Miettinen M, Kovatich AJ. HBME-1—a monoclonal antibody useful in the differential diagnosis of mesothelioma, adenocarcinoma, and soft tissue and bone tumors. *Appl Immunohistochem.* 1995;3:115–122.
50. Kennedy AD, King G, Kerr KM. HBME-1 and antithrombomodulin in the differential diagnosis of malignant mesothelioma of the pleura. *J Clin Pathol.* 1997;50:859–862.
51. Attanoos RL, Goddard H, Gibbs AR. Mesothelioma-binding antibodies: thrombomodulin, OV632, and HBME-1 and their use for the diagnosis of malignant mesothelioma. *Histopathology.* 1996;29:209–215.
52. Collins CL, Ordonez NG, Schaefer R, et al. Thrombomodulin expression in malignant pleural mesothelioma and pulmonary adenocarcinoma. *Am J Pathol.* 1992;141:827–833.
53. Ascoli V, Scalso CC, Taccogna S, Nardi F. The diagnostic value of thrombomodulin immunolocalization in serous effusions. *Arch Pathol Lab Med.* 1995;119:1136–1140.
54. Argani P, Iacobuzio-Donahue C, Ryu B, et al. Mesothelin is overexpressed in the vast majority of ductal adenocarcinomas of the pancreas: identification of a new pancreatic cancer marker by serial analysis of gene expression (SAGE). *Clin Cancer Res.* 2001;7:3862–3868.
55. Ordonez NG. Application of mesothelin immunostaining in tumor diagnosis. *Am J Surg Pathol.* 2003;27:1418–1428.
56. Hassan R, Kreitman RJ, Pastan I, Willingham MC. Localization of mesothelin in epithelial ovarian cancer. *Appl Immunohistochem Mol Morphol.* 2005;13:243–247.
57. Cao D, Ji H, Ronnett BM. Expression of mesothelin, fascin, prostate stem cell antigen in primary ovarian mucinous tumors and their utility in differentiating primary ovarian mucinous tumors from metastatic pancreatic mucinous carcinomas in the ovary. *Int J Gynecol Pathol.* 2005;24:67–72.
58. Comin CE, Novelli L, Boddi V, Paglierani M, Dini S. Calretinin, thrombomodulin, CEA, and CD-15: a useful combination of immunohistochemical markers for differentiating pleural epithelial mesothelioma from peripheral pulmonary adenocarcinoma. *Hum Pathol.* 2001;32:529–536.
59. Garcia-Prats MD, Ballestin C, Sotelo T, Lopez-Encuentra A, Mayordomo JI. A comparative evaluation of immunohistochemical markers for the differential diagnosis of malignant pleural tumors. *Histopathology.* 1998;32:462–472.
60. Roberts F, Harper CM, Downie I, Burnett RA. Immunohistochemical analysis still has a limited role in the diagnosis of malignant mesothelioma: a study of thirteen antibodies. *Am J Clin Pathol.* 2001;116:253–262.
61. Leosli H, Hurliman J. Immunohistochemical study of malignant diffuse mesothelioma of the pleura. *Histopathology.* 1984;8:793–803.
62. Battifora H, Kopinsky M. Distinction of mesothelioma from adenocarcinoma. An immunohistochemical approach. *Cancer.* 1985;55:1679–1685.
63. Pfaltz M, Odermatt B, Christen B, Rüttner JR. Immunohistochemistry in the diagnosis of malignant mesothelioma. *Virchows Arch A Pathol Anat Histopathol.* 1987;411:387–393.
64. Otis CN, Carter D, Cole S, Battifora H. Immunohistochemical evaluation of pleural mesothelioma and pulmonary adenocarcinoma. A bi-institutional study of 47 cases. *Am J Surg Pathol.* 1987;11:445–456.
65. Wharhol MJ. The ultrastructural localization of keratin proteins and carcinoembryonic antigen in malignant mesothelioma. *Am J Pathol.* 1984;116:385–390.
66. Sosolik RC, McGauhy VR, De Young BR. Anti-MOC31: a potential addition to the pulmonary adenocarcinoma versus mesothelioma immunohistochemistry panel. *Mod Pathol.* 1997;10:716–719.
67. Ordonez NG. The value of MOC31 monoclonal antibody in differentiating epithelial pleural mesothelioma from lung adenocarcinoma. *Hum Pathol.* 1998;29:166–169.
68. González-Lois C, Ballestín C, Sotelo MT, López-Ríos F, García-Prats MD, Villena V. Combined use of novel epithelial (MOC31) and mesothelial (HBME-1) immunohistochemical markers for optimal first line diagnostic distinction between mesothelioma and metastatic carcinoma in pleura. *Histopathology.* 2001;38:528–534.
69. Di Loreto C, Puglisi F, Di Lauro V, Damante G, Beltrami CA. TTF-1 protein expression in pleural malignant mesotheliomas and adenocarcinomas of the lung. *Cancer Lett.* 1998;13:73–78.
70. Bakir K, Koçer NE, Deniz H, Güldür ME. TTF-1 and surfactant-B as co-adjuvants in the diagnosis of adenocarcinoma and pleural mesothelioma. *Ann Diagn Pathol.* 2004;8:337–341.
71. Khoor A, Whitsett JA, Stahlman MT, Olson SJ, Cagle PT. Utility of surfactant protein B precursor and thyroid transcription factor-1 in differentiating adenocarcinoma of the lung from malignant mesothelioma. *Hum Pathol.* 1999;30:695–700.
72. Skov BG, Lauritzen AF, Hirsch FR, Skov T, Nielsen HW. Differentiation of adenocarcinoma of the lung and malignant mesothelioma: predictive value and reproducibility of immunoreactive antibodies. *Histopathology.* 1994;25:431–437.

73. Moch H, Oberholzer M, Christen H, et al. Diagnostic tools for differentiating pleural mesothelioma from lung adenocarcinoma in paraffin embedded tissue. II. Design of an expert system and its application to the diagnosis of mesothelioma. *Virchows Arch A Pathol Anat Histopathol.* 1993;423:493–496.
74. Brown RW, Clark GM, Tandon AK, Allred DC. Multiple-marker immunohistochemical phenotypes distinguishing malignant pleural mesothelioma from pulmonary adenocarcinoma. *Hum Pathol.* 1993;24:347–354.
75. Jordon D, Jagirdar J, Kaneko M. Blood group antigens, Lewis and Lewis, in the diagnostic discrimination of malignant mesothelioma versus adenocarcinoma. *Am J Pathol.* 1989;135:931–937.
76. Carter D, Otis CN. Three types of spindle cell tumors of the pleura. Fibroma, sarcoma, and sarcomatoid mesothelioma. *Am J Sug Pathol.* 1988;12:747–753.
77. Kannerstein M, Churg J. Desmoplastic diffuse malignant mesothelioma. In: Fenoglio CM, Wolff M, eds. *Progress in Surgical Pathology*. Vol 11. New York: Masson Publishing; 1980:19–29.
78. Cantin R, al-Jabi M, McCaughey WTE. Desmoplastic diffuse mesothelioma. *Am J Surg Pathol.* 1982;6:215–222.
79. Mangano WE, Cagle PT, Churg A, Vollmer RT, Roggli VL. The diagnosis of desmoplastic malignant mesothelioma and its distinction from fibrous pleurisy. *Am J Clin Pathol.* 1998;110:191–199.
80. Colby TV. The diagnosis of desmoplastic malignant mesothelioma. *Am J Clin Pathol.* 1998;110:135–136.
81. Henderson DW. Lymphohisticytoid mesothelioma: a rare lymphomatoid variant of predominantly sarcomatoid mesothelioma. *Ultrastruct Pathol.* 1988;12:367–384.
82. Rice D. Surgery for malignant pleural mesothelioma. *Ann Diagn Pathol.* 2009;13:65–72.
83. Harwood TR, Gracey DR, Yokoo H. Pseudomesotheliomatous carcinoma of the lung: a variant of peripheral lung cancer. *Am J Clin Pathol.* 1976;65:159–167.
84. Koss MN, Travis W, Moran C, Hochholzer L. Pseudomesotheliomatous adenocarcinoma: a reappraisal. *Semin Diagn Pathol.* 1992;9:117–123.
85. Nishimoto Y, Ohno T, Saito K. Pseudomesotheliomatous carcinoma of the lung with histochemical and immunohistochemical study. *Acta Pathol Jpn.* 1983;33:415–423.
86. Dessy E, Pietra G. Pseudomesotheliomatous carcinoma of the lung: an immunohistochemical and ultrastructural study of three cases. *Cancer.* 1991;68:1747–1753.
87. Shah IA, Salvatore JR, Kummet T, Gani OS, Wheeler LA. Pseudomesotheliomatous carcinoma involving pleura and peritoneum: a clinicopathological and immunohistochemical study of three cases. *Ann Diagn Pathol.* 1999;3:148–159.
88. Attanos RL, Gibbs AR. Pseudomesotheliomatous carcinomas of the pleura: a 10-year analysis of cases from the environmental lung disease research group. *Cardiff Histopathol.* 2003;43:444–452.
89. Koss MN, Fleming M, Przygodski RM, Sherrod A, Travis W, Hochholzer L. Adenocarcinoma simulating mesothelioma: a clinicopathological and immunohistochemical study of 29 cases. *Ann Diagn Pathol.* 1998;2:93–102.
90. Pardo J, Torres W, Martinez-Peñuela A, Panizo A, de Alava E, García JL. Pseudomesotheliomatous carcinoma of the lung with distinct morphology, immunohistochemistry, and comparative genomic hybridization profile. *Ann Diagn Pathol.* 2007;11:241–251.
91. Asa SL, Dardick I, Van Nostrand AW, Bailey DJ, Gullane PJ. Primary thyroid thymoma: a distinct clinicopathologic entity. *Hum Pathol.* 1988;19:1463–1466.
92. Martin JME, Randhawa G, Temple WJ. Cervical thymoma. *Arch Pathol Lab Med.* 1986;110:354–357.
93. Yamashita H, Murakami N, Noguchi S, et al. Cervical thymoma and incidence of cervical thymus. *Acta Pathol Jpn.* 1983;33:189–194.
94. Wadon A. Thymoma intratracheale. *Am J Pathol.* 1934;60:308–312.
95. Moran CA, Suster S, Fishback NF, Koss MN. Primary intrapulmonary thymoma. A clinicopathologic and immunohistochemical correlation of eight cases. *Am J Surg Pathol.* 1995;19:304–312.
96. Payne CB, Morningstar WA, Chester EH. Thymoma of the pleura masquerading as diffuse mesothelioma. *Am Rev Respir Dis.* 1960;94:441–446.
97. Honma K, Shimada K. Metastasizing ectopic thymoma arising in the right thoracic cavity and mimicking diffuse pleural mesothelioma. An autopsy study of a case with review of the literature. *Wien Klin Wochenschr.* 1986;98:14–20.
98. Moran CA, Travis WD, de-Christenson M, Koss MN, Rosai J. Thymomas presenting as pleural tumors: report of eight cases. *Am J Surg Pahtol.* 1992;16:138–144.
99. Vural M, Abali H, Oksuzog B, Akbulut M. An atypical presentation of thymoma with diffuse pleural dissemination mimicking mesothelioma. *Cancer Invest.* 2006;24:615–620.
100. Qing G, Ionescu DN, Colby TV, Leslie KOA. 75-year-old man with an asymptomatic pleural-based mass discovered on routine chest radiographs. Primary pleural thymoma. *Arch Pathol Lab Med.* 2006;130:e62–e65.
101. Kim HS, Lee HJ, Cho SY, et al. Myasthenia gravis in ectopic thymoma presenting as pleural masses. *Lung Cancer.* 2007;57:115–157.
102. Yamazaki K, Yoshino I, Oba T, et al. Ectopic pleural thymoma presenting as a giant mass in the thoracic cavity. *Ann Thorac Surg.* 2007;83:315–317.
103. Shin DF, Wang JS, Tseng HH, Tiao VM. Primary pleural thymoma. *Arch Pathol Lab Med.* 1997;1221:79–82.
104. Higashiyama M, Doi O, Kodama K, Yokouchi H, Tateishi R, Kuriyama K. Ectopic primary thymoma: report of a case. *Surg Today.* 1996;26:747–750.
105. Fushimi H, Tanio Y, Koth K. Ectopic thymoma mimicking diffuse pleural mesothelioma: a case report. *Hum Pathol.* 1998;29:409–410.
106. Plaza JA, Dominguez F, Suster S. Cystic adenomatoid tumor of the mediastinum. *Am J Surg Pathol.* 2004;28:132–138.
107. Ikuta N, Tano M, Iwata M, et al. A case of adenomatoid mesothelioma of the pleura. *Jpn J Thorac Dis.* 1989;27:1540–1544.
108. Kaplan MA, Tazelaar HD, Hayashi T, Schroer KR, Travis WD. Adenomatoid tumors of the pleura. *Am J Surg Pathol.* 1996;20:1219–1223.
109. Moran CA, Suster S. Primary mucoepidermoid carcinoma of the pleura: a clinicopathological study of two cases. *Am J Surg Pathol.* 2003;120:381–385.
110. Flieder D, Moran CA, Travis WD, Koss MN, Mark EJ. Pleuro-pulmonary endometriosis and pulmonary ectopic deciduosis: a clinicopathologic and immunohistochemical study of 10 cases with emphasis in diagnostic pitfalls. *Hum Pathol.* 1998;29:1495–1503.
111. Karpel JP, Appel D, Merav A. Pulmonary endometriosis. *Lung.* 1985;163:151–159.
112. Lattes R, Shepard F, Tovell H, Wylie R. A clinical and pathological study of endometriosis of the lung. *Surg Gynecol Obstet.* 1956;103:552–558.
113. Foster DC, Stern JL, Buscema J, Rock JA, Woodruff JD. Pleural and parenchyma pulmonary endometriosis. *Obstet Gynecol.* 1981;58:552–556.
114. Austin MB, Frierson Jr HF, Fechner RE, et al. Endometrioma of the lung presenting as hemoptysis and a large pulmonary mass. *Surg Pathol.* 1988;1:165–169.
115. Crotty EJ, McAdams HP, Erasmus JJ, Sporn TA, Roggli VL. Epithelioid hemangioendothelioma of the pleura: clinical and radiological features. *AJR Am J Roentgenol.* 2000;175:1545–1549.
116. Bevelaqua FA, Valensi Q, Hulnick D. Epithelioid hemangioendothelioma: a rare tumor with variable prognosis presenting as a pleural effusion. *Chest.* 1988;93:665–666.
117. Attanoos RL, Suvarna SK, Rhead E, et al. Malignant tumours of the pleura in "asbestos" workers and endothelial differentiation in malignant mesothelioma. *Thorax.* 2000;55:860–863.

118. Pinet C, Magnan A, Garbe L, Payan MJ, Vervloet D. Aggressive form of pleural epithelioid hemangioendothelioma: complete response after chemotherapy. *Eur Respir J*. 1999;14:237–238.
119. Al-Shraim M, Mahboub B, Neligan PC, Chamberlain D, Ghazarian D. Primary pleural epithelioid haemangioendothelioma with metastases to the skin. A case report and literature review. *J Clin Pathol*. 2005;58:107–109.
120. Lin BT, Colby T, Gown AM, et al. Malignant vascular tumors of the serous membranes mimicking mesothelioma. A report of 14 cases. *Am J Surg Pathol*. 1996;20:1431–1439.
121. Saqi A, Nisbet L, Gagneja P, Leslie KO. Primary pleural epithelioid hemangioendothelioma with rhabdoid phenotype: report and review of the literature. *Diagn Cytopathol*. 2007;35:203–208.
122. Falconieri G, Bussani R, Mirra M, Zanella M. Pseudomesotheliomatous angiosarcoma: a pleuropulmonary lesion simulating malignant pleural mesothelioma. *Histopathology*. 1997;30:419–424.
123. Chen L, Shih HJ, Seguerra E, Lin JH. Pathologic Quiz Case: A 39-year-old man with diffuse pleural thickening and massive hemothorax. *Arch Pathol Lab Med*. 2004;128:1299–1300.
124. Pramesh CS, Madur BP, Raina S, Desai SB, Mistry RC. Angiosarcoma of the pleura. *Ann Thorac Cardiovasc Surg*. 2004;10:187–190.
125. Maglaras GC, Katsenos S, Kakadelis J, et al. Primary angiosarcoma of the lung and pleura. *Monaldi Arch Chest Dis*. 2004;61:234–236.
126. Liu SF, Hsieh MJ. Massive hemoptysis and hemothorax caused by pleuropulmonary angiosarcoma. *Am J Emerg Med*. 2002;20:374–375.
127. Alexiou C, Clelland CA, Robinson D, Morgan WE. Primary angiosarcomas of the chest wall and pleura. *Eur J Cardiothoracic Surg*. 1998;14:523–526.
128. Roh MS, Seo JY, Hong SH. Epithelioid angiosarcoma of the pleura: a case report. *J Korean Med Sci*. 2001;16:792–795.
129. Kimura M, Ito H, Furuta T, Tsumoto T, Hayashi S. Pyothorax-associated angiosarcoma of the pleura with metastasis to the brain. *Pathol Int*. 2003;53:547–551.
130. Aozasa K, Naka N, Tomita Y, et al. Angiosarcoma developing from chronic pyothorax. *Mod Pathol*. 1994;7:906–911.
131. Del Frate C, Mortele K, Zanardi R, et al. Pseudomesotheliomatous angiosarcoma of the chest wall and pleura. *J Thorac Imaging*. 2003;18:200–203.
132. Zhang PJ, Livolvsi VA, Brooks JJ. Malignant epithelioid vascular tumors of the pleura: report of a series and literature review. *Hum Pathol*. 2000;31:29–34.
133. Witkin GB, Rosai J. Solitary fibrous tumor of the mediastinum. Report of 14 cases. *Am J Surg Pathol*. 1989;13:547–557.
134. Goodlad JR, Fletcher CDM. Solitary fibrous tumor arising at unusual sites: analysis of a series. *Histopathology*. 1991;19:512–522.
135. Dorfman DM, To K, Dickersin GR, Rosenberg AE, Pilch BZ. Solitary fibrous tumor of the orbit. *Am J Surg Pathol*. 1994;18:281–287.
136. Suster S, Nascimiento AG, Miettinen M, Sickel JZ, Moran CA. Solitary fibrous tumor of soft tissue. A clinicopathologic and immunohistochemical study of 12 cases. *Am J Surg Pathol*. 1995;19:1257–1266.
137. Scharifker D, Kaneko M. Localized fibrous "mesothelioma" of pleura (submesothelial fibroma): a clinicopathologic study of 18 cases. *Cancer*. 1979;43:627–635.
138. Dalton WT, Zolliker AS, McCaughey WT, Jacques J, Kannerstein M. Localized primary tumors of the pleura: an analysis of 40 cases. *Cancer*. 1979;44:1465–1475.
139. Briselli M, Mark EJ, Dickersin R. Solitary fibrous tumor of the pleura. Eight new cases and review of 360 cases in the literature. *Cancer*. 1981;47:2678–2689.
140. England DM, Hochholzer L, McCarthy MJ. Localized benign and malignant fibrous tumors of the pleura: a clinicopathologic review of 223 cases. *Am J Surg Pathol*. 1989;13:640–658.
141. Westra WH, Gerald WL, Rosai J. Solitary fibrous tumor: consistent CD34 immunoreactivity and occurrence in the orbit. *Am J Surg Pathol*. 1994;18:992–998.
142. Chilosi M, Facchetti F, Dei Tos AP, et al. Bcl-2 expression in pleural and extrapleural solitary fibrous tumours. *J Pathol*. 1997;181:362–367.
143. Said JW, Nash G, Banks-Schlegel S, Sassoon AF, Shintaku IP. Localized fibrous mesothelioma: an immunohistochemical and electron microscopic study. *Hum Pathol*. 1984;15:440–443.
144. Moran CA, Suster S, Koss MN. The spectrum of histopathologic growth patterns in benign and malignant fibrous tumors of the pleura. *Semin Diagn Pathol*. 1992;9:169–180.
145. McDougall A, McGarrity G. Extra-abdominal desmoid tumors. *J Bone Joint Surg Br*. 1979;61:373–377.
146. Brodsky JT, Gordon MS, Hajdu SI, Burt M. Desmoid tumors of the chest wall. A locally recurrent problem. *J Thorac Cardiovasc Surg*. 1992;104:900–903.
147. Varghese Jr TK, Gupta R, Yeldandi AV, Varghese TK, Gupta R, Yeldandi AV. Desmoid tumor of the chest wall with pleural involvment. *Ann Thorac Surg*. 2003;76:937–939.
148. Andino L, Cagle PT, Murer B, et al. Pleuropulmonary desmoid tumors: immunohistochemical comparison with solitary fibrous tumors and assessment of B-catenin and cyclin D1 expression. *Arch Pathol Lab Med*. 2006;130:1503–1509.
149. Wilson RW, Gallateau-Salle F, Moran CA. Desmoid tumors of the pleura: a clinicopathologic mimic of localized fibrous tumor. *Mod Pathol*. 1999;12:9–14.
150. Fetsch JF, Montgomery EA, Meis JM. Calcifying fibrous pseudotumor. *Am J Surg Pathol*. 1993;17:502–508.
151. Van Dorpe J, Ectors N, Geboes K, D'Hoore A, Sciot R. Is calcifying fibrous tumor pseudotumor a late sclerosing stage of inflammatory myofibroblastic tumor? *Am J Surg Pathol*. 1999;23:329–335.
152. Nascimento AF, Ruiz R, Hornick JL, Fletcher CD. Calcifying fibrous "pseudotumor": clinicopathologic study of 15 cases and analysis of its relatioship to inflammatory myofibroblastic tumor. *Int J Surg Pathol*. 2002;10:189–196.
153. Reed MK, Margraf LR, Nikaidoh H, Cleveland DC. Calcifying fibrous pseudotumor of the chest wall. *Ann Thorac Surg*. 1996;62:873–874.
154. Maeda T, Hirose T, Furuya K, Kameoka K. Calcifying fibrous pseudotumor: an ultrastructural study. *Ultrastruct Pathol*. 1999;23:189–192.
155. Soyer T, Ciftci AO, Güçer S, Orhan D, Senocak ME. Calcifying fibrous pseudotumor of the lung: a previously unreported entity. *J Pediatr Surg*. 2004;39:1729–1730.
156. Pinkard NB, Wilson RW, Lawless N, et al. Calcifying fibrous pseudotumor of the pleura. A report of three cases of a newly described entity involving the pleura. *Am J Clin Pathol*. 1996;105:189–194.
157. Hainaut P, Lesage V, Weynand B, Coche E, Noirhomme P. Calcifying fibrous pseudotumor (CFPT): a patient presenting with multiple pleural lesions. *Acta Clin Belg*. 1999;54:162–164.
158. Mito K, Kashima K, Daa T, et al. Multiple calcifying fibrous tumor of the pleura. *Virchows Arch*. 2005;446:78–81.
159. Ammar A, El Hammami S, Horchani H, Sellami N, Kilani T. Calcifying fibrous pseudotumor of the pleura: a rare location. *Ann Thorac Surg*. 2003;76:2081–2082.
160. Jang KS, Oh YH, Han HX, et al. Calcifying fibrous pseudotumor of the pleura. *Ann Thorac Surg*. 2004;78:87–88.
161. Kawahara K, Yasukawa M, Nakagawa K, Katsura H, Nagano T, Iwasaki T. Multiple calcifying fibrous tumor of the pleura. *Virchows Arch*. 2005;447:1007–1008.
162. Shibata K, Yuki D, Sakata K. Multiple calcifying fibrous pseudotumors disseminated in the pleura. *Ann Thorac Surg*. 2008;85:3–5.
163. Suh JH, Shin OR, Kim YH. Multiple calcifying fibrous pseudotumor of the pleura. *J Thorac Oncol*. 2008;3:1356–1358.
164. Erasmus JJ, McAdams HP, Patz Jr EF, Murray JG, Pinkard NB. Calcifying fibrous pseudotumor of pleura: radiologic features in three cases. *J Comput Assist Tomogr*. 1996;20:763–765.

165. Zamecnik M, Michal M, Boudova L, Sulc M. CD34 expression in calcifying fibrous pseudotumours. *Histopathology*. 2000;36:182–191.
166. Angerval L, Enzinger FM. Extraskeletal neoplasms resembling Ewing's sarcoma. *Cancer*. 1977;101:446–449.
167. Askin FB, Rosai J, Sibley R, Dehner LP, McAlister WH. Malignant small cell tumors of the thoracopulmonary region in childhood: a distinctive clinicopathologic entity of uncertain histogenesis. *Cancer*. 1979;43:2438–2451.
168. Gould V, Jannson D, Warren W. Primitive neuroenctodermal tumors (PNET) of the chest wall in adults [Abstract #681]. *Mod Pathol*. 4:1991;115A.
169. Hashimoto H, Enjoji M, Nakajima T, Kiryu H, Daimaru Y. Malignant neuroepithelioma (peripheral neuroblastoma). A clinicopathologic study of 15 cases. *Am J Surg Pathol*. 1983;7:309–318.
170. Lane S, Ironside JW. Extraskeletal Ewing's sarcoma of the nasal fossa. *J Laryngol Otol*. 1990;104:570–573.
171. Soule EH, Newton Jr W, Moon TE, Tefft M. Extraskeletal Ewing's sarcoma. A preliminary review of 26 cases encountered in the Intergroup Rhabdomyosarcoma Study. *Cancer*. 1978;42:259–264.
172. Suster S, Ronnen M, Huczar M. Extraskeletal Ewing's sarcoma of the scalp. *Pediatr Dermatol*. 1988;5:126–128.
173. Tefft M, Vawter GF, Metus A. Paravertebral "round cell" tumors in children. *Radiology*. 1969;92:1501–1509.
174. Wigger JH, Salazar G, Blanc WA. Extraskeletal Ewing's sarcoma. *Arch Pathol Lab Med*. 1977;101:446–449.
175. Fujii Y, Hongo T, Nakagawa Y, et al. Cell culture of small round cell tumor originating in the thoracopulmonary region. Evidence for derivation from a primitive pluripotential cell. *Cancer*. 1989;64:43–51.
176. Yunis EJ, Agostini Jr RM, Walpusk JA, Hubbard JD. Glycogen in neuroblastomas. A light- and electron-microscopic study of 40 cases. *Am J Surg Pathol*. 1979;3:199–208.
177. Gillespie JJ, Roth LM, Wills ER, Einhorn LH, Willman J. Extraskeletal Ewing's sarcoma. Histologic and ultrastructural observations in three cases. *Am J Surg Pathol*. 1979;3:99–108.
178. Schmidt D, Mackay B, Ayala A. Ewing's sarcoma with neuroblastoma like features. *Ultrastruct Pathol*. 1982;3:99–108.
179. Tsuji S, Hisaoka M, Morimitsu Y, et al. Peripheral primitive neuroectodermal tumour of the lung: report of two cases. *Histopathology*. 1998;33:369–374.
180. Kahn AG, Avagnina A, Nazar J, Elsner B. Primitive neuroectodermal tumor of the lung. *Atch Pathol Lab Med*. 2001;125:397–399.
181. Mikami Y, Nakajima M, Hashimoto H, et al. Primary pulmonary primitive neuroectodermal tumor (PNET). A case report. *Pathol Res Pract*. 2001;197:113–119.
182. Imamura F, Funakoshi T, Nakamura S, Mano M, Kodama K, Horai T. Primary primitive neuroectodermal tumor of the lung. Report of two cases. *Lung Cancer*. 2000;27:55–60.
183. Linnoila RI, Tsokos M, Triche TJ, Marangos PJ, Chandra RS. Evidence for neural origin and PAS-positive variants of the malignant small cell tumor of thoracopulmonary region ("Askin's tumor"). *Am J Surg Pathol*. 1986;10:124–133.
184. Tsokos M, Linnoila RI, Chandra RS, Triche TJ. Neuron-specific enolase in the diagnosis of neuroblastoma and other small, round-cell tumors in children. *Hum Pathol*. 1984;15:575–584.
185. Gonzales-Crussi F, Wolfson SL, Misugi K, Nakajima T. Peripheral neuroectodermal tumors of the chest wall in childhood. *Cancer*. 1984;54:2519–2527.
186. Ordonez NG. Application of immunohistochemistry in the diagnosis of soft tissue sarcomas: a review and update. *Adv Anat Pathol*. 1998;5(2):67–85.
187. Hill DA, Pfeifer JD, Marley EF, et al. WT1 staining reliability differentiates desmoplastic small round cell tumor from Ewing sarcoma/primitive neuroectodermal tumor. An immunohistochemical and molecular diagnostic study. *Am J Clin Pathol*. 2000;114:345–353.
188. Miettinen M, Chatten J, Paetau A, Stevenson A. Monoclonal antibody NB84 in the differential diagnosis of neuroblastoma and other small round cell tumors. *Am J Surg Pathol*. 1998;22:327–332.
189. Batsakis JG, El-Nagar A. Ewing's sarcoma and primitive neuroectodermal tumors: cytogenetic cynosures seeking a common histogenesis. *Adv Anat Pathol*. 1997;4(4):207–220.
190. Bown NP, Reid MM, Malcolm AJ, Davison EV, Craft AW, Pearson AD. Cytogenetic abnormalities of small round cell tumours. *Med Pediatr Oncol*. 1994;23:124–129.
191. Whang-Peng J, Triche TJ, Knutsen T, et al. Cytogenetic characterization of selected small round cell tumors of chlhood. *Cancer Genet Cytogenet*. 1986;21:185–208.
192. Contesso G, Llombart-Bosch A, Terrier P, et al. Does malignant small round cell tumor of the thoracopulmonary region (Askin tumor) constitute a clinicopathologic entity? An analysis of 30 cases with immunohistochemical and electron-microcopy support treated at the Institute Gustave Roussy. *Cancer*. 1992;69:1012–1020.
193. Gaertner E, Zeren EH, Fleming MV, Colby TV, Travis WD. Biphasic synovial sarcomas arising in the pleural cavity. A clinicopathologic study of five cases. *Am J Surg Pathol*. 1996;20:36–45.
194. Moran CA, Suster S, Koss MN. Smooth muscle tumours presenting as pleural neoplasms. *Histopathology*. 1995;27:227–234.
195. Smith S, Opipari MI. Primary pleural melanoma: a first reported case and literature review. *J Thorac Cardiovasc Surg*. 1978;75:827–831.
196. Wong WW, Pluth JR, Grado GL, Schild SE, Sanderson DR. Liposarcoma of the pleura. *Mayo Clin Proc*. 1994;69:882–885.
197. Gupta RK, Paolini FA. Liposarcoma of the pleura: report of a case with review of the literature and views of histogenesis. *Am Rev Respir Dis*. 1967;95:298–304.
198. Evans AR, Wolstenholme RJ, Shettar SP, Yogish H. Primary pleural liposarcoma. *Thorax*. 1985;40:554–555.
199. Adams AL, Castro CY, Singh P, Moran CA. Primary amyloidosis of the pleura mimicking mesothelioma. *Ann Diagn Pathol*. 2001;5:229–232.

14

Clinical Management of Lung Cancer

David J. Stewart

Lung cancer is the most common cause of cancer death in North America.[1] The 5-year relative survival rate among all patients with lung cancer is currently only 16%, compared with 13% in the years 1975 to 1977.[1] Thus, although progress is being made, it has been very slow, with much work still to be done. Both prognosis and management options for lung cancer depend on the disease stage and are strongly influenced by comorbid conditions. Differences in management between non–small cell lung cancer (NSCLC) and small cell lung cancer (SCLC) also have been well characterized.

NON–SMALL CELL LUNG CANCER

Surgery in Stage I and Stage II Non–Small Cell Lung Cancer

Surgical resection is the treatment of choice for patients with localized NSCLC whose pulmonary function and general medical condition permit this to be done safely. Surgical options are discussed in greater detail in Chapter 2, on the surgical staging of lung cancer.

Use of Postoperative Radiotherapy In Stage I and Stage II Non–Small Cell Lung Cancer

Postoperative radiotherapy to reduce risk of local recurrence generally is used if surgical margins are positive for tumor. In patients with clear surgical margins, randomized studies comparing outcomes with postoperative irradiation and with observation have failed to demonstrate an advantage for radiotherapy.[2] In fact, postoperative radiotherapy is associated with an increased risk of death, with absolute survival rates of 55% at 2 years without radiotherapy and 48% with radiotherapy.[2] Negative impact on survival is greatest in stage I disease and less in stage II, with no negative (or positive) impact on survival in patients with stage III disease.[2] Local tumor recurrence rates were reduced by 24% with postoperative radiotherapy, suggesting a potential positive effect on tumor control but negative effect on survival owing to radiotherapy toxicity.[2] Hence, for a majority of patients with stage I or II NSCLC, the current standard of care is not to administer postoperative radiotherapy, whereas it is frequently administered in patients after resection of stage III disease and in other patients in whom clear surgical margins could not be achieved, to reduce risk of local mediastinal recurrence.

Radiotherapy as Definitive Treatment for Medically Inoperable Stage I and Stage II Non–Small Cell Lung Cancer

A high proportion of patients with lung cancer have comorbid conditions such as chronic obstructive lung disease or coronary artery disease. In some patients, these comorbid illnesses are severe enough to preclude surgery. Although even very elderly patients may benefit from surgery if they are in good health, older patients also are more likely to have comorbid conditions that make surgery inadvisable. Radiotherapy alone may lead to long-term control in some patients with NSCLC, with overall 5-year survival rates ranging from 5% to 42% for different studies and a median 5-year survival rate across studies of approximately 15%.[3] To correct for the effect of comorbidity, cause-specific survival also has been assessed, and in most studies, cause-specific 5-year survival rates generally have been 10% to 20% higher than overall survival rates, with a median survival across studies of approximately 31 months.[3] Although no randomized comparisons of definitive radiotherapy and surgery for patients with stage I and stage II NSCLC have been conducted, median survival times for early-stage NSCLC across broad populations[4] (in which a majority of the patients had undergone surgery) are longer than the cause-specific survival noted above with radiotherapy. Although comorbid conditions could account for differences in overall survival between surgery and radiotherapy, they would be less likely to have an impact on the cause-specific survival, suggesting better local tumor control with surgery. Nevertheless, radiotherapy is a useful option for patients who are not surgical candidates.

Stereotactic Radiotherapy for Stage I and Stage II Non–Small Cell Lung Cancer

Recent studies suggest that stereotactic radiotherapy may be of value in medically inoperable patients without mediastinal node involvement. This modality typically entails delivery of radiation to a localized area in a single large treatment or as three to four fractions over 1 to 2 weeks, with a high dose each day, for a total radiation dose of approximately 45 to 60 Gy.[5] Local control rates of more than 80% have been achieved with small peripheral tumors and approximately 50% with central tumors.[5] Severe toxicity is more likely with large tumors or with centrally located tumors, whereas stereotactic radiotherapy generally is well tolerated for smaller peripheral tumors.[5] A randomized trial comparing stereotactic radiotherapy and surgery in appropriate candidates is ongoing.

Postoperative Adjuvant Chemotherapy in Stage I to Stage IIIA Non–Small Cell Lung Cancer

Patients who have undergone resection of NSCLC with curative intent often will demonstrate distant metastases a few months to a few years after surgery. Typically, large numbers of circulating tumor cells can be detected in the blood of patients with invasive malignancies, but most of these tumor cells may die or else remain quiescent after lodging in distant tissues and never form detectable metastases.[6] However, some of these surviving tumor cells also may begin to proliferate, eventually manifesting as metastases. Although chemotherapy cannot permanently eradicate tumors large enough to be seen radiologically, it may in some cases be able to eradicate micrometastases.

Recent randomized trials have demonstrated that postoperative adjuvant cisplatin-based chemotherapy may improve survival in patients after resection for stage II or III NSCLC, particularly in those with good performance status, with a 5-year absolute survival benefit of 5.4% from chemotherapy.[7] The benefit varied with stage, with a possible harmful effect seen in patients with stage IA disease (hazard ratio [HR] = 1.40; 95% confidence interval [CI], 0.95–2.06), equivocal outcome in those with stage IB disease (HR = 0.93; 95% CI, 0.78–1.10), but evidence of benefit in those with stage II disease (HR = 0.83; 95% CI, 0.73–0.95) and in stage III (HR = 0.83; 95% CI, 0.72–0.94).[7] Because prognosis worsens with increasing tumor size and with pleural or vascular invasion by tumor, adjuvant chemotherapy may in some cases also be offered to patients with stage IB disease whose tumors are larger or exhibit pleural or vascular invasion, despite the fact that no randomized clinical trials assessing benefit in this subpopulation have yet been conducted. Studies in Japanese patients with NSCLC suggested that the fluorinated pyrimidine-uracil compound UFT may be of value for adjuvant therapy in patients with resected stage I disease,[8] but this agent has not yet gained acceptance in North America or Europe, and its efficacy has been questioned.[9]

Typically, three to four cycles of adjuvant chemotherapy are administered over 9 to 12 weeks. Some clinicians substitute carboplatin for cisplatin, because it is less toxic. In advanced NSCLC, however, carboplatin is not quite as effective as cisplatin,[10] and proof of benefit of carboplatin regimens for adjuvant therapy is lacking, because only limited studies have been done. With respect to the drug added to cisplatin or carboplatin, vinorelbine, another vinca alkaloid, and etoposide each have been used with some success.[7] Taxanes such as paclitaxel and docetaxel are at least as effective as vinca alkaloids and etoposide against advanced metastatic NSCLC and also are frequently used in the adjuvant setting despite a lack of definitive testing of these agents for such therapy.

Preoperative ("Neoadjuvant") Chemotherapy in Non–Small Cell Lung Cancer

Chemotherapy may also be administered before surgery. Such neoadjuvant chemotherapy has several potential advantages over postoperative adjuvant chemotherapy, including improved drug tolerability,[11] improved drug delivery,[12] preoperative downstaging (which may improve resectability and prognosis), decreased perioperative tumor seeding, and early control of micrometastases.[12–14] In some studies, neoadjuvant chemotherapy[15,16] and chemoradiotherapy[17,18] have decreased tumor size sufficiently to render unresectable stage IIIB disease in patients with NSCLC potentially resectable, and in some small randomized studies in patients with operable stage I,[19] II,[19] or IIIA NSCLC,[20, 21] neoadjuvant chemotherapy significantly improved survival. A larger study in patients with operable stage IB to stage IIIA NSCLC found a trend toward improved progression-free and overall survival,[22] and in a meta-analysis of six randomized trials, administration of neoadjuvant chemotherapy in stage I to stage IIIA NSCLC was associated with an HR of 0.66 (95% CI, 0.48–0.93) compared with surgery alone.[23] Neoadjuvant chemotherapy is now considered an option as a standard of care for selected patients with operable stage III NSCLC. In NSCLC meta-analyses, the HR of 0.66 with neoadjuvant chemotherapy compared favorably with the HR of 0.84 (95% CI, 0.78–0.89) seen in 19 trials of postoperative chemotherapy,[23] although studies comparing neoadjuvant chemotherapy to postoperative chemotherapy in NSCLC have not yet been done.

Currently, neoadjuvant chemotherapy often is used in patients in whom preoperative staging reveals low-bulk involvement of subcarinal or ipsilateral mediastinal nodes. Patients with bulky disease involving ipsilateral mediastinal nodes or with known involvement of contralateral mediastinal nodes or of more than one mediastinal lymph node station generally are not considered to be candidates for surgery because of the high risk of later development of distant metastases despite adjuvant chemotherapy. Neoadjuvant chemotherapy also is occasionally used in patients with bulky disease in stage II NSCLC, particularly if tumor shrinkage in response to chemotherapy potentially may offer the possibility for less extensive surgery (e.g., by permitting lobectomy in a situation in which pneumonectomy would otherwise be required).

Radiotherapy for Inoperable Stage III Non–Small Cell Lung Cancer

Radiotherapy alone may be effective in a small proportion of patients with inoperable stage IIIA NSCLC and may also cure some patients with stage IIIB disease, in the absence of a malignant pleural effusion (i.e., in "dry IIIB" as opposed to "wet IIIB" disease), with long-term survival rates for patients with stage IIIA and stage IIIB NSCLC of approximately 5% to 10%.[24–26] The typical radiotherapy dosing schedule is once a day, 5 days a week, for 6 to 6.4 weeks, to deliver a total dose of 60 to 64 Gy.[25] This schedule takes advantage of the fact that normal tissues are more efficient than tumor tissues at repair of radiation damage, to maximize the therapeutic index when it is necessary to include substantial volumes of normal tissue with the radiation.

As a rule, the greater the bulk of tumor, the lower the probability of cure with radiotherapy, because more bulky disease is associated with increased risk of later distant metastases and also is associated with a higher rate of local failure.[25,27] Involvement of supraclavicular lymph nodes also increases the risk of eventual failure.[24] Outcomes with radiotherapy are somewhat better for squamous cell carcinoma than for other tumor types.[27]

The location of the primary tumor also may be relevant.[28] If a patient has a peripheral lower lobe primary tumor and nodal involvement, then the size of the radiotherapy field and the amount of lung destroyed by the radiotherapy will be relatively large, whereas the size of the radiotherapy field is much smaller and the amount of radiation damage to lung is much less if the patient has a centrally placed upper lobe tumor, and the probability of survival is higher with inoperable upper lobe tumors than with inoperable tumors in other locations.[27]

Radiation has to travel through the lung to reach the tumor and subsequently passes out of the far side of the lung; in the process, this energy destroys lung tissue in its path. Scatter to more distant lung also may occur, and the resultant exposure may be sufficient to cause extensive radiation pneumonia, which may respond to steroids but also can prove fatal in some instances.[28] Other organs and structures at risk for damage from the radiation include skin, esophagus, heart, and spinal cord. Radiation esophagitis may be severe enough to necessitate temporary placement of a feeding tube and may result in later scarring with consequent esophageal stricture formation requiring periodic esophageal dilatation. An excessive radiation dose to the spinal cord may damage blood vessels, causing irreversible transverse myelitis with paraplegia.[29] Great care is taken to limit the dose to the spinal cord, but use of the angles required to accomplish this often results in higher doses to the esophagus, with increased esophagitis.

Over the past several years, progressive improvements in radiotherapy technology have permitted delivery of higher, more effective radiotherapy doses with reduced toxicity. Orthovoltage equipment gave way to cobalt 60 equipment, which in turn was replaced by linear accelerators. Advances in radiotherapy planning methods ultimately permitted further refinement of linear accelerator techniques, first with three-dimensional conformal radiotherapy (3DCR), then with intensity-modulated radiotherapy (IMRT), and then with IMRT with mechanisms to correct for movement of the tumor with respiration. In IMRT, a relatively large number of radiotherapy beamlets with differing dose intensities are directed at the tumor from different angles. With IMRT, a very large volume of low-dose radiation is delivered with the entrance and exit of these many beamlets, but in comparison with 3DCR, a smaller volume of lung receives 20 Gy (considered to be the threshold for development of radiation pneumonitis),[30,31] and the observed rate of treatment-related pneumonitis is significantly lower with IMRT than with 3DCR.[32]

Recently, a growing experience with proton beam radiotherapy (PBR) has been the subject of study. PBR has the advantage that it deposits all of its radiation energy at the tumor; accordingly, although toxicity to tissues is incurred along the path of radiation into the tumor, toxicity resulting from radiation exiting the far side of the tumor is greatly reduced.[33] Preliminary data suggest that the observed clinical reduction in toxicity with PBR matches that anticipated in theoretical analyses.

Chemoradiotherapy for Inoperable Stage III Non–Small Cell Lung Cancer

Randomized trials showed that addition of chemotherapy to radiotherapy improved the probability of long-term control in locally advanced, inoperable NSCLC. The initial studies involved administration of a few cycles of platinum-based chemotherapy, followed by approximately 6 weeks of radiotherapy.[34,35] Subsequent studies showed that administration of low-dose chemotherapy with once-daily or once-weekly dosing during radiotherapy also improved survival by improving control of the local tumor.[36] Still later randomized studies demonstrated that administration of chemotherapy concurrently with radiotherapy is superior to sequential administration of chemotherapy followed by radiotherapy,[37–39] and this is now the standard of care for patients with stage IIIA and "dry" stage IIIB NSCLC.

Chemotherapy may help improve outcome by several different mechanisms. In addition to directly adding to tumor cell kill, cisplatin and carboplatin can act as free electron acceptors—thereby taking the place of oxygen and prolonging the half-life of DNA-damaging hydroxyl radicals produced by radiation—and can inhibit repair of radiation-induced DNA damage.[40] Both the platinums[40] and a variety of other agents such as the taxanes[41] and vinca alkaloids[42] also can increase the proportion of tumor cells that are in the radiation-sensitive G_2/M phase of the cell cycle, and various other mechanisms also may be at play.[40] Although the addition of chemotherapy to radiation therapy does increase toxicity to the esophagus, this toxicity is manageable.

Palliative Radiotherapy for Advanced Non–Small Cell Lung Cancer

Stage IV and "wet" stage IIIB NSCLC—so-called advanced NSCLC—is incurable, so the objective of therapy is symptom control. Radiotherapy (with a typical dose of 30 Gy given in 10 fractions over 2 weeks or 45 Gy given in 15 fractions over 3 weeks) may be useful for reducing the frequency or severity of a variety of cancer-induced symptoms, including pain, cough, hemoptysis, and dyspnea. It also can reduce the risk of several complications of metastases, including pathologic fractures from bone metastases, paralysis from spinal cord compression, and neurologic complications of brain metastases. Irradiation also may open up airways or esophagus obstructed by tumor, thereby facilitating breathing and eating.

First-Line Chemotherapy for Advanced Non–Small Cell Lung Cancer

In a recent meta-analysis of randomized studies, the median survival time for patients with advanced NSCLC who did not undergo chemotherapy was 4.5 months and the 1-year overall survival rate was 20%; in patients who received chemotherapy, median survival was 6.0 months and the 1-year survival rate was 29% (HR = 0.75; 95% CI, 0.67–0.84; $P < .0001$).[43] The beneficial effects of chemotherapy were observed irrespective of age, gender, histologic features, type of cytotoxic drug (although long-term alkylating agents were associated with a detrimental effect in an earlier meta-analysis[44] and were excluded from this updated report), or baseline performance status (although more than 75% of the patients had a performance status of 0 or 1).[43] Quality of life either was improved after chemotherapy or was comparable to that seen in the best supportive care group.[45–49]

Two-drug combinations are superior to single-agent chemotherapy in advanced NSCLC, although such regimens also are associated with somewhat greater toxicity.[50] Platinums (cisplatin or carboplatin) form the backbone of most NSCLC combination regimens, and meta-analyses suggest that cisplatin is slightly more effective than carboplatin, although it also is more toxic.[10] Docetaxel, paclitaxel, vinorelbine, and gemcitabine all give similar results when added to a platinum,[51] although one study suggested that docetaxel may be somewhat superior to vinorelbine when added to cisplatin, with a median overall survival of 11.3 months versus 10.1 months (HR = 1.183; 97.2% CI, 0.989–1.416; $P = .044$) and better quality-of-life scores.[52] In one study, progression-free survival was slightly longer with the use of gemcitabine than with taxane regimens.[53] However, all of these agents generally are looked upon as being equivalent in efficacy when added to a platinum, yielding response rates in the range of 17% to 32% and a median survival of 7.8 to 11.3 months. Older agents such as etoposide, vinblastine, and vindesine are somewhat less effective. The topoisomerase I inhibitor irinotecan also may be helpful when combined with a platinum in advanced disease.

The combination of cisplatin with the multitargeted antifolate pemetrexed was superior to the combination of gemcitabine with cisplatin in patients with adenocarcinoma and large cell carcinoma, whereas the gemcitabine combination was superior to the pemetrexed combination in patients with squamous cell carcinomas.[54] Adding a third chemotherapy agent to a two-drug platinum-based regimen results in increased response rate but does not improve survival.[50]

Typically, four to six cycles of chemotherapy are administered to patients who are responding. Chemotherapy is not continued for longer periods because the first few cycles of chemotherapy appear to be the most effective ones. Moreover, randomized trials have not demonstrated any benefit to proceeding with chemotherapy beyond the initial four to six cycles,[55–57] although recent studies of maintenance pemetrexed after initial chemotherapy with other agents suggest a possible benefit in patients with adenocarcinoma.[58] In some patients, rapid tumor regrowth occurs when therapy is discontinued; in others, regrowth may not occur until several months later.

Chemotherapy in Previously Treated Patients with Advanced Non–Small Cell Lung Cancer

Tumors that have previously been exposed to chemotherapeutic agents are less likely than chemo-naive tumors to respond to subsequent chemotherapy. Nevertheless, randomized studies comparing docetaxel with best supportive care in previously treated patients demonstrated that docetaxel provided a benefit, with an improvement in median life expectancy from 4.6 months to 7 months,[59] as well as an improvement in average quality of life.[60] Subsequent studies demonstrated that pemetrexed was as effective as docetaxel in the second-line setting but was less toxic.[61] Gemcitabine also may be of some value in this setting,[62] whereas vinorelbine appears to be ineffective.[63]

Targeted Therapies in Non–Small Cell Lung Cancer

Targeted therapies are based on the use of drugs or other agents that are directed specifically against a cell growth receptor or its ligands, signaling pathway components, or other effectors of function. Several such agents currently are under investigation for the treatment of lung cancer. The monoclonal antibody bevacizumab (Avastin) binds to and inactivates vascular endothelial growth factor (VEGF), thereby antagonizing the new vessel formation (angiogenesis) required by tumors for growth. Randomized trials confirmed that addition of bevacizumab to carboplatin plus paclitaxel increased both response rate (from 15% with chemotherapy alone to 35% with chemotherapy plus bevacizumab) and median survival (10.3 months and 12.3 months, respectively).[64] Preliminary assessments suggest that vandetanib, a small molecule that inhibits both the VEGF receptor and the epidermal growth factor receptor (EGFR), also may prolong progression-free survival when added to chemotherapy regimens for treatment of NSCLC.[65]

In a comparison of outcomes achieved with the EGFR tyrosine kinase inhibitor (TKI) erlotinib and with best supportive care, erlotinib treatment significantly prolonged survival of patients with NSCLC previously treated with chemotherapy, from a median of 4.7 months with best supportive care to 6.7 months with erlotinib,[66] with improvement also noted in average quality of life.[67] Treatment with erlotinib is now considered a standard of care in this setting. This agent is most effective in patients with EGFR-activating mutations or high *EGFR* gene copy number, and with K-ras wild type.[68]

The related EGFR TKI gefitinib also is effective against NSCLC in selected patients, but improvement in survival over that observed with best supportive care failed to achieve statistical significance (P = .087).[69] Gefitinib is no longer used in North America but is widely used in Asia. Of interest, however, gefitinib recently was found to be comparable in efficacy to docetaxel in the second-line setting,[70] so this agent may be assessed further.

Female patients with lung adenocarcinomas who have never smoked and are East Asian are particularly likely to have *EGFR* mutations and also are particularly likely to benefit from treatment with an EGFR TKI,[71] and in a randomized trial, gefitinib was superior to standard chemotherapy in chemotherapy-naive Asian never-smokers. Addition of an EGFR TKI to first-line chemotherapy did not result in improved survival, except in patients who had never smoked[72] and in fact was associated with decreased survival in patients whose tumors had K-ras mutations.[73] For reasons that are unclear, administration of gefitinib after completion of chemoradiotherapy for locally advanced NSCLC also worsened overall survival despite having minimal impact on progression-free survival,[74] so this protocol is not currently recommended in this setting.

Although the EGFR TKIs do not improve outcome when added to first-line chemotherapy regimens in advanced NSCLC, addition of the anti-EGFR monoclonal antibody cetuximab (C-225 [Erbitux]) resulted in modest improvement of median overall survival, from 10.1 months in the control group to 11.3 months in the cetuximab-treated patients (HR = 0.871; 95% CI, 0.762–0.996; P = .0441).[75] Additional studies combining cetuximab with chemotherapy plus bevacizumab are under way.

The Ras/Raf/VEGFR inhibitor sorafenib[76] and the proteasome inhibitor bortezomib[77] also appear to have modest activity in NSCLC but do not yet have an established role in clinical practice. Because amplification of c-Met is a potential cause of acquired resistance to EGFR TKIs,[78] clinical studies of use of c-Met inhibitors in NSCLC have recently been launched. Earlier trials of matrix metalloproteinase inhibitors yielded negative results.[79]

Management of the Patient with a Solitary Metastasis from Non–Small Cell Lung Cancer

Although widely metastatic NSCLC generally is considered to be incurable, patients with solitary metastases to one or two sites may potentially achieve long-term survival if such disease is resected. The largest experience with metastasis resection in NSCLC involves solitary brain metastases[80] and, to a lesser extent, adrenal gland metastases.[81] Randomized trials have demonstrated that brain metastasis resection is superior to cranial irradiation alone[82] and that survival is further improved by administering whole-brain radiotherapy after the brain metastasis resection.[83] Aggressive local therapy for solitary bone metastases generally does not result in long-term disease control.

SMALL CELL LUNG CANCER

Management of Limited Small Cell Lung Cancer

In patients with SCLC, "limited disease" refers to cancer confined to one hemithorax. Approximately 40% of patients present with limited disease.[84] In limited-disease SCLC, median survival time is approximately 3 months without chemotherapy[85] and 15 months with combination chemotherapy,[86] and 10% to 25% of patients with limited-disease SCLC achieve long-term survival.[86,87] Although prolonged survival occasionally is achieved with surgery alone (predominantly in patients with uncommon small peripheral lesions) or with radiotherapy alone,[87] chemotherapy is regarded as the most important component of therapy because of the aggressive nature of the disease, with rapid development of distant metastases.[87,88]

The standard chemotherapy regimen used in the treatment of SCLC consists of cisplatin (or, less commonly, carboplatin) administered on day 1 of a 3-week cycle and the topoisomerase II inhibitor etoposide administered intravenously or orally for 3 consecutive days.[84] Multiple-day administration of etoposide is more effective in SCLC than is administration of the entire dose on a single day.[89] Combining the topoisomerase I inhibitor irinotecan with cisplatin gives results comparable to those with the combination of etoposide with cisplatin.[90] Other regimens appear to be less effective.[91] As with NSCLC, no major survival benefit is derived from going beyond four to six cycles with first-line chemotherapy,[88] presumably because of the emergence of acquired resistance.

Despite the general inability of radiotherapy alone to control SCLC, addition to chemotherapy of full-dose radiotherapy directed at the intrathoracic disease improves the long-term survival rate by 5% over that achieved with use of chemotherapy alone.[86,88] Administration of the radiotherapy early in the course of chemotherapy (starting with cycle 1 or 2) appears to be superior to delaying radiotherapy until late in the course of chemotherapy,[86,88] and hyperfractionated radiotherapy with twice-daily administration may be superior to once-daily fractionation in limited-disease SCLC.[86,88]

Brain metastases develop in up to 30% of patients with SCLC who demonstrate a good response to systemic chemotherapy, and the brain may be the first or only site of relapse in these patients.[86] Prophylactic cranial irradiation (PCI) administered after completion of chemotherapy reduces the rate of brain metastases from 30% to approximately 15% and improves the probability of long-term survival by approximately 5%.[86] PCI is now the standard of care for patients who have demonstrated a good response to systemic therapy.

Management of Extensive Small Cell Lung Cancer

SCLC that has spread beyond one hemithorax is referred to as extensive disease. In patients with SCLC characterized as extensive, median survival without chemotherapy is 6 weeks,[85] whereas median survival with chemotherapy is approximately 8 to 13 months.[86] Approximately 70% of patients with extensive disease respond to chemotherapy, and 20% or more will experience complete remission,[87] but only approximately 1% to 2% achieve long-term survival.[86,87] Chemotherapy choice and number of cycles generally are the same as in limited disease. Radiotherapy generally is used only for palliation of symptoms in patients whose disease has progressed after chemotherapy, although 1-year survival rates were significantly improved from 13.3% to 27.1% by administration of PCI to patients with extensive-disease SCLC who had responded to chemotherapy.[86]

Second-Line Chemotherapy for Small Cell Lung Cancer

SCLC that worsens during first-line chemotherapy or within 3 months of its completion tends to be resistant to further chemotherapy; this clinical recurrence pattern has been termed *resistant relapse*. By contrast, SCLC that responds to chemotherapy and regrows only after more than 3 months after its completion may respond well to further chemotherapy; this pattern is termed *sensitive relapse*.[87] For patients who experience sensitive relapse, one option is to repeat the first-line chemotherapy (with a reasonable expectation of a good clinical response but shorter response duration).[92] An alternative approach is to change to another regimen such as single-agent topotecan or a combination of cyclophosphamide, doxorubicin, and vincristine.[87] These options also may be tried in resistant relapse, but with only a low probability of working. To date, targeted therapies have not proved useful in SCLC.

CONCLUSION

Lung cancer remains a major health care problem. Gradual progress has been made, but 84% of all afflicted patients in North America still die of their disease. Substantial effort is under way to identify new drugs and new therapeutic targets, with the goal of greatly improving current outcomes.

REFERENCES

1. Jemal A, Siegel R, Ward E, et al. Cancer statistics, 2008. *CA Cancer J Clin*. 2008;58(2):71–96.
2. PORT Meta-analysis Trialists Group. Postoperative radiotherapy in non-small-cell lung cancer: systematic review and meta-analysis of individual patient data from nine randomised controlled trials. *Lancet*. 1998;352(9124):257–263.
3. Zimmermann FB, Bamberg M, Molls M, Jeremic B. Radiation therapy alone in early stage non-small cell lung cancer. *Semin Surg Oncol*. 2003;21(2):91–97.
4. Groome PA, Bolejack V, Crowley JJ, et al. The IASLC Lung Cancer Staging Project: validation of the proposals for revision of the T, N, and M descriptors and consequent stage groupings in the forthcoming (seventh) edition of the TNM classification of malignant tumours. *J Thorac Oncol*. 2007;2(8):694–705.
5. Ball D. Stereotactic radiotherapy for nonsmall cell lung cancer. *Curr Opin Pulmon Med*. 2008;14(4):297–302.
6. MacDonald IC, Groom AC, Chambers AF. Cancer spread and micrometastasis development: quantitative approaches for in vivo models. *Bioessays*. 2002;24(10):885–893.
7. Pignon JP, Tribodet H, Scagliotti GV, et al. Lung adjuvant cisplatin evaluation: a pooled analysis by the LACE Collaborative Group. *J Clin Oncol*. 2008;26(21):3552–3559.
8. Hamada C, Tanaka F, Ohta M, et al. Meta-analysis of postoperative adjuvant chemotherapy with tegafur-uracil in non-small-cell lung cancer. *J Clin Oncol*. 2005;23(22):4999–5006.
9. Stewart L, Burdett S. Adjuvant UFT therapy does not increase survival in people with resected stage 1 non-small cell lung cancer. *Cancer Treat Rev*. 2005;31(6):487–490.
10. Ardizzoni A, Boni L, Tiseo M, et al. Cisplatin- versus carboplatin-based chemotherapy in first-line treatment of advanced non-small-cell lung cancer: an individual patient data meta-analysis. *J Natl Cancer Inst*. 2007;99(11):847–857.
11. Betticher DC. Adjuvant and neoadjuvant chemotherapy in NSCLC: a paradigm shift. *Lung Cancer*. 2005;50(Suppl 2):S9–S16.
12. Bunn Jr PA. Early-stage non-small-cell lung cancer: current perspectives in combined-modality therapy. *Clin Lung Cancer*. 2004;6(2):85–98.
13. Belani CP. Adjuvant and neoadjuvant therapy in non-small cell lung cancer. *Semin Oncol*. 2005;32(2 Suppl 2):S9–S15.
14. Cappuzzo F, Bartolini S, Calandri C, Crino L. Induction therapy for early-stage non-small-cell lung cancer. *Oncology (Williston Park)*. 2004;18(8 Suppl 5):32–37.
15. Cappuzzo F, De Marinis F, Nelli F, et al. Phase II study of gemcitabine-cisplatin-paclitaxel triplet as induction chemotherapy in inoperable, locally advanced non-small cell lung cancer. *Lung Cancer*. 2003;42(3):355–361.
16. Grossi F, Pennucci MC, Serrano J, et al. Phase II study of neoadjuvant chemotherapy in patients with surgically-proven, unresectable stage III non-small cell lung cancer. *Anticancer Res*. 2002;22(6B):3519–3524.
17. Ichinose Y, Fukuyama Y, Asoh H, et al. Induction chemoradiotherapy and surgical resection for selected stage IIIB non-small-cell lung cancer. *Ann Thorac Surg*. 2003;76(6):1810–1814.
18. Galetta D, Cesario A, Margaritora S, et al. Enduring challenge in the treatment of nonsmall cell lung cancer with clinical stage IIIB: results of a trimodality approach. *Ann Thorac Surg*. 2003;76(6):1802–1808.
19. Depierre A, Milleron B, Moro-Sibilot D, et al. Preoperative chemotherapy followed by surgery compared with primary surgery in resectable stage I (except T1N0), II, and iiia non-small-cell lung cancer. *J Clin Oncol*. 2002;20(1):247–253.
20. Roth JA, Fossella F, Komaki R, et al. A randomized trial comparing perioperative chemotherapy and surgery with surgery alone in resectable stage IIIA non-small-cell lung cancer. *J Natl Cancer Inst*. 1994;86(9):673–680.
21. Rosell R, Gómez-Codina J, Camps C, et al. Preresectional chemotherapy in stage IIIA non-small-cell lung cancer: a 7-year assessment of a randomized controlled trial. *Lung Cancer*. 1999;26(1):7–14.
22. Pisters K, Vallieres E, Bunn P, et al, for the Southwest Oncology Group. S9900: a phase III trial of surgery alone or surgery plus preoperative (preop) paclitaxel/carboplatin (PC) chemotherapy in early stage non-small cell lung cancer (NSCLC): preliminary results [abstract #LBA7012]. *J Clin Oncol*. 2005;23(16S):624s.
23. Berghmans T, Paesmans M, Meert AP, et al. Survival improvement in resectable non-small cell lung cancer with (neo)adjuvant chemotherapy: results of a meta-analysis of the literature. *Lung Cancer*. 2005;49(1):13–23.
24. Govindan R, Bogart J, Vokes EE. Locally advanced non-small cell lung cancer: the past, present, and future. *J Thorac Oncol*. 2008;3(8):917–928.
25. Choi N, Baumann M, Flentjie M, et al. Predictive factors in radiotherapy for non-small cell lung cancer: present status. *Lung Cancer*. 2001;31(1):43–56.
26. Payne DG. Non-small-cell lung cancer: should unresectable stage III patients routinely receive high-dose radiation therapy? *J Clin Oncol*. 1988;6(3):552–558.
27. Hayakawa K, Mitsuhashi N, Saito Y, et al. Impact of tumor extent and location on treatment outcome in patients with stage III non-small cell lung cancer treated with radiation therapy. *Jpn J Clin Oncol*. 1996;26(4):221–228.
28. Mehta V. Radiation pneumonitis and pulmonary fibrosis in non-small-cell lung cancer: pulmonary function, prediction, and prevention. *Int J Radiat Oncol Biol Phys*. 2005;63(1):5–24.
29. Lester JF, Macbeth FR, Toy E, Coles B. Palliative radiotherapy regimens for non-small cell lung cancer. *Cochrane Database Syst Rev*. 2006;4: CD002143.
30. Liu HH, Balter P, Tutt T, et al. Assessing respiration-induced tumor motion and internal target volume using four-dimensional computed tomography for radiotherapy of lung cancer. *Int J Radiat Oncol Biol Phys*. 2007;68(2):531–540.
31. Murshed H, Liu HH, Liao Z, et al. Dose and volume reduction for normal lung using intensity-modulated radiotherapy for advanced-stage non-small-cell lung cancer. *Int J Radiat Oncol Biol Phys*. 2004;58(4):1258–1267.
32. Yom SS, Liao Z, Liu HH, et al. Initial evaluation of treatment-related pneumonitis in advanced-stage non-small-cell lung cancer patients treated with concurrent chemotherapy and intensity-modulated radiotherapy. *Int J Radiat Oncol Biol Phys*. 2007;68(1):94–102.
33. Goitein M, Cox JD. Should randomized clinical trials be required for proton radiotherapy? *J Clin Oncol*. 2008;26(2):175–176.
34. Dillman RO, Seagren SL, Propert KJ, et al. A randomized trial of induction chemotherapy plus high-dose radiation versus radiation alone in stage III non-small-cell lung cancer. *N Engl J Med*. 1990;323(14):940–945.
35. Le Chevalier T, Arriagada R, Quoix E, et al. Radiotherapy alone versus combined chemotherapy and radiotherapy in nonresectable non-small-cell lung cancer: first analysis of a randomized trial in 353 patients. *J Natl Cancer Inst*. 1991;83(6):417–423.
36. Schaake-Koning C, van den Bogaert W, Dalesio O, et al. Effects of concomitant cisplatin and radiotherapy on inoperable non-small-cell lung cancer. *N Engl J Med*. 1992;326(8):524–530.
37. Furuse K, Fukuoka M, Kawahara M, et al. Phase III study of concurrent versus sequential thoracic radiotherapy in combination with mitomycin, vindesine, and cisplatin in unresectable stage III non-small-cell lung cancer. *J Clin Oncol*. 1999;17(9):2692–2699.
38. Curran Jr WJ, Scott C, Langer C, et al. Phase III comparison of sequential vs concurrent chemoradiation for patients with unresected stage III non-small cell lung cancer (NSCLC): initial report of Radiation Therapy Oncology Group (RTOG) 9410 [Proc ASCO Abstract #1891]. *J Clin Oncol*. 2000;19:484A.

39. Zatloukal P, Petruzelka L, Zemanova M, et al. Concurrent versus sequential chemoradiotherapy with cisplatin and vinorelbine in locally advanced non-small cell lung cancer: a randomized study. *Lung Cancer*. 2004;46(1):87–98.
40. Douple EB, Richmond RC. A review of interactions between platinum coordination complexes and ionizing radiation: implications for cancer therapy. In: Prestayko AW, Crooke ST, Carter SK, eds. *Cisplatin: Current Status and New Developments*. New York: Academic Press; 1980:125–147.
41. Toiyama Y, Inoue Y, Hiro J, et al. The range of optimal concentration and mechanisms of paclitaxel in radio-enhancement in gastrointestinal cancer cell lines. *Cancer Chemother Pharmacol*. 2007;59(6):733–742.
42. Fukuoka K, Arioka H, Iwamoto Y, et al. Mechanism of the radiosensitization induced by vinorelbine in human non-small cell lung cancer cells. *Lung Cancer*. 2001;34(3):451–460.
43. NSCLC Meta-Analyses Collaborative Group. Chemotherapy in addition to supportive care improves survival in advanced non-small-cell lung cancer: a systematic review and meta-analysis of individual patient data from 16 randomized controlled trials. *J Clin Oncol*. 2008;26(28):4617–4625.
44. Non-Small Cell Lung Cancer Collaborative Group. Chemotherapy in non-small cell lung cancer: a meta-analysis using updated data on individual patients from 52 randomised clinical trials. *BMJ*. 1995;311(7010):899–909.
45. Brown J, Thorpe H, Napp V, et al. Assessment of quality of life in the supportive care setting of the Big Lung Trial in non-small-cell lung cancer. *J Clin Oncol*. 2005;23(30):7417–7427.
46. Helsing M, Bergman B, Thaning L, Hero U. Quality of life and survival in patients with advanced non-small cell lung cancer receiving supportive care plus chemotherapy with carboplatin and etoposide or supportive care only. A multicentre randomised phase III trial. Joint Lung Cancer Study Group. *Eur J Cancer*. 1998;34(7):1036–1044.
47. Cullen MH, Billingham LJ, Woodroffe CM, et al. Mitomycin, ifosfamide, and cisplatin in unresectable non-small-cell lung cancer: effects on survival and quality of life. *J Clin Oncol*. 1999;17(10):3188–3194.
48. Anderson H, Hopwood P, Stephens RJ, et al. Gemcitabine plus best supportive care (BSC) vs BSC in inoperable non-small cell lung cancer—a randomized trial with quality of life as the primary outcome. UK NSCLC Gemcitabine Group. Non-Small Cell Lung Cancer. *Br J Cancer*. 2000;83(4):447–453.
49. Ranson M, Davidson N, Nicolson M, et al. Randomized trial of paclitaxel plus supportive care versus supportive care for patients with advanced non-small-cell lung cancer. *J Natl Cancer Inst*. 2000;92(13):1074–1080.
50. Delbaldo C, Michiels S, Syz N, Soria JC, Le Chevalier T, Pignon JP. Benefits of adding a drug to a single-agent or a 2-agent chemotherapy regimen in advanced non-small-cell lung cancer: a meta-analysis. *JAMA*. 2004;292(4):470–484.
51. Kelly K, Crowley J, Bunn Jr PA, et al. Randomized phase III trial of paclitaxel plus carboplatin versus vinorelbine plus cisplatin in the treatment of patients with advanced non–small-cell lung cancer: a Southwest Oncology Group trial. *J Clin Oncol*. 2001;19(13):3210–3218.
52. Fossella F, Pereira JR, von Pawel J, et al. Randomized, multinational, phase III study of docetaxel plus platinum combinations versus vinorelbine plus cisplatin for advanced non-small-cell lung cancer: the TAX 326 study group. *J Clin Oncol*. 2003;21(16):3016–3024.
53. Bonomi P, Kim K, Fairclough D, et al. Comparison of survival and quality of life in advanced non-small-cell lung cancer patients treated with two dose levels of paclitaxel combined with cisplatin versus etoposide with cisplatin: results of an Eastern Cooperative Oncology Group trial. *J Clin Oncol*. 2000;18(3):623–631.
54. Scagliotti GV, Parikh P, von Pawel J, et al. Phase III study comparing cisplatin plus gemcitabine with cisplatin plus pemetrexed in chemotherapy-naive patients with advanced-stage non-small-cell lung cancer. *J Clin Oncol*. 2008;26(21):3543–3551.
55. Smith IE, O'Brien ME, Talbot DC, et al. Duration of chemotherapy in advanced non-small-cell lung cancer: a randomized trial of three versus six courses of mitomycin, vinblastine, and cisplatin. *J Clin Oncol*. 2001;19(5):1336–1343.
56. von Plessen C, Bergman B, Andresen O, et al. Palliative chemotherapy beyond three courses conveys no survival or consistent quality-of-life benefits in advanced non-small-cell lung cancer. *Br J Cancer*. 2006;95(8):966–973.
57. Socinski MA, Schell MJ, Peterman A, et al. Phase III trial comparing a defined duration of therapy versus continuous therapy followed by second-line therapy in advanced-stage IIIB/IV non-small-cell lung cancer. *J Clin Oncol*. 2002;20(5):1335–1343.
58. Ciuleanu T, Brodowicz T, Belani C. Maintenance pemetrexed plus best supportive care (BSC) versus placebo plus BSC: a phase III study [abstract 8011]. *J Clin Oncol*. 2008;26(Suppl):426s.
59. Shepherd FA, Dancey J, Ramlau R, et al. Prospective randomized trial of docetaxel versus best supportive care in patients with non-small-cell lung cancer previously treated with platinum-based chemotherapy. *J Clin Oncol*. 2000;18(10):2095–2103.
60. Dancey J, Shepherd FA, Gralla RJ, Kim YS. Quality of life assessment of second-line docetaxel versus best supportive care in patients with non-small-cell lung cancer previously treated with platinum-based chemotherapy: results of a prospective, randomized phase III trial. *Lung Cancer*. 2004;43(2):183–194.
61. Hanna N, Shepherd FA, Fossella FV, et al. Randomized phase III trial of pemetrexed versus docetaxel in patients with non-small-cell lung cancer previously treated with chemotherapy. *J Clin Oncol*. 2004;22(9):1589–1597.
62. Coskun U, Kaya AO, Buyukberber S, et al. Single agent gemcitabine in the second-line treatment of advanced non-small cell lung cancer after treatment with taxane + platinum regimens. *Med Oncol*. 2008;25(2):133–136.
63. Wozniak AJ. Single-agent vinorelbine in the treatment of non-small cell lung cancer. *Semin Oncol*. 1999;26(5 Suppl 16):62–66.
64. Sandler A, Gray R, Perry MC, et al. Paclitaxel-carboplatin alone or with bevacizumab for non-small-cell lung cancer. *N Engl J Med*. 2006;355(24):2542–2550.
65. Heymach JV, Paz-Ares L, De Braud F, et al. Randomized phase II study of vandetanib alone or with paclitaxel and carboplatin as first-line treatment for advanced non-small-cell lung cancer. *J Clin Oncol*. 2008;26(33):5407–5415.
66. Shepherd FA, Rodrigues Pereira J, Ciuleanu T, et al. Erlotinib in previously treated non-small-cell lung cancer. *N Engl J Med*. 2005;353(2):123–132.
67. Bezjak A, Tu D, Seymour L, et al. Symptom improvement in lung cancer patients treated with erlotinib: quality of life analysis of the National Cancer Institute of Canada Clinical Trials Group Study BR.21. *J Clin Oncol*. 2006;24(24):3831–3837.
68. Zhu CQ, da Cunha Santos G, Ding K, et al. Role of K-ras and EGFR as biomarkers of response to erlotinib in National Cancer Institute of Canada Clinical Trials Group Study BR.21. *J Clin Oncol*. 2008;26(26):4268–4275.
69. Thatcher N, Chang A, Parikh P, et al. Gefitinib plus best supportive care in previously treated patients with refractory advanced non-small-cell lung cancer: results from a randomised, placebo-controlled, multicentre study (Iressa Survival Evaluation in Lung Cancer). *Lancet*. 2005;366(9496):1527–1537.
70. Kim ES, Hirsh V, Mok T, et al. Gefitinib versus docetaxel in previously treated non-small-cell lung cancer (INTEREST): a randomised phase III trial. *Lancet*. 2008;372(9652):1809–1818.
71. Tamura K, Fukuoka M. Gefitinib in non-small cell lung cancer. *Expert Opin Pharmacother*. 2005;6(6):985–993.
72. Herbst RS, Prager D, Hermann R, et al. TRIBUTE: a phase III trial of erlotinib hydrochloride (OSI-774) combined with carboplatin

and paclitaxel chemotherapy in advanced non-small-cell lung cancer. *J Clin Oncol*. 2005;23(25):5892–5899.
73. Eberhard DA, Johnson BE, Amler LC, et al. Mutations in the epidermal growth factor receptor and in K-RAS are predictive and prognostic indicators in patients with non-small-cell lung cancer treated with chemotherapy alone and in combination with erlotinib. *J Clin Oncol*. 2005;23(25):5900–5909.
74. Kelly K, Chansky K, Gaspar LE, et al. Phase III trial of maintenance gefitinib or placebo after concurrent chemoradiotherapy and docetaxel consolidation in inoperable stage III non-small-cell lung cancer: SWOG S0023. *J Clin Oncol*. 2008;26(15):2450–2456.
75. Pirker R, Szczesna A, von Pawel J, et al. FLEX: a randomized, multicenter, phase III study of cetuximab in combination with cisplatin/vinorelbine (CV) versus CV alone in the first-line treatment of patients with advanced non-small cell lung cancer (NSCLC) [abstract #3]. *J Clin Oncol*. 2008;26(18S):1006s.
76. Blumenschein Jr G. Sorafenib in lung cancer: clinical developments and future directions. *J Thorac Oncol*. 2008;3(6 Suppl 2):S124–S127.
77. Fanucchi MP, Fossella FV, Belt R, et al. Randomized phase II study of bortezomib alone and bortezomib in combination with docetaxel in previously treated advanced non-small-cell lung cancer. *J Clin Oncol*. 2006;24(31):5025–5033.
78. Engelman JA, Janne PA. Mechanisms of acquired resistance to epidermal growth factor receptor tyrosine kinase inhibitors in non-small cell lung cancer. *Clin Cancer Res*. 2008;14(10):2895–2899.
79. Auberger J, Loeffler-Ragg J, Wurzer W, Hilbe W. Targeted therapies in non-small cell lung cancer: proven concepts and unfulfilled promises. *Curr Cancer Drug Targets*. 2006;6(4):271–294.
80. Shahidi H, Kvale PA. Long-term survival following surgical treatment of solitary brain metastasis in non-small cell lung cancer. *Chest*. 1996;109(1):271–276.
81. Tanvetyanon T, Robinson LA, Schell MJ, et al. Outcomes of adrenalectomy for isolated synchronous versus metachronous adrenal metastases in non-small-cell lung cancer: a systematic review and pooled analysis. *J Clin Oncol*. 2008;26(7):1142–1147.
82. Patchell RA, Tibbs PA, Walsh JW, et al. A randomized trial of surgery in the treatment of single metastases to the brain. *N Engl J Med*. 1990;322(8):494–500.
83. Patchell RA, Tibbs PA, Regine WF, et al. Postoperative radiotherapy in the treatment of single metastases to the brain: a randomized trial. *JAMA*. 1998;280(17):1485–1489.
84. Ganti AK, Zhen W, Kessinger A. Limited-stage small-cell lung cancer: therapeutic options. *Oncology (Williston Park)*. 2007;21(3):303–312.
85. Green RA, Humphrey E, Close H, Patno ME. Alkylating agents in bronchogenic carcinoma. *Am J Med*. 1969;46(4):516–525.
86. Lally BE, Urbanic JJ, Blackstock AW, Miller AA, Perry MC. Small cell lung cancer: have we made any progress over the last 25 years?. *Oncologist*. 2007;12(9):1096–1104.
87. Jackman DM, Johnson BE. Small-cell lung cancer. *Lancet*. 2005;366(9494):1385–1396.
88. Kurup A, Hanna NH. Treatment of small cell lung cancer. *Crit Rev Oncol Hematol*. 2004;52(2):117–126.
89. Sinkule JA. Etoposide: a semisynthetic epipodophyllotoxin. Chemistry, pharmacology, pharmacokinetics, adverse effects and use as an antineoplastic agent. *Pharmacotherapy*. 1984;4(2):61–73.
90. Hanna N, Bunn Jr PA, Langer C, et al. Randomized phase III trial comparing irinotecan/cisplatin with etoposide/cisplatin in patients with previously untreated extensive-stage disease small-cell lung cancer. *J Clin Oncol*. 2006;24(13):2038–2043.
91. Chua YJ, Steer C, Yip D. Recent advances in management of small-cell lung cancer. *Cancer Treat Rev*. 2004;30(6):521–543.
92. Vincent M, Evans B, Smith I. First-line chemotherapy rechallenge after relapse in small cell lung cancer. *Cancer Chemother Pharmacol*. 1988;21(1):45–48.

15

Handling and Grossing of Larger Cases

The correct procedures for handling resected tissue and preparing gross specimens for histologic evaluation of thoracic tumors are of great importance not only for diagnostic purposes but also for staging of the various neoplasms occurring in the lung and pleura. In every case, therefore, resected specimens must be handled with the utmost care, and the sections submitted for histologic evaluation must be representative of the different areas involved in disease.

The nature of the clinical case often necessitates special considerations in obtaining and preparing surgical specimens. Although the entire gamut of different forms and shapes that may appear in tumors of the lung and pleura is beyond the scope of this discussion, a selected group of cases that may pose problems in macroscopic evaluation are presented in this chapter, to provide some guidance for proper sectioning. The following cases are considered:

- Extrapleural pneumonectomy
- Resections with staple line
- Neoplasms obstructing the airway

EXTRAPLEURAL PNEUMONECTOMY

Extrapleural pneumonectomy has become a commonly used procedure for the surgical treatment of malignant mesothelioma. Resected specimens usually comprise the following anatomic structures: (1) lung, (2) visceral pleura, (3) parietal pleura, (4) diaphragm, and (5) pericardium. Each of these structures must be properly identified and sampled, and it also is imperative to obtain appropriate lymph nodes to complete the required staging of these tumors. Figures 15-1 to 15-8 illustrate many of the considerations and techniques involved.

SPECIMENS WITH STAPLE LINE

It is a common surgical practice to submit specimens in which the parenchymal margin has a staple line. In many instances these specimens are submitted for frozen section, which raises the issue of the "true" margin of resection. The recommended process for handling these specimens includes the following:

1. Measure the specimen.
2. Remove all of the tissue incorporated in the staple line.
3. Ink the parenchymal margin exposed.
4. Ink the pleural margin closer to the tumor mass.
5. Cross section the tumor mass and measure the tumor to the closest margin of resection.
6. Submit sections, keeping the surgical margin.

Figs. 15-9 to 15-14 illustrate the clinical application of this approach.

BRONCHIAL OBSTRUCTING TUMORS

With tumors that obstruct the airway, it is essential to document the presence of an uninvolved bronchial margin of resection, to permit proper dissection of the airway with conservation of its anatomic structure. The suggested procedure is as follows (Figs. 15-15 and 15-16):

1. Carefully dissect the airway.
2. Separate the airway without destroying the anatomic structure.
3. Measure the tumor and determine the extent of invasion.
4. Cross section the specimen to determine the extent of tumor invasion.
5. Obtain lymph nodes for staging.
6. Sections from the bronchus should be radial sections.

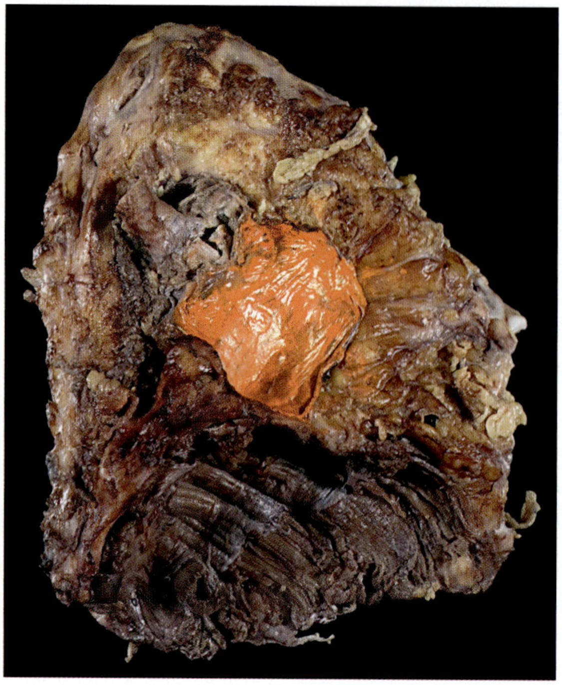

Figure 15-1 Extrapleural pneumonectomy specimen. Note the orange color identifying pericardium.

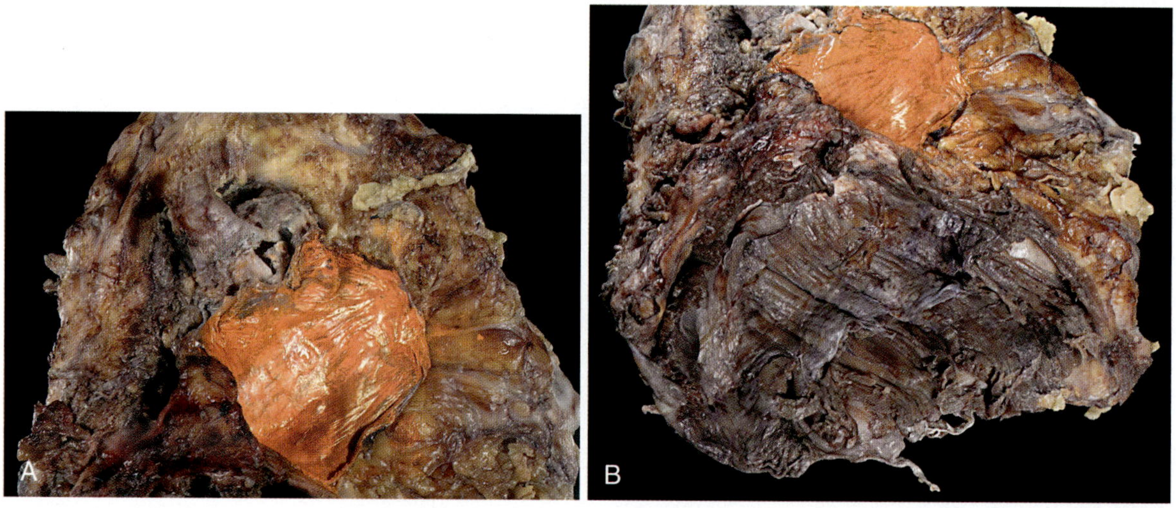

Figure 15-2 **A**, Pericardium *(orange)* and airway. Sections from the pericardium must be submitted in order to determine the extent of tumor invasion. **B**, Different view of the specimen, as seen from the diaphragm.

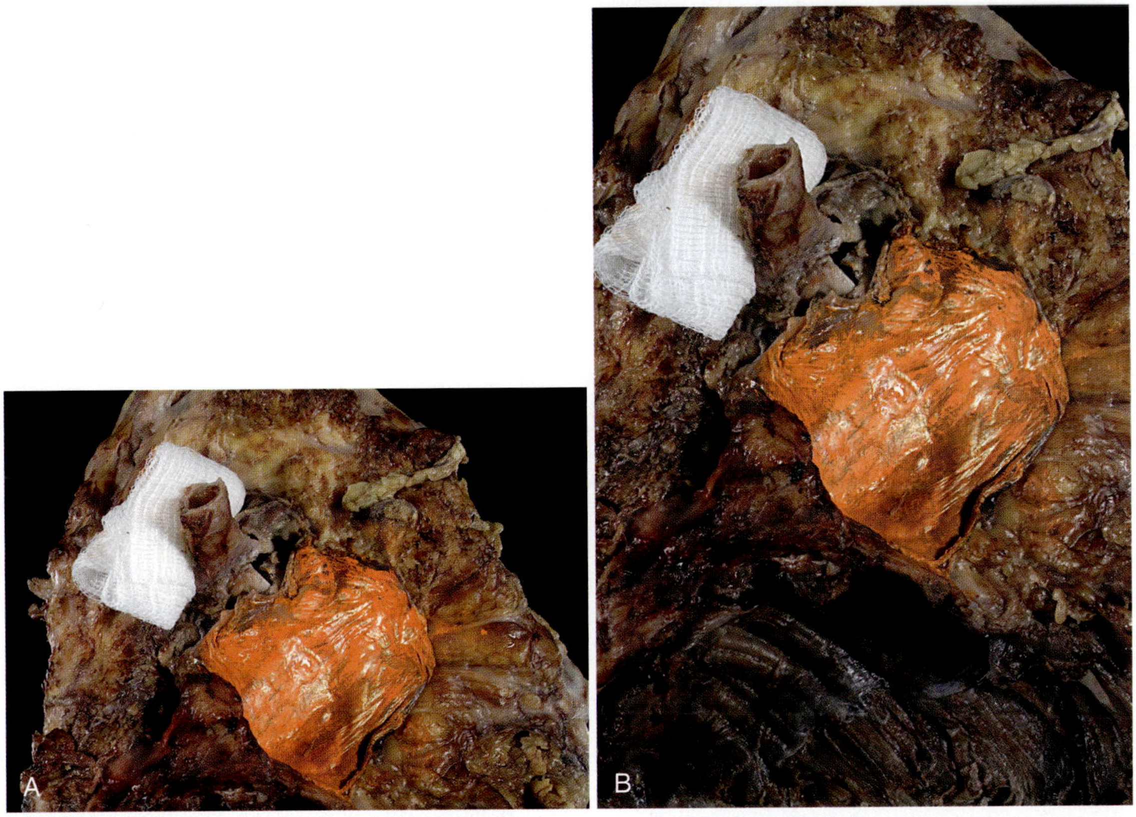

Figure 15-3 **A**, Main bronchus has been exposed. The surgical bronchial margin of resection must be documented. **B**, Close-up view of greater depth showing the patent airway and the pericardial aspect.

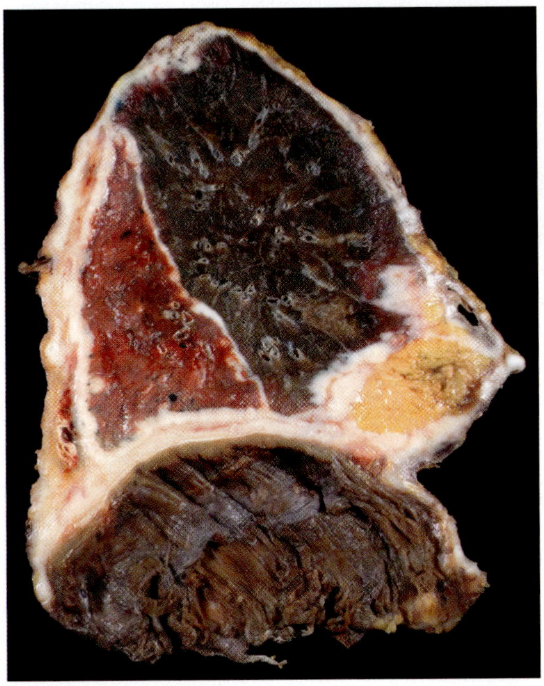

Figure 15-4 Cross section of the entire specimen showing thickened pleura encasing the lung parenchyma. Sections from the pleura must be submitted for histologic evaluation.

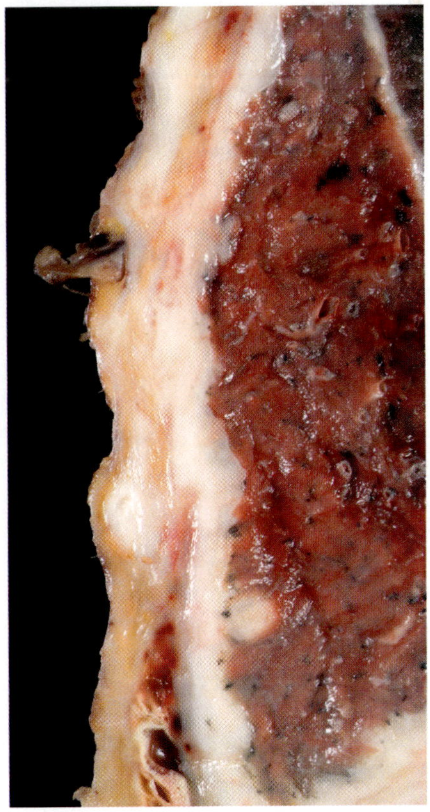

Figure 15-5 Thickened pleura with superficial invasion into lung parenchyma. This finding must be documented, and sections must be submitted for histologic evaluation.

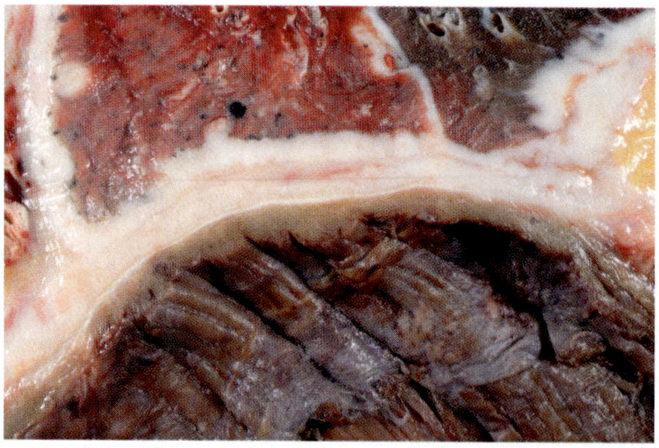

Figure 15-6 Close-up view of the thickened pleura and the diaphragm. Presence or absence of gross invasion into the diaphragm needs to be recorded. In addition, sections from the diaphragm must be submitted for histologic evaluation.

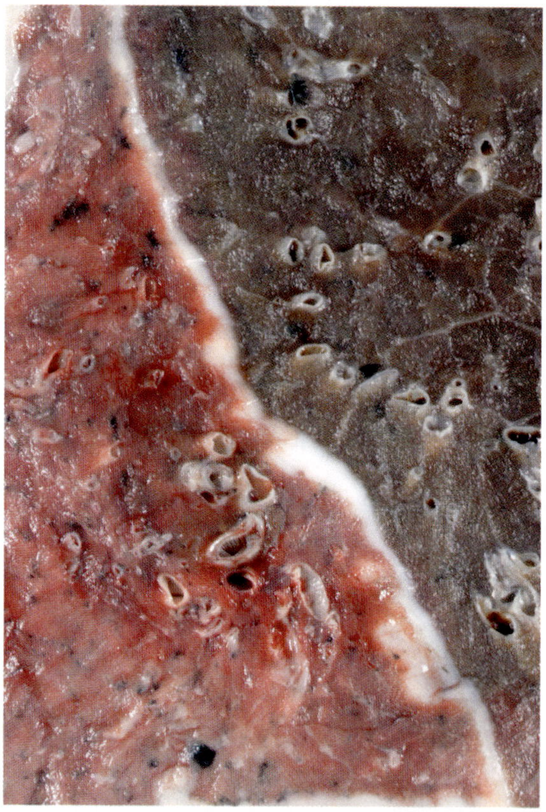

Figure 15-7 Thickened fissures. This finding needs to be documented and the involved tissue sectioned for histologic evaluation.

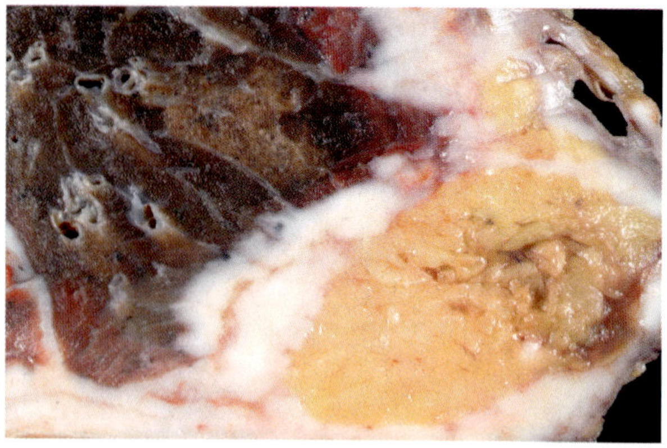

Figure 15-8 It is important to identify any other area in which the tumor has infiltrated into adjacent tissue (adipose tissue). Such infiltration needs to be documented, and appropriate sections must be submitted for histologic examination.

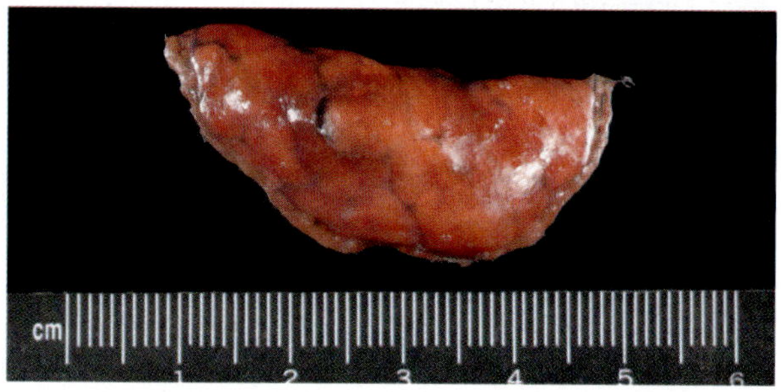

Figure 15-9 Segment of lung with an identifiable staple line.

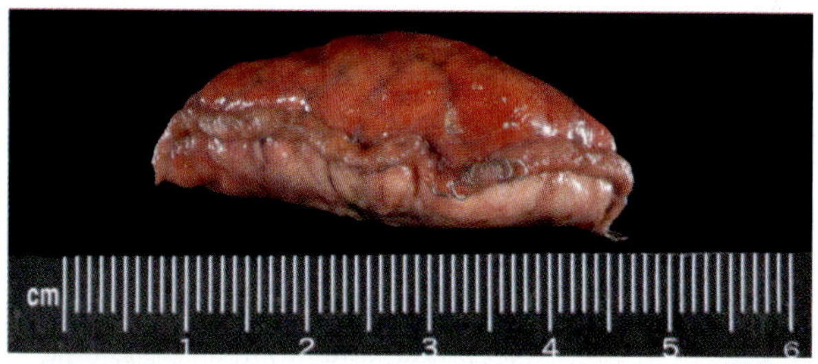

Figure 15-10 The specimen has been turned to show the staple line more clearly.

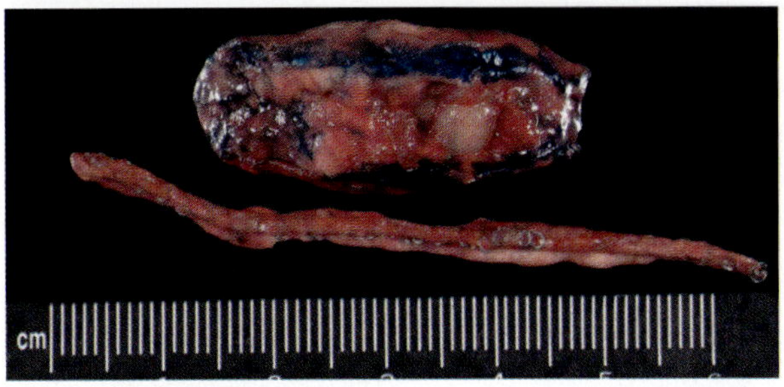

Figure 15-11 Removal of the tissue included in the staple line with exposure of the tumor mass. Note that the specimen also has been inked.

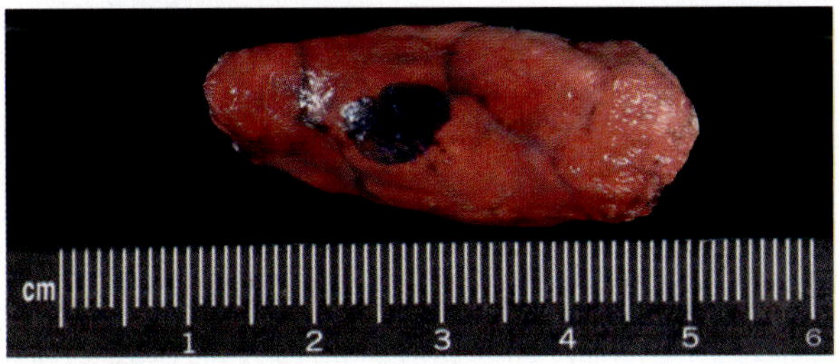

Figure 15-12 Different view of the specimen showing the inked pleura.

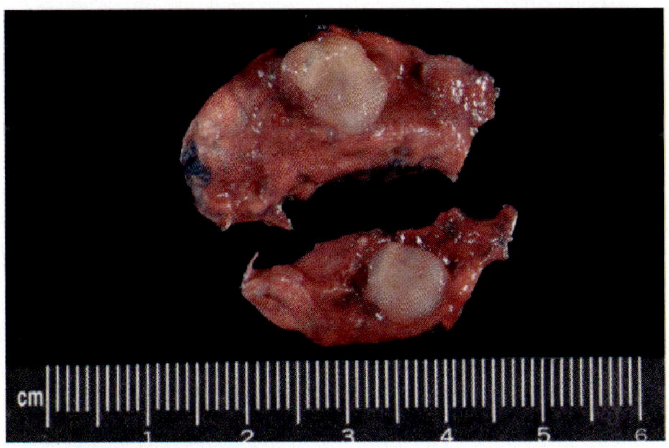

Figure 15-13 Cross section of the tumor mass clearly showing the margins of resection.

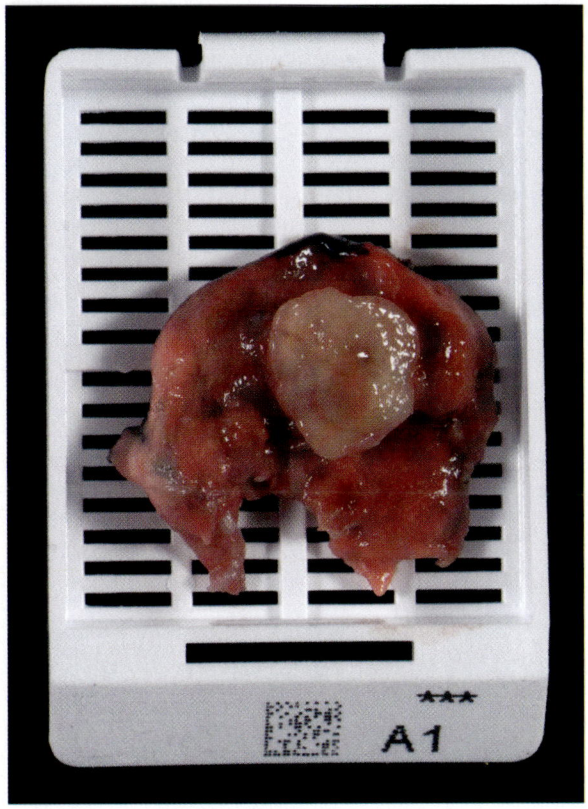

Figure 15-14 Submitted section for histologic evaluation.

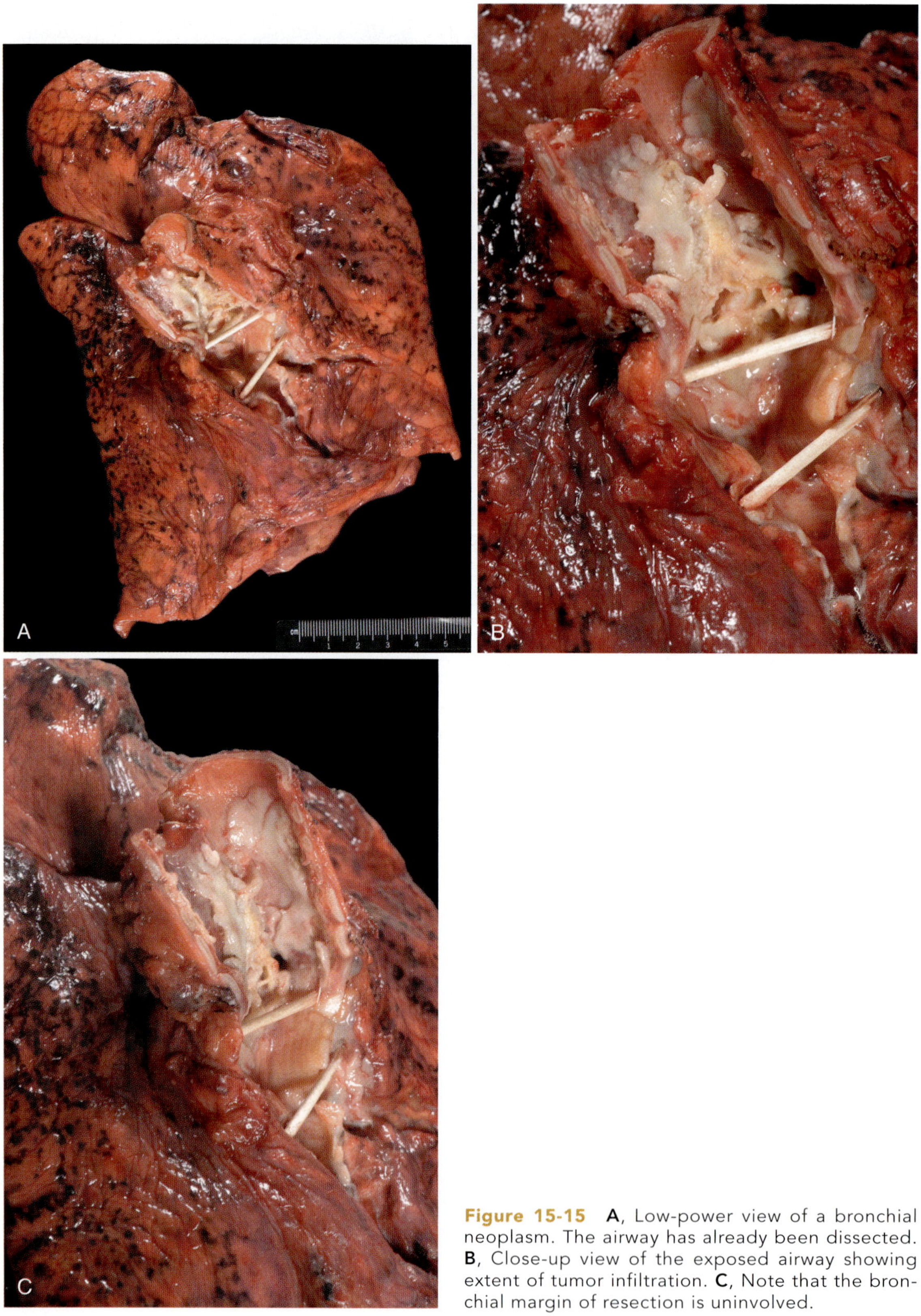

Figure 15-15 **A**, Low-power view of a bronchial neoplasm. The airway has already been dissected. **B**, Close-up view of the exposed airway showing extent of tumor infiltration. **C**, Note that the bronchial margin of resection is uninvolved.

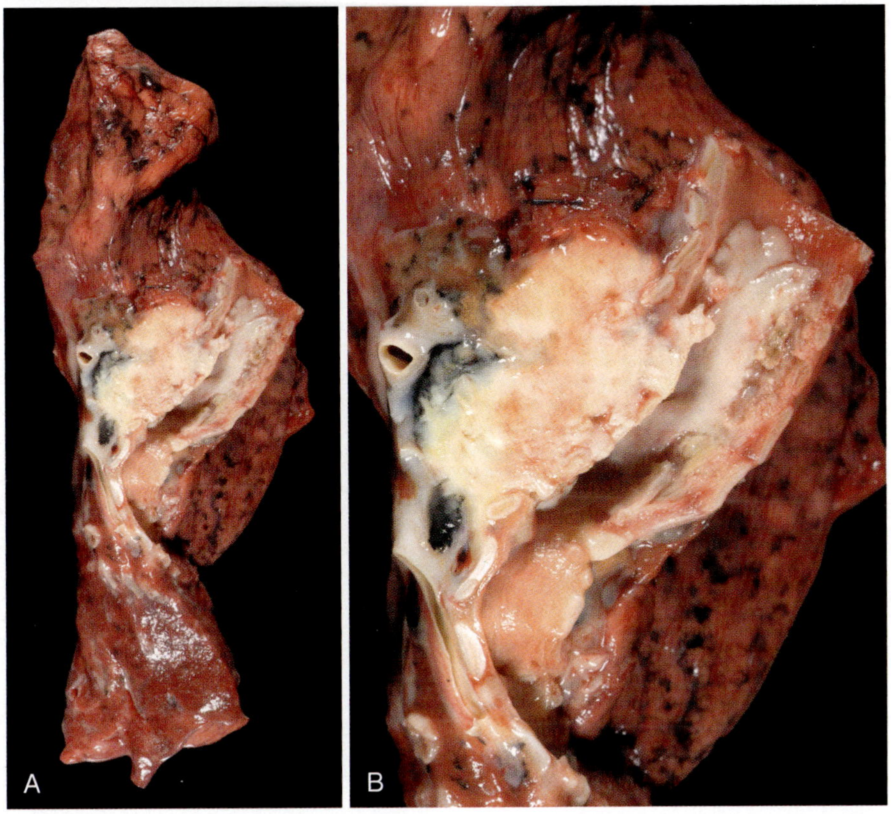

Figure 15-16 **A**, Low-power view of a cross section of the tumor showing depth of infiltration within lung parenchyma. **B**, Close-up view showing matted lymph nodes overrun by the tumor mass.

INDEX

Note: Page numbers followed by *f* refer to figures, and those followed by *t* refer to tables.

B

C

H

I

N

R

S

T

U

V

W

X

Z